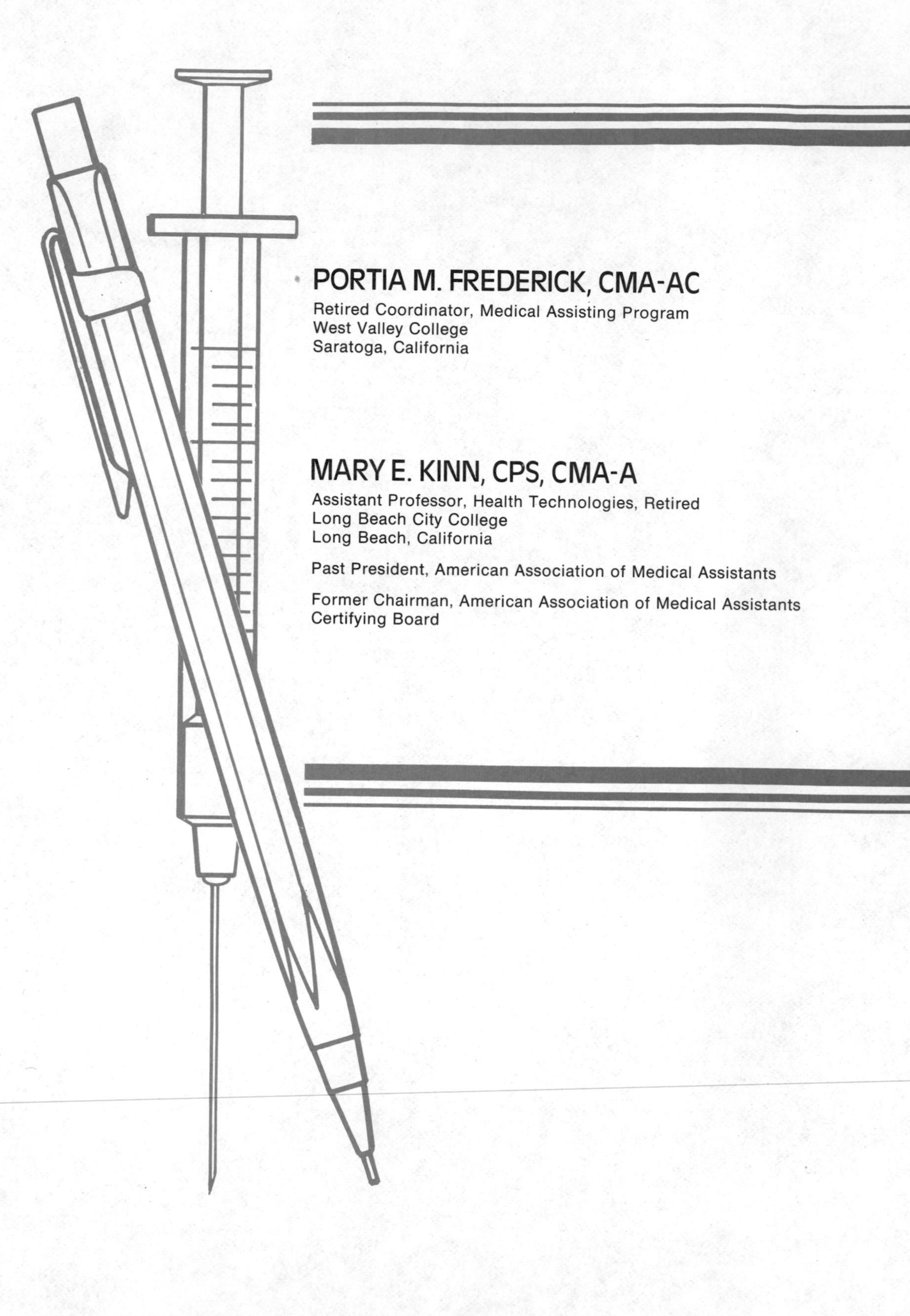

PORTIA M. FREDERICK, CMA-AC
Retired Coordinator, Medical Assisting Program
West Valley College
Saratoga, California

MARY E. KINN, CPS, CMA-A
Assistant Professor, Health Technologies, Retired
Long Beach City College
Long Beach, California

Past President, American Association of Medical Assistants

Former Chairman, American Association of Medical Assistants
Certifying Board

5th Edition

The medical office assistant

Administrative and Clinical

W.B. Saunders Company
Philadelphia
London
Toronto
Mexico City
Rio de Janeiro
Sydney
Tokyo

W. B. Saunders Company: West Washington Square
Philadelphia, PA 19105

1 St. Anne's Road
Eastbourne, East Sussex BN21 3UN, England

1 Goldthorne Avenue
Toronto, Ontario M8Z 5T9, Canada

Apartado 26370—Cedro 512
Mexico 4, D.F., Mexico

Rua Coronel Cabrita, 8
Sao Cristovao Caixa Postal 21176
Rio de Janeiro, Brazil

9 Waltham Street
Artarmon, N.S.W. 2064, Australia

Ichibancho, Central Bldg., 22-1 Ichibancho
Chiyoda-Ku, Tokyo 102, Japan

Library of Congress Cataloging in Publication Data

Frederick, Portia M.

The medical office assistant.

Second-3d ed. published in 1960 and 1967 under title: The office assistant in medical practice.

Includes index.

Bibliography: p.

1. Medical assistants. I. Kinn, Mary E., joint author. II. Title. [DNLM: 1. Medical secretaries. W 80 F852o]

R728.8.F7 1981 610.73'7 80-53368

ISBN 0-7216-3863-5

The Medical Office Assistant ISBN 0-7216-3863-5

Last digit is the print number: 9 8 7 6 5 4 3

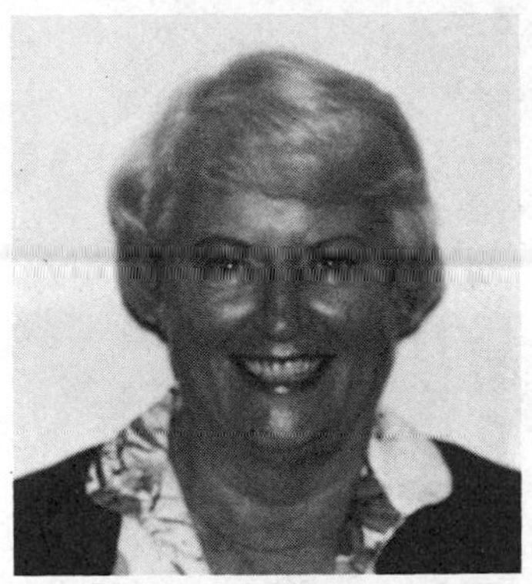

IN MEMORIAM
PORTIA M. FREDERICK, CMA-AC

Shortly after completion of the manuscript for this Fifth Edition Portia Frederick died suddenly at her home in Los Altos, California. It is impossible to estimate the impact of her thirty-one years of teaching medical assisting in the California Community College system. I do know that she was loved and highly respected by her students and colleagues at Long Beach City College, Foothill College, and West Valley College. I also know that her modest self image would not have permitted this public recognition, but after a friendship of nearly thirty years I take the privilege of acknowledging this loss on behalf of all those whose lives she touched.

MARY E. KINN

PREFACE
To The Fifth Edition

In the 25 years since the first edition of this book, many changes have taken place within the practice of medicine, the management of the medical office, and the responsibilities of medical office personnel. With each revision the authors have attempted to keep pace with the times by adding new material, deleting those portions that no longer seemed applicable, and updating every chapter. Eliminating reference to the medical office assistant as the "girl" or "aide" in the doctor's office is indicative of the current professional standing of the medical assistant.

The 5th edition again has a change of format with the addition of a second color to make the volume more attractive to the reader and simplify the locating of specific information. The many new illustrations will aid the instructor as well as enhance the students' understanding of the material. This edition includes a new chapter on electrocardiography, a new chapter on the assistant's management responsibilities, a completely rewritten microbiology chapter, an expanded chapter on finding a suitable position, and additional instruction on written communications. Detailed instruction for implementing the pegboard system of bookkeeping has also been added. Responding to changes in medical care and the language of medicine, the appendix of common abbreviations, acronyms, and symbols has been completely revised. The new glossary of words that appear in bold print within the text will be a valuable assist to the student.

This book is designed primarily as a teaching aid in training programs for medical assistants. A companion workbook and review for students emphasizes the salient points. Its use by the student will aid in retaining the essence of the instruction.

Not all medical assistants have the opportunity to attend formal classes of instruction. Many have learned through on-the-job training supplemented by reading articles in medical journals, studying books on medical assisting, and attending workshops and seminars. Practicing medical assistants who have a previous edition of this book in their office library say they refer to it frequently in performing their daily tasks. In addition to offering suggestions for the most efficient ways to complete routine tasks, the book may provide those already working in the medical field with a new perspective of their responsibilities. In fact, the objectives of the book may be summed up by quoting the first paragraph of the objectives of the American Association of Medical Assistants: "To inspire its members to render honest, loyal, and more efficient service to the profession and to the public which they serve."

The medical assistant who plans to take the national examination for Certified Medical Assistant will find this book and its companion workbook useful in reviewing areas covered by the examination. However, the book has not been sponsored or officially approved by the American Association of Medical Assistants or its Certifying Board.

The preparation of a book such as this seemed at times an awesome task, involving the assistance and cooperation of many. Sincere thanks is extended to the

American Medical Association, the California Medical Association, and the American Association of Medical Assistants; to Baxter Venable, Medical Editor, Allied Health Sciences, W. B. Saunders Company, and to the myriad of other individuals of the W. B. Saunders Company who were involved in bringing the book to the point of publication.

Special recognition is given to the assistance of the contributing authors: Dr. Lee Weller Callaway for her chapter on Nutrition and Diet Therapy; Dr. Donald J. Reinhardt for his chapter on Basic Medical Microbiology; and the late Mary W. Falconer for the chapter on Pharmacology and Preparation of Medications, revised for this edition by Edward A. Gustafson.

Appreciation is also due the many supply companies, pharmaceutical firms, professional organizations, and publishers who have shared their wealth of materials and illustrations. Appropriate recognition is given throughout the book.

Individually, I wish to thank Robert A. Mantovani, Coordinator of Career Planning at Long Beach City College who reviewed the material on Finding the Right Position; Jack Jackson, of Custom Recovery Systems, Santa Ana, for his help in preparing the chapters on credit and collections; Linda Warsek Woods, Market Administrator, Pacific Telephone Company; Marcia Cook, Product Representative, Bibbero Systems; and Catherine C. McCandless, CMA-AC, Coordinator of Medical Assisting, Cypress College, who acted as my mentor throughout the entire revision and who must have been as glad as I to see the task completed. There are doubtless other individuals who would have been acknowledged by my co-author had she lived to share the writing of this Preface.

The countless students, educators, paramedical practitioners, and physicians with whom the authors have associated over a span of many years in the profession have all, directly or indirectly, contributed to the knowledge and experience contained in this volume. It has been said that an expert is one who has written a book on the subject; an authority is one who has read the books and shares the information with others. The number of both experts and authorities in the realm of medical assisting continues to proliferate and we all rejoice in the recognition of medical assisting as a viable profession. The authors of this text have been relentless in their attitude that medical assisting requires intelligence, training, and a caring heart. There is no substitute for quality in the learning or the performing.

Medical assisting instructors are rightfully proud of their students who perform well. The authors, both of whom were medical assistants before becoming educators, are proud to have been contributing members of this growing profession.

MARY E. KINN, CPS, CMA-A
San Clemente, California
February 1, 1981

CONTENTS

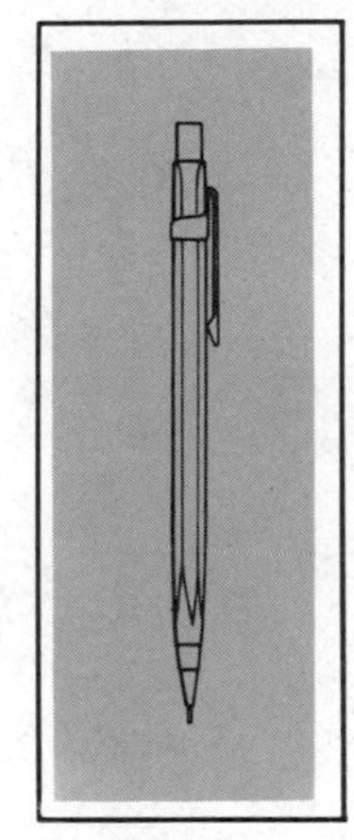

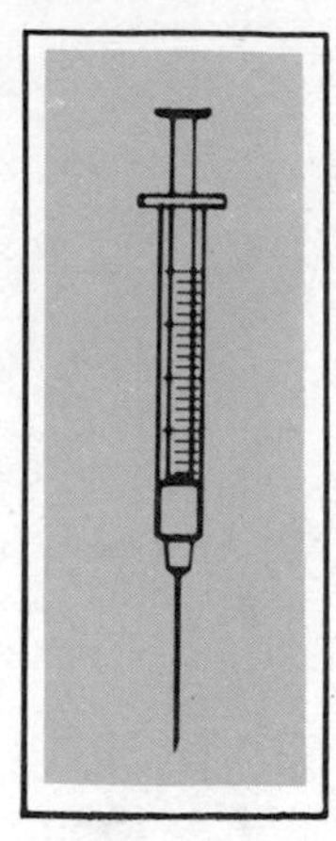

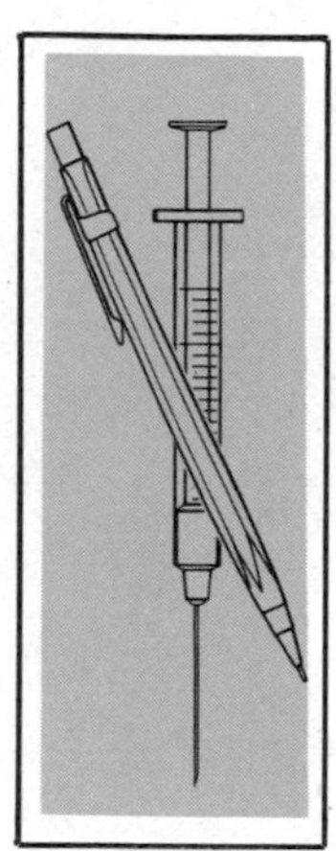

The medical office assistant

Administrative and Clinical

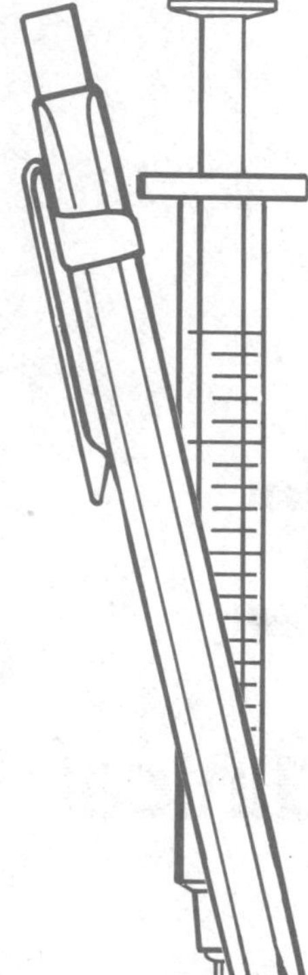

CHAPTER OUTLINE

BEHAVIORAL OBJECTIVES

The medical office assistant should be able to:

- **Explore a variety of job possibilities that require knowledge of medical assisting**
- **List the expected qualifications of a medical office assistant**
- **Compare the duties of an administrative assistant with those of a clinical assistant**
- **State the possible avenues for acquiring necessary and approved training**

1

A CAREER AS A MEDICAL OFFICE ASSISTANT

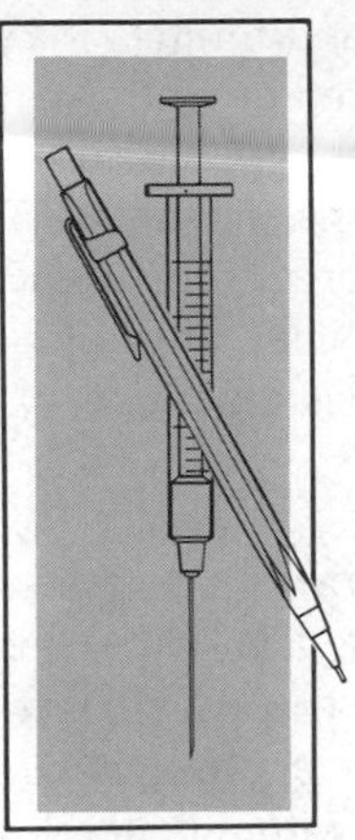

A career as a medical office assistant offers variety, excitement, job satisfaction, opportunity for service, opportunity for advancement, and fair financial reward. Both men and women enter into this career. Because most medical assistants are female, however, the feminine pronoun will be used throughout this volume.

Although doctors have employed assistants in their offices for many years, the role of *medical assistant* has become more than just a job — it is a career. As the qualifications for the position have become more clearly defined, formal training programs have been developed to train competent assistants. Medical office assisting has become an important allied health profession.

Employment opportunities abound in the health field and are increasing every day because of the growing concern for health protection for every individual in the nation. It is estimated that for every physician there are at least 12 persons engaged in an allied health career. Each year thousands become medical assistants, nurses, laboratory and x-ray technicians, physical or occupational therapists, speech pathologists, medical technologists, medical record administrators, or medical transcriptionists, or serve in other capacities in the health field. There is a shortage of adequately trained people to fill these challenging positions.

The advantages of a career in medicine rarely need to be "sold" by enumerating specific benefits. Medicine is of great interest to everyone; it is front-page news. Most Americans are better informed on health and medical subjects than ever before. New discoveries push back the frontiers of medical science so rapidly that a new drug may be obsolete before druggists get it on their shelves. The continuing battle of physicians, researchers, and allied health personnel to defeat illness and prolong life is a never-ending, exciting one.

4 A CAREER AS A MEDICAL OFFICE ASSISTANT

A woman who had worked in a physician's office for more than ten years wrote: "I get a wonderful sense of satisfaction from my work. It's still a thrill to share the joy of the young woman who finds she's going to have a baby or share the victory of the young man over a serious disease. I see quiet bravery every day. We do our best to make people well and cheer them up a little in the process. I know that even the little things I do in the office are worthwhile, and it's a real joy to know you are helping others."

The medical field holds many opportunities for youth. Yet it is one career that usually does not have mandatory retirement. Many medical assistants are still employed beyond the usual retirement age because physicians realize the value of the experienced mature employee. The person who trains for medical assisting is equipped with a flexible, adaptable career. The medical assistant acquires skills that she can carry with her all through life, and she can readily find employment anywhere in the world that medicine is practiced.

CAREER OPPORTUNITIES

Opportunities for the person who trains as a doctor's assistant are extremely varied. She can work as a medical assistant, a medical secretary, a medical or hospital receptionist, a medical transcriptionist, a psychiatric aide, or a hospital admitting officer. She may choose to work for a physician in solo practice or for several physicians in a group. She may work with a general practitioner or with a specialist in one of the many medical specialties, which include **surgery, internal medicine, dermatology, obstetrics, pediatrics, psychiatry,** and **radiology.**

There are career opportunities in public health work, in hospitals, laboratories, medical schools, research institutions, colleges, or with voluntary health agencies or medical firms of all kinds. There are also opportunities for work with such federal agencies as the Veterans Administration, the United States Health Service, or Armed Forces clinics or hospitals.

Although her training may equip her for work in the fields listed above, this book is designed primarily for the person who wishes to become a medical office assistant or who is already employed as a medical office assistant.

Today's medical office assistant must be *trained.* Ideally she should have both administrative and clinical training even though she may have a personal preference for one or the other. The physician's staff should be able to handle all responsibilities of the office except those requiring the services of a physician or other licensed personnel. Where there are several assistants, each should be able to substitute in an emergency for any of the others. Few physicians in private practice attempt to get along without at least one assistant. The great majority have at least two, and many have five or more.

A line of authority must be established. If there is only one assistant, she reports directly to the physician. In a larger staff, usually one is designated as supervisor or office manager. This individual should have management skills and the ability to deal with personnel matters.

While the career of the medical office assistant is more challenging than it may have been in years past, it also offers more opportunities for advancement. The recent graduate whose first position is as a receptionist may gradually be given more responsibilities and eventually become office manager of a large staff. Of course, the position of "boss" must always be reserved for the physician.

The job turnover among medical assistants is surprisingly low, a fact that may indicate that assistants who work in doctors' offices derive a high degree of satisfaction from their work. Many cases have been reported of women who were hired when a physician started practice and remained with him until his retirement.

What kind of earnings can the medical assistant expect? As in any other field of work, salaries vary in different parts of the country. There is also usually some difference between earnings in rural and urban areas. However, the office assistant generally gets a satisfactory return on her investment in training, experience, and skill. Medical organizations encourage physicians to pay better-than-average salaries to their office assistants, and most have come to realize that a good office assistant is worth a good salary. Many have learned through bitter experience that bargain-basement help is often the most expensive in the long run.

QUALIFICATIONS FOR OFFICE ASSISTANT

PERSONAL ASSETS. The services performed by a medical assistant are extremely personal. For this reason, her personality can actually affect the health and welfare of the patient. Physicians rank intelligence, dependability, and personality as top qualifications for the ideal office assistant.

The American Medical Association, in a public relations booklet for physicians' assistants entitled *Winning Ways with Patients,* compares the duties of the doctor's assistant with those of the airline stewardess, who greets passengers in a friendly, tactful manner and cares for their needs during flight. The booklet contains this little personality test for the office assistant:

1. Do you like people?
2. Do you enjoy helping people?
3. Are you cheerful?
4. Are you friendly?
5. Are you polite?
6. Do you try to be tactful in every situation?
7. Are you kind and sympathetic toward the doctor's patients?

The key to a good office personality is consideration, human kindness, and sympathy. The good assistant learns to view a situation from the patients' standpoint and to give her attention to their problems, no matter how insignificant they may seem.

A pleasant, friendly disposition is as necessary to the medical office assistant as are secretarial or clinical skills. She must combine sympathy, friendliness, and graciousness with calm efficiency.

She must be neat, accurate, dependable, and have a good head for details. Because the assistant often must assume charge of the office when the doctor is out, she must not hesitate to accept responsibility. Should an emergency arise, she must be able to meet it with composure. **Discretion** and good judgment also are important requirements for the man or woman who works in a doctor's office.

SKILLS. Every profession or trade has its special language, and the language of medicine must be understood by anyone who expects to work in a physician's office. The medical office assistant must also have a basic knowledge of law and ethics as they apply to the medical profession. To qualify for secretarial duties, the medical assistant must be a good typist and have basic skills in English and mathematics. Shorthand is helpful, but in many medical offices the dictation-transcription machine has become standard equipment. Some training in records management is desirable for both the administrative and clinical assistant. The clinical assistant must be skilled in certain nursing arts and must have training necessary to do some common medical tests.

PUBLIC RELATIONS RESPONSIBILITIES. Even though she may not serve as office receptionist, every assistant comes into daily contact with the doctor's patients. For this reason she is of tremendous importance in helping the doctor create either favorable or unfavorable personal public relations. The kind of impression the assistant makes upon patients often affects their opinions of the doctor and the care they can expect. An assistant can attract or **repel** patients by her very personality. She is the front door to the physician's practice, his office hostess and, often, his receptionist.

A manual published by the American Medical Association points up the public relations importance of the medical assistant in these words:

> If you employ an assistant . . . , she is a key person in determining what people think of you and your office. Into her hands you entrust the good will of your patients.
>
> A neat, attractive assistant is "good medicine" for any patient. As your goodwill ambassador she should have a nice personality, combining friendliness, courtesy, graciousness, and sympathy. A girl who dislikes or becomes impatient with people should not work in a doctor's office. A sad-faced gal with a mournful mien, a bored miss with a perpetual sneer, or a dragon who strikes terror into the hearts of patients is no asset to a physician. His assistant should be cheerful, tactful and efficient, prepared to meet any emergency with cool-headed composure.

Any person employed in a medical facility should be professional in both appearance and manner. This is evidenced in good grooming, proper dress (be it a uniform or appropriate street clothes), respect for the feelings of others, and appropriate conduct with both her employer and his patients. The physician may address his assistant by her first name, but usually she should not reply in kind. Patients tend to look with suspicion on any such informality in the professional office.

The medical assistant will be very cautious, too, about any laughter or **frivolity** with other members of the office staff in situations where the cause for the laughter is not entirely evident to waiting patients. A person who is not well or who has any obvious personal defect could quite easily get the idea that the laughter is about him. The medical assistant will observe this caution out of respect for the patients.

DUTIES OF THE OFFICE ASSISTANT

The duties of the office assistant will vary from one office to another since the schedule must be geared to the working habits and type of practice of the individual physician. In the office with only one employee the assistant will divide her time between administrative and clinical duties. In the multiple-employee office the assistant may be strictly limited to either administrative or clinical duties.

ADMINISTRATIVE DUTIES. The administrative duties of the medical office assistant will be similar to those of any responsible secretary to a top executive but will

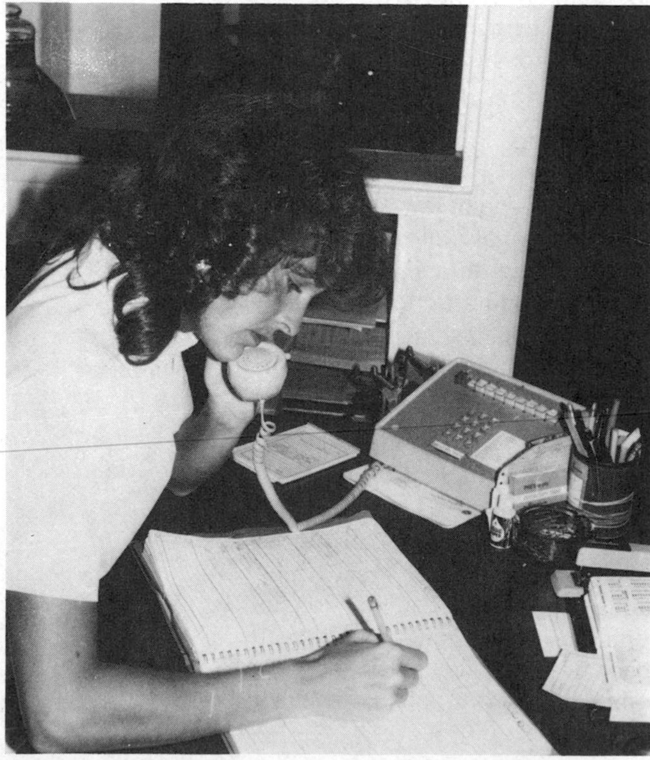

FIGURE 1–1 One of the administrative duties of the medical office assistant is to schedule patient appointments.

have specific medical aspects. She will answer telephones, schedule appointments, interview new patients to complete a registration form, screen nonpatient visitors and salesmen requesting to see the doctor, explain the doctor's fees to patients, open and sort mail, answer routine correspondence, pull medical charts for scheduled appointments and file reports and correspondence in patients' charts. She may make arrangements for patient admission to a hospital and instruct the patient regarding admission (Fig. 1–1).

She will make financial arrangements with patients, complete insurance claim forms, maintain the financial records and files, prepare and mail statements, prepare checks for doctor's signature, maintain a file of paid and unpaid invoices, prepare and maintain employees' payroll records, or submit payroll information to an outside accountant.

Sometimes she serves as an informal editorial secretary to the doctor, helping him in the preparation of manuscripts or speeches, or clipping articles from professional journals and assisting him with the maintenance of his personal medical library (see Chapter 18).

The secretary-assistant in the professional office probably will assume more responsibilities than other secretaries in the business world, since the busy doctor depends upon her to manage his everyday affairs and also requires her assistance with certain professional duties as well.

CLINICAL DUTIES. The clinical duties of the medical office assistant will also vary. Generally speaking, she helps patients prepare for examinations and other office procedures, stands by to assist the doctor when he requests her to do so, cleans and **sterilizes** instruments and equipment, and keeps the supply cabinets well-stocked. She may collect specimens from patients and either send them to a laboratory or perform certain **diagnostic** tests for which she has been trained (Fig. 1–2). She may assist with electrocardiography and radiography, take and record the patient's temperature, pulse, and respiration, prepare treatment trays, and assist with minor surgery. She may be called upon to administer emergency first aid.

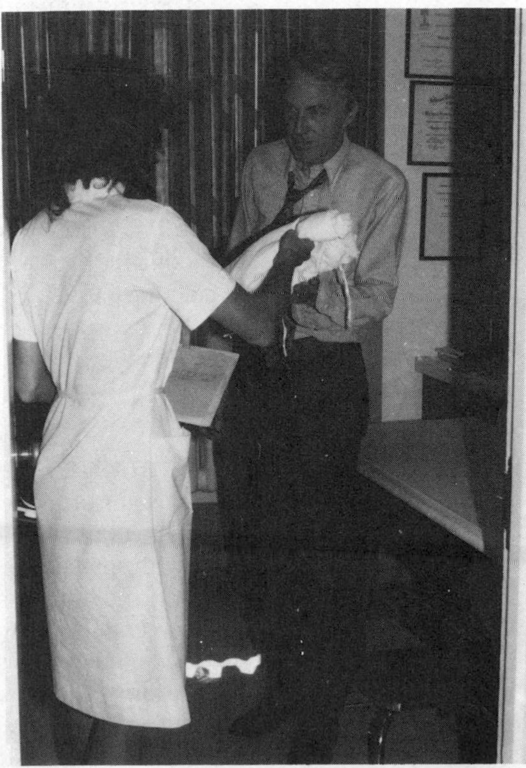

FIGURE 1–2 A medical office assistant helps prepare a patient for the physical examination.

TASK ANALYSIS. In 1971 the Division of Vocational Education of the University of California at Los Angeles, under a grant from the U.S. Department of Health, Education, and Welfare, concluded a three-year research and demonstration project instituted to develop curricula and instructional materials in the allied health occupations. The medical office assistant occupation was included in this study. The task inventory developed for this project encompassed 122 tasks related to clerical, secretarial, office management, and business functions, and 108 tasks classified as clinical and technical tasks. The task inventory was arranged in four major groups with 22 subclassifications:

Clerical, Secretarial, and Management
(a) Reception of patients and visitors
(b) Public relations
(c) Secretarial
(d) Scheduling patients
(e) Medical records
(f) Office management and housekeeping

Business Office
(a) Billing and bookkeeping
(b) Cashiering and banking
(c) Credits and collection
(d) Payment of vendors' bills
(e) Payroll

Diagnostic Tests and Procedures
(a) Specimens: obtaining and handling
(b) Urinalysis
(c) Hematology
(d) Microbiology, pathology, and sterilization
(e) Electrocardiograms
(f) X-ray procedures

Examination and Treatment Room Procedures
(a) Preparation of patient and assistance to doctor
(b) Injections
(c) Physical therapy
(d) First aid and emergency
(e) Specialty practice procedures

The 210 respondents whose questionnaires were used reported 45 different occupational titles. These 45 titles were consolidated into five categories:

Registered Nurse (RN)
Licensed Professional or Vocational Nurse (LPN)
Medical Office Assistant (technical) (MOA-T)
Medical Office Assistant (generalist) (MOA-G)
Administrative and Clerical (ADM-CL)

With the exception of **hematology,** x-ray and physical therapy, all of the 22 subclassifications of duties were performed by more than 25 per cent of the MOA-G group, the audience for which this text is designed.

TRAINING

GETTING STARTED. How does a man or woman who wishes to become a medical office assistant get started? Formal training for medical assistants was practically nonexistent until about 30 years ago. It was customary for physicians to hire a woman with some business training or perhaps a registered nurse, and then allow her to learn on the job. This is almost unheard of today.

Many community colleges throughout the nation are now offering vocational courses for medical assistants leading to a certificate or associate degree. One of the authors of this volume taught what is believed to be the first community college program for medical assistants in the nation. There are also **proprietary** schools that train assistants for medical offices. Medical assistants already employed in the field were among the first to recognize the need for more trained personnel for doctors' offices. Through chapters of the American Association of Medical Assistants (AAMA) and aided by medical societies, they have been instrumental in rapidly accelerating the development of such training programs. The community college programs include medical terminology, anatomy and physiology, biology, psychology, medical law and ethics, human relations, nutrition, first aid, medical laboratory procedures, elementary nursing arts, accounting practices, medical shorthand, filing and records management, typing and transcription, business English, and written and oral communications. Many of the college courses require in-service training in the offices of local physicians. Instructors for these courses have been recruited from the ranks of those with practical experience in the field.

CONTINUING EDUCATION THROUGH AAMA. The medical assistant on the job must continue her education, just as her employer does. For the assistant this can best be done through membership and participation in the local, state, and national levels of the American Association of Medical Assistants.

Although random organizations of medical assistants had been in existence since the 1930s, it was not until the founding of the American Association of Medical Assistants in 1956 that these groups became a real force in the education of the medical office assistant (Fig. 1–3).

At regular meetings, medical assistants' groups hear speakers on a variety of educational topics related to medicine and their work in the doctor's office. Many times these speakers are physicians. Through bulletins, conventions, symposia, workshops, and other media, AAMA members exchange ideas on more efficient ways to perform office responsibilities and keep abreast of the nonscientific subjects of interest to their employers.

Physician advisers to these groups as well as the American Medical Association have commended AAMA aims, which are to inspire the assistant to render more loyal, efficient service to the medical profession and to educate their members. The American Medical Association, in encouraging such groups to continue their educational programs, said: "The medical assistant is not only the doctor's ally in bringing the people of the community better medical care, but is tremendously important in the overall medical public relations picture."

Every chapter of the American Association of Medical Assistants has an advisory board of physicians. Several past presidents of the American Medical Association have served as advisers to the national group. At its clinical meeting in November 1962, the AMA House of Delegates passed the following resolution:

> Whereas, The American Association of Medical Assistants has as its objectives basically the same purposes as the American Medical Association; and
>
> Whereas, the American Association of Medical Assistants has, in its short span of six years' growth, rendered inestimable services not only to the people of America but also to the medical profession; and
>
> Whereas, The potential for growth and service of the American Association of Medical Assistants is recognized by the American Medical Association; therefore be it
>
> Resolved, That the American Medical Association express to the American Association of Medical Assistants its sincere appreciation for the dedicated and unselfish assistance and work in the combined goal of the two organizations in continually striving to improve the character of medical standards; and be it further
>
> Resolved, That the American Medical Association wholeheartedly endorse the program and functions of the American Association of Medical Assistants and encourage every physician who has in his employ or under his supervision medical assistants who are eligible for membership in the American Association of Medical Assistants to urge all these assistants

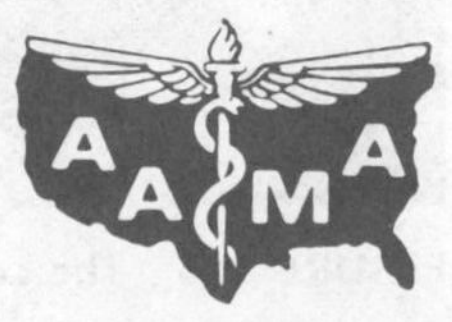

FIGURE 1–3 Insignia of the American Association of Medical Assistants. (Courtesy of the American Association of Medical Assistants, Inc., Chicago, Illinois.)

not only to join the American Association of Medical Assistants but to actively participate in their programs.

IMPORTANCE OF PROFESSIONAL ORGANIZATION. In 1959 the American Association of Medical Assistants established an executive office in Chicago, Illinois, with only one employee. The activities and responsibilities of this professional organization continued to expand year after year and by 1981 AAMA required a paid staff of over 20 employees in addition to the countless hours of volunteer work contributed by AAMA members and friends. The association publishes a bimonthly journal, *The Professional Medical Assistant* (PMA), which goes to its approximately 18,000 members as a benefit of membership. The PMA keeps the members abreast of current developments in medical office practices, offers useful hints for increasing the assistant's efficiency and includes original articles by experts in the fields of health insurance, medical law, clinical procedures, and a wide range of activities of interest to medical assistants. In the fall of each year, AAMA holds a week-long convention where members can participate in workshops, learn of educational advances in their field, hear renowned speakers on medical and management problems, and perhaps most importantly of all, develop personal friendships with medical assistants throughout the nation (Fig. 1–4).

CERTIFICATION FOR MEDICAL ASSISTANTS. In 1962, after a three-year study, the AAMA established a Certifying Board to encourage and assist in the continuing education of medical assistants by administering a qualifying examination and recognizing those who meet the standards. Those who are successful in passing the basic examination are awarded a certificate and recognition as a Certified Medical Assistant (CMA) (Fig. 1–5). Additional specialty examinations are offered in two categories, Administrative (CMA-A) and Clinical (CMA-C). The examination is not restricted to members of AAMA, and study outlines may be obtained upon request to the headquarters office in Chicago.

The first annual examination was given in October 1963 at three test centers. The certification examination is now given two times a year in January and June at more than 100 centers throughout the United States. The National Board of Medical Examiners oversees the construction and administration of the examination. Twenty-three of the 110 medical assistants who took the first examination in 1963 received certificates. Approximately 3500 applicants took the examination in 1979 with about 80 percent being successful. This increase in interest and successful completion reflects the professional advancement of medical assisting, the increased availability of training, and the continued elevation of standards by AAMA.

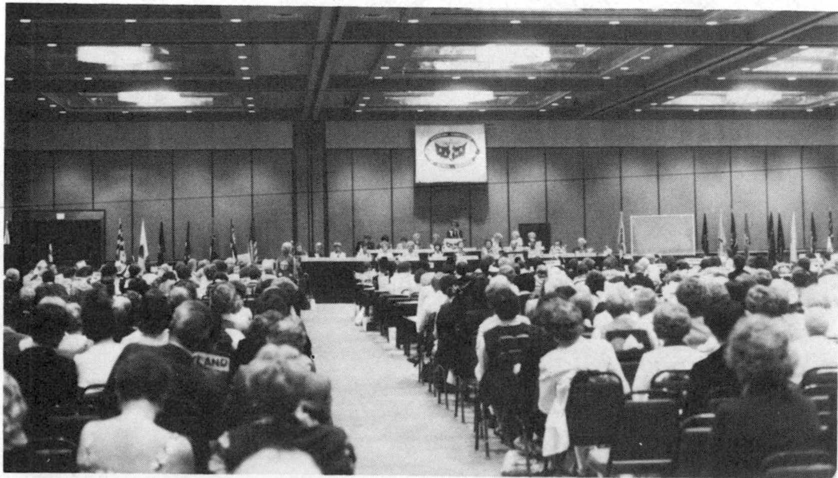

FIGURE 1–4 The convention floor of a recent meeting of the AAMA.

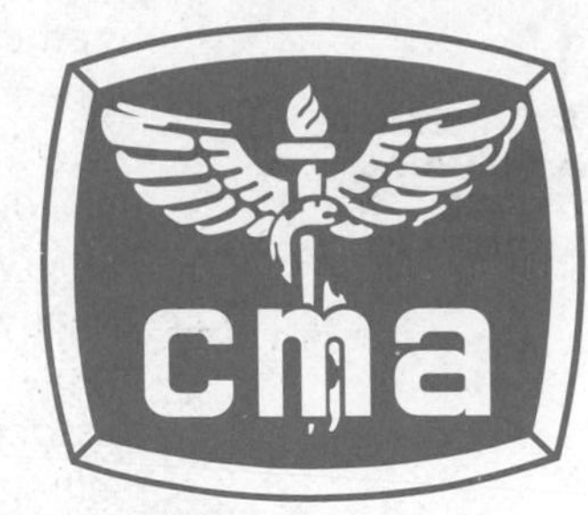

FIGURE 1–5 Pin worn by the Certified Medical Assistant. (Courtesy of the American Association of Medical Assistants, Inc., Chicago, Illinois.)

The American Association of Medical Assistants grants a number of scholarships each year for worthy students who are in need of financial aid in order to train for a medical assisting career. The Maxine Williams Scholarship Fund, named for the association's charter president, is supported by voluntary contributions.

The American Association of Medical Assistants is also instrumental in the accreditation of medical assisting programs in proprietary and community colleges. Formerly the accrediting was accomplished by the American Medical Association's Council on Medical Education. In January 1977 all accreditation responsibilities of the Council were transferred to an **autonomous** body, the Committee on Allied Health Education and Accreditation (CAHEA). Programs are evaluated by a joint AMA/AAMA survey team and its recommendations for accreditation are presented to CAHEA, which is the accrediting body for 28 organizations.

Inquiries regarding any of the association activities may be directed to a local chapter or to the national headquarters located at One East Wacker Drive, Suite 2110, Chicago, Illinois 60601.

Medical assisting has come a long way since the first edition of this book and the organizational meeting of AAMA, both of which occurred in 1956.

REWARDS OF A HEALTH CAREER

There are rewards above and beyond those of salary and job security for the office assistant. There is the stimulation of growing with the job, and there is a justifiable pride and humility that result from participation in the professional partnership. The role of assistant is a demanding but rewarding one. It is stated in *Partners for Health* that:

> Compared job for job with like occupations in other fields, health occupations are generally above average so far as surroundings and working conditions are concerned. But as far as time and energy, alertness and dependability, patience and determination, skill and accuracy, responsibility and integrity, courage and character are concerned — for all of these qualities, there is no denying that health careers make demands beyond the call of duty.
>
> Choosing a health career is a big decision because working for health is more than just a job. It is a point of view, a way of looking at life — your own life and the lives of the people you see and serve and work with every day.

Anyone who decides to become a medical office assistant makes that important decision. It is one that few ever regret having made — and a decision that thousands will make in the future as the career of medical office assistant is more widely publicized and its rewards cited.

MEMBERS OF THE TEAM

The man or woman who seeks employment in a medical office must be prepared to function as a member of a team. A solo practitioner may hire only one assistant, the "girl Friday," in which case the team will comprise only the assistant and the doctor. The trend, however, is toward a multiple number of employees, even in those offices where there is only one physician. There is a strong possibility, too, that the assistant will be employed in a group practice or clinic where there are many members of the team.

The medical office assistant needs some acquaintance with the scope of duties and the training required of other paramedical employees. These may include a nurse, an x-ray technologist, **inhalation therapist,** EKG technician, **EEG** technician, omit

medical transcriptionist, insurance clerk, bookkeeper, and office manager, as well as others.

A *licensed practical nurse* (LPN) or, in some states, *licensed vocational nurse* (LVN), is prepared to work in almost all fields of nursing. She works under the direct supervision of the physician or a registered nurse. Since the LPN/LVN is licensed, she legally may be capable of performing some clinical duties in the doctor's office that may not be performed by the unlicensed medical assistant. The *registered nurse* (RN) (associate degree or baccalaureate degree) will more likely be found in a hospital setting rather than in a physician's office.

omit

The *physician's assistant* (PA) is a relatively new member of the medical office team. The PA has taken special academic training that includes clinical practice in providing medical services under the responsibility and supervision of the physician. The PA may do well-patient physicals, make house calls, perform routine medical services such as changing dressings, removing **sutures,** or other duties assigned by the physician. The range of duties will depend to a great degree upon the practice specialty and the disposition of the physician to delegate duties. The term physician's assistant should not be confused or used interchangeably with the term medical assistant.

The medical profession is making more and more use of x-rays and other sources of radioactive energy. Therefore, the *radiologic technologist* may be found in the physician's office. The x-ray technologist works under the direct supervision of the physician in taking the films that are required for radiographic examination of disease and injury. The technologist has usually completed at least 24 months of specialized education and experience in a hospital, followed by successful completion of the certifying examination conducted by the American Registry of Radiologic Technologists. In some states the medical assistant may have state sanction to perform certain x-ray procedures for which she is trained. In California this is called a limited x-ray permit.

The *medical technologist* (MT) is an allied health professional, and is often referred to as the detective of the health care team. Usually they work in a medical laboratory, helping to determine the nature and causes of disease, but group practices often employ an MT on the team. With the help of microscopes and precision instruments they examine and analyze samples of tissues and body fluids to assist in the diagnosis of disease. MTs bring important skills and knowledge of chemistry, physics, and biology to the health care team.

Inhalation therapy (now sometimes referred to as *respiratory care*) is an allied health specialty in the treatment, management, control, and care of patients with difficulties and abnormalities associated with the process of breathing. It is used primarily in the treatment of heart and lung ailments, such as cardiac failure, **asthma, pulmonary edema, emphysema, cerebral thrombosis, hemorrhage,** and **shock.** The therapist must be fully capable, under medical supervision, of operating inhalation therapy equipment, and administering to patients the therapeutic and diagnostic procedures of inhalation therapy.

The electrocardiograph is an instrument that records a patient's heart action. An *EKG technician* is employed in the offices of many physicians, especially cardiologists and internists. The technician prepares the patient and makes the recording of the patient's heart action. The tracings are then "read" and interpreted by the physician.

The **electroencephalograph** is an instrument that records brain waves. The *EEG technician* might be employed in the office of a neurologist.

A *medical transcriptionist* may be employed by a physician who dictates a great deal of correspondence, reports, records, and so forth. The transcriptionist has a thorough knowledge of medical terminology, grammar, and spelling, is a good typist, and must be familiar with the use of dictating equipment. Hospitals employ many medical transcriptionists in their records departments.

Most multiple-doctor practices will employ someone specialized in processing insurance claim forms. The *insurance clerk* may have had on-the-job training or she may have attended special classes to familiarize herself with local insurance plans. She needs an understanding of medical diagnoses and procedures and the coding books that are used to designate them, as well as knowledge of the numerous insurance plans and their requirements.

Larger practices will probably employ a full-time *bookkeeper* with advanced training and experience in accounting practices.

In the one-doctor, one-assistant office, delegation of duties and responsibilities goes hand in hand. When there is more than one employee there usually must be one individual designated as *office manager,* on whom final responsibility must fall for the smooth operation of the office. When there are many employees, the managerial responsibility becomes greater, and someone specially trained in management techniques may be needed for this position.

Large or small, the medical facility must function as a unit with each person assuming full responsibility for her own duties, but with an awareness that the cooperation of every member of the team is vital to the best care of the patient.

References

American Medical Association: *Winning Ways with Patients*. Chicago, American Medical Association, 1966.

DiCicco, O., and Earl, B. S.: *Occupational Analysis, Medical Office Assistant.* University of California, Los Angeles, Division of Vocational Education, Allied Health Professions Project, 1971.

National Health Council, *Partners for Health.*

New York Times Encyclopedic Almanac, New York Times, 1971.

Shaffer, H. B.: *Medical Ethics: Editorial Research Reports on Medical Issues*. Washington, D.C., Congressional Quarterly, Inc., 1972.

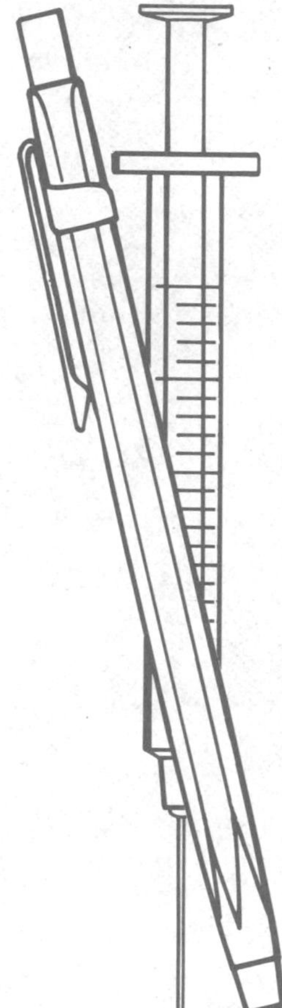

CHAPTER OUTLINE

BEHAVIORAL OBJECTIVES

The medical office assistant should be able to:

- **Plan the appropriate strategy for applying for a position as a medical office assistant.**
- **Prepare an effective personal data sheet and letter requesting an interview.**
- **Assist her employer in screening applicants for a job.**
- **Assist her employer in evaluating a new employee.**

2

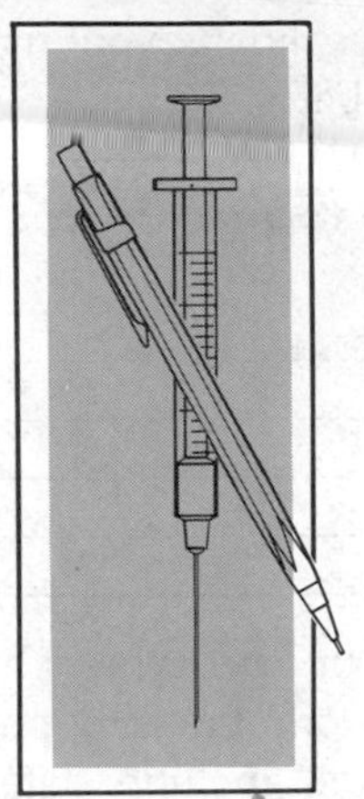

FINDING THE RIGHT POSITION

THE MEDICAL ASSISTANT AS AN APPLICANT

After the medical office assistant has been trained for employment in a doctor's office, the next step is to match her capabilities with the requirements of a physician who is seeking an employee. It may be the assistant's first position, she may be returning to the field after an absence of several years, or an employed assistant may be planning to change employers. The essential steps in applying for a position will be similar in all of these situations:

Step One: Preparation for the Interview
Step Two: Locating Prospective Employers
Step Three: The Interview

PRELIMINARY STEPS. Before seeking an interview, ask yourself some pertinent questions:

What type of work do I really want?
Do I prefer clinical or administrative duty?
Do I prefer to work in a solo practice or in a large medical group?
Do I prefer general practice or a specialty?
How important to me are salary, hours, and location?

You may not get exactly what you want, and if you have very definite answers to all of these questions, you may be too inflexible to find suitable employment in medical assisting. On the other hand, if you are absolutely certain of something that would make you dissatisfied, that is a different matter. Remember, though, that your attitude can also alert an interviewer to whether you are favorably motivated or to the likelihood that you are just looking for a paycheck.

PREPARATION FOR THE INTERVIEW

Personal Inventory. It may be that when you are ready to go to work, someone will offer you an ideal position that you will accept and stay in for the remainder of your working years. More likely, though, you will have to search for employment and will make several changes of employment during your lifetime. A *personal inventory,* to which you will add as you gain additional experience and education, will prove invaluable to you later as well as now. The personal inventory is for your own information and reference. It will be a ready source of information in preparing and updating your **resume**. The personal inventory is *complete* information about yourself; a resume is *selected* information tailored to the position you are seeking.

1. Start with a page for biographical data: your name, birth date, social security number, address and telephone number.

BIOGRAPHICAL DATA

Name ______________________________ Birth Date ____________
__________________________________ Soc. Sec. No. __________
Address ____
__________________________________ Tel. No. ______________

2. Prepare a separate page for your employment history. If you have never been employed but have done volunteer work requiring personal responsibility, list that here. The employment history should include dates of employment, name of employer, type of business, your position title and major duties. List all employment in **chronological** order starting with the first major job you held.

EMPLOYMENT HISTORY

June 1978 to June 1980 Employer Looking Good
Month Year Month Year

Type of Business: Women's clothing

Position Held: part-time sales clerk

Major Duties: Assisting customers in their selections, registering sales, closing out register at end of day

Satisfactions: Enjoyed personal contacts
Learned to accept responsibility

Dissatisfactions: Not related to my goals

3. Next, record your educational data beginning with high school. List the dates, the institution attended, and the year of graduation plus diploma or degree earned. Make note of the areas of study you enjoyed most, special competencies, awards, or honors. As time goes by it may be difficult to recall these details and you never know what will be important to an employer in the future. Remember, you are starting a permanent record for your own information and as a handy reference tool when needed.

EDUCATIONAL DATA

Dates	Institution Attended	Yr Graduated/Degree
1976–1978	Valley High School Ola Vista	1978 Diploma
1978–1980	Ola Vista Community College	1980 Associate in Science, Medical Assisting

Special Competencies:
Typing Certificate (70 WPM)
Limited X-ray permit, 1980
CPR Certificate, 1977, renewed annually
Fluency in Spanish
Awards:
Dean's List, all four semesters in college

4. You may wish to include a page for your **avocational** interests. List organization memberships and activities and any positions of leadership you held. Your volunteer activities might be included here if they are not in your employment record.

AVOCATIONAL INTERESTS

Organization Membership	Year	Personal Activities
Associated Women Students	1978–1980	Secretary
American Association of Medical Assistants	1978–	Convention page, 1979

5. Finally, have a page for your personal goals. What are your immediate goals? your long-term goals? What concessions are you willing to make in order to reach your goals?

PERSONAL GOALS

Date	Immediate Goals	Long-Term Goals
1980	Medical assistant position, preferably in pediatric practice	Bachelor of Science in Business Administration Administrative position in large group practice or HMO

Hobbies: Oil painting, backpacking, Brownie group leader

Personal Data Sheet (Resume). The most important step in preparing for an interview is making a personal data sheet that will arouse the interest of a prospective employer (Figs. 2–1 and 2–2). Using your personal inventory, select the information that applies to the position you have in mind. Choose an attractive **format,** and type the information on one sheet of paper with absolutely no errors or misspelled words. Tinted paper will make it more distinctive.

If you do not feel confident in doing this yourself, get help. If you are a student in a two-year college there is probably a career center on campus where you can ask for assistance. There are also many commercial establishments that offer this service. Look under Resume Service in the yellow pages of your telephone directory.

The purpose of the resume is to get an interview, not to get a job. Keep this in mind as you decide what to include. The resume gives you an opportunity to display the qualifications that enhance your appeal to prospective employers. Omit anything that cannot help you or anything that would detract from your image. Once you are in the interview, you can clarify any item not entirely explained on the resume.

There is no standard form for a resume. At the top of your paper, so that it stands apart (may be centered), place the necessary personal information: name, address, and telephone number. Display this prominently for easy identification.

1. State your **objective.** Be as specific as you can without narrowing your possibilities too much. The objective tells the prospective employer what kind of position you are seeking.

2. and 3. Education and experience. If you are a recent graduate with little or no experience, list your education first and then your employment, if any. Those of you with a good history of recent employment should make this the first item, followed with education. In both cases, start with the most recent and list in reverse time order.

4. List any **extracurricular** or avocational interests that would be applicable to the position sought.

5. State on your resume that references will be furnished upon request. Be prepared to furnish the names of at least three references at the time of your interview. These should have been typewritten on a separate page in the same style as your resume. Don't forget to obtain permission from the persons you are listing.

THERESA O'SULLIVAN
233 West Wentworth Street
San Diego, CA 92184
714-239-2345

OBJECTIVE:	To secure a challenging position in a medical facility where I can use my training as a clinical medical assistant	
EDUCATION:	Associate in Science Medical Assisting Ola Vista Community College	June 1980
	Dean's List, 4 semesters	
	Diploma, Valley High School	June 1978
SPECIAL COMPETENCIES:	Speak Spanish fluently Hold Limited X-ray Permit CPR Certificate (renewed annually)	
EMPLOYMENT:	William O. Madden, M.D. Duties included: preparing patients for examination in general practice office; handling front desk 3-6 p.m. four afternoons a week	Part-Time June 1979 to Sept 1980
	Looking Good Part-time sales clerk Duties included: assisting customers in their selections, registering sales, closing out register at end of day	June 1978 to June 1980
AVOCATIONAL INTERESTS:	Student member, American Association of Medical Assistants Secretary, Associated Women Students OVCC	
REFERENCES:	Furnished upon request	

FIGURE 2–1 Sample resume.

LOCATING PROSPECTIVE EMPLOYERS. If you are a student in an accredited school, your instructor or the school may be able to give you names of prospective employers. Other good sources for leads are the local medical society, other medical office assistants, and branches of the United States Employment Service and state-operated employment offices. You may also wish to check the classified advertisements in your local newspaper, or place your name with an employment agency. Private employment agencies generally charge a fee equivalent to two to four weeks' salary to successful applicants.

REQUESTING AN INTERVIEW. You may either telephone an employer asking for an interview, or write a letter requesting an interview (Fig. 2–3). Send your personal data sheet along with the letter. Each interviewer is to be given a copy of the data sheet. This should be either an original or a good quality copy. Do not use carbon copies or poor photocopies. Never ask the interviewer to return the copy of your data sheet.

THERESA O'SULLIVAN, CMA-A

STATEMENT OF EMPLOYMENT ASSETS FOR A CAREER IN ADMINISTRATIVE MEDICAL ASSISTING

233 West Wentworth Street, San Diego CA 92184 714-239-2345

EDUCATION

June 1980 Associate in Science Medical Assisting
Ola Vista Community College

Dean's List, 4 semesters

June 1978 Diploma, Valley High School

Goal: Degree in Business Administration
Southern California College

SPECIAL COMPETENCIES

Speak Spanish fluently
CPR Certificate, renewed annually since 1977
Typing Certificate 70 WPM
Experience in machine transcription and telephone reception in office of College President
Certified Medical Assistant, Administrative

EMPLOYMENT

June 1979–June 1980 William O. Madden, M.D.
Duties included: preparing patients for examination in general practice office; handling front desk 3-6 p.m., four afternoons a week

AVOCATIONAL INTERESTS

Student member, American Association of Medical Assistants
Secretary, Associated Women Students OVCC

REFERENCES

Furnished upon request

FIGURE 2–2 Sample resume.

At the suggestion of M ______________________________,
my medical assisting instructor at ______________________________
College, I am writing to inquire whether you have an opening for a medical assistant on your staff.

In a few weeks, I will be graduating with an A.S. Degree and a certificate in medical assisting. As you will see from the enclosed resumé, my training has included both the administrative and the clinical skills necessary for employment in a physician's office. If you will require a replacement or addition to your staff in the near future, may I be considered as an applicant for this job?

Please call me at 123-4567 and suggest a time when I may come to your office for an interview.

Sincerely yours,

FIGURE 2–3 Letter requesting an interview.

DAY OF THE INTERVIEW. Appearance is extremely important, whether you are wearing street clothes or a uniform. Your hair should be neat and worn in a professional looking style. Makeup should be carefully applied and in good taste. Do not go to an interview with bare legs or wearing an extreme shoe or dress style. Carry a modest purse that is not bulging with unnecessary items. Take a critical look at yourself in the mirror before leaving home. An employer may attach importance to some careless detail. Your appearance at the time of the interview is the only way of judging how you will look as an employee.

Arrive promptly for the interview. Under no circumstances should you be even so much as a minute late and then have to make a weak excuse. *Go alone.* You may want moral support, but you will be more relaxed if there is no one waiting for you. *Enter the office confidently,* without appearing rushed. Introduce yourself to the receptionist, then thank her when she asks you to be seated. If you must wait, relax but maintain a ladylike posture. *Do not smoke or chew gum!*

When you are ushered into the interviewer's room, wait to be seated until you are invited to do so. Let the interviewer lead the conversation. Be prepared to answer such questions as "Tell me about yourself," and "Why do you want to work here?" Remember, the interviewer will be observing your manners, poise, speech, alertness,

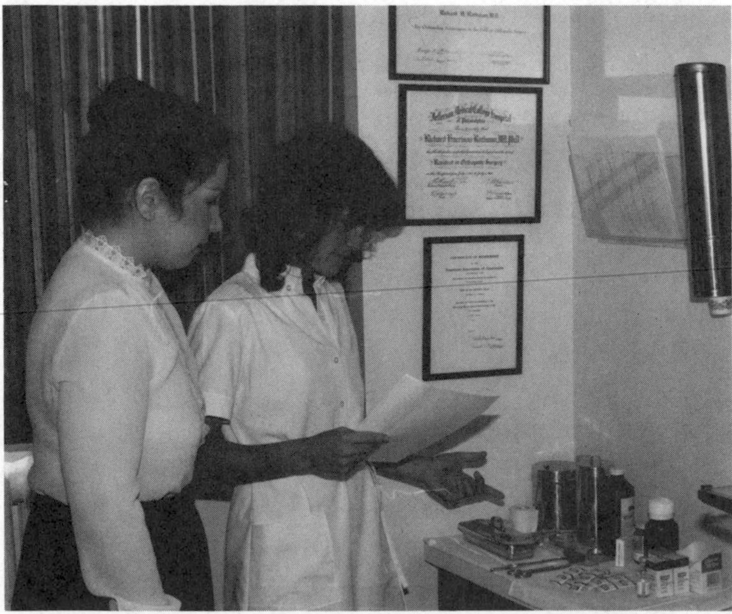

FIGURE 2–4 The medical office assistant is often required to give a prospective employee a tour of the facilities.

and ability to give direct answers. Your sense of humor may be tested as well, and questions may be directed to you that will test your common sense and frankness. You can promote yourself honestly and graciously by showing that you enjoy others, are willing to work and accept responsibility, and that you have an open mind about the position and are willing to learn. Recent legislation in fair employment practices has influenced hiring practices nationwide. Employers are restricted in the information that can be required on an application or asked in an interview. But while you may not be *required* to answer questions regarding your age, birthplace, marital status, and so forth, you may be inclined to mention them in conversation. Remember your objective — a position. A straightforward attitude may be appreciated.

At the end of the interview, if the interviewer has not mentioned hours and salary, you may properly inquire at this time. If you are not really interested in the position, do not bother to ask, but if it sounds satisfactory and is one that you would like to accept, you may then ask if the interviewer wishes to discuss the salary. This should be enough of a lead, since it was probably an oversight on the interviewer's part. If the interviewer seems reluctant to discuss it, though, do not press the issue since he may not be interested in your qualifications and does not wish to pursue the interview further.

If you have been given a tour of the office (Fig. 2–4), you may make some pleasant observations and comments, but do not be falsely overenthusiastic. When you are introduced to the staff be gracious and friendly. Try to remember their names so that you can thank them later. Show enthusiasm, but do not overdo it because it may appear to others that you are "putting on an act."

CLOSING THE INTERVIEW. The interviewer will usually take the initiative in closing the interview. He may slide back his chair and ask if you have further questions. Do not show disappointment if the position is not offered to you at the time of the interview. The interviewer may have other applicants to see, or he may wish to check your references before making a commitment. Thank him for the interview as you leave. Remember, too, to thank the receptionist and say a friendly goodbye.

FOLLOW-UP ACTIVITIES. A brief, well-worded letter of thanks sent to the interviewer immediately after the interview makes a good impression. After a few days you may call the office and ask if the position has been filled, and tell them you are interested because you enjoyed your interview and the office. If the position is still open, and if it is one you really want, then inquire again in a few days. Always be brief, and thank the person with whom you speak. Even if you are not hired, you should never feel that an interview is a waste of time. You learn from each experience, and with experience you are better able to promote your qualifications in future interviews.

SURVEY OF DESIRABLE QUALITIES. An extensive survey* conducted by several college students in January 1972 reported maturity, compatibility, and personality as highly rated qualities. Ambition and initiative were also mentioned by all employers. This survey found the following qualities to be the ones most widely looked for by employers:

1. Good appearance
2. Common sense
3. Ability to think
4. Ability to take criticism
5. Interest in job (and company)
6. Pleasing personality

Most surveys have shown that many people fail to get or keep jobs because of personality problems. Technical skills are usually considered less important than the ability to work **amicably** with others.

*Qualities of the Industrial Office Worker, National Business Education Association, November, 1972, Volume 27, No. 2.

Also listed here are some "pet peeves" of employers. Read them carefully so that you will not be guilty of similar actions:

1. Lack of eye contact during interview
2. Came on too strong
3. Talked of salary and hours immediately
4. Wiggled in chair and fidgeted with hands
5. Had to dig too hard for information
6. Used poor grammar or too much slang
7. Was chewing gum
8. Too much makeup and perfume
9. Was late
10. Too much chatter, tried too hard to explain
11. Was too **aggressive** or too **blasé**
12. Answers were unclear, tried to hide something
13. No enthusiasm
14. Poor data sheet
15. Poor grooming, showed lack of respect for interviewer

THE MEDICAL ASSISTANT AS AN INTERVIEWER

LOOKING FOR A MEDICAL ASSISTANT? Many times a physician will ask his experienced medical assistant to aid in finding someone to fill an opening either to increase the staff or to replace someone who is retiring or moving away. The assistant who is given this responsibility must use great care and judgment, and remain objective in her search for a prospective employee. If an applicant for the position is a friend or former classmate, she must still meet the qualifications set by office needs. The individual you recommend to the doctor may be working with you and the other members of the staff for a long while.

PRELIMINARY STEPS. First, ask the doctor to state (a) what personal qualifications the applicant should have, (b) what her duties will be, (c) what salary he is willing to pay, and (d) how soon he expects the job to start. Next, add your own suggestions to the list. Then, set forth these requirements in an outline to guide you in selecting prospective applicants. Here are some suggested guidelines:

1. What age range would probably blend best with present office personnel?

2. Is the applicant's appearance satisfactory? Is weight an important consideration? Is personal grooming up to expectations?

3. Work experience: Has she had previous employment? What were her duties on her last job? In what skills is she proficient? How long was she on her last job? Did she enjoy her work? Does she accept and enjoy responsibility?

4. Why did she leave her last job? The manner in which she describes her last employer and the office staff may provide a clue to her general attitude or disposition.

5. Educational background: What has been her formal education? Is she a Certified Medical Assistant? If not, is she planning to take the certifying examination? Does she attend medical assisting workshops? Is she a member of the local chapter of the A.A.M.A.? An assistant who thinks she knows all there is to running an office may be less satisfactory than one who is inexperienced but willing to learn.

6. What are her family responsibilities? Is she married or single? If she has young children, has she made adequate child care arrangements?

7. Check the applicant's references. Can she give the names of responsible persons? References from close friends or neighbors are virtually useless. Has she provided full name, title, address, and telephone number so that you can easily check with these individuals?

ARRANGING THE PERSONAL INTERVIEW. If the applicant sent a letter asking for an interview, you probably noted whether the letter was correctly typed, included the essential information, and enclosed a personal data sheet. You cannot be certain that the applicant personally prepared the letter and data sheet; ask her at the time of the interview. Forget the applicant who sends a letter handwritten with pencil!

If the applicant telephoned for an interview appointment, then you had the opportunity to hear her telephone voice. If her telephone voice is poor, you may not wish to consider her further.

Set a time for the personal interview when you most likely will be able to give the applicant your undivided attention. However, the applicant should have an opportunity to see your office when there is a fairly normal amount of activity. The prospective employee who is interviewed in a peaceful, quiet office on the doctor's day out may have a rude awakening when she appears for work on a normal day.

THE INTERVIEW. Before interviewing any applicant, make certain you are thoroughly familiar with the federal, state and local fair-employment practice (FEP) laws affecting hiring practice. The purpose of such laws is to prevent **discrimination** in the hiring of minority-group members, women, older people, the handicapped, and others. Unless you are up-to-date on these regulations, you could find yourself involved in an expensive lawsuit or settlement with a disappointed applicant claiming discrimination. These laws also determine what information you may request on an employment application. Check with the Department of Labor for current regulations.

Either send the applicant an application form to be completed and brought in at the time of the interview, or allow ample time for its completion on the day of the interview. The application form can serve as a check of the applicant's penmanship and thoroughness as well as a permanent record for your files. If you do wish it completed in the applicant's own handwriting be sure to state this on the instructions. The applicant should be **meticulous** about following instructions and filling in *all* the blanks. As you speak with the applicant, make a mental note of these observations: Does she converse easily? Is she a good listener? Is she free of annoying mannerisms? Does she have a ready smile? Is she interested enough to ask, as well as to answer questions? Does she appear interested in the office and the doctor's specialty?

An interview should not be a one-way flow of information from applicant to interviewer. If the applicant appears to be one who will receive serious consideration, you have the responsibility of telling her what will be expected of her in the way of duties; office policies regarding appearance, working hours, overtime, time off, and vacations; what initial salary is offered, any fringe benefits, and the office policy on increases. Often the interviewer fails to mention these items, and the applicant may be too timid to inquire.

FOLLOW-UP ACTIVITIES. When the interview is over, take a few moments to immediately rate the applicant on your checklist. Jot down some notes to refresh your memory when you refer this applicant to the doctor for the final interview. Do not trust to memory, especially if several applicants will be interviewed. The following is a suggested checklist which may be modified to suit your own circumstances.

Name ______________________ **Date** __________ **Time** __________

	Superior	Above Average	Average	Poor	Remarks
Appearance and grooming					
General Health					
Voice and diction					
Mannerisms					
Poise					
Friendliness					
Interest in work					
Did applicant ask questions?					
Overall impression					

If your employer is a member of a credit bureau, it may be advisable to check the applicant's credit rating, especially if she will be expected to handle the office finances. It can be safely assumed that one who is unable to handle her own financial affairs will be a poor risk in handling office finances. The ability to handle one's financial affairs may also be considered a mark of maturity.

If you had no telephone contact with the applicant, find a reason to call her on the telephone. You might ask a question about her data sheet or application form; you may call to say you are still interviewing and wondered if she were still available; or you may be completely candid and say you wanted to hear her telephone voice.

CHECKING REFERENCES. It is always advisable to carefully check all references, and follow through on any leads for information. Sometimes certain names have been omitted, and this could be important. It is best to use the telephone in checking references, because people are sometimes less than candid in a letter; furthermore, letter writing is time-consuming and you may not get a reply. Prepare a check list before you place the call, and then when you talk with the person called be sure to "listen between the lines." Note the tone of the replies to your questions. Here are some questions you might ask in your inquiry:

Applicant's name ____________________

Name of Reference Called ____________________ **Telephone No.** __________

1. When did ____________________ work for you? How long?
2. What were her duties? Did she seem to enjoy the work?
3. Why did she leave? (listen carefully)
4. Would you rehire her under the right circumstances?
5. Was she frequently absent or late?
6. Was she in good health?
7. Did she assume responsibility well?
8. How was her rapport with other staff members?
9. Do you have any suggestions or advice about hiring this person?

Do not recommend an applicant to the doctor for his final approval and interview until you have completed your share of the investigation and have prepared a report for him. This preliminary screening may save an embarrassment for the doctor and for you as well. It may also prevent having to start the process all over again within a few months.

THE OTHER APPLICANTS. When a decision has been reached to hire someone, remember to notify others who have applied. They may have hesitated to accept other interviews in hope of hearing from you. It is unfair to keep individuals who are seeking employment "on the string." Good etiquette requires that you drop them a note or call by telephone, and say the position is filled. Thank the individual for applying, and say that you will keep her application on file.

EVALUATING THE NEW EMPLOYEE. A new employee should be granted a probationary period. Sixty to 90 days has been traditional, but many employers feel that two weeks is sufficient to determine whether the employee will be able to learn and adapt to the position. A definite date for a performance review at the end of the probationary period should be set at the time of employment. This review should not be squeezed in between patient visits, or be given a token few minutes at the end of a day. There should be ample time to relax and talk. At this time the new employee is told how well she has met expectations and whether there are any deficiencies in her work. She should be given the opportunity to ask questions. Sometimes an employee does not perform as expected because she was never told what she was supposed to do.

If, at the time of the performance review, her work has not been satisfactory and there is little hope that she will work out, her employment should be terminated then and there. In all fairness, an individual should be told why the employment is ended, and not be given weak excuses or untruths that do not give her the opportunity to correct her deficiencies. Many times an employee never knows the true reason for termination and does not know whether the employer can be used as a future job reference.

Although the probationary period does not allow time to fully train an individual for a specific office, it is fair to assume that her potential for being a satisfactory employee can be judged at this time. Now is the time to talk out any problems and make suggestions for improvement. The assistant who is doing fine should be told so, then a raise and a welcome to the staff will do wonders for her and the office. It is encouraging to any employee, but especially so for the new employee, to hear "You are doing a great job and we are glad to have you with us."

References

Bolles, R. N.: *The Three Boxes of Life, and How to Get Out of Them.* Berkeley, Cal., Ten Speed Press, 1978.

Bolles, R. N.: *What Color is Your Parachute?* Berkeley, Cal., Ten Speed Press, 1978.

Gootnick, D.: *Getting a Better Job.* New York, McGraw-Hill Paperbacks, 1978.

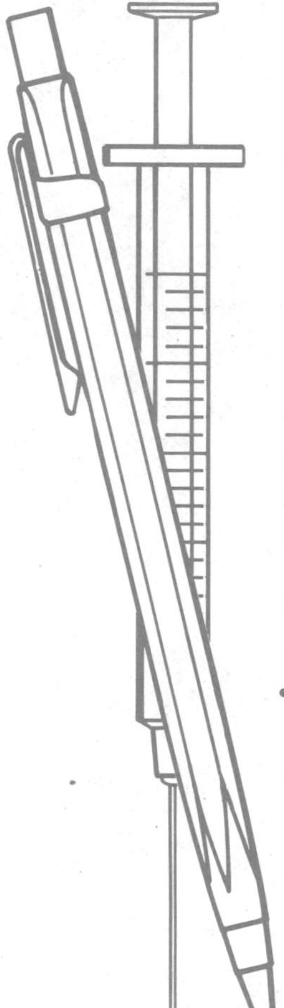

CHAPTER OUTLINE

Medical Language and Mythology
Medicine in Ancient Times
Pioneers in Modern Medicine

BEHAVIORAL OBJECTIVES

The medical office assistant should be able to:

- **Identify the contributions to medicine made by important historical figures.**

3

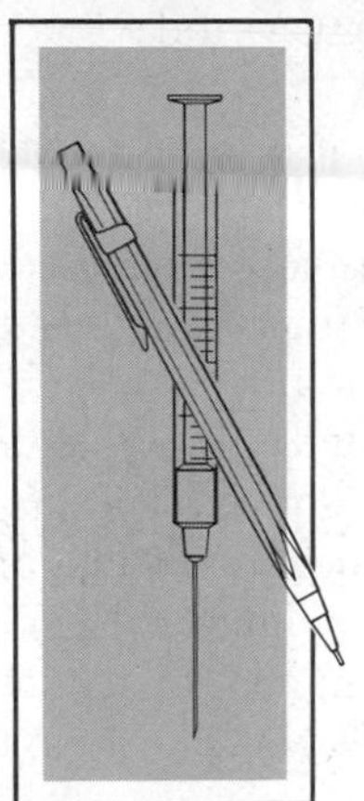

A BRIEF HISTORY OF MEDICINE

Modern medicine reflects its history in the names given to anatomy, physiology, medications, diseases, instruments and specialties. Even the latest medical discoveries often have names drawn from the ancients. It is impossible to live in the world of medicine and to talk its language without being constantly touched by this fascinating past. The rich cultural heritage of medicine is interesting to study and to draw upon, but it is also a process filled with hardships and disappointments that were pushed aside by determined men and women who wanted to pursue their dreams and goals. It can be inspiring to think of these pioneers and realize that we too are part of the heritage of caring and discovery that continues to improve health care throughout the world.

MEDICAL LANGUAGE AND MYTHOLOGY

It may seem strange for modern medicine to borrow so liberally from ancient mythology, and to use so actively the classical languages that most men abandoned centuries ago. Yet today's medicine uses words whose origins stem from the romance and fantasy of this long "dead" world. Anatomy, especially, seems to reach back to the dawn of history and, although some terms are today erroneous when translated literally because the ancients did not correctly understand body functions, many early anatomic terms have reached modern times almost unchanged.

Greek and Roman mythology has contributed a major portion of our medical terms, but we have also borrowed liberally from Arabic, Anglo-Saxon, and German sources, with a heavy dash of the Bible added. Here are a few of the many examples from the classical past: the anatomic name for the first cervical vertebra upon which the head rests is aptly named Atlas, the famous Greek Titan, who, according to mythology, was condemned by Zeus to bear the heavens on his shoulders. The tendon of Achilles reminds us of the story of the youth whose mother held him by the heel and dipped him into the river Styx to make him invulnerable. This particular tendon was not immersed and later a mortal wound was inflicted in Achilles' heel. The dubious honors given in medicine to Venus, the Roman Goddess of Love, are paid to her not so much as the goddess of love but of lust. She has a portion of the female anatomy, the mons veneris, dedicated to her memory. Venereal diseases are also named after her. Aphrodite, the Greek Goddess of Love and Beauty, gave her name to the sex-exciting drugs known as aphrodisiacs.

Aesculapius, the son of Apollo, was revered as the God of Medicine. The early Greeks worshipped the healing powers of Aesculapius and built temples in his honor, where patients were treated by trained priests. His daughters were Hygeia, Goddess of Health, and Panacea, Goddess of All Heal and Restorer of Health. These two names are prominent in our language today.

MEDICINE IN ANCIENT TIMES

Though religion and myth were the basis of care for the sick for millennia, there is evidence of drugs, surgery, and other treatments based on theories about the body from as early as 5000 to 2000 BC. In the well-developed societies of the Egyptians, Babylonians, and Assyrians, certain men acted as physicians, using their scant knowledge to try to treat illness and injury.

Around 1205 BC Moses incorporated rules of health into the Hebrew religion. He was thus the first advocate of preventive medicine and could even be called the first "public health officer." Moses knew that some animal diseases may be passed on to man and that contamination may linger on unclean dishes. Thus, it became a religious law that no one was permitted to eat animals that were not freshly slaughtered or to eat or drink from dirty dishes, lest they become defiled and lose their souls.

Hippocrates (460–377 BC) is the most famous of the ancient Greek physicians and is known as the "Father of Medicine." He did much to separate medicine from mysticism and gave it a scientific basis. He is best remembered for the "Hippocratic Oath" of medical ethics which has been administered to physicians for more than 2000 years. Hippocrates' astute clinical descriptions of diseases and his voluminous writings on epidemics, fevers, epilepsy, fractures, and instruments were studied for centuries. He believed that the body tends to heal itself and it is the physician's responsibility to help nature.

There were many Greek physicians who practiced, studied, and taught in Rome in the time after Hippocrates. One was Galen (131–201 AD), who came to Rome in 162 AD and became known as the "Prince of Physicans" (Fig. 3–1). Galen is said to have written 500 treatises on medicine. He was also appointed physician to the Emperor Marcus Aurelius. He wrote an excellent summary of anatomy as it was known at that time, and is considered to be the father of experimental physiology.

The profound influence of the writings of Hippocrates and Galen on the course of medicine gives praise to these great thinkers, but their unquestioned authority actually had a negative effect on the progress of science throughout the "Dark Ages." Their theories and descriptions were held to as law, so innovation was rarely attempted. Experimenters were scoffed at by their contemporaries. It was not until the 16th century that Andreas Vesalius (1514–1564) began to correct some of Galen's errors (Fig. 3–2).

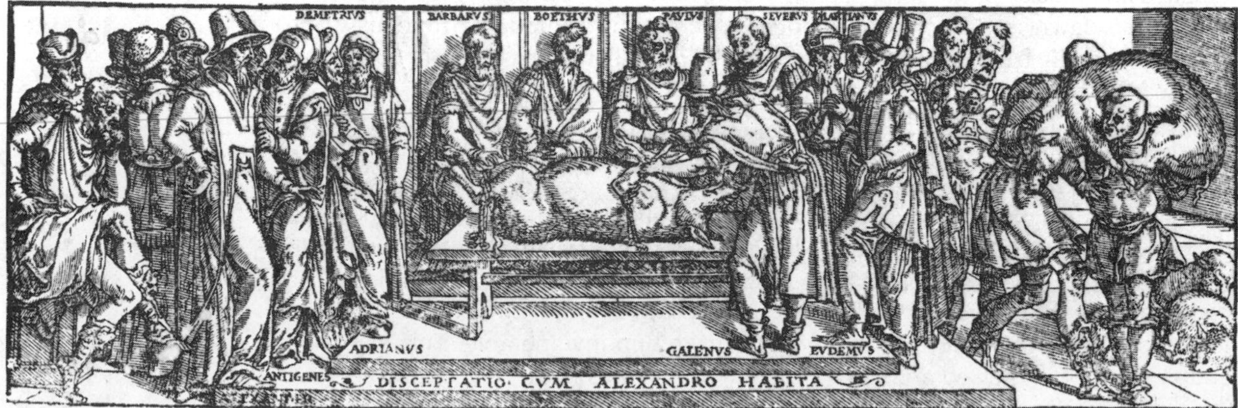

FIGURE 3–1 Galen. (Courtesy of the National Library of Medicine.)

Vesalius, a Belgian anatomist, is known as the "Father of Modern Anatomy." At the age of 29 he published his great *De Corporis Humani Fabrica,* in which he described the structure of the human body. Vesalius introduced many new anatomic terms but, despite his great contributions to the science of anatomy, his name does not appear with any important anatomic structures. A student of Vesalius, Gabriele Fallopius, was also an accurate and detailed dissector and described and named many parts of the anatomy. He gave his own name to the oviducts, known as the **fallopian tubes.** He also gave the **vagina** and the **placenta** their present names.

In 1628, William Harvey (1578–1657) made his pronouncement, based on experimentation and brilliant reasoning, that blood circulates through the body (Fig. 3–3). The work of this English physician was not fully recognized until 1827, when the full importance of his work was substantiated. Harvey's writings were recognized in Germany before the English permitted their publication at home. Modern England now considers Harvey to be its "medical Shakespeare."

Great advances in medicine were somewhat stilled for a century or so, but the unseen world of microorganisms was opened as Anton van Leeuwenhoek (1632–1723) pursued his hobby of grinding lenses. In grinding lenses, Leeuwenhoek discovered how to make use of a simple biconvex lens to magnify the minute world of organisms and structures never seen before. Leeuwenhoek was a Dutch draper and custodian of the city hall of Leyden and, although he was an amateur scientist, his work was not conducted according to the strictest of scientific plans. He was considered to be rather temperamental and eccentric. His writings on his discoveries and theories were rambling and not accepted by the learned men of his time, nor was he very willing to share the viewing of his "tiny little beasties," as he called the microorganisms. In 1677 he described his findings to the Royal Society in London, but there was considerable variation in acceptance of his report.

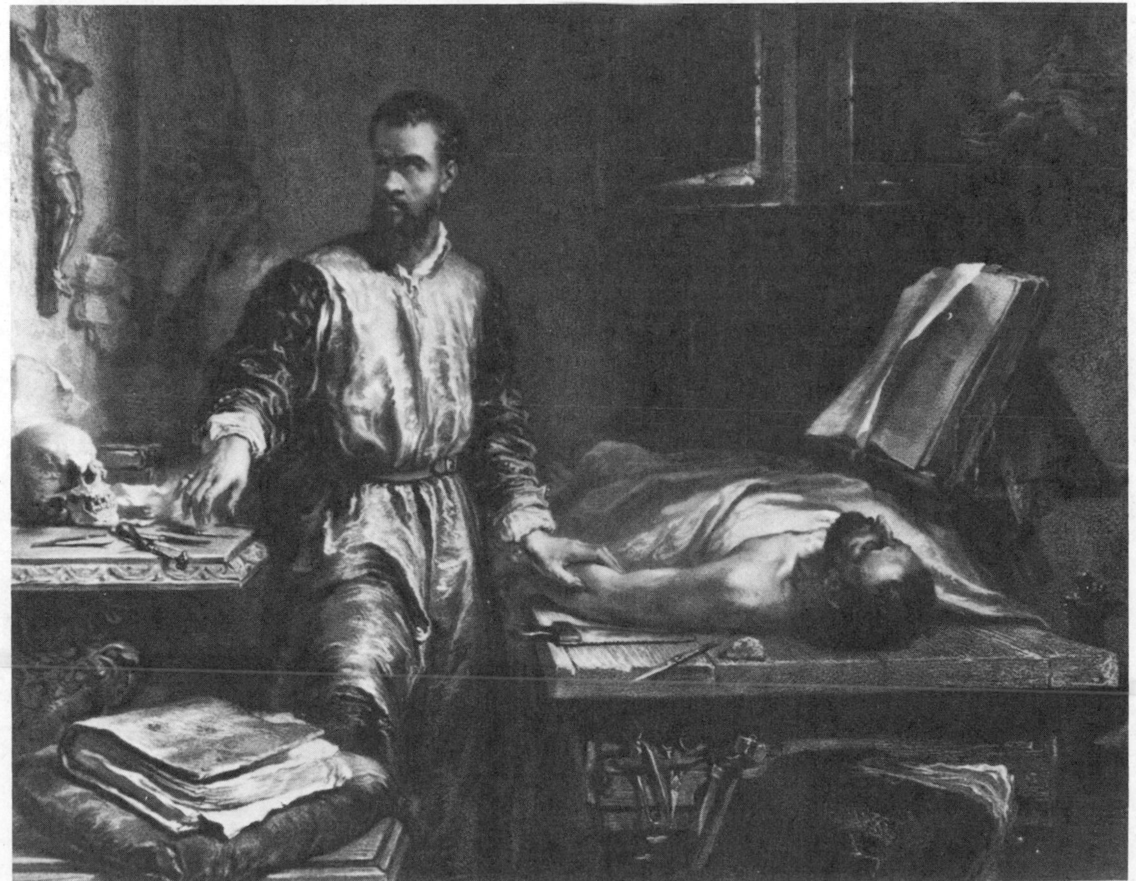

FIGURE 3–2 Andreas Vesalius. (Courtesy of the National Library of Medicine.)

A few years after Leeuwenhoek's death, a famous English surgeon and anatomist, John Hunter (1728–1793), was born (Fig. 3–4). Hunter has been given the title of "Founder of Scientific Surgery" because his surgical procedures were based on sound **pathologic** reasons. He was the first to classify teeth in a scientific manner. In 1778 he introduced artificial feeding by means of a flexible tube passed into the stomach. His description of the syphilitic chancre is classic, and the lesion is sometimes called the "Hunterian chancre." In an unsuccessful attempt to differentiate gonorrhea from syphilis, Hunter inoculated himself with what he thought was gonorrhea, but acquired syphilis. His great collection of anatomic and animal specimens formed the basis for the museum of the Royal College of Surgeons. He was also a member of the Royal Society of Medicine and the Royal Academy of Surgery at Paris. Hunter wrote many papers on anatomy and physiology; he was a brilliant lecturer and teacher. Among his many students was one who would become famous and well-loved — Edward Jenner.

Edward Jenner (1749–1823) was a country physician in Dorsetshire, England (Fig. 3–5). He is listed among the immortals of preventive medicine for his discovery of the smallpox vaccine. The story goes that one day, while Jenner was serving as an apprentice in the office of Daniel Ludlow, his preceptor, a dairy maid was being given treatment. Smallpox was mentioned, and she said, "I cannot take that disease, for I have had cowpox." Smallpox at that time was the deadliest of pandemics. Jenner observed that farmers and dairy maids who once had cowpox never contracted smallpox. Later, as a practicing physician, Jenner continued investigating the relationship between cowpox and smallpox, to the extent that other medical society members felt bored and threatened to expel him from their ranks.

On May 14, 1796, Dr. Jenner took some purulent matter from a pustule on the hand of Sarah Nelmes, a dairy maid, and inserted it through two small superficial incisions into the arm of James Phipps, a healthy boy of eight. This was the first vaccination. Later, on July 1, a virulent dose of smallpox matter was given to young Phipps in the same arm. It had no effect: Phipps had been vaccinated and was safe from the dreaded disease. Edward Jenner's method of vaccination spread throughout the world to all people. The results of his methods and experiments were published in 1798. He called this method of protection "vaccination" because the Latin word *vacca* means cow. Cowpox was called "vaccinia." Pasteur applied the term "vaccine" to suspensions of dead bacteria or attenuated bacteria. This term has come to be used in reference to other immunizing antigens not derived from cows.

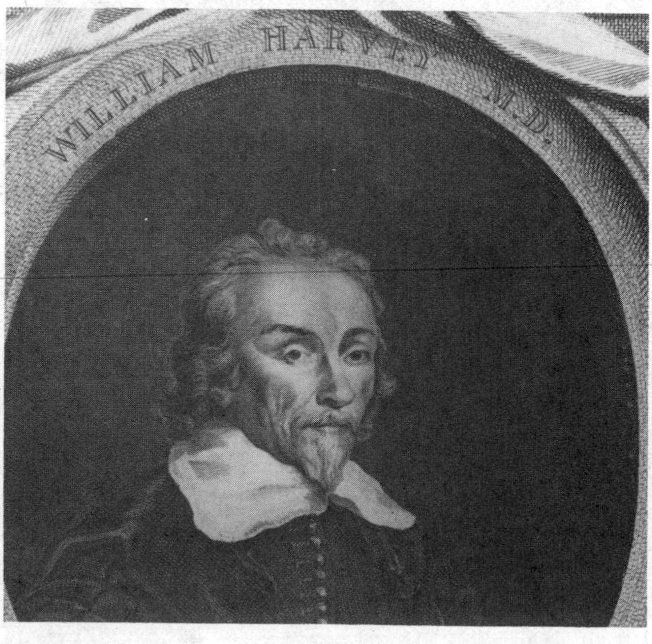

FIGURE 3–3 William Harvey. (Courtesy of the National Library of Medicine.)

Victor Robinson, in *Pathfinders in Medicine,* said of Dr. Jenner, "He died where an intellectual man should die — in his library. The village which gave him birth received his illustrious ashes. When his worn out body was laid to rest, it would not be surprising if some humble woman, whose child he had saved from smallpox, imagined that Edward Jenner had gone to heaven — to vaccinate the angels."

In the early 1800s there were several men who are remembered for their fight against puerperal fever and for their concern for women's health. Puerperal fever, an infectious disease of childbirth, is also known as puerperal sepsis or childbed fever. This term is from *puerpera,* denoting a woman in childbed, from the Latin *puer*, a child, and *pario,* to bring forth. The word "puerperium" now designates the period from delivery to the time the uterus returns to normal size.

The best known of these men is Ignaz Philipp Semmelweis (1818–1865). History has called him the "Savior of Mothers." His fight against puerperal fever is a sad story of hardships and resistance, especially from his instructor, Professor Klein. Semmelweis noted the terrible results of puerperal fever in lying-in hospitals and observed that it occurred with special frequency in cases delivered by medical students who came directly from the autopsy or dissecting room. Semmelweis directed that in his wards the students were to wash and disinfect their hands with a solution of chloride of lime after leaving the dissection room and before going to the wards to examine a woman and deliver her child. This brought about a marked reduction of cases of childbed fever on his ward, but violent opposition was given by the hospital's medical men, and especially by Dr. Klein. As his theories were proven correct, Semmelweis began to feel the horror of the deaths he had caused in the past.

At the age of 47 Semmelweis died, ironically from the infection he had fought, brought on by a cut in his finger while he was doing an autopsy. His grave had hardly been closed when Pasteur and Lister began to reveal the secrets that had caused this deadly disease. A monument to Semmelweis in Budapest is given great care and it has been said that if people had been as tender to the man as they are to his statue, his career would have been happier. Surely Semmelweis' death was a matter of tragic timing, for the year of his death was to introduce the great works of Pasteur and a physician in Edinburgh and Glasgow named Joseph Lister.

Louis Pasteur, a Frenchman, did brilliant work as a chemist, but it was his studies in bacteriology that made him one of the most famous men in medical history and earned him the title of "Father of Bacteriology" (Fig. 3–6). He has also sometimes been honored with the name "Father of Preventive Medicine." His skills and studies reached far beyond the outermost boundaries of the knowledge of the time. He pursued everything with the fire of genius. His adventures included studying the difficulties in the fermentation of wine. He saved the most important industry of France at that time from disaster by a process now called pasteurization. By this

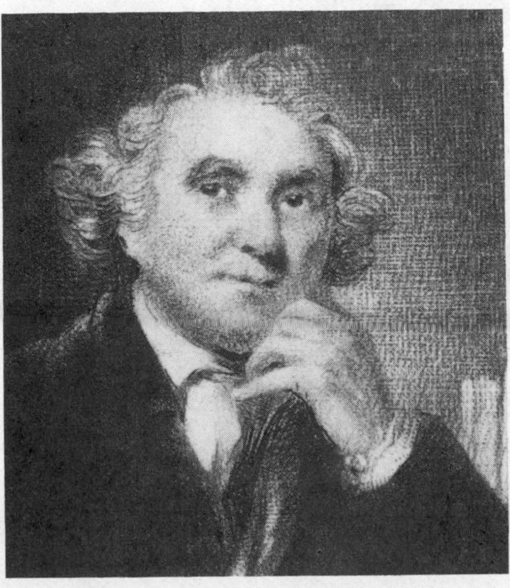

FIGURE 3–4 John Hunter. (Courtesy of the National Library of Medicine.)

process of supplying enough heat to destroy microorganisms, wine was prevented from turning into vinegar. This made great improvements in spirit and malt liquors. The French people called on Pasteur again to help the ailing silkworm industry. The silkworm epidemic in the south of France had reached such proportions that whole plantations were ruined. Pasteur devoted five years to the conquest of the two diseases that infected the silkworm. His work was interrupted only when he was stricken with hemiplegia. But after a long, difficult recovery time, when his mind was always fully active, he continued his work with a stiff hand and a limping foot.

With the conviction that the "infinitely small" world of bacteria held the key to the secrets of contagious diseases, he again left chemistry, this time to become a medical man. Many renowned scientists denied the germ theory of disease and devoted themselves to degrading Pasteur. In the midst of all this "controversy" he became involved in the prevention of anthrax, which threatened the health of the cattle and sheep of France, as well as of the world. Pasteur's name was also honored for work on many other diseases, such as rabies, chicken cholera, and swine erysipelas.

Pasteur died in 1895, with his family at his bedside. His last words were said to be "There is still a great deal to do."

Joseph Lister (1827–1912) was to revolutionize surgery through the application of Pasteur's discoveries. He saw the similarity between the infections that were taking place in postsurgical wounds and the processes of putrefaction which Pasteur had proven were caused by microorganisms. Before this time surgeons accepted infection in surgical wounds as inevitable. Lister reasoned that microorganisms must be the cause of infection and must, therefore, be kept out of wounds. His own colleagues were quite indifferent to Lister's theories since they felt infections were God-given and natural. Lister had once seen pain quelled by the administration of an anesthetic, and pain had been thought to be God-given and inevitable also. He developed antiseptic methods by using carbolic acid for sterilization. By spraying the room with a fine mist of the acid, by soaking the instruments and ligatures, and by washing his hands in carbolic solutions, Lister proved his theory. He is honored with the title of "Father of Sterile Surgery."

Pasteur and Joseph Lister met at the Sorbonne after years of great mutual admiration. The meeting was filled with emotion, and Robinson, in *Pathfinders in Medicine,* has said that "a new star should have appeared in the heavens to commemorate the event. Only a small percentage of the human race entertains any adequate realization of how much we really owe to the combined labors of Louis Pasteur and Joseph Lister."

The name Robert Koch (1843–1910) is familiar to all bacteriologists, for the first law learned as a neophyte in this microscopic world is Koch's Postulates, which state rules that must be followed before an organism can be accepted as the causative agent in a given disease.

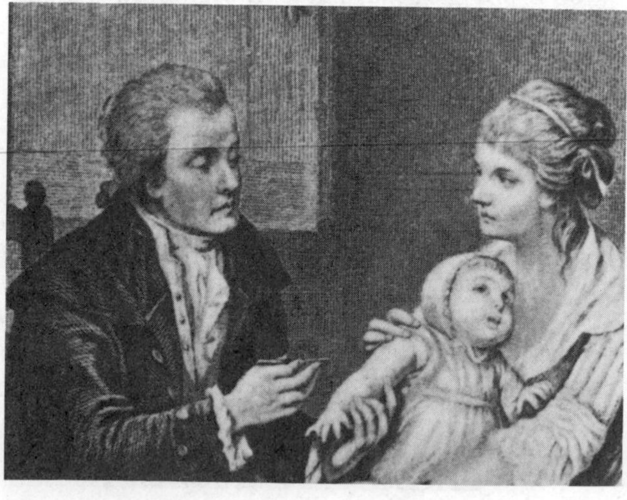

FIGURE 3–5 Edward Jenner. (Courtesy of the National Library of Medicine.)

Robert Koch was a German physician who truly earned great honors in bacteriology and public health. He gave the bacteriology laboratory many of its "tools," such as the culture-plate method for isolation of bacteria. He discovered the cause of cholera and demonstrated its transmission by food and water. This discovery completely transformed health departments and proved the importance of bacteriology. It also established a place of great respect for Koch in the scientific world. A great disappointment in Koch's career was his failure to find a cure for tuberculosis. In this attempt, however, he isolated tuberculin, the substance produced by tubercle bacteria. Its use as a diagnostic aid proved to be of immense value to modern medicine.

Koch's work took him throughout the world. He traveled to America, Africa, Bombay, Italy, and anywhere nations sought his help in ridding themselves of feared diseases. He was investigating anthrax at the same time as Pasteur, but the ill-concealed animosity between the two men prevented any cooperative effort.

In 1885 the University of Berlin created the Chair of Hygiene and Bacteriology in his honor. He became the Nobel Laureate in 1905.

While Robert Koch's brilliant career was nearing an end because of age and illnesses, the work of Paul Ehrlich (1854–1915) was reaching its zenith (Fig. 3–7). Ehrlich had been greatly honored when Koch had invited him to work in his laboratory. Koch had known Ehrlich well, since he had been a distinguished student of his and had already made a place for himself in scientific circles.

Ehrlich was a German physician, and one of the pioneers in the fields of bacteriology, **immunology,** and especially **chemotherapy,** a fairly new science. He was only 28 years old when he wrote his first paper on typhoid, but his greatest gift to mankind was to be called his "magic bullet," or "606," and was designed to fight the terrible disease, syphilis. Only three years before, Bordet and Wasserman had identified the organism and devised a test that would smoke it out of hiding. With the offending germ identified, Ehrlich set out to find a chemical that would destroy the organism but not harm the germ's host, the human body. The search was long and tedious, and history tells us it was the 606th drug that Ehrlich tried that finally did the healing. He called the drug salvarsan because he felt it offered mankind salvation from this disease. This also was the beginning of injecting chemicals into the body to destroy a specific organism.

Later, in 1912, Ehrlich discovered a less toxic drug, called neosalvarsan, to replace the original 606. The new drug bore the number 914. In 1908 Ehrlich shared the Nobel prize with Eli Metchnikoff, who is remembered for his theory of **phagocytosis** and immunology.

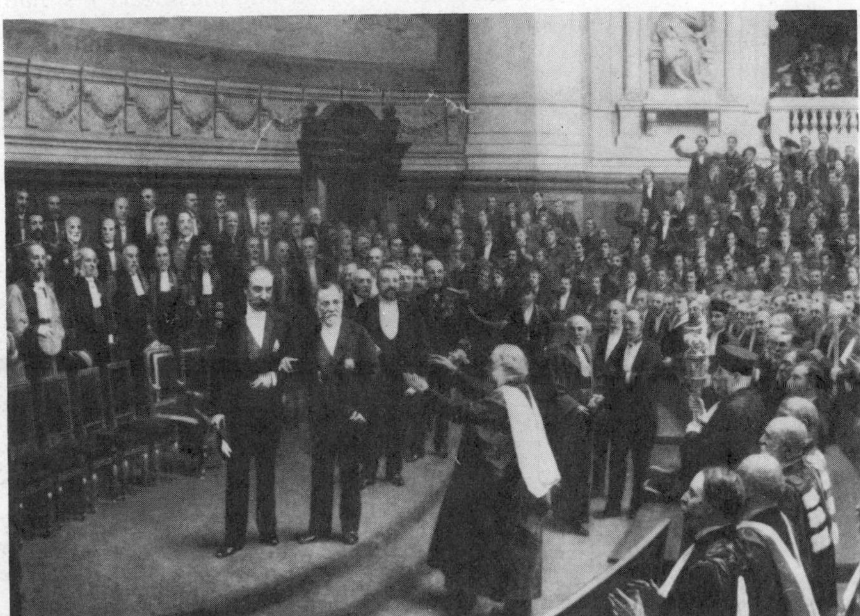

FIGURE 3–6 Louis Pasteur. (Courtesy of the National Library of Medicine.)

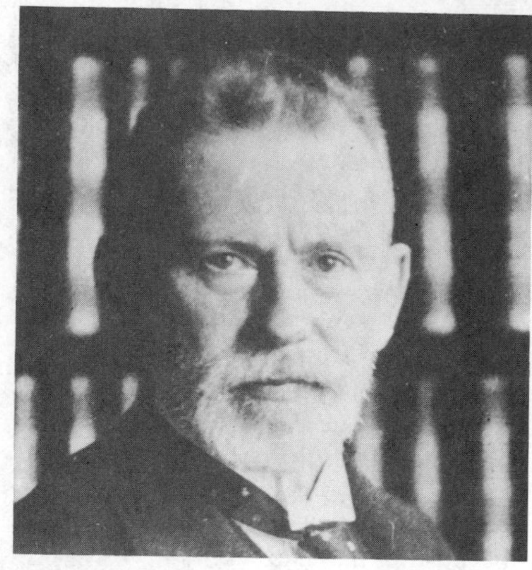

FIGURE 3–7 Paul Ehrlich. (Courtesy of the National Library of Medicine.)

Much time is spent with honoring great men in medical history, but women have also played important roles, which during those times was not an easy thing to do. Two famous women, in particular, are Florence Nightingale (1820–1910) and Clara Barton (1821–1912). You may notice that their careers overlap almost to the year.

Florence Nightingale has been honored and known far and wide as "The Lady with the Lamp" and is immortalized as the founder of nursing (Fig. 3–8). She was of noble birth, and somewhat late in life she sought nurse's training in both England and Europe. By the time of the Crimean War in 1854 she already had a reputation for her work in hospital organization. She was invited by the Secretary of War to visit the Crimea to correct the terrible conditions that existed in caring for the wounded. She created the Women's Nursing Service at Scutari and Balaklava. The doctors at Scutari regarded Florence Nightingale as a troublesome female intruder and treated her and her nurses quite shabbily. Only a crisis that brought thousands of wounded and sick soldiers to army hospitals persuaded the doctors to accept help from her and her nurses.

Miss Nightingale ruled her nurses with an iron hand. Aside from the practical work she did, it was she who insisted the nursing profession get public recognition, and that nursing required special training and experience. From donated funds she organized a school of nursing that bears her name. The modern conception of nursing is based largely on the foundations she laid.

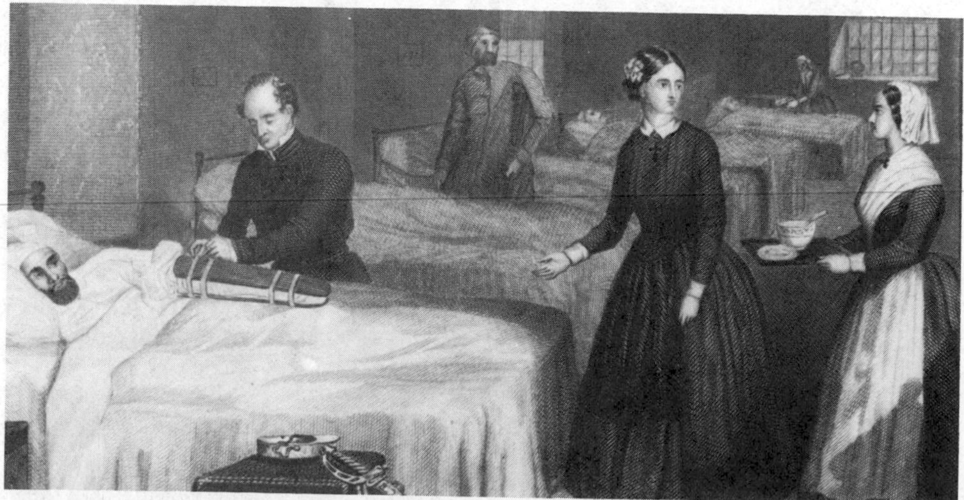

FIGURE 3–8 Florence Nightingale. (Courtesy of the National Library of Medicine.)

The American counterpart to Florence Nightingale's story is the one of Clara Barton (Fig. 3–9). She was a nurse and philanthropist whose work during the American Civil War led her to recognize that very poor records, if any at all, were kept in Washington to aid in the search for missing men wounded or killed in combat. This led to the formation of the Bureau of Records. Clara Barton's fame spread as a result of her organization and recruitment of supplies for the wounded. In 1870 she observed the work of the Red Cross in the Franco-Prussian War, and in 1881 she organized a Red Cross Committee in Washington, forming the American Red Cross, of which she served as the first president from 1881 to 1904.

Anyone who has ever been spared the pain of surgery through the sleep of an anesthetic can give thanks to the memory of two dentists, Dr. Horace Wells and Dr. William T. G. Morton; and a physician, Dr. Crawford Williamson Long. There has been considerable controversy as to whom should be given final credit for the actual discovery of anesthesia, but it now seems to be established that Dr. Long (1815–1878) was the first to employ ether as an anesthetic agent. Early in 1842, after lectures on chemistry, a group of students would have a social gathering and inhale ether as a form of amusement. At one of these so-called "ether frolics" Dr. Long observed that people under the influence of ether did not seem to feel pain. After considerable thought, Dr. Long decided to use ether for a surgical operation. On March 30, 1842, he removed a tumor from the neck of James M. Venable after placing him under the influence of ether. Long did not report this operation or his discovery until 1848. Wells reported his discovery in 1844, and Morton his in 1846, when he extracted a tooth after the patient had been given ether, and he also used it at Massachusetts General Hospital for a surgical procedure.

The list goes on and on. Patients who have had an x-ray or received radium therapy should know the long struggle of Marie and Pierre Curie. Diabetics should give thanks to Frederick Banting, the Canadian physician who discovered insulin in 1922. The vaccines developed by Jonas Edward Salk and Albert Sabin almost eradicated polio, once the killer or crippler of thousands, from the United States. The work of Dr. Christiaan Barnard inspired transplantation of hearts and other organs.

And the work continues. Bypass surgery has made thousands of hearts more functional. Great advances have been made in the treatment of cancer — who will find a real breakthrough? Dialysis machines allow people with nonfunctional kidneys, who would have died a few decades ago, to lead relatively normal lives. Countless unnamed people are engaged in research, or are implementing new developments. Let us not forget those who are involved in organizing public health services and have thus contributed to bettering the availability and distribution of health care. It is tremendously exciting to simply be open to such advancements and aware of their potential. The supportive role of medical assisting is very important in maintaining the quality of medical service today and in making today a strong foundation for the progress of tomorrow.

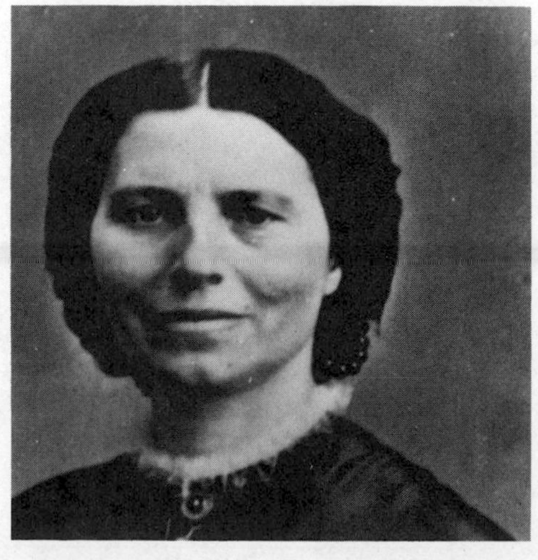

FIGURE 3–9 Clara Barton. (Courtesy of the National Library of Medicine.)

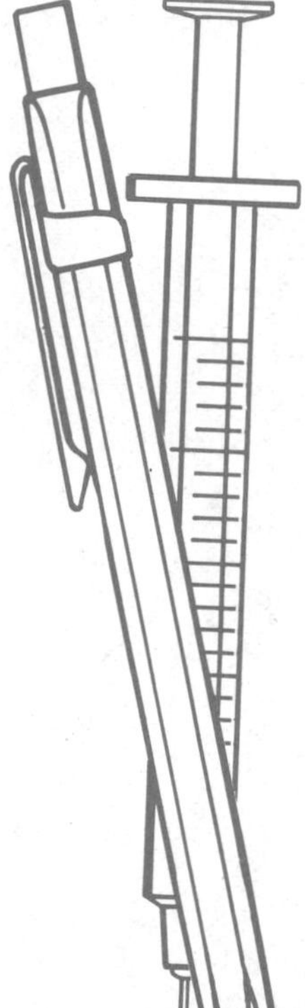

CHAPTER OUTLINE

Historical Codes
Oath of Hippocrates
Principles of Medical Ethics
- Hospital-Physician Relations
- Interprofessional Relations
- Office Practices
- Patient Records
- Patient Relations and Medical Responsibilities
  - Artificial Insemination
  - Clinical Investigation
  - Euthanasia
  - Neglect of Patient
  - Professional Courtesy
  - Ownership and Availability of Records
  - Ghost Surgery and Unnecessary Services
- Public Responsibilities
  - Communications Media
  - News in the Public Domain
  - Discipline and Medicine
  - Nonexploitation of Patients
  - Fee Splitting and Rebates
  - Patents and Secret Remedies
  - Community Responsibilities

AAMA Code of Ethics

BEHAVORIAL OBJECTIVES

The medical office assistant should be able to:

- **Define medical ethics.**
- **Trace the evolution of the modern code of medical ethics.**
- **Apply the code as set forth in the Principles of Medical Ethics of the American Medical Association.**
- **Apply the code of ethics of the American Association of Medical Assistants.**

4

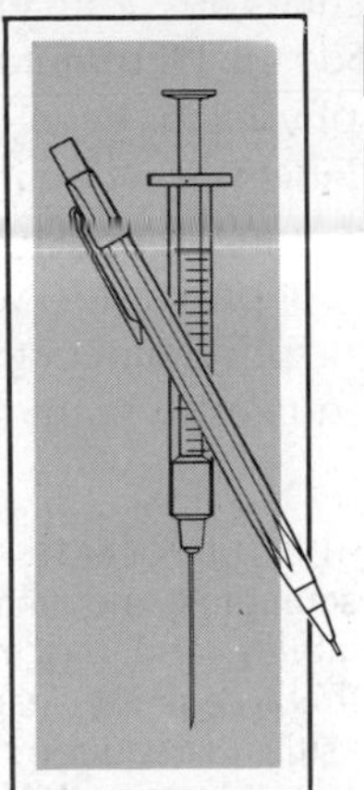

MEDICAL ETHICS

Ethics concerns the thoughts, judgments, and actions on issues that have the greater implications of moral "right" and "wrong." A "morally right" attitude is usually understood to be directed toward an ideal form of human character or action, which should culminate in the "highest good" for humanity. From the desire to achieve this good comes the sense of moral duty and a system of interpersonal moral obligations.

(Medical) ethics should not be confused with (medical) etiquette. Etiquette deals with courtesy, customs, and manners; ethics concerns itself with the underlying philosophies in the ideal relationships of humans. These relationships are often formally set forth in social contracts and codes.

The Preamble to the present Principles of Medical Ethics of the American Medical Association says that, "These principles are intended to aid physicians individually and collectively in maintaining a high level of **ethical** conduct. They are not laws but standards by which a physician may determine the **propriety** of his conduct in his relationships with patients, with colleagues, with members of allied professions, and with the public."

They are not laws but standards . . . laws vary from state to state, from community to community. Ethical standards do not. The Judicial Council of the AMA emphasizes that "there is but one code of ethics for all, be they group, clinic, professional corporation, or individual and be they great and prominent or small and unknown." Ethical standards are never less than the standards required by law; frequently they may be higher. Violation of the ethical standards of an association or society may result in **censure, expulsion,** or **suspension** of membership. Violation of a law followed by conviction may result in punishment by fine, imprisonment, or **revocation** of license.

HISTORICAL CODES

Ethics, judgments of right and wrong, have always been a concern of human beings. It is not surprising that for centuries, the medical profession has set for itself a rigid standard of ethical conduct toward patients and colleagues. The earliest written code of ethical conduct for medical practice was conceived around 2250 BC by the Babylonians and was called the Code of Hammurabi. It went into much detail regarding the conduct expected of a physician, even prescribing the fees that could be charged. Probably because of its length and detail it did not survive the ages.

About 400 BC Hippocrates, the Greek physician known as the Father of Medicine, developed a brief statement of principles, which has come down through history and remains an inspiration to the physician of today. The Oath of Hippocrates has been administered to medical graduates in many European universities for centuries.

THE OATH OF HIPPOCRATES

I swear by Apollo, the physician, and Aesculapius, and Health, and Allheal, and all the gods and goddesses, that, according to my ability and judgment, I will keep this oath and stipulation, to reckon him who taught me this art equally dear to me as my parents, to share my substance with him and relieve his necessities if required; to regard his offspring as on the same footing with my own brothers, and to teach them this art if they should wish to learn it, without fee or stipulation, and that by precept, lecture and every other mode of instruction, I will impart a knowledge of the art to my own sons and to those of my teachers, and to disciples bound by a stipulation and oath, according to the law of medicine, but to none others.

I will follow that method of treatment which, according to my ability and judgment, I consider for the benefit of my patients, and abstain from whatever is deleterious and mischievous. I will give no deadly medicine to anyone if asked, nor suggest any such counsel; furthermore, I will not give to a woman an instrument to produce abortion.

With purity and holiness I will pass my life and practice my art. I will not cut a person who is suffering with a stone, but will leave this to be done by practitioners of this work. Into whatever houses I enter I will go into them for the benefit of the sick and will abstain from every voluntary act of mischief and corruption; and further from the seduction of females or males, bond or free.

Whatever, in connection with my professional practice, or not in connection with it, I may see or hear in the lives of men which ought not to be spoken abroad, I will not divulge, as reckoning that all such should be kept secret.

While I continue to keep this oath unviolated, may it be granted to me to enjoy life and the practice of the art, respected by all men at all times, but should I trespass and violate this oath, may the reverse be my lot.

PRINCIPLES OF MEDICAL ETHICS

The practice of medicine today is guided by a more modern code, known as the Principles of Medical Ethics, which contains the same underlying philosophy as the Oath of Hippocrates. An English physician, Sir Thomas Percival, wrote the first Principles of Ethics in 1803 to provide a model statement of what a doctor should be. In 1847 the newly organized American Medical Association patterned its code of ethics upon Percival's *Code of Medical Ethics*. The AMA Principles of Medical Ethics has been revised at least six times since 1900 to keep it consistent with the times, but there has never been a change in its moral intent or overall idealism. In 1957 the Principles of Medical Ethics of the American Medical Association was condensed to a preamble and ten sections (Fig. 4–1). The Judicial Council of the AMA is charged with interpreting the Principles of Medical Ethics as adopted by the House of Delegates of the American Medical Association. The Council periodically publishes a compilation of its **interpretations,** opinions and statements. The format of the 1977 edition was revised to follow an outline based on subject matter, in contrast to previous editions which were presented in eleven parts corresponding to the Preamble and the ten sections of the Principles of Medical Ethics. We shall discuss some of the interpretations of the Principles set forth in the Judicial Council Opinons and Reports, 1977 Revision, in the following pages. The Code and the interpretations are directed specifically toward physicians. However, the medical assistant, as a

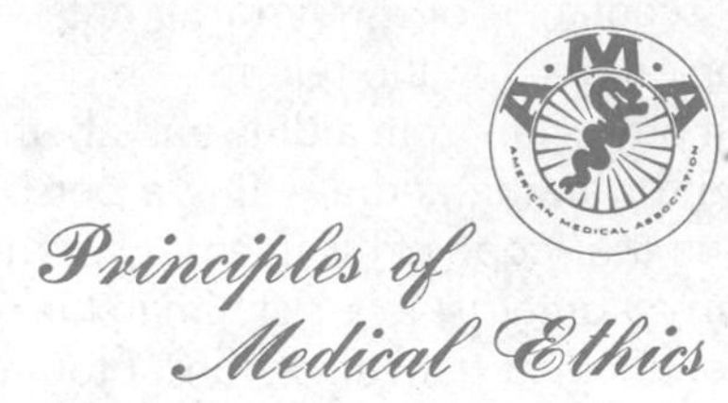

Principles of Medical Ethics

Preamble: These principles are intended to aid physicians individually and collectively in maintaining a high level of ethical conduct. They are not laws but standards by which a physician may determine the propriety of his conduct in his relationship with patients, with colleagues, with members of allied professions, and with the public.

Section 1—The principal objective of the medical profession is to render service to humanity with full respect for the dignity of man. Physicians should merit the confidence of patients entrusted to their care, rendering to each a full measure of service and devotion.

Section 2—Physicians should strive continually to improve medical knowledge and skill, and should make available to their patients and colleagues the benefits of their professional attainments.

Section 3—A physician should practice a method of healing founded on a scientific basis; and he should not voluntarily associate professionally with anyone who violates this principle.

Section 4—The medical profession should safeguard the public and itself against physicians deficient in moral character or professional competence. Physicians should observe all laws, uphold the dignity and honor of the profession and accept its self-imposed disciplines. They should expose, without hesitation, illegal or unethical conduct of fellow members of the profession.

Section 5—A physician may choose whom he will serve. In an emergency, however, he should render service to the best of his ability. Having undertaken the care of a patient, he may not neglect him; and unless he has been discharged he may discontinue his services only after giving adequate notice. He should not solicit patients.

Section 6—A physician should not dispose of his services under terms or conditions which tend to interfere with or impair the free and complete exercise of his medical judgment and skill or tend to cause a deterioration of the quality of medical care.

Section 7—In the practice of medicine a physician should limit the source of his professional income to medical services actually rendered by him, or under his supervision, to his patients. His fee should be commensurate with the services rendered and the patient's ability to pay. He should neither pay nor receive a commission for referral of patients. Drugs, remedies or appliances may be dispensed or supplied by the physician provided it is in the best interests of the patient.

Section 8—A physician should seek consultation upon request; in doubtful or difficult cases; or whenever it appears that the quality of medical service may be enhanced thereby.

Section 9—A physician may not reveal the confidences entrusted to him in the course of medical attendance, or the deficiencies he may observe in the character of patients, unless he is required to do so by law or unless it becomes necessary in order to protect the welfare of the individual or of the community.

Section 10—The honored ideals of the medical profession imply that the responsibilities of the physician extend not only to the individual, but also to society where these responsibilities deserve his interest and participation in activities which have the purpose of improving both the health and the well-being of the individual and the community.

FIGURE 4–1 A.M.A. Principles of Medical Ethics. (Reprinted with permission of the American Medical Association.)

member of the medical team, must be familiar with these principles and cooperate with the physician in practicing within their concepts.

Hospital-Physician Relations (2.00–2.70 Judicial Council Opinions & Reports)

The AMA regards these practices as ***unethical:***

a) charging a separate fee for nonmedical services in admitting a patient to a hospital;

b) **compulsory** assessments which if not paid would cause physicians to lose staff membership;

c) payment to a hospital by a physician of a percentage of the fees the physician receives from patients who are cared for in the hospital;

d) unnecessary or prolonged hospitalization of a patient in a for-profit hospital owned totally or in part by the physician;

e) a physician billing or being paid for a service which the physician did not perform; mere referral does not constitute a professional service.

Interprofessional Relations (3.50–3.71 JCO & R)

Section Three of the Principles of Medical Ethics states:

A physician should practice a method of healing founded on a **scientific basis;** and he should not voluntarily associate professionally with anyone who violates this principle.

According to the Judicial Council, "A physician is deemed to be associating 'professionally' when he serves as a consultant or shares responsibility jointly in treating a patient." A physician may, however, treat a patient no matter what the source of his referral. Acceptance of a referral is not interpreted as a professional relationship with the person making the referral.

State laws prohibit a physician from aiding and abetting an unlicensed person in the practice of medicine, or aiding and abetting a person with a limited license in providing services beyond the scope of his license. For instance, an *ophthalmologist* may choose to employ an *optometrist* to assist him in his office. This is ethical as long as the optometrist is identified to patients as an optometrist and does not perform services beyond the scope of his license. The same principle applies to the referral of patients. It is ethical for a physician to refer a patient for diagnosis or treatment to any other provider of health care services permitted by law to furnish such services whenever he believes that this may benefit the patient. Physicians are free to engage in any teaching permitted by law for which they are qualified.

Office Practices (4.00–4.31 JCO & R)

Medical assistants will have a particular interest and concern with medical ethics as applied to office practices.

a) Missed appointments can create scheduling problems as well as financial loss. If the patient has been fully advised that a charge will be made for a missed appointment or for one not cancelled 24 hours in advance, A.M.A. does not consider it unethical to make the charge. However, under most circumstances it is not advisable and if the patient refuses to pay, the doctor may be placed in the position of having to prove that the time was in fact lost and not used for another patient or purpose.

b) Group practices, clinics, and professional corporations are subject to the same principles of ethics as their participating members would be if practicing as individuals.

c) Since the principal objective of the medical profession is to render service to humanity, the levying and collection of fees must remain a secondary consideration. Section 7 of the Principles states that the physician's fee should be **commensurate** with the services rendered and the patient's ability to pay. When an account is delinquent, the Judicial Council urges physicians to:

1. first give due consideration to the patient's ability to pay the fee which is due;
2. not utilize the services of a collection agency whose tactics and methods of collection might be unfair or abusive;
3. not "sell" his delinquent accounts to a collection agency; and
4. not enter into any arrangement under which the physician would lose complete control of the delinquent account or the method of collection.

The medical assistant frequently is given the responsibility of discussing fees

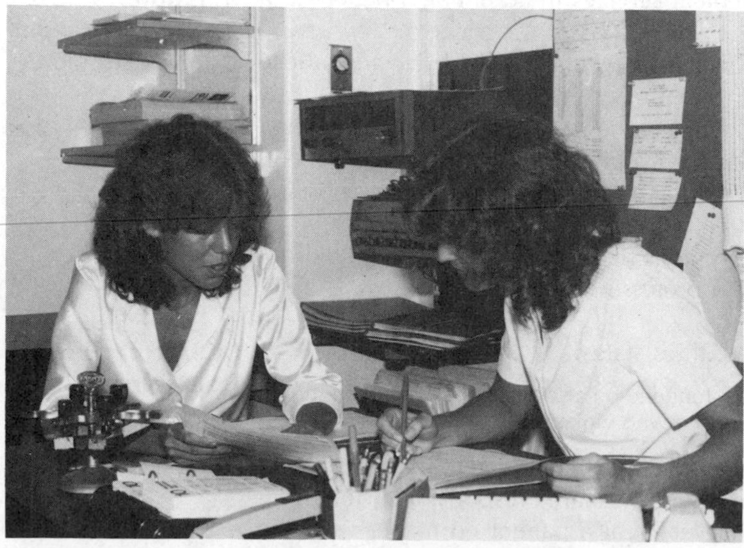

FIGURE 4–2 One of the medical office assistant's duties is to discuss fees with the patient.

with the patient and the duty of collecting the fees (Fig. 4–2). Many potential fee complaints can be eliminated by advance discussion with patients, with a clear understanding of what the fees will be and how they are expected to be paid.

d) Local customs will probably dictate whether a charge will be made for completion of insurance claim forms. The Judicial Council believes that the attending physician should complete without charge the simplified Health Insurance Council forms and similar insurance claim forms as a part of his service to the patient to enable the patient to receive his benefits, but the physician may make a charge for more complex forms if this is the local custom.

The Judicial Council also believes it is not in the best interest of the public or the profession to charge: (1) interest on an unpaid bill or note, (2) a penalty on fees for professional services not paid within a prescribed period of time, or (3) a flat collection fee if it becomes necessary to refer the account to an agency for collection.

If the patient is notified in advance, it is not improper to add a service charge equal to the actual administrative cost of rebilling on accounts not paid within a reasonable time.

Patient Records

The handling and disposition of patient records are often subjects of concern for medical assistants. Two prime considerations are: the best interest of the patient and the confidentiality of the records. For instance, two physicians who are partners in the practice of medicine decide to terminate that partnership. Who will retain possession of the patients' records? This should be decided on the basis of what is best for each individual patient.

If a physician is practicing in the capacity of an employee of another and decides to terminate this relationship, there may be contractual arrangements that

Form D-5

AUTHORIZATION FOR EXAMINATION OF PHYSICIAN'S RECORDS

To Dr. ____________________:

I authorize you to furnish a copy of the medical records of ______________________________, covering the period from
(state name of patient or "myself")

____________, 19____ to ____________, 19____ or to allow those records to be inspected or copied by ____________________. I release you from all legal responsibility or liability that may arise from this authorization.

Signed ____________________

Date ____________________

Witness ____________________

FIGURE 4–3 (From *Medicolegal Forms with Legal Analysis. 3rd Ed.* Office of the General Counsel, 1973, p. 11. Copyright © 1973 American Medical Association.)

regulate ownership of the records. Still, availability of the records should be on the basis of the best interests of the patient. If the physician who terminated his employment should have need for the records in the best interest of a patient under his care, the contents of the record should be available to him, with the consent of the patient.

According to Section 9 of the Principles, a physician may not reveal the confidences entrusted to him in the course of medical attendance. The physician's records summarize these confidences and thus may not be transferred without the patient's consent (Fig. 4–3). Consequently, it is unethical to either purchase or sell a patient's records. If a patient moves or decides to change doctors, his records may be transferred to another doctor upon request or consent of the patient. When a physician retires from practice, he may not sell his patients' records to another physician. For the patient's benefit, but only with his consent, the records may be transferred to a physician designated by the patient. A reasonable charge for secretarial or duplicating service connected with such transfer is not improper.

Patient Relations and Medical Responsibilities (5.01–5.71 JCO & R)

ARTIFICIAL INSEMINATION. Special emphasis is put upon the preservation of confidentiality by the physician and his staff concerning the procedure of **artificial insemination.** The competence of the physician, concern for the patient, spouse and child, and the need for voluntary and informed consent are also stressed. The assistant shares especially the responsibility for preserving confidentiality.

CLINICAL INVESTIGATION. "Physicians should strive continually to improve medical knowledge and skill, and should make available to their patients and colleagues the benefits of their professional attainments." Medical progress is made through scientific research. The ethical participation in clinical investigation must be under accepted standards of scientific research as part of a systematic program to produce data which are scientifically valid and significant.

> In conducting clinical investigation, the investigator should demonstrate the same concern and caution for the welfare, safety, and comfort of the person involved as is required of a physician who is furnishing medical care to a patient independent of any clinical investigation . . . Voluntary, written consent must be obtained from the patient or from his legally authorized representative if the patient lacks the capacity to consent.

Prior to the consent, the investigator must:

a) disclose the fact that an investigational drug or procedure is to be used;
b) give a reasonable explanation of the nature of the procedure to be used and the risks to be expected; and
c) offer to answer any inquiries concerning the drug or procedure.

In clinical investigation *primarily for the accumulation of scientific knowledge,* minors or mentally incompetent persons may be used only if the nature of the investigation is such that mentally competent adults would not be suitable subjects. In clinical investigation *primarily for treatment,* the subject must, in addition, be told the possible **therapeutic** benefits, as well as the alternative drugs or procedures that may be available. No person may be used as a subject against his will.

The Principles of Medical Ethics place great emphasis on **confidentiality,** always with the greater good of the patient uppermost. A modern note is a reference to computers — the ethical principle of confidentiality applies to computerized medical records as it applies to any other medical records. With the consent of the patient or his lawful representative, the patient's history, diagnosis, treatment, and prognosis may be discussed with the patient's lawyer or with his insurance company representative. In the case of a patient who has been diagnosed as having a venereal disease, if the medication prescribed might reveal the nature of the disease, the physician may ethically dispense the drugs directly to the patient rather than send the patient to a pharmacy with a prescription.

EUTHANASIA. The AMA does not condone **euthanasia,** or "mercy killing." Any decision to discontinue the use of "extraordinary means to prolong the life of the body where there is irrefutable evidence that biological death is imminent" must be made by the patient and/or his immediate family.

NEGLECT OF PATIENT. Section 5 of the Principles clearly states that although a physician is free to choose whom he will serve, once he initiates care of a patient, he must do so to the best of his ability. If a doctor-patient relationship is established, he cannot withdraw from the case without giving notice to the patient (Fig. 4–4), his relatives, or his responsible friends sufficiently in advance to allow them to secure another physician. If a letter of withdrawal from a case is necessary, it should be sent by certified mail, return receipt requested, and a copy of the letter with the receipt kept in the patient's record.

ORGAN TRANSPLANTATION. Guidelines are set forth for ethical conduct in the transplantation of human organs: (5.51)

omit

Care must be taken to protect the rights of both the donor and the recipient, and no physician may assume a responsibility in organ transplantation unless the rights of both donor and recipient are equally protected.

PROFESSIONAL COURTESY. **Professional courtesy** is a tradition that applies to the relationship that exists among physicians. It is generally accepted that a physician should not attempt to treat members of his own family or himself. Consequently, a physician cheerfully and without compensation gives his professional services to another physician or his immediate family. There are situations in which exceptions to this courtesy may be made:

a) Where professional courtesy is offered but "the recipient of services insists

Form A-1

LETTER OF WITHDRAWAL FROM CASE

Dear Mr.__________________:

I find it necessary to inform you that I am withdrawing from further professional attendance upon you for the reason that you have persisted in refusing to follow my medical advice and treatment. Since your condition requires medical attention, I suggest that you place yourself under the care of another physician without delay. If you so desire, I shall be available to attend you for a reasonable time after you have received this letter, but in no event for more than five days.

This should give you ample time to select a physician of your choice from the many competent practitioners in this city. With your approval, I will make available to this physician your case history and information regarding the diagnosis and treatment which you have received from me.

Very truly yours,

__________________, M.D.

FIGURE 4–4 (From *Medicolegal Forms with Legal Analysis. 3rd Ed.* Office of the General Counsel, 1973, p. 3. Copyright © 1973. American Medical Association.)

upon payment, the physician need not be embarrassed to accept a fee for his services."

b) "If a physician or his dependents have insurance providing benefits for medical or surgical care, a physician who renders such service may accept the insurance benefits without violating the traditional practice of physicians caring for the medical needs of their colleagues and their dependents without charge."

c) If service is rendered "with such frequency as to involve a significant proportion of his professional time, or in cases of long-term extended treatment," an adjusted fee may be charged.

d) "Professional courtesy should always be extended without qualification to the physician in financial hardship and members of his immediate family who are dependent upon him."

Some physicians extend professional courtesy to clergymen, teachers, nurses, medical assistants and other health care personnel. This is a matter of private determination and not based on traditional medical ethics.

OWNERSHIP AND AVAILABILITY OF RECORDS. There is a common misconception on the part of many patients, and some medical assistants, that the medical record belongs to the patient because he paid for it. It is important that the medical assistant understand ownership of the record and the extent of the patient's rights because sooner or later the question will arise. Some interpretations of the Judicial Council follow:

a) "When a colleague who is presently treating a patient requests records from another physician who has formerly treated the patient, that former physician should promptly make his records available to the attending physician." It is unethical to refuse such a request.

b) Medical notes made by a physician "are the personal property of the physician, although the patient (or his legal representative) has certain legal rights to the information contained in the record about the patient's diagnosis and treatment."

c) The patient record is confidential and "should not be communicated to a third party without the patient's prior written consent, unless it is required by law or is necessary to protect the welfare of the individual or the community."

d) Medical reports should not be withheld because of an unpaid bill for medical services.

A special situation presents when a physician is considering retirement or relocation to another community. Although he is under no obligation to turn his records over to his patients, he should notify the patients on his active list of his plans and encourage them to seek the services of some other physician to whom the records can be transferred.

GHOST SURGERY AND UNNECESSARY SERVICES. When a patient is arranging surgery with a physician, he is entering into a contractual relationship. The physician obtains from the patient a written informed consent agreeing that a specific surgeon may perform a specific procedure.

The surgeon's obligation to the patient requires him to perform the surgical operation: (1) within the scope of authority granted him by the consent to the operation; (2) in accordance with the terms of the contractual relationship; (3) with complete disclosure of all facts relevant to the need and the performance of the operation; and (4) to utilize his best skill in performing the operation.

If the surgeon merely assists or supervises another surgeon, and the patient is not informed as to the identity of the operating surgeon, the situation is **"ghost surgery."** The surgeon can properly utilize the services of an assistant, but it must be remembered that it is the operating surgeon to whom the patient grants consent and with whom he has contracted to perform the operation.

Public Responsibilities (6.00–6.70 JCO & R)

The American Medical Association has a long-standing policy of opposing the **solicitation** of patients, which is interpreted as the attempt to obtain patients by persuasion or influence. It does not prohibit advertising, which is the action of making information or intention known to the public. The *Judicial Council Opinions and Reports* points out, however, that

Local, state, or specialty medical associations, as autonomous organizations, may have ethical restrictions on advertising, solicitation of patients, or other professional conduct of physicians that exceed the Principles of Medical Ethics. Furthermore, specific legal restrictions on advertising or solicitation of patients exist in the medical licensure laws of at least 34 states. Other states provide regulation through statutory authority to impose penalties for unprofessional conduct.

Prepaid medical care plans and health maintenance organizations generally seek members through advertising, such advertising informing the public of the nonprofessional aspects of their services and facilities. Ethical plans do not laud the skills or make extravagant claims on the qualifications of their practitioners.

COMMUNICATIONS MEDIA. The physician whose patient is a public figure carries unusual responsibility. The public looks for, and may be entitled to, frequent reports on the patient's condition. The physician's first obligation is to his patient, but the patient may have an obligation to others. In discharging that obligation the patient must depend upon the physician to ensure the medical accuracy of any authorized report.

A patient or his lawful representative may authorize a physician to disclose certain health information to the press. Under these circumstances, the release of information by the physician does not violate any ethical principle. However, a physician may release only authorized information or that which is public knowledge.

There is great temptation for the inexperienced medical assistant to tell her family or close friends when she has inside information regarding the treatment of a prominent public figure. She should remember at all times that this is not her privilege and even the physician must have the patient's consent to divulge any information.

It is customary for local medical societies to appoint a responsible individual or individuals through which the communications media may clear all medical matters of interest to the public. In some cases the executive director of the medical society serves in this capacity. The purpose of such appointments is to ensure the accuracy of information to the public and therefore if the spokesman's name and title is mentioned, this is not regarded as solicitation and is entirely ethical.

NEWS IN THE PUBLIC DOMAIN. Certain news is a part of the public record or is a matter of concern to civil authorities and consequently is readily available for publication. This includes: births, deaths, accidents, and police cases. This is known as news in the **public domain.** In such cases the following information can be released by the physician without the patient's consent:

a) personal information (patient's name, address, age, sex, race, marital status, employer, occupation, name of parents in case of births, name of next-of-kin in case of deaths)
b) nature of accident
c) diagnosis and **prognosis**
d) patient's general condition

Physicians who are interviewed by the communications media (newspapers, magazines, radio, TV) quite naturally are judged as representatives of the medical profession and are cautioned to use "sound judgment and good common sense." They should refrain from sponsoring products directly or by implication and should not make promises of radical cures or boast of extraordinary skill or success.

DISCIPLINE AND MEDICINE. It is always difficult to take responsibility for exposing the unethical behavior of a colleague. Yet the statements of the Judicial Council are quite clear on the physician's responsibility:

A physician should expose, without fear or favor, incompetent or corrupt, dishonest or unethical conduct on the part of members of the profession . . . An ethical physician will observe the laws regulating the practice of medicine and will not assist others to evade such laws.

When questions of ethical conduct do occur, they should first receive a fair and objective hearing before a proper medical tribunal.

The basic principles of a fair and objective hearing should always be accorded to the physician whose professional conduct is being reviewed. The fundamental aspects of a fair hearing are: a listing of specific charges, adequate notice of the right to a hearing, the opportunity to be present and to rebut the evidence, and the opportunity to present a defense. These principles apply when the hearing body is a medical society tribunal or a hospital committee composed of physicians.

NONEXPLOITATION OF PATIENTS. Some physicians own or have a financial interest in a pharmacy, nursing home, or optical company. This in itself is not unethical. However, it is unethical if it involves **exploitation** of the patient. It is unethical for a physician to be influenced in the prescribing of drugs or devices by his financial interest in a pharmaceutical firm or other supplier. Sometimes a pharmacy will offer to provide local physicians with free prescription blanks bearing the name of the pharmacy. On the premise that the patient should have free choice of pharmacy, the use of such prescription blanks by the physician is considered unethical. For the same reason "the Council looks with disfavor upon the use of direct telephone lines between a physician and a pharmacist."

FEE SPLITTING AND REBATES. **Fee splitting** means the sharing by two or more persons, without the knowledge of the patient, in a fee which has been given by the patient supposedly as payment for the service of one person alone. Fee splitting is unethical conduct. This includes situations such as the following:

a) Doctor F refers a patient to Doctor G for surgery. Doctor G shares the fee with Doctor F as an assistant when in fact it was only a referral.

b) Doctor M refers a patient to XYZ Optical Company for glasses. XYZ Optical Company **rebates** part of the patient's payment for glasses to Doctor M for the referral.

c) A pharmaceutical firm gives expensive gifts to a physician who prescribes its products. The acceptance of such gifts is unethical.

In cases where two or more physicians actually are participating in the care of the patient, they should render separate bills. If they are associates in the same office and they send a combination statement to the patient, the billing should itemize each physician's charges separately to eliminate any question of secrecy.

Sometimes a physician has an agreement with a laboratory by which the physician will pay the laboratory and request reimbursement from the patient. The request for reimbursement (statement) should show the amount charged by the laboratory and include the name and address of the laboratory.

In a group practice the division of income among the members may take into consideration other services and contributions to the group as well as the professional medical services. For instance, one partner or group member may have strong administrative skills and agree to assume management responsibilities for which the practice will pay him.

PATENTS AND SECRET REMEDIES

It is not unethical for a physician to patent a surgical or diagnostic instrument he has discovered or developed. The laws governing patents are based on the sound doctrine that one is entitled to protect his discovery.

Once the physician has obtained the patent, however, it would be unethical for him to use this patent right to retard or inhibit research or in any way restrict the benefits that might be derived from the use of such instrument. Imagine a situation where

Doctor X has perfected an instrument for performing a common surgical procedure that would greatly reduce the risk to the patient. He allows the manufacture of only enough instruments for his own use or the use of a small select group. This would not be in the best interests of the public welfare and would be an unethical practice.

The AMA considers it unethical for a "physician to prescribe, dispense, administer, or promote the use of any drug whose content or effect is unknown to him or to refuse to inform the patient (or his legal representative) about the identity and purpose of any drug which he has prescribed, dispensed, or administered to the patient."

COMMUNITY RESPONSIBILITIES. Physicians, as good citizens, are urged to advise concerning the health of their communities and to help enforce those laws and sustain the institutions that advance the interest of humanity. Whereas the standards of the medical profession forbid that physicians exploit their ability or achievements to the laity, they are encouraged to cooperate with medical society requests to write, act or speak for general readers or audiences. The medical assistant may be called upon to aid her employer in carrying out these civic responsibilities. She should accept these duties cheerfully and feel proud that her employer has this commitment to his profession and to the community.

AAMA CODE OF ETHICS

A code of ethics specifically for medical assistants is set forth in the Bylaws of the American Association of Medical Assistants.

CODE OF ETHICS

The Code of Ethics of this Association shall set forth principles of ethical and moral conduct as they relate to the medical profession and the particular practice of medical assisting.

Members of this Association dedicated to the conscientious pursuit of their profession, and thus desiring to merit the high regard of the entire medical profession and the respect of the general public which they serve, do pledge themselves to strive always to:

(a) Render service to humanity with full respect for the dignity of person.
(b) Respect confidential information gained through employment unless legally authorized or required by responsible performance of duty to divulge such information.
(c) Uphold the honor and high principles of the profession and accept its disciplines.
(d) Seek to continually improve our knowledge and skills of medical assisting for the benefit of patients and professional colleagues.
(e) Participate in additional service activities which aim toward improving the health and well-being of the community.

Note that paragraph (a) of the AAMA Code closely resembles the first section of the AMA Code. The first concern of both the physician and the medical assistant is to render service. The medical assistant code also stresses the importance of respecting the confidentiality of information learned from or about patients in the course of employment. It is *not* all right to reveal confidences to anyone — this includes your family, your spouse, your best friend, your beauty operator, other medical assistants, anyone at all! The medical assistant must avoid even mentioning the names of patients, for sometimes the doctor's specialty reveals the patient's reason for consulting him.

In *Winning Ways With Patients,* the AMA tells doctors' assistants: ". . . never discuss another patient's case; if you are asked questions by a curious patient, change the subject. When a patient asks about his own case, refer him to the doctor for information. Patients may ask for your advice on personal matters, but you should refrain from answering. Patients tend to identify your remarks as those of the doctor. By staying mum in all instances, you'll be protecting the physician, yourself and the patient." Confidential papers, case histories, and even the appointment book should be kept out of reach of curious eyes — to protect the patient, as well as the doctor and his assistants (Fig. 4–5).

Like Section 4 of the AMA Principles, paragraph (c) of the AAMA Code reminds medical assistants to uphold the honor and high principles of the profession and accept its disciplines. Patients, naturally, associate medical assistants with medicine and if they see the medical assistant outside the office, her appearance and actions

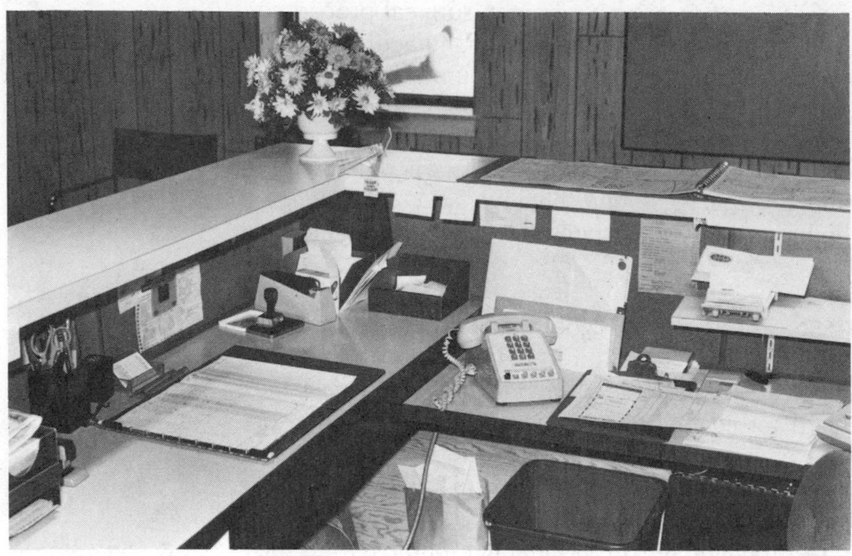

FIGURE 4–5 Desk with shoulder-high shield for privacy.

will reflect either positively or negatively on the medical profession. The medical assistant has a greater responsibility in this regard than does the average office employee. The medical assistant accepts this discipline as part of her responsibility.

In paragraph (d) the medical assistant recognizes the need to continually improve her knowledge and skills for the benefit of patients and professional colleagues, just as the physician does in the Principles, Section 2. Fortunately for modern day medical assistants they can accomplish this through attending regular meetings of the American Association of Medical Assistants, by subscribing to guided study programs developed by the Association, and through classes offered in many community colleges and private schools.

The concluding paragraph (e) suggests participation in service activities which aim toward improving the health and well-being of the community (Fig. 4–6). Chapters of the AAMA encourage their members to donate blood through the Red Cross, participate in health fairs and career days, sponsor classes in cardiopulmonary resuscitation, hold fund raising events for various charities, address envelopes for

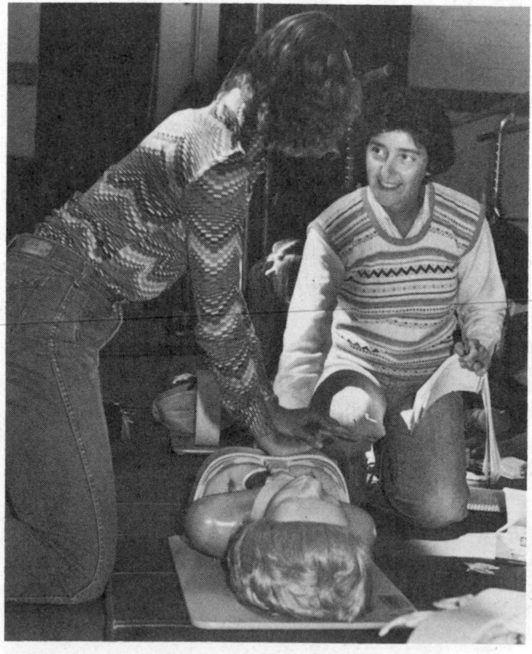

FIGURE 4–6 The medical office assistant learns cardiopulmonary resuscitation — one aspect of continuing education.

fund raising drives, etc. These activities generate respect for the profession and personal growth for the individual.

Occasionally a medical assistant is faced with the discovery that her employer's conduct appears to fall short of the ethical standards she has learned. Before making any judgments she must be absolutely sure of all the facts and circumstances. If there has, in fact, been a history of unethical conduct, the assistant must then make a decision as to whether she will remain in the physician's employ. This is a difficult situation, particularly if the relationship and employment conditions have been congenial. In some cases, a decision to stay may adversely affect future opportunities for employment in another physician's office.

References

American Medical Association: *Judicial Council Opinions and Reports*. Chicago, American Medical Association, 1977.

American Medical Association: *Medicolegal Forms with Legal Analysis*. Chicago, American Medical Association, 1973.

American Medical Association: *Winning Ways with Patients*. Chicago, American Medical Association, 1979.

American Association of Medical Assistants Bylaws. Chicago, American Medical Assistants Association, 1979.

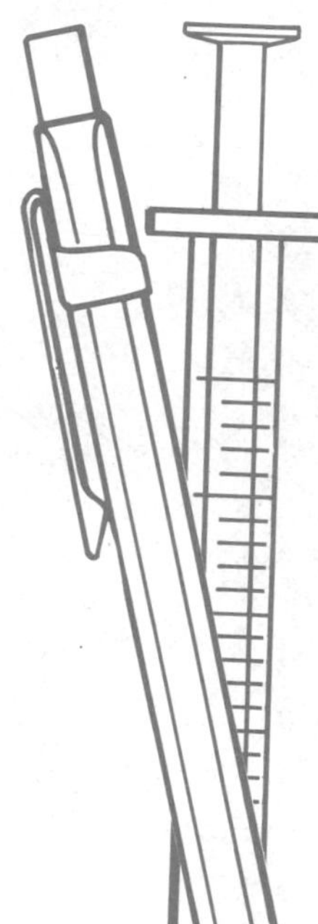

CHAPTER OUTLINE

Licensure and Registration
- Medical Practice Acts
- Licensing
- Registration
- Revocation or Suspension

Certification
- Approved Specialty Boards

Professional Liability
- Definition
- Assistants' Role in Claims Prevention
- Malpractice and Negligence
- Four D's of Negligence
- A B C D's of Negligence

Arbitration

Law of Contracts

Statute of Frauds

Good Samaritan Act

Controlled Substances Act of 1970
- Records under the Act

Uniform Anatomical Gift Act

Securing Patients' Informed Consent

Legal Responsibilities of the Medical Assistant
- Agent of Employer
- Need for Extreme Care
- Rechecking Equipment
- Illegal Practice of Medicine
- Instructions to Patient
- Examinations of Women
- Emergency Aid
- Claims Prevention

Glossary of Legal Terms

BEHAVIORAL OBJECTIVES

The medical office assistant should be able to:

- State the purpose of medical practice acts.
- List the methods and requirements for licensing physicians.
- State the requirements for registration.
- Define continuing education units.
- List three general grounds for revocation or suspension of license.
- State the purpose and function of specialty boards.
- Define professional liability in medicine.
- List the four components of negligence.
- Explain the medical office assistant's role in claims prevention.
- List four advantages of arbitration.
- State the requirements for record-keeping under the Controlled Substances Act.
- Briefly explain the Uniform Anatomical Gift Act.
- State the requirements for informed consent.
- Practice the principles of claims prevention.
- Recall and recognize the definitions of legal terms included in the Chapter Glossary.

5

MEDICINE AND THE LAW

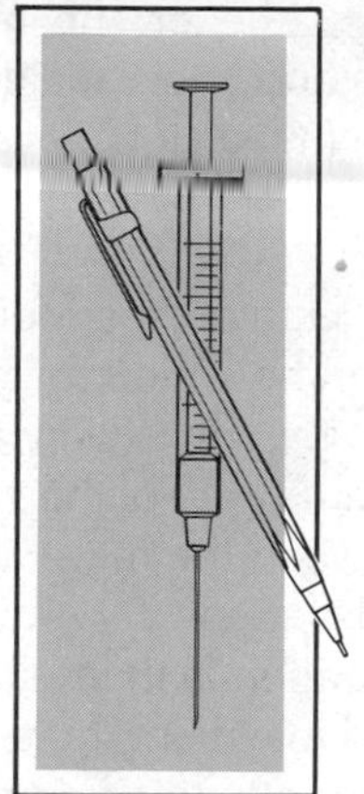

Closely allied with medical ethics are certain medicolegal principles that must be considered in the daily operation of the doctor's office. A book of this nature can touch only the surface of such a complex subject.

LICENSURE AND REGISTRATION

MEDICAL PRACTICE ACTS. Medical practice acts are established by *statute* in each of the 50 states. They define what is included in the practice of medicine within that state and govern the methods and requirements of licensure and the grounds for *suspension* or *revocation* of license.

Although medical practice acts existed as early as colonial days, these were later repealed, and in the mid-nineteenth century practically none of the states had laws governing the practice of medicine. As might be expected, there was a rapid decline in professional standards. The general welfare of the people was endangered by medical **quackery** and inadequate care; by the beginning of the twentieth century, medical practice acts were again in effect in every state.

LICENSING. A Doctor of Medicine degree (MD) is conferred upon the graduate from medical school. Some graduates may not wish to actually engage in the practice of medicine; their interests may lie in research or administration, or even in the practice of law with a special interest in medical **liability.** In such cases it is not necessary for them to be licensed. However, before an MD can engage in the practice of medicine, he or she must be licensed and must meet additional requirements, which will vary from state to state but will generally relate to age, moral character, internship, and residence. The Supreme Court has ruled that American citizenship can no longer be required for license to practice medicine.

The license is granted by a state board, frequently known as the Board of

Medical Examiners or Board of Registration. In California the name of this body has been changed to the Board of Medical Quality Assurance; in Kansas the agency is the State Board of Healing Arts. Licensure may be by *examination,* by **reciprocity,** or by **endorsement.** State *examinations* are prepared and graded by physicians. Some states grant a license to practice medicine by *reciprocity;* that is, they recognize that the requirements of another state in which the physician is already licensed meet or surpass their own requirements. If an applicant has passed the examination of the National Board of Medical Examiners, he or she may be granted a license by *endorsement.* All states except Florida and Louisiana grant licenses by endorsement, and the majority of medical school graduates now take the National Boards. The license to practice medicine is a privilege, not a right.

REGISTRATION. After a license is granted, periodic re-registration is necessary annually or biennially. A physician can be concurrently registered in more than one state. The issuing body will notify the physician when re-registration is due; however, not all states do this at the same time of the year. The medical assistant can aid the physician by being aware of when the registration fees are due and thereby prevent a possible lapsing of the registration.

A recent development in re-registration in many states is the requiring of proof of continuing education in addition to payment of a registration fee. **Continuing education units (CEUs)** are granted for attending approved seminars, lectures, and scientific meetings, as well as formal courses in accredited colleges and universities. Fifty hours a year is the average requirement. The medical assistant may be expected to remind the physician and help make arrangements for completing the necessary units for license renewal.

REVOCATION OR SUSPENSION. Under certain conditions the license to practice medicine may be revoked or suspended. Grounds for revocation or suspension of a medical license generally fall within three categories: (1) conviction of a crime, (2) unprofessional conduct, and (3) personal or professional incapacity.

CERTIFICATION

Most physicians have a special interest in a particular branch of medical practice and eventually direct their interests to becoming expert in that field. The physician who decides to limit his or her practice to a specialized field will probably seek

TABLE 5–1 Approved Specialty Boards of the United States

American Board of Allergy and Immunology
American Board of Anesthesiology
American Board of Colon and Rectal Surgery
American Board of Dermatology
American Board of Family Practice
American Board of Internal Medicine
American Board of Neurological Surgery
American Board of Nuclear Medicine
American Board of Obstetrics and Gynecology
American Board of Ophthalmology
American Board of Orthopaedic Surgery
American Board of Otolaryngology
American Board of Pathology
American Board of Pediatrics
American Board of Physical Medicine and Rehabilitation
American Board of Plastic Surgery
American Board of Preventive Medicine
American Board of Psychiatry and Neurology
American Board of Radiology
American Board of Surgery
American Board or Thoracic Surgery
American Board of Urology

certification by one of the specialty boards. At present there are 22 specialty boards under the umbrella of the American Board of Medical Specialties. These specialty boards assist in improving the quality of medical education by elevating the standards of graduate medical education and approving facilities for specialty training. The primary function of each approved specialty board is to determine the **competence** of candidates in its field who appear voluntarily for examination and to certify as **diplomates** those who are qualified. To accomplish this function, specialty boards determine if candidates have received adequate preparation in accordance with established educational standards; they provide comprehensive examination to determine the competence of such candidates, and they certify to the competence of those physicians who have satisfied the requirements. Those physicians who are certificated are known as diplomates of a specific specialty board, for example, William F. Donovan, MD, Diplomate of the American Board of Surgery. A listing of the 22 specialty boards is found in Table 5–1. The American Board of Medical Specialties is located at 1603 Orrington Avenue, Suite 1160, Evanston, Illinois 60201. It regularly publishes a directory listing all physicians certified as diplomates by the specialty boards with biographic sketches detailing their educational qualifications. Many physicians consult the directory in making referrals.

PROFESSIONAL LIABILITY

DEFINITION. The term "medical professional **liability**" encompasses all possible **civil liability** which a physician can incur as a result of any of his professional acts. It is preferred over the term "medical **malpractice**" because the latter carries some negative overtones. Medical professional liability is more easily prevented than defended.

ASSISTANT'S ROLE IN CLAIMS PREVENTION. The competent medical assistant, with **empathy** for the patient's problems, has an important role in claims prevention. For instance, a patient who is kept waiting for what he considers an inexcusably long time, without explanation or reassurance, has developed some feeling of hostility before he ever sees the doctor. A few words from the receptionist at the proper time may forestall hostility and promote understanding. Any time a medical assistant has reason to believe that a patient is dissatisfied, it is the assistant's duty to pass along such information to the physician. The assistant must be very careful in the choice of words while reassuring an apprehensive patient. Instead of saying, "I'm sure you will soon be entirely well," a gentle touch or a friendly smile will comfort the patient but be noncommittal.

MALPRACTICE AND NEGLIGENCE. **Negligence,** when applied to the medical profession, is called malpractice. It is generally defined as the doing of some act which a reasonable and **prudent** physician would not do, or the failure to do some act which such a person should or would do. The standard of prudent conduct is not defined by law but is left to the determination of a judge or jury.

When injury results to a patient through a doctor's negligence, the patient can legally initiate a malpractice **suit** to recover financial damages. Experience has shown, however, that the incidence of malpractice claims is directly related to the *personal relationship* existing between the physician and the patient. A person seldom sues someone whom he regards as a true friend.

A physician who performs an operation carelessly or contrary to accepted standards, for example, is guilty of negligence or malpractice. If the state prescribes by law that drops be placed in the eyes of all newborn infants and a physician does not do it, he is guilty of *statutory negligence*. If an illegal **abortion** is performed, the physician is guilty of criminal negligence and is also liable for prosecution under the **penal** statutes. A nurse is guilty of negligence if she fails "to exercise reasonable and ordinary care and the application of her knowledge and exert her best judgment" in the care and treatment of the patient. For instance, if the nurse is instructed to **administer** medication **hypodermically,** she may be expected to know whether the medication prescribed should be injected **subcutaneously** or **intramuscularly.**

If a physician were held legally responsible for every unsuccessful result occurring in treatment, no person would undertake the responsibility of practicing medicine. The courts hold that a physician must use reasonable care, attention, and diligence in the performance of his professional services, follow his best judgment in treating his patients, and possess and exercise the skill and care that are commonly possessed and exercised by other reputable physicians in the same or a similar locality. If he calls himself a specialist, he must meet the standards of practice of his specialty. Whether or not he has met these requirements in treating a particular case is generally a matter for the court to decide upon the basis of **expert testimony** provided by another physician. *Negligence is not presumed; it must be proved.*

No doctor is required to possess extraordinary learning and skill. But he must keep abreast with medical developments and techniques and he cannot experiment. He also is bound to advise his patients if he discovers that the condition is one beyond his knowledge or technical skill.

The Committee on Medicolegal Problems of the American Medical Association stated in a 1963 report that

The Four D's of Negligence

> To obtain a judgment against a physician for negligence, the patient must present evidence of what have been referred to as the "four D's." He must show: (1) that the physician owed a *duty* to the patient, (2) that the physician was *derelict* and breached that duty by failing to act as the ordinary, competent physician in the same community would have acted under the same or similar circumstances, (3) that such failure or breach was the *direct cause* of the patient's injuries, and (4) that *damages* to the patient resulted therefrom.

Duty exists when the physician-patient relationship has been established. That is, the patient has sought the assistance of the physician and the physician has knowingly undertaken to provide the needed medical service.

Derelict (neglectful of obligation). Proof of **dereliction,** or proof of negligence of an obligation, must be shown in obtaining a **judgment** for malpractice.

Direct cause. "There must be a proof of a direct and uninterrupted chain of causation from the wrongful act or omission of the physician to the injury suffered by the patient. There must be no independent intervening cause capable of producing the injury."

Damages. There are three kinds of **damages** recognized by the law: (1) nominal, (2) punitive or exemplary, and (3) compensatory or actual. *Nominal* (existing in name only) damages are a token compensation for the invasion of a legal right where no actual injury was suffered. *Punitive* (inflicting punishment) or *exemplary* (serving as a warning) damages require allegations and proof of willful misconduct and are unusual in suits against physicians. It is the *compensatory* or actual damages that are most frequently involved in professional liability cases. Compensatory damages may be *general* or *special*.

Compensation for injuries or losses which are the natural and necessary consequences of the physician's negligent act or omission is called "general damages." General damages include compensation for pain and suffering, for loss of a bodily member or faculty, for disfigurement, and other similar direct losses or injuries. The *fact* of the losses must be proved — the *monetary value* need not be proved.

Special damages are those injuries or losses that are not a necessary consequence of the physician's negligent act or omission. This may include the costs of medical and hospital care, loss of earnings, cost of travel, and so forth. *Both* the fact of these injuries or losses and the monetary value must be proved.

The Committee on Professional Liability of the California Medical Association in 1971 called these same four elements the "A B C D's" of negligence in medical practice:

- **A** Acceptance of a person as a patient.
- **B** Breach of the physician's duty of skill or care.
- **C** Causal connection between the breach by the physician and the damage to the patient.

D Damage of foreseeable nature — that is, injury, pain, loss of earnings, and so on, which could reasonably have been foreseen to result.

ARBITRATION

5

Arbitration, the settlement of a dispute by a third party or parties, selected because of their familiarity with the practices involved, is commonplace in modern business life. It has only recently been implemented in the medical profession. Arbitration is an alternative method of resolving legal disputes between doctor and patient. Many physicians and lawyers see it as one way to help solve the malpractice crisis. Instead of taking the disagreement through the long and expensive process of court **litigation**, which may take as long as seven or eight years, the patient and the doctor (or hospital) agree in advance to submit the dispute informally to a neutral person or persons.

An arbitration agreement is a contract and is subject to judgment of the courts only as to the fairness of the agreement. The agreement is precisely worded by an attorney and should not be paraphrased in explaining it to a patient (Fig. 5–1). Signing the agreement is a voluntary act on the part of the patient, who has a period of grace in which to revoke the agreement if he later decides against it. Both the patient and the doctor have the opportunity to agree on who will arbitrate the case, so it does not favor one side over the other. By prior agreement, the **arbitrator**(s) may be appointed by or from the American Arbitration Association, which is a neutral, private, nonprofit association dedicated solely to the advancement of out-of-court remedies. Its panels of arbitrators are made up of persons from business, the professions, and public interest groups.

After an informal hearing the arbitrator(s) then renders a binding decision, based on very specific rules of arbitration, as to any award. Arbitration is established by statute and applies essentially the same **substantive law** and the same measure of damages as a court. Arbitration is fair, it is less expensive, it is faster, and it is more confidential than court litigation.

If an arbitration statute exists in your state, you should get details of the procedure from your state or local medical society. If a physician elects to implement the procedure, every member of the physician's staff should know the details of the agreement, how to sign patients up, and how to answer the patient's questions. The fairness with which the physician's personnel present the program to the patient and the willingness with which the personnel answer the patient's questions will largely determine whether or not the court will uphold the arbitration agreement. Furthermore, when the physician's personnel "speak for the physician," any representations made by the personnel could be held against the physician.

LAW OF CONTRACTS

Although we do not give it much thought, the law of contracts touches us in many ways, practically every day of our lives. For instance, when you order medications or supplies for the office, you have entered into a **contract.** In fact, your employment is in itself a contract, though not necessarily in writing.

A contract, to be valid, must have these four basic requisites: (1) manifestation of assent (an offer and an acceptance), (2) legal subject matter, (3) parties must have legal capacity to contract, and (4) consideration.

A contract may be written or oral, express or implied. The party making the offer is known as the *offeror* and the party to whom the offer is made is the *offeree*. Let us illustrate how this would apply to the doctor-patient relationship, which is generally held by the courts to be a contractual relationship. When the doctor "hangs out his shingle" he is inviting an offer. The patient, in presenting himself for treatment, is making an offer. The doctor accepts the offer when he undertakes treatment of the patient.

Until he accepts the offer, the doctor is under no obligation, and no contract exists. Once he has accepted the patient, however, an implied contract does exist that he will treat the patient, using reasonable care, and that he possesses the degree of knowledge, skill, and judgment which might be expected of another physician in

Patient's Copy

PATIENT-PHYSICIAN ARBITRATION AGREEMENT

1. It is understood that any dispute as to medical malpractice, that is as to whether any medical services rendered under this contract were unnecessary or unauthorized or were improperly, negligently or incompetently rendered, will be determined by submission to arbitration as provided by California law, and not by a lawsuit or resort to court process except as California law provides for judicial review of arbitration proceedings. Both parties to this contract, by entering into it, are giving up their constitutional right to have any such dispute decided in a court of law before a jury, and instead are accepting the use of arbitration.

2. I voluntarily agree to submit to arbitration any and all claims involving persons bound by this agreement (as set forth in Article 3) whether those claims are brought in tort, contract or otherwise. This includes, but is not limited to, suits for personal injury, actions to collect debts, or **any kind of civil action.**

3. I understand and agree that this Patient-Physician Arbitration Agreement binds me, my heirs, assigns, or personal representative and the undersigned physician, his/her professional corporation or partnership, if any, his/her employees, partners, heirs, assigns, or personal representative, and any consenting substitute physician. I also hereby consent to the intervention or joinder in the arbitration proceeding of all parties relevant to a full and complete settlement of any dispute arbitrated under this agreement, as set forth in the Medical Arbitration Rules included in this booklet.

4. I agree to accept medical services from the undersigned physician and to pay therefor. I UNDERSTAND THAT I DO **NOT** HAVE TO SIGN THIS AGREEMENT TO RECEIVE THE PHYSICIAN'S SERVICES, AND THAT IF I DO SIGN THE AGREEMENT AND CHANGE MY MIND WITHIN 30 DAYS OF TODAY, THEN I MAY REVOKE THIS AGREEMENT BY GIVING WRITTEN NOTICE TO THE UNDERSIGNED PHYSICIAN WITHIN THAT TIME STATING THAT I WANT TO WITHDRAW FROM THIS ARBITRATION AGREEMENT. After those 30 days, this agreement may be changed or revoked only by a written revocation signed by both parties.

5. I agree to be bound by the Medical Arbitration Rules of the California Hospital Association and California Medical Association and the CHA-CMA Rules for the Arbitration of Hospital and Medical Fee Disputes hereby incorporated into this Agreement.

6. I have read and understood the attached explanation of the Patient-Physician Arbitration Agreement and I have read and understood this Agreement, including the Rules, and this writing makes up the entire arbitration agreement between me and the undersigned physician.

NOTICE: BY SIGNING THIS CONTRACT YOU ARE AGREEING TO HAVE ANY ISSUE OF MEDICAL MALPRACTICE DECIDED BY NEUTRAL ARBITRATION AND YOU ARE GIVING UP YOUR RIGHT TO A JURY OR COURT TRIAL. SEE ARTICLE 1 OF THIS CONTRACT.

DATED: ____________________, 19____

____
(PATIENT)

Physician's Agreement to Arbitrate

In consideration of the above-named patient's promise to be bound by this Patient-Physician Arbitration Agreement, I likewise agree to be similarly bound by its terms, as set forth in this Agreement and in the Rules specified in paragraph 5 above.

DATED: ____________________, 19____

____
(PHYSICIAN)

____
(TITLE—e.g. PARTNER, PRESIDENT, ETC.)

____
(NAME OF PARTNERSHIP OR PROFESSIONAL CORPORATION)

FIGURE 5–1 Arbitration agreement used in the state of California.

the same locality and under similar circumstances. It is extremely important that no *express* promise of a cure be made, for this then becomes a part of the contract.

The patient's part of the agreement includes the liability for payment for services and a willingness to follow the advice of the doctor.

STATUTE OF FRAUDS

In 1677, a statute was adopted in England aimed at reducing the evil of **perjured testimony** by providing that certain contracts could not be enforced if they depended upon the testimony of witnesses alone and were not evidenced in writing. The provisions of this English statute have been closely followed by statutes adopted in the various states of this country. Under the *Statute of Frauds* some contracts, in order to be enforceable, must be in writing. One of these is the promise to pay the debts of another. Thus, if a third party, not legally responsible, agrees to pay a patient's medical bills, the agreement cannot be enforced unless it is in writing.

GOOD SAMARITAN ACTS

The physician is sometimes reluctant to fulfill his ethical obligation to render aid in an emergency to someone who is not his patient, for fear he may later be charged with negligence or abandonment by a total stranger. In 1959, California passed the first **Good Samaritan Act,** and many other states have followed suit (Fig. 5–2). Although there are minor variations in the state statutes, their purpose is to protect the physician from liability for any civil damages as a result of rendering emergency care, provided such care is given in good faith and with due care under the circumstances. In some states the law applies to nurses as well as to physicians. There is no creation of a contract in giving emergency care.

CONTROLLED SUBSTANCES ACT OF 1970

Prior to April 1968, physicians practiced their professions primarily under the Narcotic Acts and the Drug Abuse Control Amendments. Under the Harrison Narcotic Act, physicians registered with the Internal Revenue Service, which issued narcotic stamps with the physician's registration number and also issued the order form books to physicians.

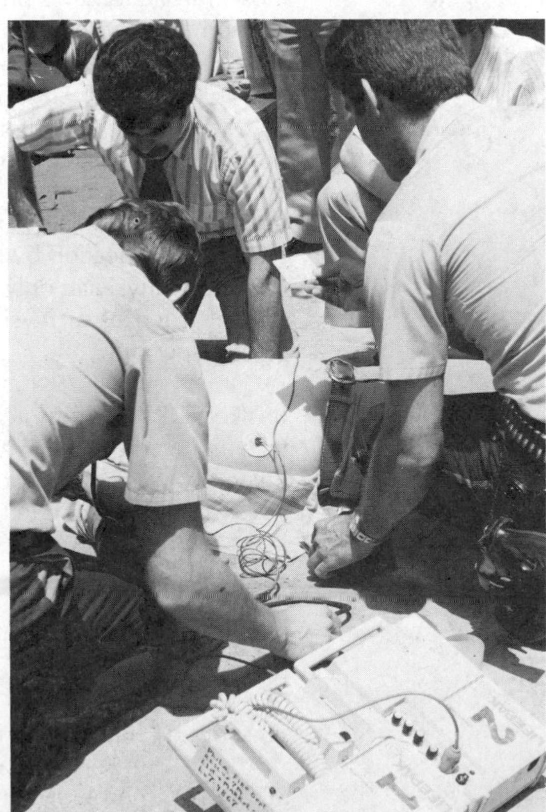

FIGURE 5–2 Physician treating at the scene of an accident. The Good Samaritan Act protects the physician from liability for any civil damages as a result of rendering emergency care. (Courtesy of H. Armstrong Roberts.)

On April 8, 1968, the Federal Bureau of Narcotics in the Treasury Department and the Bureau of Drug Abuse Control in the Food and Drug Administration merged into a new agency known as the Bureau of Narcotics and Dangerous Drugs (BNDD), located in the Department of Justice. From April 1968, to May 1971, the new Bureau operated under the laws and regulations of the two former agencies.

On May 1, 1971, the Controlled Substances Act of 1970 became fully effective, replacing the former Narcotic Acts and the Drug Abuse Control Amendments. In October 1973, the regulatory agency became known as the Drug Enforcement Administration. The Internal Revenue Service no longer registers physicians, nor do they issue order forms. Both of these functions are now carried out by the Drug Enforcement Administration (DEA). Physicians are required to register with the Registration Branch, Drug Enforcement Administration, P.O. Box 28083, Central Station, Washington, D.C. 20005, or the nearest regional office. If a physician has more than one office in which he administers and/or dispenses any of the drugs listed in the five Schedules, he is required to register at each office. However, if he only **administers** or **dispenses** at his principal office and only writes prescriptions at the other office or offices, he then is only required to register at his principal office where he administers or dispenses. (NOTE: The word "physician," as used in this Act, means any physician, dentist, veterinarian, or other practitioner authorized to administer, dispense, and prescribe controlled substances.)

Under the Controlled Substances Act, drugs are categorized into Schedules I, II, III, IV, and V. Schedule I drugs are those that have *no* accepted medical use in treatment in the United States. A physician will have no concern with Schedule I unless he is involved in conducting research with such drugs. Regulations regarding the writing, telephoning, and refilling of prescriptions vary according to which Schedule is involved. The physician and his assistant must keep abreast of regulations as they are issued.

Records Under the Act

NARCOTIC DRUGS. A physician who **prescribes** and/or **administers narcotic drugs** in the course of his professional practice *is not* required to keep records of those transactions. If a physician *dispenses* a narcotic drug to a patient, he *is* required to keep a record of such dispensing.

NON-NARCOTIC DRUGS. A physician who regularly engages in dispensing any of the non-narcotic drugs listed in the Schedules to his patients as a regular part of his professional practice, and for which he charges his patients either separately or together with other professional services, must keep records of all such drugs received and dispensed. The records must be kept for a period of two years and are subject to inspection by the DEA.

If the physician only occasionally dispenses a non-narcotic controlled drug to a patient (such as a physician's sample) he is not required to maintain a record of such dispensing.

INVENTORY. A physician who is required to keep records as stated above must take an inventory every two years of all stocks of controlled drugs on hand. The first inventory was required on May 1, 1971. A physician who registered after May 1, 1971 should take the initial inventory when he first engages in dispensing. He must keep this record for two years; he is *not* required to submit a copy to the DEA.

ORDER FORMS. A physician who has need for controlled drugs in Schedule II for use in his office or medical bag must obtain these drugs by the use of a triplicate order form. Order forms are obtained from the DEA at no charge to the physician. The Federal Triplicate Order Forms should not be confused with the triplicate prescription blanks that are required by some states.

SECURITY. A physician who has controlled substances stored in his office or clinic must keep these drugs in a locked cabinet or safe. Any loss of controlled drugs by theft must be reported to the regional office of the DEA at the time the theft is discovered. The local police department should also be notified.

DISCONTINUANCE OF PRACTICE. A physician who discontinues his practice must return his Registration Certificate and any unused order forms to the nearest office of the DEA. The regional office of the DEA in his area will advise him on how to dispose of any controlled drugs still in his possession.

UNIFORM ANATOMICAL GIFT ACT

A Uniform Anatomical Gift Act was approved by the National Conference of Commissioners on Uniform State Laws on July 30, 1968. Although many states had passed laws prior to this time that permitted a living person to make a gift of his body or portions of it after death, the laws were so different from state to state that arrangements for a donation in one state might not be recognized in another.

Essentially, the model law for donation states that: (1) any person of sound mind and 18 years of age or over may give all or any part of his body after death for research, transplantation, or placement in a tissue bank; (2) a donor's valid statement of gift is paramount to the rights of others except where a state autopsy law may prevail; (3) if a donor has not acted during his lifetime, his survivors, in a specified order of priority, may do so; (4) physicians who accept organs or tissues, relying in good faith on the documents, are protected from law suits. The physician attending at

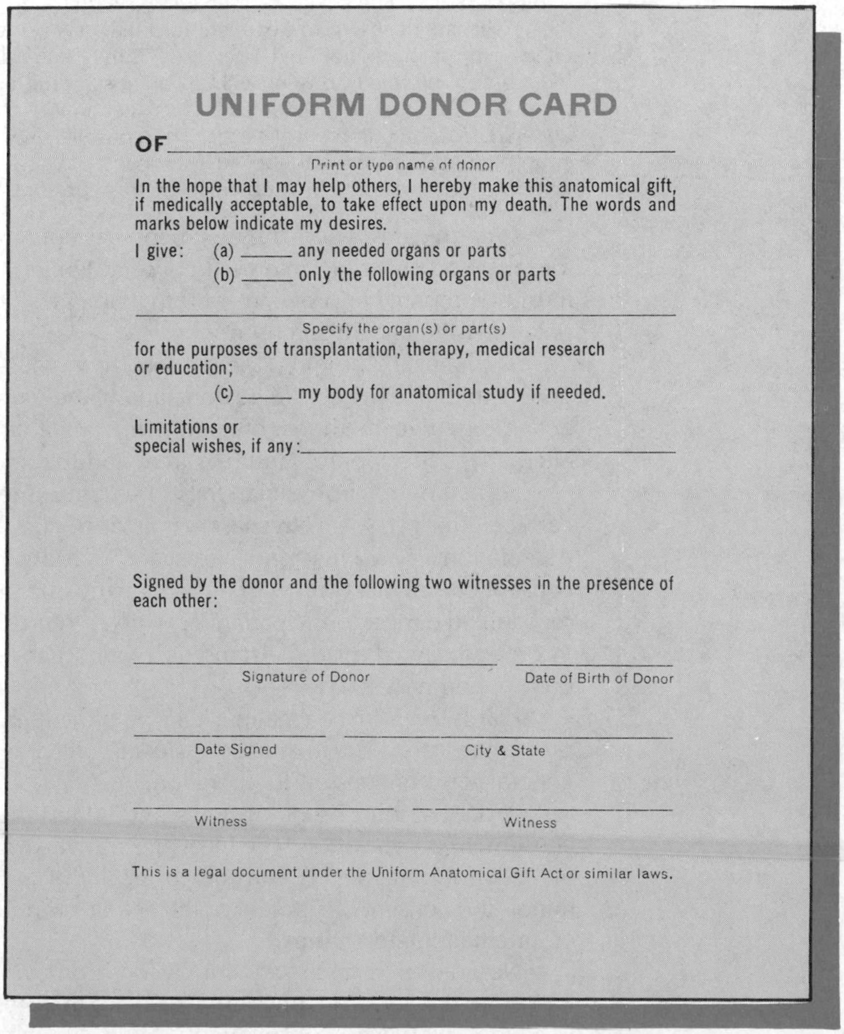

UNIFORM DONOR CARD

OF ______________________________

Print or type name of donor

In the hope that I may help others, I hereby make this anatomical gift, if medically acceptable, to take effect upon my death. The words and marks below indicate my desires.

I give: (a) _____ any needed organs or parts
(b) _____ only the following organs or parts

____

Specify the organ(s) or part(s)

for the purposes of transplantation, therapy, medical research or education;

(c) _____ my body for anatomical study if needed.

Limitations or special wishes, if any: ______________________________

Signed by the donor and the following two witnesses in the presence of each other:

______________________________ Signature of Donor

______________ Date of Birth of Donor

______________ Date Signed

______________ City & State

______________ Witness

______________ Witness

This is a legal document under the Uniform Anatomical Gift Act or similar laws.

FIGURE 5–3 Uniform Donor Card.

the time of death, if acquainted with the donor's wishes, may dispose of the body under the Uniform Anatomical Gift Act; (5) the time of death must be determined by a physician who is not involved in the transplantation, and the attending physician cannot be a member of the transplant team; (6) the donor may revoke the gift or the gift may be rejected. The most important clause permits the donation to be made by a will (without waiting for **probate**) or by other written or witnessed documents, such as a card designed to be carried on the person (Fig. 5–3). The Uniform Donor Card is considered a legal document in all 50 states.

The provisions of the Uniform Anatomical Gift Act are so designed that the offer is exercised only after death. Therefore, the donor should reveal his intentions to as many of his relatives and friends as possible, including his physician. Also, since the human body or its parts are not commodities in commerce, no money can be exchanged in making an anatomical donation. Additional details about organ and tissue donations and donor cards may be obtained from the National Kidney Foundation, 315 Park Avenue South, New York 10010.

SECURING PATIENT'S INFORMED CONSENT

A physician must have consent to treat a patient, even though this consent is usually implied by virtue of the fact that the patient chooses a particular physician to treat him. Consent may be express or implied, oral or written.

In *Medicolegal Forms with Legal Analysis,* the American Medical Association explains some of the implications of consent in this way:

> Usually authority to treat or operate arises from the valid consent of the patient or someone authorized to act in his behalf. A statute in Georgia (Georgia Code, Chapter 88–29) enumerates those who may consent to treatment for themselves or for others. The consent given may be either express or implied and, if express, it may either be written or oral. The consent given must be an informed consent with an understanding of what is to be done and of the risks involved. The procedure involved and its attendant risks should be explained to the patient in understandable nontechnical terms. The consent given may be invalid (a) because the act consented to is unlawful, (b) because the consent was given by one who had no legal right to give it, or (c) because it was obtained by misrepresentation or fraud.

Even in cases where the treatment was not negligent, the physician can be sued for failing to obtain an informed consent. Under such circumstances, the physician must be prepared to prove in court that he gave the patient a full explanation before obtaining the patient's consent.

To be legally binding, the consent given must be an **informed consent** with an understanding of what is to be done and of the risks involved, why it should be done, and alternative methods of treatment available and their attendant risks. The alternatives include the failure to treat and the attendant risk.

Sometimes, if a physician fails to secure some formal expression of consent, he can be charged with **trespass** or **assault** and **battery.** The American Medical Association's Law Division states that "a prudent physician will demand a written consent or authorization with respect to any operation which involves an element of recognized danger to the patient or which requires hospitalization." This is desirable in order to avoid misunderstandings which can lead to lawsuits; it also facilitates proof when necessary.

Forms on which a patient can grant written consent for operations or other procedures are kept in most physicians' offices. Figures 5–4 and 5–5 illustrate a general form of consent to operation.

A patient must be of legal age and be in full possession of his faculties to give consent for an operation. The legal age will vary from state to state; sometimes a girl of 18 who is married is considered legally of age, for example. If the patient is a minor, the consent of a parent or the acting guardian is necessary, except in the case of an **emancipated minor.**

No consent is necessary if a person is dangerously ill and unconscious and his life is in danger. The physician can use his best judgment in proceeding with treatment. However, consultation is advisable in such cases.

Birth control through voluntary surgical sterilization procedures such as **vasectomy** or **tubal ligation** is lawful in some states. It is recommended that for every such procedure the physician should obtain from the patient and the spouse, if any, a signed, written informed consent (see Fig. 5–6).

KEEPING COMPLETE RECORDS

To protect the doctor from malpractice actions, it is important to keep ideal medical records that could be taken to court if necessary to show that the care and treatment given fully met standards of law and medical practice. For this reason details should be fairly complete on medical records and dates upon which treatment was given

Form P-1

CONSENT TO OPERATION, ANESTHETICS, AND OTHER MEDICAL SERVICES

Date__________ Time__________ A.M. / P.M.

1. I authorize the performance upon ____________________
(myself or name of patient)

of the following operation ____________________
(state nature and extent of operation)

to be performed by or under the direction of Dr.______________.

2. I consent to the performance of operations and procedures in addition to or different from those now contemplated, whether or not arising from presently unforeseen conditions, which the above-named doctor or his associates or assistants may consider necessary or advisable in the course of the operation.

3. I consent to the administration of such anesthetics as may be considered necessary or advisable by the physician responsible for this service, with the exception of ________________
(state "none," "spinal anesthesia," etc.)

4. The nature and purpose of the operation, possible alternative methods of treatment, the risks involved, the possible consequences, and the possibility of complications have been explained to me by Dr.______________ and by______________.

5. I acknowledge that no guarantee or assurance has been given by anyone as to the results that may be obtained.

6. I consent to the photographing or televising of the operations or procedures to be performed, including appropriate portions of my body, for medical, scientific or educational purposes, provided my identity is not revealed by the pictures or by descriptive texts accompanying them.

7. For the purpose of advancing medical education, I consent to the admittance of observers to the operating room.

8. I consent to the disposal by hospital authorities of any tissues or body parts which may be removed.

9. I am aware that sterility may result from this operation. I know that a sterile person is incapable of becoming a parent.

10. I acknowledge that all blank spaces on this document have been either completed or crossed off prior to my signing.

(CROSS OUT ANY PARAGRAPHS ABOVE WHICH DO NOT APPLY)

Signed ____________________
(Patient or person authorized to consent for patient)

Witness________________

FIGURE 5–4 **(From *Medicolegal Forms with Legal Analysis. 3rd Ed.* Office of the General Counsel, 1973, p. 57. Copyright © 1973. American Medical Association.)**

Form P-2

CONSENT TO OPERATION, ANESTHETICS, AND OTHER MEDICAL SERVICES (ALTERNATE FORM)

Date____________Time________A.M. P.M.

1. I authorize the performance upon ________________
(myself or name of patient)

of the following operation ____________________
(state name of operation)

to be performed under the direction of Dr. __________.

2. The following have been explained to me by Dr.______:

A. The nature of the operation ________________
(describe the operation)

____

____

B. The purpose of the operation________________
(describe the purpose)

____

C. The possible alternative methods of treatment ______

____
(describe the alternative methods)

D. The possible consequences of the operation ______

____
(describe the possible consequences)

E. The risks involved ____________________
(describe the risks involved)

____

F. The possibility of complications ____________

____
(describe the possible complications)

3. I have been advised of the serious nature of the operation and have been advised that if I desire a further and more detailed explanation of any of the foregoing or further information about the possible risks or complications of the above listed operation it will be given to me.

4. I do not request a further and more detailed listing and explanation of any of the items listed in paragraph 2.

Signed ____________________
(Patient or person authorized to consent for patient)

Witness________________

FIGURE 5–5 (From *Medicolegal Forms with Legal Analysis. 3rd Ed.* Office of the General Counsel, 1973, p. 59. Copyright © 1973. American Medical Association.)

indicated. Sometimes it is necessary to make a correction or change in a record. This should be done by lightly crossing out the part to be changed and inserting the correction. If any patient fails to keep an appointment, discontinues treatment before he should, or fails to follow advice, the medical record should show this information. The doctor should write to these patients, advising of the importance of continued medical treatment, and include copies of all such letters in the patient's record. Samples of these letters are reproduced in Figures 5–7, 5–8, and 5–9.

LEGAL RESPONSIBILITIES OF THE MEDICAL ASSISTANT

What is the responsibility of the medical assistant for any acts that she performs while working for a physician? This is a question of vital importance to anyone who is employed in a doctor's office.

AGENT OF EMPLOYER. The medical assistant, while acting within the scope of her employment, is considered an **"agent"** of her employer. If she would say to a patient, "Go right to the hospital; Dr. White will see you there," then Dr. White is bound by contract to do so.

Generally, the law holds that every person is liable for the consequences of his own negligence when another person is injured as a result. In some situations this liability also extends to the employer. Physicians may be held responsible for the mistakes of those who work in their offices and sometimes must respond in damages for their negligent acts.

The physician is legally responsible for the acts of his assistant or employees

Form P-17

REQUEST FOR STERILIZATION

Date____________ Time__________ A.M. / P.M.

We, the undersigned husband and wife, each being more than twenty-one years of age and of sound mind, request Dr.

________________, and assistants of his choice, to perform upon

________________, the following operation: ________________.
(name of patient) *(state nature and extent of operation)*

It has been explained to us that this operation is intended to result in sterility although this result has not been guaranteed. We understand that a sterile person is NOT capable of becoming a parent.

We voluntarily request the operation and understand that if it proves successful the results will be permanent and it will thereafter be physically impossible for the patient to inseminate, or to conceive or bear children.

Signed________________
(Husband)

Signed________________
(Wife)

Witness________________

FIGURE 5–6 (From *Medicolegal Forms with Legal Analysis. 3rd Ed.* Office of the General Counsel, 1973, p. 69. Copyright © 1973. American Medical Association.)

Form B-1

LETTER TO CONFIRM DISCHARGE BY PATIENT

Dear Mr. ________________:

This will confirm our telephone conversation of today in which you discharged me from attending you as your physician in your present illness. In my opinion your condition requires continued medical treatment by a physician. If you have not already done so, I suggest that you employ another physician without delay. You may be assured that, at your request, I will furnish him with information regarding the diagnosis and treatment which you have received from me.

Very truly yours,

________________, M.D.

FIGURE 5–7 (From *Medicolegal Forms with Legal Analysis. 3rd Ed.* Office of the General Counsel, 1973, p. 5. Copyright © 1973. American Medical Association.)

Form B-3

STATEMENT OF PATIENT LEAVING HOSPITAL AGAINST ADVICE

This is to certify that I am leaving ________________ Hospital at my own insistence and against the advice of the hospital authorities and my attending physician. I have been informed by them of the dangers of my leaving the hospital at this time. I release the hospital, its employees and officers, and my attending physician from all liability for any adverse results caused by my leaving the hospital prematurely.

Signed________________ 2

I agree to hold harmless the ________________ Hospital, its employees and officers, and the attending physician from all liability, with reference to the discharge of the patient named above.

____

(Husband, wife, parent, etc.)

Date ________________

Witness________________

FIGURE 5–8 (From *Medicolegal Forms with Legal Analysis. 3rd Ed.* Office of the General Counsel, 1973, p. 6. Copyright © 1973. American Medical Association.)

when they are acting within the scope of their duties or employment. He is also responsible for the acts of those who assist him, even though they are not directly employed by him, if they commit acts of negligence while under his immediate supervision and in his presence. For example, a nurse who is a hospital employee makes an error in a procedure while acting under a physician's direction. The court

Form B-5

LETTER TO PATIENT WHO FAILS TO KEEP APPOINTMENT

Dear Mr. ________________:

On __________, 19____, you failed to keep your appointment at my office. In my opinion your condition requires continued medical treatment. If you so desire, you may telephone me for another appointment, but if you prefer to have another physician attend you, I suggest that you arrange to do so without delay. You may be assured that, at your request, I am entirely willing to make available my knowledge of your case to the physician of your choice.

I trust that you will understand that my purpose in writing this letter is out of concern for your health and well-being.

Very truly yours,

________________, M.D.

Form B-7

LETTER TO PATIENT WHO FAILS TO FOLLOW ADVICE

Dear Mr. ________________:

At the time that you brought your son, William, to me for examination this afternoon, I informed you that I was unable to determine without X-ray pictures whether a fracture existed in his injured right arm. I strongly urge you to permit me or some other physician of your choice to make this X-ray examination without further delay.

Your neglect in not permitting a proper X-ray examination to be made of William's arm may result in serious consequences if in fact a fracture does exist.

Very truly yours,

________________, M.D.

FIGURE 5–9 (From *Medicolegal Forms with Legal Analysis. 3rd Ed.* Office of the General Counsel, 1973, p. 7. Copyright © 1973. American Medical Association.)

may determine that she came so completely under the direction and supervision of the physician that the physician is **liable** for her negligence. This is known as the doctrine of **respondeat superior** (let the master answer). A special nurse is employed by the patient; therefore, the physician is not usually held liable for her acts. When doctors practice as partners, each partner is liable not only for his own acts and those of his partner but also for the negligent acts of any agent or employee of the partnership.

If a physician properly writes a prescription, he is not liable for a pharmacist's negligence in **compounding** it, but he may be liable where there is misunderstanding as to the ingredients when the prescription is ordered over the telephone.

NEED FOR EXTREME CARE. A medical assistant who is guilty of negligence is liable for her own actions, but the injured party generally sues the physician since there is a better chance of collecting from him. However, even if the assistant has no money, she can still be liable for her actions. This fact should indicate the continuing importance of exercising extreme care in performing all duties in the professional office. While working under pressure there is always the danger she may interchange blood, serum, or medications, or mix names or improperly prepare labels. Never proceed with administration of a medication or treatment without checking all details at least twice, and preferably three times.

RECHECKING EQUIPMENT. The doctor and his staff should frequently check the condition of all office equipment and make use of every available safety installation to prevent accidents to patients. Each assistant should be alert for potential hazards, such as slipping rugs, exposed telephone and light cords, highly waxed floors, and protruding objects, since patients who are harmed as a result of these things can sue for damages (Fig. 5–10).

ILLEGAL PRACTICE OF MEDICINE. There are certain other medicolegal aspects of her work which the assistant must understand. The doctor goes to school many years to learn his profession; he is licensed by his state to practice medicine. *The assistant is not licensed to practice medicine.* She must never prescribe, even though she feels she knows what the doctor would order. This is unlawful. She must never try to *diagnose* a patient's ailment. This, too, is the illegal practice of medicine. As a result, it is not good policy for the assistant to discuss patients' ailments with them. Patients tend to identify the assistant's every remark with the doctor himself.

INSTRUCTIONS TO PATIENT. Both the doctor and his staff must be extremely careful in giving instructions to patients. If the patient misunderstands the instruc-

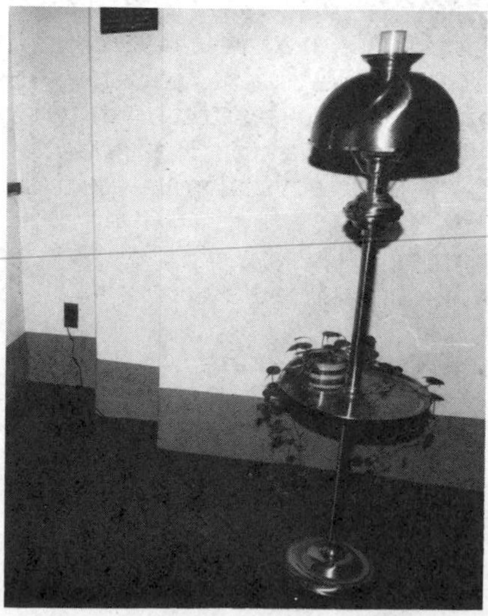

FIGURE 5–10 Example of a hazardous area that may cause the patient to trip.

tions, the physician may have a malpractice suit on his hands. When written instructions can be provided, this should be done.

EXAMINATIONS OF WOMEN. Except in an actual emergency, the male physician should not examine a female patient unless a third person is present. The charge of undue familiarity against a doctor is very damaging. That is why the assistant generally will stand by when the doctor performs such examinations.

EMERGENCY AID. The question sometimes arises: should the assistant give emergency care to a patient brought into the office while the doctor is away? The assistant, as any other layman, in a medical emergency may do whatever is reasonably necessary provided that the action taken is within her skill and competence. The physician should instruct his assistant regarding what course of action he wishes her to take in such instances. She must immediately get in touch with the doctor or another physician to care for the patient, once she has performed any emergency measures.

CLAIMS PREVENTION. It is not expected that the medical assistant will know all the legal ramifications of the practice of medicine; nor should she develop an attitude of skepticism. The majority of patients never entertain the thought of legal action against their physicians. She should be aware, however, of her role in "claims prevention."

The American Medical Association Committee on Medicolegal Problems in 1963 set forth 21 prevention "commandments." Many of these commandments require the active cooperation of the medical office assistant. They are set forth here for your study and frequent review:

1. The physician must care for every patient with scrupulous attention given to the requirements of good medical practice.
2. The physician must know and exercise his legal duty to the patient.
3. The physician must avoid destructive and unethical criticism of the work of other physicians.
4. The physician must keep records which clearly show what was done and when it was done, which clearly indicate that nothing was neglected, and which demonstrate that the care given met fully the standards demanded by the law. If any patient discontinues treatment before he should, or fails to follow instructions, the records should show it; a good method is to preserve a carbon copy of the physician's letter advising the patient against an unwise course.
5. The physician must avoid making any statement which constitutes, or might be construed as constituting, an admission of fault on his part. He should instruct employees to make no such statements.
6. The physician must exercise tact as well as professional ability in handling his patients and should insist on a professional consultation if the patient is not doing well, if the patient is unhappy and complaining, or if the family's attitude indicates dissatisfaction.
7. The physician must refrain from overly optimistic prognoses.
8. The physician must advise his patients of any intended absences from practice and recommend, or make available, a qualified substitute. The patient must not be abandoned.
9. The physician must unfailingly secure an "informed" consent (preferably in writing) for medical and surgical procedures and for autopsy.
10. The physician must carefully select and supervise assistants and employees and take great care in delegating duties to them.
11. The physician must keep abreast of general medical and scientific progress.
12. The physician should limit his practice to those fields which are well within his qualifications.

13. The physician must frequently check the condition of his equipment and make use of every available safety installation.

14. The physician should make every effort to reach an understanding with his patient in the matter of fees, preferably in advance of treatment.

15. The physician must realize that it is dangerous to diagnose or prescribe by telephone.

16. The physician should not sterilize a patient solely for the patient's convenience, except after a reasonably complete explanation of the procedure, its risks and possible complications, and after obtaining a signed consent from the patient and the patient's spouse, if the patient is married. Such sterilization is a crime in Connecticut, Kansas, and Utah, and should not be performed in those states. **Eugenic** sterilization should be performed only in conformity with the law of the state, if any exists. Sterilization for therapeutic purposes may lawfully be performed with the informed consent of the patient and preferably with the informed consent of the patient's spouse, if the patient is married.

17. Except in an actual emergency situation which makes it impossible to avoid doing so, a male physician should not examine a female patient unless an assistant or nurse, or a member of the patient's family, is present.

18. The physician should exhaust all reasonable methods of securing a diagnosis before embarking upon a therapeutic course.

19. The physician should use conservative and less dangerous methods of diagnosis and treatment whenever possible, in preference to highly **toxic** agents or dangerous surgical procedures.

20. The physician should read the manufacturer's brochure accompanying a toxic agent to be used for diagnostic or therapeutic purposes, and, in addition, should ascertain the customary dosage or usage in his area.

21. The physician should be aware of all the known toxic reactions to any drug he uses, together with the proper methods for treating such reactions.

GLOSSARY OF LEGAL TERMS

Burden of Proof — The necessity or duty of affirmatively proving a fact or facts in dispute on an issue raised between the parties in a cause.

Civil Law — That division of municipal law occupied with the exposition and enforcement of civil rights as distinguished from criminal law.

Common Law — Law derived from court decisions, judge-made law.

Contributory Negligence — The act or omission amounting to want of ordinary care on the part of the patient, which, concurring with defendant's negligence, is proximate cause of injury.

Criminal Case — An action suit, or cause instituted to punish an infraction of the criminal laws.

Criminal Law — Law that deals with conduct offensive to society as a whole, or the state.

Defamation Offense of injuring another's reputation by false and malicious statements.

Defendant The person defending or denying; the party against whom relief or recovery is sought in an action or suit.

Deposition Sometimes used as a synonym for oath, but the term is specifically applicable to the testimony of a witness taken in writing, under oath or affirmation, before a judicial officer, in answer to oral or written interrogation.

Feasance The doing of an act; a performing or performance.

Malfeasance. The doing of an act which is wholly wrongful and unlawful.

Misfeasance. The improper performance of some act which a man may lawfully do.

Nonfeasance. The omission of an act which a person ought to do.

Felony A crime of a graver or more atrocious nature than those designated as misdemeanors; generally, an offense punishable by imprisonment in a penitentiary.

Grievance Committee A committee established by a local medical society to hear and investigate the complaints of patients respecting professional care rendered by an attending physician or allegedly excessive fees charged by him.

Invasion of Privacy An encroachment on the right of privacy, the right to be "left alone" or to live in seclusion without being subjected to unwarranted or undesired publicity. Thus, without the knowledge and authorization of the patient, there should be no publication of his medical case record and no showing of a photograph or motion picture from which the identity of the patient is determinable.

Judicial Relating to or connected with the administration of Justice.

Jurisprudence The philosophy of law, or the science which treats of the principles of positive law and legal relations.

Libel	Defamatory words that are printed, written or published which injure the character or reputation of another by holding him up to ridicule, contempt, shame, disgrace or degrade him in the estimation of the community. (See **Slander**.)
Locum Tenens	"Holding the place." A deputy, substitute, lieutenant, or representative.
Medical Audit	A study of the patient's medical record for the purpose of determining the quality of medical care the patient received.
Non Compos Mentis	Not sound of mind; insane. This is a very general term, embracing all varieties of mental derangement.
Plaintiff	The person who brings an action; the party who complains or sues in a personal action and is so named in the record.
Proximate Cause	That which, in a natural and continuous sequence, unbroken by any efficient intervening cause, produces the injury, and without which the result would not have occurred.
Que Facit per Alium Facit per se	"He who acts through another acts himself."
Quid pro Quo	Something for something.
Res Gestae	"Things done." Res gestae is considered as an exception to the hearsay rule. In its operation it renders acts and declarations which constitute a part of the things done and said admissible in evidence, even though they would otherwise come within the rule excluding hearsay evidence or self-serving declarations.
Res Ipsa Loquitur	"The thing speaks for itself."
Res Judicata	A matter adjudged; a thing judicially acted upon or decided; a thing or matter settled by judgment.
Rule of Discovery	Statute of limitations does not begin to run until the patient knew or should have known of the injury.

Slander Oral defamation; speaking falsely about another with resulting injury to his reputation. (See **Libel**.)

Statute of Limitations A legal limit on the time one has to file suit in civil matters, usually measured from the time of the wrong or from the time a reasonable person would have discovered the wrong.

Subpoena A writ or order directed to a person and requiring his attendance at a particular time and place to testify. It may also require him to bring with him any books, documents, or other things under his control which he is bound by law to produce in evidence (subpoena duces tecum).

Tort A private or civil wrong or injury.

References

American Medical Association: *Professional Liability and the Physician.* Chicago, American Medical Association, 1963.

American Medical Association: *Medicolegal Forms with Legal Analysis.* Chicago, American Medical Association, 1973.

Black's Law Dictionary, Revised 4th edition, 1968.

California Medical Association: *Arbitration for Physicians in Private Practice.* San Francisco, California Medical Association, 1975.

California Medical Association: *Professional Liability.* San Francisco, California Medical Association, 1971.

Hayt, E., and J. Hayt: *The Law of Hospital and Nurses.* New York, Hospital Textbook Company, 1958.

Hemelt, M. D., and M. E. Mackert: *Dynamics of Law in Nursing and Health Care.* Reston, Virginia, Reston Publishing Company, Inc., 1978.

Moritz, A. R., and R. Crawford Morris: *Handbook of Legal Medicine,* 4th ed. St. Louis, C. V. Mosby Company, 1975.

Stetler, J., and A. R. Moritz: *Doctor and Patient and the Law,* 4th ed. St. Louis, C. V. Mosby Company, 1962.

U.S. Dept. of Justice, Bureau of Narcotics and Dangerous Drugs: *Practitioner's Informational Outline of the Controlled Substances Act of 1970,* 1972.

CHAPTER OUTLINE

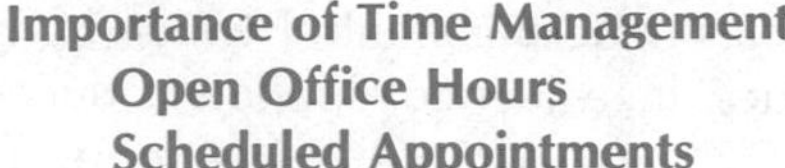

- Importance of Time Management
  - Open Office Hours
  - Scheduled Appointments
- The Appointment Book
  - Selection
  - Advance Preparation
- Guidelines for Scheduling
  - Patient Need
  - Doctor's Preferences
  - Available Facilities
  - Individualizing the System
  - Wave Scheduling
  - Double Booking
  - Grouping Procedures
  - Advance Booking
- Exceptions to Appointment System
  - Emergency Patients
  - Acutely Ill Patients
  - Physician Referrals
  - Failed Appointments
- Handling Cancellations and Delays
  - When the Patient Cancels
  - When the Doctor is Delayed
  - When the Doctor is Called Out on Emergencies
- Making the Appointment
  - In Person
  - By Telephone
  - Appointments for New Patients
  - Special Problems
- Mechanics of the Appointment Book
- Appointment Cards and Reminders
- Appointments Outside the Office
  - Scheduling Surgeries
  - House Calls
  - Laboratory and X-ray Appointments for Patients
- Other Callers
  - Pharmaceutical Representatives
  - Physicians
  - Salesmen
  - Miscellaneous

BEHAVIORAL OBJECTIVES

The medical office assistant should be able to:

- Compare the utilization of time in offices using (a) scheduled appointments and (b) open office hours.
- List advantages of realistic scheduling.
- Select a suitable appointment book.
- Apply efficient guidelines for scheduling appointments.
- Describe wave scheduling and grouping procedures.
- Adjust a schedule interrupted by an emergency or delay.
- Control failed appointments within legal boundaries.
- Handle cancellations and delays.
- Explain and apply the mechanics of appointment scheduling.
- Use appointment cards and reminders correctly.
- Determine appropriate procedures for handling callers who do not have appointments.
- Schedule appointments for procedures required outside the office.

6

SCHEDULING APPOINTMENTS

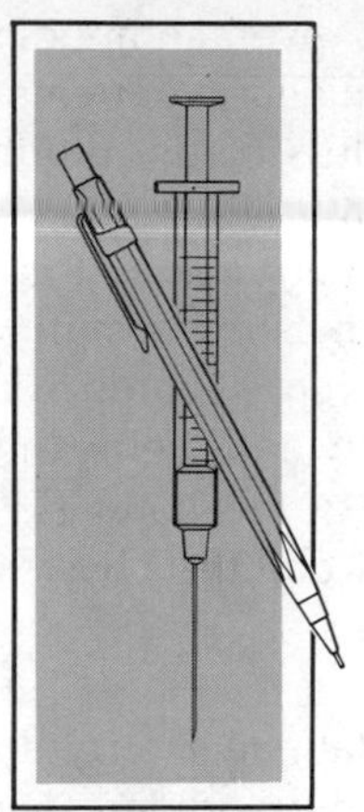

One of the most important duties that the doctor delegates to his assistant is the scheduling of appointments. In most offices, the appointment book is the hub around which all activity revolves. Properly controlled, the appointment book can be a highly useful device for running the office smoothly. Improperly controlled, it can become either an overly stern taskmaster or an ineffectual mechanism of little or no consequence in the operation of the office. The effectiveness of the appointment book is determined by the skill the medical assistant develops in using it and the effort the doctor himself exerts in abiding by the schedule.

IMPORTANCE OF TIME MANAGEMENT

When the physician delegates responsibility for his appointment book to his assistant, he is in effect saying, "Here, manage my time, a precious commodity which must be used well but never wasted."

Management of the schedule is a two-pronged responsibility; first, arranging the schedule; second, keeping the schedule operating smoothly. The first part will be dealt with in this chapter; the second in Chapter 7 on reception techniques.

There are two opposing views among physicians on the utilization of office time — *open office hours* with no appointments vs. *scheduled appointments*.

OPEN OFFICE HOURS. A minority of physicians prefer to keep open office hours rather than schedule appointments. This tendency is more common in rural areas where the general population, although consisting of busy people, is not governed so much by the clock as by the sun and the weather. It is made generally known that the doctor is in his office at given hours of the day. He most probably "schedules" his patients by saying something like "come back in a couple of weeks." On a day convenient for the patient, he comes in and waits his turn to see the doctor. The patient knows ahead of time that he may have a considerable wait and takes it in his stride. Physicians who use this method say that it eliminates the annoyance of broken appointments and "running late." The assistant in this kind of office need not worry much about how much time to allow per individual patient.

SCHEDULED APPOINTMENTS. Studies have shown that physicians are able to see more patients with less pressure when they schedule appointments. It does have its hazards, however. The patient who is given an appointment may feel that if only a few minutes were needed for the examination or treatment, he is entitled to the "rest of the time allotted to him," regardless of the number of people waiting in the reception room. Some patients need *more* time than was planned. They may have told the assistant of one complaint when making the appointment, but "discover" additional complaints when they are being examined by the doctor. Judicious scheduling will keep most of the inherent hazards to a minimum.

Planning appointments realistically and seeing that the physician starts on time and sticks to the schedule will please the patients, bring economic gain to the physician, and give both the assistant and the physician a better chance of getting home in time for dinner.

THE APPOINTMENT BOOK

SELECTION. Office suppliers and stationers carry a variety of appointment book styles, and at least one of the standard preprinted styles will be satisfactory for the physician who is just starting a practice. As the practice develops, the physician may find the preprinted books too restrictive. When this happens, it is time to look for an appointment book that more closely suits the practice, or, failing this, to personally design one. In either case, there are certain basic features to consider. The appointment book should:

1. Conform to the size of desk space available
2. Be large enough to accommodate the practice
3. Open flat for easy writing and reference
4. Allow space for *when, who,* and *why*

In addition, one might wish to consider:

1. A book that shows an entire week at a glance
2. Color coding with a special color for each day of the week
3. Multiple columns corresponding with the numbers of doctors in a group practice
4. Division into time units more suitable to the practice

Professional stationery companies will furnish planning kits and work with you to develop what is best for the practice. Some of these suppliers are listed in the references at the end of the chapter.

ADVANCE PREPARATION. Having chosen an appropriate book, some advance preparation should be done. This is sometimes called "establishing the **matrix**." Block off, in pencil, those periods when the doctor is routinely not available to see patients (days off, holidays, hospital rounds, lunch, meetings, and so forth). In the space where you would ordinarily write the patient's name, write a memo showing the reason for blocking off these spaces. Always try to account for every time period in each day.

If your employer keeps you informed of social or family engagements, make a note of these also so that you can remind him of them as necessary.

GUIDELINES FOR SCHEDULING

Failure to keep appointment times is still the most frequent complaint heard from patients. There can be no hard and fast rules for scheduling appointments efficiently. The system to be used must be individualized to the specific office and the doctor's own preferences and habits. There are, however, certain general basic considerations to be observed in every practice: patient need, doctor's preferences, and available facilities.

PATIENT NEED. Time must be allotted to patients on the basis of each one's particular needs. What is the purpose of the visit? What is the age of the patient? A teenager will probably not require as much time as his grandparent will. Will the patient require the *doctor's* time for the entire visit or will another member of the staff be performing part or all of the service? Is the patient the mother of several schoolchildren who likes to schedule her appointments during the school hours? If an attempt is made to make the appointment suit the convenience of the patient, one possible cause for complaint is eliminated.

DOCTOR'S PREFERENCES. Is the doctor methodical and careful about being in the office when patient appointments are scheduled to begin? Or must you allow for his being late? Does he move easily from one patient to the next or must you allow a "break" time for him? If he would rather see fewer patients and spend more time with each one, then that is his **prerogative** — but it must be taken into account in the scheduling. Some doctors become restless if the reception room isn't packed with waiting patients; others worry if one patient is kept waiting. All these personal preferences and habits become an **integral** part of the scheduling problem.

AVAILABLE FACILITIES. There's no point in getting a patient into the office at a time when no facilities are available for the service he needs. For instance, suppose in a two-physician office that there is only one room which can be used for minor surgery. You wouldn't schedule two patients requiring minor surgery to come in at the same time, even though both doctors could be available. If there is only one sigmoidoscope, the intelligent medical assistant will not book a second **sigmoidoscopy** immediately following a similar examination. She will provide time for cleaning and sterilization procedures, and for readying the examination room. With some knowledge of the patients' needs, the medical office assistant attempts to pair those needs with the available facilities in an open time slot.

INDIVIDUALIZING THE SCHEDULING SYSTEM. Ideally, the scheduling system should provide for "same-day" service for *sick* patients and for seeing all scheduled patients on time. One big advantage of same-day service for sick patients is that it eliminates the problem of cancellations that often occur when the sick patient shows improvement prior to the time of an advance appointment. Every doctor's schedule should have at least one appointment slot open each day. A family practitioner may want to leave as much as 25 per cent of the time open for emergencies and work-in patients. Many doctors find that reserving the time slot at the end of the morning and at the end of the afternoon works well and causes the least **disruption** of schedule. Two facts are clear: (1) there must be a system, and (2) the system must fit the practice.

WAVE SCHEDULING. Many schedules are too inflexible. Wave scheduling is an attempt to correlate a time schedule with the variables brought about by patients who need more time or less time than planned for, the patient who arrives late, and other unavoidable **deviations** from the schedule such as no-show and work-in patients.

What happens when all patients are assigned the same length of time? The schedule might look like this, with a patient scheduled every 20 minutes.

10:00 Alicia Barker
10:20 Colleen Davis
10:40 Edna Farber

11:00 Gertrude Havens
11:20 Irene Jackson
11:40 Katherine Lambert

Mrs. Barker, the first patient, arrives at 10:15. The physician has already lost 15 minutes. The patient needs 25 minutes instead of the allotted 20 minutes. Mrs. Davis, the second patient, also arrived at 10:15, five minutes early for her appointment, but is kept waiting until 10:40, the time that Mrs. Farber, the third patient, was to have been seen. Mrs. Farber is on time but will also be kept waiting. Fortunately, Mrs. Davis actually needs only 10 minutes, so Mrs. Farber can be seen at 10:50, but if she requires the allotted 20 minutes, Mrs. Havens, the fourth patient, will also have to wait, and so on throughout the day.

Wave scheduling assumes that the actual time needed will average out. If the average time is 20 minutes per patient, three patients will be scheduled for each hour, and seen in order of arrival. Thus, one person's late arrival will not disrupt the entire schedule. The appointment schedule would then look like this:

10:00	Alicia Barker
	Colleen Davis
	Edna Farber
11:00	Gertrude Havens
	Irene Jackson
	Katherine Lambert

Given the circumstances illustrated above, Mrs. Davis would have arrived first (five minutes early), Mrs. Farber would be next (on time), and Mrs. Barker would be third (fifteen minutes late). All could have been seen within the hour, with no delay affecting the patients scheduled for the next hour.

Modified Wave Schedule. There are several ways of modifying the wave schedule. One method is to have two patients scheduled to come in at 10:00 and the third at 10:30, with this hourly cycle repeated throughout the day. Another application is to have patients scheduled to arrive at given intervals during the first half of the hour, and none scheduled to arrive during the second half of the hour.

DOUBLE BOOKING. The office assistant who books two patients concurrently, both of whom are to be seen by the doctor, is fooling only herself. Of course, if each is expected to take only five minutes or so, there is no harm in telling both to come at 2:00 and reserve a 15-minute period for the two. This is an application of wave scheduling. But if each one will require 15 minutes, two will require 30 minutes no matter how their names are written in the book.

It is not "double booking" if a patient comes to the office for a treatment or injection from the nurse. In a case such as this, the office assistant should briefly say, when she calls this patient in from the reception room, "You may come in now; the nurse can take care of you," or "You were not to see the doctor today; the nurse will take care of you." A comment such as this reveals no medical information about the patient but does let the waiting patients know that this patient is not being shown preference in seeing the doctor.

GROUPING PROCEDURES. Another method of time management that appeals to some practitioners is grouping of procedures. An internist, for example, might reserve all morning appointments for complete physicals; a surgeon whose practice depends upon referrals might reserve one day a week or specific hours on each day for new patients; a pediatrician might have well-baby hours, and so forth. Experimentation with different groupings may help in arriving at the best arrangements. In applying a grouping system of appointments, the assistant may find it helpful to lightly color code those sections of the appointment book being reserved for special procedures.

ADVANCE BOOKING. When booking appointments weeks or months ahead, make it a policy to leave some open time during each day's schedule. Then, if a patient calls with a somewhat acute problem that is not an immediate emergency, you won't have to tell him, "We don't have any time open until next month." The busy doctor will always be able to fill these appointments, and no time will be lost, but his patients will appreciate that it is possible to see their doctor within a reasonable time when the circumstances warrant.

It may be a good idea, if possible, to set time aside in the morning and afternoon for a breather. Even 15 or 20 minutes will give the doctor an opportunity to return calls from patients, verify prescription calls, or answer questions you may have that were not an emergency; this is especially necessary in pediatrics and obstetrics.

EXCEPTIONS TO APPOINTMENT SYSTEM

The day that goes along according to schedule, without having to make any adjustments in the plan, is the exception in some offices rather than the rule. The medical office assistant realizes there are certain situations that will require an immediate adjustment in the schedule.

EMERGENCY PATIENTS. If someone telephones to report an emergency that can be seen or treated in the office, the medical office assistant will have no hesitancy in having the patient come immediately. However, she must be sure it really is an emergency, and not just a patient who has suddenly decided this is the day he wants to see a doctor. Before such a situation arises, the assistant should have reached some agreement with her doctor on what kinds of emergencies he will see in the office, his **criteria** for determining whether it is an emergency, and what steps the assistant should take. Until you have had a chance to discuss this with your doctor here are some questions you might ask:

Is there bleeding?
Where is the blood coming from?
What is the patient's temperature?
Are there chills?
Is there nausea or vomiting?
If there is pain, is it steady or **intermittent**?
Is it severe? sharp? dull?
How long have the symptoms been present?

The application of first aid and emergency care for cases that present in the office is discussed in Chapter 33. Here we are concerned mainly with the telephone caller who reports an emergency and requests to be seen.

ACUTELY ILL PATIENTS. Patients can't always give advance notice of when they will need a doctor. There is a fine line that can be drawn between an emergency patient and the acutely ill patient, but the latter should be seen as soon as possible. At the very least, let the physician decide whether the patient should be seen immediately or whether he can safely wait. The 15- to 20-minute breather time you saved in the middle of the morning and afternoon may save your schedule.

PHYSICIAN REFERRALS. If another physician telephones and requests that a patient be seen by your doctor today, this is another exception you will have to make. Most physicians recognize the importance of keeping a schedule and will not be inconsiderate in this respect (you'll soon learn to recognize the few who are).

FAILED APPOINTMENTS

Some patients are forgetful about appointments. If you detect this tendency in a patient, form the habit of telephoning him the day before his appointment to remind him, or send a postcard timed to arrive a day or two in advance of his appointment. If your office consistently runs behind schedule, with patients being kept waiting for an hour or two, the patient whose own time is well planned may simply decide he doesn't have time today to come and sit in your office. Perhaps you gave him an appointment at a time that really was not agreeable to him. Or if you have been pressing a patient for payment he may stay away because he is unable to pay on that day. Try to determine the reason for failed appointments and do what you can to remedy it. Anyone can forget an appointment once, but if broken appointments occur frequently, you will be wise to reexamine your appointment system to see where the problem lies.

A busy practice must have a very specific policy on appointment "no-shows" and enforce it effectively. Michael Silver, Practice Management Consultant of Williamsville, New York, makes these suggestions in *Physician's Management* October, 1978.

> The first time a patient fails to show, note the fact on the medical record or ledger card. The second time this happens, you'll have a warning, and if the patient is more than a half hour late, call his or her home. The third time a patient fails to show without good reason, I suggest dropping the patient by using the customary methods that avoid legal problems.
>
> Incidentally, a patient with a major appointment — physical exams, counseling or the like — should be reminded by phone 24 to 48 hours before the appointment.

Legally a patient may be charged for an uncanceled appointment which he has not kept if it can be shown that this time was not used for another patient. However, few doctors attempt to collect for such occasions. The risk of poor public relations such a procedure engenders is too great; it generally results in a lost patient. Some other way must be found to handle failed appointments if they become a problem.

A notation should be made in the patient's record if an appointment is not kept and the patient is seriously ill. The doctor should also be told of this unkept appointment. This may be a legal consideration at some later date. In some cases it may be necessary for the doctor or the assistant to call and remind the patient that an unkept appointment may have serious results on the patient's health.

HANDLING CANCELLATIONS AND DELAYS

WHEN THE PATIENT CANCELS. If the patient cancels an appointment on a day that is heavily booked and you're already behind schedule, you'll probably just feel grateful. But suppose it's a fairly light day and you don't want to let that time be wasted. If you've formed the habit of keeping a list of patients with advance appointments who wanted to come in sooner, get busy on the telephone and try to get one of them in to fill that available time.

WHEN THE DOCTOR IS DELAYED. Inevitably, there are days when the doctor is delayed in reaching the office. If you have advance notice of this you can start calling those patients with early appointments and suggest they come later. If some have already arrived before you learn of the delay, you will have to explain that an emergency has prevented the doctor from getting in. You must show concern for the patient, but avoid being over-apologetic. This would imply some degree of guilt feeling. Most patients realize that a doctor has certain priorities, and that the patient who is able to be in the office may be inconvenienced but it is not a life-and-death matter. If this kind of situation occurs frequently, though, you may have to devise a different scheduling system or have a talk with your doctor about it.

WHEN THE DOCTOR IS CALLED OUT ON EMERGENCIES. All physicians are conscious of their responsibilities for responding to medical emergencies. Most patients will be sympathetic to such occurrences if the assistant will take time to explain what has happened. You may say something like this: "Dr. Wright has been called away to answer an emergency. He asked me to tell you he is very sorry to keep you waiting. He will be gone at least an hour. Do you wish to wait? If it is inconvenient, I'll be glad to give you another appointment that will be more convenient. Or perhaps you'd like to have some coffee or do some shopping and return in an hour."

In the meantime, head off patients scheduled for a later hour. In many offices, especially those of obstetricians, surgeons, and general practitioners, it is sometimes necessary to cancel a whole day's appointments. For this reason it is particularly important that you have the telephone number of each patient available so that you can cancel the appointment and make a new one. If it is at all possible, cancel appointments before the patients arrive in the office to find that the doctor is not in.

THE DOCTOR IS ILL OR IS CALLED OUT OF TOWN. Although it comes as a shock to most patients, physicians do get ill, too. The patients who are scheduled to be seen during the course of the doctor's expected absence must be informed of this. They need not be told the nature of his illness. It is customary to provide the patient with the name of another physician, or possibly a choice of several, who will take care of the doctor's patients during his absence. The physician may be called out of town for personal or professional reasons, and his appointments will have to be canceled.

MAKING THE APPOINTMENT

Many return appointments are arranged while a patient is in the office. The patient's first appointment, though, was probably made by telephone. Pleasantness on the part of the assistant who sets up the appointment is extremely important, whether the encounter is in person or by telephone.

IN PERSON. As the patient is leaving the office, the physician will probably ask him to stop by the desk and make his next appointment. While you reach for your pencil and the appointment book, *look* at the patient and say something like this: "Will next Thursday, the 8th, at 10:00 be satisfactory?" Avoid asking the question, "When would you like to come in?" Chances are this will only open up a debate and the patient will finally decide on a time that you don't have available anyway. Write his name in the book, in pencil, followed by his telephone number, and hand the patient a completed appointment card (after you have double checked the date and time with your book), along with your best smile.

BY TELEPHONE. It is as important for the assistant to express pleasantness and her desire to be helpful when she uses the telephone as it is when she meets patients face to face. This is particularly essential in the arranging of appointments, since it is often the manner in which the booking is made rather than the actual time of appointment which is important to the patient.

Study the principles of telephone technique as set forth in Chapter 8, Effective Telephone Practices. Be especially considerate if you must refuse an appointment for the time requested. Explain why and offer a substitute time and date. Comply with the patient's desires as much as possible and do not show impatience if a few patients are not understanding of the problems involved in scheduling appointments. Most people do appreciate the need for a well-managed office and are willing to cooperate. End the conversation pleasantly with something like this: "Thank you for calling, Mrs. Albright. Dr. Wright will see you next Wednesday, the 18th, at 2:30. Goodbye." This little courtesy adds to the patient's feeling of esteem, along with reinforcing the time of the appointment. While you are saying this, you should be rechecking your appointment page to be certain you have written it in the right time slot on the right day.

APPOINTMENTS FOR NEW PATIENTS. Arranging the first appointment for a new patient requires a bit more time and attention to detail. Check carefully the correct spelling of the name by repeating or spelling it back. Obtain the address, the telephone number where the patient can be reached, the patient's age, and the name of the referring doctor or individual. If possible, determine the nature of the visit so that the proper amount of time can be allotted on the appointment book.

If another physician has referred the patient, the assistant may need to call his office and obtain additional information for her employer. This information should be typed and given to the doctor in advance of the patient's arrival.

SPECIAL PROBLEMS. Probably every doctor has a few patients who are habitually late for appointments. This seems to be a problem for which no cure has yet been found; consequently, you must find a way of booking this patient without disrupting your entire schedule. One way of handling this is to book the patient as the last appointment of the day. Then if closing time arrives before he does, you need feel no obligation to wait for him. Some assistants simply tell the patient to come in a half hour earlier than the time they actually write in the book. The point to remember is

DAY: MON 8/1 · TUES 8/2 · WED 8/3 · THUR 8/4 · FRI 8/5 · SAT 8/6

Time	DR. BLACK	DR WHITE	DR. GREEN
9:00	TOM JONES		ELLY ADAMS ↓
9:15		MARY BANKS	
9:45	CHARLES THOMAS		
10:15	RITA LOPES ↓		
10:30		PETER GAINS	DORIS LONG
10:45		JEFF BARTS	
11:00			MIKE VANS
1:30		BONNIE REED	
2:00	SUSAN PIPP ↓	KATE FOGG	MARK McCALL
2:30		JOHN MOSBY ↓	

FIGURE 6–1 An office appointment schedule.

that you must learn to work around this patient, with the realization that in all likelihood he is not going to change.

When a former patient returns after a lengthy absence, the medical assistant should recheck the address, telephone number, insurance and employment information. If the appointment is made by telephone, be sure to ask for the patient's telephone number. You may need to call him, and you cannot safely assume that he still has the same number. You should also inquire into the nature of the current complaint.

MECHANICS OF THE APPOINTMENT BOOK

Use a pencil for making entries in the appointment book. Trying to change an entry made in ink is difficult and messy. At the end of the day the names may be written over in ink for a permanent record, if desired (Fig. 6–1).

Always write the patient's name *in full,* last name first, together with the reason for the appointment, *immediately*. DO NOT TRUST TO MEMORY. Be sure to cross off sufficient time for the appointment. It's a good idea to write the patient's telephone number after every entry in the appointment book. You may have to cancel or rearrange that day's schedule in a hurry, and many precious minutes can be saved if you don't have to look up each patient's telephone number.

Sometimes changes must be made in the appointment schedule. For instance, the patient who has a 3 PM appointment next Monday calls and asks to have this changed to one week later. You find an opening at 3 PM on the following Monday and write in the patient's name, but in your haste you fail to cross out the first appointment. Someone else looking at the appointment book (or possibly even yourself a couple of days later) will either expect the patient on both days or be unable to determine *which* day she is expected. Avoid this embarrassing situation by making it a habit to cross out or erase the first appointment *before* writing in the new one.

You may have a patient who requires a series of appointments, say at weekly intervals. Try to set up the appointments on the same day of each week, at the same time of day if possible. This considerably reduces the risk of a forgotten appointment. A calendar that shows the dates several months in advance at a glance is useful to have on or near the appointment desk.

At the end of each day, type a daily schedule listing the appointments for the following day, showing each patient's name and reason for visit, to place on the doctor's desk. If changes occur during the day, be sure to correct the daily schedule sheet as well as your appointment book.

APPOINTMENT CARDS AND REMINDERS

Most offices use appointment cards to remind patients of appointments, as well as to eliminate misunderstandings about dates and times. There are many styles of such cards.

Make a habit of reaching for an appointment card while making an entry in the appointment book. After you have written the date and time on the appointment card, double check with the book to see that the entries agree. Some offices mail cards to patients who have made appointments several weeks in advance. Patients who telephone for appointments also can be sent reminder cards.

Some patients like to be sent reminders of when they are to return to see the doctor. A simple way of handling this is to have a supply of postal cards on hand; while he is still in the office, have the patient write his name and address on one; then file it in your **tickler** under the date it is to be mailed.

APPOINTMENTS OUTSIDE THE OFFICE

There are other appointments that the assistant will make and which will appear on the appointment book, such as scheduled surgery at the hospital, consultations at the hospital or at another physician's office, house calls at extended care facilities or in the home. The doctor must have time to get from one place to another, so be sure to allow for traveling time when arranging these appointments.

SCHEDULING SURGERIES. You may be responsible for scheduling surgeries. In most hospitals you should call the secretary in surgery *first* when your doctor plans an operation. Give the surgical secretary the date and time the doctor prefers, the type of surgery to be performed, and the approximate time he will require. After the date and hour have been established, give the patient's full name, sex, age, and telephone number; also any special requests the doctor may have, such as the amount of blood to have available. Be sure you have all this information at hand before placing the call. It may be the responsibility of the assistant to arrange for the surgical assistant, the anesthesiologist, and the bed reservation.

Procedures vary in different areas and different hospitals, but the assistant will soon learn how her doctor's surgeries are to be handled. Some hospitals request the patient to complete a preadmittance form so that all records can be processed before the patient is admitted. Be sure the patient receives adequate admitting instructions.

HOUSE CALLS. If your doctor regularly makes house calls you probably set aside a special block of time for this on your appointment schedule. If it's only an occasional event, though, be sure to check with the doctor before committing him to make the call. He may decide after learning all the details that the patient can come into the office, or that the patient should go to the hospital. In speaking with the patient be sure to get all the pertinent details — name and address of patient, telephone number, best way to reach the home, nearest cross street, and name of person making the request. Again, traveling time must be allowed for.

OUTSIDE APPOINTMENTS FOR PATIENTS. Your doctor may ask you to arrange laboratory or x-ray appointments for patients. Before calling the laboratory or x-ray facility, determine from the physician the exact procedure he wants done, whether expediency is a factor, and whether he wants a **stat report**. Also ask the patient if there is any time he *cannot* have the procedure done. With this information before you, you can set up the appointment with confidence. When you inform the patient of the time, you can also give him any special instructions that may be necessary. Then be sure to note these arrangements on the patient's chart, and place a follow up reminder on your tickler or desk calendar.

PATIENTS WITHOUT APPOINTMENTS

The assistant often is faced with the question: What shall I do about patients who arrive without an appointment? There are a number of suggested procedures, but the policy in your office must be agreed upon by the doctor and then carried out by the assistant.

If the patient requires immediate attention, he must be fitted into the schedule somehow. If his case does not need immediate care, he can be given a short visit with the doctor and asked to schedule an appointment at a time when the doctor can devote more attention to his complaints.

The assistant should always make it clear, even when sending patients without appointments in to see the doctor, that the office runs on an appointment basis. She can say, for example:

"The doctor will be able to see you, but we would appreciate it very much if you would make an appointment for your next visit." Or,

"The doctor can see you now. I'm sorry you had to wait so long. Perhaps it would be possible for you to make an appointment the next time."

Patients should be told as gently as possible that appointments save not only the doctor's time but theirs as well. Emphasize to these patients that the doctor will be able to give them his full attention and more time on the next visit if an advance appointment is made.

It is important to remember one thing, however. Don't play favorites in sending patients in to see the doctor. If you're "found out" by the other waiting patients, their esteem for the doctor, as well as for you, will decline rapidly.

OTHER CALLERS

PHYSICIANS. When another physician calls at your doctor's office, he should be ushered in to see the doctor as soon as possible. He should not be kept waiting, regardless of your previous appointment schedule. If the physician arrives when your doctor is seeing a patient, explain the situation and, if possible, take him into an inside room so that the doctor can see him as soon as he is finished with the patient. If this is not convenient for the visiting doctor, make arrangements for him to see the doctor at an acceptable time. When another doctor has been ushered into an inside room or is waiting in the reception room, tell your employer at once. The visits of other physicians are usually brief, since they have heavy schedules of their own to maintain.

PHARMACEUTICAL REPRESENTATIVES. Also known as "detail persons," representatives from leading **pharmaceutical** houses are frequent visitors to physicians' offices and are generally welcomed by the doctor if his schedule permits. They are well trained and bring the doctor valuable information on new drugs. The assistant is often able to screen such visitors and turn away those who would have nothing to offer her employer. If the assistant does not know the caller, she may ask for his card, then check with the doctor and let him decide whether or not he wishes to see the caller.

If the doctor is in a specialty practice or limits his callers to a few selected pharmaceutical houses, the medical assistant can ask him to help her prepare a list of the representatives whom he will see, time permitting. Then, when a detail person arrives at the office, she can quickly tell, by consulting her list, whether she should try to work him in. The detail person who knows he is not on the list for a particular doctor will also appreciate the saving in time for him. Most representatives say they would rather be told outright if the doctor does not wish to see them than to be given some evasive reply.

The pharmaceutical representative is willing to wait patiently a long while for just a brief visit with the doctor. The assistant can tell him whether or not the doctor can see him that day, give him an idea of how long he will have to wait, or suggest a later time at which he can return. He can then make his own decision as to whether he wishes to wait or return later. The pharmaceutical representative is usually quite understanding and cooperative. The assistant should in turn treat him with courtesy and give him as much cooperation as possible. In some cases, she herself can accept the literature or materials for the doctor and make sure he receives it.

SALESPERSONS. Salespersons from medical and surgical supply houses call regularly at physicians' offices. Sometimes they will want to see the doctor, but if the assistant is in charge of ordering supplies she may be able to handle this herself. Unwelcome salespersons sometimes present a problem in the professional office. If the physician does not wish to see such a caller, the assistant must firmly but tactfully send him away. She can suggest to such callers that they leave their literature and cards for the doctor to study and say that the doctor will contact them if he desires further information. Persistent callers can be dispatched with alacrity if they ignore a polite "no" merely by suggesting that perhaps they would like to schedule an appointment — at the doctor's customary fee!

MISCELLANEOUS. From time to time, other callers appear in the doctor's office. Some are civic leaders seeking the doctor's aid in community projects. Others may be church leaders, insurance representatives, solicitors for fund drives, and so forth. Most doctors inform their assistants of their general policy in regard to seeing such callers. Check with your employer in advance on procedure to follow in such instances.

Civic leaders should be treated with courtesy and consideration when they telephone or enter the office. Every doctor has a real responsibility to take an active part in community affairs. However, no doctor can participate in *all* activities. Often, he delegates to his assistant the responsibility for accepting or refusing such community appointments for him. In this event, she must use discretion and exercise complete tact and courtesy. Disgruntled community leaders who are turned away with a terse refusal do not help create good medical public relations. If it is necessary to refuse such callers, be sure to explain that the doctor would be happy to cooperate but that he is already participating in such community projects as the Boy Scouts, Kiwanis, and the Health Council, and his schedule does not permit him to accept additional responsibilities. The same rule regarding the exercise of tact, courtesy, and consideration should always apply to every caller in a doctor's office.

References

American Medical Association: *Winning Ways with Patients.* Chicago, American Medical Association, 1979.
Beck, Leif C.: *The Physician's Office.* Princeton, NJ, Excerpta Medica, 1977.
Colwell Company, 275 Kenyon Road, Champaign, IL 61820.
Patient Care Systems, 16 Thorndal Circle, Darien, CT 06820.
VISIrecord Systems, 160 Gold Star Boulevard, Worcester, MA 01606.

CHAPTER OUTLINE

First Impressions
- The Assistant
- The Reception Room

Before the Patient Arrives
Enter the Patient
Patient Flow
Soothe the Waiting Patient
Problem Patients
- The Talker
- Children
- The Angry Patient
- The Patient's Relatives

Friendly Farewell

BEHAVIORAL OBJECTIVES

The medical office assistant should be able to:

- **Maintain professional appearance and manner.**
- **Assist in maintaining appearance of reception area.**
- **Replenish supplies as necessary.**
- **Annotate daily schedule.**
- **Scrutinize patient charts for current entries.**
- **Greet arriving patients.**
- **Manage patient flow effectively.**
- **Escort patients to examining room.**
- **Direct smooth operation of an appointment schedule.**
- **Control interpersonal relations in the reception area.**

7

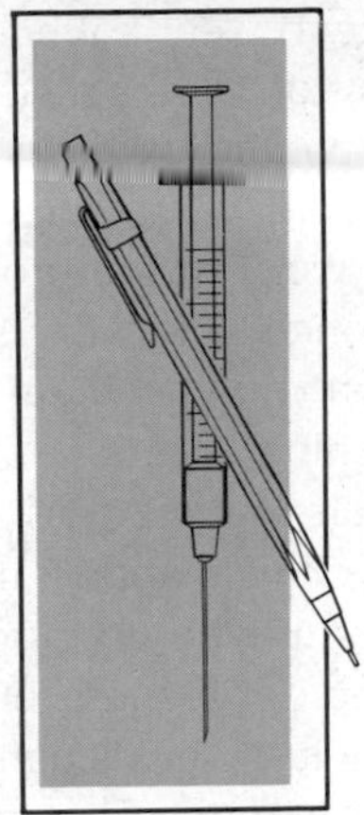

YOUR ROLE AS RECEPTIONIST

Appearances and first impressions mean a great deal in any situation. This is especially true in the physician's office, where an atmosphere of cleanliness and order must prevail. The kind of impression that the doctor's assistant makes upon his patients often colors their impressions about the doctor himself or his office. The patient who feels friendly toward the assistant will probably feel friendly toward the doctor.

FIRST IMPRESSIONS

THE ASSISTANT. A neat, attractive assistant has a good **psychologic** effect upon patients. The three most essential aspects of an attractive appearance are good health, good grooming, and good taste.

Good health means getting plenty of sleep, eating balanced meals, and getting sufficient exercise to keep fit. No crash diets or all-night orgies for the medical assistant, just a sensible **regimen** of healthful living and a regular checkup at least once each year.

The medical assistant usually wears a uniform. The uniform not only gives a professional look but identifies the assistant as a member of the team. Uniforms are no longer limited to the traditional white. Modern fabrics and styling in uniforms have made it possible for the office assistant to be attractive, as well as practical. The assistant's "uniform" may be a pantsuit, in white or color, or perhaps with contrasting top and pant; a two-piece dress-type uniform in white or color, or an attractive design in the traditional white dress uniform. Some physicians, particularly pediatricians, often prefer that their assistants wear pastels. Today's fabrics are so easy to care for, there should be no temptation to wear a uniform a second day without laundering. Even spills and spots that occur during the course of the working day can usually be washed out immediately.

Whatever style of uniform the assistant chooses, it should be one that is personally becoming, worn over appropriate undergarments and without extraneous ornamentation. Keep jewelry to a minimum, only an engagement ring, wedding band, and professional pin — no fluffy handkerchiefs or other adornments.

If there is more than one assistant in the office, name pins worn by everyone in the office help the patient to identify each assistant by name. There are commercial organizations that sell so-called professional pins for medical assistants and grant meaningless certificates of competence. It is best to check with your medical society or the American Medical Association before investing in such items. At present the American Association of Medical Assistants is the only professionally recognized group of medical assistants (see Chapter 1).

Some medical office assistants like to wear a white cap. Unless an assistant is a registered nurse or is entitled by graduation from a medical assisting school to wear a special assistant's cap, she should not violate professional etiquette by doing so.

The shoes the assistant wears should be appropriate for a uniform, spotlessly clean, and comfortable! White shoes worn in the professional office must be *kept* white by daily cleaning. A damp sponge and Ivory soap will take care of quick cleanups during the working day; when you give them a thorough cleaning at night, don't forget that shoestrings need cleaning, too, if you wear a tie shoe.

In some offices the physician prefers that his assistant not wear a uniform. Some psychiatrists, for example, feel that the clinical appearance of a uniform may have an adverse effect upon patients. The assistant who does not wear a uniform should still follow the dictates of good taste and appropriateness in choosing an office wardrobe. The high style dress that looked great at last week's party will do nothing to enhance the appearance of the medical assistant at work. The garments worn on the job must be comfortable, becoming, allow easy movement, and still look good at the end of a busy day.

The medical assistant's makeup should be carefully selected and applied. There's no need for the assistant to appear drab, but harsh or exaggerated makeup is definitely out of place in the professional office. Subtle eye makeup and discreet shades of nail polish enhance the assistant's appearance; the boldly artificial detracts. The hair should be clean, neatly styled, and off the collar, never falling untidily around the shoulders.

Good grooming is little more than attention to the details of personal appearance. Personal cleanliness, which includes the daily bath, a good deodorant, and **oral hygiene,** is vital. The assistant who is well groomed looks her best from top to toe: her shoes are polished; stockings are of neutral shade or white; her hemline is even; the costume is well chosen and in good condition; nails are clean; makeup is carefully applied; and her hair is attractively arranged. The personal drawer in her desk should hold extra hose, a clothes brush, spot remover, and a small mirror for checking her appearance occasionally. The assistant who will take that extra few minutes each day to attend to the details of her appearance will make a better impression upon the people with whom she comes in contact.

THE RECEPTION ROOM. Take an objective look around the reception room in your doctor's office every once in a while. Could it use a little brightening or freshening up? Try to look at it as if you were seeing it for the first time. The reception room is just that — a place to receive patients. It should be planned for the patient's comfort, made as attractive and cheerful as possible, then kept tidy and clean (Fig. 7–1).

Elaborate furnishings, expensive carpeting or draperies are not necessary to achieve the desired effect. Fresh harmonious colors and cleanliness are the basis of an attractive room. Add comfortable furniture, adequate to accommodate the peak load of patients seen each day, and arrange it in conversational groupings. Individual chairs are usually best. People will sometimes stand rather than sit next to a stranger on a sofa. Provide good lighting, ventilation, and a regulated temperature for additional comfort, and you have the essentials of an attractive reception room that tells the patient you care. A place to hang coats, rainwear, and umbrellas will help reduce reception room clutter. The overall effect should be bright and cheerful, or subdued and restful, but never gaudy or depressing.

Plants, pictures, travel posters, and bulletin board displays can add charm and individuality to a reception room. Indoor plants are suitable but fresh flowers may cause **allergic reactions.** Artificial flower arrangements and plants are now so attractive and realistic it seems impractical to spend time in the care of fresh ones. In some areas, a rental service will provide new flower arrangements at regular intervals. One word of caution is in order — don't allow those artificial arrangements to collect dust. Either wipe them off regularly or take time to "dunk" them occasionally.

Most physicians' offices are well supplied with recent magazines in washable plastic covers. Many patients, especially women, like to clip or copy recipes from magazines. Try placing an exotic cookbook or two in the reception area (well identified with your doctor's name) and be sure you have some 3 by 5 cards handy. Another popular diversion is the pictorial travel book. Patients seem to enjoy looking at pictures rather than at something that requires concentrated reading. The reception room, incidentally, is not the proper place for the professional journals your doctor receives.

Some doctors place writing desks and writing paper in the room for the convenience of patients; others play restful music over a concealed speaker. In practices with a large number of children as patients, a children's corner, equipped with small-scale furniture and some playthings, is a good idea. It helps keep youngsters occupied who might otherwise get into mischief. Toys should be easily cleanable; plastic washable ones are especially good. Be scrupulously careful that the toy has no sharp corners that could injure a child or small parts that could be swallowed. Also, in selecting toys, make sure they will not stimulate the child to make loud noises or create an uproar in the office. And no rubber balls.

Even such additions as a television set, a lighted aquarium, or an educational

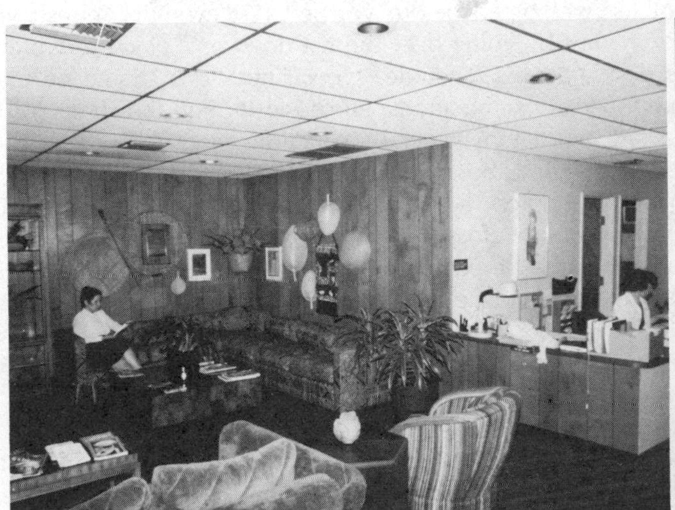

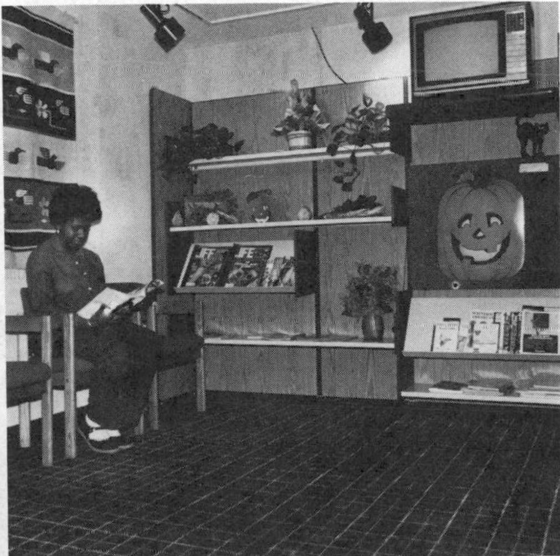

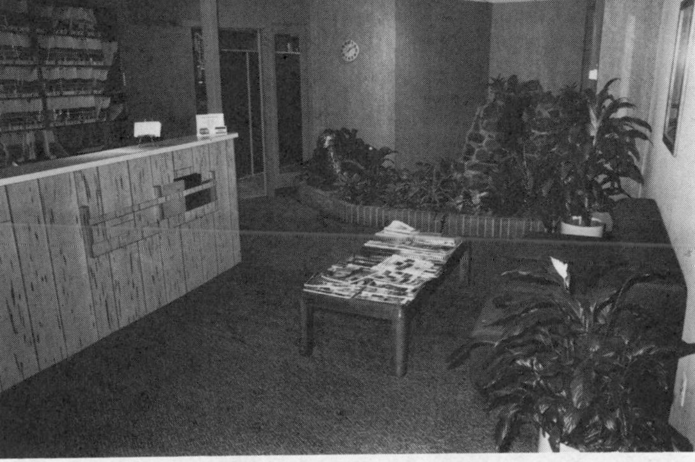

FIGURE 7–1 Three examples of reception room decor. (Upper righthand figure courtesy of Ferris State College, Michigan.)

display of some sort enhance the attractiveness and individuality of the "front door to the doctor's practice."

The assistant is at least partly responsible for the appearance of the reception room. She sometimes has to exert her efforts or enlist the help of the doctor's wife to make reception room improvements that add to the patient's comfort and enjoyment. It is her responsibility to make sure that the room remains neat and orderly throughout the day. A quick check at intervals during the day and a minute or two devoted to putting the room back in order help keep it looking its best.

If the assistant's desk is in the reception room or in open view of the patients, she should keep it free of clutter. In particular, patients' charts or financial cards should not be in sight. Personal articles, coffee cups, and ashtrays should not be on the receptionist's desk.

BEFORE THE PATIENT ARRIVES

When the patients start arriving, you want to have everything ready for the day so that you and the doctor can give undivided attention to their needs. If the previous day was a busy one, the supplies in the treatment rooms may have been **depleted** and instruments may need sterilizing. Your doctor may have had to return to the office to care for a patient during the evening. Check the rooms to make certain that everything is clean, the cabinets well stocked, and everything ready for the first patient of the day. If reserve supplies are kept in another room, you may wish to obtain a hand basket or a cart on wheels so that everything can be carried at one time rather than having to make numerous trips to and fro.

Supplies at your desk should also be checked periodically. Stationery, appointments cards, charge slips, sharpened pencils, and any items you are likely to use during the day should be on hand to avoid needless trips to the supply closet.

If the appointment list was typed before you left last evening, refresh your memory of the patients' names by going over the list now, and place a duplicate copy on your doctor's desk. On this schedule, special notations should be made concerning new patients, special examinations, and so forth. Pull the charts for the patients to be seen that day, noting any special instructions, and place them in the order they are expected to be seen. Laboratory reports, x-ray readings, and any other data concerning the patient's records should also be placed with the history. The assistant should check each history before the physician sees it to make certain that all information has been correctly entered and is up to date. The physician may want the charts placed on his desk, or he may expect the assistant to hand the chart to him as the patient arrives.

This advance preparation will make your day smoother and will contribute toward a more relaxed atmosphere for all who enter.

ENTER THE PATIENT

Every patient has a right to expect courteous treatment in the doctor's office. No matter what his economic status, each individual who enters the reception room should receive a cordial, friendly greeting.

The assistant can do a great deal to give each patient reassurance and a feeling of importance by the manner in which she receives him. Contrast the closed opaque window over a sign that reads "Ring Bell and Be Seated" with the friendly greeting of the assistant: "Good morning, Mr. Barker. I see you are right on time! The doctor will see you in just a few minutes. Won't you sit down? There are some new magazines on the table."

Ideally, the assistant's desk is placed so that she can see all visitors who come into the office. If there is only one assistant, it is sometimes impossible for her to be on hand to welcome personally each new caller. In this event some announcement system must be worked out. The patient who enters an empty reception room doesn't know whether to sit down or to try to announce his presence in some way. Sometimes a register is placed in the reception room with a sign above it reading: "Please sign the register when you arrive. Doctor will see you shortly." This is a makeshift arrangement, as is the bell advising the patient to ring and be seated. Either of these arrangements is better than no reception at all, but cannot compare with the personal greeting of the assistant.

The importance of the personal touch in receiving patients should not be overlooked. A good receptionist cultivates the habit of greeting each patient in a friendly, self-assured manner, yet guards against appearing too **effusive,** since this sometimes implies insincerity or overfamiliarity. She can introduce herself if the patient is new or greet him with friendliness, calling him by name, if he is a patient she has met before. She tries to become acquainted with each patient by name and to remember something personal about each one, so that on his return visit she can inquire about his garden or the activities of his children. She is careful to learn how to pronounce each patient's name correctly, since incorrect pronunciations offend and irritate people. If the name is unusual it is a good idea to write the **phonetic** spelling on the history card. This may save embarrassment at future visits.

It isn't wise to appear over-curious about patients' personal lives, but each individual appreciates the interest of the doctor and his staff in his family, hobbies, or work. Sometimes the assistant can jot down key words on the patient's history card that provide her and the doctor with subjects for future conversations. She can get other valuable "conversation pieces" from the pages of the local newspaper.

PATIENT FLOW

The patient's first question, once he has been received, almost always is "When can I see the doctor?" The assistant should get the patient in to see the doctor as near his appointment time as possible or explain why he must wait. It is her responsibility to convey both her own and the doctor's concern if there will be a delay. Consideration for the patient's time is extremely important.

Most experts agree that in a well-managed, busy office there are never more than three to five patients in the reception room. When long waits in the doctor's office are eliminated, one of the major sources of complaints by the public about doctors is also eliminated. "Too long a wait in the doctor's office" is one of the most frequently heard condemnations of the medical profession. When a patient complains about medical fees or care he may really be complaining about the long wait or discourteous service.

The claim that a crowded waiting room is an indication of a doctor's popularity may not be true. It may reveal, instead, that the doctor or his assistant is inefficient in scheduling patients. In some rare instances it is a haughty disregard for the patient. Patients don't seem to mind waiting 20 to 30 minutes to see the doctor, but they do consider a wait of more than a half hour excessive.

The experienced medical assistant will keep the appointment schedule operating smoothly by tidying each examination room immediately and moving the next patient in so that the doctor need have no idle moments waiting for a patient to be prepared (Fig. 7–2). It is very inconsiderate, however, to place a patient in an examining room just to get him out of the reception area, and then keep him waiting a long time. Avoid placing a patient on a table, draped in an uncomfortable position, only to be "forgotten" for an hour while the doctor is doing something else. If you think there might be some delay, suggest that the patient take along a magazine or something to occupy his time during the additional wait. Avoid an assembly line atmosphere.

When you do direct a patient to an examining room, take him at least to the door if you can. If the patient is to disrobe, be specific about how much clothing to remove and where to hang it.

You may have to rescue your doctor sometimes from an over-talkative patient. This should be done with the greatest possible tact, by reminding the doctor that his "3 o'clock appointment is here now" or his "next patient must leave in half an hour to meet another appointment." Once you learn the patients who take extra time, then you can book them for the end of the day or simply allow more time for them.

SOOTHE THE WAITING PATIENT

When prolonged waiting is unavoidable, the assistant can help the patients pass the time as pleasantly as possible. This is something of a challenge since most people do not like to wait. Businessmen, for example, who are in the habit of making the most of their time, are particularly resentful at what may appear to them to be inefficient scheduling of appointments.

The assistant can often suggest a particularly good story or article in a magazine to a patient who wants to read. She sometimes can chat briefly with a restless patient. It should, however, be the patient's decision in regard to whether or not he wants to talk. Select conversational subjects that interest the patient — his hobbies, family, business, profession, or recreational interests — and steer clear of controversial subjects such as religion and politics.

The assistant can sometimes increase patients' esteem for the physician by mentioning his hobby or telling about his forthcoming trip to a medical meeting to present a scientific paper. She should also be well versed on such subjects as health insurance, new medical discoveries, local health agencies, and other topics pertaining to medical care which patients may raise during conversation. She can often distribute literature on these subjects from medical organizations to answer patients' questions. Active members of medical assistants' groups keep well informed on such subjects by attending local meetings regularly.

Some personal attention, such as offering a drink of water, presentation of a new magazine, or a brief conversation, sometimes will quiet a patient who is becoming visibly irritated at waiting. If possible, he should be taken into an inner office. Usually one patient can be placed in an examining room and another in a treatment room, while the doctor talks to a third in his office.

Many patients are fearful and tense, but a good assistant can often put them in a better frame of mind merely by a friendly smile and show of concern.

PROBLEM PATIENTS

THE TALKER. There are certain "problem patients" in any professional office. The talker, for example, takes up far more of the doctor's time than is justified. An alert assistant can usually spot these individuals during her initial conversation with them. She can check such a patient's card with a symbol to alert the doctor. A prearranged agreement to buzz the doctor on the **intercom** at the end of the appointment time, telling him his next patient has arrived, gives him an opportunity to conclude the interview.

CHILDREN. Children sometimes present special management problems. It is often advisable for young patients to come into the treatment room without their parents. This, of course, should be at the discretion of the physician.

While this technique of separating children from their parents to treat their needs is not always feasible in every professional office, it sometimes can be applied with great success. In some offices a token of the doctor's friendship, such as a trinket or toy, is given the child at the completion of the visit.

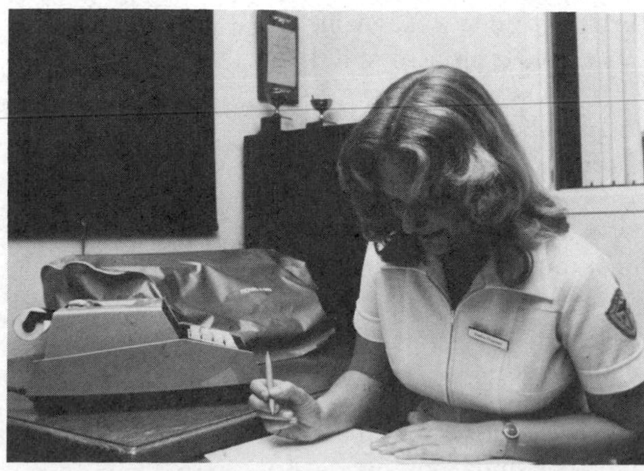

FIGURE 7–2 Medical assistant working on patient accounts. (Courtesy of Long Beach City College, Long Beach, California.)

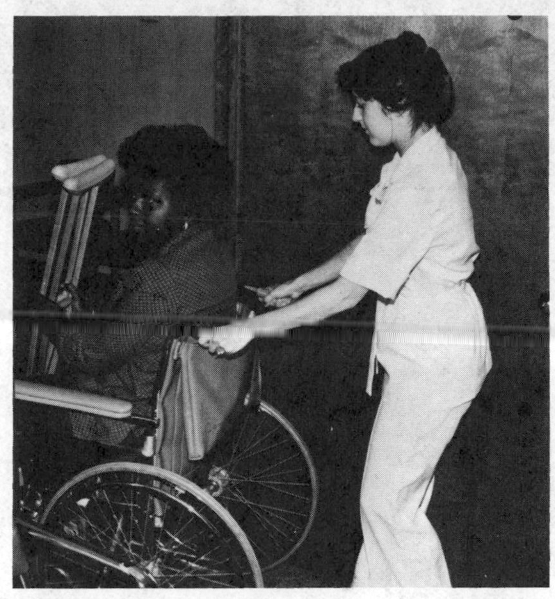

FIGURE 7–3 The medical office assistant walks a departing patient to the door. (Courtesy of Ferris State College, Michigan.)

7

THE ANGRY PATIENT. Every office assistant at some time is confronted with the angry patient. The anger may be simply a reflection of the patient's pain or his fear of what the doctor may discover on his examination. It is usually best to let him talk out his anger. A calm attitude on the part of the medical assistant, with a few remarks interjected in a low voice, will often quiet the patient. Under no circumstances should the assistant return the anger or become argumentative.

THE PATIENT'S RELATIVES. A patient will sometimes be accompanied by a relative or well-meaning friend who may become restless while waiting for the patient and attempt to discuss the patient's illness. The assistant should side-step any discussion of a patient's medical care, except by direction of the physician. She should also avoid a too-casual attitude, such as, "I'm sure there's nothing to worry about." A show of moderate concern, offering reassurance that "the patient is in good hands," will usually take care of the situation.

FRIENDLY FAREWELL

The assistant should be ready to take over the patient as soon as the physician has finished. She can assist the patient in dressing, if necessary, or show him to the rest room. Ask the patient whether he is to have another appointment and, if so, be sure the appointment time is arranged before the patient leaves the office.

If a patient seems hesitant to leave, there may be some problem still on his mind. A friendly offer on the part of the assistant to help or explain a problem will often relieve anxiety and save a telephone call later. The assistant can help convey the impression of friendliness by terminating the patient's visit with the same cordiality she would use with guests in her own home. If she has time, she can walk to the door with the patient (Fig. 7–3). She should make certain there are no unanswered questions. If the patient is returning for another visit, the assistant can say, "See you next week." If it is the patient's last visit, say something like "I certainly hope you'll be feeling fine from now on." The assistant may want to tell a patient on his last visit that he has been a fine patient and that it has been a pleasure to serve him. Whatever words of goodbye she chooses, each patient or caller should leave the doctor's office feeling that he or she has received top quality care and has been treated with friendliness and courtesy.

Reference

American Medical Association: *Winning Ways with Patients.* Chicago, American Medical Association, 1979.

CHAPTER OUTLINE

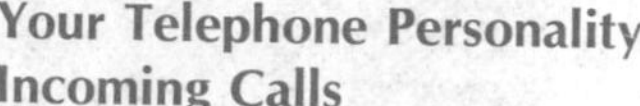

Your Telephone Personality
Incoming Calls
- Receiving Calls
- Summary of Office Telephone Rules
- The Telephone Message
- Incoming Calls the Assistant Can Handle
- Calls Requiring Transfer or Call Back
- Special Telephone Problems
- Routine but Troublesome Calls
- Telephone Answering Services

Outgoing Calls
- Using The Telephone Directory
- Organizing Telephone Numbers
- Pre-Planning the Call
- Placing the Call
- Calling Etiquette
- Long Distance Calls
- Wrong Numbers
- Conference Calls
- Special Equipment
- Telegraph Services

BEHAVIORAL OBJECTIVES

The medical office assistant should be able to:

- **Utilize the principles of good telephone etiquette.**
- **Receive, transmit, and record telephone messages.**
- **Recognize the kinds of telephone calls the assistant can appropriately handle.**
- **Recognize the kinds of calls requiring the attention of the physician.**
- **Describe available kinds of telephone answering services.**
- **Plan and place outgoing telephone calls.**
- **List the major features of special telephone equipment.**
- **List the classes of available telegrams and related services.**

8

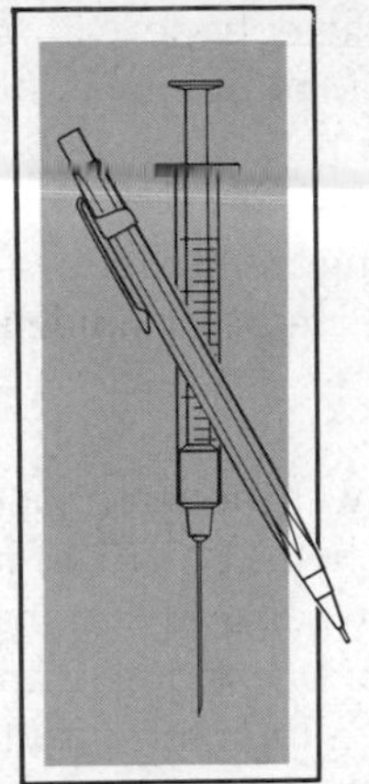

EFFECTIVE TELEPHONE PRACTICES

The telephone is a powerful public relations instrument. Its *proper* use can build a beginning medical practice; its *improper* use can do much to destroy a flourishing one. The physician's office without one or more telephones is difficult to imagine, and the assistant who regards the telephone as a nuisance has no place in the doctor's office.

To the seasoned medical assistant, the ringing telephone is not an unwelcome interruption — it is the lifeline of the office. A patient previously treated may be calling for an appointment or to seek advice; another may be reporting an emergency; a physician may be calling to make a referral; the laboratory may be reporting vital information regarding one of the doctor's patients; a new patient may be making his first contact.

The telephone responsibilities of the medical assistant CANNOT BE OVEREMPHASIZED.

YOUR TELEPHONE PERSONALITY

To a telephone caller, your voice constitutes your entire personality. He can't see you, your smile, or your facial expression. His impressions of you and the office you represent will be formed only from your voice. What impression *will* you create with your telephone personality? If your voice is warm and friendly, if it sounds confident, if your conversation is courteous and tactful, you will be practicing good public relations and creating a favorable impression with each telephone call you handle. Try to visualize the person to whom you are talking. A small mirror, placed near the telephone, will remind you to smile. Now pretend that each caller is a new patient meeting you for the first time.

Every caller should be made to feel that you have time to attend to his wishes, regardless of how tedious some telephone requests may be. If you are rushed when you pick up the receiver, wait a few seconds until you are able to answer graciously. The person calling does not know you were assisting the doctor or at work in the laboratory; he only infers from your impatient, breathless tone that you resent being bothered by his call.

The assistant should always remember that the office telephone is for business use only, not for personal use. If a friend calls, it is best to take down the number and graciously say that you will return the call in the evening from your own home. The privilege of monopolizing the office telephone with personal calls does not apply even during lunch hours. The lines of the doctor's office should be clear to receive emergency calls and other calls from patients.

INCOMING CALLS

You will be receiving many calls during the course of a single day. Each one deserves your most competent attention. Here are a few guidelines to follow in answering all telephone calls.

Receiving Calls

ANSWER PROMPTLY. Always answer the telephone promptly, on the first ring if possible. An answer on the first ring helps create an image of efficiency. If you are unable to complete the conversation when you first answer the telephone, you might say, "Will you please hold the line for one moment and I will be with you." Do not pick up the receiver and snap, "Just a minute!" or "Doctor's office, hold please!" When you return to the telephone, make certain you thank the caller for waiting. Of course you would not delay completing a call unless it were absolutely necessary.

HOLD THE INSTRUMENT CORRECTLY. Hold the handset around the middle, with the mouthpiece about one inch from the lips, and directly in front of the teeth. Never hold it under your chin. You can check the proper distance by taking your first two fingers and passing them through sideways in the space between your lips and the mouthpiece. If your fingers just squeeze through, your lips are the correct distance from the telephone and your voice will go over the wires as close to its natural tone as possible. Speak directly into the telephone immediately after removing it from the cradle. If you turn to face a window or another part of the room, make sure the telephone transmitter moves too, or your voice will be lost.

DEVELOP A PLEASING TELEPHONE VOICE. What are the qualities of a good telephone voice? And how do you cultivate good voice quality? Here are some tips from the Bell Telephone system:

(1) STAY ALERT. Give the impression you are wide-awake and alert, interested in the calling person. Let him know he has your full attention.

(2) BE PLEASANT. Build a pleasant, friendly image for you and your office. Be the "voice with a smile."

(3) TALK NATURALLY, BE YOURSELF. Use your own words and expressions. Avoid repetition of mechanical words or phrases. Do not use slang. Avoid the temptation to use those impressive medical terms you've recently learned.

(4) SPEAK DISTINCTLY. Clear, distinct **pronunciation** and **enunciation** are vital. Move the lips, tongue, and jaw freely. Talk directly into the transmitter. Never answer the telephone when you are eating or chewing gum.

(5) BE EXPRESSIVE. A well-modulated voice carries best. Use a normal tone of voice, neither too loud nor too soft. Talk at a moderate rate, neither too fast nor too slow. Vary your tone. It will bring out the meaning of sentences and add color and vitality to what you say.

To develop a good voice, your facial muscles must be trained. These muscles should not be tense, nor should they sag. Do not set your teeth or jaws. The lips should move freely. Proper breathing also contributes to a good voice and helps in enunciation.

Everyone should have the experience of hearing his own voice; it reveals immediately the importance of careful **diction**. Try putting your voice on tape and listening to a playback. Each word and each sound must be given individual attention in order to achieve clarity. Slurring your words or dropping your voice too much at the end of a sentence can place a strain on your listener. Try to avoid the habit of allowing "ers," "uhs," and long pauses in your conversation. Remember, though, it is seldom necessary to *raise* the pitch of your voice in order to be heard. If a person has trouble being heard, it is generally because he speaks too fast, does not enunciate clearly, or does not speak into the transmitter.

GUIDES TO GOOD DICTION

NUMERAL OR LETTER	SOUNDED AS	PRINCIPAL SOUNDS
0	oh	Round and long O
1	wun	Strong W and N
2	too	Strong T and long OO
3	th-r-ee	A single roll of the R and long EE
4	fo-er	Strong F, long O, and strong final R
5	fi-iv	I changing from long to short, strong V
6	siks	Strong S and KS
7	sev-en	Strong S and V, well-sounded EN
8	ate	Long A and strong T
9	ni-en	Strong N, long I, well-sounded EN
10	ten	Strong T and N
J	jay	Strong J and long AY
R	ahr	Strong R
M	em	Short E and strong M
W	dubble-yoo	Full value given to every syllable
F	ef	Short E and strong F

Do not over-accentuate; it causes you to sound artificial. Use a friendly natural style. Few words need to be spelled over the telephone if a person speaks slowly and clearly. Below are key words you can use when it is necessary to verify letters in spelling back over the telephone:

A as in Adams
B as in Boston
C as in Charles
D as in David
E as in Edward
F as in Frank
G as in George
H as in Henry
I as in Ida
J as in John
K as in Katie
L as in Lewis
M as in Mary
N as in Nellie
O as in Oliver
P as in Peter
Q as in Queen
R as in Robert
S as in Samuel
T as in Thomas
U as in Utah
V as in Victor
W as in William
X as in X-ray
Y as in Young
Z as in Zebra

A telephone conversation necessarily involves two persons. We put a great deal of stress upon rules for speaking, but we often neglect the importance of good listening. The same attention should be given a telephone conversation that would be given a face-to-face conversation. Concentration is not always easy; it must be practiced. It is annoying to a caller to have to repeat himself because the assistant did not listen closely to his original statement.

IDENTIFY YOURSELF. The telephone should never be answered with just "Hello." Your response should identify first the office, and then yourself. There are several variations of telephone greetings that can be used, which you will probably wish to discuss with the doctor, but your response might be something like this: "Dr. Black's office — Miss Anderson." If the doctor's surname is fairly common to your area, you may wish to use his given name also to provide further identification, saying, "Dr. Sherman Black's office — Miss Anderson."

The use of salutations in telephone identifications is optional. Sometimes the addition of "Good morning" or "Good afternoon" to the identification is awkward. A rising inflection or a questioning tone in your voice will indicate interest and a willingness to assist, and eliminate the need for an additional greeting.

If there are two doctors in the office, both names should be included in the identification. Say "Drs. Smith and Taylor," or "Drs. Taylor and Smith's office." Some names will not blend smoothly; then you must modify the identification so that it will be easy to say and easy to understand. Keep in mind the reason for answering the phone by using the doctor's name. You are telling the caller he has reached the correct number. If callers frequently ask you to repeat, you must analyze the failure to communicate and modify your response in some way. Some authorities suggest preceding the identification with the words "This is. . ." by saying "This is Dr. Black's office," theorizing that the first two words are probably lost on the listener, and he will only begin to hear you when you have reached ". . . . Dr. Black's office."

Answering an office telephone merely by repeating the telephone number is even less desirable than saying "Hello." The caller will invariably ask, "Is this Dr. Black's office?" Rarely can a person immediately recall the number he has just dialed. Time is wasted, the caller is psychologically rebuffed, and you have lost another opportunity to create a favorable impression of your office.

There are some legal regulations that apply to the manner of identification to use when answering the telephone of a medical corporation. If yours is a corporate practice, check with the physician's attorney for clarification.

When you have decided upon the greeting to be used, practice it until you can say it easily and smoothly without thinking about what you are saying.

IDENTIFY THE CALLER. If the caller does not identify himself, you must always ask to whom you are speaking. It is a good idea to repeat the name by using it in the conversation as soon as possible, *unless* there are other patients within the range of your voice and the caller's privacy should be respected.

OFFER ASSISTANCE. Always offer assistance, both in the tone of your voice and in your conversation. The phrase "May I help you?" or "How may I help you?" helps start the conversation and assures the caller you are both willing and capable of being of service.

SCREEN INCOMING CALLS. Most employers expect the assistant to **screen** all telephone calls. Good judgment in deciding whether or not to put calls through to the doctor comes only with experience.

Put through calls from other physicians at once. If your doctor is busy and cannot possibly come to the telephone, explain this briefly and politely and say that you will have him return the call the moment he is free. Make sure he does.

Most callers will ask, "Is the doctor in?" You should never answer the question with a simple "Yes" or "No" or respond with the question, "Who is calling, please?" If the doctor is *not* in, say so before asking the identity of the caller. Otherwise the person calling may suspect the doctor is simply not willing to talk to him.

If the doctor is not in the office, the rule of offering assistance still holds. You can say, "No, I am sorry, Dr. Black is not in. May I take a message?" or "No, I am sorry, but Dr. Black will be at the hospital most of the morning. May I ask him to return your call after 12 o'clock?"

If the doctor *is* in, and available for the telephone, a typical response would be, "Yes, Dr. Black is in; may I tell him who is calling, please?" If your doctor prefers to keep his calls to a minimum, you might say, "Yes, Dr. Black is here, but I'm not sure he's free to come to the phone. May I tell him who is calling, please?" That way, if it's someone he does not wish to speak with, you have given him an out.

If the doctor is with a patient, he probably will not wish to be disturbed for a routine call. In this case, you might say, "Yes, Dr. Black is in, but he is with a patient right now. May I help you?" or "Yes, Dr. Black is in but he is with a patient right now. Is there anything you want me to ask him?"

You must guard against being overprotective. A patient has a right to talk with his doctor; however, unless it is an emergency, he is probably willing to do so at the doctor's convenience. Don't let it be said of your doctor, "He's a good doctor, but you can never get to talk to him." The assistant who answers the telephone should act as a screen — not as an impenetrable wall.

Find out exactly how your doctor wishes calls to be handled when he is out of the office and under what circumstances he is willing to be interrupted when he is in the office; be firm in your commitment to his preferences; and cultivate a reputation for being helpful and reliable. You will save the doctor many trips to the telephone if patients develop confidence in your ability to help them, and have faith in your promise to take their messages and deliver them properly.

MINIMIZE WAITING TIME. If a caller asks to speak with the doctor when he is talking on another line, or if it will take a few minutes for him to accept the call, ask, "Will you wait, or shall I call you back when he is free?"

If the caller elects to wait, remember that waiting with a silent telephone can be irritating. The waiting time, no matter how brief, always seems long. Let no more than one minute pass without breaking in with some reassuring comment, for instance, "I'm sorry, Dr. Black is still busy."

Sometimes if the waiting is longer than expected, the caller will want to reconsider and call back another time or have the call returned, but he wants you to know this. By going back on the line at frequent intervals, you give the caller an opportunity to express his wishes. In fact, you may ask him if he wishes to continue waiting. Say something like this: "I'm sorry to keep you waiting so long, Mr. Hughes. Would you prefer to have me return your call when Dr. Black is free?" Try to give the caller some estimate of when he may expect the return call. In any event, irritation can be lessened by your consideration in saying, "Thank you for waiting, Mr. Hughes."

Sometimes it is necessary for you to leave the telephone to obtain information. Ask the caller, "Will you please wait while I get the information?" and then *wait for a reply*. When you return to the telephone, thank the caller for waiting. If it will take longer than a few seconds to get the information, give some estimate of the time required and offer to call back.

TRANSFERRING A CALL. Always identify the caller when transferring a call to the doctor. Any person who refuses to give his name should not be put through unless your doctor instructs you otherwise.

If it is a patient calling, the doctor will presumably want the patient's history in front of him when he is talking. If there is no concern about others hearing your conversation, you can announce the caller's name on the intercom and tell the doctor you will bring the history. If there are other persons within hearing, you might simply take the history to the doctor and say, "Dr. Black, this party is waiting on the telephone to speak with you." In this way, the patient's right to privacy is protected even in regard to his telephone calls.

ANSWERING A SECOND CALL. If your office has several incoming lines, or more than one telephone, it will sometimes be necessary for you to interrupt a conversation to answer another ring. Excuse yourself by saying, "Pardon me just a moment, the other line is ringing." Answer the second call, determine who is calling, and ask that person to hold while you complete the first call. Return to your first call as soon as possible, and apologize briefly for the interruption.

Do not make the mistake of continuing with the second call while the first one waits. Think what you would do if there were a face-to-face conversation. You would not allow a second person to just interrupt a conversation and then ignore the one you were speaking with first.

If the second call is an emergency, you can still take a moment to return to the first line and alert the caller that you will have to keep him waiting or call back. NEVER answer a call by saying, "Hold the line, please," without first finding out who is calling. It could be an emergency. It takes only a moment to be courteous — this courtesy could save a life.

ENDING A CALL. When a caller's requests have been satisfied, do not encourage needless chatting or permit him to monopolize your time unnecessarily. The telephone lines should be cleared for other calls.

End the call pleasantly. It is considered good telephone etiquette to allow the person who placed the call to hang up first. It is a gracious gesture to thank a person for calling. Always close the conversation with some form of goodbye; do not just hang up abruptly. Replace the telephone on the cradle as gently as if you were closing a door in the office; do not slam it.

Summary of Office Telephone Rules

memorize

1. Answer promptly.
2. Visualize the person to whom you are talking.
3. Hold the instrument correctly.
4. Develop a pleasing telephone voice.
5. Identify your office and yourself.
6. Identify the caller.
7. Offer assistance.
8. Screen incoming calls.
9. Minimize waiting time.
10. Identify the caller when transferring a call.
11. When answering a second call, identify the caller, then return to first call.
12. End each call pleasantly and graciously.
13. Let the caller hang up first

The Telephone Message

BE PREPARED. NEVER answer the telephone without a pen or pencil in your hand and a message pad nearby. You may be answering several calls before you have an opportunity to relay a message or carry out a promise of action. Therefore, the *written* message is vital.

What kind of message pad will you use? Probably the most satisfactory is an ordinary spiral-bound stenographer's notebook. It is inexpensive, sturdy, well-proportioned, will lie flat on your desk, and can be filed for future reference if desired. Do not be guilty of using small scraps of paper for messages. They are too easily lost. Date the bottom of the first blank page in your notebook at the beginning of each day. You will then have a permanent record that can be referred to later if the need arises. If you will draw a half-inch column down one side of each page, you can use this area to check off each message as it is delivered or taken care of. This is a good reminder system for yourself.

MINIMUM INFORMATION REQUIRED. The minimum information you will need from each call includes: the caller's name, telephone number, the reason for the call, and the action to be taken.

TRANSMITTING AND RECORDING THE MESSAGE. Messages that are to be transmitted to another person may be rewritten on individual slips and delivered or posted on a message board later. Message pads that provide for a carbon copy of each page are good insurance that no message will be forgotten. The nature of the message will determine whether you must report it immediately or not. The American Medical Association, in *The Business Side of Medical Practice*, presents a model message form (Fig. 8–1), which can be adapted to the practice by inserting the patient symptoms and requests you hear most often. The person who completes the call must sign and date it. It is also possible to get message forms with a self-adhesive back that can be placed permanently in the patient's case history (Fig. 8–2). If the call is from a patient and relates in any way to his medical history, or if any instructions were given, or queries answered, this information should be recorded in the patient's chart.

TAKING ACTION. The message procedure is not complete until the necessary action has been taken. Notations on the memo pad should be carried over to the following day if they have not been attended to. Just place an X in front of the item and move it onto the next page. Sometimes a notation will be carried over for several days until action can be completed. Do not trust to memory in regard to messages unattended to from previous days; always carry them forward in writing.

Make brief notations of patients' reactions while you are talking to them on the telephone. The doctor does not require a character study, but it certainly is helpful to him if he learns from his assistant that a patient revealed extreme fear, apprehension, or nervousness. If a patient shows such symptoms, it may be wise to transfer the call to the doctor himself.

When your employer is talking to another physician in regard to a referral, he sometimes may ask you to take down a brief outline of the patient's case history by listening on the extension telephone. This information can be typed and placed on the doctor's desk just before the patient arrives in the office.

PHONE CALL/Line # 1 for Dr.

Date	Time	Taken by
1/26/81	10 a.m.	Louise

Ernest Dinero
Patient's name ______ New pat. ______ Est. pat.

643 - 2319
Phone number Home Work Ext.

420 Baker, City
Patient's address

✓	Fever		Lab/X-ray results
	Chest pain		Rx refill
	Vomiting		Insurance
✓	Sore throat		Statements
	Abdominal pain		Appointment

☑ Please call ☐ Will call back

Message Symptoms for two days.

Action taken and recorded: ______ Date ______ Sign ______

FIGURE 8–1 Telephone message form. (From *The Business Side of Medical Practice*. American Medical Association, Chicago, Illinois, 1979; reprinted with permission.)

Date 4-23	Time 2:40	Who Called Peter Herndon			Phone 494-8330
About Whom self		Age 47	Temp. N	Physician JBM	
Address 436 West Mariposa				Urgent	Call Back ✓

MESSAGE:	DISPOSITION:
wants report of X-rays taken last week.	
	Chart ☐ Chart #
Medication Allergy / Rec'd by: MK	Handled by:

FIGURE 8–2 Message form with self-adhesive backing. © 1971 Patient Care Systems, Inc.)

PITFALLS TO AVOID

1. Having too few telephone lines. The telephone company will do a traffic survey to determine how many busy signals are occurring and advise you as to whether you need additional lines. If collections and insurance processing require extensive use of the telephone, a special line just for this purpose may be advisable.

2. Having too few assistants to handle the existing lines. One assistant can handle two incoming lines, but three lines are probably too many for one person. Another assistant should be assigned to pick up the phone after a specified number of rings.

3. Wasting time looking up frequently called numbers. Keep these in a personal directory where they can be quickly and easily located.

4. Incoming or outgoing personal calls by employees, except in emergencies. Most doctors have an unlisted private line to take care of their own personal and priority calls.

5. Using the telephone to give travel directions to new patients (except for short notice appointments). This information should be included in a Patient Information Sheet or Folder sent to every new patient.

6. Taking extensive patient histories over the telephone when this can be done more efficiently at the time of the patient visit.

7. Diagnosing or giving medical advice without authorization from the physician.

8. Releasing patient information without authorization.

Incoming Calls the Assistant Can Handle

One reason for having the office assistant answer the incoming calls is to spare the physician unnecessary interruptions during his time with patients. Additionally, many calls relate to the administrative aspects of the office and can actually be better handled by the assistant. The doctor's policy regarding how calls are to be handled by the assistant should be set forth in the office procedure manual. Figure 8–3 shows how the instruction page might be arranged in the manual. Listed below are some kinds of calls that can be handled by the assistant in most offices.

APPOINTMENTS FOR NEW PATIENTS. As mentioned in the chapter on scheduling appointments, the first appointment for a new patient requires more time and attention to detail. The assistant who is in charge of scheduling appointments should handle these calls. It is well to remember that you are in a sense "opening the door." The patient will form a first impression of the office, of you, and of the doctor from his first telephone contact. Follow all the prescribed rules of telephone courtesy in offering your friendly assistance.

Take the patient's full name, age, complete address and telephone number, name of person who referred him, and the general type of examination required. This helps decide how much time to allot the patient on the appointment schedule. Your doctor also may ask you to give general instructions to patients seeking care for specific complaints; for example, to request the patient to bring in a urine specimen.

STANDARD PROCEDURE FOR TELEPHONE CALLS IN THE OFFICE OF

____________________________:

CALLS THE ASSISTANT CAN HANDLE:

Appointments for New Patients

Office Administration Problems

CALLS TO BE PUT THROUGH IMMEDIATELY:

Calls from Other Physicians

Emergency Calls

CALLS TO BE REFERRED TO PHYSICIAN:

Unsatisfactory Progress Reports

Third Party Requests for Information

FIGURE 8–3 Page from procedure manual.

When you have recorded the necessary data, you may ask the patient, "Do you prefer morning or afternoon?" and then offer the first available date. Make certain the patient knows where the office is located and, if necessary, how to get there. If there are special parking conveniences, tell the patient. Ideally, transportation and parking instructions would be described in a Patient Information Folder to be mailed to the patient prior to a first visit if time permits. Before hanging up, repeat the appointment date and time agreed upon and thank the person for calling.

RETURN APPOINTMENTS. Usually it will only be necessary to determine when the patient was expected to return, then find a suitable time on the schedule. It will not be necessary to give extensive explanations about the location of the office and parking facilities. However, if it has been some time since he has been in the office, it is advisable to ask whether his address and telephone number remain the same. You may also wish to inquire whether the patient wants to see the doctor about a condition similar to his former one. He may have a different complaint which might require a longer or shorter visit than previously.

INQUIRIES ABOUT BILLS. A patient may telephone and say he has received a bill and wants to talk to the doctor about it. The assistant may ask the caller to "Hold" for a moment while she pulls the ledger. If she finds nothing irregular noted on the ledger, she can return to the telephone and say, "I have your account in front of me now. Perhaps I can answer your inquiry." The chances are the patient will have some simple inquiry such as "Is that my total bill?" "Has my insurance paid anything?" or "May I wait until next month to make a payment?" Not all patients realize that it is the assistant who usually takes charge of these matters.

INQUIRIES ABOUT FEES. In many offices the assistant is instructed not to quote fees. A caller who inquires, "How much does Dr. Arnold charge for an examination?" may not be pleased with "That's impossible to say — it depends entirely on how extensive an examination is necessary." The following response is equally noncommittal but far more satisfying to the caller: "Mr. Barker, that naturally varies with the nature of the problem. A simple physical examination without any laboratory tests or x-rays might run as little as $________. On the other hand, it could run considerably more if special tests were required."

REQUESTS FOR INSURANCE ASSISTANCE. Again, it is the office assistant who is in a better position to answer inquiries about insurance. Oftentimes patients find insurance claims very confusing and think they must answer questions with precise medical terminology. A simple statement to "just put it in your own words" may take care of this kind of inquiry. It is best to steer clear of interpreting insurance coverage by telephone. If the patient has a complicated problem that will tie up the telephone for a long while, the assistant can ask him to mail in the pages so that she can review them.

RECEIVING X-RAY AND LABORATORY REPORTS. Many physicians have x-ray and laboratory reports telephoned to their offices on the day the test is completed. The assistant can take these reports. Her task will be greatly simplified if she has blank forms on which she can just fill in the results rather than having to write down the names of all the tests, particularly on laboratory reports. If it is impossible to get blank forms from the laboratory, she can type up her own and run it through the copy machine. By typing four or six to a page, the expense of duplication will be cut considerably. They can then be cut to size.

SATISFACTORY PROGRESS REPORTS FROM PATIENTS. Doctors sometimes ask a patient to "phone and let me know how you're feeling in a few days." The assistant can take this call and relay the information to the doctor if it is a satisfactory report. Say something to the patient that will assure him that you will inform the doctor about the call, for example, "I'll give this information to the doctor as soon as he arrives in the office."

ROUTINE REPORTS FROM HOSPITALS AND OTHER SOURCES. There may be routine calls from the hospital and other sources reporting a patient's progress. If it is only a reporting procedure, take the message carefully, make sure that the doctor sees it, and then place it in the patient's history.

OFFICE ADMINISTRATION MATTERS. Not all calls concern patients. There may be calls from the accountant or auditor, or calls regarding banking procedures, office supplies, office maintenance, and so forth, all of which the assistant can either handle immediately or get the necessary information and call back.

REQUESTS FOR REFERRALS. Doctors who are liked and respected by their patients frequently receive requests from patients for referrals to other specialists, for themselves or for friends. If the physician has furnished the assistant with a list of doctors to whom he usually refers certain types of cases, she can handle these inquiries without referring them to the physician. She should, however, tell the physician about the calls.

PRESCRIPTION REFILLS. If the physician has placed a note upon the patient's chart indicating that a prescription may be filled a certain number of times, the assistant can give an OK to the pharmacist after double-checking with him on the number of times it has already been filled. This information should appear on the patient's chart, but it is always best to double-check. If there is any question, tell the pharmacist you will have to check with the doctor and call back.

Calls that Require Transfer to the Doctor or Call Back

CALLS FROM OTHER PHYSICIANS. As stated earlier, calls from other physicians should be put through immediately. If it is impossible for the doctor to take the call at once, be sure to offer to call back as soon as possible.

PATIENTS WHO WILL NOT REVEAL SYMPTOMS. Sometimes a patient will call and wish to talk with the doctor about symptoms that he is reluctant to discuss with an assistant. Do not make the mistake of pressing for details. Even though you may not be embarrassed, the patient has the right to some privacy. Put these calls through to the doctor or offer to have him call back.

UNSATISFACTORY PROGRESS REPORTS. If the patient reports that he "still is not feeling well," or the "prescription the doctor gave me makes me feel sick," do not try to practice medicine by telling the patient "this is to be expected." Even if you think the doctor will say the same thing, the patient should hear it from the doctor himself for reassurance.

REQUESTS FOR TEST RESULTS. When the physician orders special tests for the patient, he may tell him to call the office in a couple of days for the results. Be sure the physician has seen the results and has given you permission to tell the patient before giving out any information. Particularly if the result is unfavorable, the physician should be the one to inform the patient and give him further instructions. This call must be handled tactfully; otherwise, the patient may get the feeling that you are hiding something from him. Some patients do not understand that the assistant does not have the privilege of giving out information without permission of the physician. You might answer the inquiry like this: "The doctor has not seen the report yet; will you please call back after 2:00? I will try to have the information for you then." Or offer to call the patient as soon as you have the necessary information.

THIRD PARTY REQUESTS FOR INFORMATION. Remember, if there is no legal requirement for disclosure of information, you must have the written permission of the patient before giving information to third-party callers. This includes insurance companies, attorneys, relatives, neighbors, employers, or any other third party.

COMPLAINTS ABOUT CARE OR FEES. You may be able to offer a satisfactory explanation to a patient who complains about the care he received or the fee charged. If the patient is angry when he calls, you may tell him it will take a few moments to pull his chart, and offer to call him back. This reassures him that someone is willing to talk to him about his problem, and also gives him a chance to "cool off." If you are unable to appease the patient easily, though, your doctor would probably prefer to talk to the patient himself.

CALLBACK SYSTEM. The transfer of nonemergency calls as they occur may cause needless interruption in the physician's daily schedule. Some offices set aside a special time once or twice a day when the physician will accept or return calls — for instance, at the end of the morning office hours and again at the end of the afternoon. The person answering the telephone logs each caller's name, telephone number, and reason for calling. Patients' charts are pulled and given to the physician along with the log. When calls are handled in this manner, the physician is better prepared to answer questions and the caller is better assured of undivided attention to the call.

Special Telephone Problems

EMERGENCY CALL PROCEDURES. The procedures for handling emergencies that present in the office are discussed in a later chapter. At this point we are concerned only with handling the telephone call involving a possible emergency situation. According to the American Medical Association's *The Business Side of Medical Practice*, "Many emergency calls are judgment calls on the part of the person answering in the physician's office. Good judgment only comes from proper training by the physician as to what constitutes a real emergency in his/her type of practice and how such calls should be handled. If you are not immediately available, what should your assistant do?" The person answering the telephone should first determine, "Is it urgent?" If the physician is in, the call should probably be transferred immediately. Some plan for action should be agreed upon for the situation when the physician is not present (Fig. 8–4). It is estimated that less than 10 per cent of assistants in doctors' offices have such guidance.

The physician and assistant may also jointly develop typical questions to ask the caller, to determine the validity and disposition of an emergency. For example, What are the chief symptoms? When did they start? Has this happened before? Are you alone? Do you have transportation? What is the telephone number where you can be reached?

UNIDENTIFIED CALLERS. Although it will happen rarely, you will sometimes encounter an individual who refuses to give you his name or business but is rudely insistent upon speaking to the doctor. Such callers usually are sales persons who are fully aware that if their identity is revealed they will never get the opportunity to speak to the doctor. Your own course in such instances is to say firmly, "Dr. Jones is very busy with a patient and has asked me to take all messages. If you will not give me a message, I suggest you write the doctor a letter. I'm sure he will give it his immediate attention."

CALLS FROM FAMILY AND FRIENDS. Every doctor receives a certain number of personal calls at his office from his family and friends. As you become acquainted with the doctor and his practice, you will soon know how to handle these calls. However, some persons abuse the telephone privilege. If a friend of the doctor calls too often and the doctor does not wish to speak with him, the assistant must deal

EMERGENCY CALL PROCEDURES

If the physician is not in the office, the following calls should be handled as indicated.

Danger Signal	Call Physician Below	Call RN	Call Ambul.	Have Patient Go to Hosp.	Have Patient Come to Ofc.
Heavy Bleeding					
Head Injury					
Severe Chest Pain					
Broken Limb					
Unconscious					
High Fever					
Difficulty in breathing					

FIGURE 8–4 Emergency call procedures. (From *The Business Side of Medical Practice*. American Medical Association, Chicago, Illinois, 1979; reprinted with permission.)

politely with him. She can say, "Dr. Wilson is with a patient now and I cannot disturb him. He is booked rather heavily this afternoon, and you may have more time to talk with him if you call him at home this evening. His home telephone number is. . . ."

ANGRY CALLERS. No matter how efficient you are at the telephone or how well-liked your employer may be, sooner or later you will have an angry caller on the other end of your line. There may be a legitimate reason for the anger, or it may have resulted from a misunderstanding. It is a real challenge to handle such a call. You must avoid getting angry yourself; then, try to find out what the problem is and provide the answers if possible. If answers are not readily available, a friendly assurance that you will find the answer and call back will usually soothe the angry feelings. Be sure to really *listen* while you let the caller talk, express interest and understanding, do not "pass the buck," take careful notes, maintain your own poise, and then take the required action, even if it is to say that you will take the matter up with your employer as soon as possible and call back later.

MONITORING CALLS. Occasionally you may be asked by your employer to **monitor** a telephone call. You will be expected to listen from an extension phone and take notes on the conversation. It is possible to record both sides of a telephone call by placing a dictating machine close to the telephone receiver. However, you should be aware that this is illegal unless the other person is told that his conversation is being recorded.

REQUESTS FOR HOUSE CALLS. Scheduling house calls was discussed briefly in Chapter 6. In response to a telephone request for a home visit, be sure to inquire the nature of the illness. There are certain conditions that are impossible to treat at home, and time will be saved if the patient is sent directly to the hospital, where the doctor can meet him. Or urge the patient to come to the office. It can be pointed out that facilities for giving the best medical treatment are available there and office calls are more economical. This also conserves the doctor's time.

Consult the doctor, if possible, before obligating him to a house call. In most cases you can explain to the patient that you will check with the doctor and call back immediately. If he cannot visit the patient, you must see that another doctor is sent out. It is easier for you to call another physician than it is for the distraught patient. One of the most common complaints about the medical profession is that you cannot get a doctor in an emergency. It is particularly difficult for newcomers to get a doctor to make a house call. Your medical society may operate an emergency answering panel which can be of service in such cases.

If your doctor agrees to make a house call and the area is unfamiliar to him, it is a good idea to have a local map on which you can pinpoint the location of the house for him. This is a little extra service that your doctor will greatly appreciate, since it may save him precious moments he might spend uselessly hunting for the house.

Routine but Troublesome Calls

Many of the so-called "routine calls" coming into the physician's office will be difficult for a new assistant to handle (Fig. 8–5). Though no stock answer can be phrased for these calls, a gracious and prompt answer paves the way for a quicker handling of the call, since it tells the patient the assistant is capable, pleasant, and willing to offer assistance.

Here are a few typical calls that any medical assistant may receive:

1. The Call — "I have an appointment with the doctor this morning and cannot keep it. May I come in this afternoon instead?"

   The Answer — Even though this type of call throws the appointment book into confusion, showing irritation with the patient won't help the situation. Make a sincere effort to help the caller make a new appointment. Explain that appointments are made in order that the doctor can give the very best care without rushing his patients and that consequently keeping appointments is to each patient's personal benefit.

AMA Call Check

Patient Symptoms	Refer immediately to doctor	Doctor will call back	Refer to Clinical personnel, i.e., R.N., L.P.N., C.M.A., P.A., N.P.,	Other
Unconscious — in shock				
Fever — Vomiting				
Severe pain				
Heavy Bleeding				
Reaction to medication — injection				
Routine				
New patient — ill, wants to talk to doctor				
Patient under treatment — wants to talk to doctor				
Patient — request for lab results				
Family — request for patient information				
Patient or pharmacy — regarding Rx refill				
Another physician — wants to talk to doctor				
Hospital — regarding a patient				
Insurance Co. or attorney — request for patient information				
Business calls for physician's attention — CPA, Attorney, Broker, Medical Society				
Personal calls for physician: Family: Friends:				

If doctor not available:

Send patient to emergency room ______________________ Hospital

Phone ______________ Address ______________________

Non-emergency refer to Dr. ______________________

Ambulance: ______________________

Poison control: ______________________

Other: ______________________

FIGURE 8–5 AMA Call Check Chart. (From *Handling Patient Telephone Calls Effectively.* American Medical Association, Chicago, Illinois, 1979; reprinted with permission.)

2. The Call — "I received my statement this morning and I don't understand why it is so high."

   The Answer — When this type of call comes in, politely ask the patient to hold the line while you pull the financial card. When you return to the line, thank the patient for waiting and explain the charges carefully. If there is an error, apologize and say a corrected statement will be sent out at once. Thank the patient for calling. If patients are properly advised about charges at the time services are rendered, the number of these calls will be considerably reduced.

3. The Call — "Last time I had an office call, Doctor gave me a prescription for some sleeping tablets. I want you to call the druggist and okay a refill."

   The Answer — Remember that the medical assistant is *not* licensed to practice medicine. Ask the patient for the prescription number, the date, the name, address and telephone number of the druggist, and obtain the patient's phone number. Explain that you will give the message to the doctor as soon as he returns to the office. At this point it may be advisable to pull the patient's history card and have it ready with the message when the doctor comes in. If he okays the refill, he may ask the assistant to phone the patient with the information.

4. The Call — "Does the doctor treat stomach trouble?"

   The Answer — It depends upon the doctor's field of practice. Many people don't understand the various medical specialties, and this call may come from a person referred to the doctor by a friend who didn't explain that the doctor is a specialist. If your doctor is unable to handle the case, you may have to refer the patient to another doctor. Always give the patient the names of at least three physicians when possible; these should only be names which your employer has had you place on the referral list. Never presume to make a diagnosis when a patient calls in with bizarre complaints; transfer the call to the doctor himself or take the caller's name and number and have the doctor return the call later.

5. The Call — "My next door neighbor is a patient of the doctor and I am quite concerned about her. Could you tell me what is wrong with her?"

   The Answer — Professional ethics is involved here. It is not the role of the medical assistant to give out any information about a patient's condition, except that information the physician has specifically okayed for "release." The caller in this case may be merely curious, or may actually be a kindly neighbor who wishes to help her friend. Generally, refer such calls to the doctor.

Telephone Answering Services

Because a physician's telephone is an all-important tool of his practice, it must be constantly "covered"—that is, there must be someone to answer it at all times—day and night, Sundays and holidays. This presents no problem during weekdays, but nights and weekends present special problems. Most doctors subscribe to telephone answering services that assume around-the-clock coverage. Some telephone answering services are privately owned; others are owned and operated by the local medical society. Or the doctor may own an automatic answering device.

OPERATOR-ANSWERED SERVICES. There are two types of operator-answered services: (1) doctor-subscribers leave messages with, or obtain patients' messages from, a service whose number appears in the local telephone directory in this way: "After ____________ p.m., call ____________ (number)," or "If no answer, call__________(number)." Such listings are found immediately following the doctor's own telephone number. This form of service offers some inconvenience for the patient but is far better than no coverage at all. (2) The answering service has a direct connection with the office telephone. When the telephone rings in the physician's office or at home, it also signals on the switchboard of the answering service. As long as the telephone is ringing, it will continue to signal at the answering service. If the doctor or someone in his office or home does not answer within a certain agreed upon number of rings, the answering service operator takes the call. This method provides constant telephone coverage.

Even during the day, such an answering service can function effectively. There may be times when you are assisting the doctor and it is impossible for you or anyone else to answer the telephone. An unanswered telephone is extremely poor policy; but, if you have an agreement with the answering service, its operators will accept calls for you in such situations. With this direct-wire answering method, the operator answers the telephone in your employer's name, as you would in the office, explaining, "This is Dr. Wilson's exchange. May I take a message?" The operators on the exchange switchboards are usually exceptionally well trained, especially if the service is owned by the medical society.

The answering service will greatly appreciate your cooperation if you call them every evening before leaving the office, telling them where the doctor will be during the evening or giving them other special messages. Then, in the morning when you return to the office, call the exchange and ask for any messages they may have. Invariably, there will be messages from patients who called during the night but whose calls were not important enough to merit an emergency call to the doctor. An exchange can act as a buffer for your doctor and help eliminate too frequent, unnecessary calls during the night. Here's how the system works.

During the night and on weekends and holidays, the exchange will answer the doctor's office telephone, take a message, and immediately relay it to the doctor. If the doctor feels it is necessary, he will then return the call to the patient; if not, the exchange will call the patient and explain that the doctor will call first thing in the morning. Of course, the exchange does not tell the patient about its recent conversation with the doctor but reports he is not available. Emergency calls, however, are immediately put through by the exchange to the doctor.

Occasionally, it is a good idea to check up on your answering service by placing a few calls at various hours. It may be that now and then the service does not answer the call or the response is gruff and rude, offering absolutely no cooperation to the "patient." Such poor service can deal a bad blow to the doctor's reputation.

AUTOMATIC ANSWERING DEVICES. Many doctors use an automatic answering device after office hours. Callers who dial the office hear a recorded message either telling them how to reach the doctor (or a colleague who may be covering the practice for him) or inviting the caller to leave a message. The caller's message is recorded for later checking by the doctor or his staff.

One type of telephone-answering device is equipped with a remote control with which the doctor can call his office from any telephone and, by simply holding the remote control near the mouthpiece of the telephone he is calling from, receive the messages that have been recorded during his absence.

The automatic telephone-answering devices are particularly useful in areas where no competent answering service is available.

OUTGOING CALLS

USING THE TELEPHONE DIRECTORY. The primary purpose of the telephone directory, of course, is to provide lists of those who have telephones, with their numbers and in most cases their addresses. In addition, the directory is an aid in checking the spelling of names and in locating certain types of businesses through the yellow pages. Directories are usually organized in three sections: (1) introductory pages, (2) alphabetical pages (white pages), and (3) yellow pages. In large metropolitan areas the yellow pages appear in a separate volume. The introductory pages are sometimes entirely overlooked by the subscribers. This section precedes the white alphabetical pages and provides basic information concerning the telephone services in the area, including: emergency services (fire, police, ambulance), service calls, dialing instructions for local and out-of-town calls, and area codes for some cities. The introductory pages may also include a survival guide, community service numbers, prefix locations, rates, long distance calling information, time zones, and money-saving tips. Some directories include zip code maps for the local area. Take a few moments to familiarize yourself with your local directory; then use it frequently for getting information fast.

ORGANIZING TELEPHONE NUMBERS. Organize your telephone numbers in an indexed 3 by 5 inch desktop file or a rotary file. Emergency numbers might be typed on a colored card or flagged with a color tab. Your procedure manual should include lists of:

1. specialists to whom your employer sometimes refers patients,
2. physicians who will take house calls if your doctor does not find it possible to accept them or is unable to make such calls on a particular day,
3. professional facilities, such as hospitals, the Poison Control Center, pharmacies, ambulance companies, laboratories,
4. special duty nurses — registered, practical, and general duty — along with their ages, specialties, and other information,
5. administrative contacts, such as stationers, equipment dealers and repair services, laundry and maintenance services, surgical supply houses, and
6. personal numbers, such as doctor's family, special friends, his insurance agent, stock broker, accountant, lawyer.

PRE-PLANNING THE CALL. Before placing a call, make certain you have the correct telephone number. If you are not absolutely sure about it, look it up in the directory. Have the information you will need during the call at your fingertips. If you are reporting a patient's history, have the complete record before you, including all the latest laboratory and x-ray reports. If you are placing a call to order supplies, have the catalog in front of you with any previous order sheets or invoices. Also have a list of the items desired, the specifications for them, and any questions you may have regarding them. Apply this rule to every call you make. The called party will be impressed with your competence, and you will save a great deal of time.

PLACING THE CALL. Lift the receiver, listen for the dial tone, then start dialing your number. It sometimes happens that just as you pick up the telephone to place a call, an incoming call has reached your line but you lifted the receiver before the telephone had a chance to ring. If you start dialing without listening for the dial tone, you will not only fail to reach your number, you will have offended the ear of the party trying to reach you. If your telephone has a rotary dial, use the index finger or a special dialing instrument for dialing your call. Do not use the eraser end of a pencil and do not let your finger remain in the dial openings on the return of the dial. It is the return of the dial that determines the number you reach, and if it is not allowed to return freely you may reach a wrong number.

CALLING ETIQUETTE. When placing a call to another doctor or to a patient at the doctor's request, your employer should be ready to receive the call. Doctors, because of their busy schedules, sometimes are negligent in this respect. The telephone company's courtesy rule is that the person placing the call should be on the wire ready to speak when the called party answers. You may have to ask your doctor when he requests you to place a call for him if he is ready to answer the telephone while you are putting through the call. Promptness is one of the first rules of telephone etiquette.

If you are calling a patient to change an appointment, be ready to offer a new appointment time. Also, give the patient a logical reason for the inconvenience of having to change his original appointment. This change may cause considerable disruption in his plans, and he is fully entitled to an explanation. Your employer may ask you to call a patient and change a medication instruction. Or it may be your duty to call a patient and instruct him to go to the hospital or laboratory for a special test or x-ray. Make certain you have the correct instructions written down carefully and that you have checked these instructions. This is of particular importance when you are changing medication instructions. Remember that if your telephone is within hearing distance of office patients you should be careful in mentioning names or diagnoses.

LONG DISTANCE CALLS. Long distance calls are no longer reserved for special occasions. The calls are simple to place and not exorbitant in cost. It is certainly much easier to telephone to obtain information than it is to wait for an exchange of letters.

Before placing a long distance call, have the correct number ready. This number often may be obtained from a letterhead or from other records. The telephone company also has a collection of major city telephone directories in every town. If you do not have the number, you can dial the area code, then 555–1212 for information service.

It is important to keep in mind the different time zones when you are calling long distance (Fig. 8–6). The continental United States is divided into four standard time zones: Pacific, Mountain, Central, and Eastern. When it is 12 noon Pacific time, it is 3 PM Eastern time. If you are calling from Los Angeles to New York, you will probably want to make the call no later than 2 PM if you are calling a business or professional office, because it will already be 5 PM on the East coast.

Dialing Direct. By dialing your own long distance calls, you will pay the lowest rate and pay for only the minutes you talk (minimum one minute). Use this approach when you are willing to talk with anyone who answers the phone and you want the call charged to the number from which you are calling.

"800" WATS (Wide Area Telephone Service) Numbers. Some businesses and people have "800" WATS numbers, to which long distance calls can be made without charge. To call an "800" number, dial 1 + 800 + the 7-digit telephone number. You can get the telephone numbers of those businesses and people who have 800 numbers by dialing 1 + 800 + 555–1212.

Operator-Assisted Calls. Some long distance calls require the assistance of an operator. For instance, if you wish to place a collect call, a credit card call, or a person-to-person call you will need the assistance of an operator. This service is more expensive than dialing direct and the minimum charge is for three minutes. To place an operator assisted call, dial 0 + area code + 7-digit telephone number. After you have dialed the number, the operator will come on the line for information as to what service is required.

WRONG NUMBERS. One slip in direct long distance dialing can give you Los Angeles instead of Dallas. If you reach a wrong number when dialing long distance, be sure to obtain the name of the city, state, and central office you have reached. By reporting this information promptly to the operator in your own city, you will not be charged for this wrong number. If you are cut off before terminating your call, this too should be reported to the operator, who will either reconnect your call or make an adjustment of the charge.

CONFERENCE CALLS. Conference telephone service is of great value to the medical profession. This service is used in special postgraduate course presentations,

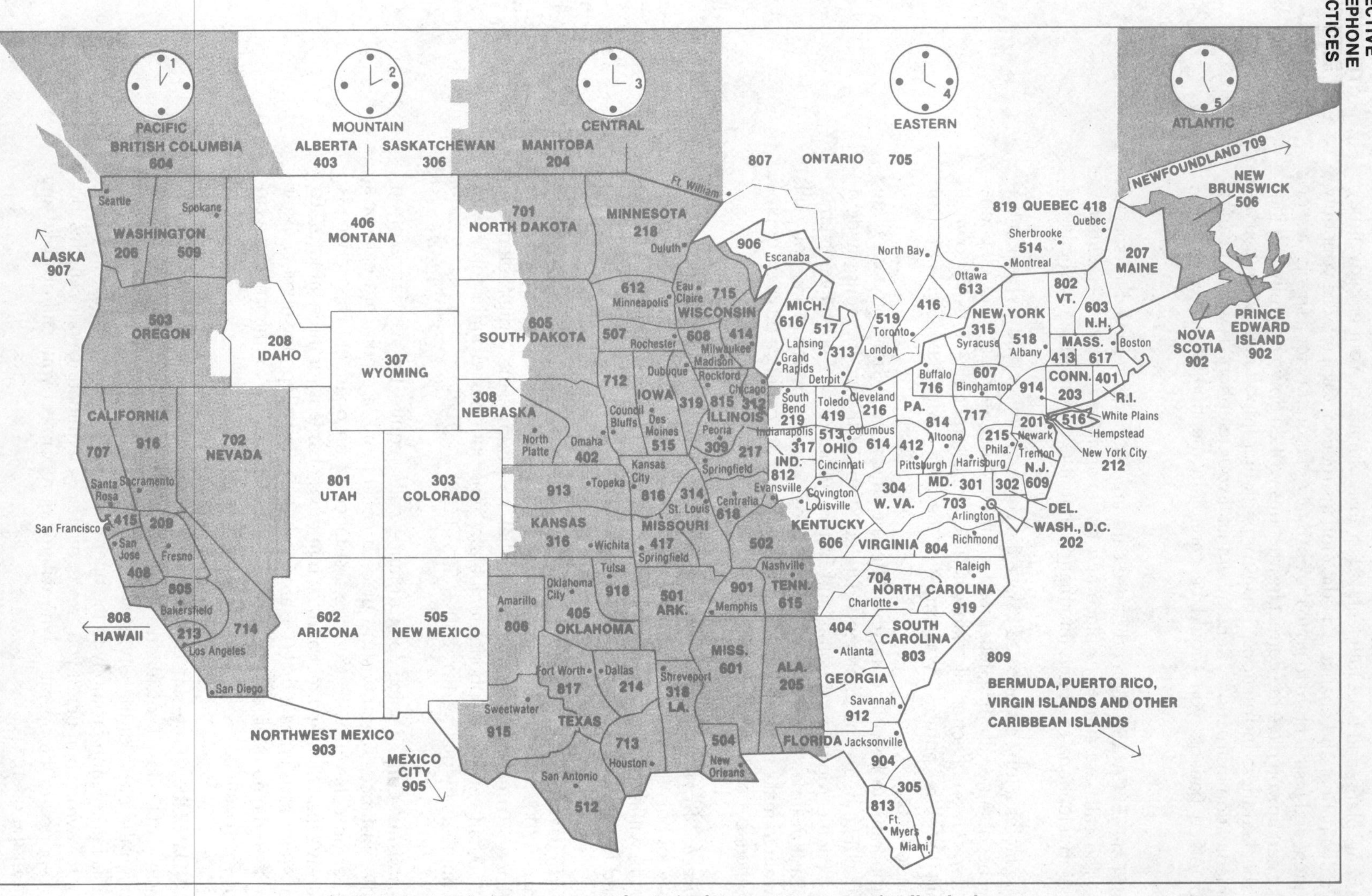

FIGURE 8–6 Time zones across the United States. (Courtesy of Bell Telephone.)

in consultations, and in notifying and explaining to a family how a patient is progressing. This service may connect from 3 to 14 long distance points for a two-way conference. Each person can hear or talk to all others participating. Up to 49 points can be connected for a one-way conference call in which only the voice of the caller is heard. This service is available through the long distance operator; call her and ask for the conference operator. The charges are based on person-to-person rates to the two farthest points, plus a lower rate for each additional telephone used in the conference. This service has exceptional value in family conferences requiring a quick decision by the entire family in regard to a patient's condition.

By following these suggested techniques the assistant will be able to use the telephone wisely and efficiently. Correct use of the telephone really is an art which can be developed only through actual practice. It is one of the most important skills the medical assistant should possess.

Special Equipment

Much research and development has taken place in recent years to improve the efficiency and capabilities of telephone communications. The new doctor just opening a practice will be wise to consult with telephone specialists to set up the system best for the practice. As the practice grows, additional conveniences may be added. Familiarity with a multiple-line telephone is a must for the medical office assistant. The multiple-line instrument allows holding one or more calls while answering another, or while speaking with another person within the office on an intercom line.

SIX-BUTTON KEY SET. The most common telephone instrument in the doctor's office is the six-button key set. It can have several outside lines, can hold calls, and can be used as an intercom or for signaling. Lights within the buttons flash for incoming calls and wink rapidly to remind of calls being held. A steady light indicates that the line is in use. Although many rotary dial telephones are still in use, they are gradually being phased out and replaced with the speedier touch-tone instrument (Fig. 8–7).

SPEAKERPHONE. Some doctors like the Speakerphone, a small receiver-transmitter which sits on the desk and picks up and amplifies normal conversation, freeing the hands for note-taking. This same device can be very useful to the secretary or receptionist who may receive frequent calls that require her to leave her

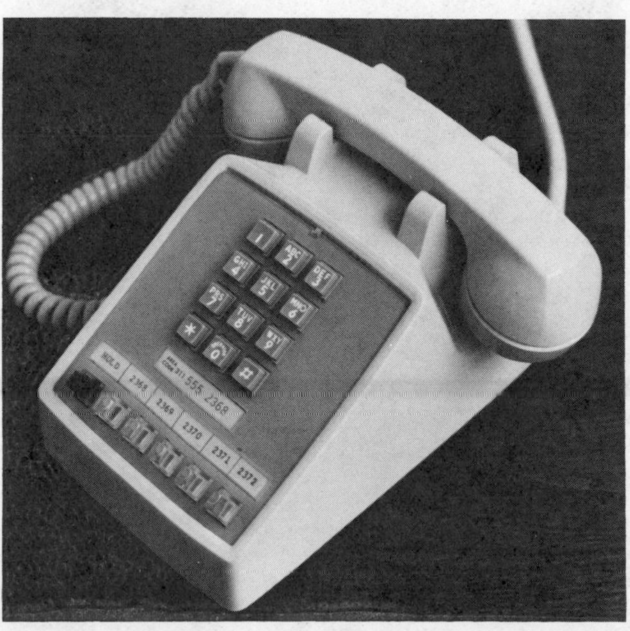

FIGURE 8–7 Key Set Touch-Tone. The Key Set features one "hold" button and five others for calling, signalling, or access to other extensions. (Courtesy of American Telephone and Telegraph.)

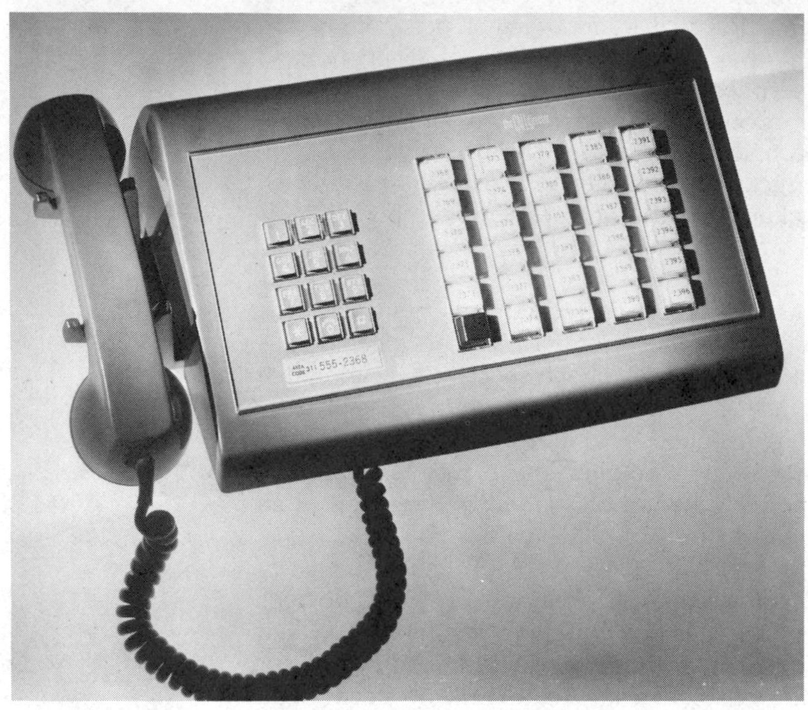

FIGURE 8–8 Call Director Touch-Tone. Thirty-button Call Director with self-designating keys. (Courtesy of American Telephone and Telegraph.)

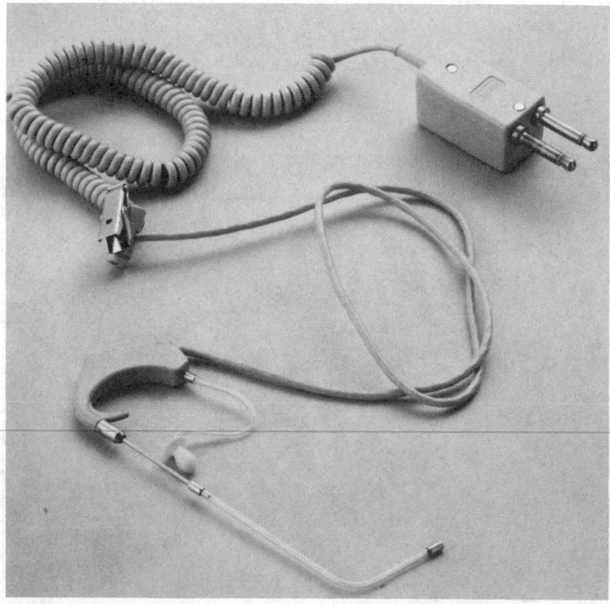

FIGURE 8–9 StarSet telephone. (Courtesy of American Telephone and Telegraph.)

desk to refer to charts or financial records. With the Speakerphone there is no break in communication while she goes to the files for information. The Speakerphone is convertible; at the touch of a button it changes from a regular telephone to a hands-free communications system.

10-BUTTON PHONE. As the practice grows, it may become necessary to add additional telephone lines. The 10-button phone handles as many as nine lines, with the subscriber choosing the appropriate number and "mix" of outside and inside lines serving each phone.

COM KEY. Ideal for the larger office is the flexible Com Key, which utilizes 10-button phones. It provides up to seven incoming lines, plus built in equipment for multi-line intercom conferencing as well as one-way voice signaling on the intercom. A built in loud speaker system is an added convenience. A simple control switch at each phone allows the selection of which phones will ring on any combination of outside lines — ideal for "after hours" assignments or reduced staff situations.

11- AND 20-BUTTON DESK TELEPHONE SETS. The office that has frequent need for outside conferencing will find this instrument convenient. Up to 7 lines of the 11-button set and up to 15 lines of the 20-button set may be used as conferencing lines by simultaneously depressing the line buttons on the lines to be used without going through an operator. These instruments also have a special recall button that lets you flash your operator without losing a call or breaking a conference connection.

CALL DIRECTOR OR CALL COMMANDER TELEPHONE. This piece of equipment may have 18 or 30 buttons. One button is reserved for "Hold" and the remainder may be a mix of outside and inside lines. It is a compact desk-top instrument and may be thought of as a desk-sized switchboard offering many optional features (Fig. 8–8).

TOUCH-A-MATIC. The Bell System refers to its Touch-a-Matic telephone as "the telephone that remembers." It has the ability to store up to 31 telephone numbers electronically and can dial any one of them for you at the touch of a single button. The names of the people or places you call most frequently are displayed on the face of the instrument, eliminating the need for an index or cards to insert. A very attractive feature of this instrument is its *last number dialed* button. If you want to call back someone you've just spoken to, or try a number that was busy a few minutes ago, the number is re-dialed for you electronically by simply touching the *last number dialed* button. By following simple recording instructions you can add to, delete, or change the numbers assigned to the memory system.

TELEDIALER 32. The same features that are found in the Touch-a-Matic may be added to your present phone by installing the auxiliary TeleDialer 32.

DESIGN LINE TELEPHONES. Not too many years ago almost all office telephones were black and heavy. Then came the lightweight plastic instruments in decorator colors. Today it is possible to have a telephone that blends with any decor, or possibly serves as a decorative accessory. Models range from the playful to objets d'art.

HEADSETS. A new development in headsets is a very light plastic earphone and microphone combination that allows the receptionist or the doctor to move about the room and to have the hands free. One brand name is StarSet (Fig. 8–9). It was originally designed for the astronauts and weighs less than one ounce. Instead of being worn over the head, it is worn behind the ear or clipped to your glasses. It can be equipped with a cord up to ten feet long for easy movement about the room. There is also an optional quick-disconnect feature that allows the user to separate the headset even during a call without breaking the connection.

CALL FORWARDING. Though not yet available in all areas, Call Forwarding may be something your employer will want to investigate. This is a particularly attractive feature for the doctor who has two offices and does not want to confuse the patients with different numbers for different days of the week. With the Call Forwarding feature all you do is dial a special code followed by the number of the other office (or, the number where the doctor can be reached). Then all phone calls will be automatically transferred to the new location.

MOBILE SERVICE. To guarantee continual availability to patients, some doctors have telephones in their automobiles. Others use a pocket radio receiver which signals with a tone that he is to call his office or answering service. The Bell System's unit is called Bell Boy.

TELEPHONE DICTATION. In hospitals, dial dictation and recording services are quite common. A doctor can dictate a case history or report by telephone into a centrally located recording machine. The report will then be transcribed by typists at the central location. In a group practice, the recording machine may be in the doctor's office, where the office personnel will do the typing.

New concepts in telecommunications are being developed continually. A call to the marketing division of your local telephone company will help keep you informed of what is available in your locality.

Telegraph Services

Although most long distance communications from the physician's office will be via the telephone, there are instances in which the telegraph message is the one of choice. The projected delivery time and the urgency of the message would determine the type of service to be used. There are two basic classes of domestic telegraph service: the *regular telegram* and the more economical *overnight telegram*.

REGULAR TELEGRAM. The regular telegram is accepted at any time and transmitted immediately. Usually delivery may be expected within two hours. The minimum charge is based on 15 words, and an extra charge is made for each additional word.

OVERNIGHT TELEGRAM. The overnight telegram may be sent up until midnight for delivery the next morning. The minimum charge is based on 100 words, and an extra charge is made for each additional word.

MAILGRAM. The mailgram is a variation of the overnight telegram. It is wired to the office of the US Postal Service nearest the recipient, where it is placed in a special Mailgram envelope and delivered by the regular letter carrier.

The secretary should be familiar with the methods used in counting the chargeable words and characters. One address and one signature are free. Punctuation marks are not charged for; however, if such words as *stop, period,* or *quote* are used, they are considered chargeable words. Three of the characters on your typewriter cannot be transmitted and must be written as words in a telegram: these are ¢, @, and ° (for degree).

Telegrams may be telephoned to the telegraph company and charged on your telephone bill. However, before telephoning, the message should be carefully composed and a copy typed for the office files, including the date and time sent. Telegrams may be addressed to airports, to sailing or arriving ships, to ships at sea, and even to isolated places if there is a telephone there.

TYPES OF EQUIPMENT. The private practitioner will ordinarily have no need for telegraph transmitting equipment in his office. However, with the growing tendency toward more complex practices, in clinical group practice and hospitals, the medical assistant should familiarize herself with the more commonly used equipment: Desk-fax, Intrafax, Wirefax, Telex Service, and Tieline.

OTHER SERVICES FROM WESTERN UNION. Your Western Union office will make and confirm hotel or motel reservations. They will sometimes call as many as eight hotels or motels in the same city in order to get the accommodations you wish.

It is possible to send money by telegraph and cable to all parts of the world. Payments in foreign countries are made in the currency of that country. In addition to the amount of money being wired, you must pay for the cost of a 15-word telegram or a 100-word overnight telegram, plus a service charge based on the amount of money to be sent.

Western Union offers many additional services, although there would be little need for most of them in the average doctor's office.

References

What Every Telephone User Should Know, General Telephone System
Your Telephone Personality, Bell Telephone System
Your Voice is You, Bell Telephone System
The Business Side of Medical Practice, American Medical Association, 1979.

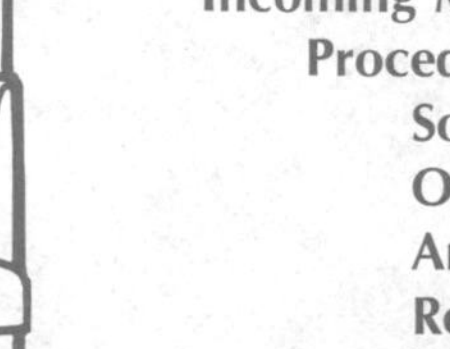

CHAPTER OUTLINE

- Incoming Mail
  - Procedure for Handling
    - Sorting
    - Opening
    - Annotating
    - Responding
  - Mail the Assistant Can Handle
    - Cash Receipts and Insurance Forms
    - Drug Samples
- Outgoing Mail
  - Classifications of Mail
  - Size Standards for Domestic Mail
  - Postal Services
    - Air Mail
    - International Mail
    - Priority Mail
    - Special Delivery
    - Special Handling
    - Express Mail Service
    - Mailgram
    - Certificate of Mailing
    - Certified Mail
    - Registered Mail
    - Insured Mail
    - Postal Money Orders
  - Handling Special Problems
    - Forwarding Mail
    - Change of Address
    - Recalling Mail
    - Returned Mail
    - Tracing Lost Mail
  - Preparing the Outgoing Mail
    - Sealing and Stamping Hints
    - Sorting and Banding
    - Getting Faster Mail Service
  - Postage Meters
    - Postage Economy
  - Vacation Mail

BEHAVIORAL OBJECTIVES

The medical office assistant should be able to:

- **Open, sort, and annotate incoming mail.**
- **Prepare newly arrived correspondence for response.**
- **Handle cash receipts, insurance forms, and drug samples.**
- **Select correct class of postage.**
- **Select appropriate special postal services as required.**
- **Prepare outgoing mail for posting.**
- **Operate and monitor postage meter.**
- **Post mailing.**
- **Plan appropriate procedure for handling vacation mail.**

9

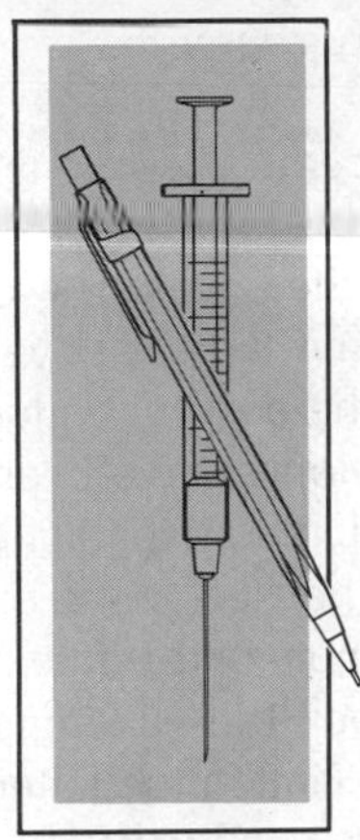

PROCESSING THE MAIL

Probably no other business or professional person receives more mail than a physician. Into his office each day pours a variety of mail: letters from patients and other physicians, payments for services, bills for office purchases, laboratory reports, hospital reports, medical society mailings, flashy promotional pieces and samples from drug houses, advertisements from equipment houses, requests for contributions, professional periodicals, and other personal mail.

In large clinics the mail is opened by specially delegated persons in some central department to speed up this daily task. But in the average professional office, the assistant or secretary opens the mail, using the tried and true letter-opener method.

INCOMING MAIL

Procedure for Handling

Before opening any mail, a new assistant in a doctor's office should ask her employer what procedure she should follow in regard to incoming mail. In other words, what letters should the assistant open and what pieces does the doctor prefer to open himself? If there is any doubt in the assistant's mind in regard to opening a letter, the best rule to follow is, Don't! Treat your doctor's mail with the same consideration you expect others to exercise toward your own. Assuming you have been instructed to sort and open all except personal items, here are some suggestions for proceeding efficiently.

SORTING. When mail arrives, usually early in the morning, it should be separated according to importance and urgency. Before settling down to this daily task, assemble the tools and supplies you will need: a letter opener, paper clips, stapler, transparent tape, and date stamp. Here is a rule-of-thumb sorting guide:

1. Mailgrams or special delivery letters
2. Checks from patients
3. Doctor's personal mail
4. Ordinary first class mail
5. Periodicals and newspapers
6. All other classes, including drug samples

OPENING. Even such a simple procedure as opening the day's mail can be done with more efficiency if a good system is followed (Fig. 9–1). Have a clear working space on your desk or counter. Stack the envelopes so that they are all facing in the same direction. Pick up the top one and tap the envelope so that when you open it you will not cut the contents. Open the envelope along the top edge for easiest removal of contents. When all the envelopes have been opened, start removing their contents. As each envelope is emptied, hold it to the light to see that nothing remains inside, then discard it after you have checked to see that there is a return address on the message contained inside. Make a note of the date of postmark if this is important. (Some offices make it a policy to attach the envelope to each piece of correspondence until it has received attention.) Flatten the letter and attach any enclosures. If there is an enclosure notation at the bottom of the letter, check to be sure the enclosure was included. Should it be missing, indicate this on the notation by writing the word "no" and circling it. After all the envelopes have been emptied, date stamp each letter or write the date in pencil at the top. Sometimes the letter bears no date, or possibly one which does not correspond closely to the date received. It may be that this is as far as your employer will want you to proceed with handling the correspondence.

ANNOTATING. You can be of far greater service if you are permitted to read each letter through, underlining the significant words and phrases, and noting in the

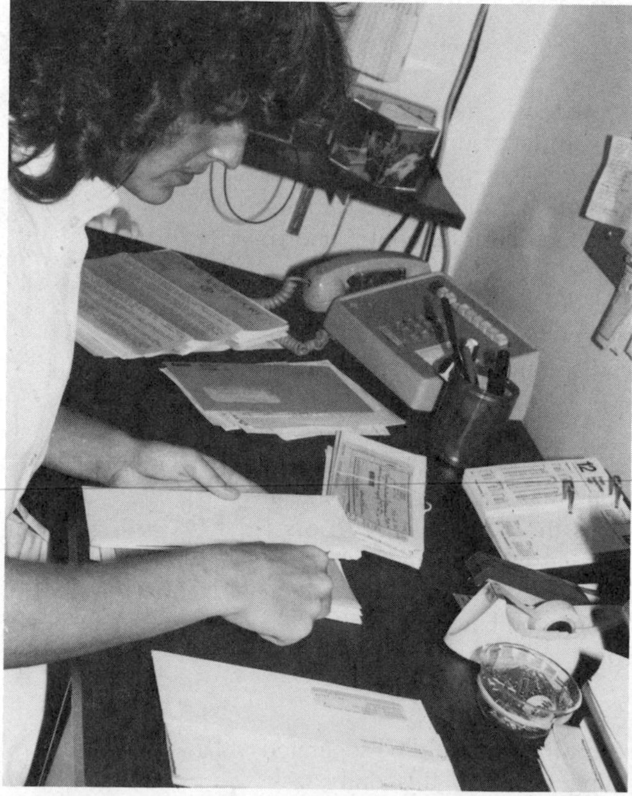

FIGURE 9–1 The medical office assistant opening the mail.

margin any action required. This is called **annotating.** If it is a letter that needs no reply, you can code it for filing at this time. A non-print pencil that does not photocopy may be used for the annotating if desired.

When mail refers to previous correspondence, secure this from the file and attach it. Or if a patient's chart is needed in replying to an inquiry, pull the chart and place it with the letter.

A definite place should be agreed upon for placing the opened mail for your doctor's perusal. This will probably be some spot on his desk. When you have completed the sorting, opening, and annotating of mail, place those items that the doctor will wish to see in the established place, with the most important mail on top. Personal mail, of course, is unopened. Should you in error open a piece of personal mail addressed to your employer, fold and replace it inside the envelope, and write across the outside "Opened in error," followed by your initials. Use the same procedure with a piece of mail addressed to another office that may have been opened in error. In that case, reseal the envelope with transparent tape, and hand it to your carrier.

RESPONDING TO THE MAIL. In some offices the doctor and the assistant go over the pieces of mail together. As you gain confidence, you will find that you can draft a reply to some inquiries. Most doctors are very pleased to relinquish this responsibility, especially on matters that do not relate to patient care.

Letters of referral from other physicians should be carefully noted so that an answer may be sent after the doctor has seen the patient and can give a report. If considerable time may pass before such information can be sent, it is a nice policy to write a note to the referring physician thanking him and advising him that a detailed letter will follow. Some physicians send printed cards expressing thanks for referrals; others prefer to write thank-you letters to professional colleagues.

Mail the Assistant Can Handle

CASH RECEIPTS AND INSURANCE FORMS. There will be some mail that the assistant can handle alone, for instance, payments from patients and insurance forms to be completed. All cash and checks should be separated and recorded immediately in the day's receipts. Insurance forms should be placed with the patient's history on your desk for attention at a time during the day when it is convenient for you to handle them. Do not place them where they may be covered with other papers, and misplaced or forgotten; have a specific place where you will keep insurance forms. If there is an insurance clerk or other individual who processes the claims, they should be passed along to that person immediately or to a predetermined place for pick-up.

DRUG SAMPLES. Frequently the mail brings in samples and related literature. The assistant should learn from the doctor what types of literature and samples he wishes to have placed on his desk for review. For example, a psychiatrist probably would not be greatly interested in a new vitamin preparation for expectant mothers. Most physicians keep pertinent new samples in their desks, along with the accompanying literature for immediate reference. Other samples are placed in the sample cabinet in their respective categories. Many offices maintain a "catch-all" box for samples that are of no interest. Contents of these boxes are generally given to a medical charity clinic or a medical missionary. In some areas the woman's auxiliary to the medical association makes this its project. Samples should never be tossed into the trash. Too many people who are in need of care can make use of these valuable preparations. There is also the danger that youngsters may find the discarded samples and experiment with them; the result could be disastrous.

Pharmaceutical companies have drastically reduced the distribution of unrequested drug samples to physicians. However, many companies will provide specific medications when requested in writing, either for the physician's own use or for a poor patient, not on public assistance, who is financially unable to otherwise obtain necessary medications.

OUTGOING MAIL

Mail also pours out from the professional office. The mailing costs for even a small office are a sizable item in the annual budget. The greater the assistant's knowledge of the U. S. Postal Service, the more the doctor will get for his postage dollar. In addition to saving postage dollars, the knowledgeable assistant can utilize many special postal services. But first she must be aware of what services are available, what type of service best fits each situation, and how to handle unusual postal problems. *The Postal Manual* may be purchased from the Superintendent of Documents, U. S. Government Printing Office, Washington, DC 20402. Smaller publications that contain basic postal information are available without charge from local post offices. A summary of the most common services are described in this chapter.

Classifications of Mail

Mail is classified according to type, weight, and destination. The ounce and pound are the units of measurement. Here are types of mail commonly handled in a medical office.

FIRST CLASS MAIL. Sealed or unsealed handwritten or typed material, such as letters, postal cards, post cards, and business reply mail.

SECOND CLASS MAIL. Newspaper and periodical publications. Publishers who mail in bulk lots and who have been granted second class mail privileges pay a special second class rate. Copies mailed unsealed by the public go by *transient rate,* ten cents for the first two ounces and six cents for each additional ounce, or the fourth class rate, whichever is lower.

THIRD CLASS MAIL. Printed matter or merchandise weighing up to but not including 16 ounces not included in first or second class. Third class mail includes such things as catalogs, circulars, books, photographs, and other printed matter, and even seeds, bulbs, keys, and so forth. Pieces should be sealed or secured so that they can be handled by machine but must be clearly marked with the two words "Third Class." Mailing of sealed articles at the third class rate carries the implied consent of the mailer to postal inspection of the contents.

FOURTH CLASS MAIL (PARCEL POST). Merchandise, books, printed matter, and so forth not included in first or second class, and weighing 16 ounces or more but not exceeding 70 pounds. There are also size limitations on fourth class mail; check with your post office regarding regulations on very large parcels. Rates are determined on the basis of weight and destination. Such mail may be sealed or unsealed.

COMBINATION MAILING. A first class letter may be sent along with a parcel, either by placing the letter in an envelope and attaching it to the outside of the package or by enclosing it within the parcel and writing on the outside, just below the space for postage, "Letter Enclosed." In either case, separate postage is paid for the letter. This method is often used in the physician's office when mailing x-rays and an accompanying letter. This type of mailing travels with the appropriate class for the package, not with first class letters.

EDUCATIONAL MATERIALS. A special rate, lower than regular fourth class, is applicable for educational materials. This includes bound books of 24 or more pages, manuscripts for books, sound recordings and films, and printed tests. The package must be marked "Educational Materials." This was formerly called the *book rate.*

Size Standards for Domestic Mail

NONSTANDARD MAIL. The Postal Service assesses a surcharge on each piece of nonstandard mail in addition to the applicable postage and fees. The following material is considered nonstandard mail. First class mail weighing one ounce or less and single piece third-class mail weighing two ounces or less which:

(1) Exceeds any of the following:
Height — 6-1/8 inches
Length — 11-1/2 inches
Thickness — 1/4 inch

(2) Has a height-to-length ratio that does not fall between 1:1.3 and 1:2.5 inclusive.

MINIMUM MAIL SIZES. All mail must be at least .007 of an inch thick and mail which is 1/4 inch or less in thickness must be:

(1) at least 3-1/2 inches in height and at least 5 inches long, and
(2) rectangular in shape.

Postal Services

Different types of mail require different handling by the post office. Make sure you classify your mail appropriately.

Mail traveling long distances may be given special treatment.

AIR MAIL. Most domestic mail to distances greater than 300 miles travels by air, but it is no longer necessary to use special air mail postage.

INTERNATIONAL MAIL. Sending mail to distant points of the globe has become quite commonplace. In almost all cases, letters will be sent air mail and can be expected to reach their destination within a very few days. First class mail to Canada and Mexico travels at the same rate as within the United States. A table of international rates can be obtained from your local post office. The rate of international mail is based on one-half ounce. Aerogrammes, a thin air mail-weight sheet of paper which can be folded for mailing and which does not require an envelope, can be purchased at the post office (currently 22 cents) and used for sending messages anywhere in the world. In some cases this is a considerable savings. Writing can be on only one side and no enclosures are permitted. Aerogrammes are convenient as well as inexpensive. If you wish to supply a foreign correspondent with reply postage, international reply coupons may be purchased at the post office and sent to other countries.

PRIORITY MAIL. Heavy pieces weighing over 12 ounces may be sent by air for a fee somewhat higher than parcel post. The rate is determined by weight and destination. The minimum fee is $1.71 to $2.25 for up to one pound, depending upon destination.

SPECIAL DELIVERY. Any class mail that has been so marked will be charged the special delivery rate. Such pieces may be regular first or second class mail, registered, insured, or COD (Collect on Delivery) pieces. Special delivery instruction generally does not speed up the normal travel time between two cities but does assure immediate delivery of the item when it arrives at the designated post office. Special delivery stamps may be purchased at the post office or the equivalent value in regular stamps may be placed upon the envelope, which should always be clearly marked "Special Delivery." The current (1980) rate is $2.00 plus regular postage. Use Special Delivery when you need delivery the same day the item is received at the addressee's post office, including weekend delivery not available with regular mail. Do not use for mail addressed to a Post Office Box or military installation.

SPECIAL HANDLING. Applied only to third and fourth class mail. For a small additional fee, these two classes will receive the fastest handling and ground transportation practicable, about the same as first class mail. This does not include insurance or special delivery at the destination, but special delivery, if desired, is available at an added fee. If a parcel is sent by priority mail, special handling is of no additional advantage because it is already traveling at the greatest possible speed. Fees are determined according to weight; currently 70 cents for up to 10 pounds, $1.25 for more than 10 pounds, in addition to regular postage.

EXPRESS MAIL SERVICE. This service is based on a high-speed delivery network linking all major cities in the United States as well as many smaller communities. One of its features is a Downtown-to-Downtown service which guarantees that if you mail by 5 p.m. at the designated window, your urgent communication or parcel will be ready for pickup at the receiving post office at 10 a.m. the next business day or will be delivered by 3 p.m. Five other service options are available on a contract basis under Express Mail: (1) door to door, (2) your door to a destination airport, (3) originating airport to addressee, (4) airport to airport, and (5) United States to England. Check with your local post office for the availability of Express Mail service in your area.

MAILGRAM. A popular service offered jointly by the Postal Service and Western Union. Described in Chapter 8 under Telegraph Services.

There are also ways to insure proper delivery of valuable or important pieces of mail.

CERTIFICATE OF MAILING. If a sender needs proof of mailing but is not especially concerned with proof of receipt of an item, the most economical method is to obtain a Certificate of Mailing. Fill in the required information, attach a ten-cent stamp, and hand it to the postal clerk along with the piece of mail. The clerk will postmark the receipt, initial it, and hand it back as acknowledgment of having received the piece of mail at the post office. This is sometimes used when mailing income tax reports or other items that must be posted by a certain date.

CERTIFIED MAIL. This provides the sender of domestic mail with a receipt of delivery if requested and fee paid. A record of delivery is kept at the post office of delivery for two years. However, no record is kept at the post office at which it is mailed, and this type of mail does not provide insurance coverage. Anything without intrinsic value you wish to mail on which postage is paid at the first class rate will be accepted as certified mail. Such items as contracts, deeds, mortgages, bank books, checks, passports, insurance policies, money orders, and birth certificates, which are not valuable intrinsically but would be hard to duplicate if lost, should be certified. Certified mail can be sent special delivery if the prescribed additional fees are paid. The assistant should keep a supply of certified mail forms and return receipts on hand (Figs. 9–2 and 9–3). These may be obtained at any post office. The current fee for certified mail, in addition to regular postage, is 80 cents. If a return receipt is desired, an additional fee of 45 cents is necessary. Other services are available for additional fees, such as restricted delivery, address of delivery, and date of delivery. Full instructions are included on the forms. Fees and postage may be paid by ordinary postage stamps, meter stamps, or permit imprint. Certified mail can be mailed at any post office, station, or branch, or can be deposited in mail drops or in street letter boxes if you follow specific directions. Certified mail is often used as an aid in collections.

REGISTERED MAIL. All classes of mail, particularly those of unusually high value, can be given additional protection, together with evidence of having been delivered, if registered. Registering mail also helps trace delivery. When sending a registered letter it is necessary to go to the post office and fill in the required forms. All articles to be registered must be thoroughly sealed (do not use cellophane tape) and postage paid at first class rates. Upon receipt of the item, the recipient is required to sign a form, acknowledging receipt of delivery. A registered letter may be released to the person to whom it is sent or to his agent. For an additional fee, a personal receipt may be requested. This assures that the letter will be released only to the individual to whom it is addressed. Such pieces bear the label "To Addressee Only." Registered mail is accounted for by number from time of mailing until delivery and is transported separately from other mail under a special lock. In case of loss or damage the customer may be reimbursed up to $10,000, provided the value of the registered articles has been declared at the time of mailing and the appropriate fee has been paid. Minimum registry fee is $3.00 in addition to postage, and is based upon declared value of up to $100. Fees increase based on value declared.

INSURED MAIL. Third or fourth class mail that has been insured against loss. All packages valued at more than $25 and not registered should be insured. Parcel post packages may be *registered* with postage paid at the first class rate, but generally they are insured instead of registered. Indemnity on insured mail is limited to $400.

POSTAL MONEY ORDERS. Postal money orders are a convenient way of mailing money, especially for the individual who does not have a personal checking account. Postal money orders may be purchased in amounts as high as $400. If a sum greater than $400 is needed, additional money orders must be purchased in

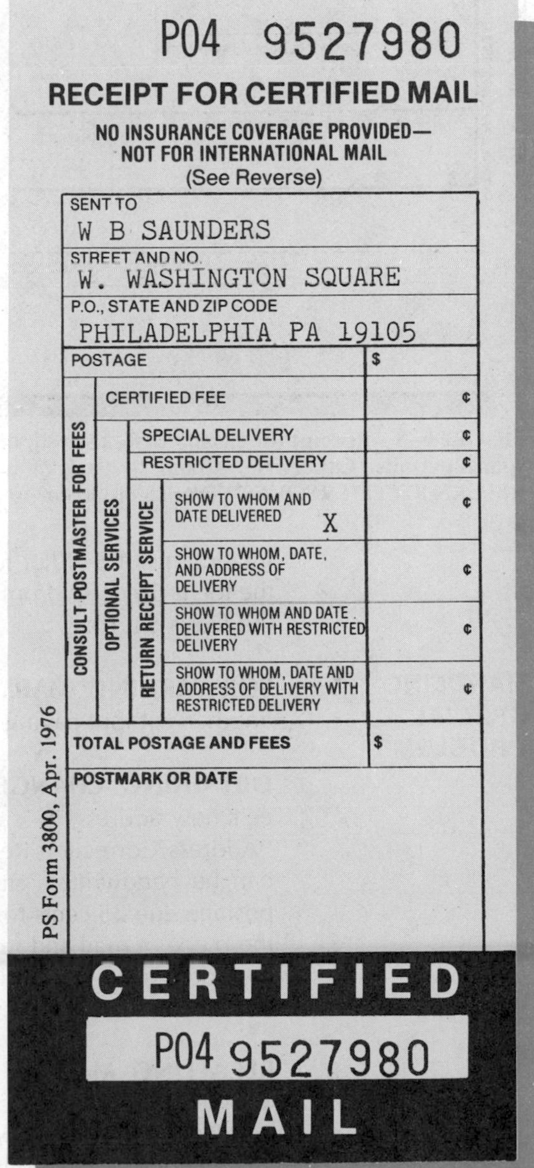
P04 9527980

RECEIPT FOR CERTIFIED MAIL

NO INSURANCE COVERAGE PROVIDED—NOT FOR INTERNATIONAL MAIL
(See Reverse)

SENT TO W B SAUNDERS				
STREET AND NO. W. WASHINGTON SQUARE				
P.O., STATE AND ZIP CODE PHILADELPHIA PA 19105				
POSTAGE				$
CONSULT POSTMASTER FOR FEES	CERTIFIED FEE			¢
	OPTIONAL SERVICES	SPECIAL DELIVERY		¢
		RESTRICTED DELIVERY		¢
		RETURN RECEIPT SERVICE	SHOW TO WHOM AND DATE DELIVERED X	¢
			SHOW TO WHOM, DATE, AND ADDRESS OF DELIVERY	¢
			SHOW TO WHOM AND DATE DELIVERED WITH RESTRICTED DELIVERY	¢
			SHOW TO WHOM, DATE AND ADDRESS OF DELIVERY WITH RESTRICTED DELIVERY	¢
TOTAL POSTAGE AND FEES				$
POSTMARK OR DATE				

PS Form 3800, Apr. 1976

CERTIFIED
P04 9527980
MAIL

FIGURE 9–2 **Attach to front of envelope on the left of the address.**

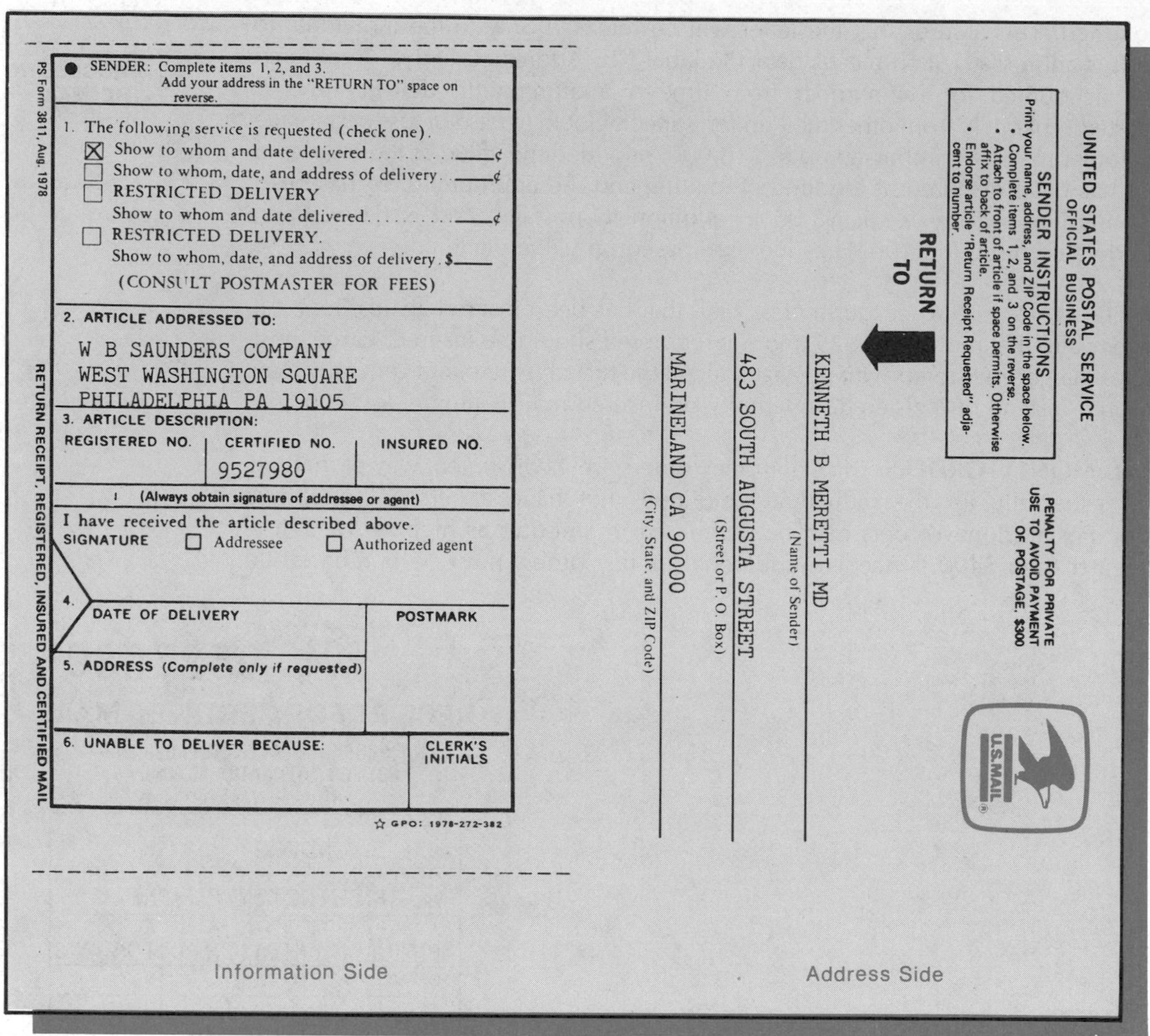

PS Form 3811, Aug. 1978 — RETURN RECEIPT, REGISTERED, INSURED AND CERTIFIED MAIL

● SENDER: Complete items 1, 2, and 3.
Add your address in the "RETURN TO" space on reverse.

1. The following service is requested (check one).
[X] Show to whom and date delivered .... ¢
[ ] Show to whom, date, and address of delivery .. ¢
[ ] RESTRICTED DELIVERY
Show to whom and date delivered .... ¢
[ ] RESTRICTED DELIVERY.
Show to whom, date, and address of delivery . $
(CONSULT POSTMASTER FOR FEES)

2. ARTICLE ADDRESSED TO:
W B SAUNDERS COMPANY
WEST WASHINGTON SQUARE
PHILADELPHIA PA 19105

3. ARTICLE DESCRIPTION:

REGISTERED NO.	CERTIFIED NO.	INSURED NO.
	9527980	

(Always obtain signature of addressee or agent)

I have received the article described above.
SIGNATURE [ ] Addressee [ ] Authorized agent

4. DATE OF DELIVERY — POSTMARK

5. ADDRESS (Complete only if requested)

6. UNABLE TO DELIVER BECAUSE: — CLERK'S INITIALS

☆ GPO: 1978-272-382

UNITED STATES POSTAL SERVICE
OFFICIAL BUSINESS

SENDER INSTRUCTIONS
Print your name, address, and ZIP Code in the space below.
• Complete items 1, 2, and 3 on the reverse.
• Attach to front of article if space permits. Otherwise affix to back of article.
• Endorse article "Return Receipt Requested" adjacent to number.

PENALTY FOR PRIVATE USE TO AVOID PAYMENT OF POSTAGE, $300

RETURN TO

KENNETH B MERETTI MD
(Name of Sender)
483 SOUTH AUGUSTA STREET
(Street or P. O. Box)
MARINELAND CA 90000
(City, State, and ZIP Code)

U.S.MAIL

Information Side — Address Side

FIGURE 9–3 Receipt for Certified, Registered, or Insured Mail. Attach to front of article if space permits. Otherwise, attach to back of article and endorse front of article with RETURN RECEIPT REQUESTED adjacent to the number.

increments of $400 or less. The rates are reasonable. Currently (1980) for up to $10 the fee is 55 cents; from $10.01 to $50 the fee is 80 cents; and from $50.01 to $400 the fee is $1.10.

HANDLING SPECIAL PROBLEMS

FORWARDING MAIL. First class mail only may be forwarded from one city to another without paying additional postage.

OBTAINING CHANGE OF ADDRESS. If the mailer wants to know an addressee's new address, he can get this service from the post office by placing the words "Address Correction Requested" beneath the return address on the envelope. This can be handwritten, stamped, typewritten or printed. The post office will charge postage due 25 cents for this service. For first class mail, the post office will forward the piece of mail and return a card to the sender showing the forwarding address of the addressee. The card will have a postage due stamp on it for the amount of the required fee.

RECALLING MAIL. If you have dropped a letter in the mailbox and want it back, do not ask the mail collector to give it to you; he is not permitted to do this. Mail can be recalled, however, by making written application at the post office, together with an envelope addressed identically to the one being recalled. If your letter has already left the local post office, the postmaster, at the sender's expense, can telephone or telegraph the postmaster at the destination post office to return the letter.

RETURNED MAIL. If a letter is returned to the sender after an attempt has been made to deliver it, it cannot be remailed without new postage. It is best simply to prepare a new envelope with the correct address, affix the proper postage, and re-mail.

TRACING LOST MAIL. Receipts issued by the post office, whether for money orders, registered mail, or insured mail, should be retained until receipt of the item has been acknowledged. If after an adequate time elapses no acknowledgement of receipt for such mailing arrives, notify the post office to trace the letter or package. Regular first class mail is not easily traced, but the post office will make every attempt to find it for you. In tracing a lost letter or package, the post office requires that a special form be filled out, on which data from any original receipt should be written, along with any other identifying information.

PREPARING THE OUTGOING MAIL

SEALING AND STAMPING HINTS. Here's a suggestion for speeding up the sealing of a number of envelopes. At statement time, for example, many envelopes will be going into the mail at once. Fan out unsealed envelopes, address side down, in groups of six to ten. Then draw a damp sponge over the flaps and, starting with the lower piece, turn down the flaps and seal each one. Do not use too much moisture as this will cause the glue to spread and several letters will stick together.

A similar process simplifies stamping several letters at a time. If possible, purchase your stamps by the roll. Tear off about ten stamps. Fanfold them on the perforations so that they will separate easily. Again fan the envelopes, this time address side up. Wet a strip of stamps with the sponge and, starting at one end of the fanned envelopes, attach the stamp at the end of the strip, tear it off, and proceed to the next envelope.

SORTING AND BANDING. For large mailings, local letters should be separated from out-of-town letters and foreign letters that require special postage. Keep a supply of mail banding tapes on hand. The post office will supply these free of charge upon request — blue bands for local mail, red for out-of-town mail. The tapes are self-sealing and require no glue or rubber bands. Sort the mail according to destination and put a tape around each bundle before dropping it in a pickup box or taking it to the post office. This presorting greatly assists the postal clerks in the rapid routing of your mail.

GETTING FASTER MAIL SERVICE. Post offices that handle a large volume of mail will appreciate your mailing early in the day whenever possible. Place a letter tray on your desk or some other convenient place so that you can keep all outgoing mail together until you are able to send it on its way. Letters or packages that need to be rushed should be taken directly to the post office for mailing. Others can be placed in street boxes or your own building mail chute for pickup. Never leave packages on top of public mail boxes; these should always go to the post office.

POSTAGE METERS

Metered mail does not have to be canceled or postmarked when it reaches the post office. This means that it can move on to its destination faster. The postage meter is the most efficient way of stamping the mail in a business office (Fig. 9–4). Meters vary in size and capabilities. Consult your office equipment dealer for your own needs.

In order to use a postage meter, the user applies to the post office for a license, indicating the make and model of the meter he plans to use. The postage meter machine is purchased, but the meter itself is leased from the manufacturer. The meter must be taken to the post office, where the user pays in advance for a specified amount of postage. This is recorded by the post office on the dials of the postage

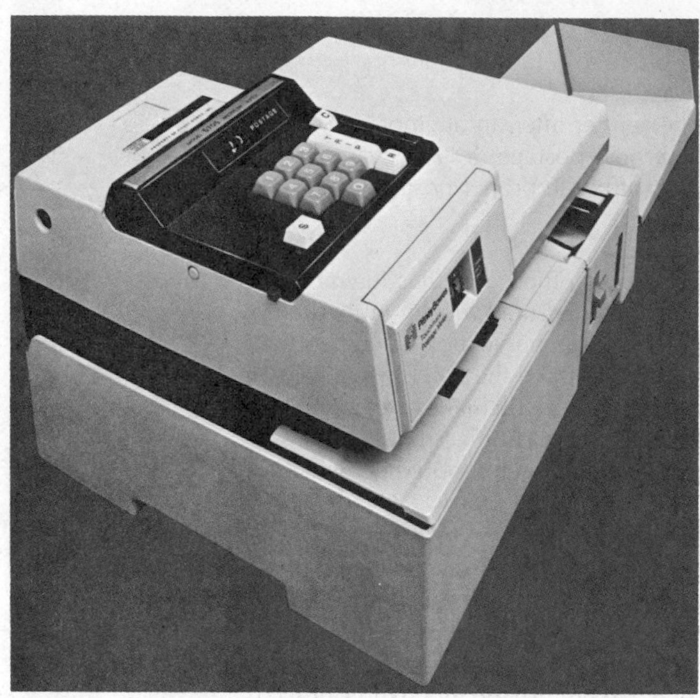

FIGURE 9–4 Example of one type of postage meter-mailing machine. (Courtesy of Pitney Bowes Company.)

meter. When the meter is in operation it records the amount of postage used and the amount remaining. Before the postage is exhausted the meter should be taken to the post office and more purchased. If the postage is entirely used up the meter locks until it is again taken to the post office and more postage purchased. Planning can avoid this inconvenience.

A WORD ABOUT POSTAGE ECONOMY. Although mailing fees are still one of our better bargains, carelessness can cause them to soar. If your office does not have a postage meter that dispenses postage exactly, then be sure that you are not putting too many stamps on your outgoing mail. A one-ounce letter costs 18 cents; a two-ounce letter costs 30 cents, not 36 cents. The first ounce of the letter is the only one that costs 18 cents. Frequent overpaying can add considerably to the annual postage expense. Check the accuracy of your postal scale periodically, too.

VACATION MAIL

When the doctor is away from the office, it is generally the responsibility of his assistant to handle all mail. In this event, all pieces should be studied carefully. The assistant must then make her decision in regard to handling each piece on the basis of these questions:

1. Is this important enough that I should call or wire the doctor?
2. Shall I forward this to him for his immediate attention?
3. Shall I answer this myself or send a brief note explaining that there will be a slight delay because the doctor is out of his office?
4. Can this wait for attention until the doctor returns without appearing negligent?

If you are unable to contact your employer or to forward important mail to him, always answer the sender immediately, explaining the delay and asking his cooperation. Most offices have some kind of copy machine as part of the office equipment. Instead of forwarding the original of important pieces of mail to your employer when he is away, and risking possible loss, make a copy for forwarding. Then if he wishes you to answer the letter he can make notations on the copy and return it to you without defacing the original letter.

If your employer is traveling from place to place, each envelope you send him should be numbered consecutively. By doing this he can easily determine whether any mail has been lost or gone astray. By keeping your own record of each piece of mail sent out, with its corresponding number, anything that does not reach him can be identified and remailed if necessary.

Correspondence that does not require immediate action, but which the assistant is unable to answer until the doctor returns, should be placed in a special folder on the doctor's desk, marked "Requires Attention." Mail that the assistant can answer, but which requires the doctor's approval before mailing, should be put into another special folder, marked "For Approval." When the doctor returns, he can then rapidly check and sign these letters for mailing.

Letters marked "Personal" which you hesitate to open and are unable to forward may be acknowledged to the return address on the envelope. The brief acknowledgment should state that the doctor is out of town for a certain length of time and will give the letter his attention upon his return. Your acknowledgment should also offer your help in any way possible in the meantime.

Discard any mail which it is unnecessary for the doctor to see, if at all possible. Some promotional literature will fall into this class. (Make certain, however, that mailings from his professional organizations, whether they are first, second, third, or fourth class, reach his desk.)

Although it is rare, there may be occasions when the entire office is closed. In such cases, the local post office should be notified to forward all first class mail to an address supplied by the doctor, if possible. Your postal carrier cannot accept an oral request that he leave the mail with the person next door for a few days. A formal request must be made. If forwarding is out of the question, place a request with the post office to hold the mail until your return. Never leave mail unattended to gather outside a mailbox or clutter up a doorway in a hall. Even mail slots may become filled or magazines become stuck in them, causing important mail to pile up outside the slot. There is far too much money sent to doctors' offices to take chances on mail theft. In addition, other important pieces of mail for the doctor may become lost under such circumstances.

Systematizing your routine for processing all incoming and outgoing mail can put you in control of the paper blizzard!

Reference

The Postal Manual, Superintendent of Documents, U. S. Government Printing Office, Washington, D.C.

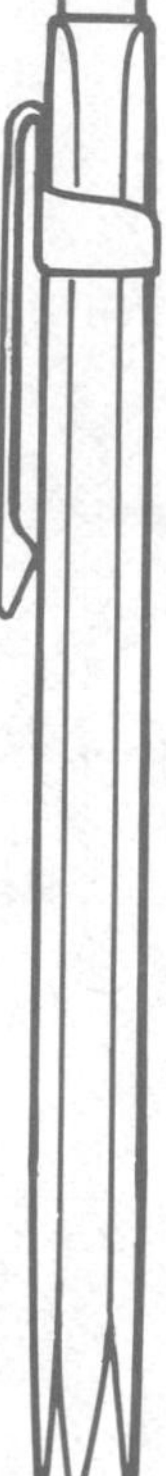

CHAPTER OUTLINE

Equipment
Stationery
Language Skills
- Spelling
- Transcription
- Editing and Proofreading

Letter Styles and Punctuation
Parts of Letters
Signature
Composing Responsibilities
Writing Style
Addressing the Envelope
Folding and Inserting Letters

BEHAVIORAL OBJECTIVES

The medical office assistant should be able to:

- **Produce mailable copy from dictation.**
- **Compose original letters.**
- **Initiate routine letter response.**
- **Demonstrate knowledge of correct letter styles.**
- **Edit and proofread.**
- **Demonstrate knowledge of grammar and spelling.**
- **Demonstrate knowledge of medical terminology.**
- **Develop time-saving skills in composing.**
- **Write instructions for patients.**
- **Address envelopes for optical scanning.**
- **Correctly fold letters.**

10

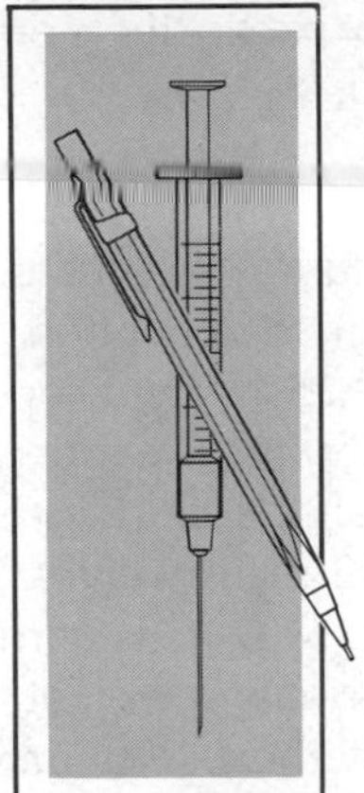

WRITTEN COMMUNICATIONS

Written communications offer a beautiful opportunity for making a good impression on others — but it won't just happen automatically. It takes thought, preparation, skill, and a caring attitude. Written communications take many forms in the medical office. The assistant may be required to transcribe from machine or shorthand dictation, compose original letters, reply to inquiries, respond to requests for information, write collection letters, order supplies, write instructions for patients, type consultation and surgical reports, as well as process a variety of other communications. Written communications should be *courteous* to the reader, *correct* in content, and *concise* without being *curt*. In order to create a good impression, one must begin with good equipment and quality stationery.

EQUIPMENT

The typewriter used should be one that will produce good copy; the typewriter ribbon should be dark enough that the letters will be easily read but not so heavily inked as to result in smudged copy. The keys to the typewriter must be kept clean. This is easily accomplished by the regular use of a commercial cushion sheet made especially for this purpose that cleans the keys as you type on it. If the typewriter is equipped with a carbon ribbon, the type will be uniform, never lighter or darker, and the keys will not fill with ink from the ribbon.

Many of the newer typewriters are single element typewriters — that is, the type is on a ball or element, rather than on keys. The carriage is immovable, and consequently quieter, and requires less desk space. This seems ideal for the professional office. A variety of type styles are available, and the element can be changed in a moment to what is best suited for the kind of copy being produced. If, in addition, the typewriter is dual-pitch, it can be changed from pica type, with 10 characters to the linear inch, to elite type, with 12 characters to the linear inch, by the flip of a switch. The single element typewriter with dual-pitch allows great versatility in the appearance of written communications. Professional correspondence usually looks best when done with the smaller elite type; reports may preferably be done with the larger pica type. Both elite and pica produce the standard six vertical lines to the inch.

The typewriter may also have a correction device that lifts an incorrect character off the paper, allowing the typist to put in the correct character with no visible evidence of an error having occurred.

STATIONERY

The quality of paper used unquestionably affects the total impression on the reader. Your stationer or printer is qualified to advise on the selection of paper, which can range from all-sulfite (a wood pulp) to all-cotton fiber (sometimes called rag). Letterhead paper is usually made of 25 percent, or more, cotton fiber bond. The weight of paper is described by a substance number. This number is based on the weight of a ream consisting of 500 sheets of 17 by 22 inch paper. The larger the number, the heavier the paper. If the ream weighs 24 pounds, the paper will be referred to as Sub 24 or 24-pound weight. Letterhead stationery and matching envelopes are usually 16-, 20-, or 24-pound weight.

There are three basic sizes of letterhead: Standard; Monarch or Executive; and Baronial. Standard letterhead, 8-½ × 11 inches, is used for general business and professional correspondence. Some executives and professional persons also have letterheads in Monarch (Executive) size, 7-¼ × 10-½ inches, for informal business and social correspondence. The third size, which is a half-sheet called Baronial, 5-½ × 8-½ inches, is used for very short letters or memoranda. Each size letterhead should have its matching envelope.

Continuation pages of a letter or report are typed on plain bond that matches the letterhead in weight and fiber content. Paper has a "felt" side and a "wire" side. Printing and typing is done on the felt side. Pick up a sheet of letterhead, hold it to the light, and you will see a design or letters than can be read from the printed side. This design is called a watermark and is an indication of quality. The side from which you can read the watermark is the "felt" side of the paper and is the side on which typing should be done. Always have the watermark read across the page in the same direction as the typing.

LANGUAGE SKILLS

Most persons, before they reach adulthood, have been exposed to considerable instruction in language skills. Unfortunately, through lack of use, much of the basic information is forgotten. A little book published by The Macmillan Company, *The Elements of Style*, by William Strunk, Jr. and E. B. White, is probably the most interesting and best refresher manual available. In its 78 pages, one can find practical information regarding punctuation, elementary principles of composition, explanations of many words and expressions commonly misused, and some very pointed hints on developing style in writing.

The medical office assistant needs a basic knowledge of composition, including sentence structure, spelling, and punctuation. An up-to-date standard dictionary, a medical dictionary, and a secretary's reference manual should be her constant companions.

SPELLING. If the assistant has difficulty with spelling, she may wish to keep a personal notebook or card index of words that are troublesome. Whenever it is necessary to look up a word in the dictionary for spelling, record it in the notebook or card index where it will be easy to refer to next time. If the assistant will purchase a small looseleaf notebook and index it alphabetically, she will find this a very convenient way to jot down words that give difficulty, and a handy way to find them in a hurry. The doctor or an assistant who is familiar with the practice might compile

TABLE 10–1 150 English Words Frequently Misspelled or Misused

absence	disastrous	newsstand	repetition
accede	discreet	noticeable	rheumatism
accessible	discrete	occasion	rhythmical
accommodate	discriminate	occurrence	ridiculous
achieve	dissatisfaction	oscillate	sacrilegious
affect	dissipate	paid	seize
agglutinate	drunkenness	pamphlet	separate
all right	ecstasy	panicky	siege
altogether	effect	parallel	similar
analyze	eligible	paralyze	sizable
analyses (pl.)	embarrass	pastime	stationary
analysis (s.)	exceed	perseverance	stationery
anoint	exhilaration	persistent	subpoena
argument	existence	personal	succeed
assistant	February	personnel	suddenness
auxiliary	forty	possession	superintendent
balloon	grammar	precede	supersede
believe	grievous	precedent	surprise
benefited	height	predictable	tariff
brochure	incidentally	predominant	technique
bulletin	indispensable	predominate	thorough
category	inimitable	prerogative	tranquility
changeable	inoculate	prevalent	transferred
clientele	insistent	principal	truly
committee	irrelevant	principle	tyrannize
comparative	irresistible	privilege	unnecessary
concede	irritable	procedure	until
conscientious	judgment	proceed	vacillate
conscious	labeled	professor	vacuum
coolly	led	pronunciation	vicious
corroborate	leisure	psychiatry	warrant
definitely	license	psychology	Wednesday
description	liquefy	pursue	weird
desirable	maintenance	questionnaire	
despair	maneuver	rearrange	
development	miscellaneous	recede	
dilemma	mischievous	receive	
disappear	misspell	recommend	
disappoint	necessary	referring	

TABLE 10–2 Medical Words Frequently Misspelled

abscess	epistaxis	metastasis	pneumonia
additive	eustachian	neurilemma	polyp
aerosol	fissure	neuron	prophylaxis
agglutination	flexure	occlusion	prostate
albumin	glaucoma	optic chiasm	prosthesis
anastomosis	gonorrhea	oscilloscope	pruritus
aneurysm	graafian	osseous	psoriasis
anteflexion	hemorrhage	palliative	pyrexia
arrhythmia	hemorrhoids	parasite	respiratory
bilirubin	homeostasis	parenteral	rheumatic
bronchial	humerus	parietal	roentgenology
cachexia	idiosyncrasy	paroxysmal	sagittal
calcaneus	ileum	pemphigus	sciatica
capillary	ilium	percussion	scirrhous
cervical	infarction	perforation	serous
chromosome	intussusception	pericardium	sessile
cirrhosis	ischemia	perineum	sphincter
clavicle	ischium	peristalsis	sphygmomanometer
curettage	larynx	peritoneum	squamous
cyanosis	leukemia	petit mal	staphylococcus
defibrillator	malaise	pharynx	suppuration
desiccate	malleus	pituitary	trochanter
ecchymosis	melena	plantar	venous
effusion	mellitus	pleura	wheal
epididymis	menstruation	pleurisy	xiphoid

a basic list of medical terms and abbreviations used in the practice, for the trainee. On page 133 there is a list of 150 frequently misspelled or misused English words (Table 10–1); above is a list of 100 frequently misspelled medical terms (Table 10–2). The individual assistant's list may be entirely different, depending upon her capabilities and the branch of medicine involved.

TRANSCRIPTION. Much of the doctor's correspondence is dictated either to a machine for later transcription (Fig. 10–1) or directly to the assistant who writes shorthand. In transcribing such dictation, it is the assistant's responsibility to check for errors in sentence structure, punctuate sentences correctly, and spell every word correctly. The transcriber should check the finished typewritten page *twice* — once for typing accuracy and once to be sure it makes sense. Never present material for signature unless it makes sense to you and is free of errors.

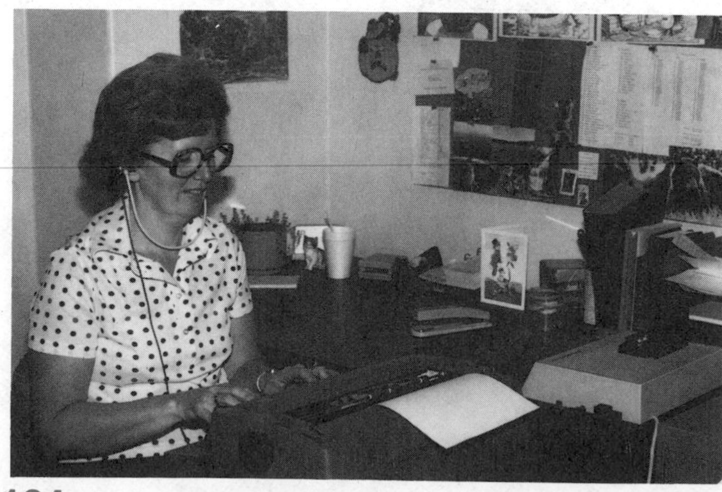

FIGURE 10–1 The medical office assistant using transcribing equipment.

EDITING AND PROOFREADING. Whether you are transcribing from shorthand or machine dictation, the material will probably need some editing. This involves proper placing of insertions, checking dates and spelling of names, sentence structure, and making all dictated changes. Many machine transcriptionists first type a rough draft on which they make corrections, and then retype for the final copy. Shorthand transcriptionists usually read over their notes for editing before typing the finished product. In making corrections, be certain not to change the meaning. When in doubt, ask! Before taking the final copy from the machine, check for any typographical errors. Corrections are more easily made before the paper is removed from the typewriter.

LETTER STYLES

A business letter is usually arranged in one of three styles: blocked, semiblocked, or full-blocked. A fourth, simplified style, is occasionally used. The blocked and semiblocked are most commonly used in the physician's office.

BLOCKED STYLE. The date line, the complimentary closing, and the typewritten signature all begin at the center. All other lines begin at the left margin (Fig. 10–2).

MEDICAL ARTS PROFESSIONAL ANNEX
3578 North Willow Avenue
Palm Beach, FL 33480

January 29, 1983

Elizabeth Blackwell, M.D.
223 Orange Avenue, N.W.
Cottonwood, UT 84121

Dear Doctor Blackwell:

We have two remaining street-level suites available for occupancy about July 1. These are marked on pages 3 and 4 of the enclosed descriptive brochure. If either of these suites appeals to you, we will be pleased to customize it for your practice.

Please feel free to call me collect at the number on the brochure for further discussion of your needs.

Sincerely yours,

Richard Fluege
Business Manager

RF:mk

Enc.

FIGURE 10–2 Blocked letter style.

WILLIAM OSLER, M.D.
1000 South West Street
Park Ridge, NJ 07656

January 26, 1983

Robert Koch, M.D.
398 Main Street
Park Ridge, NJ 07656

Dear Doctor Koch:

Mrs. Elaine Norris

Thank you for referring your patient, Mrs. Elaine Norris, for consultation and care. She was examined in the office today.

FINDINGS: The patient complained of pain in the left lower quadrant and some abdominal tenderness. She had a temperature of 100.2 degrees.

RECOMMENDATIONS: The patient was placed on a soft, low-residue, bland diet, antibiotics, and bedrest for a few days. Upper and lower gastrointestinal X-rays will be performed next week.

TENTATIVE DIAGNOSIS: Diverticulitis of large bowel.

Mrs. Norris has been asked to return here for re-evaluation in about ten days.

Sincerely yours,

William Osler, M.D.

WO:mk

FIGURE 10–3 Semi-blocked letter style.

ELIZABETH BLACKWELL, M.D.
223 Orange Avenue, N.W.
Cottonwood, UT 84121

January 26, 1983

Mr. Richard Fluege
3578 North Willow Avenue
Palm Beach, FL 33480

Dear Mr. Fluege:

Please send me full particulars on the professional suites you expect to offer for sale or rent in the Medical Arts Professional Annex.

In about six months I will be ready to open my practice, and I am interested in locating in Florida. My preference is a street-level suite of approximately 2,000 square feet.

After I have had an opportunity to study the information you send me, I will write or telephone you if I have further questions.

Very truly yours,

Elizabeth Blackwell, M.D.

EB:mk

FIGURE 10–4 Full blocked letter style.

SEMIBLOCKED STYLE. This is identical to the blocked style except that the first line of each paragraph is indented five spaces (Fig. 10–3).

FULL BLOCKED STYLE. All lines start flush with the left margin. This is considered more efficient but is less attractive on the page (Fig. 10–4).

SIMPLIFIED STYLE. All lines begin flush with the left margin. The salutation is replaced with an all-capital subject line on the third line below the inside address. The body of the letter begins on the third line below the subject line. The complimentary closing is omitted. An all-capital typewritten signature is typed on the fifth line below the body of the letter (Fig. 10–5).

PUNCTUATION

In dealing with letters we speak specifically of open punctuation, close punctuation, and mixed punctuation patterns. Traditionally, the punctuation pattern is selected on the basis of letter style. The message within the body of the letter is always punctuated with normal punctuation. The other parts follow one of the three following patterns.

OPEN PUNCTUATION. No punctuation is used at the end of any line outside the body of the letter unless that line ends with an abbreviation. This pattern is often used with the full-block and always in the simplified letter styles.

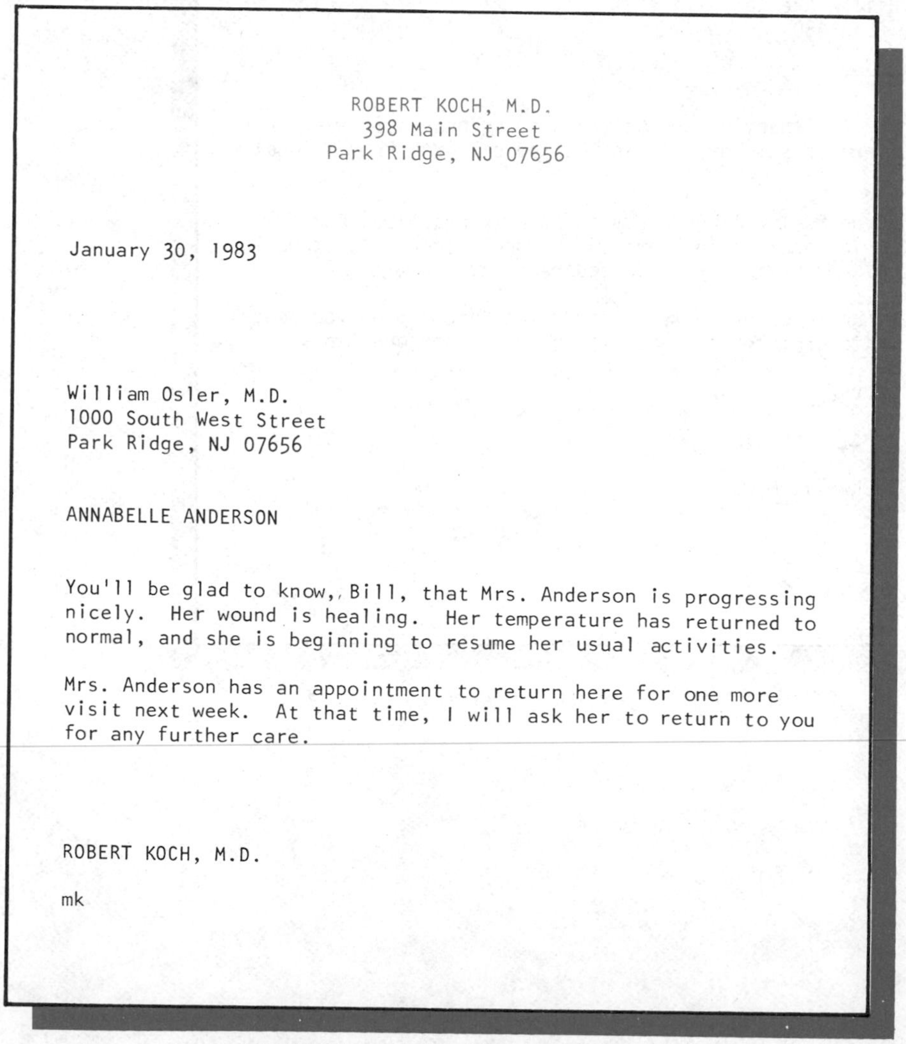

ROBERT KOCH, M.D.
398 Main Street
Park Ridge, NJ 07656

January 30, 1983

William Osler, M.D.
1000 South West Street
Park Ridge, NJ 07656

ANNABELLE ANDERSON

You'll be glad to know, Bill, that Mrs. Anderson is progressing nicely. Her wound is healing. Her temperature has returned to normal, and she is beginning to resume her usual activities.

Mrs. Anderson has an appointment to return here for one more visit next week. At that time, I will ask her to return to you for any further care.

ROBERT KOCH, M.D.

mk

FIGURE 10–5 Simplified letter style.

CLOSE PUNCTUATION. Each line outside the body of the letter ends with a comma or a period. Close punctuation is rarely used today.

MIXED (STANDARD) PUNCTUATION. A colon is placed after the salutation and a comma after the complimentary closing. This is the punctuation pattern most commonly used and is appropriate with the full-block, block, and semiblock letter styles.

PARTS OF LETTERS

The parts of letters and their placement are fairly standard but there is some degree of flexibility and some variation in published guidelines. Just remember the objective — an attractively arranged communication that reflects dignity and clarity and says to the reader what you want it to say.

LETTERHEAD. The printed letterhead is usually centered at the top of the page and includes the name of the physician or group and the address. It may include the telephone number and the medical specialty (specialties). In a group or corporate practice, the names of the physicians may also be listed.

DATE LINE. On standard stationery the date line is typed two to three lines below the last line of the letterhead or on line 15, whichever is lower. The name of the month is written in full, followed by the day and year. The date should not be abbreviated, nor should ordinal numbers such as 1st, 2nd, and 3rd be used following the name of the month.

INSIDE ADDRESS. The inside address has two or more lines, starts flush with the left margin, and contains at least the name of the individual or firm to whom the letter is addressed, and the post office address. When the letter is addressed to an individual the name is preceded by a courtesy title, such as Dr., Mr., Mrs., Miss, or Ms. When addressing a letter to a physician, omit the courtesy title and type the physician's name followed by his academic degree. Do not use a courtesy title and a degree that mean the same thing, such as *Dr.* Herbert H. Long, *M.D.*

ATTENTION LINE. The attention line, if used, is placed on the second line below the inside address. The current trend, however, is to avoid using an attention line. If you know the name of the person for whom the letter is intended, use that person's name in the inside address, and address him/her personally. Use the same procedure if the letter is being directed to a division or department within a company.

SALUTATION. The salutation is the letter writer's introductory greeting to the person being addressed. It is typed flush with the left margin on the second line below the last line of the inside address. It is followed by a colon unless open punctuation is used. The words used in the salutation will vary depending upon the degree of formality of the letter. In addressing a physician, spell out the word "Doctor" (Dear Doctor Long).

SUBJECT LINE. Often in medical office correspondence, the subject of a letter is the patient. The patient's name is used as the subject line. Because the subject line is considered a part of the body of the letter it is typed on the second line below the salutation. It may start flush with the left margin, at the point of indentation of indented paragraphs, or be centered. The word *Subject*, followed by a colon, may be used or may be omitted entirely.

BODY OF LETTER. Begin typing the body of the letter (the message) on the second line below the subject line or the second line below the salutation if there is no subject line. The first line of each paragraph may be indented 5 or 10 spaces, or may start flush with the left margin, depending upon the letter style being used.

COMPLIMENTARY CLOSE. The complimentary close is the writer's way of saying goodbye. The words used are determined by the degree of formality in the salutation. For instance, if the salutation is "Dear Herb:" the close might be "Cordially" or "Sincerely." If the letter is addressed to a business firm, the complimentary close generally used is "Very truly yours." The complimentary close is typed on the second line below the last line of the body of the letter, and followed by a comma unless open punctuation is used. Only the first word is capitalized.

TYPEWRITTEN SIGNATURE. Typing the name of the signer of the letter is a courtesy to the reader, especially if the name does not appear on the printed letterhead. Type the signature on the fourth line directly below the complimentary close.

REFERENCE INITIALS. The reference initials identify the dictator and the transcriptionist, and are typed flush with the left margin on the second line below the typed signature. If the secretary composes the letter, she uses only her own initials. There are variations in typing the reference initials, but the form most generally used has the dictator's initials in caps followed by a colon and the typist's initials in lower case (PF:mk).

ENCLOSURE AND CARBON COPY NOTATIONS. If the letter indicates an enclosure, type the word *Enclosure* or *Enc.* on the first or second line (authorities differ) below the reference initials. If there is more than one enclosure specify the number (Enclosures 3). If carbon copies are to be sent to others, type this notation in the same manner as the enclosure notation, or following it if both notations are needed. The carbon copy notation is usually written *cc: E. F. Duggan, M.D.* If more than one carbon copy is to be distributed, list the names of the individuals either alphabetically or according to rank.

SECOND PAGE HEADING. If the letter requires one or more continuation pages, the heading of the second and subsequent pages must contain three bits of information: the name of the addressee, the page number, and the date. Three accepted forms for the heading follow.

Elizabeth Blackwell, M.D. -2- March 14, 19xx

William Osler, M.D.
Page 2
March 14, 19xx

William S. Halsted, M.D.
Page 2
March 14, 19xx
Subject: Susan Barstow

The heading should be typed on the seventh line from the top of the page; continuation of the body of the letter begins on the tenth line or the third line below the heading.

Always carry at least two lines of the body of the letter over to the second page. Do not use a continuation page just to type the closing section of a business letter.

SIGNATURE

Some physicians prefer to sign all letters leaving their offices, but the majority do delegate to the assistant the responsibility of composing and signing some letters.

Although not all authorities agree on the form to be followed, most recommend that a woman's typewritten signature include a title, *Miss* or *Mrs.*, and that the title *not* be enclosed in parentheses. It is not necessary to include the title in the handwritten signature.

How will you know which letters to sign? In general, the doctor should sign all letters that deal with medical advice to patients, letters to officials of his medical society or chairmen of committees, referral and consultation reports to colleagues, medical reports to insurance companies, personal letters, and any other letters dictated for his personal signature.

The assistant usually signs letters of a strictly routine or business nature, such as arranging or rescheduling appointments, ordering office supplies, reserving hotel accommodations, notifying patients of surgery or hospital arrangements, collecting delinquent accounts, ordering subscriptions, and so forth.

COMPOSING RESPONSIBILITIES

Many doctors have said, when queried about the skills they most desire in an administrative assistant, "Send me an assistant who can write a good letter." When the physician delegates to the assistant the responsibility for composing letters (which will certainly reflect positively or negatively on his practice) this is a mark of confidence, a "plus" that increases the assistant's value to her employer.

Letter composition can be speeded up by developing a portfolio of sample letters to suit the various situations that arise. Suppose, for instance, you need to write a patient to change an appointment. Compose the very best letter you can — clear, concise, and courteous — and make an extra copy to place in your portfolio of letters. Do this each time you write a new kind of letter and soon you will be able to select a letter from your samples, change it slightly to suit the current situation, and you have letters written in no time. Watch for sample letters that appear from time to time in the doctor's journals that arrive regularly in your office, and clip them for your portfolio. Scan the textbooks and office manuals on the market or in your public library for additional help.

Written communications include more than letter writing. Those telephone messages you take, for instance. Are you sure they are clearly stated and convey to the reader what you intended? You may need to mail a prescription to a patient, with instructions from the doctor. Will the patient "read" what you intended to say? Communication is an art, as well as a skill. The ability to communicate effectively is extremely important to the medical assistant on the way "up the ladder."

COMPOSING TIPS. If your only experience in letter writing has been social correspondence, you'll have a new set of rules to learn. Social letters tend to be long and chatty, "I" oriented, and do not necessarily follow any organized plan. Most business letters should be less than one page long, "You" oriented, and carefully organized. This takes practice and preparation.

GETTING READY TO WRITE. If you are asked to answer a letter, first organize your facts.

1. Read carefully the letter you are to answer.
2. Make note of or underline any questions asked or materials requested.
3. Decide on the answers to the questions and verify your information.
4. Draft a reply, using the tools you're most comfortable with — typewriter, longhand, or shorthand.
5. Rewrite for clarity.

Keep most of your sentences short. Put only one idea in each sentence. Eliminate the superfluous words. Be careful about using medical terms in correspondence; use only language that the reader will understand.

There's a well-known expression, "I wrote a long letter because I didn't have time to write a short one."

WRITING STYLE

Every person who writes letters develops his/her own personal style. Most physicians conform to a highly professional, dignified style in their dictation. The assistant who is given the responsibility of composing some of the correspondence for the medical office should strive for the same degree of formality as the physician does. It would be inappropriate for the assistant to write in a breezy, informal style when she is acting as the representative of an employer who is strictly formal in approach. The main thing to remember is that every letter produced in your office should project the personality of the physician, irrespective of who signs it.

ADDRESSING THE ENVELOPE

By 1984 the Postal Service expects to have all mail (in No. 10 and No. 6-¾ envelopes) read, coded, sorted, and cancelled automatically at regional sorting stations where mail will be processed at the rate of 30,000 letters per hour. The success of automatic sorting depends upon the cooperation of mailers in preparing envelopes in the format that can be read by automatic equipment.

1. Type all envelope addresses in the blocked format and in the area on the envelope that the scanner is programmed to read:
   No. 10 envelope — Type the address 12 lines from the top of the envelope and four inches from the left edge of the envelope.
   No. 6-¾ envelope — Type the address 12 lines from the top of the envelope and 2-½ inches from the left edge of the envelope.
2. Capitalize everything in the address.
3. Eliminate all punctuation in the address.
4. Use the standard two-letter state code instead of the spelled out name of the state (Fig. 10–6).
5. The last line of the address must contain the city, state code, and Zip Code and it must not exceed 22 digits. The digits should be distributed so they will not exceed the following limits:

Allowance for city name	13
Space between city name and state code	1
Allowance for state code	2
Space between state code and Zip Code	1
Allowance for Zip Code	5
	22

If a city name contains more than 13 digits you must use the approved code for that city as shown in the Abbreviations Section of the National Zip Code Directory.

The Postal Service provides three special sets of abbreviations: (1) state names; (2) long names of cities, towns, and places; and (3) names of streets and roads and general terms like University or Institute. By using these abbreviations it is possible to limit the last line of any domestic address to 22 strokes (See Postal Service Publication 59.) The next-to-last line in the address block should contain a street address or post office box number.

MEDICAL ASSOCIATES INCORPORATED
4444 WILSHIRE BOULEVARD
LOS ANGELES CA 90013

HENRY B TURNER MD
PO BOX 845
ALBANY NY 12210

Leave a bottom margin of at least ⅝ inch and a left margin of at least 1 inch. Nothing should be written or printed below the address block or to the right of it.

Any notations on the envelope directed toward the addressee, for example "personal" or "confidential," should be typed two lines below the return address

TWO-LETTER ABBREVIATIONS

UNITED STATES AND TERRITORIES

Alabama	AL	Montana	MT
Alaska	AK	Nebraska	NE
Arizona	AZ	Nevada	NV
Arkansas	AR	New Hampshire	NH
California	CA	New Jersey	NJ
Canal Zone	CZ	New Mexico	NM
Colorado	CO	New York	NY
Connecticut	CT	North Carolina	NC
Delaware	DE	North Dakota	ND
District of Columbia	DC	Ohio	OH
Florida	FL	Oklahoma	OK
Georgia	GA	Oregon	OR
Guam	GU	Pennsylvania	PA
Hawaii	HI	Puerto Rico	PR
Idaho	ID	Rhode Island	RI
Illinois	IL	South Carolina	SC
Indiana	IN	South Dakota	SD
Iowa	IA	Tennessee	TN
Kansas	KS	Texas	TX
Kentucky	KY	Utah	UT
Louisiana	LA	Vermont	VT
Maine	ME	Virgin Islands	VI
Maryland	MD	Virginia	VA
Massachusetts	MA	Washington	WA
Michigan	MI	West Virginia	WV
Minnesota	MN	Wisconsin	WI
Mississippi	MS	Wyoming	WY
Missouri	MO		

CANADIAN PROVINCES AND TERRITORIES

Alberta	AB	Nova Scotia	NS
British Columbia	BC	Ontario	ON
Manitoba	MB	Prince Edward Island	PE
New Brunswick	NB	Quebec	PQ
Newfoundland	NF	Saskatchewan	SK
Northwest Territories	NT	Yukon Territory	YT

FIGURE 10–6 Two-letter abbreviations for states and territories should be used only with ZIP Codes in addresses.

and three spaces from the left edge of the envelope in all capitals. Any notations directed toward the post office, such as "special delivery" or "certified mail," should be typed in all capital letters in the upper right corner of the envelope immediately below the area where the stamp will be placed. If an address contains an attention line, it should be typed as the second line of the address.

FOLDING AND INSERTING LETTERS

Standard ways of folding and inserting letters are used so that the letter will fit properly into the envelope and so that it can be removed easily without damage. Three different methods may be useful (Fig. 10–7):

1. To fold a standard size letter for a No. 10 envelope, bring the bottom third of the letter up and make a crease. Fold the top of the letter down to within about ⅜ inch of the creased edge and make a second crease. The second crease goes into the envelop first.

2. To fold a standard size letter for a No. 6-¾ envelope, bring the bottom edge to within about ⅜ inch of the top edge and make a crease. Then, folding from the right edge, make a fold a little less than one-third the width of the sheet and crease it. Folding from the left edge, bring the edge to within about ⅜ inch of the previous crease. Insert the left creased edge into the envelope first.

3. To fold a letter for insertion into a window envelope: bring the bottom third of the letter up and make a crease, then fold the top of the letter *back* to the crease you made before. (The inside address should now be facing you.) This method is often followed for mailing statements.

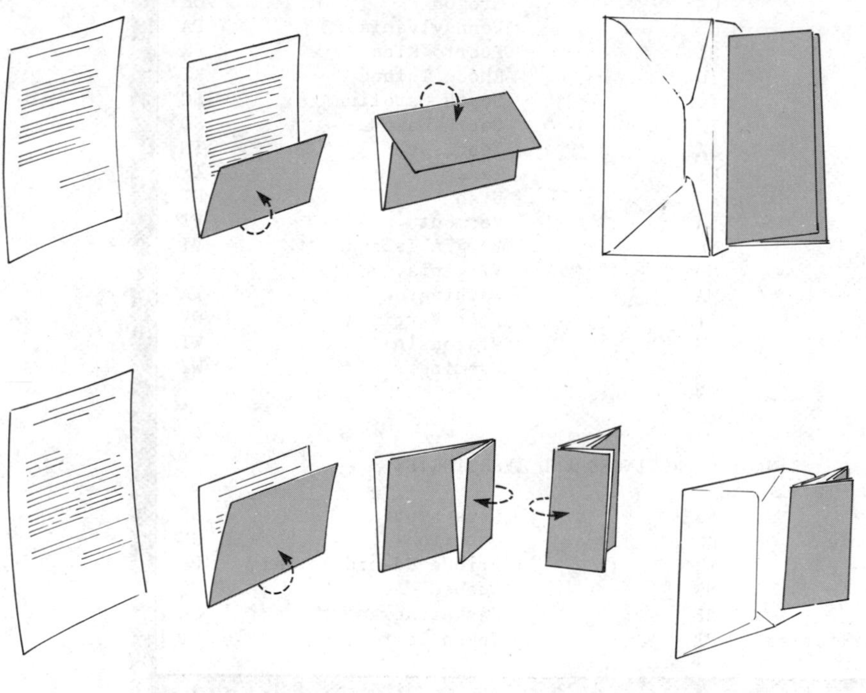

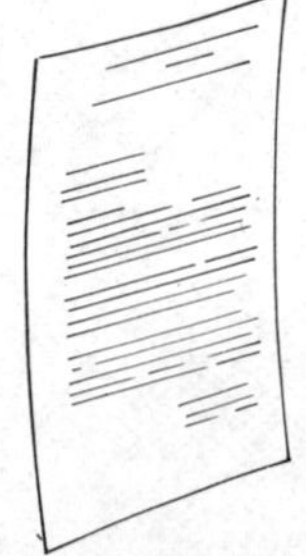

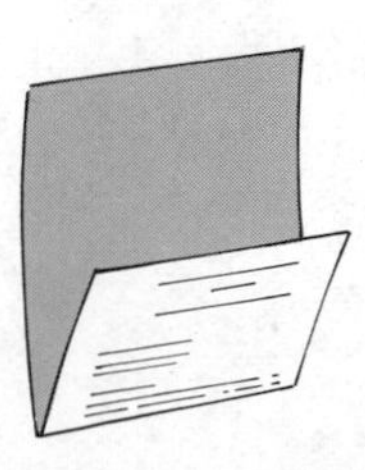

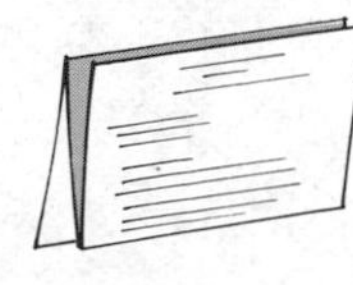

FIGURE 10–7 Correct methods for folding letters.

Hanna, J. M., Popham, E. L., and Tilton, R. S.: *Secretarial Procedures and Administration*, 6th ed. Cincinnati, South-Western Publishing Co.
Sabin, W. A.: *The Gregg Reference Manual,* 5th ed. New York, Gregg Division/McGraw-Hill Book Company, 1977
Strunk, W., Jr., and White, E. B.: *The Elements of Style,* 2nd ed. New York, The Macmillan Company, 1972.

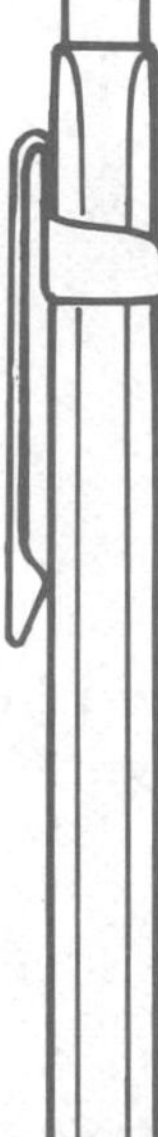

CHAPTER OUTLINE

Reasons for Medical Records
Types of Case Histories
Content of the Complete Case History
  Subjective
  Objective
Obtaining the History
Making Additions and Corrections
Keeping Records Current
The Problem-Oriented Medical Record

BEHAVIORAL OBJECTIVES

The medical office assistant should be able to:

- **State the reasons for keeping patient records.**
- **Request essential subjective information for the record from the patient.**
- **Correctly make necessary additions or corrections to the patient record.**
- **Keep the record orderly, in correct form, and current.**
- **Understand the concept of the problem-oriented medical record.**

11

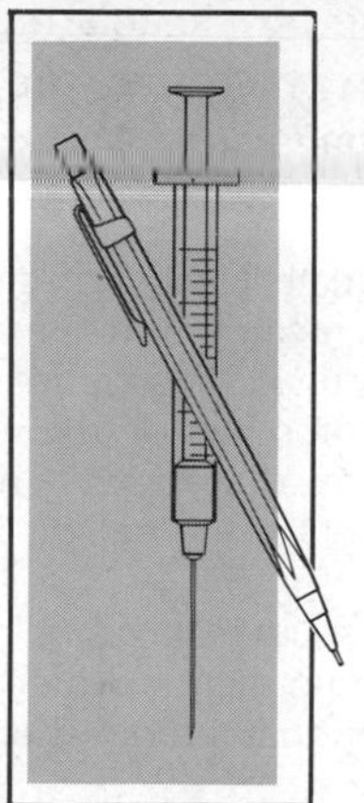

THE PATIENT RECORD

Complete and accurate records are essential to a well-managed medical practice. They provide a continuous story of a patient's progress from the date of his first visit to his last. The treatment and therapy prescribed are noted, along with regular reports on the patient's condition; when a patient is discharged, the degree of improvement is placed upon the record.

REASONS FOR MEDICAL RECORDS

There are three important reasons for carefully recording medical information:

1. **To Provide the Best Medical Care.** The doctor examines the patient and reports his findings on the medical record. These are the clues to diagnosis. Sometimes the doctor orders many types of tests to confirm or augment his clinical findings. As the reports of these tests come in, the findings fall into place like the pieces of a jigsaw puzzle. The physician, on the basis of his diagnosis and the confirmation data, now can prescribe treatment and form his opinion about the patient's chances of recovery, assured that he has utilized every technique to arrive at a correct judgment.

Keeping good medical records helps a physician provide continuity in his patients' medical care. Earlier illnesses and difficulties that appear on the patient's record may supply the key to current medical problems. For example, the information on a patient's record that he was treated for rheumatic fever when he was a child can be extremely important in determining the course of treatment the doctor prescribes when he develops an illness a number of years later.

2. **To Supply Statistical Information.** Medical records may be used to evaluate the effectiveness of certain kinds of treatment or to determine the incidence of a given disease. Correlations of such statistical information may result in a new outlook

on some phases of medicine and can lead to revised techniques and treatments. The statistical data from medical records also are valuable in the preparation of scientific papers, books, and lectures.

3. **To Avoid Legal Difficulties.** Sometimes a physician must produce case histories and medical records in court. For example, a patient may wish to substantiate his claims to an insurance company for damages resulting from an accident in which he was injured and required medical treatment. A patient may involve a physician in **litigation.** The physician's records can be a help or a hindrance, depending on the care with which they are kept. In an article appearing in the October 1969 *Physician's Management* (Would Your Records Survive Cross Examination?), the author states:

> A proper patient record to furnish adequate legal protection should include the patient's medical history, results of examinations, records of treatment, copies of laboratory reports, notations of all instructions given, copies of all prescriptions, and any other pertinent data.
>
> When a patient fails to follow instruction or refuses to undergo a recommended treatment, a letter should be sent containing a "warning" and a carbon copy retained in your files. A similar type of letter should be sent if the patient leaves your care or if you feel it necessary to withdraw your services.
>
> Sometimes a record introduced in court may be of more significance because of an omission than for what was included. If information which should have been included in a record is not, a jury may form the opinion that the omission was deliberate and intended to conceal the truth.

TYPES OF CASE HISTORIES

The style and form which a physician will select to record his case histories will depend partly upon the nature of his practice. General practitioners and some specialists keep very detailed records. The specialist who sees patients only on a consultant basis, or the specialist who is likely to see a patient only once, such as the dermatologist, the radiologist, or the anesthesiologist, need not keep complex records. The nature of the patient's complaint is also a factor determining just how detailed a record should be. If a patient comes into a physician's office to have a foreign body removed from his eye or to have some minor injury treated, a detailed report on his past medical history or that of his family is unnecessary. However, the cardiac, hypertensive, or diabetic patient seeking medical attention should provide a complete history.

In some medical offices where detailed histories are not required, a simple patient registration slip (Fig. 11–1) can be used to record personal data and a plain sheet of paper used to record the complaint and treatment given. In the great majority of offices, however, a more complete record and an individual folder for each patient, is preferable.

The physician who uses just a plain sheet of paper for the patient record generally develops an outline which serves as a guide to taking down the information he requires for a history. He then dictates the history and the secretary types it according to the established format and places it in the patient's folder.

There are many different types of forms available from printing companies: forms for general practice, obstetrics, surgery, pediatrics, internal medicine, or any other of the established specialties. Some physicians design their own forms which they feel are best suited to their particular practice and have them printed to order. Companies that specialize in medical forms will sometimes provide a planning kit for the physician to use. Local printers, too, often can be very helpful in form design. Regardless of the form it takes, the case history will contain certain basic information.

CONTENT OF THE COMPLETE CASE HISTORY

Recordkeeping in the hospital medical records department is deemed important enough that it is entrusted only to specially trained individuals. The job of medical record librarian requires a Master's degree; a medical record technician requires an associate degree with specialization in the specifics of cataloging and recordkeeping in the hospital medical records department. Although it is not necessary for the medical assistant to be a trained medical record librarian or technician, she must be familiar with some of the basic essentials of the work.

The medical case history is the most important record in a doctor's office. For completeness each patient's record should contain:

Subjective Information Provided by the Patient

(1) Routine personal data about the patient
(2) Patient's personal and medical history
(3) Patient's family history
(4) Patient's complaint (in the patient's own words) and date of onset

Objective Information Provided by the Doctor

(5) Physical examination and findings, laboratory and x-ray reports
(6) Diagnosis and prognosis
(7) Treatment prescribed and progress notes
(8) Condition at time of termination of treatment

PATIENT INFORMATION FOR MEDICAL RECORDS *(Please Print)* DATE: 4-20-82

PATIENT — MR. MRS. MISS

LAST NAME	FIRST NAME	MIDDLE
MORRIS	SAMUEL	ALBERT

PATIENT ADDRESS: STREET	CITY	STATE	ZIP	HOME PHONE
3810 Commonwealth Avenue	Los Angeles	CA	90056	213-862-9917

SOCIAL SECURITY NUMBER	DATE OF BIRTH	AGE	DRIVER'S LICENSE NO.
012-34-5678	04-05-40	42	Z80037

PATIENT EMPLOYER	OCCUPATION
Morris Appliances	Merchant

EMPLOYER'S ADDRESS: STREET	CITY	STATE	ZIP	BUS PHONE
5400 Hollywood Blvd.	Los Angeles		90036	213-462-8122

SPOUSE'S NAME	MARITAL STATUS	REFERRED BY	
Louise Marie	(M) S D W SEP.	Dr. F. Gentry	714-635-4300

SPOUSE'S EMPLOYER	STREET	CITY	STATE	ZIP	BUS. PHONE
Morris Appliances (see above)					

IN CASE OF EMERGENCY CONTACT: NAME	ADDRESS	CITY	STATE	ZIP	TELEPHONE
(Daughter) Ellen Spivak	486 Vine Street	Los Angeles		90036	213-536-4142

MEDICAL INSURANCE INFORMATION

COMPANY	POLICY NUMBER
Occidental Insurance Company	SD 4305

IF SOMEONE OTHER THAN PATIENT IS RESPONSIBLE FOR PAYMENT PLEASE COMPLETE THIS SECTION

RESPONSIBLE PARTY — MR. MRS. MISS

LAST NAME	FIRST NAME	MIDDLE	RELATION

ADDRESS: STREET	CITY	STATE	ZIP	TELEPHONE

OCCUPATION	EMPLOYED BY

EMPLOYER'S ADDRESS: STREET	CITY	STATE	ZIP	BUS. PHONE

I hereby authorize Dr. Theodore Wilson to furnish to the above insurance company(s) or to a designated attorney, all information which said insurance company(s) or attorney may request. I hereby assign to Dr. Wilson all money to which I am entitled for medical and/or surgical expense relative to the service rendered by him, but not to exceed my indebtedness to said physician and/or surgeon. It is understood that any money received from the above named insurance company, over and above my indebtedness will be refunded to me when my bill is paid in full. I understand I am financially responsible to said doctor(s) for charges not covered by this assignment. I further agree in the event of non-payment, to bear the cost of collection, and/or Court cost and reasonable legal fees should this be required.

INSURED OR GUARDIAN SIGNATURE ____________ Samuel A. Morris — PATIENT'S SIGNATURE

MDP 8409 © 1976 BIBBERO SYSTEMS, INC., SAN FRANCISCO

FIGURE 11–1 Patient registration form. (Courtesy of Bibbero Systems, Inc., San Francisco, California.)

If these entries are completed, the case history will stand the test of time. No branch of medicine is exempt from the necessity of keeping records. Records aid the physician in the practice of medicine, as well as provide for his legal protection.

Subjective Information

1. **Routine Personal Data About the Patient.** The patient's case history begins with routine personal data which the patient usually supplies on his first visit. The basic facts needed are: (a) patient's full name, spelled correctly; (b) if patient is child, names of parents; (c) date of birth, marital status, name of spouse, number of children; (d) home address and telephone number; (e) occupation; (f) business address and telephone number; (g) source of referral; (h) health insurance information. When a new patient comes into the doctor's office, certain additional information should be secured for the financial record. This is described more completely in Chapter 13, Medical Fees: Credit Arrangements.

2. **Patient's Personal and Medical History.** This portion of the medical record, which is often obtained by having the patient complete a questionnaire, provides information about any past illnesses or surgical operations that the patient may have had, and includes data about injuries or physical defects, congenital or acquired. It also furnishes information about the patient's daily health habits.

3. **Patient's Family History.** The physical condition of the various members of the patient's family, any past illnesses or diseases that individual members may have suffered, and a record of the causes of death comprise the patient's family history. This information is important, since a definite hereditary pattern is often present in the case of certain diseases.

4. **Patient's Complaint.** This is a concise account of the patient's symptoms, explained in his own words. It should include nature and duration of pain, if any, the time when patient first noticed his symptoms, his opinion as to the possible causes for his difficulties, any remedies he may have applied, or other medical treatment he has already had for the same condition.

Objective Information

5. **Physical Examination and Findings; Laboratory and X-ray Reports.** This section of the case history varies greatly with the specialty of the physician and the complaint of the patient. After the physician has completed his examination of the patient, his findings are recorded on the history. Results of other tests or requests for these tests are then recorded or, if they appear on separate sheets, attached to the history.

6. **Diagnosis.** The physician, on the basis of all evidence provided by the patient's past history, the physician's examination, and any supplementary tests, places his diagnosis of the patient's condition upon the medical record. If there is some doubt, it may be termed "Provisional Diagnosis."

7. **Treatment Prescribed and Progress Notes.** The physician's suggested treatment is listed following the diagnosis. Generally, instructions to the patient to return for follow-up treatment in a specific period of time are noted here too.

On each subsequent visit, the date must be entered on the chart, and information about the patient's condition and the results of treatment added to the history, on the basis of the physician's observations. Notations of all medications prescribed or instructions given, as well as the patient's own report about his condition and progress, should be placed upon the record. Any home visits are noted. If the patient is hospitalized, record the name of the hospital, the reason for admission, the dates of admission and discharge. Much of this information may be obtained from the hospital discharge summary.

8. **Condition at Time of Termination of Treatment.** When the treatment is terminated, the physician will record that information. For example,

"August 18, 1984. Wound completely healed. Patient discharged."

OBTAINING THE HISTORY

It has been pointed out that four kinds of subjective information must be secured from the patient in order to prepare the initial history: (1) routine personal data; (2) patient's personal and medical history; (3) patient's family history; and (4) patient's complaint. The assistant usually secures the routine personal data. The personal and medical history and the patient's family history may be secured by asking the patient to complete a questionnaire, with the physician augmenting this during his interview with the patient.

If the doctor delegates the taking of patients' histories to his assistant, care must be exercised to assure that the patient's answers are not heard by others in the reception room. If privacy is not possible, it is better to give the patient a form which he can fill out himself and then transfer this information to permanent records later. If convenient, it is timesaving to ask the patient questions and at the same time type the answers directly on the record. This method offers you an opportunity to become better acquainted with the patient as you complete the necessary records. In some offices, where lengthy questionnaires are to be completed by the new patient, the questionnaire is mailed to the patient with a request that it be completed and returned to the doctor's office prior to the appointment.

The patient may have indicated his chief complaint to the assistant, but the physician will question the patient in more detail on this. The majority of doctors write their own entries on the chart in longhand. Others may dictate the material, either to the assistant or to a recording device. If the material is dictated and typed, each entry should be checked by the physician for accuracy and then initialed by him. Although the physician may find this a bother, it should be encouraged. For a chart to be admissible as evidence in court, the person dictating or writing the entries should be able to attest that they were true and correct at the time they were written. The best indication of that is the physician's signature or initials on the typed entry.

MAKING ADDITIONS AND CORRECTIONS

As long as the patient is under the physician's care, his medical history will be building. Each laboratory report, x-ray report, and progress note is added to the record, in **chronological order,** with the latest information always on top. Although each item is important, it is usually the most recent which is of greatest significance to the patient's care.

LABORATORY REPORTS. Different colors are often used for different procedures. For example, urinalysis report forms may be yellow, blood count forms pink, and so forth. Laboratory slips are usually smaller than the history form and should be placed on a standard size sheet of colored paper. Type the patient's name in the upper righthand corner, then, with transparent tape, fasten the first report even with the bottom of the page. The second laboratory report will be taped or glued in place on top of and about ½ inch above the first slip, allowing the date to show on the first report. By this method, called "shingling," the latest report always appears on top. When checking previous reports, it is only necessary to run your finger down the slips until you find the desired date; then flip up the slips above. Fifteen to twenty slips may be kept on one sheet by using this method, which is illustrated in Figure 11–2. Laboratory report carrier forms with adhesive strips may be purchased (Fig. 11–3).

X-RAY REPORTS. X-ray reports are usually typed on standard letter-size stationery. X-ray reports are placed in the patient's history folder with the most recent report on top. All x-ray reports may be stapled together or kept behind a special divider in the chart.

PROGRESS NOTES. Reports on the patient's progress are continually being added to the case history. Each visit of the patient should be entered on the chart, with the date preceding any notations about the call. The assistant can type or stamp the date on the chart when she pulls the folder. Every instruction, prescription, or telephone call for advice should be entered with the correct date. If there are several persons handling and making entries on a patient's record, it is advisable to initial each entry. This aids in tracing entries about which there may be some question.

CORRECTIONS. Sometimes it is necessary to make corrections on medical records. Erasing and obliteration must be avoided. If an error is made in a handwritten entry, it should be struck out by drawing a line through it and the correction written above or immediately following. The word "correction" or "Corr." is then written in the margin and the initials of the person making the correction are placed on the record, along with the date. Errors made while typing are corrected in the usual way. An error discovered in a typed entry at a later date, however, is corrected in the same manner as described above for a handwritten entry.

GENERAL INSTRUCTIONS. The appearance of the case history is important. Keep all information orderly and in correct form. Type reports and entries whenever possible with a typewriter that is kept clean and has a fresh ribbon. Although completeness is important in medical records, the information should be concise.

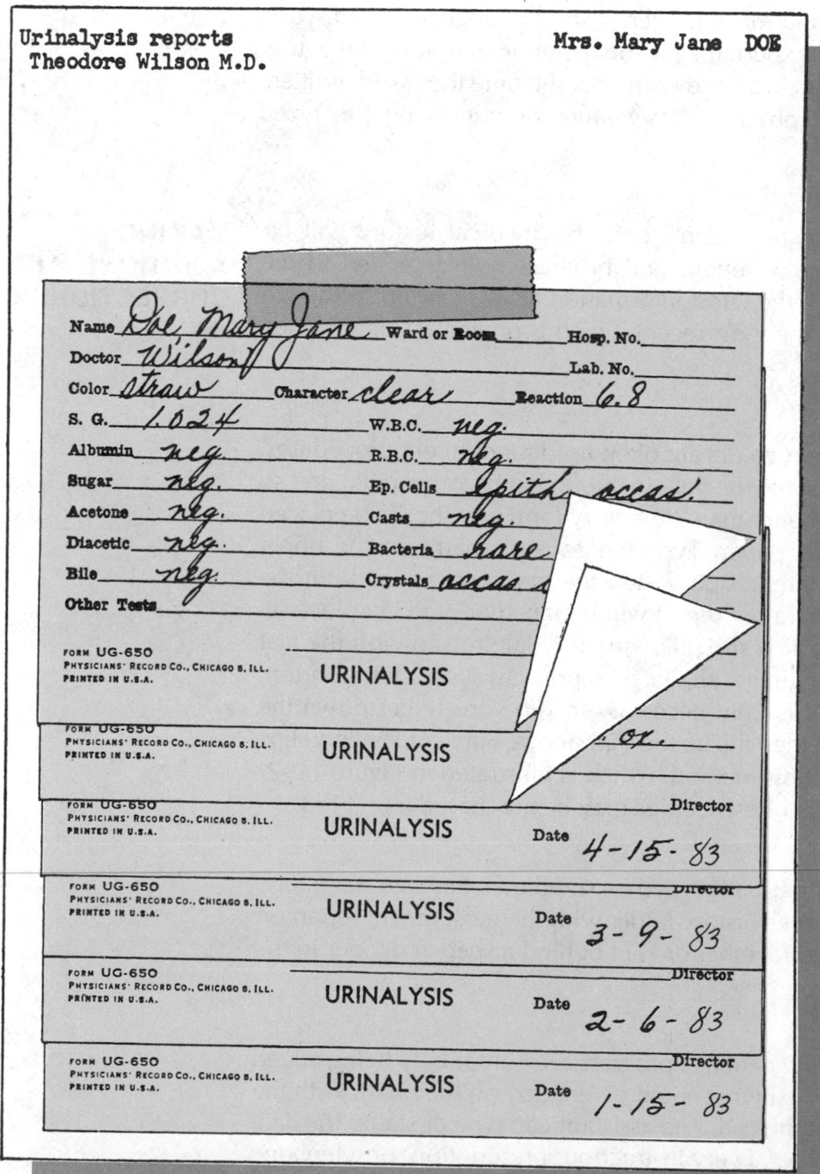

Urinalysis reports
Theodore Wilson M.D.

Mrs. Mary Jane DOE

Name Doe Mary Jane Ward or Room Hosp. No.
Doctor Wilson Lab. No.
Color straw Character clear Reaction 6.8
S. G. 1.024 W.B.C. neg.
Albumin neg. R.B.C. neg.
Sugar neg. Ep. Cells Epith. occas.
Acetone neg. Casts neg.
Diacetic neg. Bacteria rare
Bile neg. Crystals occas.
Other Tests

FORM UG-650
PHYSICIANS' RECORD CO., CHICAGO 8, ILL.
PRINTED IN U.S.A.
URINALYSIS

FORM UG-650
PHYSICIANS' RECORD CO., CHICAGO 8, ILL.
PRINTED IN U.S.A.
URINALYSIS

FORM UG-650
PHYSICIANS' RECORD CO., CHICAGO 8, ILL.
PRINTED IN U.S.A.
URINALYSIS
Director
Date 4-15-83

FORM UG-650
PHYSICIANS' RECORD CO., CHICAGO 8, ILL.
PRINTED IN U.S.A.
URINALYSIS
Director
Date 3-9-83

FORM UG-650
PHYSICIANS' RECORD CO., CHICAGO 8, ILL.
PRINTED IN U.S.A.
URINALYSIS
Director
Date 2-6-83

FORM UG-650
PHYSICIANS' RECORD CO., CHICAGO 8, ILL.
PRINTED IN U.S.A.
URINALYSIS
Director
Date 1-15-83

FIGURE 11–2 Laboratory reports arranged chronologically on a page. (Courtesy of Bibbero Systems, Inc., San Francisco, California.)

Coding of information on records is sometimes a helpful shortcut, but any coding system used should be a standard one — not some system that you as a secretary may invent. It must be understood by anyone who needs to consult the chart. If the coding in an office does vary somewhat from the standard methods, a key should be prepared and placed in the front of the files for immediate reference.

Every doctor has certain technical terms that he uses frequently. When in doubt about the spelling, be sure to check with your dictionary. Because of close similarity in some medical words, it is wise to also check the definition to be sure the word fits the context in which it is used. You may find it helpful to get a small, alphabetized notebook and write the words in it that give you trouble most frequently (see Chapter 10, "Written Communications"). There are many excellent books on medical terminology that include lists of standard abbreviations. A list of the more common abbreviations will be found in the appendix on Medical Terminology.

Correspondence relating to the patient's medical history may be stapled together in chronologic order with the latest on top and placed in a pocket in the patient's folder or kept in the back of the folder.

KEEPING RECORDS CURRENT

One of the greatest dangers to good record keeping is procrastination. The record must be kept current methodically. Many physicians are predisposed to putting off paper work, and the assistant must be relentless in her reminders.

The case histories and reports will probably accumulate on the doctor's or the assistant's desk at the end of the day. After the last patient has left, check each history to make certain all necessary material has been recorded and that each entry is sufficiently clear for future understanding. Give your employer all extra reports, such as laboratory and x-ray, to read. After he has read them, ask him to initial each one so that it may be filed in the patient's case history folder.

While the doctor is reviewing these reports, you can pull the histories of the patients he has seen outside the office that day, as well as those of patients who have been given special instructions by telephone or for whom prescriptions were sent out. These entries are made in the same manner as for an office visit, but the type of

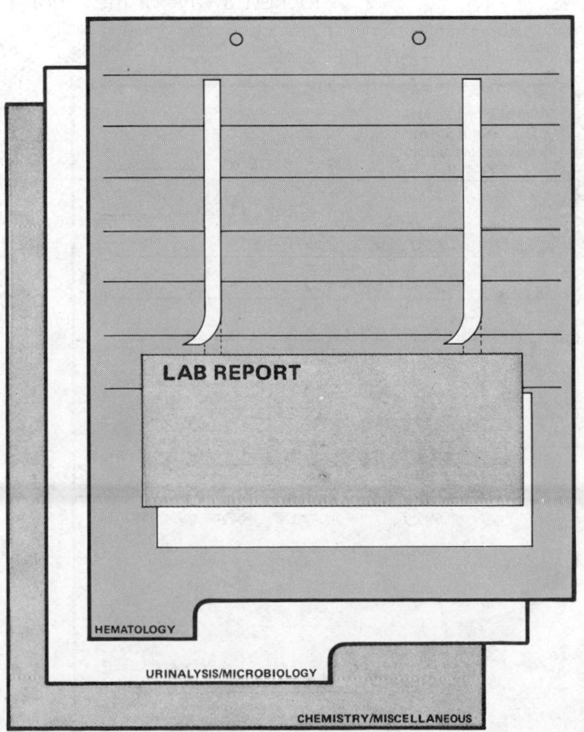

FIGURE 11–3 Quick-Stick color coded lab carriers. Reports are affixed to proper carrier in chronological order by shingling from bottom of page to top. Remove zip tape from designated spot and press down on report. Be sure to indicate Problem Number on each report for future reference. (Courtesy of Bibbero Systems, Inc., San Francisco, California.)

call is explained in parentheses after the date. For example, here's what the history might include about a home visit to see a patient:

> "May 16, 1983 (Res.) Routine ph. ex. Temp. 98.6. Chest clear. Cont. Rx. May now eat semi-bland diet."

When a patient telephones the doctor, the entry should be made on his record as follows:

> "June 26, 1983. (Tel.) To change Rx (Vit. B Comp) to one b.i.d. Force fluids. Feeling much better."

If tests are ordered for a patient, they should be charted in detail on the medical record.

> April 10, 1983. Consultation. Scheduled with Dr. Abbot for consultation at her office on April 26.
> Bilateral mammograms scheduled at SJH on April 17.

Prescriptions should be charted:
April 15, 1983. Refill Tylenol c̄ Cod. #25

A new kind of prescription pad, printed on no-smear, spot carbon paper, is available for a time-saving write-it-once system. By placing the prescription blank over the patient's record, the Rx is automatically copied on the record as it is written (Fig. 11–4). Prescription carriers with adhesive strips are also available if the doctor uses duplicate prescription blanks (Fig. 11–5).

The patient record should not leave the office. A Physician's Pocket Call Record, as shown in Figure 11–6, can be used for outside calls, and the information transferred to the chart in the office.

Also, at the end of the day notations should be made of any unkept appointments or of refusals to cooperate with instructions.

After all records have been reviewed, they should be placed in a file tray and locked away for the night, if the assistant does not have time to file them before she

August Grayson, MD
101 George Street
Crossville, Ind. 90911
721-4110

BNDD No. ______

Date 2/12/77

Patient JOHN W. BATES

Address 723 NORTH AVE.
CROSSVILLE

℞

ESIDRIX 25 mgm
TABS # 2̄

TABS i̅ AFTER BREAKFAST
AND DINNER

August Grayson, MD

Renew PRN IN 100s

FIGURE 11–4 Prescription pad for write-it-once system. (Courtesy of Bibbero Systems, Inc., San Francisco, California.)

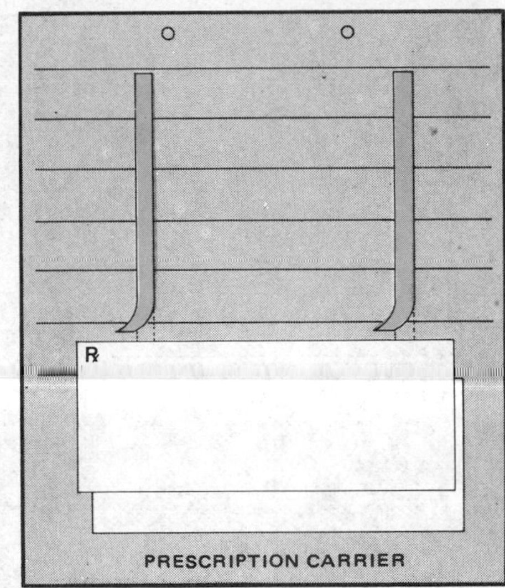

FIGURE 11–5 Quick-Stick Prescription Carrier for shingling copies of prescriptions in patient record. (Courtesy of Bibbero Systems, Inc., San Francisco, California.)

leaves. Do not leave histories out in view at night, especially if the office has a night cleaning service.

When the office assistant arrives the next morning she can index the histories for filing. Attach extra reports and information sheets; don't just drop them into the folders. It is best to attach them to the case histories with tape or rubber cement. When this is done, the records are ready for filing.

The doctor may prefer to dictate his notes rather than write them in longhand. At appropriate moments during the day he dictates everything: patient histories, physical examination findings, medications prescribed, follow-up findings, summaries of telephone conversations. At the end of the day the recorded information is handed to the typist for transcribing onto the records.

A great deal of time may be saved in transcribing these notes if the typist will use a continuous roll or pages of self-adhesive strips (Fig. 11–7). When the transcription is completed, the doctor may wish to check the notes, underline important points, and initial each entry before returning them to the assistant for insertion in the charts. The use of self-adhesive strips saves removing the sheet from a chart which may be bound with metal fasteners, inserting the sheet in the typewriter, and putting the sheet back into the folder. It also simplifies the doctor's part in checking and initialing the notes, because he handles only the transcribed material instead of bulky charts.

PHYSICIANS POCKET CALL RECORD DATE ______

NAME	ADDRESS OR REMARKS	SYMBOL	MONEY RECEIVED	HOME CHARGES	HOSPITAL CHARGES
Donald Jones	out home	H.			5 –
Mrs. Mary L. Lent	Chest exam. inj.	Res	15 00	15	
John James	Chickenpox (report to P.H.D)	"		7 –	
Mr. Ronald White	Surgery St. Luke's Blue Cross # 512-8669	H.			350 –
After posting totals to Office Book file this card by date in BANCO PROFESSIONAL SYSTEM filing box.	Post these TOTALS to office book daily				

FORM 834 BANCO-PRINTERS S.F. REG. U. S. PAT. OFF.

FIGURE 11–6 Physician's Pocket Call Record for patient visits outside office. (Courtesy of Banco Printers, San Francisco, California.)

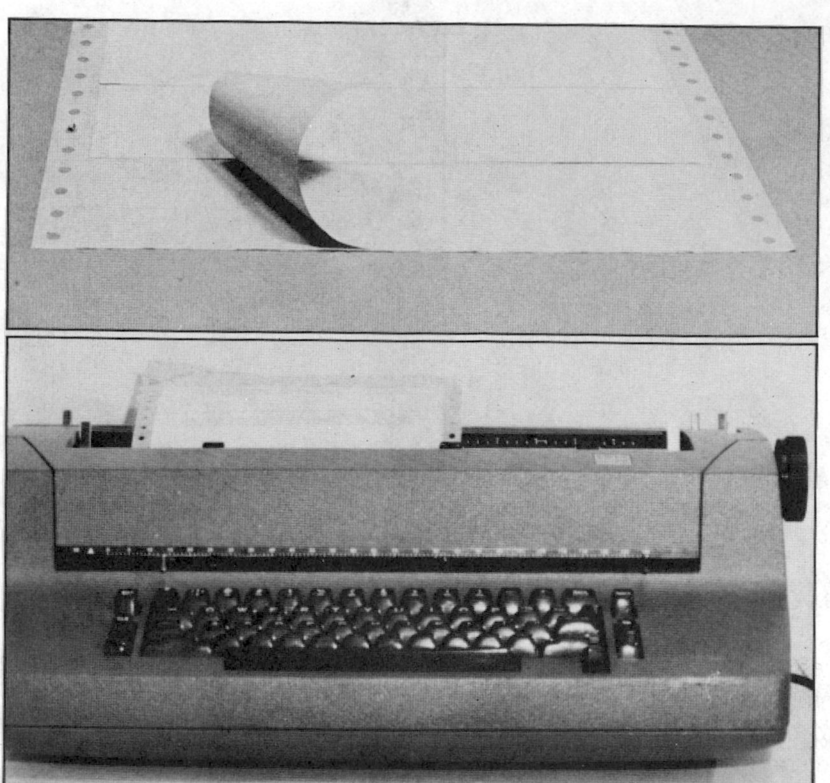

FIGURE 11–7 Adhesive transcription strips. Simply insert this continuous form of pressure sensitive, adhesive-backed strips into the typewriter for easy dictation typing. Then peel off the strip and affix on Progress Notes or any other form. (Courtesy of Bibbero Systems, Inc., San Francisco, California.)

THE PROBLEM-ORIENTED MEDICAL RECORD

Read only

A chapter on the patient record would be incomplete without some discussion of the problem-oriented medical record (POMR), sometimes referred to as the "Weed System." The POMR, originated by Lawrence L. Weed, MD, a professor of medicine at the University of Vermont's College of Medicine, is a major innovation and a radical departure from the traditional system of keeping patient records. The traditional record is "source-oriented;" that is, observations and data are catalogued according to their source — physician, laboratory, x-ray, nurse, technician — with no recording of a logical relationship between them. In an article appearing in the February, 1973, issue of *Medical Opinion* (Who is Dr. Weed — and Why is He Saying All Those Nasty Things About My Charts?), the editors describe the POMR:

> This is a record of clinical practice that divides medical action up into four bases. First you put down information for a carefully defined, standardized data base. That includes chief complaint, present illness, patient profile; and also a review of systems, physical examination, and lab reports. Next you write out a numbered and titled list of every problem the patient has had that requires management or work-up. We believe this should include social and demographic troubles as well as strictly medical or surgical ones.
>
> Then you write a treatment plan for each problem. That is, " What am I going to do to make this patient well?" This includes management, additional workups needed, and therapy. Each plan is titled and numbered with respect to the problem. Finally, you write progress notes, each also labelled according to these problems. This is the universe of information.

It is not the intent of this text to provide comprehensive instruction in using the problem-oriented medical record, but merely to introduce the concept. During the years since the Weed system was first conceived there have been ongoing research, development, field testing, and modification.

One designer (The Andrus/Clini-Rec Charting System)* has developed a file folder for its recommended organization of patient data. The folder is preprinted on the front for age dating and easy access to basic information. With the calendar years printed on the cover it is simple to keep track of when the patient was last seen.

*Available through Bibbero Systems, Inc., 109 Stevenson, San Francisco, CA 94105

On the patient's initial visit, the year, say 1980, is checked on the cover. If he appears again in 1982, and the year 1981 is not checked, you know immediately that more than a year has elapsed since the last visit (Fig. 11–8). It has suggested dividers for lab reports, consultations and hospital reports, and X-ray and EKG reports (all scientific information) on the left side; and data base and progress notes (communication and supervision) on the right side.

The chart is begun by obtaining a patient-completed data base system record, which contains family and past medical history together with 135 carefully selected screening questions. It is so designed that the page that goes into the chart shows only the positive answers (Fig. 11–9). There are also questionnaires designed for screening problems in specialty practices — **cardiovascular, gastrointestinal, gynecologic,** pediatric, and **respiratory.**

The problem list is entered on the divider cover for lab reports. Special sections are provided for current major and chronic problems, and for inactive major or chronic problems. The divider cover for progress notes is a chart for listing medications and other therapeutic modalities. Progress notes take the SOAPing approach: (Fig. 11–10).

S Subjective impressions
O Objective clinical evidence
A Assessment or diagnosis
P Plans for further studies, treatment or management

The problem-oriented medical record has the advantage of imposing order and organization on the information added to a patient's medical record. The records are more easily reviewed, and the likelihood of overlooking a problem is greatly

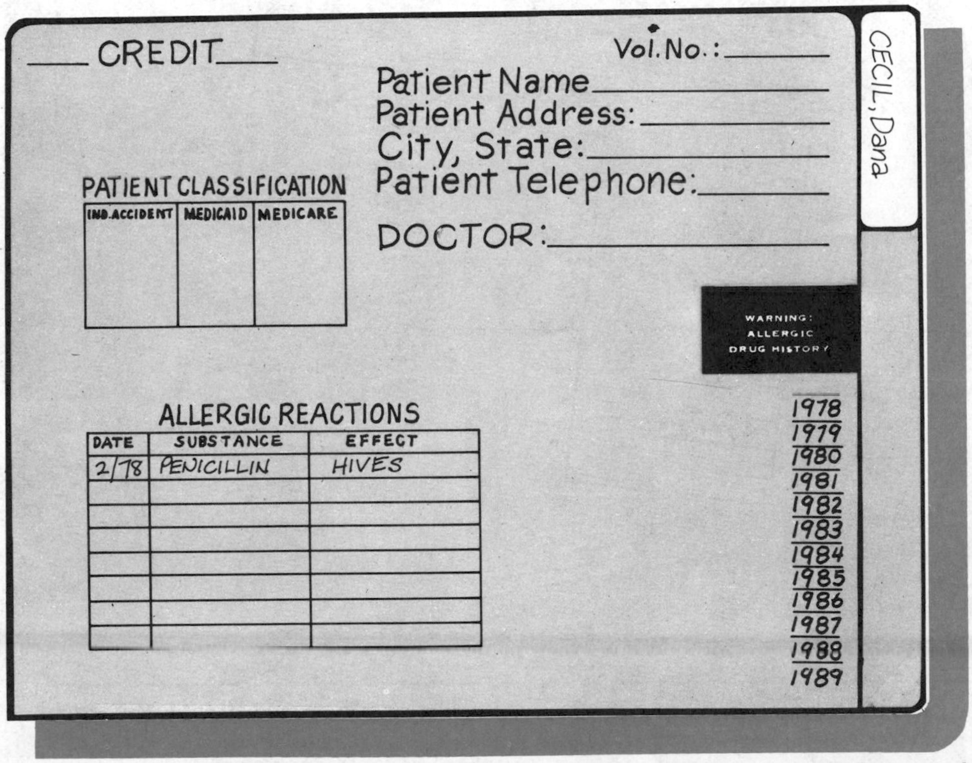

FIGURE 11–8 **Andrus/Clini-Rec File Folder, preprinted on the front for age dating and easy access to basic information. (Courtesy of Bibbero Systems, Inc., San Francisco, California.)**

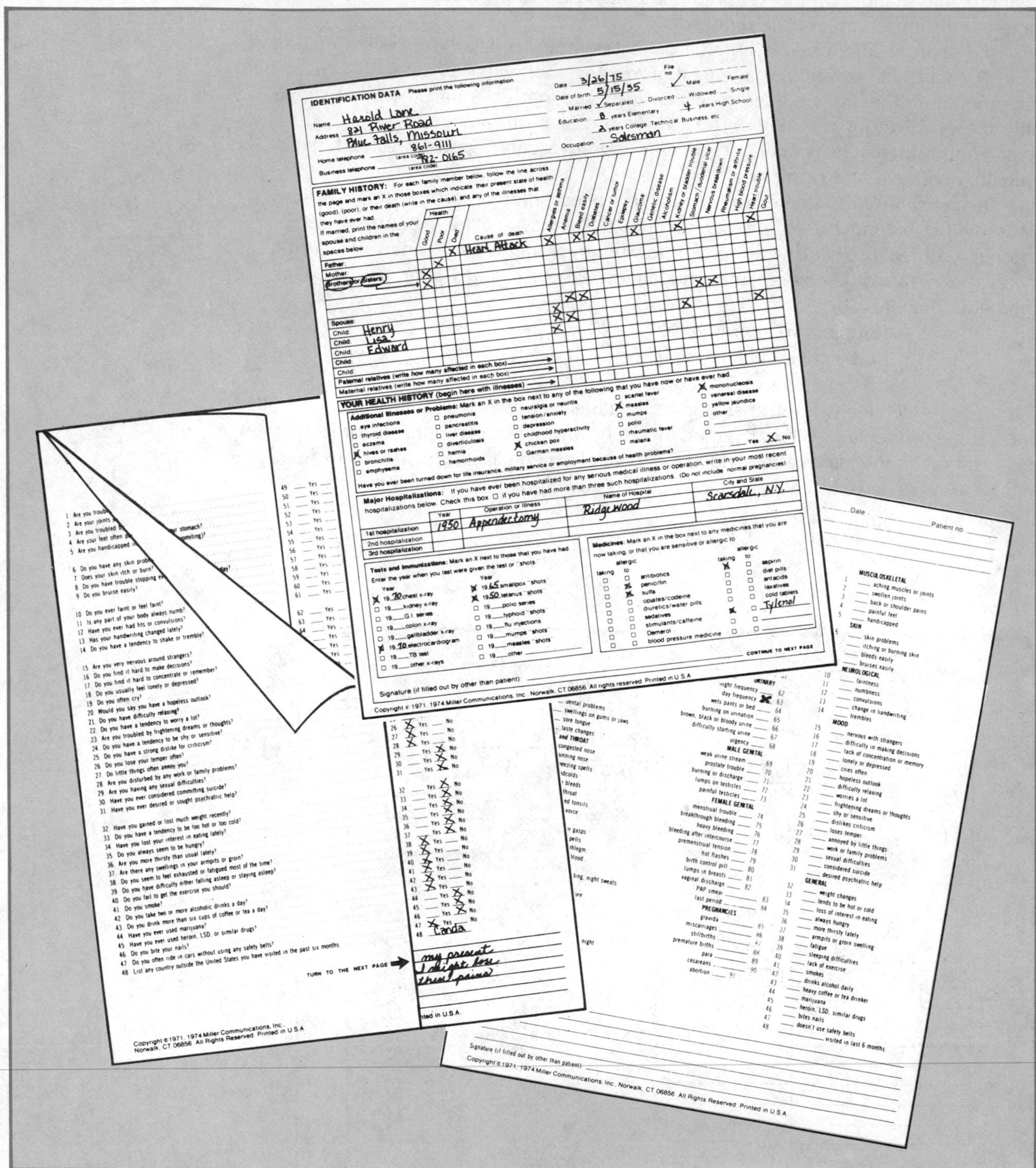

IDENTIFICATION DATA Please print the following information

Name Harold Lane
Address 821 River Road
Blue Falls, Missouri
Home telephone 861-9111
Business telephone 782-0165

Date 3/26/75
Date of birth 5/15/35
File no.
✓ Male __ Female
__ Married ✓ Separated __ Divorced __ Widowed __ Single
Education 8 years Elementary 4 years High School 2 years College Technical Business etc.
Occupation Salesman

FAMILY HISTORY: For each family member below, follow the line across the page and mark an X in those boxes which indicate their present state of health (good), (poor), or their death (write in the cause), and any of the illnesses that they have ever had. If married, print the names of your spouse and children in the spaces below.

Health: Good, Poor, Dead; Cause of death; Allergies or asthma; Anemia; Bleed easily; Diabetes; Cancer or tumor; Epilepsy; Glaucoma; Genetic disease; Alcoholism; Kidney or bladder trouble; Stomach/duodenal ulcer; Nervous breakdown; Rheumatism or arthritis; High blood pressure; Heart trouble; Gout

Father: X Heart Attack
Mother
Brothers or Sisters
Spouse
Child: Henry
Child: Lisa
Child: Edward
Child
Child
Paternal relatives (write how many affected in each box)
Maternal relatives (write how many affected in each box)

YOUR HEALTH HISTORY (begin here with illnesses)

Major Hospitalizations: 1st hospitalization 1950 Appendectomy Ridgewood Scarsdale, N.Y.

Tests and Immunizations

Medicines: Tylenol

CONTINUE TO NEXT PAGE

Signature (if filled out by other than patient)

Copyright © 1971, 1974 Miller Communications, Inc., Norwalk, CT 06856 All rights reserved Printed in U.S.A.

FIGURE 11–9 Data Base Self-Administered General Health History Questionnaire. (Courtesy of Bibbero Systems, Inc., San Francisco, California.)

Progress Notes Forms

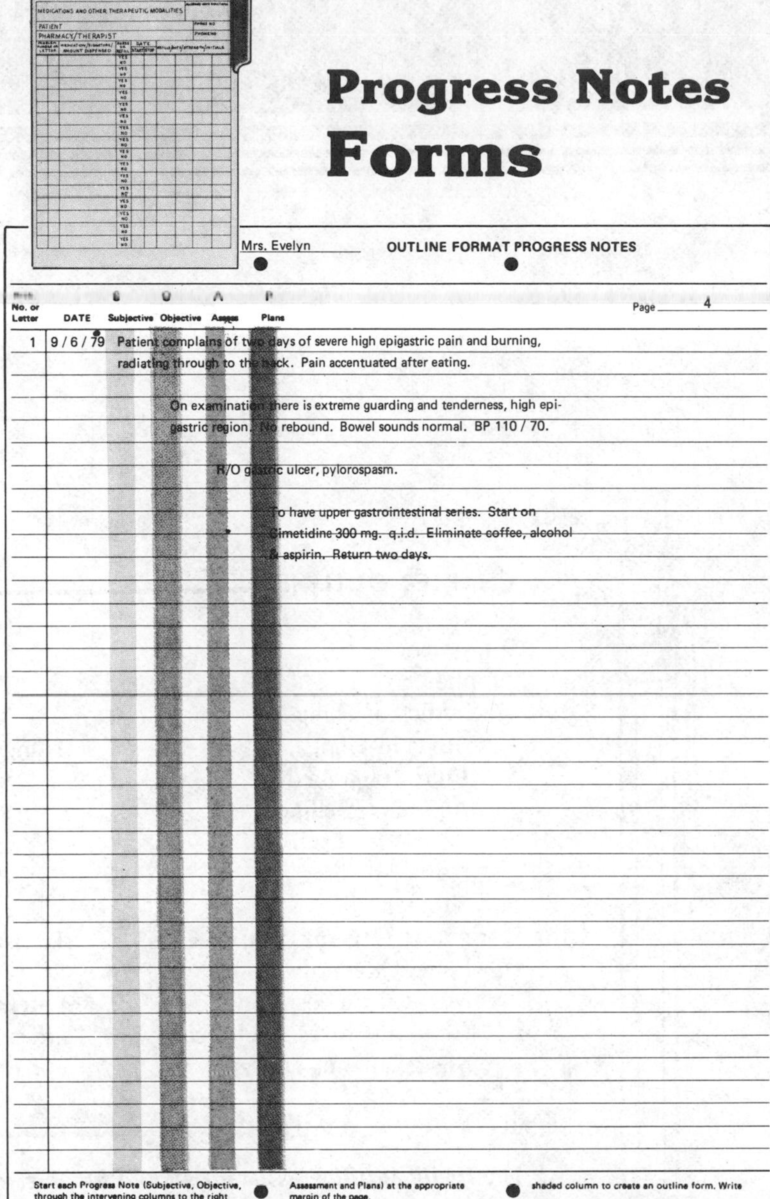

Mrs. Evelyn — OUTLINE FORMAT PROGRESS NOTES

Page 4

No. or Letter	DATE	S Subjective O Objective A Assess P Plans
1	9/6/79	Patient complains of two days of severe high epigastric pain and burning,
		radiating through to the back. Pain accentuated after eating.
		On examination there is extreme guarding and tenderness, high epi-
		gastric region. No rebound. Bowel sounds normal. BP 110/70.
		R/O gastric ulcer, pylorospasm.
		To have upper gastrointestinal series. Start on
		Cimetidine 300 mg. q.i.d. Eliminate coffee, alcohol
		& aspirin. Return two days.

Start each Progress Note (Subjective, Objective, Assessment and Plans) at the appropriate shaded column to create an outline form. Write through the intervening columns to the right margin of the page.

ANDRUS/CLINI-REC® PRIMARY CARE CHARTING SYSTEM, MDP 7115, © 1976 BIBBERO SYSTEMS, INC., SAN FRANCISCO, CA

FIGURE 11–10 The S.O.A.P. Progress Note Form. The four columns on the left indicate *S*ubjective impressions, *O*bjective clinical evidence, *A*ssessment or diagnosis, and *P*lans for further studies. (Courtesy of Bibbero Systems, Inc., San Francisco.)

reduced. SOAPing essentially forces a rational approach to patient problems and assists in formulating a logical and orderly plan of patient care.

While the POMR was practically unheard of before 1970, by 1973 a majority of the medical schools in the United States were either teaching or preparing to teach the problem-oriented system. It has continued to grow in popularity and is used not only in private practices but may be even more valuable in clinics and hospitals where more than one person must be able to find essential information in the chart. Although the long-established physician may continue to use the source-oriented record, clearly the assistant working with the recent medical school graduate will need to be acquainted with the POMR.

References

American Medical News, published by American Medical Association, 535 North Dearborn Street, Chicago, Illinois 60610

Medical Opinion, published by Weston Communications, Inc., 575 Madison Avenue, New York, New York 10022

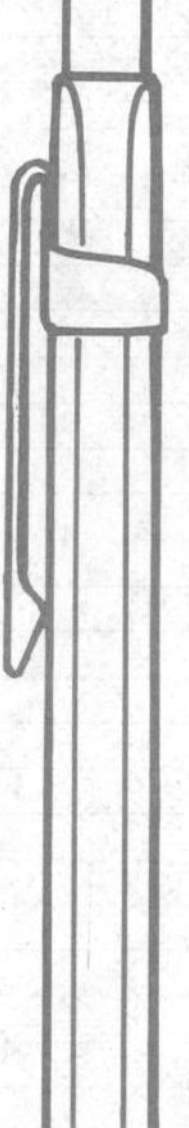

CHAPTER OUTLINE

Equipment
Supplies
Mechanics of Filing
- Steps in Filing
- Rules for Indexing
- Alphabetic Filing
  - Color Coding
- Numeric Filing
- Subject Filing

Systematic Organization of Files
- Patient Records
- Medical Correspondence
- General Correspondence
- Miscellaneous Folders
- Business and Financial Records
- Follow-up or Tickler File
- Transitory or Temporary File

Filing Procedures
- Sorting
- Placing in Folders
- Indexing
- Preventing Accidents
- Locating Misplaced Files

Transfer of Files
Records Protection
Retention and Destruction
Storage
Personal Records

BEHAVIORAL OBJECTIVES

The medical office assistant should be able to:

- **Select suitable equipment and supplies for records management.**
- **Organize the files in a physician's office.**
- **Utilize the advantages of color coding.**
- **Apply the rules of indexing to records management.**
- **File and retrieve correspondence and records.**
- **Establish a retention and destruction schedule for office records.**

12

RECORDS MANAGEMENT

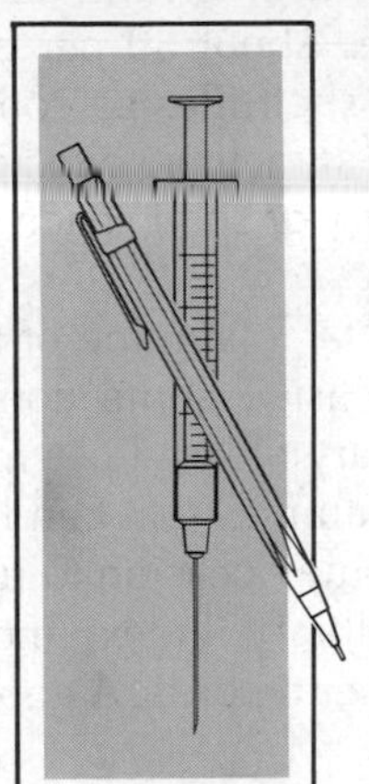

Unless the medical office assistant has had formal secretarial training or extensive experience in secretarial procedures, she may find filing to be her Waterloo. Assembling the medical record is important, as was stressed in the previous chapter. But this record must be filed so that it can be easily and quickly found when needed. A filing system is only as good as the "findability" of everything in the files.

The point of view of the person in charge of the files often makes the difference between efficiency and chaos. Some persons equate "filing" with "storing"; the term "records management" is more appropriate to the medical assistant's filing responsibility. Management of the records will include filing, finding, transferring, protection, and retention, storage, and destruction. A modern filing system, according to Michael Silver, Practice Management Consultant (*How to Tailor Your Filing System to Your Own Needs*, Physician's Management/November 1979) should have three key components:

1. A way to tell if the record is active or inactive from the outside of the jacket or folder, so that updating is continuous and easy,
2. Safeguards to prevent misfiling, and
3. A filing technique that allows quick, accurate retrieval and refiling.

The first component was discussed in the previous chapter (Fig. 11–8). Discussion of the second and third components follows.

EQUIPMENT

The four-drawer steel filing cabinet has been standard equipment for years. In offices where space is limited the trend is toward shelf filing (Fig. 12–1). The rotary circular file is also increasing in popularity. Some kinds of records will be kept in card or tray files. Regardless of the type or style of equipment, the best quality is always an economy.

Drawer files should be full-suspension; they should roll easily, close securely, and be equipped with a locking device. The best cabinets will have a center trough at the bottom of each drawer with a rod for holding divider guides. Floor space of twice the depth of the drawer must be allowed so that the drawer can be pulled out to its full extent.

Shelf files should have doors to protect the contents. A popular type of shelf file has doors which slide back into the cabinet; the door from a lower shelf may be pulled out and used for work space. About 50 per cent more material per square foot of floor space may be filed in shelf files as compared with the usual drawer file. Shelf files are available in many attractive colors and can add a decorative note to the business office. Special storage or shelf space should be provided for x-rays if many films are stored.

Rotary circular files can hold a large volume of records. They save space and clerical motion. The files revolve easily; some come with pushbutton controls. Several persons can work at one rotary file and use records at the same time. They afford less privacy and protection than files that can be closed and locked.

Almost every office will have some occasion to use a card file. This may be for patient ledgers, a patient index, library index, index of surgical tray set-ups, telephone numbers, or numerous other records. A good quality steel box or tray is a sound investment.

SPECIAL ITEMS. Metal framework is available which will convert a regular drawer file into suspension-folder equipment. The assistant with a great deal of filing may wish to purchase a portable filing shelf that fits on the side of an opened drawer and can be moved from place to place as needed. A sorting file can be a great timesaver. A portable suspense file cart for temporary filing of unbilled insurance claims may be quite useful. Such a file cart may also be used for the preliminary sorting of charts to be refiled (Fig. 12–2).

SUPPLIES

Filing supplies include guides, OUTguides or OUTfolders, folders, vertical pockets, and labels.

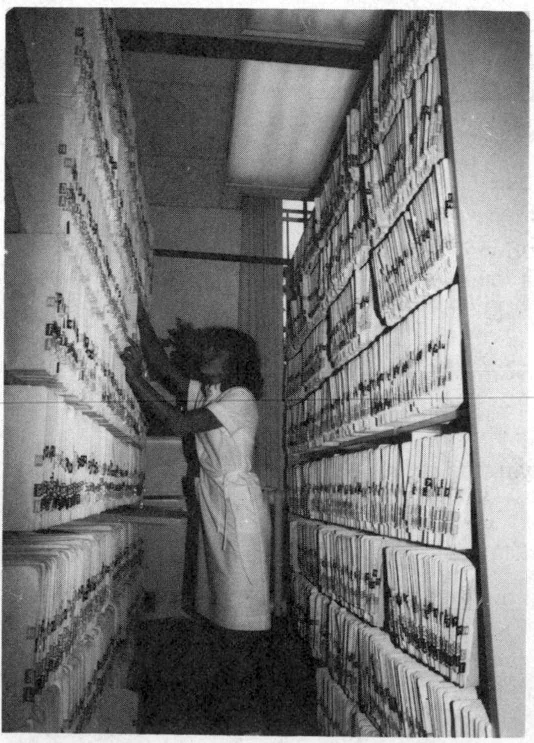

FIGURE 12–1 The medical office assistant at patient files in a physician's office.

DIVIDER GUIDES. Each file drawer or shelf should be equipped with plenty of dividers or guides. Some authorities recommend one guide for approximately each inch and a half of material, or every 8 to 10 folders. Guides should be of good quality pressboard. "Economy" guides will soon become bent and frayed and have to be replaced. Divider guides have a protruding tab, which may be either an integral part of the card or may be made of metal or plastic. The guides reduce the area of search and serve as supports for the folders. They are available in single, third, or fifth cut (one, three, or five different positions). The guide may have a projection at the bottom edge with a ring or hole through which a rod may go. This type of guide card is used in drawers that have a trough for the projection and a rod to hold the guides in place.

OUTguides. An OUTguide is a heavy guide that is used to replace a folder that has been temporarily removed. It may be of a distinctive color for quick detection. This makes refiling simpler and alerts the file clerk that a file is missing. The OUTguide may have lines for recording information, or it may have a plastic pocket for inserting an information card.

FOLDERS. Most records to be filed are placed in tabbed folders. The most commonly used is a general-purpose third-cut manila folder that may be expanded to ¾ inch. These are available with a double thickness reinforced tab that will greatly lengthen the life of the folder. Folders kept in drawers will have tabs at the top; those kept on shelves will have tabs at the side. There are many variations of folder styles obtainable for special purposes. One example is the classification folder, which will separate the papers in one file into six categories yet keep them all together. The OUTfolder is used like the OUTguide but provides space for temporary filing of

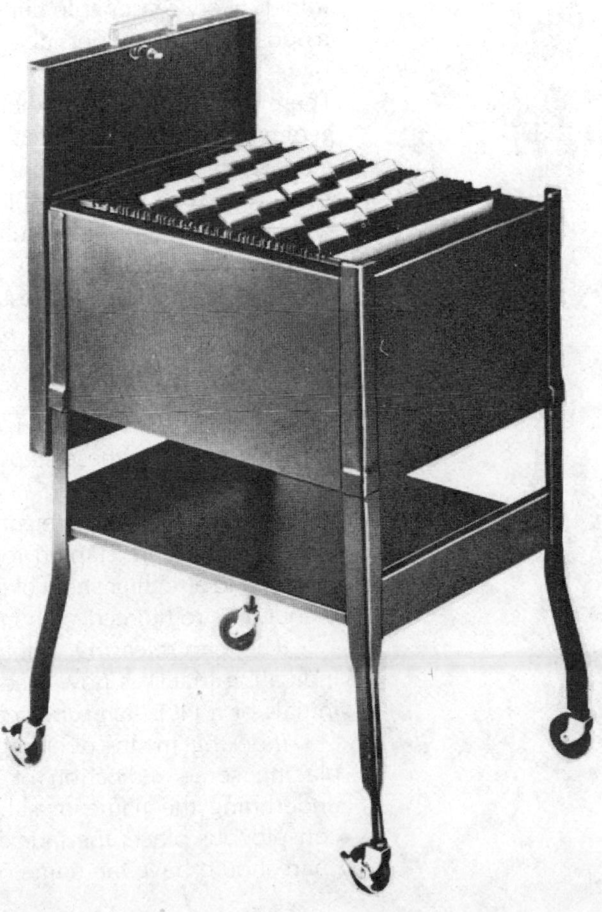

FIGURE 12–2 Suspense file cart, Bibbero Systems.

materials. Another example is the vertical pocket, which is heavier weight than the general purpose folder, has a front which folds down for easy access to contents and is available with up to 3½ inch expansion. These are used for bulky histories or correspondence. Hanging or suspension folders are made of heavy stock and hang on metal rods at the side of a drawer. They can be used only with files equipped with suspension drawers. Binder folders have fasteners with which to bind papers within them. These offer some security for the papers but are time-consuming in filing the materials.

LABELS. Each shelf, drawer, divider guide, and folder will have a label. The label is a necessary "filing and finding" device. Labels may be prepared with a mechanical tapewriter or the typewriter. Paper labels may be purchased in rolls of gummed tape, or they may have adhesive backs that are peeled from a protective sheet after typing. Labels are available in almost any size, shape, or color to meet the individual needs of any office. Visit your stationer and study the catalogs to find the best product for you.

The label on the drawer or shelf identifies the nature of its contents. It should also indicate the range (alphabetic, numeric, or chronologic) of the material filed in that space. For example:

A. PATIENT HISTORIES (Active)
A–F
B. GENERAL CORRESPONDENCE
1980–1984

The label should be easy to read. The tapewriter is probably preferable to the typewriter for these labels.

The final step in locating a record in the file is identification of the individual folder. Every reasonable filing aid should be used to ensure reaching this as speedily as possible. The folder label must be descriptive and legible.

MECHANICS OF FILING

There are four basic methods of filing: (1) alphabetic by name, (2) numeric, (3) geographic, and (4) subject. A fifth method, chronologic, is sometimes used. In the management of records in the physician's office, the assistant will probably be concerned with only three filing methods — alphabetic, numeric, and subject. These will be described more fully. Geographic filing is used in businesses that are interested in information by location rather than by name, such as sales organizations, mailing houses, real estate firms, and so forth. Chronologic filing refers to filing according to date and is used in a follow-up or tickler file, as described on page 169.

STEPS IN FILING. All materials to be filed will involve several steps. In the language of filing, these steps are called *conditioning, releasing, indexing,* and *coding*.

Papers to be filed are *conditioned* by removing all pins, brads, and paper clips; related papers are stapled together; clippings or items smaller than page size are attached to a regular sheet of paper with rubber cement or tape; damaged records are mended or reinforced with tape.

The term *releasing* simply means that some mark has been placed on the paper indicating that it is now ready for filing. This will usually be either the secretary's initials or a FILE stamp placed in the upper left corner.

Indexing means deciding where to file the letter or paper, and *coding* means placing some indication of this decision on the paper. This may be done by underlining the name or subject, if it appears on the paper, or writing, in some conspicuous place, the indexing subject or name. Every paper placed in a patient's chart should have the name of the patient on it, usually in the upper right corner. If

Read

the material could logically be filed in more than one place, it may be necessary to prepare a cross-reference sheet.

RULES FOR INDEXING. Indexing rules are fairly well standardized based on current business practices. The American Records Management Association takes an active part in updating the rules. Recent changes have affected the indexing of hyphenated names, names containing an apostrophe, and names containing seniority terms. For the average physician's office, the following basic rules will be all that is needed.

1. Last names of persons are considered *first* in filing; given name (first name), *second*; and middle name or initial, *third*. Compare the names from the first letter to the last. The first letter that is different in two names is the letter that determines the order of filing. Example: abe, abi, abx, acl, acm, ada, ade, adi, and so one.

2. Initials precede a name beginning with the same letter. Example:

Smith, J.
Smith, Jason

This illustrates the librarian's rule, "Nothing comes before something."

3. Hyphenated names, whether first names, middle names, surnames of people, or business names, are considered to be one unit.

4. The apostrophe is disregarded in filing. Anderson's Surgical Supply is filed as Andersons Surgical Supply. Before the recent revision, anything *after* the apostrophe was not considered in filing.

5. Unusual names of individuals, such as Ah Hop Akee, should be filed under the last name and cross-indexed.

Akee, Ah Hop
Ah Hop Akee (see Akee, Ah Hop).

6. Names with prefixes are filed in the usual alphabetic order. DeLong is filed as Delong; LaFrance as Lafrance; von Schmidt as Vonschmidt.

7. Abbreviated names are indexed as if spelled in full: St. John as Saintjohn; Wm. as William; Edw. as Edward; Jas. as James.

8. Mac and Mc are filed in their regular place in the alphabet:

Maag
Mabry
MacDonald
Machado
MacHale
Maville
McAulay
McWilliams
Meacham

If your files contain a great many names beginning with Mac or Mc you may, for convenience, wish to file them as a separate letter of the alphabet.

9. The name of a married woman is indexed by her legal name (her husband's surname, her given name, her middle name or maiden surname). For example:

Doe, Mary Jones (Mrs. John L.)
NOT
Doe, Mrs. John L.

10. Titles, when followed by a complete name, are disregarded in indexing:

Breckenridge, John J. (Prof.)

Titles without complete names are considered the first indexing unit:

Madame Sylvia
Sister Mary Catherine

Degrees are disregarded in filing but placed after the name, in parentheses:

Wilson, Theodore (MD)

11. Articles such as "The" or "A' are disregarded in indexing:

Moore Clinic (The)

12. Terms of seniority, such as Junior, Senior, or Second are not considered in indexing. If two names are otherwise identical, the address is used to make the indexing decision (State, City, Street).

ALPHABETIC FILING. Alphabetic filing of names is the method of choice for filing patient records in the majority of physicians' offices. If you can find a word in the dictionary or a name in the telephone directory, you already know some of the rules. Some people have difficulty all their lives with remembering the sequence of letters in the alphabet. This can play havoc with alphabetic filing!

Alphabetic filing is traditional and simple to set up. It is a *direct* system in that one need only know the name in order to find the desired file. The only requirements are a file cabinet or shelf, folders, and some divider guides. However, it does have some drawbacks. As the files grow in number, more space will be required for each section of the alphabet. This will require periodic shifting of folders from drawer to drawer, or shelf to shelf, to allow for expansion. As the files expand, more time is required for filing each folder as well as for retrieving a file because of the additional folders involved in the search. This can be somewhat alleviated by increasing the number of divider guides to break down the alphabet or, better still, by color coding.

Color Coding. When a color coding system is used, both filing and finding are easier and misfiled folders are kept to a minimum. There are a number of ready-made systems available (e.g., Bibbero, VisiRecord, Tab, Ames, Acme, Colwell, Remington Rand). If the files are extensive and strict economy is a consideration, ordinary manila folders can be color coded by using labels with color strips or self-adhesive colored dots over the edge of the folders.

The purpose of color coding is to make it possible through the use of color to visually restrict the area of search for the location of a specific record. This is done by selecting a color to identify each letter of the alphabet and applying this selection to the *second* letter of the name. The application of the principle may be through using colored folders, adhesive colored identification labels, or various combinations of these. The primary function of color coding is to prevent misfiling. Any selection of colors may be used and the division of the alphabet determined by one's own needs. However, studies have shown that there is wide variation in the frequency with which different letters occur. The following division is one that has been used successfully. Experience has proven that this breakdown results in almost equal representation of the five colors.

Color of Label	*Letters of Alphabet*	*Example*
Red	A B C D	Canfield Eberhart O'Connor Adams

Yellow	E F G H	D*e*cker
		E*f*fron
		I*g*awa
		T*h*ill
Green	I J K L M N	H*i*sted
		B*j*ork
		A*k*ron
		U*l*lman
		I*m*hoff
		A*n*derson
Blue	O P Q	G*o*rdon
		E*p*perley
		A*q*uino
Purple	R S T U V W X Y Z	G*r*einer
		O*s*terberg
		A*t*herton
		A*u*er
		U*v*ena
		O*w*sley
		O*x*ford
		N*y*e
		A*z*zaro

There are many other ways to make color work for you. Small self-adhesive tabs in a variety of colors may be used to identify certain types of insured patients. For example, a patient on Medicaid may have a red tab over the edge of his folder; a Champus patient may be identified by a blue tab; a worker's compensation patient by a green tab and so on. Matching tabs may be attached to the ledger cards. Research cases may be identified by a special color tab. In a partnership practice, it may be desirable to use a different color folder or label for each doctor's patients. Self-adhesive tabs are easily removed, less bulky than metal or plastic tabs, and not so likely to be inadvertently pulled from the record.

The business records files may also utilize color coding. Main divider guide headings may be of one color, subheadings in a second color, and subdivisions in a third color. For example:

Main Heading	DISBURSEMENTS	Red label
Subheading	Equipment	Blue label
Subdivisions	Typewriter	Yellow label
	Copier	Yellow label
	Calculator	Yellow label

A fourth color might be used for personal items. The use of color in the files is limited only by the imagination. One word of caution, though. Every person in the office who uses the files should know the key to the coding, and the key should also be written in your procedures manual.

NUMERIC FILING. Numeric filing is an **indirect** system, requiring the use of an alphabetic cross-reference in order to find a given file. Some people object to this added step and overlook the advantages. Management consultants differ in their recommendations, some recommending numeric filing only if there are more than

5,000 charts, or in some cases more than 10,000. Others recommend nothing but numeric filing. This is an individual choice.

Some form of numeric filing combined with color and shelf filing is used by practically every clinic or hospital of any size. In numeric filing each new patient is assigned a sequential number, and an alphabetic cross-index card is prepared to identify the name. It is possible to use the patient's ledger (financial) card for this purpose by simply writing the patient's number at the top of the card. This does have a disadvantage since ledger cards customarily are taken from the active file when the account is paid in full. Small 3 by 5 cards attached to a Rolodex or Wheelodex system on the receptionist's desk are usually more convenient and more efficient. Some clinics give each new patient an identification card with his/her assigned number. The patient is instructed to give the receptionist the number each time he/she telephones or comes in. Numeric filing allows unlimited expansion without periodic shifting of folders. It provides additional confidentiality to the chart. The greatest advantage is the time saved in retrieving and refiling records quickly. One knows immediately that the number 978 falls between 977 and 979. By contrast, an alphabetic system, even with color coding, requires a longer search for the exact spot.

SUBJECT FILING. Subject filing is used for general correspondence. All correspondence dealing with a particular subject is filed together. The subject headings are placed on the tabs of the folders and filed alphabetically. This is further described in the following section on Systematic Organization of Files.

SYSTEMATIC ORGANIZATION OF FILES

PATIENT RECORDS. It is very difficult for a physician to study a disorganized history. Some systematic method must be followed in placing the material in the patient folder. Details of the patient record were discussed in the preceding chapter. From the filing standpoint, it should be stressed that when a patient record is not in actual use, there is only one place it should be — in the filing cabinet. Many precious hours can be lost in searching for misplaced or lost records that were carelessly left unfiled. The patient's full name, in indexing order, should be typed on a label and attached to the folder tab. The patient's full name should also be typed on each sheet within the folder. A strip of transparent tape can be placed over the label to prevent smudging if this is a problem.

MEDICAL CORRESPONDENCE. Correspondence pertaining to patients' medical records should be filed with the case history. Other medical correspondence will probably be filed in a *subject* file.

GENERAL CORRESPONDENCE. The physician's office must be operated as a business, as well as a professional service. There will be correspondence of a general nature pertaining to the operation of the office. In all likelihood a special drawer or shelf will be set aside for the general correspondence. The correspondence will be indexed according to subject matter or names of correspondents. The *guides* in a subject file may appear in one, two or three positions, depending upon the number of headings, subheadings, and subdivisions. Examples were shown in the section on color coding above.

MISCELLANEOUS FOLDER. Papers that do not warrant an individual folder are placed in a *miscellaneous* folder. Within the folder, all papers relating to one subject, or with one correspondent, are kept together in chronologic order, the most recent on top, and then filed alphabetically with other miscellaneous material. Related materials may be stapled together. *Never* use paper clips for this purpose. When as many as five papers accumulate with one correspondent or subject, a separate folder should be prepared.

BUSINESS AND FINANCIAL RECORDS. The most active financial record is, of course, the ledger. In most offices this will be a card or vertical tray file and the accounts will be arranged alphabetically by name. There will be at least two divisions: *active* and *paid* accounts. Special categories may be set up, for example: (1) government-sponsored insurance; (2) worker's compensation; (3) delinquent accounts; (4) collection accounts, and so forth.

Other business files include records of income and expense, financial statements, income and payroll tax records, canceled checks, and insurance policies. These papers may be filed chronologically.

FOLLOW-UP FILE. The most frequently used follow-up method is that of a *tickler* file. It "tickles" the memory that something needs to be done or followed up on a particular date. The tickler file is always a chronologic arrangement. In its simplest form it consists of notations on the daily calendar. If information concerning a patient who has an appointment to come in is expected, such as an x-ray report or laboratory report, the medical assistant might make a note on her calendar or tickler file a day ahead to check on whether the report has arrived. The tickler file is often a card file with 12 guides for the names of the months, and 31 guides printed with numbers 1 through 31 for the days of the month. The guide for the current month, followed by the 31 day guides, is placed at the front of the file. Notations of actions to be taken are placed behind the guides for specific days of the current month. Notations for future months are placed behind the guide for that month. In order to be effective, the tickler file must be checked the first thing each day. It is a useful reminder for recurring events, such as payments, meetings, and so forth. On the last day in each month, all the notations from behind the next month's guide are distributed behind the daily numbered guides and the guide for the completed month is placed at the back of the file.

TRANSITORY OR TEMPORARY FILE. Many papers are kept longer than necessary because no provision is made for segregating those that have a limited usefulness. For instance, if the secretary writes a letter requesting a reprint, the carbon may be placed in the transitory folder. When the reprint is received, the request letter is destroyed. This file is used for materials having no permanent value. The paper may be marked with a "T' and destroyed when the action involved is completed.

FILING PROCEDURES

Filing should be done daily. Try to establish a definite time for this. You may think you don't have time, but searching for records that have not been filed is even more time-consuming and costly.

SORTING. Sorting is arranging the papers in order for filing. Sort papers before going to the file cabinet. Do any necessary stapling of papers at your desk or filing table. If possible, invest in a desk sorter with a series of dividers between which papers are placed in filing sequence. One general purpose sorter has six means of classification: alphabetic sections, numbers 1 to 31, days of the week, months of the year, numbers in groups of five, and space on the tabs for special captions to be taped when desired (Fig. 12–3).

You can make your own desk sorter by stapling together a series of four or five folders, leaving about one inch of each folder visible for labeling. The folders may be labeled A-E, F-K, L-R, S-Z, and SPECIAL. In the preliminary sorting you will place the

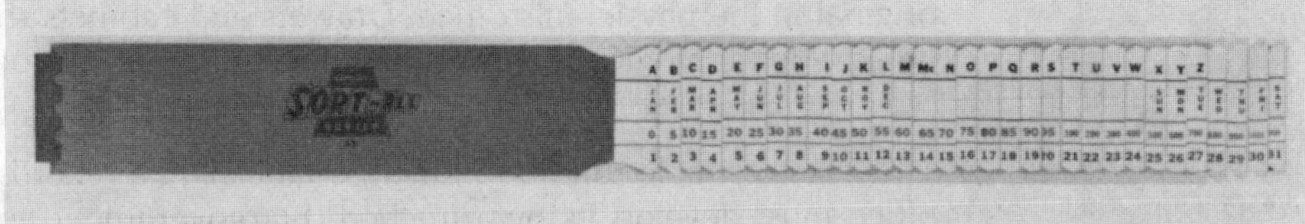

FIGURE 12–3 Sort-Aid sorter (MDP A-31), Bibbero Systems.

papers in the appropriate folder in the sorter. Then it is comparatively simple to arrange these groups into the proper sequence for filing.

PLACING IN FOLDERS. Items should be placed face up, top edge to the left, with the most recent date to the front of the folder. Lift the folder an inch or two out of the drawer before inserting material so that the sheets can drop down completely into the folder.

INDEXING. Arrange all folders to be filed in indexing order before going to the file cabinet.

PREVENTING ACCIDENTS. File drawers are heavy and can tip over, causing serious damage, unless reasonable care is observed. Open only one file drawer at a time and close it when the filing has been completed. A drawer left even slightly open can cause injury to a passerby.

LOCATING MISPLACED FILES. Unless files are promptly replaced after use, they may become lost. Papers may be misfiled, requiring a thorough search to find them. After you have made a methodical and complete search through the proper folder, there are several places you may look for a misplaced paper: in the folder in front of and behind the correct folder; between the folders; on the bottom of the file under all the folders; in a folder of a patient with a similar name; in the sorter.

TRANSFER OF FILES

Some system should be established for regular transfer of files. In most medical offices, records are filed according to three classifications: active, inactive, or closed. Active files are those of patients currently receiving treatment. Inactive files generally are histories of patients whom the doctor has not seen for six months or more. When such individuals return for care, their folders are replaced in the active file. Closed files are records of patients who have terminated their relationship with the physician, died, or moved away.

Charts for patients who are currently hospitalized may be kept in a special section for quick reference, then placed in the regular active file when the patient is discharged from the hospital.

In a surgical practice, there is frequently a specific date on which the patient is discharged from the doctor's care and the notation made on the chart, "Return prn." This record may safely be placed in the inactive file.

In a general practice office, the outside of the folder may be stamped with the date of the patient's visit each time he is seen. It will then be a simple matter to determine when the chart should be transferred to the inactive status. In the parlance of filing, this is called the perpetual transfer method.

RECORDS PROTECTION

Occasions may arise when records are temporarily out of the office. Some physicians release case histories to their colleagues, or a record may be subpoenaed by the courts. In such instances, an OUTfolder should be placed in the drawer in place of the regular folder, and a notation made of the name, date, and to whom the record was released. Interim papers may be placed in the OUTfolder until the original is returned.

The sending out of actual case histories should be avoided if possible. Instead, prepare a resume, or photocopy the materials needed for reference, and retain the original in the physician's office. Drawers and cabinets should be kept closed at all times when the office is unattended, for further protection of the records.

RETENTION AND DESTRUCTION

There is no simple rule to follow in establishing a records-retention schedule. Each office must develop its own method, but government and legal requirements will have some influence.

CASE HISTORIES. Space permitting, these will probably be kept permanently, or at least as long as the doctor is in practice. Then, if the patient is still living, his records may be made available to another doctor of his own choosing. The record would not be given to the patient himself because of the possibility of misinterpretation.

TAX RECORDS. Income tax returns are kept indefinitely; the last three returns are retained in a fireproof filing cabinet or safe; older returns are filed in dead storage.

INSURANCE POLICIES. Keep current policies in a fireproof cabinet or safe. When superseded by a new policy, throw away the old one UNLESS a claim is pending. *Professional liability policies are kept permanently.*

CANCELLED CHECKS. Keep in a fireproof file three years, then indefinitely in dead storage.

RECEIPTS FOR BUSINESS EQUIPMENT. Keep until item is fully **depreciated.**

GENERAL CORRESPONDENCE AND BUSINESS RECORDS. These should be reviewed periodically, as time permits, and any papers which are no longer of value destroyed. If the slightest doubt exists as to whether a paper should be destroyed, be sure to check with the doctor or retain the paper in the file.

MISCELLANEOUS. Many papers that are filed should instead be destroyed. Examples of these are letters of acknowledgment, announcements of meetings, duplicate copies, and letters of transmittal. Any document that is superseded by another in the file should be removed. For instance, when a new catalog is filed, destroy the old one; when a new fee schedule is received, destroy the old one. Blue Cross and Blue Shield representatives say that retaining old copies of fee schedules and claim forms causes countless problems. The Army has developed the technique of discarding papers to the highest level, and every document receives a date of destruction notation before it goes into the file.

STORAGE

Large clinics and offices may find it advisable to microfilm records for storage. This permits storage of a considerable number of histories in a small space, saves time in searching, offers protection, and eliminates loss and misfiling. However, the cost is high, microfilm is hard to read for prolonged study, it is difficult to produce film in court, and if a patient returns, it is too small for refiling.

Some papers which should be kept but which need not be readily accessible may be placed in storage. Sturdy storage file boxes may be obtained from your stationery supply house. These boxes should be labeled to identify their contents in case it should be necessary to reclaim a file or refer to a record. The boxes are uniform in size and are available with a lift-off lid or in a drawer model. These can be kept in some out-of-the-way place. If no room is available in the office, they can be placed with a storage company for a low monthly rental. In this case, a record of the contents of each box should be kept in the office. A telephone call to the storage company will produce the record within a very short time.

Can't Find Things?*

Usually, it's because you've permitted your desk — or closet — to become a catch-all for outdated papers. Mountains of old correspondence, cartoons yellowing with age, magazines never referred to, advertisements, half-finished crossword puzzles, old receipts, outdated manuals, 1958 Christmas cards, wedding announcements — are just some of the papers that add confusion to our lives.

---

*Reprinted by permission of *Physician's Management* (Vol. 2, No. 9) Sept, 1962, p. 26

Except for canceled checks and old receipts (which belong in an expanding envelope against the day you figure out your income tax), these space wasters are time-killers, for they force you to spend hours every month searching for the papers you do need.

It has been estimated that 90 per cent of the collection of papers of both a business and an individual is worthless. The word: get rid of them.

Sound ruthless? So's a clock!

Many times the medical office assistant is required to file or otherwise dispose of documents, receipts, and other records of her employer's personal affairs. An article appearing in *Medical Economics* (November 29, 1965)* gives some valuable guidelines for retention of personal records.

PERSONAL RECORDS

THE RIGHT PLACE FOR YOUR PERSONAL PAPERS. The aforementioned article tells why and how you should keep such personal papers as income tax returns, canceled checks, records of gifts and bequests received, inventory lists and appraisals, contracts and insurance policies. The list below covers other personal records and tells where to store them and how long to keep them.

Keep in safe or safe-deposit box

WHAT	HOW LONG
Birth certificates, marriage and divorce records, passports, professional certificates, licenses	Permanently
Real-estate deeds, leases, registration receipts, title abstracts, surveyors' reports, auto titles, original of burial plot deed	Until sale of property or settlement of estate; then to dead storage
Stocks, bonds, promissory notes, mortgages	Until sold, paid, or collected
Originals of wills, powers of attorney or appointment	Until revised, probated, or exercised

Keep in desk or filing cabinet

WHAT	HOW LONG
Current bank statements	Three years; then to dead storage
Bank deposit slips	Three years; then to dead storage
Receipts for paid bills	Three years if needed for tax purposes; otherwise two months to cover crediting errors; then to dead storage or (if trivial amounts are involved) discard

Medical Economics, November 29, 1965.

Keep in dead storage

WHAT	HOW LONG
Old bank statements	Permanently
Old family health records	Permanently
Old partnership and other business agreements	Permanently
Old real-estate deeds, major property records	Permanently
Old receipts for major paid bills	Until purchased item has been sold or discarded

References

Jennings, L. M.: *Secretarial and Administrative Procedures*. Englewood Cliffs, NJ, Prentice-Hall, 1978.

Johnson, M. M., and Kallaus, N. F.: *Records Management*, 2nd ed. Cincinnati, South-Western Publishing Company, 1974.

Stewart, J. R., and Kahn, G.: *Gregg Quick Filing Practice*. New York, Gregg, McGraw-Hill Co., 1979.

CHAPTER OUTLINE

BEHAVIORAL OBJECTIVES

The medical office assistant should be able to:

- **Explain how medical fees may be determined.**
- **Avoid the pitfalls of fee adjustments.**
- **State the advantages of advance discussion of fees.**
- **Obtain necessary information from patient before extending credit.**
- **Assist patient in planning financing of medical care.**

13

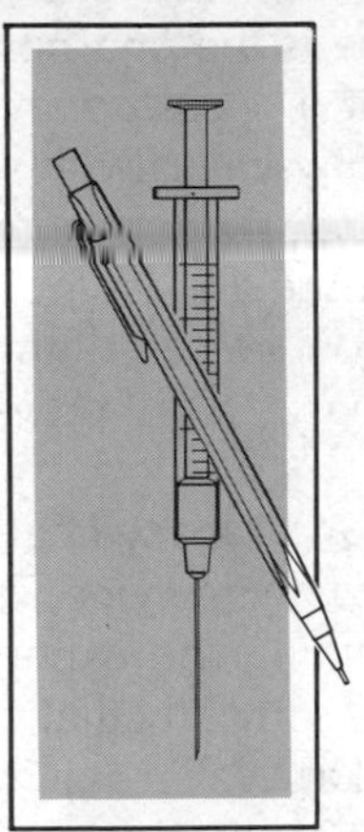

PROFESSIONAL FEES AND CREDIT ARRANGEMENTS

PROFESSIONAL FEES

The doctor is trained to view his profession from the standpoint of *service*. Little attention is given to the business side of medicine. But the doctor must charge and collect for his services in order to continue providing medical care to all his patients.

The assistant, too, has some inhibitions to overcome in relation to professional fees. She probably has not given much thought to finances from the viewpoint of the physician; her experience has been from the viewpoint of the patient.

The tasks of charging fees and collecting money from patients in exchange for medical services are often viewed by both the doctor and his assistant as unpleasant and difficult. These duties must be placed in their proper perspective, and a positive attitude toward the financial side of medical practice cultivated in the minds of the doctor, the assistant, and the patient.

How Fees are Determined

It is not easy to set a "fair fee." A doctor sells his time, his judgment, and his services — yet the value of these commodities is never exactly the same to two different individuals. Medical care has little value except to the patient himself, and the value to that patient may not be consistent with his ability to pay. In every case, the doctor himself must place an estimate upon the value of his services. This value may then be modified by other considerations.

PREVAILING RATE IN THE COMMUNITY. One of the bases for determining medical fees is the nature of the community itself. In some communities the entire cost of living scale is much higher than in other communities. This situation is reflected in medical fees, too. Consequently, the prevailing rate in the community —

the average composite fee—must be taken into consideration by each individual doctor. Strangely enough, fees that are too low drive patients away just as quickly as do fees that are too high.

USUAL AND CUSTOMARY FEE. Some insurance plans do not publish a fee schedule but agree to pay all or a percentage of the *usual and customary fee* for any given procedure. Some include the word *reasonable*, that is, *usual, customary*, and *reasonable.* The physician's *usual* fee is the one he most frequently charges for a given procedure, say, a first office visit. The *customary* fee is a range of the usual fees charged for that same procedure by physicians with similar training and experience practicing in the same geographic and socioeconomic area. The term *reasonable* usually applies to a service or procedure that is unusually difficult or complicated, requiring extraordinary time or effort on the part of the physician. It should be noted that under Medicare Part B, "customary" and "prevailing" correspond to "usual" and "customary" as defined here.

To illustrate, let us suppose that Dr. Wallace charges his private patients $30 for a first office visit. This is his *usual* fee for this service. The usual fees charged for a first visit by other doctors with similar training and experience in the same community range from $18 to $35. The insurance company that pays a usual and customary fee would then allow payment of $30 to Dr. Wallace. If, on the other hand, the range of usual fees in the community is from $12 to $25, the insurance company would allow only the maximum within the range, or $25, to Dr. Wallace.

DOCTOR'S FEE PROFILE. The fiscal agents for certain government-sponsored insurance programs keep a continuous record of the usual charges submitted for specific services by each individual doctor. By compiling these fees over a given period the doctor's *fee profile* is established. This fee profile is then used by the fiscal agent in determining the amount of third party liability for services under the program. One of the objections voiced by doctors is the lag between the time of a private fee increase and the time it is reflected in payments by an insurance carrier. It may be as long as two to three years.

INSURANCE ALLOWANCE. In some individual cases, the physician may feel that he does not wish to charge the patient in addition to what will be allowed by his insurance coverage. The full fee should be quoted to the patient and charged to his account, with the understanding that after the insurance allowance has been received, the balance will be discounted. If a smaller fee is quoted and charged several problems may arise: (1) the lower fee will disturb the doctor's fee profile; (2) if it should become necessary to bring suit for payment of the fee, only the reduced fee can be recovered; and (3) if the insurance allowance is paid on the basis of a certain percentage of the doctor's fee and a lower fee is charged, the insurance allowance will be correspondingly lower. If the physician does this with many of his patients, however, the insurance company may take the position that the reduced fee is his usual fee, and base its payments accordingly. It may even be considered *fraudulent* in some instances.

RELATIVE VALUE STUDIES. The Relative Value Study (RVS) was pioneered by the California Medical Association in 1956 to help physicians establish rational, relative fees. Other states soon followed suit. Hundreds of the most commonly performed procedures were compiled, assigned procedure numbers similar to those in Current Procedural Terminology (CPT) published by the American Medical Association, and assigned a unit value. The assigned unit value represented the value of that procedure in relation to other procedures commonly performed. Although no monetary value was placed on the units, many insurance companies, including Medicaid and Worker's Compensation, used the RVS to determine benefits by applying a conversion factor to the unit values. In 1978 the Federal Trade

Commission (FTC) interpreted the California RVS as a fee-setting instrument and prohibited its publication and distribution. The FTC is attempting to make medical practice more competitive by ruling against the setting of fees and by encouraging physicians to advertise.

Advance Discussion of Fees

It is natural for the patient, once he has seen the doctor, to wonder, "How much is this going to cost?" He may be reluctant, however, to voice this concern. The patient who seems least concerned about the fee may very likely be the patient who creates the biggest collection problem.

It is the responsibility of the doctor or his assistant to raise the discussion of fees if the patient does not do so. Clyde T. Hardy, Jr., associate dean for Private Patient Services and director of the Department of Clinics, Bowman Gray School of Medicine, Wake Forest University, Winston-Salem, NC, writing in *Medical Economics* (Feb. 7, 1977) states, "Be prepared to discuss fees with any patient who's interested, but don't assume you *must* do so with everyone." Mr. Hardy suggests opening the discussion of fees with something like this: "Mr. Willardson, do you have any questions about the costs of your operation? If you do, I'll be glad to review them." On the other hand, in this preliminary discussion of fees, the doctor must not sidestep the issue by saying "Don't worry about the bill, let's just get you well first." He must also avoid an attempt to calm a worried patient about to undergo surgery by saying, "There's really nothing to it." He may find that the patient later complains loudly about the bill since the doctor himself said it was a simple procedure. Even in those cases where the doctor quotes a fee, the assistant is often charged with the responsibility of explaining the doctor's fees to the patient. She must know how fees are determined and why charges vary. She must have special knowledge of her own employer's practice and policies in order to handle perplexing situations involving fees.

The neophyte assistant is in the position of having to educate her viewpoint to that of the doctor. She can be something of a "salesperson" for the doctor's services by gently convincing patients that money spent for medical care is an excellent investment in the future. Sometimes it is impossible for a patient to see or understand the intricate procedures involved in diagnosis and treatment. He rarely is aware of the long years of training and study and the heavy expenses that a doctor incurs in securing his education. Furthermore, he does not always realize that running a modern professional office is a costly process relying upon day-to-day income in return for services. These are factors which the assistant can point out to patients and thus convince them that money paid for care is well spent.

When a doctor frankly discusses fees in advance with his patients, even to the point of describing how he arrives at a fee, misconceptions about overcharging and fee frictions are usually eliminated. One doctor wrote the American Medical Association that, with 95 per cent of his patients, three minutes at the end of the visit spent in explaining the medical bill ensures financial success.

Advance fee discussions help the patient to plan ahead for his medical expenditures. Most patients want to pay their financial obligations but rightly insist upon an accurate estimate of those obligations before they contract for purchase of goods or services. Because many physicians and patients are reluctant to broach the subject of fees, the American Medical Association sells, for a very modest price, an attractive office plaque which encourages fee discussions, with this message:

TO ALL MY PATIENTS — I INVITE YOU TO DISCUSS FRANKLY WITH ME ANY QUESTIONS REGARDING MY SERVICES OR MY FEES. THE BEST MEDICAL SERVICE IS BASED ON A FRIENDLY, MUTUAL UNDERSTANDING BETWEEN DOCTOR AND PATIENT.

This plaque should be placed in the physician's office, not in the reception room.

SURGICAL COST ESTIMATE

Name of Patient ______________________________ Date __________

Procedure ____

Your surgery has been scheduled at ____________________ Hospital on ____________. You should report to the Admitting Office between the hours of ____ (a.m.) (p.m.) and ____ (a.m.) (p.m.).

Although medical and hospital expenses are seldom welcomed, knowing in advance what expenses to expect and how to plan for them can lessen the burden. This estimate is prepared to assist you in budgeting your surgical costs.

PROFESSIONAL FEES

When you have major surgery, the surgical team includes the operating surgeon, the assistant surgeon, and the anesthetist. Each has an important part in your care, and each will render a separate statement for services. While each doctor will independently set his/her own fee, it is usually possible to estimate in advance an approximate range of fees. Assuming an uncomplicated course for your surgery, the charges are estimated as follows:

Operating surgeon	$________	to	$________
Assistant Surgeon	________	to	________
Anesthetist	________	to	________

The assistant surgeon and the anesthetist usually base their fees on the operating time; consequently, if a surgical procedure turns out to be more complicated than was expected, their fees may be correspondingly increased.

The estimated duration of your hospital stay is _____ days at $_______ a day for a (semi-private) (private) room. During your hospital stay there will be charges for laboratory tests, medications as required, and other services. It is impossible to estimate in advance what these charges will be; they will be itemized on your hospital bill. If you have health insurance, please take the appropriate forms and I.D. information with you on the day of your admittance.

PLEASE KEEP IN MIND THIS IS ONLY AN ESTIMATE

FIGURE 13–1 Form for surgical cost estimate.

Explanations of medical costs should extend beyond the doctor's own charges. For example, if a patient is to undergo surgery, the doctor should explain the costs of the operation, the anesthetist's and radiologist's charges, the laboratory fees, and the approximate hospital bill, as well as his own charges. The importance of calling in another physician for consultation should be explained to patients when consultation becomes necessary. It should be made clear, in advance, that there will be a separate bill submitted by the consulting physician. Patients do not always understand that the consultation is for the benefit of the patient, not the physician.

The public is inclined to blame doctors for all medical costs — even hospital charges. (In 1970, doctors' fees accounted for only one-fifth of medical costs.) The doctor and his assistant can avoid misunderstanding by giving the patient an idea of what the entire medical procedure will cost. Some physicians give patients an estimate of medical expenses before hospitalization (Figure 13–1). A few medical societies cooperatively develop such estimate sheets with local hospitals. The American Medical Association includes an example of an estimate sheet in its publication, *The Business Side of Medical Practice*. Individual doctors occasionally work up their own estimate forms when a patient is embarking upon long-term treatment. The doctor should, however, always point out that he is providing an estimate only and that the total cost may vary somewhat.

Estimate slips should be written in duplicate so that the patient may have a copy and the other can be retained in the office files. This eliminates the danger of misquoting the fee later or forgetting the charge originally discussed. Advance estimation and explanation of medical fees simplifies collection, since it eliminates later misunderstanding and confusion over bills.

Adjusting or Canceling Fees

CARE FOR THOSE WHO CANNOT PAY. The medical profession has traditionally accepted the responsibility of providing medical care for those individuals who are unable to pay for these services. In spite of the increased scope of government-sponsored care for the medically indigent, doctors still donate thousands of dollars' worth of such medical services each year.

In many instances, medical care for the indigent is available, but those who need it may be unaware that such assistance is available through social service agencies. The doctor's assistant should acquaint herself with the various local organizations and agencies that can aid the patient in obtaining the necessary assistance. The doctor himself can furnish only his services — other agencies must provide hospitalization, for example, or arrange for paying costs of special therapy, rehabilitation, or drugs.

If a doctor accepts a case for which he will not be paid, complete records must still be kept on the patient. The only deviation in procedure is that the financial record will indicate "n/c" (no charge) in the debit column.

FEES IN HARDSHIP CASES. Sometimes a doctor is faced with the problem of deciding whether to reduce or cancel a fee in a hardship case. Before adjusting or canceling a fee, the doctor or his assistant should encourage a frank discussion of the patient's financial situation. Find out whether the patient is entitled to insurance settlement of some kind. The patient's circumstances may qualify him for local or state public assistance programs. If so, the assistant may direct the patient to the appropriate agency.

If the circumstances of hardship exist before the services are rendered, thorough discussion of what the fee will be and how it will be paid should take place at that time. In most cases it is far better to adjust a fee before rather than after treatment. The doctor may suggest that the patient who is truly medically indigent seek care at a County hospital with public assistance. A doctor should be free to choose his form of charity and not feel obligated to substantially reduce or cancel a fee when the circumstances are known in advance.

After a doctor and his patient have agreed upon a fee, special circumstances

October 28, 19__

Mr. John Jones
1234 East Street
Cincinnati, Ohio 45202

Dear Mr. Jones:

Your account in the amount of $135 is long past due. Understanding the financial circumstances that make it difficult for you to make any payment on these past services, Dr. Johnson has instructed me to consider the debt canceled. We will see that you are no longer billed for it.

The doctor wants you to feel free, however, to call on him for any future services you may require.

Sincerely yours,

CLAYTON L. SCROGGINS

Auditor for Dr. Johnson

FIGURE 13–2 Example of letter canceling fee.

may arise that constitute a hardship. If the doctor then agrees to reduce the fee, the patient should be told that the reduction will be effective only after the adjusted amount is paid in full. For instance, if a fee of $300 is reduced to $200, the full amount of the $300 charge should appear on the ledger and when $200 has been received, the remainder can be written off as an adjustment. Under some circumstances it may be better simply to write off an unpaid account. There must be some limit put on the time, effort, and expense invested in trying to collect an uncollectible account. An example of a letter that might be used to cancel the account and at the same time improve the image of the physician is shown in Figure 13–2.

PITFALLS OF FEE ADJUSTMENTS. Great care should be taken in reducing the fee for care of a patient who dies. The doctor's sympathy may be with the family in such instances, but the doctor's generosity in reducing a fee could be misinterpreted and result in a suit for malpractice.

If the doctor agrees to settle for a reduced fee in a situation in which the patient is disputing the fee, he should make certain the negotiations are "without prejudice." By taking this precaution the doctor protects his right to collect the original sum should the patient refuse to pay the lowered fee. The offer of a discount, therefore, should be made in writing, with the insertion of the words "without prejudice," and a definite time limit in which payment is to be made should be stated. Make two copies of the agreement and have the signatures witnessed. Keep the original for the doctor and give a copy to the patient.

A fee should never be reduced on the basis of a poor result or as a means of obtaining payment to avoid the use of a collection agency. A reduction for these reasons will degrade the doctor and his practice.

PROFESSIONAL COURTESY. Traditionally, doctors do not charge one another or their immediate dependents for medical care. In some areas, and especially in the case of specialists, giving of professional courtesy represents the loss of a large amount of potential income. If there is a substantial outlay in the cost of materials, the professional colleague will probably wish to reimburse the physician for the materials used. Many doctors subscribe to a health insurance plan. If the care they receive is covered by insurance, it is entirely ethical for the attending physician to accept the insurance benefits in payment for his services.

If the care involved is frequent enough to involve a significant proportion of the doctor's professional time, or in cases of long-term treatment, the doctor may wish to charge on an adjusted basis.

If professional courtesy is offered, but the recipient insists upon paying, the physician need not hesitate on ethical grounds to accept a fee for his services.

Professional courtesy is often extended beyond fellow physicians and their dependents. Most physicians treat their own assistants without charge, and grant discounts of 20 to 50 per cent to nurses and assistants not in their direct employ. In still other instances, professional courtesy is extended to others in the health care field, for instance, to pharmacists, dentists, and clergymen.

CHARGES TO AVOID. It is generally considered inadvisable to charge for *telephone calls*. Some physicians, especially pediatricians, find they must give considerable medical advice over the telephone. Many of these calls, however, are fairly routine to the office (although not to the worried mother or patient) and an able assistant can be trained to answer many of the questions, or a special time can be set aside for telephone calls.

Levying *late charges* on fees for professional services not paid within a prescribed time is not in the best interest of the public or the profession, according to the AMA Judicial Council.

Most physicians feel that charging for a *missed appointment* or for one not canceled 24 hours in advance, although not unethical if the patient is fully advised, is nevertheless not in the best interest of their patients or their practices.

If a patient has multiple insurance forms to be completed, the physician is justified in making a charge but may antagonize if he charges for the *first insurance form*.

The end of the year will find at least some of the patients requesting a *summary of their charges and payments for the year* just completed. There is a temptation to make an additional charge for this service. In most cases, it is probably unwise to do so.

CREDIT ARRANGEMENTS

Extending Credit

The word "credit" has numerous definitions and shades of meaning. A student receives educational *credit* for successful completion of a unit of study. To the accountant, *credit* means the right-hand side of an account. Credit may mean belief in the genuineness or truth of something. When the doctor "extends credit" to a patient, *credit* implies a given time limit during which payment will be made, and sometimes includes an oral or written promise to pay. When the patient makes a payment, the assistant *credits* the patient's account with the amount paid. The person extending credit (the doctor in this case) is known as a *creditor* and the person receiving credit is the *debtor*. Federal law (Equal Credit Opportunity Act of 1977) bars discrimination in all areas of credit, with the purpose of ensuring that credit is made available fairly and impartially. The law prohibits discrimination against any applicant for credit because of race, color, religion, national origin, sex, marital status, or age; or because the applicant receives income from any public assistance program; or because he has exercised rights under consumer credit laws. These are "prohibited bases" under the law.

Every collection for a doctor's services is preceded by an extension of credit. Credit arrangements are best made during the patient's initial visit; successful collection of an account may depend upon the skill and tact with which the first interview is conducted.

INFORMATION FROM THE PATIENT. Good records are essential to follow-up of collections. It is extremely important that the assistant get adequate information about the patient's ability to pay — on his first visit to the office, if possible. It is neither unprofessional nor time consuming to get full credit information from patients. The public is conditioned to supply such information, and will respect a businesslike approach if it is done tactfully and without apology. Although a patient needing medical care will rarely be turned away because of his credit risk, the information provided on the initial visit may alert the assistant to be cautious about allowing an account to fall in arrears.

Many medical assistants inform a patient when he telephones for a first appointment that new patients are expected to pay cash for their first visit, at which time credit arrangements can be established if further care is needed. She can say, for example, "Mr. Barrington, your appointment is scheduled for 9:30 AM, Tuesday, September 25, with Dr. Newhouse. The usual charge for a first office visit is about *X* dollars, and we ask that payment for a first visit be made at the time of service. If you wish to establish credit arrangements in case further care is needed, please plan to be here 15 minutes early so that the necessary papers can be completed." This approach informs the patient in advance that he will be expected to complete a credit application. Although the registration form the patient completes in the doctor's office is usually not as detailed as an application for credit in, for example, a department store, it must establish an information base, should future collection steps become necessary. The form illustrated in Figure 13–3 is typical.

Sometimes the assistant will ask questions of the patient and type his answers on the form; in other offices, the patient will be handed a form to complete himself. This affords him more privacy if there are others present and tends to eliminate the

PATIENT INFORMATION FOR MEDICAL RECORDS (PLEASE PRINT) DATE 04 01 82

LAST NAME (MISS / MR. / MRS.)	FIRST	MIDDLE	SOCIAL SECURITY NO.	DATE OF BIRTH	AGE
JONES	JOHN	ALLEN	000 00 0000	03 26 47	35

HOME ADDRESS STREET CITY STATE ZIP CODE HOME PHONE

1234 EAST STREET, CINCINNATI, OHIO 45202 513-252-0000

OCCUPATION: Accountant EMPLOYED BY: Central Financial Management

EMPLOYER'S ADDRESS STREET CITY STATE PHONE NO.

15 Main Street, Cincinnati 45010 513-212-0000

SPOUSE'S NAME: Cathleen Jones MARITAL STATUS: M S D W SEP REFERRED BY: M. A. Wilkins, M.D.

OTHER IMMEDIATE FAMILY MEMBERS WHO WILL BE PATIENTS

IN CASE OF EMERGENCY CONTACT: NAME, ADDRESS AND PHONE NUMBER OF RELATIVE OR FRIEND

Daughter: Marilyn Barker, 850 South Ortega, Baltimore MD 21201 301-586-7040

MEDICAL INSURANCE INFORMATION

COMPANY	POLICY NUMBER
Travelers	10101
COMPANY	POLICY NUMBER
COMPANY	POLICY NUMBER

IF SOMEONE OTHER THAN PATIENT IS RESPONSIBLE FOR PAYMENT PLEASE COMPLETE THIS SECTION

NAME OF RESPONSIBLE PARTY HOME ADDRESS PHONE NO.

OCCUPATION EMPLOYED BY

EMPLOYER'S ADDRESS PHONE NO.

I hereby authorize Dr. Edwin Johnson to furnish to the above insurance company(s) or to a designated attorney, all information which said insurance company(s) or attorney may request. I hereby assign to Dr. Edwin Johnson all money to which I am entitled for medical and/or surgical expense relative to the service rendered by him, but not to exceed my indebtedness to said physician and/or surgeon. It is understood that any money received from the above named insurance company, over and above my indebtedness will be refunded to me when my bill is paid in full. I understand I am financially responsible to said doctor(s) for charges not covered by this assignment. I further agree in the event of non-payment, to bear the cost of collection, and/or Court cost and reasonable legal fees should this be required.

INSURED OR GUARDIAN SIGNATURE PATIENT'S SIGNATURE J. A. Jones

"A PHOTOCOPY OF THIS FORM SHALL BE DEEMED AS VALID AND EFFECTIVE AS THE ORIGINAL".

BIBBERO SYSTEMS FORM NO. MDP 8411 © 1965 BIBBERO SYSTEMS, INC., SAN FRANCISCO

FIGURE 13–3 Patient information sheet for medical records. (Courtesy of Bibbero Systems, Inc., San Francisco, California.)

13

impression that the assistant is overly inquisitive. The medical assistant should check the form carefully to make certain that nothing was overlooked. The new patient will view these questions as reasonable, but the established patient may resent such an inquiry. Consequently, *it is important that the form be completed on the first visit.*

Irrespective of the form or techniques used, the following information should be obtained:

1. *Patient's Full Name*, correctly spelled. J. A. Brown is not sufficient if later collection follow-up is necessary. John Allen Brown would be more helpful.
2. *Date of Birth*. May be useful as identification if there are two patients with similar names. Also, you will be able to determine the patient's exact age at any future time.
3. *Social Security Number*, if any. The social security number is an increasingly important item of identification. In many states it is required in making collection efforts against bank accounts, wages, or any other personal property. Many insurance policies use the patient's social security number as his certificate number.
4. *Marital Status and Number of Dependents*. May be useful in determining ability to pay. When couples are divorced or separated, credit and collections sometimes become complicated.
5. *Current Address and Past Addresses for at Least Two Years*. From this information you can judge the person's stability. Multiple residences in a short time may indicate financial instability; the class of neighborhood may give indication of a patient's financial status.
6. *Telephone Numbers for both Residence and Work*. If patient has no home telephone, get the number of the nearest telephone. It may be necessary to call the patient or contact his employer.
7. *Name and Relationship of Person Legally Responsible for Payment*. See paragraph on third party liability, below.
8. *Patient's and Spouse's Occupation, Name and Address of Employer*. If a man lists his employer as Gord's Department Store, find out his employment title and the name of his immediate superior. He may be a shipping clerk or salesman, or he may be the vice president.
9. *Name, Address, and Telephone Number of Person* to be notified in case of emergency.
10. *Name of Neighbor or Friend in Area*. If a patient moves after receiving medical care, a friend or neighbor may be able to provide information on his whereabouts.
11. *Who Referred Patient to Doctor*. If patient is referred by another physician, you will want to send a report to the physician. If referred by another patient, the doctor may wish to thank the referring patient on his next visit to the office.
12. *Health Insurance Information*. See paragraph on page 185.

When a patient applies for credit, you *may not* ask the applicant's sex, race, color, religion, or national origin. You *may not* ask about birth control practices or plans to have children. You *may* collect this information when it is part of a medical history, but not when it is related to granting credit. Under the Equal Credit Opportunity Act, once you agree to extend credit to one patient, you must offer the same arrangement to any other patient who requests it. You can refuse to do so only based upon ability—or inability—to pay. It is interesting that one way to avoid involvement with the credit laws is to accept bank credit cards; this may be all that is needed to persuade more doctors to forget their long-time aversion to credit cards and extend this convenience to patients who wish to use it.

THIRD PARTY LIABILITY. If financial responsibility is attributed to an individual other than the patient, spouse, or parent, be sure to obtain full name, address, employment data, and other credit information about that person. Also, contact the named individual for verification of the obligation. If a third party's agreement to pay is contingent upon the patient's failure to pay, such an agreement must be in writing to be enforceable and must be made prior to treatment. Any agreement made after completion of treatment could be considered as a moral obligation only. The guarantee of a person to pay the account of another may be very simple. It may be typewritten or in longhand, stating:

I, the undersigned, do promise to pay for the medical services rendered by Theodore Wilson, M.D., to my nephew, Robert L. Smith.

Date:
Signed:

or

I, the undersigned, promise to pay the medical bill of Robert L. Smith, if his mother, Mrs. Lydia Smith, does not pay by the 15th of July, 19——.

Date:
Signed:

Accounts rendered to a wife or child should always carry full data about the party responsible, in most cases the husband or father. Generally, a husband or father pays the account for which he is obligated without any necessary follow-up collection procedures.

If you foresee legal difficulties in collecting on an account in a situation in which divorce, legal guardianships, or emancipated minors complicate the matter, it is best to contact your doctor's attorney for advice. The laws governing such matters vary according to each state. One reminder, however, is that you must always have the signature of the third party responsible for the debt if he is not obligated by law. An oral agreement is not binding.

HEALTH INSURANCE INFORMATION. The initial interview is the best time to get full information on the patient's insurance coverage. The patient registration form usually provides a place for the name of the insurance company. Ask to see the patient's identification card; if he has one, make a photocopy for your records. The card will usually show the name of the subscriber and the group and member number, and often will include a service code indicating the patient's coverage. Also obtain information on any supplementary coverage, for instance, a plan in which the spouse is the subscriber and the patient is covered as a dependent. There may also be major medical or supplementary benefits to the patient's policy.

ASSIGNMENTS. Many doctors ask the patient to execute an assignment of insurance benefits at this time. The assignment, authorizing the insurance company to pay benefits directly to the doctor, may be stamped on the insurance form or may be subsequently attached to a completed insurance form.

CONSENT FOR RELEASE OF INFORMATION. If a standard claim form is used or if the patient has brought along his own form, this is an appropriate time to have the patient sign the consent for release of information which is necessary on most claims, so that the insurance form can be processed without delay as services are performed. Some states require a special form for release of information separate and apart from the insurance claim form itself. The assistant should check local regulations.

INSTALLMENT BUYING OF MEDICAL SERVICES

Because installment buying is so much a part of our economic system today, the physician's office must be prepared to help patients budget for their medical care. Patients expect to use their credit resources and will appreciate businesslike assistance in establishing a payment plan. The medical profession has too long suffered a poor collection record because of its fear of appearing "too commercial." The doctor should be ready to arrange credit when medical bills will be high or when a patient for some reason is unable to pay his bills. Fees for routine office calls and small medical bills should be kept on a pay-as-you-go basis.

CREDIT CARDS. The acceptance of credit cards in the doctor's office is becoming more commonplace every day. A few years ago this would have been shocking to most physicians.

The AMA Code of Ethics discourages the use of a bank card in connection with the payment of large fees that might normally be paid to the physician in installments. However, it does set forth certain guidelines for physician participation in bank card programs:

> (1) The county medical society should be satisfied as to the financial and professional integrity of the plan. . .
>
> (2) The individual physician may not, because of his participation, increase his fee for medical service rendered the patient. He may not use the plan to solicit patients. He may not encourage patients to use the plan. His position must be that he accepts the plan as a convenience to patients who desire to use it. Plaques or other devices indicating participation in the plan within the physician's office should be kept to a discreet and dignified minimum. Plaques, signs, or other devices indicating such participation visible outside the physician's office are unacceptable.

BANK FINANCING. Some banks have set up plans to do the financing job for patients in a manner consistent with professional ethics. The dental profession has pioneered in this field, and many dental societies have worked out arrangements with banks to help patients meet dental expenses.

Here is how bank financing of bills works: The bank checks the patient's credit and, if it appears acceptable, agrees to take the patient's promise to pay. The bank then forwards the doctor the total sum which the patient owes him, less a small discount. This provides the doctor with the full amount due him immediately. The bank really is lending the money to patients at a small rate of interest; doctors often deduct the interest charges from their fees as a further encouragement to patients to take advantage of these budget plans. Literature and introductory cards to the bank or a similar professional budget bureau can be provided to patients who are interested in exploring these special budget and financing plans.

Before seeking outside financing help on behalf of patients, it is important that the doctor carefully investigate available plans and determine whether or not their use is justified. There are some unscrupulous organizations that press patients for payment in an unethical manner and create considerable ill will for the profession.

SPECIAL BUDGET PLANS. If a patient appears upset at the prospect of meeting his obligations, the doctor or his assistant can suggest in a tactful way: "Mr. Elwood, if you think you will have difficulty paying for your treatments at one time, we can work out some special arrangements." This allows the patient to ask what sort of plan you have in mind, and the discussion progresses very easily into various payment plans. It is good to ask the patient what arrangements will be best for him rather than to suggest a plan. If he is still reluctant, the assistant then can say, "Mr. Elwood, would you be able to pay $50 each month until the account is paid in full?" or "Usually an account of this size can be settled in three to four months. Would you be able to pay $100 down, then $50 a month until the account is paid in full?" When the amount of each installment has been agreed upon, it is then wise to establish definite dates on which the payments will be expected.

TRUTH IN LENDING ACT. Regulation Z of the Truth in Lending Act, which is enforced by the Federal Trade Commission, requires that when there is a bilateral agreement between doctor and patient to accept payment in more than four

FEDERAL TRUTH IN LENDING CONSUMER CREDIT DISCLOSURE STATEMENT FOR PROFESSIONAL SERVICES

January 13, 1982
Date

Joseph Brookhurst
Patient's Name

Name of Parent or Guardian

353 West Terry Lane
Address

Surgery
Services Rendered or to be Rendered

Birmingham, Alabama 35209
City State ZIP

12-28-81
Dates of Services

THEODORE WHITE, M.D.

1. Fee for Professional Service	$	800	00
2. Initial Fee	$	200	00
3. Unpaid Balance of Fee *(Item 1 minus Item 2)*	$	600	00
4. Amount Financed	$	600	00
5. FINANCE CHARGE *(If none, write "NONE")*	none		
6. Total of Payments *(Item 4 plus Item 5)*	$	600	00
7. Deferred Payment Price *(Item 1 plus Item 5)*	$	800	00
8. ANNUAL PERCENTAGE RATE *(If none, write "NONE")*	none		

The undersigned hereby agrees to pay the above named doctor an initial payment of $ 200.00 and six (Number of Payments) consecutive monthly (Monthly, Quarterly, etc.) payments of $ 100.00 each. These installments will be paid on the 15th day of the month of each period beginning February 15, 1982. Any fractional balance remaining at the time of the last installment will be included with that payment.

I HEREBY CERTIFY that I have read and received a copy of this Disclosure Statement.

Joseph Brookhurst
Signature of Patient or of Parent or Guardian if Patient is a Minor

January 13, 1982
Date

FIGURE 13–4 Disclosure statement.

13

installments, the doctor is required to provide disclosure of information regarding finance charges. Even if there are no finance charges involved the form must be completed stating that this is so. A copy of the form is retained by the doctor and the original is given to the patient. Specific wording is required in the disclosure. The form in Figure 13–4 meets the requirements. Have the patient sign the agreement in your presence, as you must have proof of signing. The disclosure statement must be kept on file for two years. Although the disclosure statement is designed as protection for the debtor, it can be a good collection tool for the creditor.

It is recognized that physicians generally permit their patients to pay in installments, and as long as there is no specific agreement on the part of the physician for payment to be made in more than four installments, and he does not make a finance charge, he is not subject to the regulation. If the patient chooses to pay installments instead of the full amount for which he is billed, this is considered a unilateral action and the physician, in accepting such payments, probably would not subject himself to the provisions of the regulation. The doctor's office, however, must be certain to bill for the *full balance* each time. If the statement is for only a partial payment, it then becomes a bilateral agreement and as such is subject to Regulation Z.

Helping patients budget their medical expenses is a rather new aspect of the business side of practice. However, it is a real service to patients and demonstrates that the doctor and his office staff are sincerely anxious to help patients pay their own way. From the assistant's standpoint, use of such plans solves many of her collection problems, thus making her work easier.

CREDIT IS CONFIDENTIAL

Always remember that credit information is confidential. It should be guarded as carefully as a confidential medical history and should not be disclosed to anyone. When you ask for credit information from patients in the office, make sure that you do so in a place where others cannot overhear the conversation. A desk or table away from the reception area where a patient can sit in total privacy and complete a credit application is a great asset. Credit information is personal — it should be kept that way.

CREDIT BUREAU. Some doctors, particularly in large cities where it is more difficult to gauge informally the patients' ability to pay, join a credit bureau. Credit bureaus round up credit information from many sources, pool it, and make it available to local businesses that become bureau members by paying dues. If you receive a request for credit information about one of your patients, it is permissible to furnish it because the debtor, by giving your name as a reference, has given implied consent; otherwise, the credit bureau would not have called you. According to the Fair Credit Practices Act Amendments of 1975, you can reply by giving *ledger information* only: (1) when the account was opened, (2) how much the patient now owes, and (3) the highest amount of the account at any time. The doctor's office should confine information furnished to these three items and avoid any reference to character, paying habits, or credit rating. Before joining a credit organization, it is a good idea for the doctor or his staff to check to make sure it is an ethical bureau with no unscrupulous practices.

BUREAUS OF MEDICAL ECONOMICS. In a number of localities, the medical societies maintain bureaus of medical economics which either have their own credit information service or have access to a reputable credit bureau. Such a society-operated bureau can be of great help in determining a patient's medical credit rating and also in helping develop good collection procedures. If there is a bureau of medical economics in your area, this will probably be your best source for determining a patient's medical credit. The county society-owned bureau maintains a master file on all acounts assigned and will advise you if an individual has a poor medical credit record.

MEDICAL-DENTAL-HOSPITAL BUREAUS. The Medical-Dental-Hospital Bureaus of America (MDHBA), with headquarters in Chicago, is a national organization of agencies serving physicians, dentists, and hospitals. It seeks to maintain the highest standards among its members and is committed to following the collection methods most acceptable to physicians. Doctors who use their collection services have access to credit information on accounts assigned by other clients. Member bureaus of the MDHBA frequently assist the medical office assistant by sponsoring collection seminars, as well as by providing speakers for medical assistant society meetings.

Even though your office uses the services of a credit bureau or collection agency, do not rely upon such organizations completely to supply you with credit information. Sometimes the information you obtain from patients in the office will be more up-to-date than that on the bureau records. Unfortunately, many people with an AAA rating on auto, bank, and charge accounts still do not like to pay medical bills.

CHAPTER OUTLINE

Billing Procedures
- Outside Services
  - Computerized Billing
  - Microfilm Billing
  - Copy Van or Centralized Photocopying
- Billing by Medical Office Personnel
  - Typewritten Statements
  - Photocopied Statements
  - The Superbill

Preparing Statements
- Send Correct Bills
- Itemize Bills
- Mail Bills Promptly
- Time and Frequency of Billing
  - Once-a-Month Billing
  - Cycle Billing

Billing Third Parties and Minors

Collection Procedures
- Reasons to Pursue Collections
- Assistant's Attitude
- Aging of Accounts Receivable
- Credit Policy
- Collection System
  - Immediate Payments
  - Charge Slip System
  - Why Medical Bills Are Paid Last
- Collection Letters
  - Who Signs Collection Letters?
  - Sample Letters
- Collection by Personal Interview
- Telephone Collection Techniques

Special Collection Problems
- Tracing Skips
- Claims against Estates
- Statutes of Limitations
- Bankruptcy

Suing for Recovery on Overdue Accounts

Selection of Accounts for Collection Agency

Small Claims Court

Accounts Receivable Insurance Protection

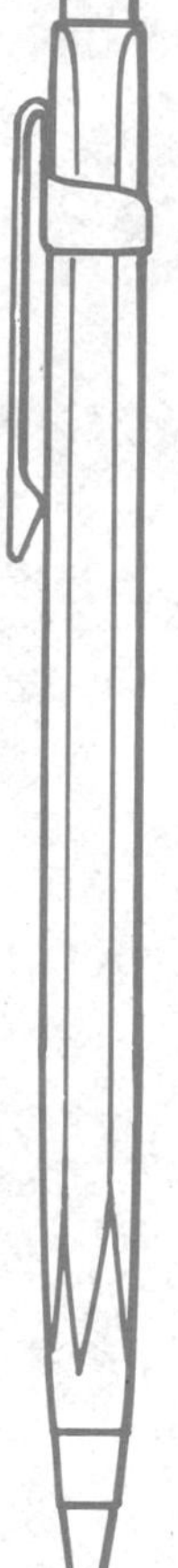

BEHAVIORAL OBJECTIVES

The medical office assistant should be able to:

- **Prepare information for an outside billing service.**
- **Select suitable statement forms for efficient billing.**
- **Prepare statements for patient billing.**
- **Prepare a superbill.**
- **Itemize charges.**
- **Observe legal regulations in billing for services.**
- **Set up cycle billing system.**
- **Explain reasons for pursuing collections.**
- **Develop a suitable attitude toward collection responsibilities.**
- **Age accounts and analyze suitable follow-up procedure.**
- **Assist in developing office credit policy.**
- **Explain credit policy to patients.**
- **Collect payments at time of visit.**
- **Prepare a charge slip for services rendered.**
- **Compose suitable and effective collection letters.**
- **Make financial arrangements with patients.**
- **Use appropriate telephone collection technique.**
- **Take initial steps in tracing a skip.**
- **Bill claims against estates.**
- **Explain statutes of limitations.**
- **Use correct procedures in bankruptcy cases.**
- **Assist in deciding which delinquent accounts to sue.**
- **Assist in selecting a collection agency.**
- **Place delinquent account with collection agency.**
- **Explain the advantages and disadvantages of collecting via small claims court.**
- **State reasons for accounts receivable insurance.**

14

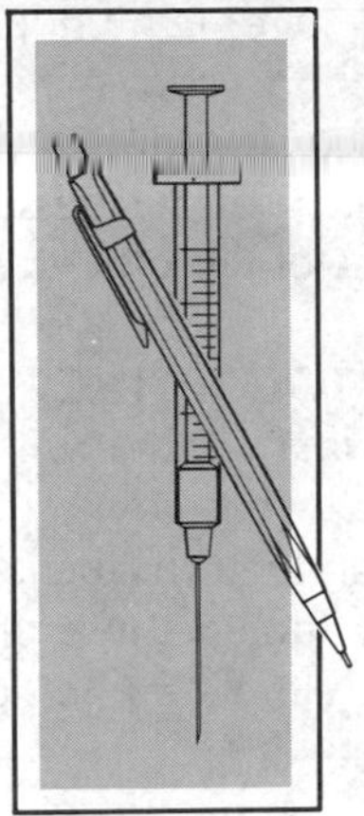

BILLING AND COLLECTION PROCEDURES

Management consultants for the medical profession say that the accounts receivable on a doctor's books should ideally equal no more than two to three months' gross charges. They also agree that a collection ratio of less than 90 per cent indicates that something is wrong with the collection procedure. Keeping accounts receivable down and collections up is neither impossible nor difficult if proper procedures are developed and consistently followed. With all financial records (including patients' account cards) kept current and a collection policy that is well-managed, collections can be a very satisfying challenge. Without such a program, however, end-of-the-month billing day can be the most psychologically difficult day of the month for the medical assistant.

The major portion of the doctor's fees will be paid without question upon presentation of a bill, provided correct procedures are being followed. Collection of professional accounts can be divided into three distinct stages:

1. Informing the patient of what the charges will be and what professional services these cover,

2. Providing an opportunity for the patient to pay at the time of service for smaller amounts and sending bills out promptly for larger fees, and

3. Conscientiously following up on uncollected accounts. In many instances, particularly if surgery or long-term treatment is involved, the first stage of collection will be done by the physician himself. The medical assistant is customarily charged with the responsibility of stages two and three, the subject of this chapter.

BILLING PROCEDURES

Direct billing from the doctor's office is the main concern of this chapter. Other choices, however, will be mentioned here.

Outside Services

COMPUTERIZED BILLING. The medical office that "has gone on computer" for accounts receivable management service has probably included a billing and insurance form completion service. These services will be discussed further in Chapter 16, Keeping Financial Records.

MICROFILM BILLING. Recommended by many management consultants, microfilm billing is particularly useful to offices with large volume billings. On a specified day of the month, a representative of the billing service brings portable camera equipment to the office and microfilms each ledger that has a balance due. This requires very little time, and the ledgers remain under the control of the office. The film is processed by the billing service, and a copy of the ledger is mailed to the patient. The mailing can include a self-addressed envelope for direct payment to the physician. An extra benefit of microfilming is that a duplicate set of ledger cards is generated, which would be useful in case of loss of the office records by fire or other causes.

COPY VAN OR CENTRALIZED PHOTOCOPYING. In some areas you may find a billing service with a copier mounted in a van that will call at the doctor's office once a month. The representative takes the ledger tray from the office to the van, runs the ledgers through a high speed copier, and returns the ledgers to the doctor's office in a matter of minutes. The service can include inserting the copy in an envelope, stamping, and mailing. For the office without a photocopy machine, this may be the most inexpensive method of outside billing.

Billing by Medical Office Personnel

When billing is done by the medical assistant there are still several choices of method: (1) typing an original statement, (2) photocopying the ledger card, and (3) preparing a superbill.

TYPEWRITTEN STATEMENTS. Twenty-five years ago almost all statements for medical services were individually typewritten — there was no choice. With the equipment available today, typing individual statements each month is practical only in the small or limited practice with few statements and an assistant whose time would not be more profitably used in other endeavors.

The appearance of the statement carries a visual impact just as a letter does, so the statement heads should be carefully chosen and the typing clean and accurate. Statement heads usually are imprinted with the same information as the doctor's letterhead. They should be of good quality and large enough to allow itemization of charges. Many offices use self-addressed return envelopes as statements. This procedure is mainly for the convenience of patients who do not always have stationery available for sending a return payment or are less likely to return a payment immediately if they must search for an envelope. Occasionally there is the complaint that when statements are sent on self-addressed return envelopes, the patient has no record of the bill once he sends in his payment. A statement form is available that allows the patient to tear the bill into two parts along a perforated line. The top half, which carries the patient's name, address, and amount owed, is returned to the doctor's office along with the payment; the bottom half, on which the bill is itemized, can be retained by the patient in his files. The return envelope statement can be mailed to the patient in a window envelope, thus avoiding duplicate typing of the patient's name and address (see Fig. 14–1).

The use of continuous form billing statements is a time-saver. The statements are printed in a roll with perforated edges for separation. The roll is fed into the typewriter for the first statement and remains until the last statement is typed, eliminating the time and energy necessary for inserting and removing each statement form from the typewriter.

Another time saver is the multiple copy statement. The Colwell Company calls its version "E–Z Statements." The E–Z Statement features three monthly statements plus one patient's ledger card in each set, all in NCR (no carbon required) paper. Services and payments are posted during the month, and at billing time the top sheet is removed, folded, and mailed in a window envelope. If more than three mailings are required, a new set must be headed and the balance forwarded.

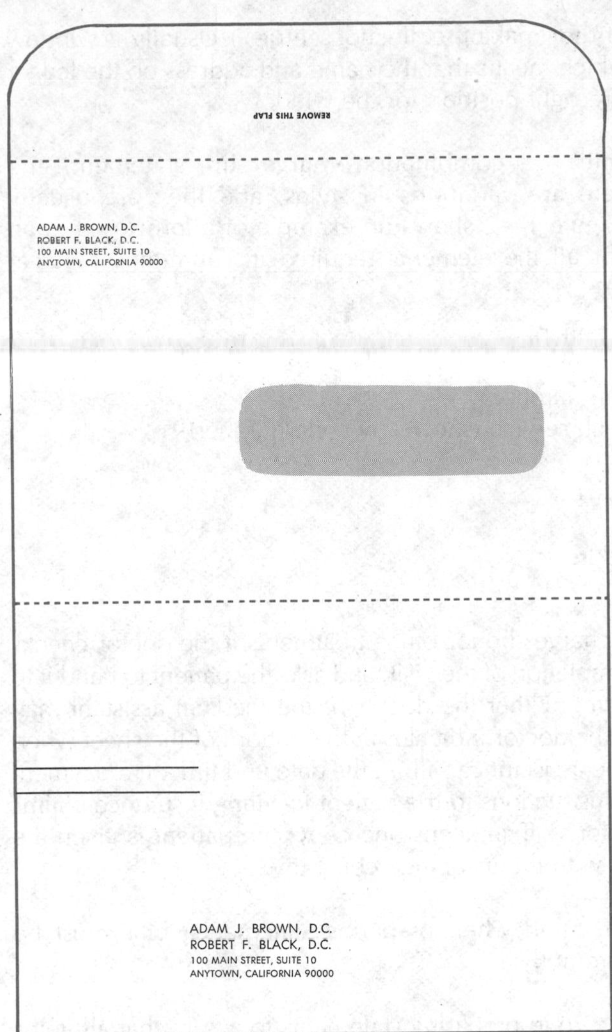

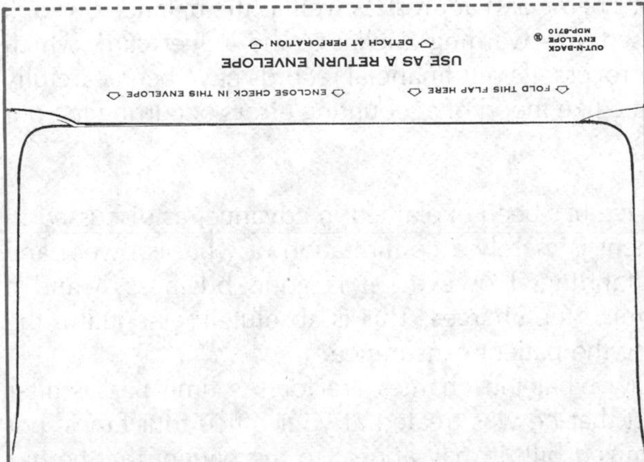

BILLING NAME	NAMES OF OTHER FAMILY MEMBERS
Paul Allan	Wife: Thelma A.
PATIENT'S NAME: same	Daughter: April
RES PHONE 492 3737 BUS PHONE 551 1797	
OCCUPATION: teacher	RELATIVE OR FRIEND
EMPLOYED BY: Anytown Unified School District	REFERRED BY: David Bucher, M.D.
INS. INFORMATION: California General	SOC. SEC. NUMBER: 111 00 2222
FORM NO. MDP 8510	© 1965 BIBBERO SYSTEMS, INC. - SAN FRANCISCO

ADAM J. BROWN, D.C.
ROBERT F. BLACK, D.C.
PALMER CHIROPRACTORS
100 MAIN STREET, SUITE 10
ANYTOWN, CALIFORNIA 90000
TELEPHONE: 399-4000

STATEMENT TO:

Mr. Paul Allan
123 Main Street
Anytown, XX 00000

TEAR OFF AND RETURN UPPER PORTION WITH PAYMENT

DATE 1981	PAYMENTS: BANK NUMBER	PAYMENTS: BY CHECK OR P.M.O.	PAYMENTS: BY COIN OR CURRENCY	PROFESSIONAL SERVICE		FEE	LAST AMOUNT IN THIS COLUMN IS BALANCE DUE
05 29				90050	Office call	25 00	25 00
				85010	CBC	10 00	35 00
06 05				90040	Office call	20 00	55 00

PROFESSIONAL SERVICE CODES:

1. CONSULTATION
2. EXAMINATION
3. DIAG. EXAM., MAJOR
4. CHIROPRACTIC ADJUSTMENT
5. ADJUSTMENT, PROLONGED
6. COMPLETE FULL SPINE X-RAYS
7. SPINE CERVICAL A-P AND LAT.
8. SPINE, CERVICAL COMP. (DAVIS)
9. SPINE, THORACIC, TWO VIEWS
10. SPINE, THORACO — LUMBAR, A-P AND LAT.
11. SPINE, LUMBOSACRAL COMPLETE
12. PELVIS, COMPLETE
13. PELVIS, SACRUM AND COCCYX, A-P AND LAT.
14. KNEE SERIES
15. SHOULDER SERIES
16. URINALYSIS
17. CERVICAL PILLOW AND CASE
18. CERVICAL COLLAR AND CASE
19. LUMBOSACRAL SUPPORT
20. NARRATIVE REPORT
21. OTHER
22. NO CHARGE
23. ADJUSTMENTS OR CORRECTIONS

ADAM J. BROWN, D.C. - LIC. #56372 ROBERT F. BLACK, D.C. - LIC. #32780

14

FIGURE 14–1 Example of a return envelope statement.

PHOTOCOPIED STATEMENTS. Photocopy equipment is almost as standard as the typewriter in today's offices. The production of photocopied statements is a natural consequence. Coordinated ledger cards and copy paper are used, and a perfect statement is ready for mailing in minimum time. Extra care must be used in posting the ledgers, however. A black pen should be used in making entries on the ledger card. Other ink colors do not reproduce well. Writing must be clear and legible. There should be no personal notes made on the ledger cards unless it is something you wish conveyed to the patient. (It is possible to get pencils with nonreproducible lead if you feel this is necessary for making collection entries.) Usually a window envelope is used for mailing, which means that the name and address on the ledger must be neat, correct, and in the right position for the window.

THE SUPERBILL. The superbill is a combination charge slip, statement, and insurance reporting form. There are variations in styles, and they are usually personalized for the practice. Figure 14–2 shows an example of a form used in an Ob-Gyn office. It has space for all the elements required in submitting medical insurance claims:

1. Name and address of patient
2. Name of insurance carrier
3. Insurance identification number
4. Brief description of each service (shown by code number)
5. Fee for each service
6. Place and date of service
7. Diagnosis
8. Doctor's name and address
9. Doctor's signature

The superbill can be used as a charge slip for office treatments if the doctor checks the services performed at the completion of the visit, and asks the patient to hand it to the medical assistant upon leaving. Either the doctor or the medical assistant may write in the amount of the fee. The doctor indicates at the bottom of the sheet when the patient should return, and the assistant can fill in the date and time. If a payment is made it can be so indicated. Instructions to the patient for filing insurance claims are on the bottom left. The doctor's office keeps one copy; the patient is given the original and one copy for filing with the insurance company.

PREPARING STATEMENTS

Three points should be kept in mind when preparing statements: bills must be correct, itemized, and mailed promptly.

SEND CORRECT BILLS. Take care in preparing statements to assure that all items are correct, including the patient's name and address as well as the balance owed. If photocopy or microfilming is used, this warning applies to the ledger card, which will be duplicated in the billing process. If your financial records have been carefully maintained each day, there is little likelihood of accounting errors occurring in your statements.

ITEMIZE BILLS. If the medical fee has been explained in advance, as discussed in Chapter 13, the monthly statement is merely a confirmation of what is owed, and there should be no misunderstanding. However, it is good business — and a courtesy to the patient — to itemize the charges. This is absolutely essential if the statement is to be used for billing the patient's insurance.

Patients are entitled to know what the charges are for. As time passes after treatment, the patient may forget that he was treated at your office four times, not three. Upon receiving an unitemized bill, it may appear to the patient that he has been overcharged. Also, remember that he may not have been told, or may have forgotten under the stress of seeking medical care, just exactly what was done to help his condition. Tests unfamiliar to the patient are sometimes ordered at his expense, without an explanation. Many physicians order tests done at outside laboratories that later bill the patient direct. The medical assistant must be sure to explain this to the patient so that there will be no surprise — or possibly indignation — when a statement arrives from the laboratory.

Itemizing bills is not difficult. The simplest method is merely to allow space on the original statement below the "For Professional Services" line on which the

RICHARD W. LANGERT, M.D.
Obstetrics, Gynecology, Infertility
647 CAMINO DE LOS MARES, SUITE 221
SAN CLEMENTE, CALIFORNIA 92672
TELEPHONE: (714) 661-0543

CAL. LIC. #G-41043
TAX ID #95-3419518
PROVIDER #OOG-410430

№ 33

☒PRIVATE ☐BLUE CROSS ☐BLUE SHIELD ☐IND. ☐MEDI-CAL ☐MEDICARE ☐GOV'T.

PATIENT INFORMATION

PATIENT'S LAST NAME	FIRST	INITIAL	BIRTHDATE	SEX	TODAY'S DATE
Albertson	Margaret	O	05 04 60	☐MALE ☒FEMALE	10 11 81

ADDRESS	CITY	STATE	ZIP	RELATIONSHIP TO SUBSCRIBER
143 W. Osborn	Anytown	XY	00000	spouse

SUBSCRIBER OR POLICYHOLDER	INSURANCE CARRIER
Donald W. Albertson	Travelers Insurance Company

ADDRESS	CITY	STATE	ZIP	INS. I.D.	COVERAGE CODE	GROUP
same				975 00 333		049

OTHER HEALTH COVERAGE ☒NO ☐YES IDENTIFY
DISABILITY RELATED TO: ☐ACCIDENT ☐INDUSTRIAL ☒PREGNANCY ☐OTHER
DATE SYMPTOMS APPEARED, INCEPTION OF PREGNANCY, OR ACCIDENT OCCURRED: LMP 08 07 81

ASSIGNMENT: I HEREBY AUTHORIZE MY INSURANCE BENEFITS TO BE PAID DIRECTLY TO THE UNDERSIGNED PHYSICIAN. I AM FINANCIALLY RESPONSIBLE FOR NON-COVERED SERVICES.
SIGNED (Patient or Parent, if Minor) *Margaret Albertson* Date *10/11/81*

RELEASE: I HEREBY AUTHORIZE THE UNDERSIGNED PHYSICIAN TO RELEASE ANY INFORMATION ACQUIRED IN THE COURSE OF MY EXAMINATION OR TREATMENT.
SIGNED (Patient or Parent, if Minor) *Margaret Albertson* Date *10/11/81*

PHYSICIAN INFORMATION

A. PROFESSIONAL SERVICE CODES	1 OFFICE VISIT		2 HOSPITAL VISIT		3 EMERGENCY ROOM		4 CONSULTATION	FEE
TYPE OF PATIENT	NEW	ESTAB.	INITIAL	REPEAT	NEW	ESTAB.	ALL	
Minimal Service		90030				90530		
Brief Service	90000	90040	90200	90240	90500	90540		
Limited Service	90010	90050		90250	90510	90550	90600	
Intermediate Service	(90015)	90060	90215	90260	90515	90560	90605	35.00
Extended Service		90070		90270		90570	90610	
Comprehensive	90020	90080	90220				90620	
Other		90088		90275		90589	90630	

✓	DESCRIPTION	CODE	FEE	✓	DESCRIPTION	CODE	FEE	✓	DESCRIPTION	CODE/MD	FEE
	B. OFFICE PROCEDURES				**C. LABORATORY (CONT.)**				**D. HOSPITAL PROCEDURES (CONT.)**		
	Total OB Care & Delivery	59400			Serology	86592			Abdominal Hysterectomy	58150	
	Total OB Care & repeat C/S	59501			Pregnancy Test - Urine	82996			Vaginal Hysterectomy	58260	
	IUD Insertion	58300			Pregnancy Test - Serum	82998			Anterior-Posterior Repair	57260	
	IUD Removal	58301			Wet Mount	87210			Vaginal Hyst. w/Repair	58265	
	Diaphragm	57170			Pap Smear	88150			Marshall - Marchetti	51840	
	Culdocentesis	57020			SMA—12	80112			Cold Cone, D & C	57521	
	Treatment, Condylomata	56500			Thyroid Panel	84251			Salpingo - Oophorectomy	58720	
	I & D, Bartholin's Abscess	56420			Rubella Titer	86171			Oophorectomy	58940	
	Biopsy, Vulva	56600			C/S - Cervix, Vagina	87070			Partial Ovarian Resection	58900	
	Biopsy, Cervix	57500			C/S - Urine	87088			Diagnostic Laparoscopy	58980	
	Biopsy, Endometrium	58100			C/S - Throat	87060			Lararoscopic Tubal Ligat.	58982	
	Cryotherapy, Cervix	57511			F.B.S.	82947			Exploratory Laparotomy	49000	
	Colposcopy	57452			Biopsy Tissue Evaluation	88304			SAb D & C	59804	
	Post-Coital Test	89300							Circumcision	54150	
	Hydrotubation	58350							Assist Surgeon	-80	
	H.A.I.	58999									
	Pessary Insertion	57160			**D. HOSPITAL PROCEDURES**				**E. MISCELLANEOUS**		
					Amniocentesis	59000			Special Supplies, Mat'ls	99070	
					Non-Stress Test	58999			Injection, Therapeutic	90730	
	C. LABORATORY				Contraction Stress Test	58999			Immunization	90721	
	(Urinalysis)	81000	7.00		Post-Partum Tubal Ligation	58605			Collection-Lab, Spec.	99007	
	CBC	85022			Primary C/S	59500			Special Reports	99080	
	Sed. Rate	85651			Tubal Ligation @ C/S	59550					
	Hematocrit	85014			Marsupialization,	56440					
	Rh & Type	86082			Bartholin's Abscess						
	(Prenatal Ab Screen)	86016	15.00		Diagnostic D & C	58120					

DIAGNOSIS:
1. *Pregnancy*
2.
3.

SERVICES PERFORMED AT:
☐ MISSION COMMUNITY HOSP. 27802 PUERTA REAL MISSION VIEJO, CA 92691
☒ OFFICE
☐ SAN CLEMENTE GEN. HOSP. 654 CAMINO DE LOS MARES SAN CLEMENTE, CA 92672
☐

ADMIT
DISCHARGE

REMARKS:

DOCTOR'S SIGNATURE/DATE *Richard W Langert MD*

RETURN APPOINTMENT INFO.:
DAYS WKS. MONS. *1* MINS.
NEXT APPOINTMENT DAY *Thursday* DATE *11-12* TIME *10*

INSTRUCTIONS TO PATIENT FOR FILING INSURANCE CLAIMS:

1. Complete upper portion of this form; sign and date.
2. Mail this form directly to your insurance company. You may attach your own insurance company's form if you wish, although it is not necessary.

PLEASE REMEMBER that our charges are due at the time the service is performed and payment is your obligation regardless of insurance or other third party involvement.

RECEIVED BY: *MK*
☐CASH
☒CHECK
☐CREDIT CARD

TODAY'S FEE	57.00
Amount Received Today	57.00
BALANCE THIS VISIT	-0-
OLD BALANCE	
NEW BALANCE	-0-

INSUR-A-BILL® • BIBBERO SYSTEMS, INC. • SAN FRANCISCO • ©3/80

FIGURE 14–2 Example of a superbill. (Courtesy of Bibbero Systems, Inc., San Francisco, California.)

assistant can list the separate charges for office, house, or hospital calls, or for treatments or tests done in the doctor's office.

Many doctors, some of them specialists, have devised their own itemized charge slips, which are given to the patient if he wishes to pay before leaving the office or which are later mailed in a combination statement-reply envelope. Use of such charge slips simplifies the itemization procedure, since filling out the slips is usually just a matter of checking procedures listed. An itemized charge slip is shown in Figure 14–3.

While the itemization of bills may seem an unnecessary waste of time, in the

PLEASE RETURN THIS SLIP TO RECEPTIONIST

FORM MDP 8241 © 1975 BIBBERO SYSTEMS, INC., SAN FRANCISCO

☐ GEORGE D. GREEN, M.D.
☐ JOHN F. WHITE, M.D.
FAMILY PRACTICE
100 MAIN STREET, SUITE 14
ANYTOWN, CALIFORNIA 90000
TELEPHONE: 399-6000

DATE 01 26 82 — 708

PATIENT'S NAME Danny McDonald — B. DATE 08 22 80

BILLING NAME John McDonald

BILLING ADDRESS 435 E. Adams, Anytown 90000

PRIVATE BLUE CROSS BLUE SHIELD IND. MEDICAID GOV'T. OTHER

PROFESSIONAL SERVICE CODES →	1 Office Visit		2 Home Visit		3 Hospital Visit		4 Emergency Room	
TYPE OF PATIENT →	Estab	New	Estab	New	Estab	All	Estab	New
MINIMAL SERVICE	90030	---	90130	---	---	---	90530	---
BRIEF	90040	90000	90140	90100	90240	90200	90540	90500
LIMITED	90050	90010	90150	90110	90250	---	90550	90510
INTERMED. EXAM	90060	90015	90160	90115	90260	90215	90560	90515
EXTENDED RE EXAM	90070	---	90170	---	90270	---	90570	---
COMP EXAM ADULT	90080	90020	---	90120	90275	90220	---	---
UNUSUALLY COMPLX	90085	90026	---	---	---	90230	---	---

5 CONSULTATION	
Limited	90600
Intermediate	90605
Extended	90610
Comprehensive	90620
Complex	90625
Unusually Complex	90630
6 IMMUNIZATIONS	
DPT, DT, Tet., Oral Polio, Flu	(90720)
Msles, Mps, Rubella, Smallpox	90721
Double Virus______	90722
Triple Virus__M-M-R	90723
7 INJECTION, THERAPEUTIC	90730
8 DRUGS SUPPLIES MAT'LS	(99070)
9 COLL. OF LAB SPECIMENS	99007
10 SPECIAL REPORTS	99080
11 OTHER SERVICES	
12 Spec. Diag. Serv. 91000-95999	
13 Spec. Ther. Proc. 96000-97799	
14 Ext. Care Facil. 90300-90370	
15 Custod. Care 90400-90470	
16 OBSTETRICAL CARE	

17 SURGICAL

18 CASTS

19 LABORATORY

20 X-RAY

21 ALLERGY TESTING

MODIFIERS:

Service Code	RVS #	TODAY'S FEE
6	90720	10.00
8	99070	6.00

REMARKS/DIAGNOSIS

5 Min. 10 Min. 15 Min. 20 Min. 30 Min. 45 Min. 60 Min.

M T W T F S DAYS WKS MOS PRN

Next Appointment Day ______ DATE TIME

TOTAL TODAY'S FEE	16—
OLD BALANCE	
TOTAL	16—
AM'T REC'D TODAY	
NEW BALANCE	-0-

Doctor's Signature: John F White — Date: 1/26/82 — ☑ Cash ☐ Check ☐ Cred. Card — Rec'd by

ACCOUNTING COPY

CONTROL COPY

FIGURE 14–3 An itemized charge slip. (Courtesy of Bibbero Systems, Inc., San Francisco, California.)

long run you will spend less time explaining services provided, clearing up misunderstandings with patients, and following up on delinquent accounts if you routinely itemize all bills. The itemization of bills is also a plus for public relations.

MAIL BILLS PROMPTLY. Most people expect to receive statements from their creditors, and they plan their budgets around first-of-the-month bills received. The bill that arrives late sometimes remains unpaid. Punctuality in billing encourages prompt payment.

TIME AND FREQUENCY OF BILLING. A regular system of rendering statements should be put into operation. Patients are entitled to know the date on which payment of their medical bill is expected. Statements should be sent at least once each month. Some doctors send bills immediately after treatment has been given; others bill at the first of each month. In other offices statements are mailed twice a month, on the first and fifteenth, or the tenth and twenty-fifth. When a billing date for an account has been established, the date of mailing the statement must not, according to the Fair Credit Practices Act Amendments of October 1975, vary more than five days without notification to the debtor. If the balance due is over one dollar, the account must be billed every 30 days.

Once-a-Month Billing. If a monthly pattern is followed, bills should leave your office no later than the last day of each month. Planning ahead for the preparation of statements can lighten the burden of once-a-month billing. The statement can be prepared at the time of service or during slack periods, postdated, and mailed at the end of the month.

Cycle Billing. Many physicians prefer to use the cycle billing system, which calls for the billing of certain portions of the accounts receivable at various times during the month instead of preparing all statements at the end of each month. Cycle billing has been used for some time in large businesses such as department stores and oil companies. The system of cycle billing has become increasingly popular in the physician's office. Its many advantages include avoiding once a month peak work loads and stabilizing the cash flow. In a small office where billing is done only once a month, the unexpected illness or absence of the assistant for any emergency can leave the doctor in a financial bind if the statements do not go out.

This is how the cycle billing system works: the accounts are separated into fairly equal divisions, the number of divisions depending upon how many times you wish to do billing during a month. If you expect to bill twice a month, divide the accounts into two equal sections; for weekly billing, divide into four groups; for daily billing, divide into 20 groups. Small alphabetical groups can be combined to keep your divisions nearly equal in the number of statements to prepare on each billing day. If your files are color-coded, you may wish to use the same alphabetical breakdown in billing. Regardless of constant changes in the accounts themselves, the mailing dates for accounts in each section remain constant. A schedule for processing and mailing of accounts is thus established, apportioning the load of work throughout the entire month.

The use of cycle billing allows an assistant to continue all her routine duties each day, handling the statements on a day-to-day or weekly schedule rather than in one intensive period at the end of the month. This means that she need never sacrifice whole days from her assisting duties in order to get statements into the mail. By spacing the billing throughout the month, she can give more time and consideration to each statement. The itemization of bills will be less burdensome, and the likelihood of error will be decreased.

Patients generally accept the cycle billing system quickly, often with enthusiasm. However, if your office decides to change from a once-a-month billing to a cycle billing system, patients should be notified in advance and the new plan explained to them. To explain the new system to established patients, enclose a notice in each statement two months prior to the transfer, describing the plan and indicating the future dates on which each patient will receive his bill.

A reasonable length of time should elapse between the new patient's first visit to the doctor's office and the mailing of a bill. It would be poor policy, for example, to see a new patient on the ninth of the month and then send him a statement on the tenth. Many would feel that the doctor is being overanxious to collect his fee. When the statement is sent, a notice explaining his future payment date should accompany it.

Before a doctor, particularly one in a small community, adopts the cycle billing system, several factors should be taken into consideration. First, what is the income of the community, and how and when does the average patient receive his pay? Do local companies pay employees at various times during the month, or are most paychecks handed out at the beginning of the month? Would cycle billing benefit patients as well as the overall operation of the office?

Regular billing and itemizing of statements not only is a service to patients but it is valuable to the doctor, since prompt payments are usually forthcoming if these practices are followed.

BILLING THIRD PARTIES AND MINORS

Many collection problems arise because the assistant fails to get the proper insurance information, particularly Medicare and Medicaid information. If these services are billed correctly and with expediency, the doctors will receive their pay. In many instances the forms are not completed correctly, and the claim is denied because of minor infractions such as failing to name the responsible party or omitting Social Security information, policy number, or group number. Time limits must also be observed in billing third parties. In cases of Medicare patients with terminal illness, it may be best to accept assignment of benefits. If the doctor does not take assignment, sometimes the doctor will receive nothing because the family is not obligated to pay and Medicare will not pay after a certain time or if proper filing has not been made.

Bills for minors must be addressed to the parents or legal guardian. If a bill is addressed to a minor, a parent could take the attitude that he is not responsible because the parent never received a bill. A minor cannot be held responsible for a bill unless he is emancipated (under legal age but not living at home). If the parents are separated or divorced, the parent who brings the child in for treatment is responsible for payment. Whatever financial agreement exists between the parents is strictly their personal business and should not concern the medical office. The responsible parent should be so informed from the beginning. If an emancipated minor appears in the office and requests treatment and you can ascertain that he is not living at home, the minor is responsible for the bill. It may be wise to make a determination either with your business manager or with the doctor himself as to whether your office wishes to treat this emancipated minor. There are many county and state aid programs for those who are unemployed or unable to suppport themselves.

COLLECTION PROCEDURES

Reasons to Pursue Collections

Collecting for professional services is a very necessary aspect of medical practice. The reasons for pursuing collections go beyond the obvious one that a physician must be paid for his services in order to meet his own expenses. Human nature operates in strange ways. A doctor often loses the good will of patients by not collecting from them. A person who owes the doctor money and is not prodded gently into payment may stay away from the doctor's office in embarrassment or may even change doctors. Noncollection of medical bills may also imply guilt. A patient may infer that the doctor felt he gave inadequate or improper care, and a malpractice suit may result. Nor is it fair to honest patients to make no attempt to collect from nonpaying patients. Abandoning accounts with no collection follow-up encourages nonpayers and, as a result, honest patients indirectly subsidize the cost of medical care for those who can pay but do not.

According to the American Medical Association, the three most common reasons for patients' failure to pay are *negligence, inability to pay,* and *unwillingness to pay*. Most patients are honest; it is estimated that probably fewer than four per cent never intend to pay. There may be a larger percentage who are financially "shipwrecked" and temporarily unable to pay. Also, a certain percentage of patients irresponsibly live beyond their incomes. The man living beyond his means can be identified by his desire to "spare no expense." When faced with questions about nonpayment, this patient says, "I'll pay it all in the near future," whereas the average honest patient says, "I'll pay you a certain amount each month."

Though it is important to pursue collections, mercenary business methods have no place in the professional world. As a result, collections must be handled in a special way and must be approached with a humanitarian but businesslike attitude. The underlying elements to success in collections are a good collection system and a good attitude on the part of the assistant.

The Assistant's Attitude

There are certain attitudes and personal qualities that will help the medical assistant meet with greater success in dealing with collection problems. She should (1) possess tact and good judgment, (2) give individual attention and personal consideration to each situation, (3) be courteous and show a sincere desire to help the patient with his financial problems by working out special payment arrangements, and (4) always try to find out the patient's reasons for nonpayment. Even though the medical assistant must be courteous and considerate, she must still balance her humanitarianism with firmness. After all, a patient has received medical services, and in exchange the doctor has justly earned his fee. However, the medical assistant must not be overzealous in her desire to boost her collection percentage. This results in ill will toward the doctor as well as toward the assistant. The assistant who is having personal budget problems will find it extremely difficult to be objective about collection problems. If at all possible, some other person should take charge of setting up payment arrangements and collection procedures until the assistant has her own budget under control.

Aging Accounts Receivable

Accounts receivable should be aged on a regular basis. *Aging* is a term used for the procedure of classifying accounts receivable by age from the first date of billing. If the patient is billed on the day of service, the aging begins on that day; if the first billing is 30 days after service, the aging begins at 30 days. Aging of accounts helps collection follow-up since it enables the assistant to tell at a glance which accounts need attention in addition to a regular statement. The form in Figure 14–4 illustrates how this may be accomplished. Some systems use a breakdown of *Current, 30 days, 60 days, 90 days,* and *90-plus days*. Looking at Figure 14–4 you see that Patient A has a balance of $450. Unless regular payments are being made, this account may be heading toward a collection problem because $350 of the balance is over three months old. Patient B presents no problem because the entire balance is current. Patient C definitely is a potential problem even though the account is small. The entire balance is over three months old, and one-fourth of it is over six months old. An established procedure should be determined for handling each situation. For example, Patient D's account should never have been allowed to reach this stage of delinquency. If there had been a good collection policy established, it would not have.

The age analysis is simply a tool to show at a glance the status of each account. There is no need to do this every month if time is at a premium. If you age the accounts quarterly you will stay on top of the problem. Usually a coding system with metal clip-on tabs or adhesive peel-off labels on the ledger cards is used in conjunction with the age analysis system. For example, after two statements have been sent, a green tab is placed on the record, indicating that a courteous reminder

ACCOUNTS RECEIVABLE AGE ANALYSIS

Dr. ____________________

Address ____________________ Date ____________

PATIENT'S NAME	TOTAL ACCOUNT RECEIVABLE	DISTRIBUTION OF ACCOUNTS RECEIVABLE BY AGE				REMARKS
		1-2-3 MONTHS	4-5-6 MONTHS	7-8-9-10-11-12 MONTHS	OVER 1 YEAR	
A	450.00	100.00	350.00			
B	50.00	50.00				
C	100.00		75.00	25.00		
D	200.00		10.00	150.00	40.00	
E	550.00		550.00			
F	42.50	42.50				
G	65.00	20.00	45.00			
H	325.00	325.00				

FIGURE 14–4 Form for accounts receivable age analysis.

was sent with the last statement. The following month the green tab is replaced with a yellow tab, showing that a second payment request was sent in the form of a polite letter. An orange tab is substituted the next month, indicating that the patient received a letter requesting prompt attention to his account. Red tabs may be reserved for accounts that, as a last resort, have been notified of a specific time limit in which payment must be made, after which sterner measures will be taken. If you reach this stage in pursuing a particular account, make certain you record the date of the time limit on the patient's card. Another code system based on letters can be used. For example, "N 1" on a patient's card indicates that one notice has been sent; "N 2," that a second notice has been sent; "L 1," that one letter has gone out, and so on.

The law requires that once you have made a statement in regard to a particular collection procedure you must follow through or be liable for the consequences under the law. If you say, for example, "I am going to turn your account over for collection unless it is paid within ten days," then you must do so. If you state in a collection letter that you are going to take the debtor to Small Claims Court if the account is not paid by a certain date, then you must do as you say. The intent of the law is to prevent the collector from making idle threats or harassing a debtor.

Fair Debt Collection Practices Act 1977 (Federal) states that the following conduct is a violation:
Section 807 (5) The threat to take any action that cannot legally be taken or that is not intended to be taken.

Credit Policy

Most offices do not have a true credit policy; thus, each account continues to be evaluated individually. It is almost impossible to judge accounts objectively and equitably under such circumstances. The doctor and his staff should think through their situation, decide what they expect of patients with respect to payment, and how they will inform the patient. Although there will always be exceptions to a rule, there should *be* a rule, which should be in writing and conveyed to the patient at the outset of the relationship. For instance, it might go something like this:

1. Charges of $25 or less are expected to be paid at the time of service.
2. We prefer that all accounts be paid in full each month.
3. A patient who cannot do so may arrange an alternate payment plan with the financial secretary.
4. Our office will assist you in filing your insurance claims. However, because

the policy is a contract between you and your insurance company, we cannot accept responsibility for collecting your claim.

There should be further provisions for how long to carry an account without a payment, at what stage a telephone call will be made or letter sent, when to turn the account to a collector, and so forth. This should all be automatic unless there are very special circumstances.

Collection System

In the introduction to this chapter, it was pointed out that the collection of professional accounts can be divided into three distinct stages, the second of which is "providing an opportunity for the patient to pay at the time of service for smaller amounts and sending bills out promptly for larger fees."

IMMEDIATE PAYMENTS. If patients get into the habit of paying their bills before they leave the office, monthly billing is lightened and bookkeeping costs are lowered. Set up a system in your office to make it easier for patients to follow this pay-as-you-go system. For example, when the patient stops at your desk to make another appointment, you can reach for your receipt book and say, "Your charge for today, Mrs. Casey, is $XX. Will that be cash or check?" Most patients are hesitant to ask about charges and are unsure whether to offer to pay or to wait until a statement is received. You will make it easier for them by offering to accept their payments, since most people are prepared to meet small bills on a cash basis. Avoid saying to the departing patient, "I don't know what the charge is today. I will have to send you a bill," or "I don't know how much it will be, but why don't you pay me $10 and, if it is more, I will bill you." In both cases, the patient leaves the office with an uneasy feeling about the unknown bill. Care should be taken to place positive reactions toward payments in the patient's mind. Compare these two statements:

1. "The charge today will be $15, Mrs. Jones. Do you want me to send you a bill?"
2. The charge today will be $15, Mrs. Jones. You may pay me now if you wish."

More often than not the second remark will lead to immediate payment.

CHARGE SLIP SYSTEM. One of the advantages of a charge slip system is that it prefaces immediate payments nicely. The doctor checks what has been done for the patient and gives the slip to the patient. The patient takes it to the assistant, who can tell at a glance exactly what the charges will be. The patient is then psychologically prepared to pay immediately.

If the patient seems reluctant, the assistant can say, "It is so much easier if you pay for each visit. Then it will not accumulate into a sizeable account." A pleasant smile and a ready receipt book are two excellent devices for encouraging on-the-spot payments.

WHY MEDICAL BILLS ARE PAID LAST. It is well known that many people pay their medical bills last. Occasionally, you hear a gracious patient say, in all good faith, "Thank goodness, we have all our bills paid off now, except the doctor. We'll start paying him as soon as we catch our breath." Strangely enough, many people do not look upon the doctor's bill as a debt in the usual sense of the word. They must be motivated to pay.

People will pay their rent because of the danger of eviction and sometimes because the landlord is frequently encountered in their daily lives. They will pay their utility bills because the service can be terminated. They will make regular payments on their automobile and furniture because these goods can be repossessed. Banks and small loan companies have a reputation for strict enforcement of contracts, and they follow up on accounts that are only a few days late, but a patient's commercial credit may be very good and his medical credit poor.

What then causes people to delay payment to the doctor? Often there is no specific arrangement made for payment. Follow-up is delayed, and in many offices the account is not even considered delinquent until at least three months have elapsed from the date of service. Even people who are educated to the necessity of paying their bills are frequently not concerned about paying them on time unless this is brought to their attention. Failure of the doctor's assistant to consistently and quickly follow up on overdue accounts may contribute to the patients' lack of concern.

Since the fee for medical services is far more intangible than any commercial account, collection efforts must not be delayed too long. Any responsible, sincere patient will call or write the doctor's office within two or three months of receiving a bill and explain why he cannot pay or ask for a payment plan. If it becomes necessary to refer the account to a collector, a good agency should have a 50 to 60 per cent recovery rate with an account that is assigned within four or five months. This may drop to 25 per cent if the account is held only a few more months.

It must be remembered that the value of medical accounts diminishes in direct proportion to the length of time that has elapsed since service was rendered. The following figures, based on a report from the United States Department of Commerce, show that the chances for recovering the full amount on a bill diminish rapidly as time passes:

After 2 months one dollar is worth 90 cents
After 6 months one dollar is worth 67 cents
After 1 year one dollar is worth 45 cents
After 2 years one dollar is worth 23 cents
After 3 years one dollar is worth 15 cents
After 5 years one dollar is worth 1 cent only

Do not fight the "law of diminishing returns." All collection activity is costly. Each notice you mail costs your doctor approximately $1 for stationery supplies, postage, and typing time. Continued efforts on the old accounts also will allow the current accounts to become delinquent. Know when to stop and call on the services of a professional agency.

Collection Letters

Current thinking is that a printed collection letter or reminder enclosed with a statement is more effective than a personal letter. The theory is that a patient is embarrassed by a personal letter and feels that he has been singled out, whereas he may be nudged into sending a payment in response to a printed message without the personal connotation. It cannot be argued that the printed form is a time saver and that sometimes the lack of time contributes to poor collection follow-up. Letters should be friendly requests for an explanation of why payment has not been made. These letters should indicate that the doctor is sincerely interested in the patient's story and wants to help him straighten out his financial obligations. The patient should be invited to visit the doctor's office to explain his reasons for nonpayment so that, if possible, special arrangements can be worked out. To give the patient an opportunity to save face, these letters can suggest that the patient may have overlooked previous statements.

Upon receipt of such a letter, most patients will make some effort to explain their delinquency. If a patient really is in financial straits, the doctor may be able to get public assistance for him. Or, if it is a temporary financial difficulty, the doctor and the patient may together be able to work out a satisfactory installment plan type of payment program as described in Chapter 13.

The doctor's assistant often is given a free hand in designing collection patterns and composing collection letters. Many assistants compose a group of such letters that they have found to be effective. Such a series usually includes a least five letters, of varying degrees of forcefulness. One would never use the same type of collection letter for a patient with good paying habits as for one who is known to neglect his financial obligations. The assistant can code the range of letters as to severity and paying habits. For example, "Rate 1, Letter 1" might indicate a first collection reminder letter sent to a patient who usually pays on time. These code symbols should be written on the patients' records so that a log can be kept of what letter was sent, and the proper sequence of mailings can be continued if payment is not forthcoming. Never use a post card or put an overdue notice of any kind on the outside of an envelope.

WHO SIGNS COLLECTION LETTERS? The question sometimes arises as to who should sign collection letters. In many medical offices the assistant signs them with the identification "Secretary to Dr. Brown" or "Financial Secretary" below her name. Other physicians feel that they should personally sign these communications. Generally, however, since financial procedures are handled by the secretary or assistant, she also signs the collection letters.

SAMPLE LETTERS. Following are some suggested reminder and personalized collection letters. These can serve as a guide for composing your own letters to suit the circumstances involved.

A gentle reminder often brings results:

> Your account has always been paid promptly in the past, so this must be an oversight. Please accept this note as a friendly reminder of your account due for $ ______

> June 1, 19___
>
> Since your care in this office in March we have had no word from you in regard to how you are feeling or your account due.
>
> If it is impossible for you to pay the full amount of $______ at this time, please call this office before June 15 so that satisfactory arrangements can be worked out.

> June 15, 19___
>
> We've sent you three statements for the care you received in March. Medical bills are payable at the time of service unless special credit arrangements are made.
>
> Please send your check in full or call this office before June 30.

For the patient who has started on a payment program and then discontinued:

> March 1, 19___
>
> We've had no word from you since January about your balance of $______ , which has been on our books since October, 19__.
>
> If you have some question about your statement, we will be happy to answer it for you. If not, may we have a payment from you before the end of this month?

> April 1, 19___
>
> Unless some definite arrangement is made to reduce your balance of $______, we can no longer carry your account on our books.
>
> Delinquent accounts are turned over to our collection agency on the 25th of the month.

When a payment plan has been established, it can be reenforced by recognizing the first remittance with a letter of acknowledgement.

> Thank you for the recent payment of $______ on your account. We are glad to cooperate with you in this arrangement for clearing your account.
>
> We will look for your next check at about the same time next month, and your final payment the following month.

When a payment schedule has been arranged by a telephone call, it can be confirmed by letter.

> January 29, 19___
>
> As agreed upon in our telephone conversation today, we will expect you to mail a payment of $50 on February 10, $50 on March 10, and the balance on April 10.
>
> If some emergency should prevent your making one of these payments on time, please notify us immediately by telephone.

If time permits, the "thank you" letter also has a place in your collection program and is a valuable public relations tool.

> Thank you for your $500 check in full payment for your recent surgery. It is much appreciated. Best wishes from the entire office staff for your continued good health.

The collection letters in this chapter will provide the medical assistant with a limited variety of styles with which to work in composing her own communications. It is important to remember that letters should sound as though each one were written personally to the individual concerned. Do not send letters with a firmer tone until you have sent one or two friendly reminders. Always imply that the patient has good intentions to pay until lack of reply over a period of time proves otherwise. Your early letters should be merely reminders of debt. Sometimes even the person with poor paying habits will pay his bill if he is treated with respect and consideration. See Figure 14–5 for a suggested collection program.

No medical assistant should ever go beyond the authority given by her employer in pursuing collections. If she has questions about special collection problems, she should always check with the doctor before proceeding. This is particularly important with patients whom she does not know personally — for example, patients the doctor has seen in the hospital or at home, and others for whom she has no credit history. It is difficult to say whether pressing collections too hard loses more good will of patients than not pursuing collections diligently enough. The doctor and the assistant together should agree upon general collection policies, and then the

1. Inform the patient, before or at the time of service, what charges he may expect.

2. For smaller fees, give him an opportunity to pay at the time of service.

3. 30 days: Send itemized statement

4. 60 days: Send statement:

   For Professional Services

   March services $ ______

5. 75 days: If there has been no response, telephone patient or send brief note.

   (Suggested wording)

   If you are unable to pay your account this month, please telephone this office (776-4900) before June 15 and let us know how you plan to take care of it.

   Balance due $100

6. 90 days: Send reminder letter requesting prompt attention

7. 120 days: Send final letter, certified mail, return receipt.

   (Suggested wording)

   Every courtesy has been extended to you in arranging for payment of your long over-due account. Our auditor suggests that it no longer be carried on our books.

   Unless we hear from you by August 15 the account will be turned over to ______ for collection.

8. 15th of next month or date mentioned in final letter: Account to collector

FIGURE 14–5 A suggested collection program.

policies should be applied. In all cases where an account is assigned for collection, be sure that the doctor is aware of it.

Collection by Personal Interview

Personal interviews with patients are usually more effective than a whole series of collection letters. By talking to a patient face to face, you can come to an understanding of his problems more quickly and reach an agreement about future payment plans.

Occasionally, a patient may undergo a long course of treatment and yet show no sign of willingness to pay anything on account. Perhaps he is only waiting for the doctor or the assistant to suggest that a payment be made. When there is advance knowledge that the patient will require extensive treatment, the matter of payment should be discussed early in the course of treatment and some agreement reached as to a payment plan.

If for some reason the doctor feels that it would be unwise to press the matter at the time the patient completes his treatments, you can make an appointment for him to come back in a month. If the patient does not keep his appointment or does not offer to make payment, then you have good reason to call or write him about the amount he owes.

Telephone Collection Techniques

A telephone call at the right time, in the right manner, is more effective than a collection letter. The personal contact of a telephone call will bring in more money. In the absence of time to make calls, the collection letter is the next best avenue. If collections are a serious problem, it may pay to hire an extra person to do the telephoning. Written notification is a must, however, if it is a final demand for payment before collection or legal proceedings are started.

GENERAL RULES TO FOLLOW IN TELEPHONE COLLECTIONS

1. Determine the identity of the person with whom you are speaking. If you ask, "Is this Mrs. Noble?" and she answers "Yes," it could be the patient's mother-in-law, who is also "Mrs. Noble." Use the person's full name.
2. Be dignified and respectful in your attitude. You can be friendly and formal at the same time.
3. Ask the patient if it is a convenient time to talk with you. Unless you have the attention of the called party, there is little to be gained by continuing. If you are told that you have called at an inopportune time, ask for a specific time when you may call back, or get a promise for the patient to call you at a specified time.
4. Do not make collection calls before 8 AM or after 9 PM. To do so may be considered harassment.
5. Assume a positive attitude. For example, convey the impression that you know the patient intends to pay, and it is only a matter of working out some suitable arrangements.
6. After a brief greeting, state the purpose of your call. Make no apology for calling but state your reason in a friendly, businesslike way. You expect payment and are interested in helping him meet his obligation. "This is Alice, Dr. Brown's financial secretary. I'm calling about your account." A well-placed pause at this point in the call sometimes gets an immediate response from the patient in regard to his nonpayment.
7. Try to get a definite commitment — payment of a certain amount on a certain date.
8. Keep the conversation brief and to the point, and avoid threats of any kind. There's a saying in collections that "the less said, the more collected."
9. Follow up on promises. This is best accomplished by a tickler file or a note on your calendar. If the payment does not arrive on the promised date, remind the patient with another call. If you fail to do this, your whole effort has been wasted.
10. Do not call patients about their accounts when there are others within hearing distance in the reception room.

There are no hard and fast rules for pursuing collections by telephone. You must handle each case individually on the basis of your own acquaintance with the person concerned.

It is poor policy to call an individual at work. If this is the only phone contact you have and you feel he must be reached, place the call without disclosing the nature of the call to others in his place of employment. You can tell the patient the reason for your call and request that he return your call at a specific time if it is not convenient for him to discuss his account now. If you do call him at work and he cannot come to the telephone, you can leave a message asking him to "call Mrs. Black at 727-5938," — not "Dr. Jones's office" or "the secretary to Dr. Jones." It should be remembered that most states have a "right of privacy law," and you are risking a lawsuit if you reveal to a third party that John Doe owes money to Dr. Jones. Therefore, be certain you have properly identified the party before talking about the account.

Whether dealing with patients by telephone or in person, do not lose your temper or your dignity. An angry patient is a poor-paying patient. Insulted patients often do not pay at all. Never proceed with telephone collections without the consent of your employer.

SPECIAL COLLECTION PROBLEMS

Tracing "Skips"

When a statement is returned marked "Moved — no forwarding address," you may consider this account as a "skip." This generally is accepted as an indication that the patient is attempting to avoid liability for his debts. Some so-called skips are innocent errors. The person may have been careless in not leaving a forwarding address. Or the mistake may have occurred in your office; the wrong name or address may have been placed on the statement. However, immediate action should be taken in regard to returned statements. Do not wait until the next billing time to attempt to trace the patient. Here are some suggestions for tracing skips:

1. Examine the patient's original office registration card.
2. Call the telephone number listed on the card. Occasionally, a patient may move without leaving a forwarding address but will transfer his old telephone number. Or the new phone number will be given when you call the old number.
3. If you are unable to contact the individual by telephone, make a few discreet calls to the references listed on the registration card to get leads.
4. Check the city directory to secure the name and telephone number of neighbors or the landlord, and contact these persons to secure information about the patient's whereabouts.
5. Do not inform the third party that the person owes you money. You can only state that you are trying to locate or verify the location of the individual.
6. Drop a note to the state motor vehicle department. In the event that the patient owns a car or has a driver's license, this department may be able to provide information. According to law, this department must be notified of changes of address.
7. Check the patient's place of employment for information. If the patient is a specialist in his field of work, the local union or similar organizations may be contacted. Although they may not give you his current address, they will relay a message to him so that he will know you are seeking to contact him. Often, a person will be stirred into paying a bill if he thinks his employer may learn of his payment failure.
8. Do not communicate with a third party more than once. This is specifically forbidden by law (Public Law 95–109 Sec. 804) unless the third party requests the collector to do so.

The tracing of skips is a challenge to any secretary. A certified letter can be sent; by paying additional fees, you can request the postal service to obtain a receipt including the address where the letter was delivered. The certified letter may be sent in a plain envelope so that the patient will not refuse to accept the letter because of the letterhead.

If all other methods fail, then turn the account over to your collection agency without delay. Do not keep a "skip" account too long — since the trail may become so cold as time elapses that even collection experts will be unable to follow it.

Claims Against Estates

A bill owed by a deceased patient may be handled a little differently from regular bills. Courtesy dictates that a bill not be sent during the initial period of bereavement, but do not delay more than 30 days. The person responsible for settling the affairs of the estate will be assembling outstanding accounts and will expect to receive the medical bills along with all others. Address the statement to:

Estate of (name of patient)
c/o (spouse or next of kin, if known)
Patient's last known address

Do not address the statement to a relative unless you have a signed agreement that that person will be responsible. If for some reason the statement cannot be addressed as suggested above — for instance, the patient was in a convalescent home, and you do not know the name of a relative — you may seek information from the county seat in the county in which the estate is being settled. A will is usually filed within 30 days of the death. A request to the Probate Department of the Superior Court, County Recorder's Office, will usually provide you with the name of the executor or administrator. The time limits for filing an estate claim are determined by the state in which the decedent resided.

After the name of the administrator or executor of the estate has been obtained, a duplicate itemized statement of the account should be sent to him by certified mail, return receipt requested, so that you will know who received it. If no response is received in ten days, you should then contact the executor or the county clerk where the estate is being settled and obtain forms for filing claim against the estate. (Some states do not have special claim forms but will accept simple itemized statements). This claim against the estate must be made within a certain length of time, varying from two to 36 months, depending upon the state in which it is filed.

The executor of the estate will either accept or reject the claim. If it is accepted, he will send an acknowledgment of the debt. Payment is often delayed, owing to the legal difficulties in settling an estate, but if the claim has been accepted you will receive your money in due time. If the claim is rejected and you have full justification for claiming the bill, then you must file claim against the executor within a limited amount of time, according to state laws. The time limit in such cases starts with the date on the letter of rejection that he sends you in response to your original claim.

Because of the various state time limits and statutes in regard to such matters, it is advisable for the assistant to contact her employer's attorney or the local court for the exact procedure to follow in such instances in her area.

Statutes of Limitations

A statute of limitations assigns a certain time after which rights cannot be enforced by action.

MALPRACTICE. In many states there are Statutes of Limitations in regard to malpractice lawsuits, which set a limit to the time during which malpractice actions can be filed. This topic is more thoroughly discussed in Chapter 5. It is usually best to wait until this time has passed before pressing the account of a patient who may feel he is entitled to sue the doctor. However, this should not be made a blanket policy; each case should be judged on its own merit.

COLLECTIONS. Statutes of Limitations in regard to collections prescribe the time within which a legal collection suit may be rendered against a debtor; the term "outlaw" is sometimes used to refer to debts on which the time limit has passed. This legal time limit varies according to the specific state in which a doctor practices. Table 14–1 lists the time limits for collections in the various states. It should be noted that if the debtor moves out of state either temporarily or permanently, the time spent out of state is not included in the time limit. Only the time during which he resides within the state is included in the statute.

Generally, accounts may be placed in one of three groups: open book accounts, written contracts, or single entry accounts.

Open book accounts are accounts on the books that are open to charges made from time to time. The bill for each illness or treatment is computed separately, and the last date of entry, debit or credit for that particular illness is the time designated by the Statute of Limitations for starting that specific debt. As you can see, it is almost impossible to have a time limit on an account of a patient with a chronic condition, since there is no actual termination of the illness or treatment unless the patient changes physician or dies. When legal time limits are set, they usually refer to these "open book accounts."

Written contracts are contracts that often have the same time limit as the open book accounts, but occasionally they vary in different states. The time limit on written contracts starts from the date due.

Single entry accounts are accounts that have only one entry or charge. These accounts are usually short-lived and are for small amounts. Some states, such as California, place a shorter Statute of Limitations span on such accounts.

In many states, even though the legal time limit set by the Statutes of Limitations

TABLE 14–1 Statute of Limitations*

Location	Open Accounts (Years)	Contracts in Writing (Years)
Alabama	3	6
Alaska	6	6
Arizona	3	6
Arkansas	3	5
California	4	4
Colorado	6	6
Connecticut	6	6
Delaware	3	3
District of Columbia	3	3
Florida	4	5
Georgia	4	6
Hawaii	6	6
Idaho	4	5
Illinois	5	10
Indiana	6	10
Iowa	5	10
Kansas	3	5
Kentucky	5	15
Louisiana	3	10
Maine	6	6
Maryland	3	3
Massachusetts	6	6
Michigan	6	6
Minnesota	6	6
Mississippi	3	6
Missouri	5	10
Montana	5	8
Nebraska	4	5
Nevada	4	6
New Hampshire	6	6
New Jersey	6	6
New Mexico	4	6
New York	6	6
North Carolina	3	3
North Dakota	6	6
Ohio	6	15
Oklahoma	3	5
Oregon	6	6
Pennsylvania	6	6
Rhode Island	6	6
South Carolina	6	6
South Dakota	6	6
Tennessee	6	6
Texas	2	4
Utah	4	6
Vermont	6	6
Virginia	3	5
Washington	3	6
West Virginia	5	10
Wisconsin	6	6
Wyoming	8	10
Puerto Rico	15	—

*From Summary of Collection Laws published in the American Collectors Association, Inc. 1980 Bonded Directory has passed, the account may be reopened and the date extended if you are able to obtain an acknowledgment of the debt due from the patient in writing. For instance, a letter from the patient stating "Yes, I know I owe you $150, but I do not intend paying Dr. Brown" is an acknowledgment of the debt. If this letter is signed and dated, keep it and contact your collector; on the basis of this letter, he can then proceed with collection. Also, a small payment on account may extend the date. Sometimes a belligerent patient will send one dollar on account, thinking it is only a teaser; he may be unaware that such a payment keeps his account open. Photocopy these small checks for proof of payment, should proof become necessary.

Sometimes a patient will ignore a bill if he does not feel responsible for the account. He may have neglected to give you the necessary information about the party responsible for the bill, and you may be billing the wrong party.

Bankruptcy

Bankruptcy laws are federal, thus eliminating the confusion of local and state laws. When you are notified that a patient has declared bankruptcy, you should no longer send statements or make any individual attempt to collect the account.

Bankruptcy laws were passed to secure equal distribution of the assets of an individual among his creditors. There are two types of bankruptcy: a straight petition in bankruptcy and a wage earner's bankruptcy, sometimes referred to as a Chapter 13 bankruptcy. In both, the debtor becomes a ward of the court and has its protection. A creditor can be fined for contempt of court if he continues to proceed against the debtor.

In a wage earner's bankruptcy, the debtor pays a fixed amount, agreed on by the court, to the trustee in bankruptcy. This is then passed on to the creditors. During this period, none of the creditors can attach his wages or bother him.

In a straight petition in bankruptcy you should file a claim on the appropriate form, which can be obtained from a stationery store or by writing the referee in bankruptcy. Although you may be notified of a creditors' meeting, it is usually a waste of time to attend. A doctor's fee is an unsecured debt and, therefore, one of the last to be paid.

SUING FOR RECOVERY ON OVERDUE ACCOUNTS

When you have done everything possible in your office to follow up on an outstanding account and have not received payment, the question arises as to what step to take next. Should the doctor sue for the amount? Should he turn the account over to a collection agency? Or should he cross it off the books as a bad debt?

Before forcing an account, you must first consider the time element. Has the patient been given a fair chance to pay this bill? Have you sent statements regularly and used a systematic method of following the account? Ask yourself if there might be a misunderstanding in regard to the fee charged. Did you fully itemize the first statement? A large unexplained bill may frighten a patient into making no payments at all because the whole thing looks too big.

If you have used correct registration forms to secure advance credit information, you should know the financial abilities of the patient in regard to payment. However, his illness may have caused a loss of salary and resulted in temporary inability to pay. A little investigation will reveal such troubles.

Could the patient have been dissatisfied with the care he received? For some unknown reason he may feel that he was not treated correctly. Perhaps he expected a complete cure too soon. Only an explanation of the condition, prognosis, and care can enlighten such patients. This is best explained by the doctor himself. If a bill is pressed too hard and the patient is dissatisfied for some reason, he may file a malpractice suit to "get even."

SHOULD WE SUE? Will a doctor lose more good will by suing for a bill than by writing it off as a loss? A management official says that, strangely enough, when a doctor-client sued two patients for large sums, the patients lost the cases, paid up, and were back in his office for treatment very shortly! However, most physicians feel it is unwise to resort to the court to collect medical bills unless there are extraordinary circumstances.

An account must be considered a 100 per cent loss to you before legal proceedings are started. Remember that you should never threaten to instigate legal proceedings unless you are prepared to carry out the threat and have the doctor's consent to issue such a warning.

If your employer decides in favor of a legal suit, then investigate thoroughly before taking action. Mr. Leslie S. Kohn, LL.B., former editor of the *New Jersey Law Journal,* says litigation to collect a bill is generally in order in the following instances:

1. When a patient can afford to pay without hardship
2. When the doctor can produce office records that support the bill
3. When the doctor can justify the size of the bill by comparison with fee practices in his community
4. When the patient's general condition after treatment is satisfactory
5. When the persuasive powers of an ethical collection agency have been exhausted, and the agency advises suing
6. When the patient can be given ample warning of the doctor's intention of collecting legally
7. When the patient (or defendant) is not judgment-proof
8. When the defendant is legally liable for the services rendered to the patient
9. When the Statute of Limitations has ruled out any possible malpractice action
10. When the doctor is not bubbling over with indignation or is not in a "he-can't-do-this-to-me" frame of mind

The experienced practitioner ticks off these ten "whens" before he plunges into costly litigation.

SELECTION OF ACCOUNTS FOR COLLECTION AGENCY

The office assistant should try every means possible within the scope of her ability and available time to collect accounts before they become delinquent. It is usually best to set up a definite collection timetable and make few exceptions (see Fig. 14–5).

As soon as the account is determined uncollectible through your office — the patient has failed to respond to your final letter or has failed to fulfill a second promise on payment — send the account to the collector without delay. Skips should be assigned immediately.

Even though collection by an agency will mean sacrificing 40 to 50 per cent of the amount owed, further delay will only reduce the chances of recovery by the professional collector. If the agency finds that the case deserves special consideration, it will probably report this for your consideration.

In the booklet entitled *Rx Public Relations* published by the American Medical Association, the following paragraph appeared in regard to use and abuse of collection agencies:

> Collections cause one of medicine's biggest public relations headaches — an unethical agency which uses unscrupulous tactics such as lumping other accounts owed by the person together for collection purposes or pursuing a threat or scare technique to recover on old bills can ruin a doctor PR-wise. An ethical agency, however, can do a real public relations job for physicians, ferreting out the patients who need special consideration and following through in collecting from people who can pay. Because a different approach is necessary in pursuing medical collections, a physician should thoroughly acquaint himself with the collection methods used by a respective bureau before making use of its services.

There are a number of agencies either owned and operated as an integral part of the county medical society or operated separately from the medical society but supervised by the medical profession. These bureaus provide specialized medical collection services.

Another type of collection agency is a division of the local credit association, recognized by the National Retail Credit Association. If the local credit association does not maintain a collection department, it will be able to recommend a reputable one. A nationally recognized credit association has considerable responsibility and a high standard to maintain. These factors act as monitors to its reliability.

The most common type of collection agency throughout the U.S. is the privately owned and operated agency. Many of these work with the local professional societies and strive to keep their work on a high ethical standard. There are a few of these bureaus that are unethical and unscrupulous in their tactics. Therefore, when a doctor chooses a collection agency, he should investigate thoroughly to determine whether it is a reliable, ethical one.

1. The best source of referral for a collection agency is the doctor's colleagues. He should check with other doctors in the same specialty, with associates in the hospitals where he practices, and so forth.

2. You may check with the Medical-Dental-Hospital Bureaus of America, 111 East Wacker Drive, Chicago, IL 60601; the American Collectors Association, 4040 West 70th Street, Minneapolis, MN 55434; or the Associated Credit Bureaus of America, Collection Division, 6767 Southwest Freeway, Houston, TX 77074 for references of local agencies.

3. Investigate the methods of collection used. Ask to see any letters, reminder notices, or follow-up literature used.

4. Investigate to determine if the agency has contacts with other services to aid in the collection of out-of-town accounts.

5. Find out the agency's collection ratio and the fees for various kinds of accounts assigned to them (large or small accounts, out-of-town accounts, skips, and so forth).

6. Find out whether the agency will report cases deserving special consideration back to the physician's office.

7. Generally speaking, one should not sign a contract. When your doctor selects a reputable agency and decides to make use of its services, the office must be prepared to provide the agency with all the necessary data to enable it to begin prompt collection procedures on overdue accounts. The agency should receive: full name of the debtor, name of the spouse, last known address, full amount of debt, date of the last entry on the account (debit or credit), occupation of the debtor, business address, and any other pertinent information.

Once an account has been turned over to a collection agency, your office makes no further collection attempts. Here are the directions for procedure in the doctor's office, once the collection agency has begun its work:

1. Send no more statements.

2. Mark the patient's card or stamp it so that you know it is now in the hands of the collector.

3. Refer the patient to the agency if he contacts you in regard to the account.

4. Promptly report any payments made directly to your office. Remember that a percentage of this payment is due to the agency.

5. Call the agency if you obtain any information that will be of value in tracing or collecting the account.

6. Do not push the agency with frequent calls. The representatives of the bureau will report to you regularly and keep you posted on collection progress.

SMALL CLAIMS COURT

Many doctors' offices find the Small Claims Court a satisfactory and inexpensive way to collect delinquent accounts. The law places a limit on the amount of the debt for which relief may be sought in the Small Claims Court. Since this varies from state to state, and in some instances even within a state, this limit should be checked locally before seeking recovery in this manner.

A party to a small claims action may not be represented by an attorney at the trial, but he may send another person to court in his behalf to produce records supporting the claim. Doctors often send their bookkeeper or office assistant with records of unpaid accounts to show the judge.

In addition to the judgment for the amount owed, the plaintiff in Small Claims Court may also recover the costs of the suit. This rarely exceeds $10. For a very small investment in time and money, the doctor who uses this method has saved the time of a regular court action; he has had no attorney's fees to pay; and he has not sacrificed the 40 to 50 per cent commission charged by most collection agencies. Remember, though, that the court has awarded only a judgment. You still do not have the money. Also, the only person in a small claims action who has the right of appeal is the defendant. An appeal may have the judgment set aside. The plaintiff (doctor) cannot file an appeal in a small claims action; the decision of the court is final.

The forms for filing action and full instructions on the course to follow may be obtained from the clerk of the Small Claims Court. The assistant who has never appeared in the Court would probably be wise to attend once as a spectator only, so that she will understand the procedure followed and feel more at ease when she appears for the doctor.

A collection agency, to whom an account may have been assigned, may not file or handle a small claims action. It must either sue in the regular municipal or justice court or attempt to collect the debt in some other way.

ACCOUNTS RECEIVABLE INSURANCE PROTECTION

The potential income represented by the doctor's accounts receivable ledger is probably considerable, and the patient ledgers may be the only record the doctor has of what is owed to him. This potential income deserves insurance protection. The doctor's general insurance representative can obtain insurance protection for these records. Most insurance companies require that the ledgers be kept in a safe place, such as an insulated file cabinet. This is a good practice to follow in any case. They will also require that the accounts receivable balance be reported monthly, for the cost of the insurance is usually based on the average balance during the year. The premium for this type of insurance is nominal. Anyone who has ever lost his records through fire or flood would say it is priceless.

In conclusion, the authors point out that to the best of their ability they have checked and verified all statements made herein pertinent to collection law and legal procedures. However, laws do change, and it is recommended that you check with your local state regulations and laws to verify points pertinent to your special area. State law will take precedence over federal law if it is stronger. For a general instruction manual of this nature, it is impossible to check each of these state requirements to determine which are stronger and which would prevail over Federal Public Law 95–109.

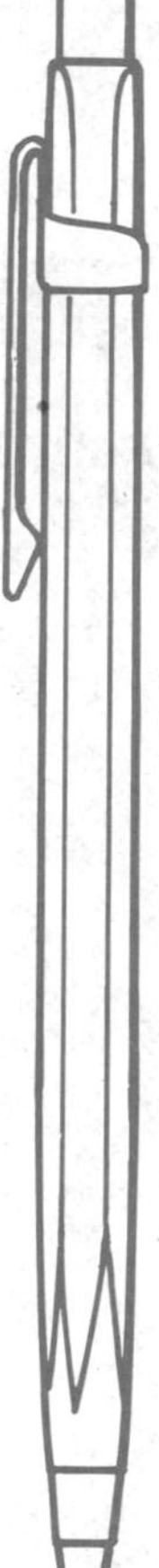

CHAPTER OUTLINE

BEHAVIORAL OBJECTIVES

The medical office assistant should be able to:

- **Recognize terms that identify individuals involved in banking exchanges.**
- **Define the various kinds of checks.**
- **Describe the principal kinds of bank accounts.**
- **Apply the rules for writing checks.**
- **Systematize the payment of bills.**
- **Observe basic rules in accepting checks.**
- **Follow proper check endorsement procedures.**
- **Prepare bank deposits.**
- **Reconcile bank balances.**

15

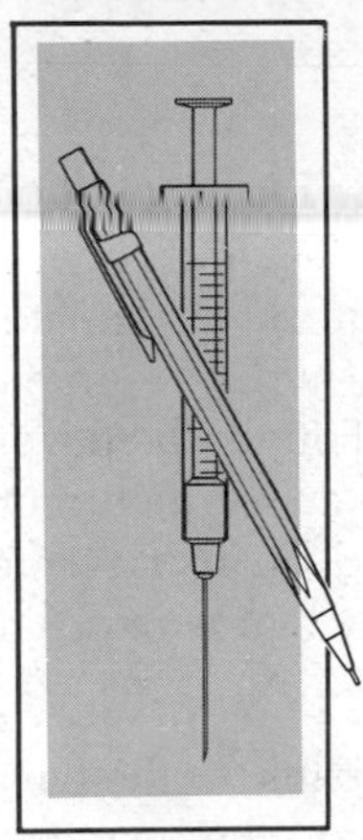

BANKING SERVICES AND PROCEDURES

Because practically every financial transaction in the professional office involves the use of checks, it is imperative that the office assistant understand basic banking terminology and procedures. There are many small differences in terminology throughout the various banks. However, the terms as defined in this chapter are fairly common. The medical office assistant must also understand the responsibilities involved in writing checks, in accepting payments, in endorsing and depositing checks, and in maintaining an accurate balance in the checking account. This chapter sets forth basic guidelines involved in these procedures.

TERMS THAT IDENTIFY INDIVIDUALS INVOLVED IN BANKING EXCHANGES

There are certain legal terms that should be understood by anyone who deals with banks. Definitions of some of these terms are provided here:

AGENT. An agent is a person authorized to represent or act for another person, called the principal, in dealing with a third party.

ENDORSER. This is the person who signs his name on the back of a check for the purpose of transferring his title to the check to another person.

MAKER. Any individual, corporation, or legal party who signs a check or any type of negotiable instrument is known as a maker.

PAYEE. The person named on a draft or check as the recipient of the amount shown is a payee. The payee's name is written after the words "Pay to the order of." The payee is the party benefiting from the payment of the instrument.

PAYER. The payer is the person who writes the check in favor of the payee. When you write a check to pay a bill at a local store, you become the payer and the store is the payee.

TELLER. A teller is an employee of a bank who is assigned the duty of waiting on the bank's customers. He is the contact between the customer and the bank. Bank tellers are directly concerned with the receiving or paying out of money by the bank.

CHECKS

The use of checks for the transfer of funds provides a number of advantages. First, when properly used, checks are both safe and convenient, particularly when making payments by mail. Second, one can quickly calculate expenditures or locate specific payments from the check record. Third, a summary of receipts can readily be determined from the deposit record. Fourth, the payer can stop payment on a check, thus protecting himself from lost, stolen, or incorrectly drawn checks. Fifth, checks provide a permanent reliable record of **disbursements** for tax purposes. Finally, checking accounts protect the money that is deposited.

What is a Check?

A check is a draft or an order upon a bank for the payment of a certain sum of money to a certain person therein named, or to the bearer, and is payable on demand. It is considered to be a *negotiable instrument.* A negotiable instrument must conform to the following requirements:

1. It must be written and signed by a maker.
2. It must contain a promise or order to pay a sum of money.
3. It must be payable on demand or at a fixed future date.
4. It must be payable to order or bearer.

Types of Checks

There are many types of checks in use in the business world. Here are descriptions of some:

BANK DRAFT. A check drawn by a bank against funds deposited to its account in another bank.

CASHIER'S CHECK. A bank's own check, drawn upon itself and signed by the bank cashier or other authorized official. It is also known as an *officer's* or *treasurer's check.* A cashier's check is obtained by paying the bank cashier the amount of the check, in cash or by personal check. Some banks charge a fee for this service. Cashier's checks are usually issued to accommodate the savings account customer who does not maintain a checking account.

CERTIFIED CHECK. This is the depositor's own check, upon the face of which the bank has placed the word "CERTIFIED" or "ACCEPTED" with the date and a bank official's signature. The check then becomes an obligation of the bank because the amount of this check is immediately drawn from the depositor's account and held. It is unlawful for a bank to certify a check for an amount that exceeds the sum the depositor has on deposit. In other words, a certified check is a depositor's own check guaranteed by the bank. Because the bank deducts the amount of the check from the depositor's account at the time it certifies the check, the bank can guarantee that the amount is available. A certified check, like a cashier's check, can be used when an ordinary personal check would not be acceptable. If not used, a certified check should be redeposited promptly, so the funds previously set aside will be credited back to the depositor's account.

COUNTER CHECK. This is a check which a depositor sometimes uses to draw funds from his own account. It is *not negotiable*. Forms for counter checks are

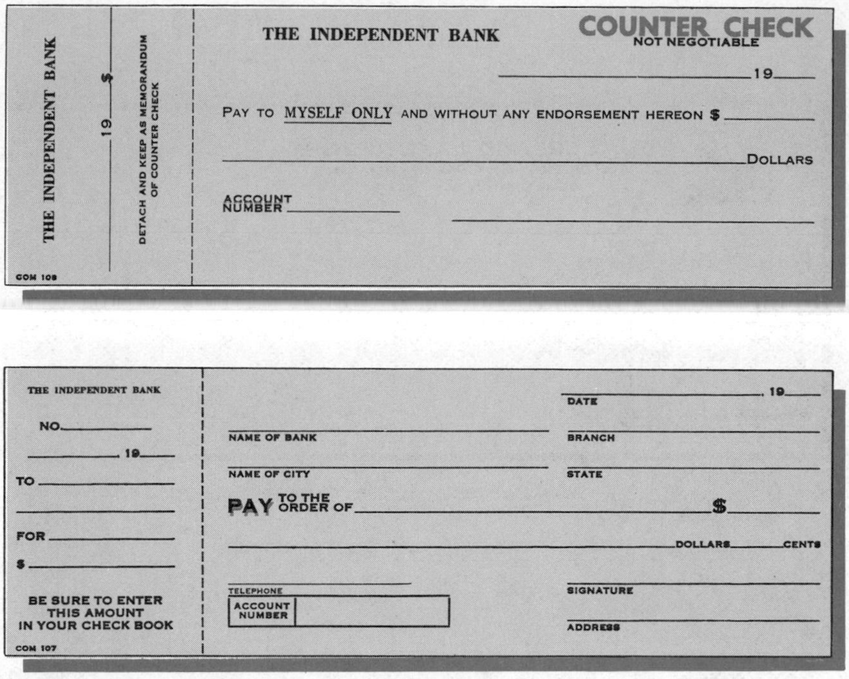

THE INDEPENDENT BANK

19___ $___

DETACH AND KEEP AS MEMORANDUM OF COUNTER CHECK

THE INDEPENDENT BANK

COUNTER CHECK
NOT NEGOTIABLE

________19___

PAY TO MYSELF ONLY AND WITHOUT ANY ENDORSEMENT HEREON $______

________DOLLARS

ACCOUNT NUMBER______

COM 108

THE INDEPENDENT BANK

NO.______

______19___

TO______

FOR______

$______

BE SURE TO ENTER THIS AMOUNT IN YOUR CHECK BOOK

COM 107

______19___ DATE

NAME OF BANK ______ BRANCH

NAME OF CITY ______ STATE

PAY TO THE ORDER OF______ $______

______DOLLARS____CENTS

TELEPHONE ______ SIGNATURE

ACCOUNT NUMBER

ADDRESS

FIGURE 15–1 Counter check *(top)* and blank check *(bottom)*. 15

available at the bank with the wording "Pay to the Order of MYSELF ONLY" upon it. It is this wording which makes a counter check non-negotiable (Fig. 15–1).

LIMITED CHECK. A check may be limited as to the amount written on it. A statement appears on such checks stating that it is void if written over a certain amount. This type of check is often used for payroll or insurance checks. A limited check may also indicate a definite time limit during which a check may be presented for payment, thus limiting the length of time it is **negotiable.**

MONEY ORDERS. Domestic money orders are sold by banks, some stores, and the United States Post Office. The maximum face value varies according to the source. Postal money orders are currently (1980) available in amounts up to $400. International money orders may be purchased for limited amounts, indicated in US dollars, for use in sending money abroad.

TRAVELER'S CHECK. This check is designed for persons traveling where personal checks may not be accepted or in cases in which it is not advisable to carry large amounts of cash. These checks usually are printed in denominations of $10, $20, $50, and $100, and sometimes $500 and $1,000. For protection against loss or theft the customer must place his signature on the face of each check, in the presence of a bank witness, at the time of purchase. He later signs his name again on the face of each check when he wishes to cash it. This item is a check and is not to be listed as cash in a deposit.

UNIVERSAL OR BLANK CHECK. Some banks and some merchants will supply the customer with a blank check form on which he can fill in the name of his bank, its branch, and its address, and the customer's account number. Because the customer is supplying all the information, the teller or the merchant will take extra precaution to identify the person and to verify the account. The universal check is sometimes called a blank check. These checks are rarely used today.

VOUCHER CHECK. This is a check with a detachable voucher form. The voucher portion is used to itemize or specify the purpose for which the check is drawn. It is used for the convenience of the payer, showing discounts and various other

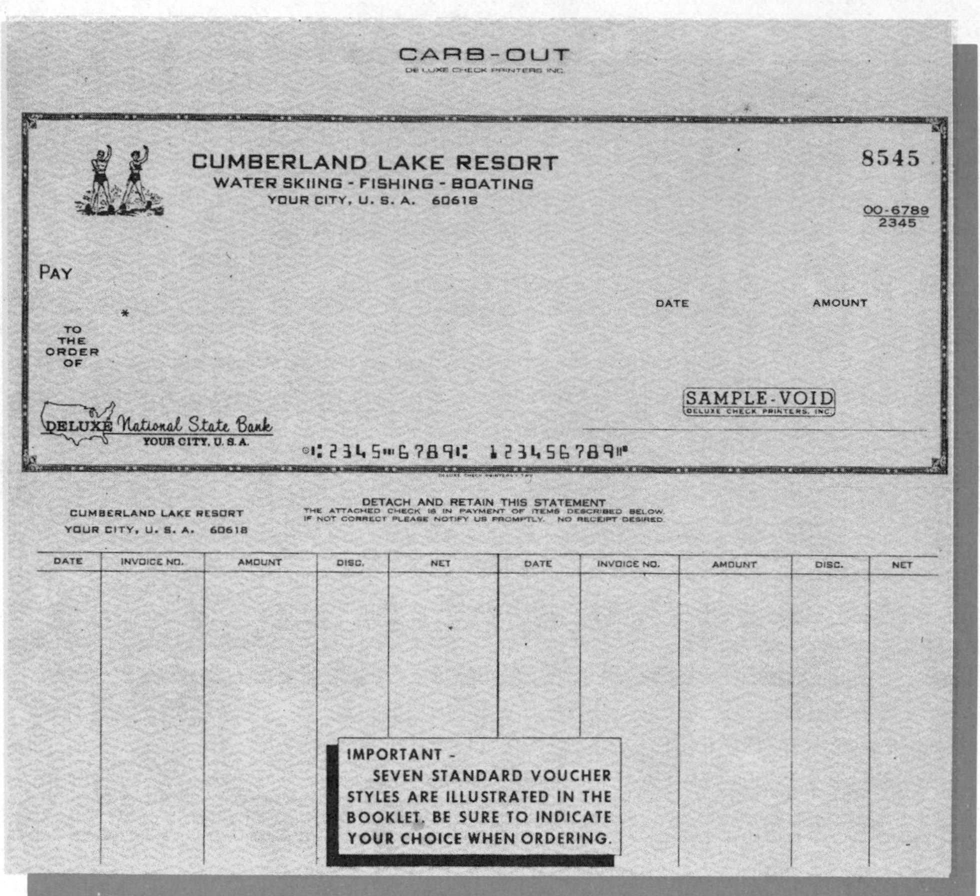

CARB-OUT
DE LUXE CHECK PRINTERS INC.

CUMBERLAND LAKE RESORT
WATER SKIING - FISHING - BOATING
YOUR CITY, U. S. A. 60618

8545

00-6789
2345

PAY

DATE AMOUNT

TO THE ORDER OF

SAMPLE-VOID
DELUXE CHECK PRINTERS, INC.

DELUXE National State Bank
YOUR CITY, U.S.A.

2345 6789 123456789

CUMBERLAND LAKE RESORT
YOUR CITY, U. S. A. 60618

DETACH AND RETAIN THIS STATEMENT
THE ATTACHED CHECK IS IN PAYMENT OF ITEMS DESCRIBED BELOW.
IF NOT CORRECT PLEASE NOTIFY US PROMPTLY. NO RECEIPT DESIRED.

DATE	INVOICE NO.	AMOUNT	DISC.	NET	DATE	INVOICE NO.	AMOUNT	DISC.	NET

IMPORTANT -
SEVEN STANDARD VOUCHER STYLES ARE ILLUSTRATED IN THE BOOKLET. BE SURE TO INDICATE YOUR CHOICE WHEN ORDERING.

FIGURE 15–2 Page from bank order book showing sample voucher check.

itemizations. This portion of the check is removed before presenting the check for payment and provides a record for the payee (Fig. 15–2).

WARRANT. This is a check that is not considered to be negotiable but can be converted into a negotiable instrument or cash. Warrants are evidence of a debt due because of certain services rendered, and the bearer is entitled to certain payment for this service. Government and civic agencies often issue such warrants. A claim draft on an insurance claim is a warrant issued by the insurance adjuster as evidence that the claim is valid. It authorizes the insurance company to pay the claim.

ABA Number

This is a coding system originated by the American Bankers Association, a voluntary association of banks and bank organizations for mutual benefit in the exchange of ideas and information. One division of the American Bankers Association is the American Institute of Banking, whose purpose it is to educate bank employees in banking procedures and banking law.

The ABA number is used on checks as a simple way to identify the area where the bank upon which the check is written is located and the particular bank within the area. The code number is expressed as a fraction: $\frac{90\text{-}2110}{1222}$ (Fig. 15–3). In the part before the hyphen, the numbers 1 to 49 designate cities in which Federal Reserve banks are located or other key cities. The numbers from 50 to 99 refer to states or territories. As the second part of the number, each bank is issued an ABA number for its own identification purposes. The number in the lower part of the fraction includes the number of the Federal Reserve District in which the bank is located and other identifying information.

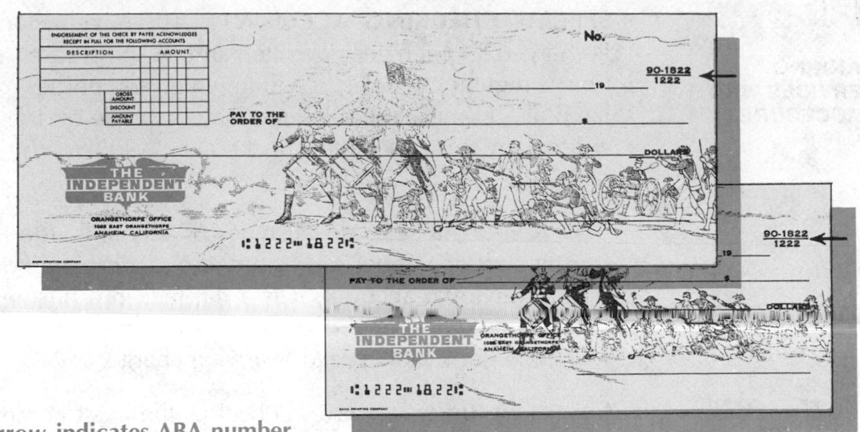

FIGURE 15–3 Sample checks. *Arrow* indicates ABA number.

MICR (Magnetic Ink Character Recognition)

Characters and numbers printed in magnetic ink are found at the bottom of most checks. They represent a common machine language, readable by machines as well as by humans. When a check is deposited, the amount of the check can also be printed in magnetic ink below the signature. MICR identification facilitates processing through a high-speed machine that reads the characters, sorts the checks, and does the bookkeeping.

15

BANK ACCOUNTS

CHECKING ACCOUNT. When an individual places an amount of money on deposit in a bank, he can set up a checking account—that is, he can draw checks upon this amount which are payable on demand. Simply stated, a checking account is a bank account against which checks may be written. Checking accounts usually do not earn interest on the balance deposited.

SAVINGS ACCOUNT. Money can also be deposited at the bank in a savings account (Fig. 15–4). In most cases, savings accounts earn interest upon the amounts deposited; that is, the bank pays the depositor a certain percentage annually for the use of the money in the savings account. When a depositor sets up a savings account, the bank issues a savings passbook in which are entered the dates, amounts deposited, interest earned, and balances on hand each time deposits are made. Withdrawals, which are made by use of special savings account checks, are also shown in the passbook. Most savings accounts are insured up to $100,000.

JOINT ACCOUNT. A joint account is owned by two or more people and is subject to check or withdrawal by the signatures of the persons who share it. It is a common practice for a husband and wife to set up a joint checking account, so that either may draw upon the account. Signatures may be placed on checks singly or jointly, depending upon the stipulations agreed upon when the original account is set up.

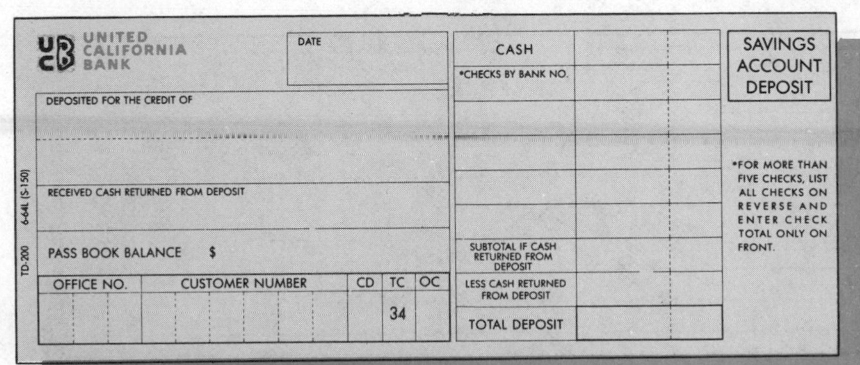

UNITED CALIFORNIA BANK

DATE

DEPOSITED FOR THE CREDIT OF

RECEIVED CASH RETURNED FROM DEPOSIT

PASS BOOK BALANCE $

OFFICE NO.	CUSTOMER NUMBER	CD	TC	OC
			34	

TD-200 6-64L (S-150)

CASH	
*CHECKS BY BANK NO.	
SUBTOTAL IF CASH RETURNED FROM DEPOSIT	
LESS CASH RETURNED FROM DEPOSIT	
TOTAL DEPOSIT	

SAVINGS ACCOUNT DEPOSIT

*FOR MORE THAN FIVE CHECKS, LIST ALL CHECKS ON REVERSE AND ENTER CHECK TOTAL ONLY ON FRONT.

FIGURE 15–4 Sample of savings account deposit slip.

SPECIAL CHECKING ACCOUNT. This is a checking account on which a fixed fee is charged for each check written and, in some cases, each deposit made. This differs from a regular checking account, which sometimes requires a minimum balance on hand at all times. The fixed fee may be made on the account before the checks are written. In this case, the checks are "sold" to the customer for a small fee per check.

SERVICE CHARGES. In all types of accounts, the bank may charge a fee against the account of a depositor for services rendered in bookkeeping. Usually in the case of an individual account, it is a flat fee; in a business account the fee is based on services rendered. If the average or minimum balance is maintained at a specific level, the bank may forego a service charge.

RULES FOR WRITING CHECKS

Checks are orders to pay. A check is the most common form of money exchange, with the exception of actual cash. Some of the advantages of making payments by check were outlined earlier in this chapter. However, the handling and writing of checks should be done with extreme care. Here are some basic rules to be remembered when writing checks:

1. Most business and personal checks are prenumbered with consecutive numbers being used with each successive checkbook. Be sure when filling in the stub that the number of the stub matches the number of the check. Business checks are usually printed three to a page.

2. *Before* you write the check, fill out the stub or the place allotted for recording your expenditures (Fig. 15–5). On the completed stub, there should appear the (a) check number, (b) date, (c) name of person or company to whose order the check is payable, (d) amount of the check, and (e) new balance to be carried forward to the next stub (Fig. 15–6). By following this procedure every time you will always know exactly where you stand concerning your balance and where your money has gone.

3. Checks should be written in ink or typewritten. The typewritten check is preferred by banks and presents a better professional image. A check-writing machine is of value in an office where many checks must be written.

4. Date the check the day it is written (not postdated). If there is an occasion when a postdated check is necessary, you must get the consent of the person accepting the check to hold it until that date.

5. Write the name of the payee after the printed words, "Pay to the order of." Always try to write the name of the payee correctly and as he writes his name (he must endorse the check exactly as his name appears on the face of the check) (Fig. 15–7). When paying bills, you will usually find a notation on the invoice stating "Make check payable to ________" with the necessary information following. Do not use abbreviations unless so instructed or unless space is limited. Write out in full, if possible. For example, Am. Med. Assn. should be written as American Medical Association.

6. Leave no space before the name, and follow it with three dashes if there is space remaining.

CHECK NO.	DATE	CHECK ISSUED TO	AMOUNT OF CHECK		✓	DATE OF DEP.	AMOUNT OF DEPOSIT		BALANCE	
									1840	57
101	8/1	Petty Cash	25	—					1815	57
102	8/2	Carson Med. Arts	600	—					1215	57
103		V.M. Surg. Supply	75	—					1140	57
						8/2	504	50	1645	07
104	8/4	Shell Oil Co.	37	54					1607	53

FIGURE 15–5 Sample depositor's record of checks and deposits.

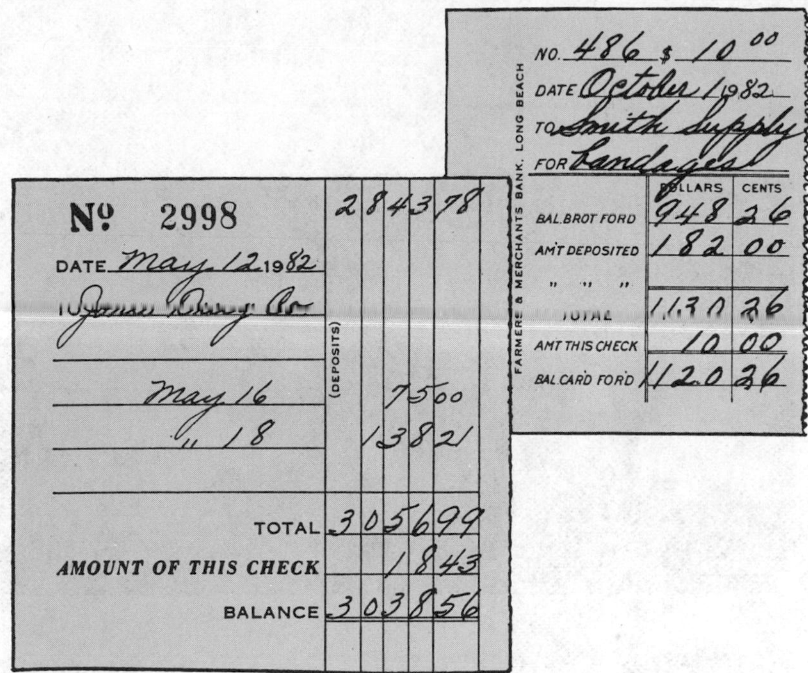

FIGURE 15–6 Methods of filling out check stubs.

15

7. Omit personal titles from the names of payees. A check should be made payable to Robert A. Jones rather than Mr. Robert A. Jones. If a married woman is using her husband's name, then it is necessary to put the Mrs. on the check, as, for example, Mrs. John L. Doe. But if the woman is using her own given name, Mary Louise Doe, then the Mrs. is omitted.

If the payee is receiving the check as an officer of an organization, then the name of the office should follow his name, such as John F. Jones, Treasurer, or Paul J. Barnes, Collector. He then accepts the check in his official capacity when he endorses it.

8. Take extreme care in stating the amount of money both in figures and in words. Make certain that the amount stated agrees in these three places: the check stub; the right side of the check close to the dollar sign ($); and the line on which the sum is written in words preceding the word "Dollars." If by chance there is a difference between the two amounts on the check, the bank generally pays the amount in words (or won't pay it at all).

9. Always start writing at the extreme left of each space on the check. Leave no blank spaces. Keep the cents close to the dollars; otherwise, there is room for alteration. If the check is typewritten, use the hyphen or asterisk key to fill in all blank spaces. Draw a line in these spaces if the check is written with pen (Fig. 15–8).

10. The amount of dollars and cents may be expressed in several different ways. Fractions of a dollar are best shown as a numerator of a fraction, i.e., as so many hundredths, when written following the dollar sign, keeping close to the dollars shown. If there are no cents in the amount, write the word "no" as the numerator instead of "00", since the "00" can easily be changed into "66" or "88." A better method is to write "Five dollars only" or "Five dollars and no cents." Double check

A. Smith
Alfred Smythe

John Doe
John B. Doe

FIGURE 15–7 Endorsement of checks. Payee's name incorrect.

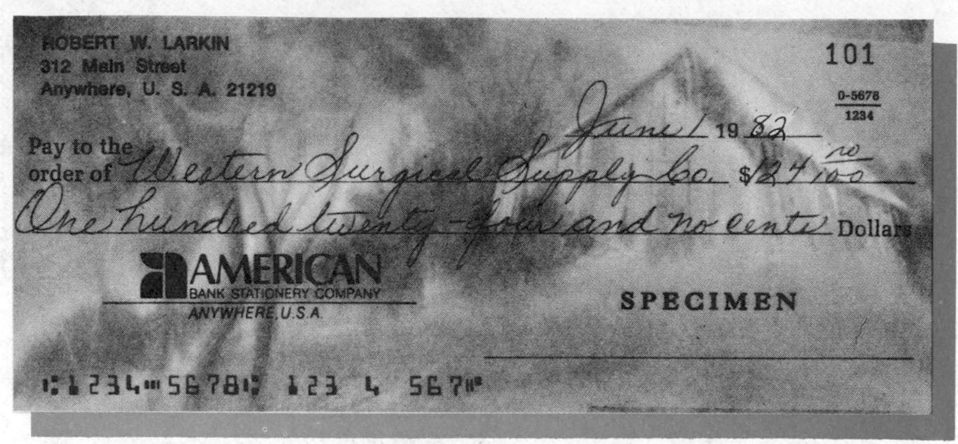
ROBERT W. LARKIN
312 Main Street
Anywhere, U. S. A. 21219
101
0-5678
1234
June 1 1982
Pay to the order of Western Surgical Supply Co. $124 no/100
One hundred twenty-four and no cents Dollars
AMERICAN BANK STATIONERY COMPANY
ANYWHERE, U.S.A.
SPECIMEN

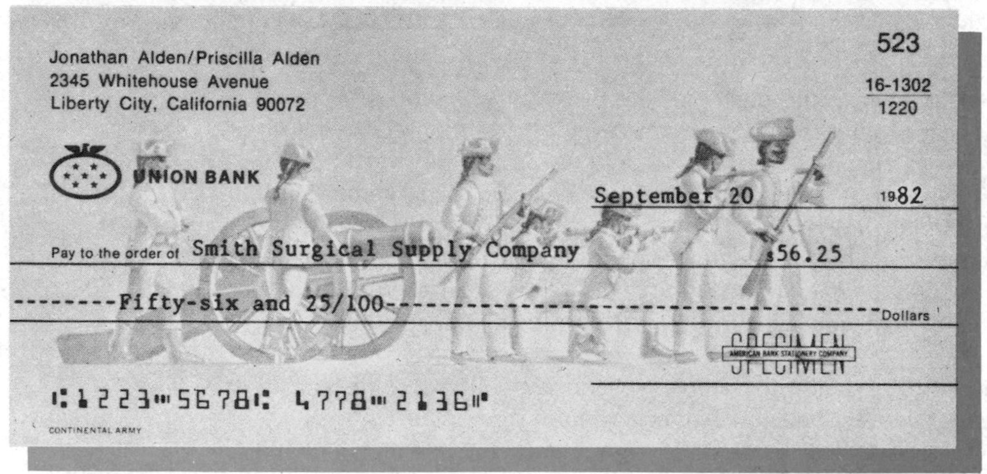

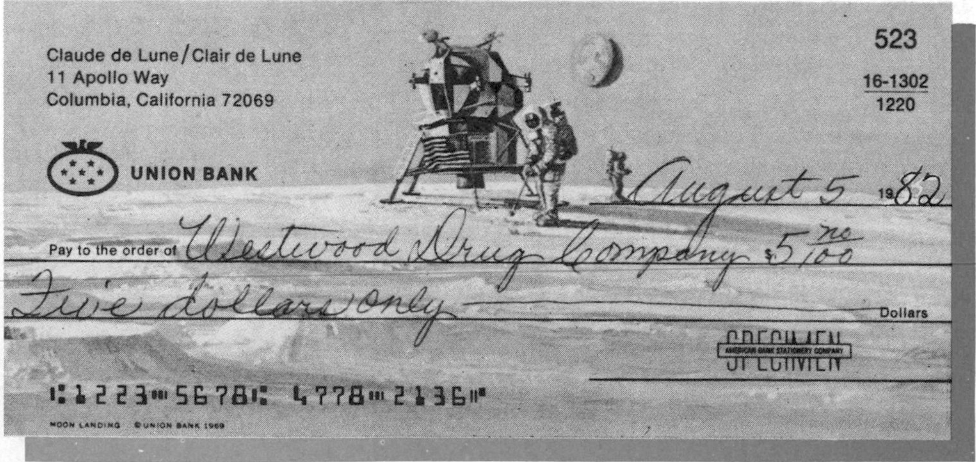

FIGURE 15–8 Correct methods of writing checks.

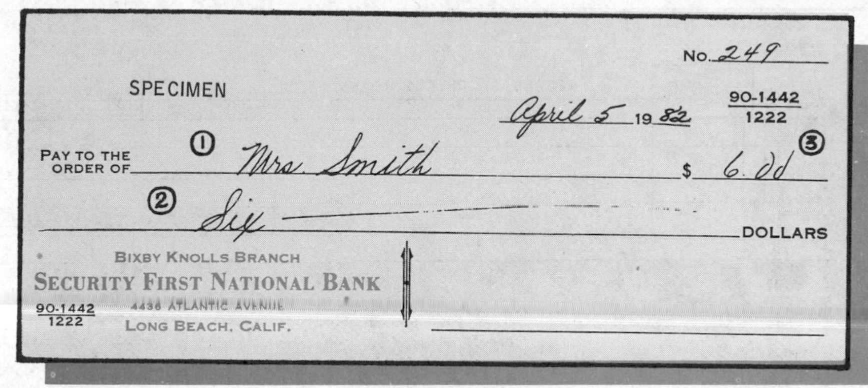

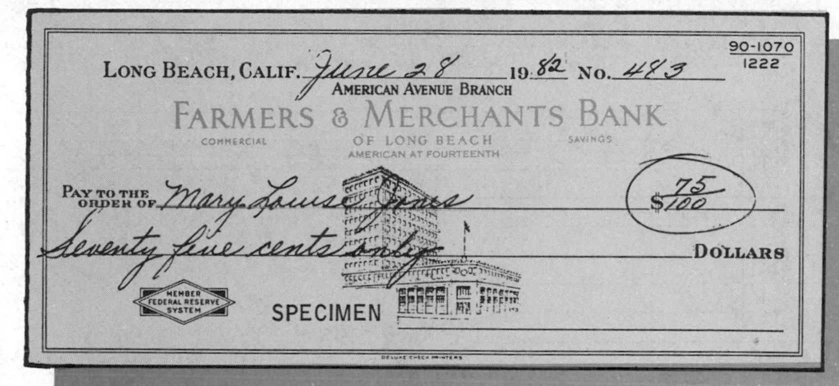

FIGURE 15–9 Incorrect check *(top): 1,* incomplete name; *2,* check could be made into $26 very easily; *3,* the "00" could be made into 88. Correct check *(bottom).*

what you've written and write so that the figures and words can be read correctly by all who need to read them. Capitalize the first word (i.e., Five).

11. If necessary, a check can be written for less than one dollar, but be very careful to emphasize the amount. The figures by the dollar sign ($) may be circled to assure proper attention, as $ (65¢) or enclosed in parentheses, as $—(65¢). The amount of money is written in full with the word "only," as "Only sixty-five cents—" (Fig. 15–9). The word *dollars* should not be crossed out. Figures 15–8 and 15–9 show examples of correct and incorrect check writing.

ONE-WRITE CHECK WRITING. A One-Write system of writing checks can save time and minimize errors in medical office disbursements. The office with a pegboard bookkeeping system (see Chapter 17) may wish to include one-write check writing. By using a combination check writing system such as the one illustrated in Fig. 15–10, one check and one record of checks drawn handle both bill paying and payroll check writing. When the bookkeeper writes the check a permanent record is created through the carbonized line of the check onto the record of checks drawn and the employee's payroll record, including a record of all deductions. Space is provided for the payee's address so that the check can be mailed in a window envelope. This not only saves time but ensures that the check goes to the right address. Suppliers of basic pegboard systems can also provide a check writing system such as the one described.

SYSTEMATIZING BILL PAYING

A systematic plan should be established for the writing of checks and the paying of bills. Check writing usually is done on the 10th or 15th of each month. An exception sometimes arises when it is possible to realize a good discount if payment of a bill is made within a specified time, for instance ten days. Such discounts usually are indicated at the bottom of invoices or billing forms.

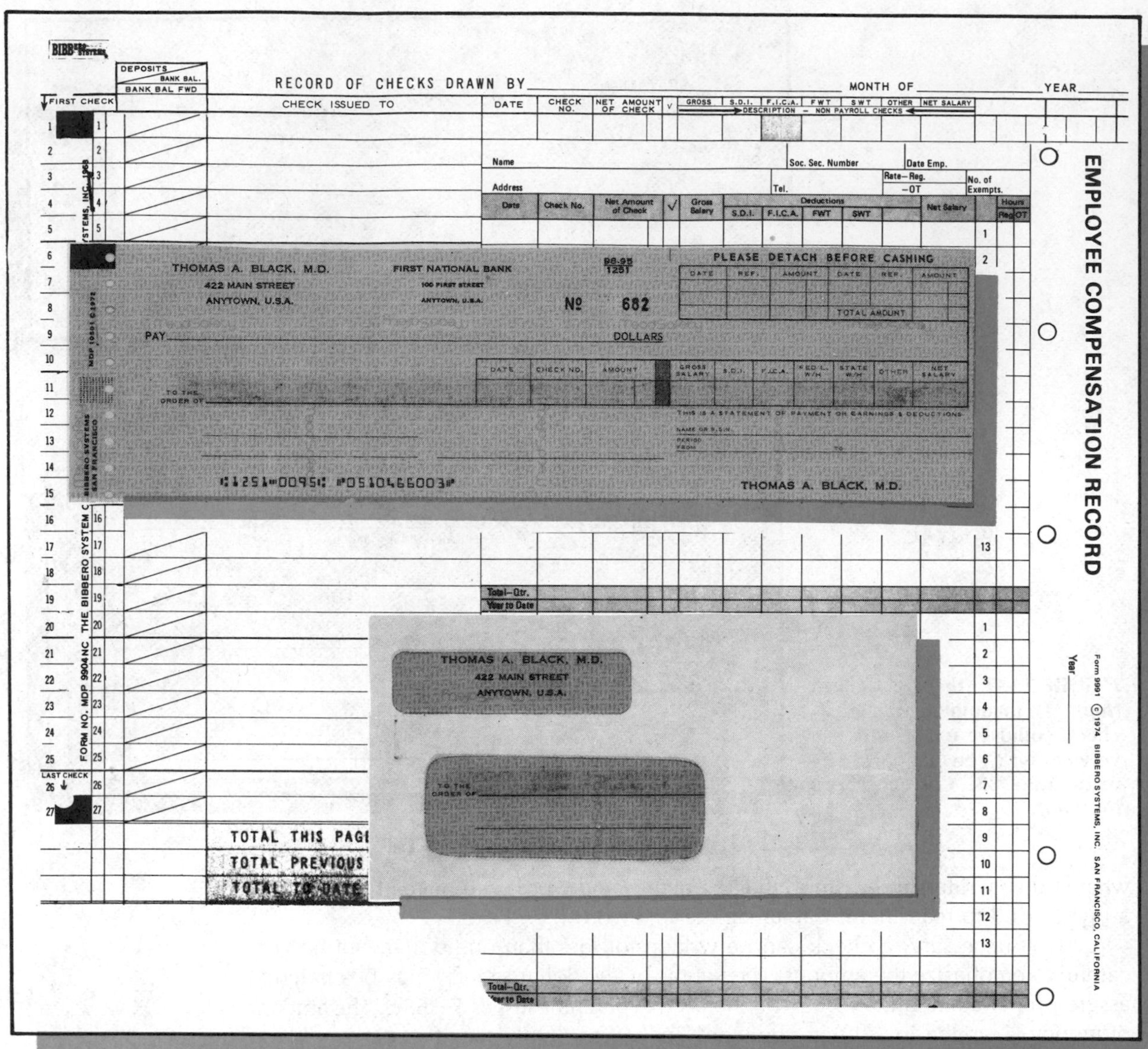

FIGURE 15–10 Pegboard system for check writing. (Courtesy of Bibbero Systems, Inc., San Francisco, California.)

When a check is written in payment of a statement or invoice, it is good practice to write on the invoice the number of the check and the date it was paid. Then if any question arises about whether the bill was paid or when it was paid, you can readily locate the check stub.

CORRECTIONS AND MISTAKES. Do not cross out, erase, or change any part of a check. Take time to be careful, so that no corrections are necessary. Checks are printed on sensitized paper so that erasures are readily noticeable, and the bank has the right to refuse to pay on any check that has been altered. If a mistake is made, write the word "VOID" on the stub and the check, but DO NOT destroy the check. It should be filed with the canceled checks so that it is available for auditing purposes. In rare cases, an error is made on a check that cannot be voided. If this situation occurs, it is necessary to strike out the error and write the correct information above. Then initial or sign your name near the correction. The bank will not accept a check in which a correction is made in regard to the name of the payee or the amount of money shown, but it may pass a correction on the date or check number.

PAYMENT IN FULL. If payment in full is to be recognized in regard to a given check, the statement "Payment in Full to Date" must appear on the back of the check above the endorsement, not on the face of the check. Canceled checks are a receipt for the maker of the check, not for the payee.

"CASH" CHECKS. A cash check is a check made payable to cash or bearer. Such checks are completely negotiable. Since these checks are easily cashed without positive identification, it is poor policy to write cash checks unless they are to be cashed at the time they are written. Banks may, however, require that the person receiving the cash endorse the check.

CHECKBOOK STUDS. The checkbook stub, the part that remains in the book after the check has been written and removed, is your own record of the checks written, date, amount, payee, and purpose of check. As mentioned earlier in this chapter, it is important that the stub be completed before the check. This prevents the possibility of writing a check and neglecting to complete the stub. If the stub is not completed and the check is sent out, you will have no record of the payee and the amount taken from the account until the canceled check is returned at a later date. Consequently, you will be unable to balance your account or determine the amount on hand until you receive those canceled checks.

If checks are to be typewritten, complete the stub first, then remove the check from the checkbook and type the necessary information on it. After typing the check, compare the amounts appearing on the stub and the check. Differences between amounts listed on check stubs and on the checks themselves are a frequent source of error in banking procedure. Always double check your check stubs against checks to avoid error, and keep the checkbook balance up to date. You will be saving yourself time and trouble in the long run.

It is good procedure to keep a separate financial disbursement record with your bookkeeping system as a double check on the status of the bank account.

SIGNING CHECKS

After all checks have been written, place them on the doctor's desk with the invoices or other information so that he can study them and sign the checks. The doctor's

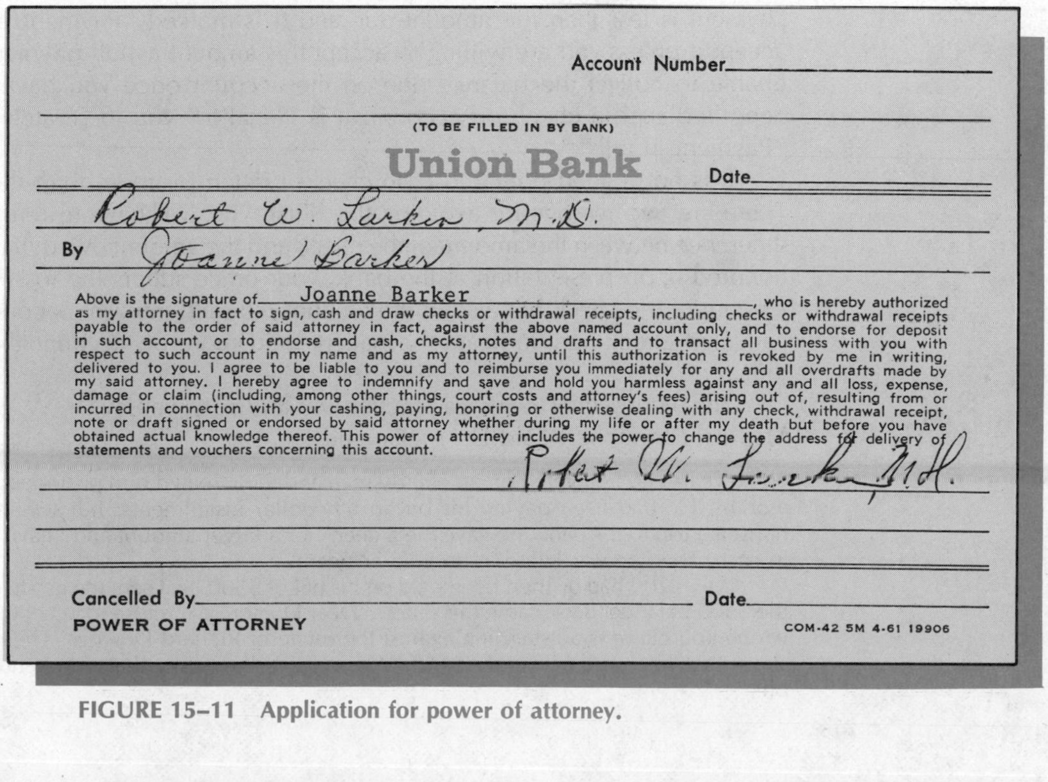

Account Number________

(TO BE FILLED IN BY BANK)

Union Bank

Date________

Robert W. Larker, M.D.

By Joanne Barker

Above is the signature of Joanne Barker, who is hereby authorized as my attorney in fact to sign, cash and draw checks or withdrawal receipts, including checks or withdrawal receipts payable to the order of said attorney in fact, against the above named account only, and to endorse for deposit in such account, or to endorse and cash, checks, notes and drafts and to transact all business with you with respect to such account in my name and as my attorney, until this authorization is revoked by me in writing, delivered to you. I agree to be liable to you and to reimburse you immediately for any and all overdrafts made by my said attorney. I hereby agree to indemnify and save and hold you harmless against any and all loss, expense, damage or claim (including, among other things, court costs and attorney's fees) arising out of, resulting from or incurred in connection with your cashing, paying, honoring or otherwise dealing with any check, withdrawal receipt, note or draft signed or endorsed by said attorney whether during my life or after my death but before you have obtained actual knowledge thereof. This power of attorney includes the power to change the address for delivery of statements and vouchers concerning this account.

Robert W. Larker, M.D.

Cancelled By________ Date________

POWER OF ATTORNEY

COM-42 5M 4-61 19906

FIGURE 15–11 Application for power of attorney.

secretary or assistant does not sign checks unless power of attorney has been delegated to her for this responsibility (Fig. 15–11).

Never ask your employer to sign a blank check. This places him in a very embarrassing situation, as he is well aware of the dangers involved. Some doctors sign several blank checks before leaving the office on an extended trip to allow the medical assistant to make certain payments during his absence. This is a dangerous procedure even though the assistant is completely trustworthy. Such checks may be misplaced or they may be stolen and cashed for any amount by anyone completing the check.

Some physicians use two different signatures in conducting the legal aspects of their practices, using one signature on prescriptions, which of course are easily available to forgers, and a second signature for banking purposes. This is an excellent precaution against forged checks on the doctor's bank account.

When checks are sent through the mail, the check should not be visible through the envelope. Either place the check within a letter or fold it into a plain sheet of paper. Checks may be folded at the right end to conceal the amount of money written. Make certain the envelopes are sealed before mailing, and mail all checks yourself as soon as possible after writing. Place these envelopes in a mailbox, not in an outgoing tray, unless you are certain the tray is a safe place in which to leave them prior to mailing.

RULES FOR ACCEPTING CHECKS

The medical assistant is frequently presented with checks by patients or others as payment for the doctor's services. In most cases these will be personal checks. Caution should be used in accepting government checks or payroll checks. Make sure the person presenting the check is known to you. Government and payroll checks sometimes are illegally secured in mailbox robberies.

Acceptance of "third-party" checks is generally unwise. A third-party check is a check made out, for example, to a patient by another person. The patient presents the check for payment on his account. It is necessary to endorse such checks, and the doctor thus becomes responsible in case the check bounces. Do not accept a postal money order for payment if the person paying you has received it from another party; postal money orders cannot be endorsed by more than two persons.

Do not accept a check marked "Payment in full" unless it does pay the account in full up to and including the date on which it is received. If the check received in payment is less than the amount due and it is marked "Payment in full," do not accept it unless you are willing to accept this amount as full payment. You will be unable to collect the balance due on the account once you have accepted and deposited such a check on account. It is illegal for you to scratch out the words "Payment in full."

It is not a good policy to cash checks written for more than the amount due. There are two reasons for avoiding this. First, you will have to return cash for the difference between the amount of the check and the amount owed. If the check is not honored upon presentation at the bank, your office suffers the loss not only of the amount of the check but also of the amount returned in cash. Second, the returned canceled check may indicate the patient paid more on account than he actually did.

The bitter sequel to such a practice was told very well by Dr. W. B. McDonald in *Medical Economics*. Said Dr. McDonald:

> Some years ago I operated on an elderly man and then treated him postoperatively for several months. He had been paying his bill in fifty-dollar installments; but several times, to save himself a trip to the bank, he gave me a check for a larger amount and I gave him the balance in cash. Then he was killed in an auto accident.
>
> Only $200 had by then been paid on his bill of $500. So I sent the estate my statement for the $300 balance. Back came this letter: "Dear Doctor: We refuse to accept the bill for $300, which you claim is outstanding against the estate of Richard Downes. The canceled checks show that he owed you only $100. We suggest, therefore, that you send us a corrected bill."

What bothered me even more than the financial loss was to have my integrity questioned. I decided then and there that the penalty for being accommodating in such cases was just too high.*

Such an experience could occur in any doctor's office, as Dr. McDonald points out. It is difficult for the assistant to tell a patient, "We never cash a check for more than the amount due." Dr. McDonald had one suggestion for making this procedure easier. He advised his assistants to explain that it is inadvisable for the office to cash such checks because of tax problems. Most people can appreciate the gravity of an income tax investigation. An alternate "escape" is simply to state that you do not keep extra cash in the office, and suggest that the patient cash the check at a bank or store where he is known and return with the correct amount.

If you do not know the individual and cannot identify his signature, ask for good identification. An honest person is always willing to show his credentials, such as credit cards or driver's license. Do not hesitate to copy the numbers of these cards on the face of the check; in case the check is returned to you, you will have a means of tracing the person who gave you the bad check. It is wise to have the person make out the check in your presence and then compare the signature with the one on the identification cards.

SUMMARY OF PRECAUTIONS TO OBSERVE IN ACCEPTING CHECKS

1. Scan the check carefully for incorrect dates or amounts which do not match.
2. Do not accept a check with corrections on it.
3. An out-of-town check, government check, or payroll check should be accepted *only* if you are well acquainted with the person presenting it.
4. If you do not know the person presenting a personal check, ask for identification and compare signatures.
5. Do not accept third-party checks unless you are willing to accept responsibility for the value of the check should it prove worthless.
6. Do not accept checks written for more than the amount due.
7. Do not accept checks marked "Payment in full" unless the check does pay the account up to and including the date the check is presented.
8. Remember that money orders cannot be endorsed by more than two persons.

ENDORSEMENT OF CHECKS

What is an Endorsement?

An endorsement is a signature plus any other writing on the back of a check by which the endorser transfers his right in the check to another party. Endorsements are made in ink, with either pen or rubber stamp, on the back of the check across the left, or perforated end.

Necessity for Endorsement

The Uniform Negotiable Instrument Act, applicable in all states, explains the need of an endorsement as follows:

> An instrument is negotiated when it is transferred from one person to another in such a manner as to pass title to another party. If payable to bearer, it is negotiated by delivery. If payable to order, it is negotiated by the endorsement of the holder completed by delivery.

The name of the last endorser of the check shows who last received the money. If a check were cashed for someone who did not endorse it and was returned for some reason, the bank would charge the check to the last endorser, not to the last person receiving the money. For this reason, it is not wise to cash a check made payable to another party without having the endorsement of the person who delivered the check to you for cashing.

Kinds of Endorsements

If a check is made payable to "Bearer" or "Cash" it is considered to be a negotiable instrument without an endorsement, because no particular party has been named.

*McDonald, W. B.: Letter to the Editor. Med. Econ., Vol. 31, Nov., 1953.

But a check made payable to a particular party must have an endorsement before it is considered negotiable.

The four principal kinds of endorsements are: blank, restrictive, special, and qualified. Blank and restrictive endorsements are most commonly used.

BLANK ENDORSEMENT. The payee signs only his name. This makes the check payable to bearer. It is the simplest and most common type of endorsement but should be used only when the check is to be cashed or deposited immediately.

RESTRICTIVE ENDORSEMENT. This specifies the *purpose* of the endorsement. You will use one kind of restrictive endorsement in preparing the doctor's checks for deposit to his checking account. An example is shown in Figure 15–12.

SPECIAL ENDORSEMENT. This includes words specifying the person to whom the endorser makes the check payable. For instance, a check naming Helen Barker as payee may be endorsed to the doctor by writing on the back of the check

Pay to the order of
Theodore F. Wilson, M.D.
Helen Barker

The check is still negotiable but requires Dr. Wilson's signature or endorsement.

QUALIFIED ENDORSEMENT. The *effect* of the endorsement is qualified by disclaiming or destroying any future liability of the endorser. Usually the words "Without Recourse" are written above the payee's signature. This kind of endorsement might be used by an attorney who accepts a check on behalf of a client but who has no personal interest in the transaction.

Endorsement Procedures

The use of a blank endorsement by the medical assistant will be more or less limited to cashing a petty cash check for the office. If the doctor writes a check to "cash" or "petty cash," the assistant will probably be asked to endorse it when she receives the cash from the bank or any party cashing the check. This endorsement should not be written until the check is actually presented for payment. Although a check made out to "cash" is immediately negotiable, the person who endorses it is verifying that he is the one who received payment.

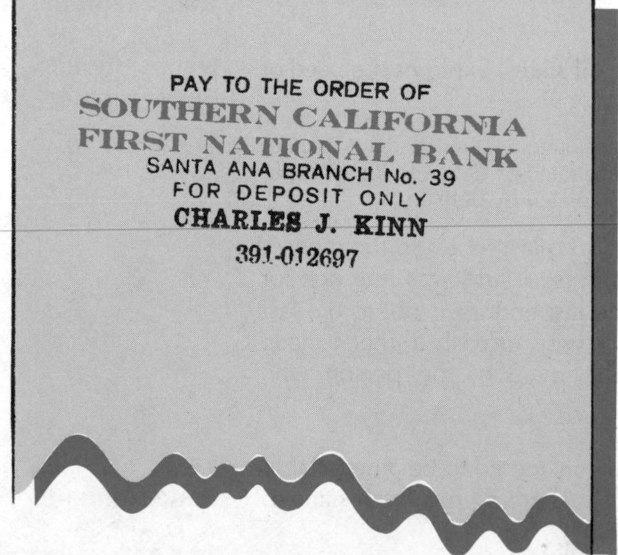
PAY TO THE ORDER OF
SOUTHERN CALIFORNIA
FIRST NATIONAL BANK
SANTA ANA BRANCH No. 39
FOR DEPOSIT ONLY
CHARLES J. KINN
391-012697

FIGURE 15–12 Example of restrictive endorsement.

It is advisable in most medical offices to deposit all receipts in the checking account. For this reason checks may be endorsed for deposit immediately upon receipt, thereby safeguarding them from being negotiable should they be lost or stolen.

Any endorsement should agree exactly with the name on the face of the check. If the name of the payee is misspelled, it is usually necessary for him to endorse the check the way the name is spelled on the face, followed by his name with the correct spelling. The Uniform Commercial Code, Section 3–203, states:

> Where an instrument is made payable to a person under a misspelled name or one other than his own he may indorse in that name or his own or both; but signature in both names may be required by a person paying or giving value for the instrument.

Most banks will accept the routine stamp endorsement that is restricted to "deposit only," if the customer is well known and maintains an established account.

Some insurance checks or drafts require a personal signature endorsement; a stamped endorsement is not accepted. This will be stated on the back of the check. In such cases, ask the payee to endorse with his signature, then stamp immediately below the signature the restrictive endorsement "for deposit only."

DEPOSITS AND BANK STATEMENTS

15

It is usually a regular duty of the medical assistant to make deposits of cash and checks received for the doctor's account. She will routinely prepare deposit slips and see that bank statements are reconciled with the checking account.

Deposit or Cash Checks Promptly

There are several reasons for processing checks promptly:

1. There is possible danger of a "stop-payment order."
2. The check may be lost, misplaced, or stolen.
3. There is the danger that if a delay occurs in presenting the check for payment, the check may be returned because of insufficient funds to cover it.
4. Some checks have a restricted time for cashing.
5. It is common courtesy to cash checks promptly so that the payer does not have checks outstanding when he receives his bank statement.

Preparing the Deposit

Deposit slips are itemized memoranda of cash or other funds which a customer presents to the bank with the money to be credited to his account. All deposits should be accompanied by a deposit slip. It is good business procedure to make a carbon or photocopy of all deposit slips to keep on file. As in check writing, the bank prefers a typed slip to one handwritten.

There are several different types of deposit slips, sometimes known as deposit tickets. The most common for the average checking account, correctly known as a commercial account, is the commercial slip (Fig. 15–13). There is also the saving slip and the deposit-by-mail slip. These slips may be obtained from your bank and should be kept on hand in your office. Checking account deposit slips are usually printed with the number of the account in Magnetic Ink Characters to correspond with the checks. The slips are frequently bound in the back of the checkbook. Some write-it-once bookkeeping systems include a deposit slip which the bank will accept as the itemization if it is attached to the customer's numbered deposit slip. The deposit slip should be prepared before going to the bank, with the money organized and ready to present to the bank teller.

Each type of money is recorded separately. The currency (paper money) is usually listed first. Organize the currency so that all of the bills are facing in the same direction — that is, the black side up and the portrait right side up. Place the larger bills on top, graduating down to the smaller ones.

The coin amount is listed next. Count the coins and place in an evelope. If there is a large quantity of a certain coin, place it in rolls provided by the bank. The depositor should sign these rolls as the rolled coins are usually not counted by the teller.

Checks are recorded by their bank number, each one individually. If the checks

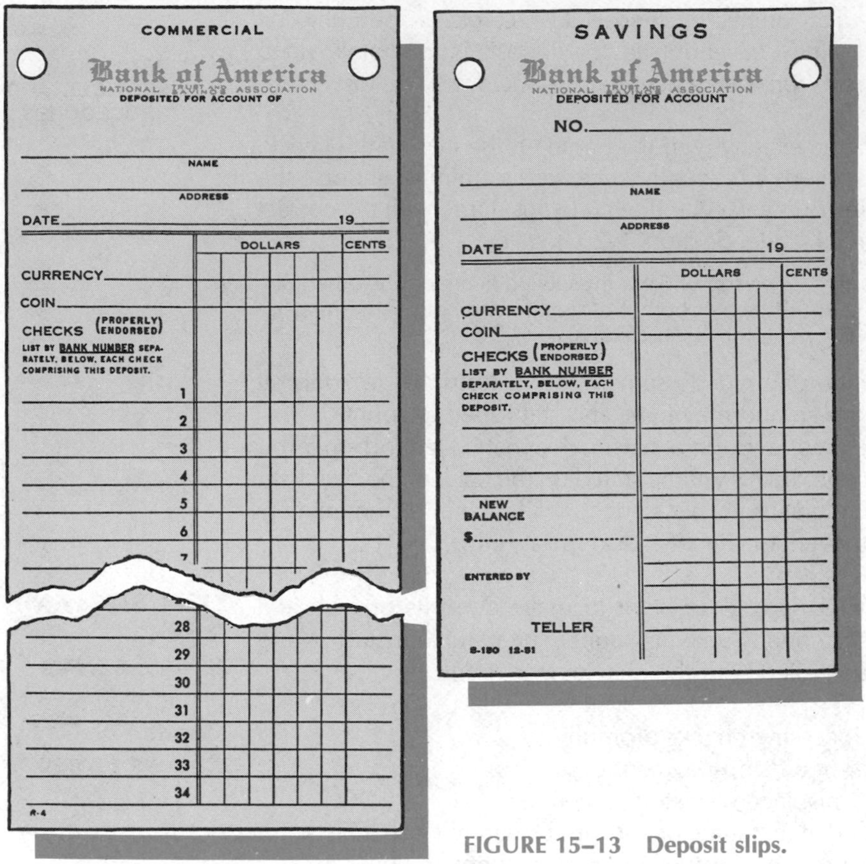

FIGURE 15–13 Deposit slips.

are arranged alphabetically by the names of the patient accounts, and these names included on your office copy of the deposit slip, you will have a ready reference of checks deposited should a question arise regarding a patient's payment.

Money orders, either postal, express, or others, are identified by "P O Money Order," or "Exp. M O." Remember that money orders cannot be endorsed by more than two persons.

The deposit slip should be carefully totaled and the total entered in the checkbook. Clip the currency together, and clip the checks in a separate packet. Then place the entire amount in a heavy envelope for taking to the bank. Deposit daily if possible. Any torn bills should be mended with transparent tape before taking to the bank.

"HOLD" ON YOUR ACCOUNT. Under certain circumstances money that is deposited to your account may not be immediately available for use. A "hold for uncollected funds (UCF)" may be placed for the full amount of a check you deposit if it is (1) for a sizable amount, (2) drawn on another bank or another branch of your bank, or (3) issued by a person or organization not known to the bank. The hold means that you cannot use the funds until the check has cleared (been processed and paid to your account).

You will be told if a hold has been placed on your account. The teller will note the hold in your deposit record by writing "UCF" and the number of days the hold will be in effect; this will appear next to the date of deposit. If you make a deposit by mail, you will either be telephoned or notified of the hold by return mail.

The hold will be for a specified number of business days and for the full amount of the check. After that time, you can begin to draw against the funds. If for some reason the check does not clear, you will be notified.

For your every banking need Look to . . .

UCB

BANK BY MAIL DEPOSIT TICKET
INSTRUCTIONS

1 - Mail checks with white and yellow copies of the form in the envelopes provided. Retain pink copy.
2 - Use registered mail when sending currency & coupons.
3 - Endorse checks using phrase "Pay to the order of United California Bank" above signature.

DEPOSITED TO THE CREDIT OF

Robert W. Larkin, M.D.

UNITED CALIFORNIA BANK

Anaheim Main Office
423 West Broadway
Anaheim, California 92805

⑆1222⑉1645⑆170170317⑈ 30

DD-206 9-69

DATE

Checks by Bank No.	DOLLARS	CENTS
TOTAL		

Note: Use registered mail when sending Currency and Coin

CUSTOMER'S COPY
REMOVE PINK COPY **ONLY** AND RETAIN

FIGURE 15–14 **Example of bank-by-mail deposit ticket.**

Depositing by Mail

Depositing by mail will save you time and is easily accomplished if there are only checks to be deposited. Banks usually supply their customers with special mailing deposit slips and envelopes, upon request (Fig. 15–14). Some mailing deposit slips have an attached portion that the bank will stamp and return as your receipt. Other banks provide the customer with a receipt card that is sent along with the deposit each time for the bank's notation. These deposits are prepared in the same manner as the regular deposits, but certain precautions should be observed:

1. Do not send cash or currency by mail. If this is absolutely necessary, then send it by registered mail.
2. Do not endorse checks in blank; use a deposit stamp or write the notation "For deposit only to the account of_____."
3. If you have not obtained mailing deposit slips or your bank does not provide them, fill out duplicate slips and mail with your deposit. The bank will stamp one copy and return it to you as a receipt.

Returned Checks

If a check is returned to your office for some reason, usually marked N.S.F. (Not Sufficient Funds), or R.T.M. (Return to Maker), do not delay in contacting the person who gave you the check (Fig. 15–15). Such situations usually arise because of carelessness on the payer's part. Many people just do not attempt to keep close track of their bank balance; they just write checks merrily until one bounces. However, it could be otherwise.

It takes considerable tact to call a patient and inform him that a check has been returned, but it is necessary that such calls be made promptly. The patient may tell you that a deposit was mailed too late to arrive before the check was presented for

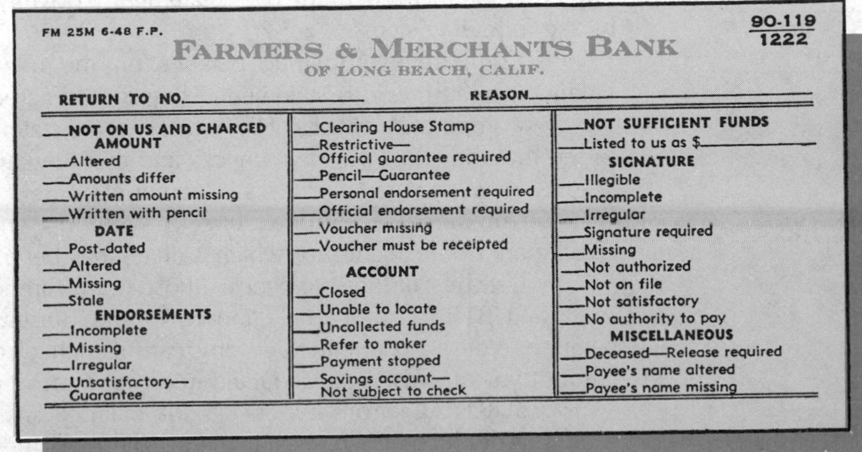

FM 25M 6-48 F.P.

90-119
1222

FARMERS & MERCHANTS BANK
OF LONG BEACH, CALIF.

RETURN TO NO.____ REASON____

__NOT ON US AND CHARGED
AMOUNT
__Altered
__Amounts differ
__Written amount missing
__Written with pencil
DATE
__Post-dated
__Altered
__Missing
__Stale
ENDORSEMENTS
__Incomplete
__Missing
__Irregular
__Unsatisfactory—Guarantee

__Clearing House Stamp
__Restrictive—Official guarantee required
__Pencil—Guarantee
__Personal endorsement required
__Official endorsement required
__Voucher missing
__Voucher must be receipted
ACCOUNT
__Closed
__Unable to locate
__Uncollected funds
__Refer to maker
__Payment stopped
__Savings account—Not subject to check

__NOT SUFFICIENT FUNDS
__Listed to us as $____
SIGNATURE
__Illegible
__Incomplete
__Irregular
__Signature required
__Missing
__Not authorized
__Not on file
__Not satisfactory
__No authority to pay
MISCELLANEOUS
__Deceased—Release required
__Payee's name altered
__Payee's name missing

FIGURE 15–15 **Returned check slip.**

payment. In that case you may simply re-deposit the check. The patient may ask you to hold the check for a few days and deposit it again. Or he may offer to send another check.

A returned check cannot serve as a receipt for the patient because it has not been "paid" by the bank. Consequently there is no harm in returning it to the maker. However, if you do return it to the maker before receiving a replacement, it is wise to photocopy the N.S.F. check for your records because it does serve as acknowledgment of the debt.

If you are unable to contact the maker of a bad check, waste no time in tracking down all leads, such as referrals, numbers you obtained from credit cards, driver's license, and so forth. There are several places to which bad checks may be reported. Credit associations are often a great help when such a problem arises. If you do not succeed in tracking down and collecting on this account yourself within a short time, turn it over to a qualified collection agency. If a check is returned to your office marked "No account," and it is a check which you had deposited promptly, you have obviously been swindled. This check should be given to the police, the local Better Business Bureau, or your collection agency.

Lost or Stolen Checks

If you lose any of your checks, report this to your bank promptly. The bank will place a warning on your account, and signatures on incoming checks will be carefully inspected to detect possible forgeries.

If you suspect that your checks have been stolen, first make a report to the police in the city or town where the theft took place. Then notify your bank and tell them the time, date, and place the police report was made. A warning will be placed on your account. In some cases, you may be asked to close your account and open a new one under a different number.

As long as you have reported your checks missing or stolen to the proper authorities, you usually will not be held responsible for losses due to forgery. The bank or merchant who accepted the forged check(s) would be charged for the loss. For this reason, anyone accepting a check from a person who is not known personally must be very careful about establishing the person's identity.

Reconciling the Bank Statement

The bank customer receives a statement from his bank each month (more often if requested) showing the activity of his account during the month and returning all checks that have cleared the bank during the month (Fig. 15–16). The bank statement balance and the customer's checkbook balance will usually be different, except in a relatively inactive account. The two balances must be "reconciled." The reconciliation will disclose any errors that may exist in the checkbook or, on rare occasions, in the bank statement (Fig. 15–17). Most banks ask to be notified within ten days of any error found in the statement. The bank statement should be reconciled as soon as received each month. You will usually find a form to follow in carrying out this procedure on the back of the bank statement. You may reconcile any bank statement by the following steps:

1. Compare the opening balance on the new statement with the closing balance on the previous statement. They should agree.

2. Compare the entries of the checks on the statement with the returned checks, to see that they are your own checks and that they are listed in the right amount.

3. Now arrange the checks in numerical order.

4. Compare the returned checks with the checkbook stubs. Place a red checkmark on each stub for which a check has been returned (Fig. 15–18).

5. List the outstanding checks (those not returned with the statement).

6. SUBTRACT the total amount of the outstanding checks from the bank balance. *Note:* Do not include any certified checks as outstanding, because the amount has already been deducted from your account.

7. SUBTRACT from the checkbook balance any bank charges (which will be shown as debits on the bank statement). These charges will include service charges, automatic withdrawals or payments, NSF checks, and so on.

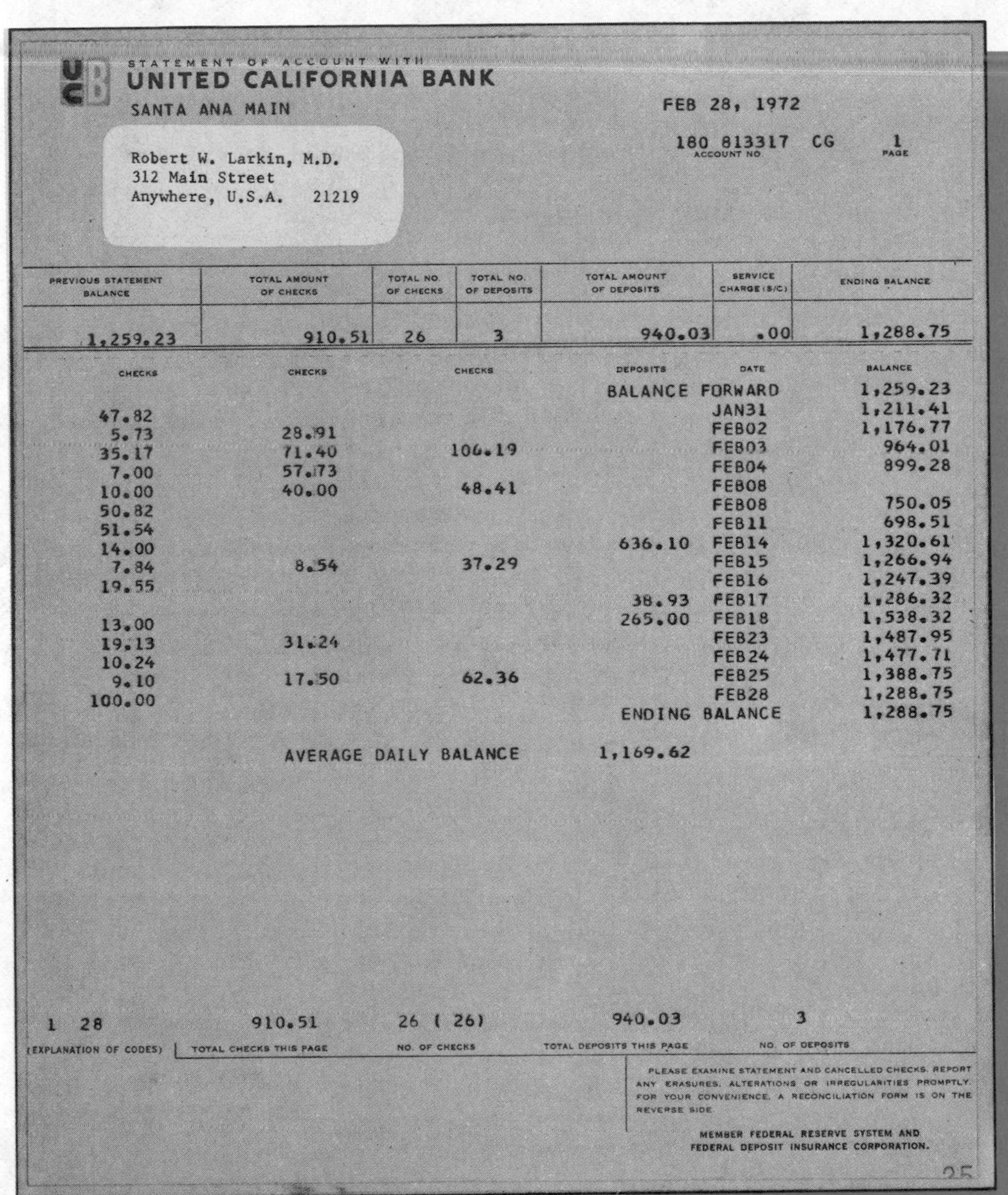

STATEMENT OF ACCOUNT WITH
UNITED CALIFORNIA BANK
SANTA ANA MAIN

FEB 28, 1972

180 813317 CG — ACCOUNT NO. — PAGE 1

Robert W. Larkin, M.D.
312 Main Street
Anywhere, U.S.A. 21219

PREVIOUS STATEMENT BALANCE	TOTAL AMOUNT OF CHECKS	TOTAL NO. OF CHECKS	TOTAL NO. OF DEPOSITS	TOTAL AMOUNT OF DEPOSITS	SERVICE CHARGE (S/C)	ENDING BALANCE
1,259.23	910.51	26	3	940.03	.00	1,288.75

CHECKS	CHECKS	CHECKS	DEPOSITS	DATE	BALANCE
			BALANCE FORWARD		1,259.23
47.82				JAN31	1,211.41
5.73	28.91			FEB02	1,176.77
35.17	71.40	106.19		FEB03	964.01
7.00	57.73			FEB04	899.28
10.00	40.00	48.41		FEB08	
50.82				FEB08	750.05
51.54				FEB11	698.51
14.00			636.10	FEB14	1,320.61
7.84	8.54	37.29		FEB15	1,266.94
19.55				FEB16	1,247.39
			38.93	FEB17	1,286.32
13.00			265.00	FEB18	1,538.32
19.13	31.24			FEB23	1,487.95
10.24				FEB24	1,477.71
9.10	17.50	62.36		FEB25	1,388.75
100.00				FEB28	1,288.75
			ENDING BALANCE		1,288.75

AVERAGE DAILY BALANCE 1,169.62

(EXPLANATION OF CODES)	TOTAL CHECKS THIS PAGE	NO. OF CHECKS	TOTAL DEPOSITS THIS PAGE	NO. OF DEPOSITS
1 28	910.51	26 (26)	940.03	3

PLEASE EXAMINE STATEMENT AND CANCELLED CHECKS. REPORT ANY ERASURES, ALTERATIONS OR IRREGULARITIES PROMPTLY. FOR YOUR CONVENIENCE, A RECONCILIATION FORM IS ON THE REVERSE SIDE.

MEMBER FEDERAL RESERVE SYSTEM AND FEDERAL DEPOSIT INSURANCE CORPORATION.

25

FIGURE 15–16 Example of monthly bank statement.

UNION BANK

RECONCILING YOUR CHECKING ACCOUNT

A STEP-BY-STEP PROCESS

1. Sort checks by number or by date.
2. Match each entry with the amount in your register. If you find an error in your register, change its **balance.**
3. Subtract from your register balance any charges deducted by the bank. Enter this **adjusted balance** on line 4 below.

You Can Figure In This Area

5. Enter ending balance of this statement. If ending balance shows OD or ¤, enter zero and include below as an outstanding check. $________

6. **Add** any deposits made after last date on the statement. ________

NEW BALANCE $

7. **Subtract** checks you have written but are not yet paid by the bank.

OUTSTANDING CHECKS		
Number or Date	AMOUNT	
TOTAL		

4. $________ ← SHOULD EQUAL → $________

Adjusted Register Balance

* SYMBOL REFERENCE

A - ACTIVITY CHARGE
B - RETURNED ITEM CHARGE
D - BANK ORIGINATED CHARGE
I - CASH RESERVE INTEREST CHARGE
L - LIST
OD - OVERDRAFT
P - PAYMENT
R - BANK ORIGINATED DEPOSIT
S - SUB-TOTAL
V - PAYMENT STOPPED
W - CHECK RETURNED
¤ - CASH RESERVE IN USE
X - CHECK REVERSAL
Y - DEPOSIT REVERSAL
* - FINAL BALANCE

FIGURE 15–17 Reverse side of bank statement. Use for reconciling your checking account.

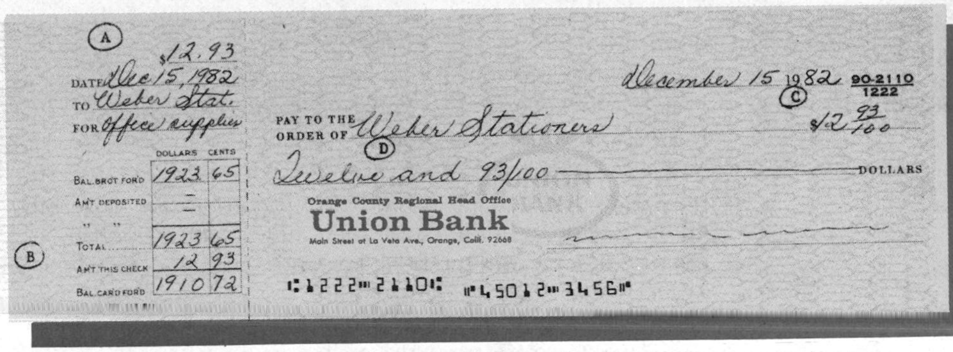

FIGURE 15–18 **Amounts in *A, B, C,* and *D* must correspond.**

8. ADD to the bank statement balance any deposits that appear on your checkbook balance but that have not been included on the bank statement.

9. The balance in your checkbook and the bank statement balance should now agree — they are *reconciled.*

The reconciliation procedure may be put in a formula as follows:

Bank statement balance	$________	
Less outstanding checks	________	
Plus deposits not shown	________	
CORRECTED BANK STATEMENT BALANCE		$________
Checkbook balance	$________	
Less any bank charges	________	
CORRECTED CHECKBOOK BALANCE		$________

If these balances agree, you may stop here. If they do not agree, SUBTRACT the lesser from the greater; the difference will usually give you a clue to locating the error.

In searching for a possible error ask yourself these questions:

- Did you forget to include one of the outstanding checks?
- Is your arithmetic correct?
- Did you fail to record a deposit or did you record it twice?
- Do all stubs and checks agree?
- Have you carried your figures forward correctly?
- Have you transposed a figure? (if the amount of your error is divisible by nine you probably did)
- Did your boss write a check without your knowledge?
- Did you fail to correct your checkbook balance at the time of the previous statement?

Once you become familiar with banking procedures, you will find that, by following prescribed procedures, you will simplify the task of "keeping books" in the doctor's office.

SAFE DEPOSIT BOX

Most commercial banks and many savings institutions have safe deposit boxes that may be rented by their customers. One need not always be a depositor in order to rent a safe deposit box.

Safe deposit boxes provide protection for valuable papers and personal property for a moderate fee. They are obtainable in various sizes to suit the need of the customer; the annual cost will range from $5 to $30 and is tax deductible. Chapter

Twelve, Records Management, lists certain items that might be placed in a safe deposit box.

The box provides protection in several ways. The box itself is a metal container which is locked with two keys into a compartment in the bank's vault. One key is in possession of the customer, the second key in possession of the bank. The bank is very strict about giving access to the safe deposit boxes. The customer must register on a special form when requesting access to the box. After signatures have been compared he is admitted to the vault, accompanied by a bank guard. The guard opens one lock with the bank key and opens the other lock with the customer's key. The box may then be removed and the customer can take it to a private room, or if he merely wishes to place something in the box he can do so and the box can be immediately replaced and locked.

The customer is given two identical keys when he rents the box. These must be guarded carefully because they cannot be duplicated, and he must return both keys to the bank when he relinquishes the box. If a key is lost the bank will charge a fee; if both keys are lost, the fee is considerably higher.

The medical office assistant may be asked to keep a perpetual inventory of the contents of the doctor's safe deposit box. An inventory faithfully kept up to date will save making useless trips to the bank only to discover that the item wanted is not there.

BANKING TERMINOLOGY

There are certain other banking terms with which the medical office assistant should be familiar, in order that she understand her duties in the handling of a physician's business affairs.

BANKBOOK (OR PASSBOOK). This is a book record prepared by the bank for the depositor, listing the amount of deposits and the dates upon which they are made. Because many businesses mail their deposits to the bank, passbooks are not used extensively. Duplicate deposit slips or mail deposit record cards are used instead. Deposit slips with MICR numbers are provided with checking accounts. In the case of a savings account, the bankbook lists deposits, withdrawals, interest paid by the bank, dates of all transactions, and the balance on hand. It must be presented with each withdrawal or deposit.

BANK STATEMENT. This is a statement sent by the bank to the customer, showing the status of the customer's account on a given date. This statement indicates the beginning balance, deposits received, checks paid, bank charges, and ending balance at the time the statement is prepared. The bank statement is accompanied by the customer's canceled checks. Such statements are prepared at regular intervals, usually each month. The bank statement is also known as a *bank reconciliation*.

COUNTERSIGN. To countersign is to have another person sign a paper that has already been signed, in order to verify the authenticity of an instrument. The person countersigning is guaranteeing for the first party and is assuming responsibility.

CURRENCY. Paper money issued by the government through an act of law is currency. This paper money has free circulation in trade and is guaranteed to be legal tender by the government.

DEPOSIT. An amount of money, either as cash, check, or draft, that is given to a bank for the purpose of establishing and maintaining a credit balance with the bank and is credited to the account of the depositor.

DEPOSIT RECORD. Machine-made receipt for a deposit, presented to customer by bank. This receipt eliminates the necessity for a pen-and-ink entry into a depositor's bankbook.

DEPOSIT SLIP. An itemized memorandum of cash or other funds that a depositor presents to the bank with the money to be credited to his account. This deposit slip also serves as a record of deposits made.

DRAFT. A drawing on money from a fund or stock, such as an account. Specifically, a draft is an order from one party to another, directing the payment of money. Draft in its broadest sense includes bills of exchange and checks, but the term is more commonly used to indicate a domestic money order. The principal difference between a draft and a check is that, in the case of a draft, the drawer is a bank; in the case of an ordinary check, the drawer is an individual.

ENDORSEMENT. The act of writing one's signature on the back of an instrument, a legal act of transferring the title of an instrument to another party. When you endorse a check with your signature, you transfer the title of the check to the bank in exchange for the sum written on the face of the check.

FLOAT. A term used to describe the amount of funds in the process of collection represented by checks in the possession of one bank but drawn on the other banks, either local or out-of-town.

INSUFFICIENT FUNDS. A term used to express the fact that the depositor's account is inadequate to cover the amount of a check drawn against his account. The abbreviation "NSF" indicates "Not Sufficient Funds."

KITE. A term used in banking circles to describe the malpractice of individuals in taking advantage of the time element of check collections by the bank. The individual either has a cohort in a distant city, or has another account in another city himself. He deposits a check drawn on a bank in a distant city, and then draws from this uncollected balance while the check is in the process of collection. The same individual also sends a check drawn upon this bank, and deposits it in the other bank, where he also draws against uncollected funds by issuing checks against this out-of-town bank. In this manner he uses both bank accounts to his advantage to draw against "nonexistent" true balances.

NOTE. This is a recognized legal evidence of debt, backed only by the promise of an individual giving the note to pay the debt; thus the term, "promissory note." It is a written promise by the maker (or borrower) to pay a given sum of money on a specific date, and it is signed by the maker (or borrower). A "collateral note" requires the pledging of marketable securities, which may be sold by the creditor if the maker of the note fails to pay within the time limit promised.

OVERDRAWN OR OVERDRAFT. When a depositor draws a check for more than the amount he has in his bank account, his account becomes overdrawn. In most states it is illegal to issue a check for more than the amount on deposit in the bank. Should this happen through error or oversight the bank may refuse to honor the check and will return it to the bank that presented it for payment. Such a check is said to "bounce." If the check is written by an established depositor, the bank may honor the check and notify the depositor that he has overdrawn his account. If the bank thus pays or "covers" the check, it issues an overdraft on the depositor's account.

POSTDATED CHECK. This is a check on which a future date of payment appears. Postdated checks cannot be presented for payment until the date specified has been reached.

POWER OF ATTORNEY. This is a legal statement in which a person authorizes another person to act as his attorney or agent. A power of attorney authorization may be

Union Bank STOP PAYMENT ORDER

OFFICE Main

ACCOUNT NUMBER	CHECK PAYABLE TO		AMOUNT OF CHECK	DATE OF CHECK
45012 3456	W. B. Saunders Company		$36.44	05/22/82
CHECK NUMBER	**CODE** / **STOP NUMBER**	**TODAY'S DATE**	**TIME**	**EXPIRATION DATE**
823		06/18/82	11 a.m.	12/18/82

REASON FOR STOP PAYMENT

Check lost in mail

THE UNDERSIGNED AGREES:
1. THAT A CHECK GUARANTEE CARD WAS NOT USED WITH THE CHECK ON WHICH THIS STOP PAYMENT ORDER IS AUTHORIZED.
2. TO INDEMNIFY AND HOLD YOU HARMLESS FROM ALL LIABILITY, DAMAGE, AND EXPENSE INCURRED ON ACCOUNT OF REFUSING PAYMENT OF SAID CHECK;
3. THAT THIS ORDER SHALL AUTOMATICALLY TERMINATE IF THE ACCOUNT ON WHICH THIS CHECK IS DRAWN IS CLOSED OR TRANSFERRED TO ANOTHER OFFICE;
4. TO NOTIFY THIS BANK TO RELEASE THIS ORDER IF AND WHEN THE REASON FOR THE STOP PAYMENT CEASES TO EXIST;
5. THAT THIS ORDER SHALL EXPIRE AND BE OF NO FURTHER EFFECT 6 MONTHS FROM DATE OF ITS RECEIPT BY THIS BANK UNLESS EARLIER RELEASED OR RENEWED BY THE UNDERSIGNED IN WRITING.

AUTHORIZED SIGNATURE T. F. Wilson PHONE 321-4567

ACCOUNT TITLE Theodore F. Wilson, M.D.

CAD-51 A (REV. 7-70)

FIGURE 15–19 Stop-payment order.

limited to the handling of certain procedures or assets listed in the power of attorney statement, or it may give full power over all assets. The person authorized to act as agent is known as an *attorney in fact.*

RECONCILIATION. (See Bank Statement.)

STALE DATE OR STALE CHECK. This term refers to an instrument that is more than six months old or for which a "reasonable time" for presentation and payment has passed. Some payers specify that a check must be presented within 90 days. Stale checks usually are returned to the bank that presented the check for payment and are not honored. This is done to protect the depositor.

STOP PAYMENT. When a depositor or maker of a check wishes to rescind or stop payment of a check he has written, he has the right to request the bank to stop payment on this check. The request to stop payment must be made in writing and must be signed by the maker. (Most banks will accept a stop payment order made by telephone or telegram for a limited time, if it is followed with a written order.) It must give all the required information, such as number of the check, date issued, name of payee, amount of check, and the reason for stopping payment. The stop payment order must reach the bank bookkeeper before the check is presented for payment. It then becomes the responsibility of the bank to refuse payment and return the check to the holder or payee. The holder must then seek his payment from the maker, who has for some reason stopped payment. The customer's account is charged a fee of several dollars for each returned check. Most banks ask a service fee for stop payment requests. Stop payment orders are void after six months unless renewed in writing. Stop payment orders should be used only in extreme emergencies. Reasons for stop payment requests are loss of a check, disagreement about a purchase, or disagreement about a payment (Fig. 15–19).

WITHDRAWAL. The term used for taking funds from a depositor's account. Withdrawal from a checking account is accomplished by writing a check. For withdrawal of funds from a savings account, the depositor must submit his passbook to the bank with a signed withdrawal slip before the bank can pay out funds from the account.

References

Anderson, R. A., Kumpf, W., and Kendrick, R. E.: *Business Law, Principles and Cases,* 5th Ed. Cincinnati, South-Western Publishing Co., 1971.

Bank of America Consumer Information Reports, 1977.

Beckner, C. J.: *Using Bank Services.* Washington, D.C., American Bankers Association, 1970.

Hutchinson, L.: *Standard Handbook for Secretaries,* 8th ed. New York, McGraw-Hill, Inc., and Gregg Publishing Co., 1969.

CHAPTER OUTLINE

What Should the Records Show?
Bases for Accounting
Who Will Keep the Records?
- Personal Qualifications
- Establishing Good Habits

Cardinal Rules of Bookkeeping
Comparison of Common Bookkeeping Systems
- Single Entry
- Write-It-Once or Pegboard
- Double Entry

Kinds of Bookkeeping Records
- Accounts Receivable Records
  - Daily Journal
  - Ledger
- Disbursements Records
  - Checkbook
  - Disbursements Journal
  - Petty Cash
  - Payroll Record

The Bookkeeping Procedure
- Terminology of Accounts
- Accounts Receivable Procedures
- Accounts Payable Procedures
- Periodic Summaries

Computer Services
Payroll Records
- Preliminary Steps
- Accounting for Payroll
- Income Tax Withholding
- Employer's Income Tax
- F.I.C.A. Taxes
- Deposit Requirements
- Quarterly Reports
- Annual Reports
- Federal Unemployment Tax
- State Unemployment Taxes
- State Disability Insurance

BEHAVIORAL OBJECTIVES

The medical office assistant should be able to:

- **State the kinds of financial records necessary in the average medical office.**
- **Define the two bases of accounting.**
- **Follow the cardinal rules of any system of bookkeeping.**
- **Briefly explain the three most common systems of bookkeeping.**
- **Keep a pegboard or single entry set of books.**
- **Prepare patient ledger for new patient.**
- **Record fees for services rendered.**
- **Make journal entries.**
- **Post patient charges to ledger.**
- **Post payments received to patient ledger.**
- **Run monthly tape of accounts receivable.**
- **Maintain file of paid and unpaid invoices.**
- **Review invoices for accuracy prior to payment.**
- **Record payments to vendors.**
- **Maintain disbursement journal.**
- **Establish and control petty cash fund.**
- **Run trial balance.**
- **Prepare and maintain employee payroll records.**
- **Prepare government forms, such as those for FICA, State and Federal Withholding, Unemployment, State Disability.**

16

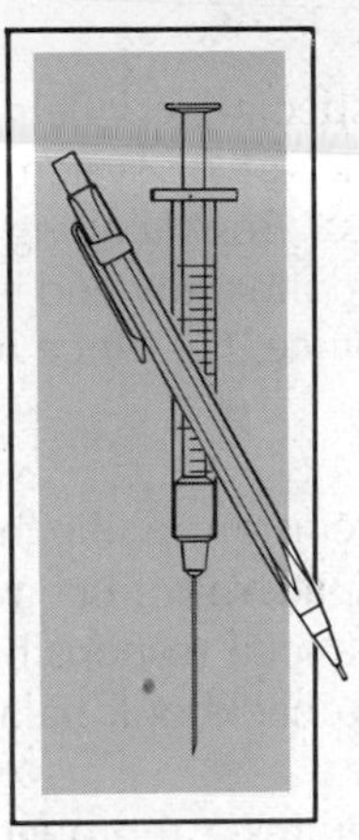

KEEPING FINANCIAL RECORDS: PAYROLL RECORDS

The medical assistant who will keep accurate financial records and who will conduct the nonmedical side of the practice in a businesslike fashion is genuinely needed and appreciated. This is reality. A doctor's business records are the key to efficient management of the practice. No one questions the necessity for keeping adequate medical records. The financial records are equally important to the doctor in private practice.

Public relations problems as well as legal problems may arise when records are poorly kept or inadequate, when statements are sent irregularly or incorrectly, and when the collection system is not handled properly.

The reporting of income to federal and state agencies and the calculating and reporting of payroll taxes require extremely careful and detailed recordkeeping.

WHAT SHOULD THE RECORDS SHOW?

The financial records of any business should, at all times, show:

1. How much was *earned* in a given period,
2. How much was *collected,*
3. How much is *owed,* and
4. The *distribution of expenses* incurred.

Monthly and annual summaries should provide a basis for comparing any given period with another similar period. Periodic analyses of the financial records can result in improved business practices, better management of time, curtailment or elimination of unprofitable services, and better budgeting of expenses.

BASES FOR ACCOUNTING

There are two bases for accounting: the cash basis and the accrual basis. Most doctors use the cash basis of accounting. Expressed simply, this means that charges for services are not recognized as income until cash is received and expenses are not recorded until they are paid.

Merchants, on the other hand, generally use an accrual basis of accounting. On the accrual basis, income is considered earned when services have been performed or goods have been sold, even though payment may not have been received. Expenses are recognized and recorded when incurred, even though they have not been paid.

WHO WILL KEEP THE RECORDS?

Bookkeeping and accounting are specialized fields, requiring special training. *Accounting* has been defined as "the art or system of recording, classifying and summarizing commercial transactions." *Bookkeeping* is mainly the *recording* part of the accounting process. This must be done daily and is the responsibility of the office assistant. In the multiple-employee office, the office manager is usually in charge of the financial records.

PERSONAL QUALIFICATIONS. Precision, willingness to pay attention to detail, ability to concentrate, and consistent patterns of behavior are all favorable qualifications for the person who assumes financial responsibility. The assistant who cannot manage her own budget or keep her checkbook balanced should not be placed in charge of the office finances.

Success in bookkeeping also requires a thorough understanding of the system and what it is expected to accomplish. Bookkeeping is not the place to be creative or take shortcuts. There is no such thing as *almost correct* financial records. The books either balance or they do not balance. The bookkeeping is either right or wrong. Some personalities find great pleasure in books that balance — others find it an abominable bore. How the assistant feels about it may determine her success.

Bookkeeping procedures are not difficult or complicated, but they do require concentration to avoid errors. The office assistant should set aside a certain time each day for bookkeeping tasks. The early morning when she is fresh and before patients start arriving is usually a good time for completing this work. Do not attempt to work on financial records while the office is full of patients, the telephone is ringing continually, or there are other distractions.

ESTABLISHING GOOD HABITS. An important part of bookkeeping is the establishment of good habits, routines, and consistent patterns.

1. Use good penmanship — no fancy letters or figures.
2. Use the same pen style and ink throughout.
3. Keep columns of figures straight.
4. Write well-formed figures. A careless "9" may look like a "7" or an open "0" may resemble a "6."
5. Carry the decimal point correctly.
6. Check arithmetic carefully; don't put blind faith in a calculator.
7. Do not erase, write over, or blot out figures. If an error is made, draw a straight line through the incorrect figure and write the correct figure above it.

CARDINAL RULES TO FOLLOW IN ANY BOOKKEEPING SYSTEM

1. Enter all fees charged and all payments received immediately in the daily record or journal.
2. Write a receipt in duplicate for any currency received. Writing receipts for checks is optional, but whatever pattern is followed should be consistent.
3. Endorse checks for deposit as soon as received.
4. Deposit all money received in the bank. Double check to be sure the total of the deposit plus the amount on hand equals the total to be accounted for on the journal page or day sheet.
5. Post all charges and receipts to the patient ledger cards daily.
6. Establish a petty cash fund so that it is never necessary to take funds from patient receipts to pay an office expense. Use the petty cash fund for only small, unpredictable expenses.

7. Pay all other expenses by check. A canceled check is the best proof of payment.

8. Check all bills for accuracy and make certain they are paid before due dates. Mark paid bills with the date of payment and the number of your check.

COMPARISON OF COMMON BOOKKEEPING SYSTEMS

There are many variations in bookkeeping systems, from simple to complex, no one of which will meet the needs of every doctor. The basic principles are the same for all — only the system of recording varies. The three most common systems found in the professional office are: Single entry; Write-it-Once or Pegboard; and Double entry.

SINGLE ENTRY. The oldest and simplest of bookkeeping systems, called single entry bookkeeping, includes at least three kinds of records:

1. General Journal, which may be called a daily log, daybook, daysheet, or charge journal (Fig. 16–1).
2. Accounts Receivable Ledger, which is a record of the amounts owed by all the doctor's patients. The accounts receivable ledger may be a bound book, a loose-leaf binder, card file, or loose pages in a ledger tray (Fig. 16–2).
3. Checkbook, which serves as a cash payment journal.

In addition, there may be auxiliary records for petty cash and payroll records.

The single entry bookkeeping system is probably the most widely used for

May 13, 1982

HOUR	NAME	SERVICE RENDERED	√	CHARGE	PAID
9:00	Brown, John	O.C. 90030		15 –	
9:20	Sullivan, Bertha	O.C 90050		20 –	
9:40	James, Ella	Dressing		N/c	
10:00	Grover, Ellen	OC 90030		15 –	15 –
10:20	Johnson, Tom	F.U.		n/c	
10:40	Taylor, Theo	O.C 90050		20 –	20 –
11:00	Sorenson, Betty	90730		15 –	
11:20	Boston, Stuart	81000		10 –	10 –
11:40	Daniger, Fred	O.C. 90030		15 –	
12:00					
12:20					
12:40					
1:00	Marlow, Eva	F.U.		n/c	
1:20	Arnold, Anne	Dressing		n/c	
1:40	Tucker, B	90015		35 –	35 –
2:00	↓				
2:20	Thompson, Dan	90015		35 –	35 –
2:40	↓				
3:00	Dunn, Beatrice	90020		60 –	60 –
3:20					
3:40	↓				
4:00	Hasted, J.B.	90000		25 –	—
4:20	Roberts, Victor	90020		60 –	60 –
4:40					
5:00					

FIGURE 16–1 Page from daily log used in single entry bookkeeping. (Courtesy of The Colwell Company, Champaign, Illinois.)

NAME TAYLOR, THEODORE
ADDRESS 1015 North Broadway, San Tomas 90077 PHONE 443-7840
EMPLOYER IBM OCCUPATION Programmer
SPOUSE Ethel AGE 45
INSURANCE Travelers S.S. # 999-00-8888
REFERRED BY Dr. Coomber
REMARKS

STATEMENT

ROBERT N. SMITH, M.D.
6117 MALT AVENUE
LOS ANGELES, CALIFORNIA 90040
(213) 724-1666

CHARGES OR PAYMENTS MADE AFTER LAST DATE SHOWN WILL APPEAR ON YOUR NEXT STATEMENT

Mr. Theodore Taylor
1015 North Broadway
San Tomas, XX 90077

BALANCE FORWARD: -0-

DATE / FAMILY MEMBER	DESCRIPTION	TOTAL FEE	CREDITS PAYMENTS	CREDITS ADJ.	BALANCE
5/13/82 Theo	#7	20 –	20 –		-0-

SAFEGUARD BUSINESS SYSTEMS Form No. LS-M-11 - WD L

PLEASE PAY LAST AMOUNT IN BALANCE COLUMN

EXPLANATION OF CHARGES

OFFICE VISIT NEW PATIENT	OFFICE VISIT ESTAB. PATIENT	PROCEDURES
1—Brief	5—Minimal	11—Immunization
2—Limited	6—Brief	12—Therapeutic Inj.
3—Intermediate	7—Limited	13—Electrocardiogram
4—Comprehensive	8—Intermediate	14—ECG Rhythm Str.
	9—Extended	
	10—Comprehensive	

ROBERT N. SMITH, M.D.
6117 Malt Avenue
Los Angeles, Ca 90040
(213) 724-1666

FIGURE 16–2 Combination account card/statement from accounts receivable ledger. (Courtesy of Safeguard Business Systems.)

doctors' offices. It is inexpensive, is simple to use, and requires very little training. It satisfies the requirements for reporting to government agencies. From a negative standpoint, it provides only for daily, monthly, and annual summaries of income and expense. Errors are not easily detected, and there are no built-in controls.

WRITE-IT-ONCE/PEGBOARD/ACCOUNTING BOARD. Generally termed "pegboard," this system generates all the necessary financial records for each transaction with one writing: (1) charge slip and receipt, (2) ledger card, and (3) journal entry. It may also include a statement and a bank deposit slip.

The board is a lightweight aluminum or masonite board with a row of pegs along the side or along the top. The accounting forms are perforated for alignment on the pegs. All of the forms used in any system must be compatible so that they may be aligned perfectly on the board.

This system is gaining in popularity with doctors. It provides up-to-date control of accounts receivable and a daily record of bank deposits and cash on hand, in addition to the record of income and expenses. The need for separate posting to patient accounts is eliminated, and the chance for error decreased. The initial cost of materials and the need for training are slightly greater than for a single entry system, but the cost is still moderate and the training is included in most medical assisting programs.

DOUBLE ENTRY BOOKKEEPING. The double entry system is based on the accounting equation:

Assets = Liabilities + Proprietorship (Capital)

The properties owned by a business, such as bank accounts, accounts receivable, buildings, equipment, and furniture, are called *assets.* Assets are *equities,* which may be subdivided into creditors' equities and owner's equity. Debts of the business, such as the mortgage on a building, installment note on equipment purchased, and amounts payable to vendors, are creditors' equities or liabilities. The owner's equity (proprietorship or capital) is what remains of the value of the assets after liabilities are subtracted. For instance, if the doctor purchased equipment for $1,000, paid $250 down, and gave a promissory note for $750, this would translate into

Assets	$1,000	=	Liabilities	$750
			+	
			Proprietorship	250
	$1,000			$1,000

The accounting terms proprietorship, capital, owner's equity, and net worth are used interchangeably.

Every transaction requires an entry on each side of the accounting equation, and the two sides must always be in balance. For this reason it is called double entry, and it is the most complete of the three systems. It provides a more comprehensive picture of the practice and its effect on the doctor's net worth. Materials are inexpensive. Errors show up more readily than in single entry bookkeeping; there are many built-in accuracy controls. The drawbacks are that it requires a specially trained and experienced bookkeeper or the regular services of an accountant, and the recordkeeping requires more time and skill. Few medical assistants are trained in accounting. If a double entry system is used, it is usually set up by a practice management consultant or the accountant who does most of the actual bookwork and reports. The medical assistant in this instance generally maintains only the daily journal, from which the accountant takes the figures once a month. An appreciation of the cardinal rules of bookkeeping and the procedures followed in the simpler bookkeeping systems described in this chapter will aid in understanding the double entry system.

KINDS OF BOOKKEEPING RECORDS

The daily journal, patient ledger, and checkbook are the general financial records. Auxiliary records for petty cash and payroll may also be kept.

ACCOUNTS RECEIVABLE RECORDS

Daily Journal. The daily journal is the chronological record of the practice—the financial diary. All information regarding services rendered, charges, and receipts is first recorded in the daily journal. The charges for which payment has not been received are called *receivables;* receivables are amounts owing but not yet received. *Receipts* are cash and checks taken in payment for professional services. It is important that every transaction be recorded. If the doctor renders a service or receives payment away from the office, this should be reported to the person responsible for keeping the records as soon as possible.

In addition there may be income from other sources, such as rental income, royalties, interest, and so forth. Usually a special place in the journal is provided for such income, and the income should be categorized to show its source. Any income that is not practice-related should be recorded separately from patient receipts.

NAME Johnson, Tom — CHARGE TO self
ADDRESS 2400 Main Street, Centerville, XX 10101 — ADDRESS
REF. BY Dr. Maltby
TELEPHONE 111-4545 Bus.300-4365 — INSURANCE Aetna Life S.S.#000-00-0000

1982		SERVICE	CHARGE	PAID	BALANCE
Feb	10	47600	800 –	—	800 –
	18	F.U.	—		800 –
Apr	2	Insur paid		620 –	180 –
	25	Pers. check		180	-0-
May	13	F.U.	n/c		-0-

NAME Dunn, Beatrice (Mrs Robert) — CHARGE TO Robert Dunn
ADDRESS 222 Center Street, Centerville, XX 10101 — ADDRESS
REF. BY sister (M. Tucker)
TELEPHONE 714-5505 — INSURANCE Mutual of Omaha(Robert Dunn Co. group) S.S.# 213-00-7536

1981		SERVICE RENDERED	CHARGE	PAID	BALANCE
May	13	New patient exam 90020	60 –	60 –	-0-

NAME JONES, JANE LILLIAN (MRS ROBERT) SS # 000-00-0000
ADDRESS 1211 East First Avenue, Anywhere, USA 10000
TELEPHONE 443-7754 Not employed Mutual Ins

1982		SERVICE RENDERED	CHARGE	PAID	BALANCE
3	4	Prenatal exam	30 –	100 –	(70 –)
4	20	"	20 –	100 –	(150 –)

FIGURE 16–3 Examples of patient account cards. (Courtesy of The Colwell Company, Champaign, Illinois.)

Ledger. The accounts receivable ledger comprises all the patients' financial accounts on which there are balances. A separate account card is prepared for each patient (or each family) at the time of the first visit or service. Several card styles are shown in Figure 16–3. The card is headed with the name and address of the person responsible for payment. The heading should include all information pertinent to collecting the account: insurance identification, Social Security number, home and business telephone numbers, name of employer, and any special instructions for billing. All charges and payments for professional services are posted to the ledger daily. The ledger then becomes a reliable source of information for answering all inquiries from patients about their accounts. Monthly statements are prepared from the ledger cards, as are insurance billings. It is extremely important to keep this information current.

DISBURSEMENT RECORDS

Checkbook. All receipts are deposited in the checking account, and a record of the deposit is entered on the check stub. A copy of each deposit slip should be kept with the financial records. All bills are paid by check, and a record of the payment is entered on the check stub and in the disbursements section of the daily journal (Fig. 16–4).

Disbursements Journal. In simplified bookkeeping systems, the disbursements journal usually comprises a section at the bottom of each daysheet and a check register page at the end of each month, plus monthly and annual summaries. *Disbursements* are funds paid out. Amounts owed to others but not yet paid are called *payables.*

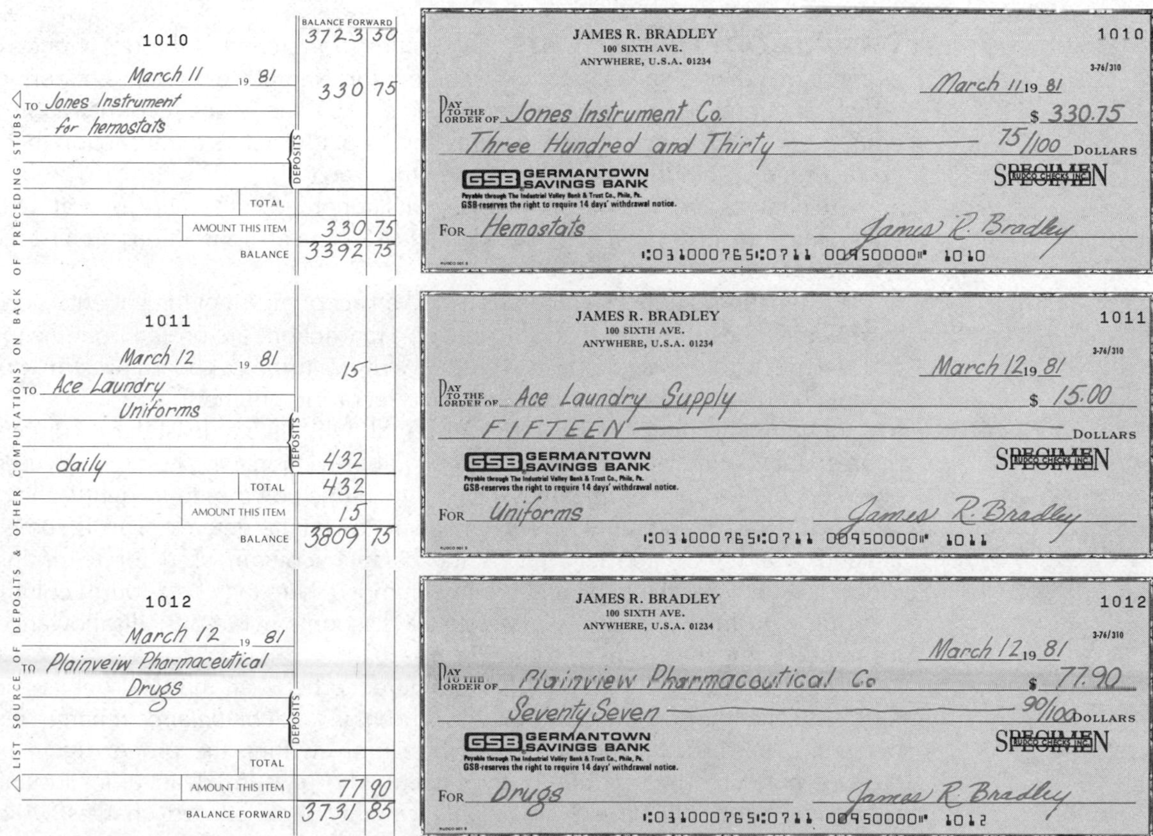

FIGURE 16–4 Page from a commercial checkbook with end stubs.

Petty Cash. A petty cash fund should be established to take care of minor incidental expenses. In the average medical office, $25 to $50 is sufficient for the petty cash fund. If a larger sum is available, there is a tendency to pay too many bills out of petty cash. When the check for this fund is exchanged at the bank for small bills and coins, the money is placed in a cashbox or drawer that can be locked or kept in the safe at night. One person only should be in charge of the petty cash fund. This person must be able to account for the full amount of the fund at any time.

Payroll Record. The payroll record is an auxiliary disbursement record. A separate page or card for each employee, as well as a summary record, should be kept. This procedure and the appropriate forms will be discussed later in the chapter.

THE BOOKKEEPING PROCEDURE

Double entry bookkeeping requires considerable training, and the assistant who needs such training should take a specific course for this purpose. Single entry and write-it-once systems, however, are easily mastered.

The basic difference between single entry and write-it-once systems is the number of steps involved in completing the process. The write-it-once or pegboard system can generate in one writing all of the required records or documents: the daily journal, patient ledger, statement, patient's receipt, and bank deposit slip. In a single entry system, the entries are made separately: first, the entry is recorded on the daily journal or log, then a patient receipt is written if payment was made, next the transaction is posted to the ledger, and from the ledger a monthly statement is produced. In each of these steps there is the chance for error. The bookkeeper may neglect to post an amount, an incorrect figure may be posted, or it may be posted to the wrong ledger.

The pegboard procedure will be explained here. The assistant who understands the pegboard will be able to adapt to the single entry easily.

TERMINOLOGY OF ACCOUNTS. A business *transaction* is the occurrence of an event or of a condition that must be recorded: for example, a service is performed for which a charge is made; a patient makes a payment on account; a piece of equipment is purchased; or the monthly rent is paid. Each is a transaction that must be recorded within the bookkeeping system.

All charges and receipts of money are first recorded in the *daily journal,* which is called the *book of original entry* because this is where all transactions are first recorded (Fig. 16–5).

Each patient's financial record is called an *account.* All of the patients' accounts together are the *accounts receivable ledger.* Transactions are posted from the journal to the ledger (this is accomplished in one writing in the pegboard system). *Posting* means the transfer of information from one record to another.

Although account cards vary in design, all will have at least three columns for figures: the column on the left, or *debit* (abbreviation *Dr.*) column, is used for entering charges and is sometimes called the charge column; to its right is the *credit* (abbreviation *Cr.*) column where payments received are entered. This is sometimes headed "Paid." On the far right is the *balance* column used for recording the difference between the debit and credit columns. There may be a fourth column for entering *adjustments,* such as professional discounts, write-offs, disallowances by insurance companies, and so forth (Fig. 16–6).

The *balance* of any account is the difference between the total debits and the total credits to the account. The balance is normally a *debit balance* (charges exceed payments). A debit balance is shown by simply writing the proper figure in the balance column. The account for the patient who pays in advance, for instance in obstetrical care, will have a *credit balance* (payments exceed charges). A credit balance is shown in one of two ways: by writing the credit entry on the card in regular ink and enclosing the figure in parentheses or encircling it, or by writing the credit entry in red ink. The latter cannot be used in pegboard unless red carbon is inserted. Discounts are also credit entries. If there is no adjustment column as

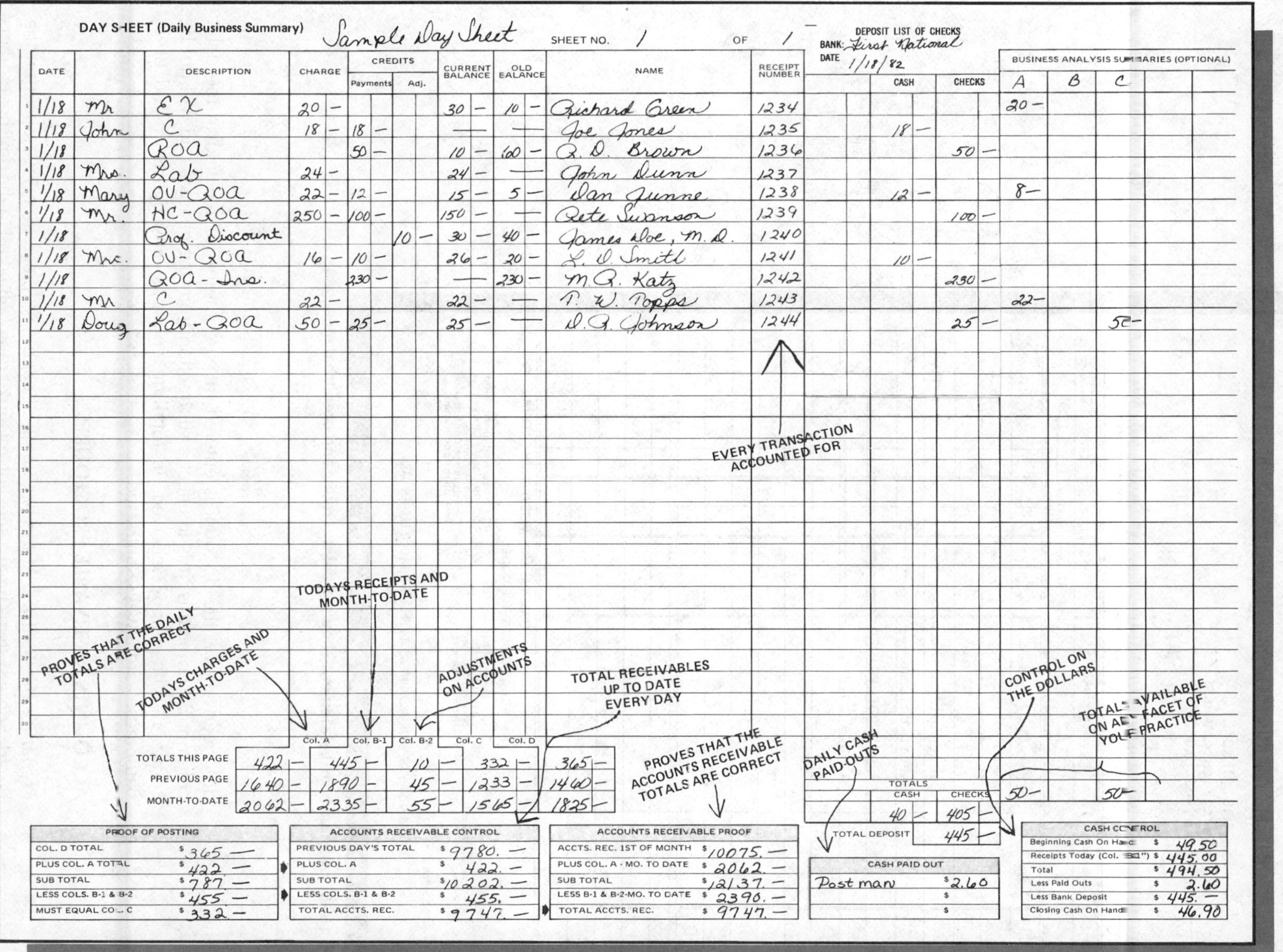

DAY SHEET (Daily Business Summary) *Sample Day Sheet* SHEET NO. *1* OF *1*

DEPOSIT LIST OF CHECKS BANK: *First National* DATE *1/18/82*

DATE		DESCRIPTION	CHARGE	CREDITS Payments	CREDITS Adj.	CURRENT BALANCE	OLD BALANCE	NAME	RECEIPT NUMBER	CASH	CHECKS	A	B	C
1/18	Mr	E X	20 –			30 –	10 –	Richard Green	1234			20 –		
1/18	John	C	18 –	18 –		—	—	Joe Jones	1235	18 –				
1/18		ROA		50 –		10 –	60 –	R. D. Brown	1236		50 –			
1/18	Mrs.	Lab	24 –			24 –	—	John Dunn	1237					
1/18	Mary	OV-ROA	22 –	12 –		15 –	5 –	Dan Dunne	1238	12 –		8 –		
1/18	Mr.	HC-ROA	250 –	100 –		150 –	—	Pete Swanson	1239		100 –			
1/18		Prof. Discount			10 –	30 –	40 –	James Doe, M.D.	1240					
1/18	Mrs.	OV-ROA	16 –	10 –		26 –	20 –	L. D. Smith	1241	10 –				
1/18		ROA-Ins.		230 –		—	230 –	M. R. Katz	1242		230 –			
1/18	Mr	C	22 –			22 –	—	T. W. Popps	1243			22 –		
1/18	Doug	Lab-ROA	50 –	25 –		25 –	—	D. R. Johnson	1244		25 –			50 –

	Col. A	Col. B-1	Col. B-2	Col. C	Col. D
TOTALS THIS PAGE	422 –	445 –	10 –	332 –	365 –
PREVIOUS PAGE	1640 –	1890 –	45 –	1233 –	1460 –
MONTH-TO-DATE	2062 –	2335 –	55 –	1565 –	1825 –

TOTALS	CASH	CHECKS	A	B	C
	40 –	405 –	50 –		50 –
TOTAL DEPOSIT		445 –			

PROOF OF POSTING	
COL. D TOTAL	$ 365 –
PLUS COL. A TOTAL	$ 422 –
SUB TOTAL	$ 787 –
LESS COLS. B-1 & B-2	$ 455 –
MUST EQUAL COL. C	$ 332 –

ACCOUNTS RECEIVABLE CONTROL	
PREVIOUS DAY'S TOTAL	$ 9780. –
PLUS COL. A	$ 422. –
SUB TOTAL	$ 10202. –
LESS COLS. B-1 & B-2	$ 455. –
TOTAL ACCTS. REC.	$ 9747. –

ACCOUNTS RECEIVABLE PROOF	
ACCTS. REC. 1ST OF MONTH	$ 10075. –
PLUS COL. A - MO. TO DATE	$ 2062. –
SUB TOTAL	$ 12137. –
LESS B-1 & B-2-MO. TO DATE	$ 2390. –
TOTAL ACCTS. REC.	$ 9747. –

CASH PAID OUT	
Post man	$ 2.60
	$
	$

CASH CONTROL	
Beginning Cash On Hand	$ 49.50
Receipts Today (Col. "B1")	$ 445.00
Total	$ 494.50
Less Paid Outs	$ 2.60
Less Bank Deposit	$ 445. –
Closing Cash On Hand	$ 46.90

FIGURE 16–5 Sample day sheet for pegboard bookkeeping system, with deposit list of checks and optional business analysis summaries. (Courtesy of Control-O-Fax Office Systems, Waterloo, Iowa.)

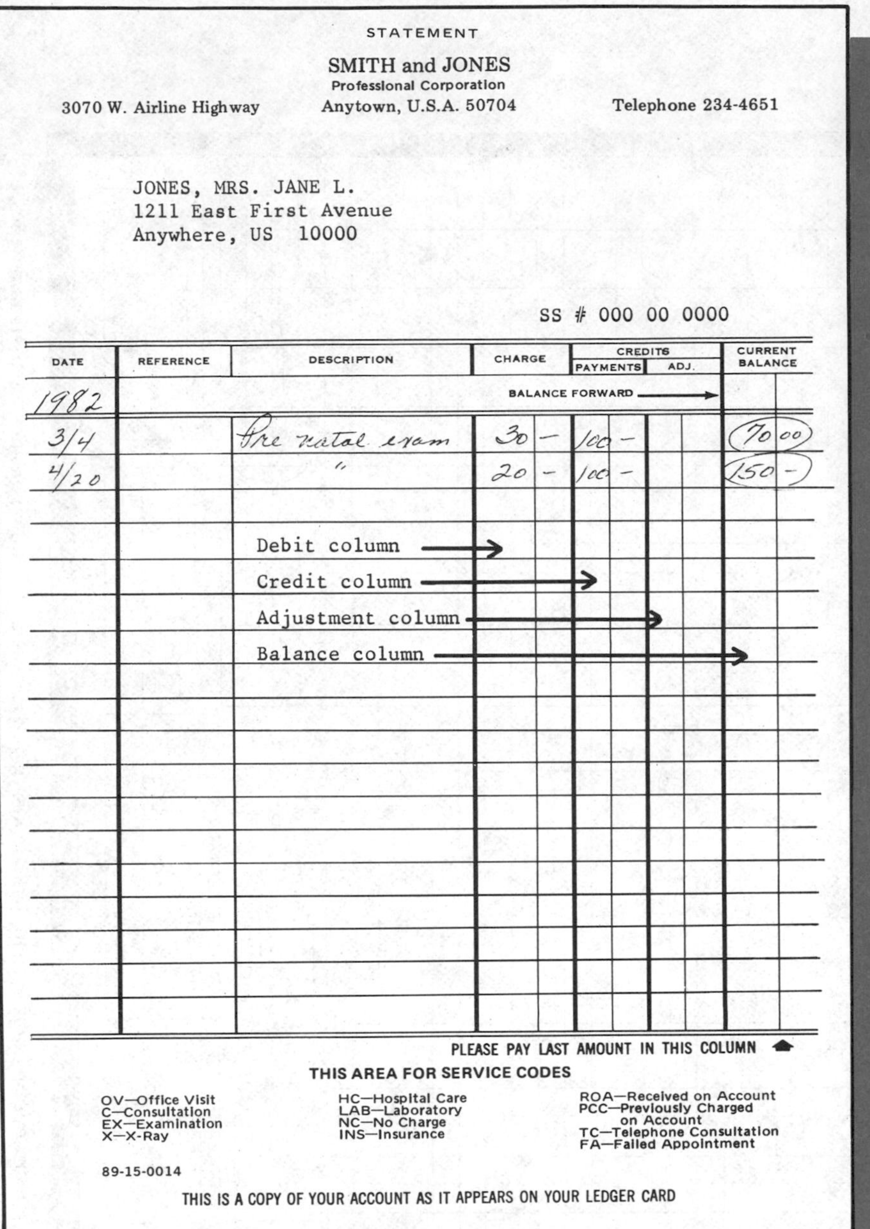

STATEMENT

SMITH and JONES
Professional Corporation
3070 W. Airline Highway — Anytown, U.S.A. 50704 — Telephone 234-4651

JONES, MRS. JANE L.
1211 East First Avenue
Anywhere, US 10000

SS # 000 00 0000

DATE	REFERENCE	DESCRIPTION	CHARGE	CREDITS PAYMENTS	CREDITS ADJ.	CURRENT BALANCE
		BALANCE FORWARD →				
1982						
3/4		Pre natal exam	30 –	100 –		(70 00)
4/20		"	20 –	100 –		(150 –)

Debit column →
Credit column →
Adjustment column →
Balance column →

PLEASE PAY LAST AMOUNT IN THIS COLUMN

THIS AREA FOR SERVICE CODES

OV—Office Visit
C—Consultation
EX—Examination
X—X-Ray

HC—Hospital Care
LAB—Laboratory
NC—No Charge
INS—Insurance

ROA—Received on Account
PCC—Previously Charged on Account
TC—Telephone Consultation
FA—Failed Appointment

89-15-0014

THIS IS A COPY OF YOUR ACCOUNT AS IT APPEARS ON YOUR LEDGER CARD

FIGURE 16–6 Account card/statement showing debit, credit, and credit balance.

described above, the discount is entered in parentheses (or red ink) in the debit column. By doing this, it is in effect a subtraction from the charges and will not be confused with money received. In totalling columns, any figures in red or in parentheses are always subtracted.

ACCOUNTS RECEIVABLE PROCEDURES

Preparing the Board. At the beginning of each day, place a new daysheet on the board. Some systems have a sheet of "clean carbon" attached to the daysheet; others use special carbon with holes for the pegs. The carbon goes on top of the daysheet. Over the carbon place the charge slip/receipt. The charge slip/receipt has a carbonized writing line which should align with the first open writing line on the daysheet. If the slips are shingled, lay the entire bank of receipts over the pegs with the top one aligned as mentioned. The remainder will be automatically in place. The slips should be kept and used in numerical order at all times.

Pulling the Ledger Cards. If a great many patients are to be seen in one day, it will save time to pull the accounts for all the scheduled patients at the beginning of the day. Keep the cards in the order in which they are scheduled to be seen.

Journal Entries. When the patient arrives, insert the ledger card under the first receipt, aligning the first available writing line of the card with the carbonized strip on the receipt. Enter the patient's name, the receipt number, and any existing balance shown on the ledger card. Detach the stub and clip it to the chart that goes to the doctor (Fig. 16–7).

After the service has been performed, the doctor can complete the stub, indicating what the service was and the amount of the charge. The doctor asks the patient to hand the slip to the assistant on the way out. This provides an opportunity for the assistant to suggest payment and to issue a receipt. At this time, reinsert the ledger card under the proper receipt, checking the number that was previously entered to make sure it is in the correct place. Indicate what the service is (usually by code number), post the charge and any payment made by the patient, and the current balance, if any. Hand the receipt portion to the patient and file the stub in numerical order. The transaction has now been fully recorded, and the ledger card is ready for refiling.

If a charge slip is used every time a medical service is provided, the slips can be an audit check at the end of the month. The total of the charge slips should equal the charges recorded for the month. They can then be cancelled and filed.

Adjustments. Adjustments may be necessary to credit professional discounts, insurance disallowances, write-offs, and so forth. If the system has an adjustment column, this is used. Otherwise, since the adjustment is actually a subtraction from the charge, enter it in the charge column with the figure enclosed within parentheses or a circle, and an explanation of the entry in the description column. When the column of figures is totalled, this figure will be subtracted rather than added. The learner has a tendency to ignore the encircled figures. This is incorrect — they must be *subtracted.*

Credit Balances. A credit balance occurs when a patient has paid in advance or when there has been an overpayment. For instance, the patient sent in two insurance checks that totalled more than the actual balance. The difference between the amount of money received and the amount owed is entered in the balance column and enclosed within parentheses or a circle. Any accountant recognizes this as a credit balance. In actuality it is money owed to the patient. If the patient has paid in advance or wishes to leave the overpayment in the account in anticipation of future charges, care must be taken in figuring the balance on future transactions. Whereas normally a charge *increases* the balance, it will *decrease* a credit balance.

Refunds. The patient may wish to have an overpayment refunded. Write a check for the amount due, enter an explanation in the description column, show the existing credit balance within parentheses, write the amount of the refund in the payment column *in parentheses* to show it is a subtraction, and show a zero balance.

NSF (Nonsufficient Funds) Checks. Sometimes a patient will send in a check without having sufficient funds in his bank account to cover it. The bank will return it to you marked NSF. You must now do two things: deduct it from your bank balance and add the amount back into the patient's balance. You can get it back into the

DAILY LOG OF CHARGES AND RECEIPTS

DATE *Mar 10, 1974* SHEET NO. *2 of 2*

RECEIPT NUMBER	DATE	PROFESSIONAL SERVICE	A CHARGE	B PAID	C NEW BALANCE	D PREVIOUS BALANCE	NAME	✓	Dr. A.	Dr. B.	Dr. C.		
		BALANCE FWD. →	280	300 –	495 –	515 –			180 –	70 –	50 –		
1030	3/10/74	P.E. wife	15 –	25 –	40 –	50 –	Mr. John Goodman	1	25 –				1
1031	3/10/74	O.C. + Lab	15 –		15 –		Mrs. Pat Maple	2					2
1032	3/10/74	O.C. wife	10 –		20 –	10 –	Ann Morris	3					3
1033	3/10/74	Ekg	25 –	15 –	10 –		Miss Virginia Black	4			15 –		4
1034	3/10/74	OL + Ekg Nell	15 –		50 –	35 –	Mrs. Don Ploeger	5					5
1035	3/10/74	O.C. + Inj. wife	15 –	15 –			Mrs. H. A. Temple	6	15 –				6
1036	3/10/74	O.C. + Lab	14 –	15 –	34 –	35 –	Wm. Tarrant	7			15 –		7
1037	3/10/74	O.C. + Inj	10 –		16 –	6 –	Mrs. Geo. Lackey	8					8
								9					9
								10					10
								11					11
								12	5 –				12
								13	10 –				13
								14	20 –		5 –		14
								15		125 –			15
								16			10 –		16
								17					17
								18					18
								19					19
								20					20
								21					21
								22					22
								23					23
								24					24
								25					25
			453 –	560 –	881 –	988 –	← TOTALS →		270 –	195 –	95 –		

RECEIPT NUMBER	DATE	PROFESSIONAL SERVICE	CHARGE	PAID	NEW BALANCE	PREVIOUS BALANCE	NAME

YOU PAID THIS AMOUNT .... $

LEONARD S. TAYLOR, M.D.
2100 WEST PARK AVENUE
CHAMPAIGN, ILLINOIS 61820
TELEPHONE 367-6671

OC - OFFICE CALL
HCD - HOUSE CALL DAY
HCN - HOUSE CALL NIGHT
HOSP - HOSPITAL CARE
L - LABORATORY
I - INJECTION
INS - INSURANCE
OB - OBSTETRICAL CARE
OS - OFFICE SURGERY
HS - HOSPITAL SURGERY
PE - PHYSICAL EXAMINATION
EKG - ELECTROCARDIOGRAM
XR - X-RAY
M - MEDICATION
NC - NO CHARGE

OFFICE CALL ....
LABORATORY ....
INJECTION ....
OBSTETRICAL CARE ....
OFFICE SURGERY ....
PHYSICAL EXAMINATION ....
ELECTROCARDIOGRAM ....
X-RAY ....
MEDICATION .... $

NEXT APPOINTMENT ________ AT ________

NO. 1038

FORM 7521 COLWELL CO., CHAMPAIGN, ILLINOIS

PROOF OF POSTING

COLUMN D TOTAL:	988. –
"PLUS" COLUMN A TOTAL:	453. –
SUB TOTAL:	1441. –
"MINUS" COLUMN B TOTAL:	560. –
EQUALS COLUMN C BALANCE:	881. –

ACCOUNTS RECEIVABLE CONTROL

PREVIOUS ACCT. REC. BALANCE:	4855. –
"PLUS" COLUMN A:	453. –
SUB TOTAL:	5308. –
"MINUS" COLUMN B:	560. –
PRESENT ACCT. REC. BALANCE:	4748. –

DAILY CASH SUMMARY

OPENING CASH ON HAND AT BEGINNING OF DAY	$ 100. –	CASH PAID OUT	$ —
CASH RECEIVED DURING DAY	$ 560. –	BANK DEPOSITS	$ 560. –
TOTAL	$ 660. –	CLOSING CASH ON HAND	$ 100. –
CASH LONG	$	TOTAL	$ 660 –
TOTAL	$	CASH SHORT	$
		TOTAL	$

FIGURE 16–7

NAME

ADDRESS

TELEPHONE INSURANCE REF BY

RECEIPT NUMBER	DATE	PROFESSIONAL SERVICES	CHARGE	PAID	NEW BALANCE

FIGURE 16–8

NAME
BROWN, JOHN S.S.# 000 00 0000
ADDRESS
429 West Market, Long Desert, XX 80056
TELEPHONE
345-6789

1980		SERVICE RENDERED	CHARGE	PAID	BALANCE
10	20	90020	60 –	30 –	30 –
11–	15	90050	20 –	—	50 –
11–	20	Pers. check		30 –	20 –
11–	28	Check Returned NSF		(30 –)	50 –

Posting Proof for Day		
Old balance		$________
Plus total charges		________
	Subtotal	$________
Less payments received		________
	Subtotal	$________
Less adjustments		________
New balance		*$________

*This figure is carried forward to next page for "old balance."

patient's balance by entering the amount in the paid column within parentheses (to indicate a subtraction) and increasing the balance by the same amount. A brief explanation of the transaction goes into the description column (Fig. 16–8).

One-Entry Cash Transactions. For the transient patient who has no ledger card, use a receipt as previously described. Enter the correct entry in the charge column and the same figure in the "paid" column, which will leave a zero balance. This places the transaction on the journal page and provides a receipt for the patient. There is no need for a ledger card.

Collection Agency Payments. When a collection agency recovers an account for the doctor, the agency is entitled to a commission, which is usually 40 to 50 per cent of the amount recovered. For instance, if the patient has a balance of $100 and pays it in full, the agency will send you $50. The patient now has a zero balance and you have only $50. To record this transaction you will enter $100 in the previous balance, $50 in the "cash received" or "paid" column, $50 in the adjustment column, and zero in the new balance column. If there is no adjustment column, the $50 commission is entered in the charge column within parentheses ($50) so that the total business is reduced by this amount and so is the accounts receivable control.

Daily Proof of Entries. At the end of the day, all columns must be totalled and proved. Although all bookkeeping is done in ink, it is a good idea to write the totals in pencil until they have been proved. If an error is discovered, you must correct the entry in which it occurred. Usually it is best to simply draw a line through the incorrect entry and make a new entry on the first open writing line. Remember that you must reinsert the ledger card for these corrections. Also, if the correction affects the receipt you have given to a patient, you must make a new receipt and notify the patient of the correction.

Pegboard systems provide several ways for proving the arithmetic on the daily journal. Some examples are:

Cash Control Proof		
Cash on hand at beginning of day		$________
Cash received		________
	Subtotal	$________
Less cash paid out		________
Less bank deposit		________
Cash on hand at end of day		*$________

*This figure is carried forward to next page for "cash on hand at beginning of day."

Accounts Receivable Control. Pegboard bookkeeping systems include a daily accounts receivable control similar to the following:

Accounts Receivable Control		
Total outstanding A/R balance (from previous day)		$______
Plus today's charges		______
	Subtotal	$______
Less today's payments		______
	Subtotal	$______
Less today's adjustments		______
Balance outstanding		*$______

*This figure is carried forward to the next page for "total outstanding A/R balance."

If a single entry bookkeeping system is used, a simple form such as the one illustrated in Figure 16–9 will be useful. Begin by adding the unpaid balances from your entire ledger on the last day of the preceding month, and enter this at the top of the card or page. When the charges and receipts are totalled each day, they are entered in columns 1 and 2. If receipts exceed charges, there is a *decrease* in the accounts receivable. The amount of the decrease is entered in column 5 and subtracted from the balance in column 6. If charges for the day exceed the receipts, there is an *increase* in the accounts receivable. The amount of the increase is entered in column 4 and added to the balance in column 6. Note that the accounts receivable figure changes at the end of any day on which there is financial activity. The balance consists of the accounts receivable figure from the day before, plus the charges for the day, minus the day's receipts and adjustments. Thus the total of the entire file of ledger card balances at the end of any day should equal the accounts receivable balance shown for that day on the control form.

ACCOUNTS RECEIVABLE CONTROL

Month of December 19XX — Accounts receivable at end of last day of preceding month: $37 506 —

Day	1 Value of Services Rendered	2 Received from Patients	3 Adjust-ments	4 Increase	5 Decrease	6 Accounts Receivable Balance
1	785	1098			313	37193
2	210	630			420	36773
3	950	510	33	407		37180
4						

FIGURE 16–9 Accounts receivable control for single entry bookkeeping system.

Trial Balance. A trial balance should be done at least once a month, preferably before preparing the monthly statements. The trial balance will disclose any discrepancies between the journal and the ledger. It does not, however, prove the accuracy of the accounts. For instance, if a charge or payment were posted to the wrong account, or if the wrong amount were entered in the journal and then posted to the ledger, the totals would still "balance" but the accounts would not be accurate.

It is best to use an adding machine or calculator with a tape for this process. All posting must have been completed before taking a trial balance. To begin, pull all the account cards that have a balance, enter each balance on the adding machine, and total them. This should equal the accounts receivable balance figure on your control. If you have not kept a daily control, you must total all the charges, payments, and adjustments for the month, then do the following computation:

Accounts receivable at first of month		$________
Plus total charges for month		________
	Subtotal	$________
Less total payments for month		
	Subtotal	$________
Less total adjustments for month		________
Accounts receivable at end of month		$________

The accounts receivable at end of month figure must agree with the figure you got by adding all the account card balances. The accounts are said to be *in balance*. If the two totals do not agree, you must locate the error.

Locating and Preventing Errors. After you have checked your tape and verified that you have not made an error in calculation, the first step in locating an error in your trial balance is to find the difference between the two totals. Then search the daily journal pages and the account cards for an entry of the identical amount. Check each one you find to verify that it was posted correctly. Of course, there may be more than one error.

If there is only one error, and the amount of the error is divisible by 9, you may have transposed a figure. For instance, if the difference is $81 (a number divisible by 9), you may find that you wrote $209 instead of $290. If the amount of the error is divisible by 2, you may have posted to the wrong column, reversing a debit and a credit.

A common error is made by entering the wrong amount in the "previous balance" column or in figuring the new balance. This kind of error will show up on the pegboard daily proof but could easily occur in the single entry system. Another common error is made by carrying forward a wrong total from one day to the next, for instance, carrying the beginning accounts receivable total rather than the ending accounts receivable total. There is always a chance of *sliding* a number, that is, writing the first digit in the wrong column, such as writing 400 for 40, or 60 instead of 600.

Many bookkeepers avoid errors in the cents column by using a line (—) instead of writing two zeros when only even dollars are involved. For instance, instead of writing $12.00, the bookkeeper will write $12. —. This eliminates the possibility of misreading zeros as other numbers. It also speeds the adding process when columns must be totalled.

ACCOUNTS PAYABLE PROCEDURES

Invoices and Statements. When time purchases are made, that is, the item is not paid for at the time of purchase, the vendor will usually include an *invoice* with delivery of the merchandise. An invoice describes the item and shows the amount due. Always check to verify that the items listed on the invoice are included in the delivery. Invoices should be placed in a special folder until paid. You may be making more than one purchase from the same vendor during the month. If the item was shipped to you, it will probably have a packing slip with it. A *packing slip* is similar to an invoice except that it does not include the purchase figures. Some vendors request that payment be made from the invoice; others expect to send a *statement* later. A statement is a request for payment.

Paying for Purchases. At the time of payment, compare the statement with the invoice(s) to verify accuracy, fasten them together, write the date and check number on the statement, and place in the "paid" file.

Recording Disbursements. Both the pegboard and the single entry daily log system provide pages for recording disbursements. This is sometimes called a check register (Fig. 16–10). On these pages, disbursements are categorized to specific expense accounts such as:

auto expense	rent and maintenance
dues and meetings	salaries
equipment	taxes and licenses
insurance	travel and entertainment
medical supplies	utilities
office expense	miscellaneous
printing, postage, stationery	personal withdrawals

Each check should be entered on the disbursement page, showing the date, to whom the check was written, the amount of the check, and the payment allocated to one or more of the expense accounts. This record is important in separating business expenses, which are tax deductible, from personal expenses, which are not deductible, in determining net income from the practice.

Recording Personal Expenditures. Some system must be established for transferring funds from the practice account to the physician's personal account. If the practice is incorporated, the physician will be paid a salary. In the unincorporated practice, the transfer is usually accomplished through what is known in accounting terms as a *drawing account.* The physican establishes a personal checking account and perhaps one or more savings accounts. Each month, or at any specified time, the assistant writes a check payable to the physician, which he signs and endorses for deposit to his personal account. In the disbursements journal, the amount of the check is posted in a special column headed "Personal" or "Drawing." Although personal expenses are not deductible in determining net income from the practice, some will qualify as personal deductions in computing income tax, so a careful accounting should be kept. Deductible expenses would include property taxes, interest on home mortgage, contributions, and so forth.

Accounting for Petty Cash. The petty cash fund is a revolving fund. It does not change in amount except to increase or decrease the established fund. To establish the petty cash fund, a check is written payable to "Cash" or "Petty Cash" and entered in the disbursements journal under Miscellaneous. This is the only time the petty cash check will be charged to Miscellaneous. Each time it is replenished, the amount of the check will be spread among the various accounts for which the money was used. This is determined from a record of expenditures such as that shown in Figure 16–11. The headings of the columns should correspond to headings in the disbursements journal to which they will be posted.

A pad of petty cash vouchers is kept in or near the box. For every disbursement from the fund, the petty cashier should either have a receipt or prepare a voucher similar to the one in Figure 16–12. The total of the petty cash vouchers and receipts plus the amount of cash in the box must always equal the original amount of the fund.

Receipt and voucher total	$14.94
Cash on hand	10.06
Amount of fund	$25.00

Figure 16–11 shows that $25 was received into the fund on April 1. This is entered in the Description column and in the Balance column. On April 2, postage

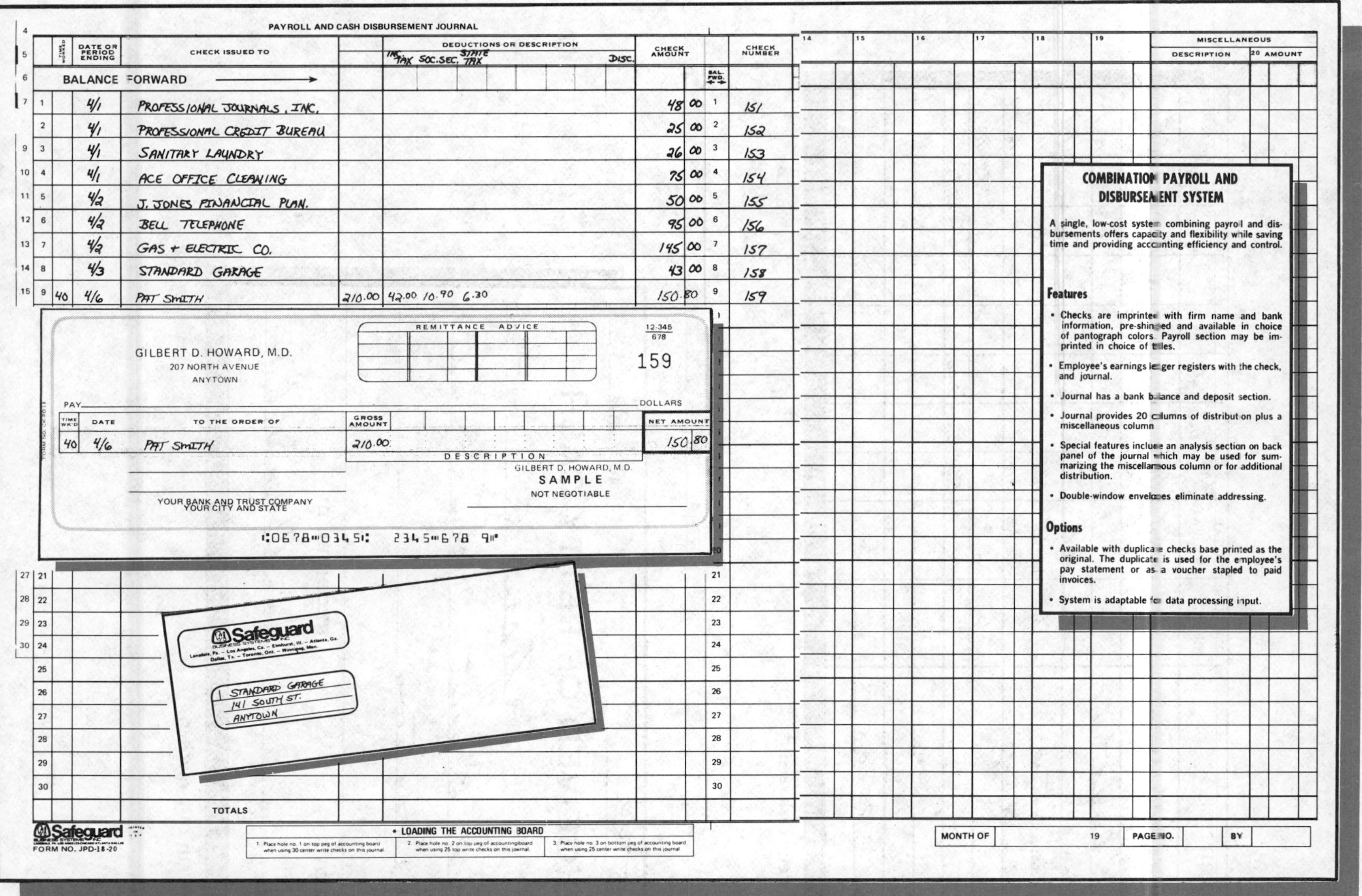

PAYROLL AND CASH DISBURSEMENT JOURNAL

	Time Wk'd	Date or Period Ending	Check Issued To	Gross	Inc. Tax	Soc. Sec.	State Tax	Disc.	Check Amount	Bal. Fwd.	Check Number
			BALANCE FORWARD ⟶								
1		4/1	PROFESSIONAL JOURNALS, INC.						48 00	1	151
2		4/1	PROFESSIONAL CREDIT BUREAU						25 00	2	152
3		4/1	SANITARY LAUNDRY						26 00	3	153
4		4/1	ACE OFFICE CLEANING						75 00	4	154
5		4/2	J. JONES FINANCIAL PLAN.						50 00	5	155
6		4/2	BELL TELEPHONE						95 00	6	156
7		4/2	GAS + ELECTRIC CO.						145 00	7	157
8		4/3	STANDARD GARAGE						43 00	8	158
9	40	4/6	PAT SMITH	210.00	42.00	10.90	6.30		150.80	9	159
			TOTALS								

14 15 16 17 18 19 MISCELLANEOUS: DESCRIPTION | 20 AMOUNT

GILBERT D. HOWARD, M.D.
207 NORTH AVENUE
ANYTOWN

REMITTANCE ADVICE

12-345
678

159

PAY ____ DOLLARS

TIME WK'D	DATE	TO THE ORDER OF	GROSS AMOUNT	NET AMOUNT
40	4/6	PAT SMITH	210.00	150.80

DESCRIPTION

GILBERT D. HOWARD, M.D.
SAMPLE
NOT NEGOTIABLE

YOUR BANK AND TRUST COMPANY
YOUR CITY AND STATE

⑆0678⑈0345⑆ 2345⑈678 9⑈

Safeguard

STANDARD GARAGE
141 SOUTH ST.
ANYTOWN

COMBINATION PAYROLL AND DISBURSEMENT SYSTEM

A single, low-cost system combining payroll and disbursements offers capacity and flexibility while saving time and providing accounting efficiency and control.

Features

- Checks are imprinted with firm name and bank information, pre-shingled and available in choice of pantograph colors. Payroll section may be imprinted in choice of titles.
- Employee's earnings ledger registers with the check, and journal.
- Journal has a bank balance and deposit section.
- Journal provides 20 columns of distribution plus a miscellaneous column
- Special features include an analysis section on back panel of the journal which may be used for summarizing the miscellaneous column or for additional distribution.
- Double-window envelopes eliminate addressing.

Options

- Available with duplicate checks base printed as the original. The duplicate is used for the employee's pay statement or as a voucher stapled to paid invoices.
- System is adaptable for data processing input.

Safeguard
FORM NO. JPD-18-20

• LOADING THE ACCOUNTING BOARD

MONTH OF ____ 19 ____ PAGE NO. ____ BY ____

FIGURE 16–10 Payroll and Cash Disbursement Journal showing payroll check being prepared for employee, and window envelope for mailing checks. (Courtesy of Safeguard Business Systems.)

DATE	DESCRIPTION	VOUCHER NUMBER	TOTAL AMOUNT	Office Exp.	Donations	Auto				Misc.	BALANCE
4-01	Fund established										25.00
4-02	Postage due	1	.26	.26							24.74
4-05	Nurse's Benefit ticket	2	5.00		5.00						19.74
4-08	Parking fee	3	2.00			2.00					17.74
4-17	Stationery items	4	1.68	1.68							16.06
4-25	Delivery charges	5	3.12	3.12							12.94
4-29	Coffee	6	2.88							2.88	10.06
			14.94	5.06	5.00	2.00				2.88	
5-01	Bal. $10.06										
	Check #376 14.94										
	Total 25.00										

FIGURE 16–11 Petty cash record.

AMOUNT $ 5.00 NO. 2

RECEIVED OF PETTY CASH

April 5 19—

FOR Nurse's Benefit, Mercy Hospital

CHARGE TO Donations

APPROVED BY MK

RECEIVED BY F. Dunn, R.N.

AICO-UTILITY Line Form No. 55-061

FIGURE 16–12 Petty cash voucher.

due was paid out, a voucher prepared, the number of the voucher and the amount of 26¢ entered, and a new balance brought down. On April 5, the doctor made a cash donation to the O.R. nurse benefit at the hospital, and told the assistant about it when he returned to the office. The amount of $5 was entered in the record, $5 taken from petty cash to reimburse the doctor, and the new balance of $19.74 brought down.

At the end of the month, or sooner if the fund is depleted, a check is written to "Cash" for replenishing the fund, but instead of being charged to Miscellaneous as previously, the amount of the check is divided among the various accounts affected. Our record shows that at the end of April we have $10.06 remaining in the fund and need $14.94 to bring it back to $25. When the check is written for $14.94, it is accounted for in the monthly distribution of expenditures by posting $5.06 as office expense, $5 as donations, $2.00 as auto expense, and $2.88 as a miscellaneous expense. In this way the expenditures from petty cash are charged to the actual accounts affected. The accounted for vouchers are clipped together and placed with paid invoices, the check for $14.94 is cashed, and the money is placed in the petty cash fund. The amount of the check is entered as being received into the fund, and the new balance of $25 is brought down.

Avoid the habit of borrowing from the petty cash fund. This admonition applies to the doctor as well as to the office assistant. If the doctor requests cash from the fund, ask him to give a personal check or an office check in exchange for cash from the fund. It is also poor policy to use the petty cash fund for making change. In offices where patients frequently pay with cash, a separate change fund should be kept.

PERIODIC SUMMARIES. Financial summaries are compiled on monthly and annual bases. They may be prepared either by the medical assistant or by the accountant (or computer). The common summary reports are (1) statement of income and expense, (2) cash flow statement, (3) trial balance, (4) accounts receivable trial balance and aging analysis, and (5) balance sheet.

The *statement of income and expense* is also known as the *profit and loss statement* and covers a specific period. It lists all the income received and all expenses paid during the period. The total income is called *gross income* or *earnings*. The income after deduction of all expenses is the *net income*.

A *cash flow statement* starts with the amount of cash on hand at the beginning of the month (or any specified period). It then lists the cash income received and the cash disbursements made throughout the period, and concludes with a statement of the amount of cash remaining on hand at the end of the period.

A *trial balance* is necessary in order to determine that the books are in balance. All of the columns on the disbursements journal must be totalled at the end of the month. The combined totals of all the expense columns must be equal to the total of the checks written. If the figures do not balance, it then becomes necessary to recheck every entry until an error is found.

The *balance sheet,* also known as a *statement of financial condition,* shows the financial picture of the practice on a specific date. Often it is done only on an annual basis. The balance sheet is set up using the accounting equation explained on page 245. The title of the statement had its origin in the equality of the elements—the balance between the sum of the assets and the sum of the liabilities and capital.

At the end of the accounting year it is very simple to combine the monthly reports to compile the annual summaries. The annual summaries simplify the reporting of income for tax returns.

COMPUTER SERVICES

There is an increasing trend toward using computer services in handling the financial recording and reporting in medical offices. A computer service can relieve the office staff of the repetitive clerical procedures necessary in the recording of charges, and in preparing and mailing of statements and insurance forms. It can produce weekly and monthly financial reports that would be too time-consuming and perhaps beyond the capabilities of the staff.

One type of computer service is based on a telephone-linked terminal on a time-share basis with other users. Second, there is the batch type in which the information is picked up at the office and taken to a computer center for processing. Third, there is the system built around a mini-computer based in the doctor's office. The decision whether to use computer services and the selection of what service to use are highly personal and require study and investigation.

A computer system can cut down on time-consuming clerical tasks, help create systematic procedures for doing work, increase the productivity of the practice, produce management information that allows the physician to be more fully informed on the economics of the practice, and protect the physician from adverse effects of staff turnover. All of these things and more can be accomplished — but not necessarily will. The system is not magic. Staff members sometimes resist conversion to a computer system because they think it is a threat to their jobs. A computer will probably not reduce the staff, but it may allow them to use their time more effectively. A computer is not a cure-all for a poorly organized office. In fact, there must be a strong front office person or team, willing to spend the time and effort to make the conversion successful. Too often the installation of a computer system is met by covert resistance on the part of the office staff and poor results follow, with unjustified blame resting on the system.

No attempt will be made here to explain the use of computer services, since there are so many variables and continuing changes. It is important to choose a service that will explain what can be expected from the computer and will provide all the instruction and supervision necessary to ensure success in using it.

PAYROLL RECORDS

If it were necessary only to write a check to each employee for the agreed upon salary for a given pay period, no discussion of payroll records would be necessary. But government regulations require the withholding of income taxes and the payment of certain other taxes by both employee and employer. In order to comply with such regulations, complete records must be kept for every employee. Such records will include the Social Security number of the employee, the number of exemptions claimed, the amount of gross salary, all deductions for Social Security taxes, federal, state, and city or other subdivision withholding taxes, state disability insurance, and state unemployment tax, where applicable.

PRELIMINARY STEPS. Each employee and each employer must have a tax identification number. The employee's Social Security number (000-00-0000) is his tax identification number. Any person who does not have a Social Security number should apply for one using Form SS-5 available from any Internal Revenue Service or Social Security office and from most post offices. The employer applies for a number for federal tax accounting purposes (00-0000000) from the Internal Revenue Service using Form SS-4. In states that require employer reports, a state employer number must also be obtained.

Before the end of the first pay period the employee should complete an Employee's Withholding Exemption Certificate (Form W-4) showing the number of exemptions claimed (Fig. 16–13). Otherwise the employer must withhold on the basis of a single person with no exemptions. The employee should complete a new form whenever changes occur in marital status or in the number of exemptions claimed. Each employee is entitled to one exemption for herself and one each for other qualified relatives she supports. She may elect to take no exemptions. In this case the tax withheld will be greater and she may qualify for a refund when her annual income tax report is filed.

A supply of all the necessary forms for filing federal returns, preinscribed with the employer's name, will be furnished to an employer if he has applied for an

Form **W-4** (Rev. October 1979)

Department of the Treasury—Internal Revenue Service

Employee's Withholding Allowance Certificate

Print your full name ▶ JOHN GREEN	Your social security number ▶ 333 33 3333
Address (including ZIP code) ▶ 28 FAIR WAY ANYTOWN, VA. 22222	

Marital status: ☐ Single ☒ Married ☐ Married, but withhold at higher Single rate

Note: *If married, but legally separated, or spouse is a nonresident alien, check the single block.*

1 Total number of allowances you are claiming (from line F of the worksheet on page 2)	8
2 Additional amount if any, you want deducted from each pay (if your employer agrees)	$
3 I claim exemption from withholding because (see instructions and check boxes below that apply): a ☐ Last year I did not owe any Federal income tax and had a right to a full refund of ALL income tax withheld, AND b ☐ This year I do not expect to owe any Federal income tax and expect to have a right to a full refund of ALL income tax withheld. If both a and b apply, enter "EXEMPT" here . . . . ▶	
c If you entered "EXEMPT" on line 3b, are you a full-time student?	☐ Yes ☐ No

Under the penalties of perjury, I certify that I am entitled to the number of withholding allowances claimed on this certificate, or if claiming exemption from withholding, that I am entitled to claim the exempt status.

Employee's signature ▶ John Green Date ▶ MARCH 15, 19 80

Employer's name and address (including ZIP code) (FOR EMPLOYER'S USE ONLY)	Employer identification number

Detach along this line

FIGURE 16–13 Form W-4 Employee's Withholding Allowance Certificate.

employer identification number. Extra forms may be obtained from the Internal Revenue office where he files returns.

ACCOUNTING FOR PAYROLL. The simplest way to prepare the payroll checks and generate the necessary accounting records is by using a write-it-once combination checkwriting system such as the one illustrated in Figure 16–14. This includes an employee compensation record (Fig. 16–15). The employee's compensation record is aligned with the first open line on the record of checks drawn, and a check with a carbonized strip is placed upon it. All information written on the check is automatically transferred to the compensation record and the record of checks drawn in one writing. The checks have a place for the address of the payee and can be mailed in a window envelope.

In situations where there are a number of employees, the summarization of the different categories for tax and reporting purposes is simplified, as the separate columns for different kinds of taxes on the record of checks drawn can simply be totalled at the end of the month (Fig. 16–16). If regular bank printed checks are used, the information for each employee must be posted to a separate record each time a payroll check is issued.

INCOME TAX WITHHOLDING. Employers are required by law to withhold certain amounts from their employees' earnings and to report and forward these amounts to be applied toward payment of income tax. The amount to be withheld is based on the total earnings of the employee, the number of exemptions claimed, the marital status of the employee, and the length of the pay period involved. Federal Publication 13, Circular E — Employer's Tax Guide, includes tables to be used in determining the amount to be withheld. Example pages are shown in Figure 16–16. There are two types of tables: one for single persons and unmarried heads of households and one for married persons. The tables cover monthly, semimonthly, biweekly, weekly, and daily or miscellaneous periods.

EMPLOYER'S INCOME TAXES. If the physician is conducting his practice as an individual, his income is not subject to withholding. Instead he will be expected to make an estimated tax payment four times a year. The accountant will prepare four copies of Form 1040-ES, Declaration of Estimated Tax for Individuals, for the ensuing year when the annual income tax return is prepared. The first form and one-fourth of the estimated tax for the next year will be filed at the same time as the tax return. The remaining three forms, with the estimated tax due, must be filed on June 15,

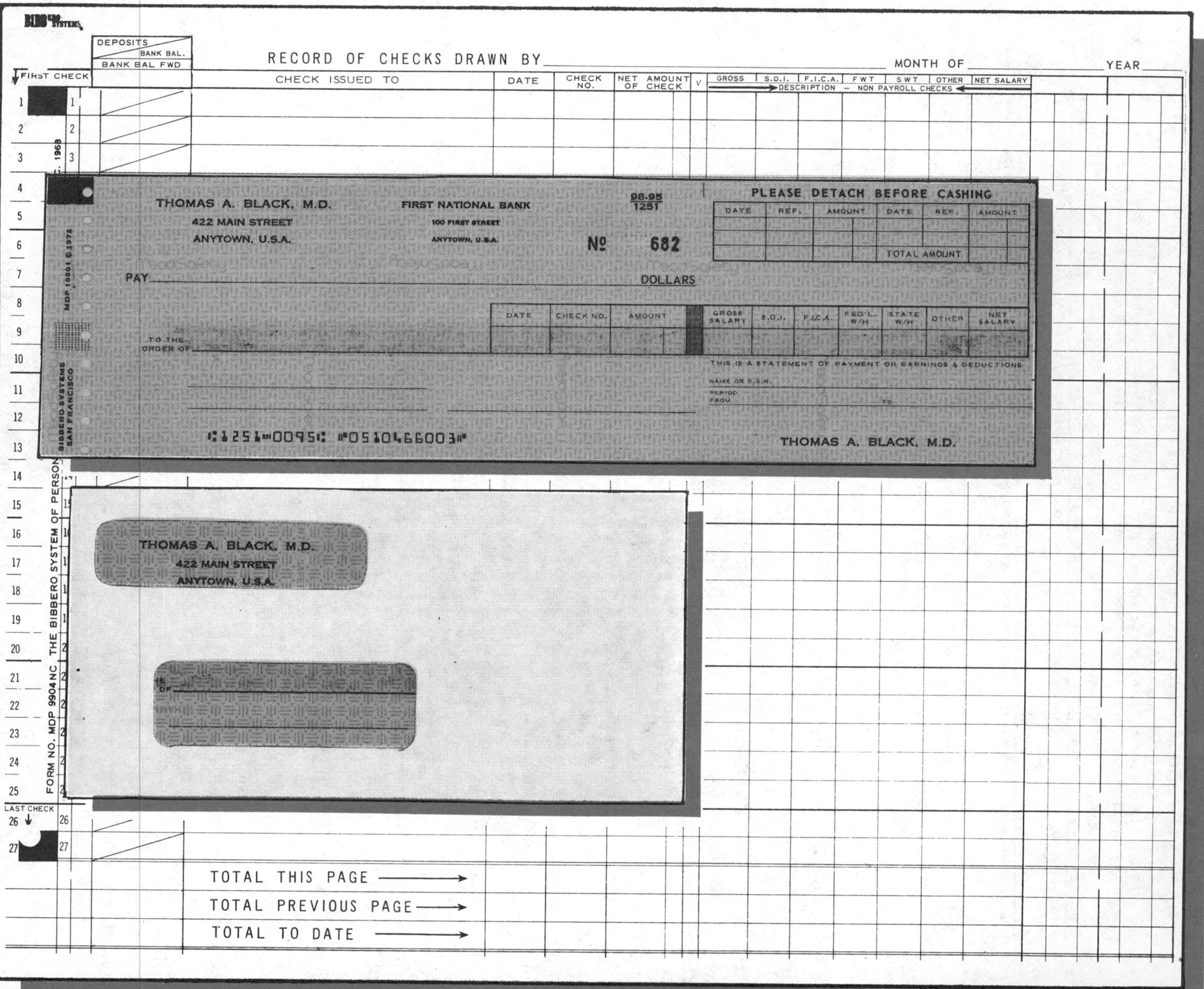

RECORD OF CHECKS DRAWN BY ____ MONTH OF ____ YEAR ____

DEPOSITS | BANK BAL. | BANK BAL FWD

FIRST CHECK	CHECK ISSUED TO	DATE	CHECK NO.	NET AMOUNT OF CHECK	V	GROSS	S.D.I.	F.I.C.A.	FWT	SWT	OTHER	NET SALARY

→ DESCRIPTION – NON PAYROLL CHECKS ←

THOMAS A. BLACK, M.D.
422 MAIN STREET
ANYTOWN, U.S.A.

FIRST NATIONAL BANK
100 FIRST STREET
ANYTOWN, U.S.A.

98-95
1251

№ 682

PAY ____ DOLLARS

TO THE ORDER OF ____

DATE	CHECK NO.	AMOUNT

PLEASE DETACH BEFORE CASHING

DATE	REF.	AMOUNT	DATE	REF.	AMOUNT
				TOTAL AMOUNT	

GROSS SALARY	S.D.I.	F.I.C.A.	FED'L. W/H	STATE W/H	OTHER	NET SALARY

THIS IS A STATEMENT OF PAYMENT OR EARNINGS & DEDUCTIONS
NAME OR S.S.N.
PERIOD FROM ____ TO ____

⑆1251⑈0095⑆ ⑈0510466003⑈

THOMAS A. BLACK, M.D.

MDP 10501 ©1972
BIBBERO SYSTEMS
SAN FRANCISCO

THOMAS A. BLACK, M.D.
422 MAIN STREET
ANYTOWN, U.S.A.

FORM NO. MDP 9904NC THE BIBBERO SYSTEM OF PERSON

LAST CHECK

TOTAL THIS PAGE →
TOTAL PREVIOUS PAGE →
TOTAL TO DATE →

FIGURE 16–14 Write-it-once Checkwriting System. (Courtesy of Bibbero Systems, Inc., San Francisco, California.)

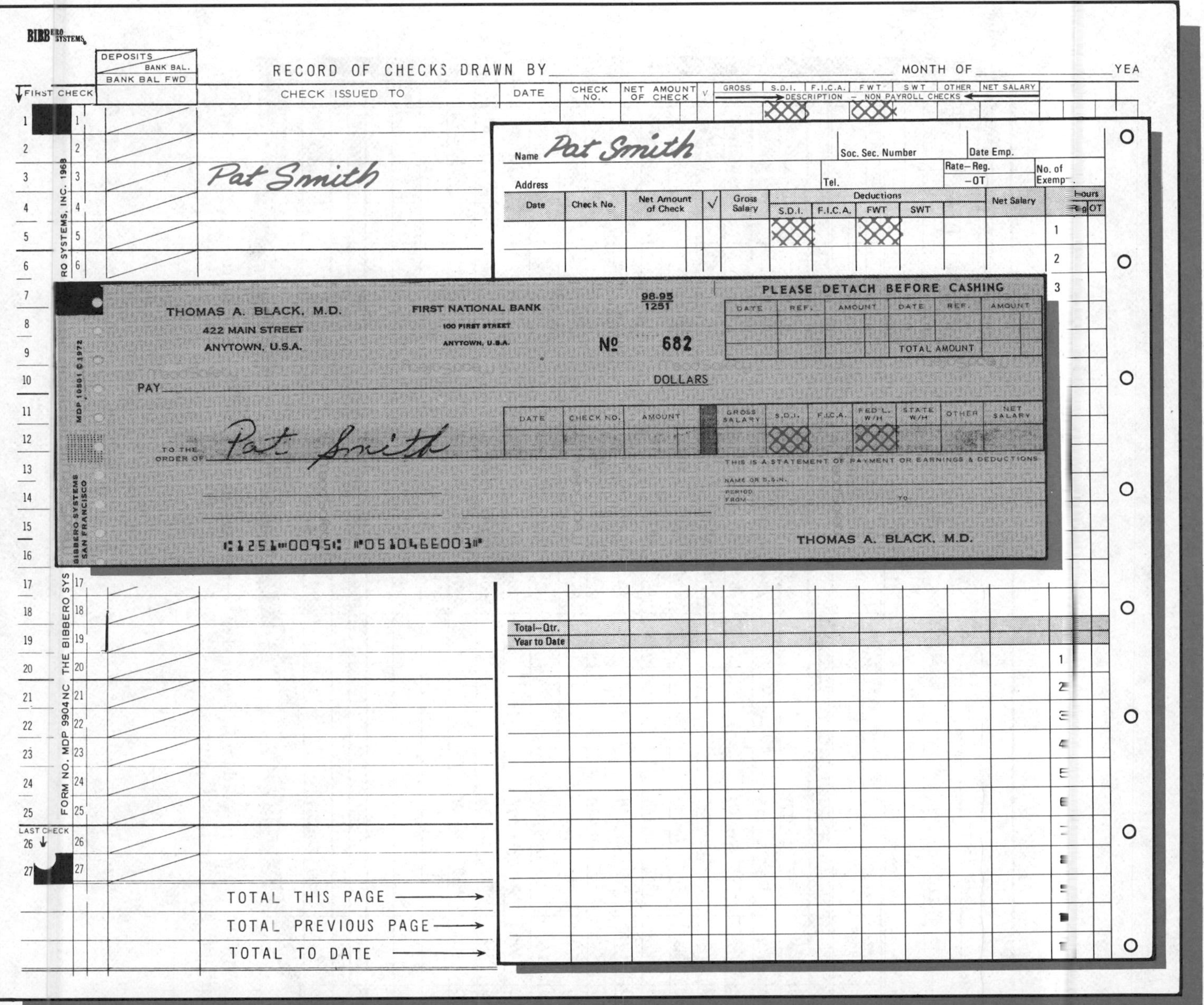

FIGURE 16–15 Employee Compensation Record for Write-it-once Checkwriting System. (Courtesy of Bibbero Systems, Inc., San Francisco, California.)

16

NAME: Pat Smith
CLOCK NUMBER:
DEPT.: Off. Mgr.
MARITAL STATUS: M
NO. OF EXEMPT.: 1
STREET: 212 South St.
SOC.SEC. NUMBER: 123-45-6789
☐ M. ☒ F.
CITY: Anytown
PHONE NO.: 876-5432
DATE STARTED: 11/5/XX
DATE LEFT:

RECORD OF PAY RATE CHANGES	
DATE	RATE
1/6/XX	5.25

YEAR ______ ENCIRCLE QUARTERS 1 (2) 3 4

TIME WORKED	DATE PAY PERIOD ENDING	TIME WORKED (SUN M TU W TH F SAT)	GROSS PAYROLL	INC. TAX	SOC. SEC	STATE TAX	NET PAY	
		BROUGHT FORWARD →						
40	1/6	PAT SMITH	210.00	42.00	10.90	6.30	150.80	1
40	1/13	PAT SMITH	210.00	42.00	10.90	6.30	150.80	2
40	1/20	PAT SMITH	210.00	42.00	10.90	6.30	150.80	3
32	1/27	PAT SMITH	168.00	33.60	8.75	5.00	120.65	4
40	2/3	PAT SMITH	210.00	42.00	10.90	6.30	150.80	5
40	2/10	PAT SMITH	210.00	42.00	10.90	6.30	150.80	6
40	2/17	PAT SMITH	210.00	42.00	10.90	6.30	150.80	7
36	2/24	PAT SMITH	189.00	37.80	9.80	5.70	135.70	8
40	3/3	PAT SMITH	210.00	42.00	10.90	6.30	150.80	9
40	3/10	PAT SMITH	210.00	42.00	10.90	6.30	150.80	10
40	3/17	PAT SMITH	210.00	42.00	10.90	6.30	150.80	11
40	3/24	PAT SMITH	210.00	42.00	10.90	6.30	150.80	12
40	3/31	PAT SMITH	210.00	42.00	10.90	6.30	150.80	13
								14
								15
								16
	QTR.		2667.00	533.40	138.46	80.00	1915.15	
	TO DATE							
40	4/6	PAT SMITH	210.00	42.00	10.90	6.30	150.80	1
								2

FIGURE 16–16 Payroll record for first quarter of year, one employee. (Courtesy of Bibbero Systems, Inc., San Francisco, California.)

September 15, and January 15. It may be the financial secretary's duty to see that these returns are filed when due.

The employer will also contribute to Social Security a self-employment tax. The rate is slightly higher than that of an employee but less than the combined employee-employer contribution. This is computed and paid as a part of the income tax return.

FICA TAXES. Taxes are imposed on both employers and employees for old-age, survivors, and disability insurance benefits (OASDI) and health insurance for the aged (HIP). Both of these taxes are under the umbrella of the Federal Insurance Contributions Act (FICA). The rate is reviewed frequently and is subject to change by Congress. It is currently (1981) 6.65 per cent on the first $29,700, with employee and employer each paying the same amount. The employee's 6.65 per cent is withheld from salary; the employer's 6.65 per cent is paid with the employer's monthly federal tax deposit or with the quarterly return. It should be noted that the *total* FICA tax on salaries paid is 13.3 per cent of the first $29,700 paid to each employee (Fig. 16–18).

DEPOSIT REQUIREMENTS. Generally, the employer must deposit withholding and Social Security taxes in an authorized financial institution or a Federal Reserve bank. A preinscribed Federal Tax Deposit Form 501 is included with each deposit. The amount of taxes owing determines the frequency of the deposits. The rules are subject to change and are set forth in Circular E previously referred to. The regulations differ, too, depending upon the amount owed: (1) less than $200 at end of the quarter, (2) $200 or more at end of the quarter, (3) $200 or more but less than $2,000 at end of first or second month of the quarter, and (4) $2,000 or more at end of the quarter-monthly period. The following guidelines will cover most physicians' offices.

1. If at the end of a quarter the total amount of undeposited taxes is less than $200, no deposit is required. The taxes may be paid directly to the Internal Revenue Service along with the quarterly Form 941.

2. If at the end of a quarter the total amount of undeposited taxes is $200 or more, the employer must deposit the entire amount on or before the last day of the first month after the end of the quarter. The required dates are April 30, July 31, October 31, and January 31.

3. If at the end of any month (except the last month of a quarter) the cumulative amount of undeposited taxes for the quarter is $200 or more, the taxes must be deposited within 15 days after the end of the month.

QUARTERLY REPORTS. The Employer's Quarterly Federal Tax Return (Form 941) must be filed on or before the last day of the first month after the end of the quarter. Due dates for this return and full payment of tax are April 30, July 31, October 31, and January 31. If deposits in full payment of taxes due have been made, the due date for the return is extended ten days. The return must show the number of employees, the names of all employees with their Social Security numbers, the total wages paid, the amount of withholding tax, the amount of wages subject to FICA and the FICA taxes paid, the total deposits for the quarter, and any undeposited taxes due.

ANNUAL REPORTS. Form W-2, Wage and Tax Statement, should be given to employees by January 31. Form W-2 must show the employer's identification number and the employee's Social Security number. It also must show the total wages and other compensation paid (whether or not they are subject to withholding), the amounts deducted for income tax and Social Security tax, including hospital insurance, and the total amount of advance earned income credit payment, if any. The employer is required to furnish two copies of Form W-2 to each employee from whom income tax or Social Security tax has been withheld, or from whom income

MARRIED Persons—**BIWEEKLY** Payroll Period

And the wages are—		And the number of withholding allowances claimed is—										
At least	But less than	0	1	2	3	4	5	6	7	8	9	10 or more
		The amount of income tax to be withheld shall be—										
$0	$92	$0	$0	$0	$0	$0	$0	$0	$0	$0	$0	$0
92	94	.10	0	0	0	0	0	0	0	0	0	0
94	96	.40	0	0	0	0	0	0	0	0	0	0
96	98	.70	0	0	0	0	0	0	0	0	0	0
98	100	1.00	0	0	0	0	0	0	0	0	0	0
100	102	1.30	0	0	0	0	0	0	0	0	0	0
102	104	1.60	0	0	0	0	0	0	0	0	0	0
104	106	1.90	0	0	0	0	0	0	0	0	0	0
106	108	2.20	0	0	0	0	0	0	0	0	0	0
108	110	2.50	0	0	0	0	0	0	0	0	0	0
110	112	2.80	0	0	0	0	0	0	0	0	0	0
112	114	3.10	0	0	0	0	0	0	0	0	0	0
114	116	3.40	0	0	0	0	0	0	0	0	0	0
116	118	3.70	0	0	0	0	0	0	0	0	0	0
118	120	4.00	0	0	0	0	0	0	0	0	0	0
120	124	4.50	0	0	0	0	0	0	0	0	0	0
124	128	5.10	0	0	0	0	0	0	0	0	0	0
128	132	5.70	0	0	0	0	0	0	0	0	0	0
132	136	6.30	.50	0	0	0	0	0	0	0	0	0
136	140	6.90	1.10	0	0	0	0	0	0	0	0	0
140	144	7.50	1.70	0	0	0	0	0	0	0	0	0
144	148	8.10	2.30	0	0	0	0	0	0	0	0	0
148	152	8.70	2.90	0	0	0	0	0	0	0	0	0
152	156	9.30	3.50	0	0	0	0	0	0	0	0	0
156	160	9.90	4.10	0	0	0	0	0	0	0	0	0
160	164	10.50	4.70	0	0	0	0	0	0	0	0	0
164	168	11.10	5.30	0	0	0	0	0	0	0	0	0
168	172	11.70	5.90	.10	0	0	0	0	0	0	0	0
172	176	12.30	6.50	.70	0	0	0	0	0	0	0	0
176	180	12.90	7.10	1.30	0	0	0	0	0	0	0	0
180	184	13.50	7.70	1.90	0	0	0	0	0	0	0	0
184	188	14.10	8.30	2.50	0	0	0	0	0	0	0	0
188	192	14.70	8.90	3.10	0	0	0	0	0	0	0	0
192	196	15.30	9.50	3.70	0	0	0	0	0	0	0	0
196	200	15.90	10.10	4.30	0	0	0	0	0	0	0	0
200	210	16.90	11.10	5.40	0	0	0	0	0	0	0	0
210	220	18.40	12.60	6.90	1.10	0	0	0	0	0	0	0
220	230	19.90	14.10	8.40	2.60	0	0	0	0	0	0	0
230	240	21.40	15.60	9.90	4.10	0	0	0	0	0	0	0
240	250	22.90	17.10	11.40	5.60	0	0	0	0	0	0	0
250	260	24.40	18.60	12.90	7.10	1.30	0	0	0	0	0	0
260	270	26.20	20.10	14.40	8.60	2.80	0	0	0	0	0	0
270	280	28.00	21.60	15.90	10.10	4.30	0	0	0	0	0	0
280	290	29.80	23.10	17.40	11.60	5.80	.10	0	0	0	0	0
290	300	31.60	24.70	18.90	13.10	7.30	1.60	0	0	0	0	0
300	320	34.30	27.40	21.10	15.30	9.60	3.80	0	0	0	0	0
320	340	37.90	31.00	24.10	18.30	12.60	6.80	1.00	0	0	0	0
340	360	41.50	34.60	27.70	21.30	15.60	9.80	4.00	0	0	0	0
360	380	45.10	38.20	31.30	24.40	18.60	12.80	7.00	1.30	0	0	0
380	400	48.70	41.80	34.90	28.00	21.60	15.80	10.00	4.30	0	0	0
400	420	52.30	45.40	38.50	31.60	24.60	18.80	13.00	7.30	1.50	0	0
420	440	56.30	49.00	42.10	35.20	28.20	21.80	16.00	10.30	4.50	0	0
440	460	60.50	52.60	45.70	38.80	31.80	24.90	19.00	13.30	7.50	1.70	0
460	480	64.70	56.60	49.30	42.40	35.40	28.50	22.00	16.30	10.50	4.70	0
480	500	68.90	60.80	52.90	46.00	39.00	32.10	25.20	19.30	13.50	7.70	2.00
500	520	73.10	65.00	56.90	49.60	42.60	35.70	28.80	22.30	16.50	10.70	5.00
520	540	77.30	69.20	61.10	53.20	46.20	39.30	32.40	25.50	19.50	13.70	8.00
540	560	81.50	73.40	65.30	57.20	49.80	42.90	36.00	29.10	22.50	16.70	11.00
560	580	85.70	77.60	69.50	61.40	53.40	46.50	39.60	32.70	25.80	19.70	14.00
580	600	90.30	81.80	73.70	65.60	57.60	50.10	43.20	36.30	29.40	22.70	17.00

FIGURE 16–17 Page from 1980 withholding tax table for married persons.

SINGLE Persons — BIWEEKLY Payroll Period

And the wages are—		And the number of withholding allowances claimed is—										
At least	But less than	0	1	2	3	4	5	6	7	8	9	10 or more
		The amount of income tax to be withheld shall be—										
$260	$270	$35.80	$28.80	$21.90	$14.90	$8.50	$2.70	$0	$0	$0	$0	$0
270	280	37.90	30.60	23.70	16.70	10.00	4.20	0	0	0	0	0
280	290	40.00	32.40	25.50	18.50	11.60	5.70	0	0	0	0	0
290	300	42.10	34.20	27.30	20.30	13.40	7.20	1.40	0	0	0	0
300	320	45.30	37.20	30.00	23.00	16.10	9.50	3.70	0	0	0	0
320	340	49.50	41.40	33.60	26.60	19.70	12.80	6.70	.90	0	0	0
340	360	53.70	45.60	37.50	30.20	23.30	16.40	9.70	3.90	0	0	0
360	380	57.90	49.80	41.70	33.80	26.90	20.00	13.10	6.90	1.20	0	0
380	400	62.10	54.00	45.90	37.80	30.50	23.60	16.70	9.90	4.20	0	0
400	420	67.10	58.20	50.10	42.00	34.10	27.20	20.30	13.30	7.20	1.40	0
420	440	72.30	62.40	54.30	46.20	38.10	30.80	23.90	16.90	10.20	4.40	0
440	460	77.50	67.50	58.50	50.40	42.30	34.40	27.50	20.50	13.60	7.40	1.60
460	480	82.70	72.70	62.70	54.60	46.50	38.50	31.10	24.10	17.20	10.40	4.60
480	500	87.90	77.90	67.90	58.80	50.70	42.70	34.70	27.70	20.80	13.90	7.60
500	520	93.10	83.10	73.10	63.10	54.90	46.90	38.80	31.30	24.40	17.50	10.60
520	540	98.30	88.30	78.30	68.30	59.10	51.10	43.00	34.90	28.00	21.10	14.20
540	560	103.70	93.50	83.50	73.50	63.50	55.30	47.20	39.10	31.60	24.70	17.80
560	580	109.70	98.70	88.70	78.70	68.70	59.50	51.40	43.30	35.20	28.30	21.40
580	600	115.70	104.20	93.90	83.90	73.90	63.90	55.60	47.50	39.40	31.90	25.00
600	620	121.70	110.20	99.10	89.10	79.10	69.10	59.80	51.70	43.60	35.60	28.60
620	640	127.70	116.20	104.60	94.30	84.30	74.30	64.30	55.90	47.80	39.80	32.20
640	660	133.70	122.20	110.60	99.50	89.50	79.50	69.50	60.10	52.00	44.00	35.90
660	680	140.00	128.20	116.60	105.10	94.70	84.70	74.70	64.70	56.20	48.20	40.10
680	700	146.80	134.20	122.60	111.10	99.90	89.90	79.90	69.90	60.40	52.40	44.30
700	720	153.60	140.60	128.60	117.10	105.50	95.10	85.10	75.10	65.10	56.60	48.50
720	740	160.40	147.40	134.60	123.10	111.50	100.30	90.30	80.30	70.30	60.80	52.70
740	760	167.20	154.20	141.10	129.10	117.50	106.00	95.50	85.50	75.50	65.50	56.90
760	780	174.00	161.00	147.90	135.10	123.50	112.00	100.70	90.70	80.70	70.70	61.10
780	800	180.80	167.80	154.70	141.60	129.50	118.00	106.50	95.90	85.90	75.90	65.90
800	820	187.60	174.60	161.50	148.40	135.50	124.00	112.50	101.10	91.10	81.10	71.10
820	840	194.40	181.40	168.30	155.20	142.10	130.00	118.50	106.90	96.30	86.30	76.30
840	860	201.20	188.20	175.10	162.00	148.90	136.00	124.50	112.90	101.50	91.50	81.50
860	880	208.30	195.00	181.90	168.80	155.70	142.60	130.50	118.90	107.40	96.70	86.70
880	900	216.10	201.80	188.70	175.60	162.50	149.40	136.50	124.90	113.40	101.90	91.90
900	920	223.90	208.90	195.50	182.40	169.30	156.20	143.20	130.90	119.40	107.80	97.10
920	940	231.70	216.70	202.30	189.20	176.10	163.00	150.00	136.90	125.40	113.80	102.30
940	960	239.50	224.50	209.50	196.00	182.90	169.80	156.80	143.70	131.40	119.80	108.30
960	980	247.30	232.30	217.30	202.80	189.70	176.60	163.60	150.50	137.40	125.80	114.30
980	1,000	255.10	240.10	225.10	210.10	196.50	183.40	170.40	157.30	144.20	131.80	120.30
1,000	1,020	262.90	247.90	232.90	217.90	203.30	190.20	177.20	164.10	151.00	137.90	126.30
1,020	1,040	270.70	255.70	240.70	225.70	210.70	197.00	184.00	170.90	157.80	144.70	132.30
1,040	1,060	278.50	263.50	248.50	233.50	218.50	203.80	190.80	177.70	164.60	151.50	138.50
1,060	1,080	286.30	271.30	256.30	241.30	226.30	211.30	197.60	184.50	171.40	158.30	145.30
1,080	1,100	294.10	279.10	264.10	249.10	234.10	219.10	204.40	191.30	178.20	165.10	152.10
1,100	1,120	301.90	286.90	271.90	256.90	241.90	226.90	211.90	198.10	185.00	171.90	158.90
1,120	1,140	309.70	294.70	279.70	264.70	249.70	234.70	219.70	204.90	191.80	178.70	165.70
1,140	1,160	317.50	302.50	287.50	272.50	257.50	242.50	227.50	212.50	198.60	185.50	172.50
1,160	1,180	325.30	310.30	295.30	280.30	265.30	250.30	235.30	220.30	205.40	192.30	179.30
1,180	1,200	333.10	318.10	303.10	288.10	273.10	258.10	243.10	228.10	213.10	199.10	186.10
1,200	1,220	340.90	325.90	310.90	295.90	280.90	265.90	250.90	235.90	220.90	205.90	192.90
1,220	1,240	348.70	333.70	318.70	303.70	288.70	273.70	258.70	243.70	228.70	213.70	199.70
1,240	1,260	356.50	341.50	326.50	311.50	296.50	281.50	266.50	251.50	236.50	221.50	206.50
1,260	1,280	364.30	349.30	334.30	319.30	304.30	289.30	274.30	259.30	244.30	229.30	214.30
1,280	1,300	372.10	357.10	342.10	327.10	312.10	297.10	282.10	267.10	252.10	237.10	222.10
1,300	1,320	379.90	364.90	349.90	334.90	319.90	304.90	289.90	274.90	259.90	244.90	229.90
		39 percent of the excess over $1,320 plus—										
$1,320 and over		[illegible]	[illegible]	353.80	338.80	323.80	308.80	293.80	278.80	263.80	248.80	233.80

FIGURE 16–17 *Continued.* **Page from 1980 withholding tax table for single persons.**

Social Security Employee Tax Table–Continued

6.13 percent employee tax deductions

Wages		Tax to be withheld	Wages		Tax to be withheld	Wages		Tax to be withheld	Wages		Tax to be withheld
At least	But less than		At least	But less than		At least	But less than		At least	But less than	
$35.16	$35.32	$2.16	$45.93	$46.09	$2.82	$56.69	$56.86	$3.48	$67.46	$67.62	$4.14
35.32	35.49	2.17	46.09	46.25	2.83	56.86	57.02	3.49	67.62	67.79	4.15
35.49	35.65	2.18	46.25	46.42	2.84	57.02	57.18	3.50	67.79	67.95	4.16
35.65	35.81	2.19	46.42	46.58	2.85	57.18	57.35	3.51	67.95	68.11	4.17
35.81	35.98	2.20	46.58	46.74	2.86	57.35	57.51	3.52	68.11	68.28	4.18
35.98	36.14	2.21	46.74	46.91	2.87	57.51	57.67	3.53	68.28	68.44	4.19
36.14	36.30	2.22	46.91	47.07	2.88	57.67	57.84	3.54	68.44	68.60	4.20
36.30	36.47	2.23	47.07	47.23	2.89	57.84	58.00	3.55	68.60	68.77	4.21
36.47	36.63	2.24	47.23	47.39	2.90	58.00	58.16	3.56	68.77	68.93	4.22
36.63	36.79	2.25	47.39	47.56	2.91	58.16	58.32	3.57	68.93	69.09	4.23
36.79	36.95	2.26	47.56	47.72	2.92	58.32	58.49	3.58	69.09	69.25	4.24
36.95	37.12	2.27	47.72	47.88	2.93	58.49	58.65	3.59	69.25	69.42	4.25
37.12	37.28	2.28	47.88	48.05	2.94	58.65	58.81	3.60	69.42	69.58	4.26
37.28	37.44	2.29	48.05	48.21	2.95	58.81	58.98	3.61	69.58	69.74	4.27
37.44	37.61	2.30	48.21	48.37	2.96	58.98	59.14	3.62	69.74	69.91	4.28
37.61	37.77	2.31	48.37	48.54	2.97	59.14	59.30	3.63	69.91	70.07	4.29
37.77	37.93	2.32	48.54	48.70	2.98	59.30	59.47	3.64	70.07	70.23	4.30
37.93	38.10	2.33	48.70	48.86	2.99	59.47	59.63	3.65	70.23	70.40	4.31
38.10	38.26	2.34	48.86	49.03	3.00	59.63	59.79	3.66	70.40	70.56	4.32
38.26	38.42	2.35	49.03	49.19	3.01	59.79	59.96	3.67	70.56	70.72	4.33
38.42	38.59	2.36	49.19	49.35	3.02	59.96	60.12	3.68	70.72	70.89	4.34
38.59	38.75	2.37	49.35	49.52	3.03	60.12	60.28	3.69	70.89	71.05	4.35
38.75	38.91	2.38	49.52	49.68	3.04	60.28	60.45	3.70	71.05	71.21	4.36
38.91	39.08	2.39	49.68	49.84	3.05	60.45	60.61	3.71	71.21	71.38	4.37
39.08	39.24	2.40	49.84	50.00	3.06	60.61	60.77	3.72	71.38	71.54	4.38
39.24	39.40	2.41	50.00	50.17	3.07	60.77	60.93	3.73	71.54	71.70	4.39
39.40	39.56	2.42	50.17	50.33	3.08	60.93	61.10	3.74	71.70	71.86	4.40
39.56	39.73	2.43	50.33	50.49	3.09	61.10	61.26	3.75	71.86	72.03	4.41
39.73	39.89	2.44	50.49	50.66	3.10	61.26	61.42	3.76	72.03	72.19	4.42
39.89	40.05	2.45	50.66	50.82	3.11	61.42	61.59	3.77	72.19	72.35	4.43
40.05	40.22	2.46	50.82	50.98	3.12	61.59	61.75	3.78	72.35	72.52	4.44
40.22	40.38	2.47	50.98	51.15	3.13	61.75	61.91	3.79	72.52	72.68	4.45
40.38	40.54	2.48	51.15	51.31	3.14	61.91	62.08	3.80	72.68	72.84	4.46
40.54	40.71	2.49	51.31	51.47	3.15	62.08	62.24	3.81	72.84	73.01	4.47
40.71	40.87	2.50	51.47	51.64	3.16	62.24	62.40	3.82	73.01	73.17	4.48
40.87	41.03	2.51	51.64	51.80	3.17	62.40	62.57	3.83	73.17	73.33	4.49
41.03	41.20	2.52	51.80	51.96	3.18	62.57	62.73	3.84	73.33	73.50	4.50
41.20	41.36	2.53	51.96	52.13	3.19	62.73	62.89	3.85	73.50	73.66	4.51
41.36	41.52	2.54	52.13	52.29	3.20	62.89	63.06	3.86	73.66	73.82	4.52
41.52	41.69	2.55	52.29	52.45	3.21	63.06	63.22	3.87	73.82	73.99	4.53
41.69	41.85	2.56	52.45	52.62	3.22	63.22	63.38	3.88	73.99	74.15	4.54
41.85	42.01	2.57	52.62	52.78	3.23	63.38	63.54	3.89	74.15	74.31	4.55
42.01	42.17	2.58	52.78	52.94	3.24	63.54	63.71	3.90	74.31	74.47	4.56
42.17	42.34	2.59	52.94	53.10	3.25	63.71	63.87	3.91	74.47	74.64	4.57
42.34	42.50	2.60	53.10	53.27	3.26	63.87	64.03	3.92	74.64	74.80	4.58
42.50	42.66	2.61	53.27	53.43	3.27	64.03	64.20	3.93	74.80	74.96	4.59
42.66	42.83	2.62	53.43	53.59	3.28	64.20	64.36	3.94	74.96	75.13	4.60
42.83	42.99	2.63	53.59	53.76	3.29	64.36	64.52	3.95	75.13	75.29	4.61
42.99	43.15	2.64	53.76	53.92	3.30	64.52	64.69	3.96	75.29	75.45	4.62
43.15	43.32	2.65	53.92	54.08	3.31	64.69	64.85	3.97	75.45	75.62	4.63
43.32	43.48	2.66	54.08	54.25	3.32	64.85	65.01	3.98	75.62	75.78	4.64
43.48	43.64	2.67	54.25	54.41	3.33	65.01	65.18	3.99	75.78	75.94	4.65
43.64	43.81	2.68	54.41	54.57	3.34	65.18	65.34	4.00	75.94	76.11	4.66
43.81	43.97	2.69	54.57	54.74	3.35	65.34	65.50	4.01	76.11	76.27	4.67
43.97	44.13	2.70	54.74	54.90	3.36	65.50	65.67	4.02	76.27	76.43	4.68
44.13	44.30	2.71	54.90	55.06	3.37	65.67	65.83	4.03	76.43	76.60	4.69
44.30	44.46	2.72	55.06	55.23	3.38	65.83	65.99	4.04	76.60	76.76	4.70
44.46	44.62	2.73	55.23	55.39	3.39	65.99	66.16	4.05	76.76	76.92	4.71
44.62	44.78	2.74	55.39	55.55	3.40	66.16	66.32	4.06	76.92	77.08	4.72
44.78	44.95	2.75	55.55	55.71	3.41	66.32	66.48	4.07	77.08	77.25	4.73
44.95	45.11	2.76	55.71	55.88	3.42	66.48	66.64	4.08	77.25	77.41	4.74
45.11	45.27	2.77	55.88	56.04	3.43	66.64	66.81	4.09	77.41	77.57	4.75
45.27	45.44	2.78	56.04	56.20	3.44	66.81	66.97	4.10	77.57	77.74	4.76
45.44	45.60	2.79	56.20	56.37	3.45	66.97	67.13	4.11	77.74	77.90	4.77
45.60	45.76	2.80	56.37	56.53	3.46	67.13	67.30	4.12	77.90	78.06	4.78
45.76	45.93	2.81	56.53	56.69	3.47	67.30	67.46	4.13	78.06	78.23	4.79

FIGURE 16–18 Page from 1980 Social Security Employee Tax Table.

tax would have been withheld if the employee had claimed no more than one withholding exemption.

If employment ends before December 31, the employer may give the W-2 to the terminated employee any time after employment ends. If the employee asks for Form W-2, the employer should give him or her the completed copies within 30 days of the request or the final wage payment, whichever is later (Fig. 16–19).

To help employers in states where both federal and state taxes must be withheld, a combined form, for use in states or cities authorizing its use, is available on request. This form also may be used where city or other subdivision taxes are withheld. It is printed in sets of six copies so that copies are available for filing and for the records of the employee.

Employers must file Form W-3, Transmittal of Income and Tax Statement, annually to transmit wage and income tax withheld statements (Forms W-2) to the Social Security Administration. These forms are processed by the Social Security Administration, which then furnishes the Internal Revenue Service with the income tax data that it needs from those forms. Form W-3 and its attachments must be filed separately from the Form 941 on or before the last day of February following the calendar year for which the Forms W-2 are prepared (Fig. 16–20).

FEDERAL UNEMPLOYMENT TAX. If an employer paid wages of $1500 or more in any calendar quarter, or had one or more employees for some portion of at least one day during each of 20 different calendar weeks, he is subject to Federal Unemployment Tax. The 20 weeks do not have to be consecutive. Individuals on vacation or sick leave are counted as employees in determining the employer's status.

The Federal Unemployment Tax is imposed on the employer; it must not be collected or deducted from the wages of the employee. The rate is 3.4 per cent on the first $6000 of wages paid to each employee during the calendar year. The employer may receive credit for up to 2.7 per cent of the wages for State Unemployment taxes he paid or for having been granted a favorable experience rate by the state. For this reason, the net Federal liability may be as low as 0.7 per cent.

Federal Unemployment Tax Deposits. If the liability for undeposited Federal unemployment tax exceeds $100 for any calendar quarter and any preceding quarter, the employer must deposit the tax with an authorized financial institution or a Federal Reserve bank within one month following the close of the quarter. The deposit must be accompanied by a Federal Unemployment Tax Deposit form (Form 508).

Annual Return. An annual federal unemployment tax return must be filed on Form 940 on or before January 31, following the close of the calendar year for which the tax is due. Any tax still due is payable with the return. Form 940 may be filed on or before February 10, following the close of the year if all required deposits were made on time and if full payment of the tax due is deposited on or before January 31 (Fig. 16–21).

STATE UNEMPLOYMENT TAXES. All of the states and the District of Columbia have unemployment compensation laws. In most states the tax is imposed only on the employer, but a few states require employers to withhold a percentage of wages for unemployment compensation benefits. An employer may be subject to Federal Unemployment tax and not subject to state unemployment tax. In some states, for instance, the employer with fewer than four employees is not subject to the state unemployment tax. The office assistant should check the requirements in her own state in regard to state unemployment taxes.

☆ U.S. GOVERNMENT OFFICE: 1980—283-030 EI-362441915

1 Control number	22222	

2 Employer's name, address, and ZIP code	3 Employer's identification number	4 Employer's State number
	5 Stat. employee ☐ Deceased ☐ Pension plan ☐ Legal rep. ☐ 942 emp. ☐ Subtotal ☐ Correction ☐ Void ☐	
	6 *	7 Advance EIC payment

8 Employee's social security number	9 Federal income tax withheld	10 Wages, tips, other compensation	11 FICA tax withheld
12 Employee's name (first, middle, last)		13 FICA wages	14 FICA tips
		16 Employer's use	

	17 State income tax	18 State wages, tips, etc.	19 Name of State
15 Employee's address and ZIP code	20 Local income tax	21 Local wages, tips, etc.	22 Name of locality

Form **W-2 Wage and Tax Statement 1980** Copy A For Social Security Administration * See Instructions for Forms W-2 and W-2P Department of the Treasury Internal Revenue Service

Do NOT Cut or Separate Forms on This Page

☆ U.S. GOVERNMENT OFFICE: 1980—283-030 EI-362441915

1 Control number	22222	

2 Employer's name, address, and ZIP code	3 Employer's identification number	4 Employer's State number
	5 Stat. employee ☐ Deceased ☐ Pension plan ☐ Legal rep. ☐ 942 emp. ☐ Subtotal ☐ Correction ☐ Void ☐	
	6 *	7 Advance EIC payment

8 Employee's social security number	9 Federal income tax withheld	10 Wages, tips, other compensation	11 FICA tax withheld
12 Employee's name (first, middle, last)		13 FICA wages	14 FICA tips
		16 Employer's use	

	17 State income tax	18 State wages, tips, etc.	19 Name of State
15 Employee's address and ZIP code	20 Local income tax	21 Local wages, tips, etc.	22 Name of locality

Form **W-2 Wage and Tax Statement 1980** Copy A For Social Security Administration * See Instructions for Forms W-2 and W-2P Department of the Treasury Internal Revenue Service

Do NOT Cut or Separate Forms on This Page

☆ U.S. GOVERNMENT OFFICE: 1980—283-030 EI-362441915

1 Control number	22222	

2 Employer's name, address, and ZIP code	3 Employer's identification number	4 Employer's State number
	5 Stat. employee ☐ Deceased ☐ Pension plan ☐ Legal rep. ☐ 942 emp. ☐ Subtotal ☐ Correction ☐ Void ☐	
	6 *	7 Advance EIC payment

8 Employee's social security number	9 Federal income tax withheld	10 Wages, tips, other compensation	11 FICA tax withheld
12 Employee's name (first, middle, last)		13 FICA wages	14 FICA tips
		16 Employer's use	

	17 State income tax	18 State wages, tips, etc.	19 Name of State
15 Employee's address and ZIP code	20 Local income tax	21 Local wages, tips, etc.	22 Name of locality

Form **W-2 Wage and Tax Statement 1980** Copy A For Social Security Administration * See Instructions for Forms W-2 and W-2P Department of the Treasury Internal Revenue Service

FIGURE 16–19 Form W-2 Wage and Tax Statement.

1 Control number	33333				
☐ Kind of Tax Statements Transmitted	2 941/941E ☐ Military ☐ 943 ☐ CT-1 ☐ 942 ☐ Section 218 ☐	3 W-2 ☐ W-2P ☐	4 Original ☐ Corrected ☐	5 With TIN ☐ Without TIN ☐	
6 State SSA number	7 Advance EIC payments	8 Number of statements attached			
9 Federal income tax	10 Wages, tips, and other compensation	11 FICA tax withheld			
12 Employer's State number	13 FICA wages	14 FICA tips			
15 Employer's identification number		16 Establishment number			
17 Employer's name		18 Gross annuity, pension, retired pay, or IRA payment			
		20 Taxable amount			
19 Employer's address and ZIP code (If available, place label over boxes 15, 17, and 19.)					

Under penalties of perjury, I declare that I have examined this return, including accompanying documents, and to the best of my knowledge and belief, it is true, correct, and complete. In the case of documents without recipients' identifying numbers, I have complied with the requirements of the law by requesting such numbers from the recipients, but did not receive them.

Signature ► Title ► Date ►

Form **W-3** **Transmittal of Income and Tax Statements** **1980**

Department of the Treasury
Internal Revenue Service

Please return this entire page.

FIGURE 16–20 Form W-3 Transmittal of Income and Tax Statements.

Form **940**
Department of the Treasury
Internal Revenue Service

Employer's Annual Federal Unemployment Tax Return

1979

T	
FF	
FD	
FP	
I	
T	

If incorrect, make any necessary change ▶

Name (as distinguished from trade name): PETER CONE
Trade name, if any
Address and ZIP code: 362 MAIN ST. ANYTOWN, YOURSTATE 99999

Calendar Year: 1979
Employer identification number: 71-6788123

A Have you paid all required contributions to your State unemployment fund by the due date of Form 940? . . . . . . ☒ Yes ☐ No
If you check the "Yes" box, enter amount of contributions timely paid to your State unemployment fund . . . ▶ $810

B Are you required to pay contributions to only one State? . . . . . . ☒ Yes ☐ No
If you check the "Yes" box: (1) Enter the name of the State that you are required to pay contributions to . . ▶ YOURSTATE
(2) Enter your State experience rate(s) for 1979 (see instructions for Part V, columns 4 and 5) . ▶ 2.7 %. %. %

Part I Computation of Taxable Wages (To Be Completed by All Taxpayers)

	Exempt Payments	Amount paid	
1	Total payments (including exempt payments) during the calendar year for services of employees		60,000
2	Exempt payments. (Explain each exemption shown, attaching additional sheets if necessary) ▶	-0-	
3	Payments for services in excess of $6,000. Enter only the excess over the first $6,000 paid to individual employees exclusive of exempt amounts entered on line 2. Do not use State wage limitation	30,000	
4	Total exempt payments (add lines 2 and 3)		30,000
5	**Total taxable wages** (subtract line 4 from line 1). (If any portion is exempt from State contributions, see instructions) . . ▶		30,000

Part II Tax Due or Refund (Complete if You Checked the "Yes" boxes in Both Items A and B Above)

1	FUTA tax. Multiply the wages on line 5, Part I, by .007 and enter here	210
2	(a) Delaware wages included on line 5, Part I . . ▶ $........ multiplied by .003 . . .	-0-
	(b) Pennsylvania wages included on line 5, Part I . ▶ $........ multiplied by .003 . . .	-0-
3	Total FUTA tax (add lines 1, 2a, and 2b)	210
4	Less: Total FUTA tax deposited from line 5, Part IV	210
5	**Balance due** (subtract line 4 from line 3—this should not be over $100). Pay to Internal Revenue Service . . ▶	-0-
6	**Overpayment** (subtract line 3 from line 4) . . . . . ▶	

Part III Tax Due or Refund (Complete if You Checked the "No" Box in Either Item A or Item B Above)

1	Gross FUTA tax. Multiply the wages on line 5, Part I, by .034		
2	Maximum credit. Multiply the wages on line 5, Part I, by .027		
3	Enter the smaller of the amount on line 11, Part V, or line 2, above		
4	(a) Delaware wages included on line 5, Part I . . ▶ $........ multiplied by .003		
	(b) Pennsylvania wages included on line 5, Part I . ▶ $........ multiplied by .003		
5	Credit allowable (subtract lines 4a and 4b from line 3)		
6	Net FUTA tax (subtract line 5 from line 1)		
7	Less: Total FUTA tax deposited from line 5, Part IV		
8	**Balance due** (subtract line 7 from line 6—this should not be over $100). Pay to Internal Revenue Service . . ▶		
9	**Overpayment** (subtract line 6 from line 7) . . . . . ▶		

Part IV Record of Federal Tax Deposits for Unemployment Tax (Form 508)

	a. Quarter	b. Liability by period	c. Date of deposit	d. Amount of deposit
1	First	105	4-27-79	105
2	Second	91		
3	Third	14	10-31-79	105
4	Fourth			

5 **Total FUTA tax deposited** (add column d, lines 1 through 4) (do not include contributions paid to State) . . ▶ 210

If you will not have to file returns in the future, write "Final" here (see general instruction "Who Must File") . . ▶

Under penalties of perjury, I declare that I have examined this return, including accompanying schedules and statements, and to the best of my knowledge and belief, it is true, correct, and complete, and that no part of any payment made to a State unemployment fund claimed as a credit was or is to be deducted from the payments to employees.

Date ▶ 1-18-80 Signature ▶ Peter Cone Title (Owner, etc.) ▶ OWNER

Form **940** (1979)

FIGURE 16–21 Form 940 Employer's Annual Federal Unemployment Tax Return.

STATE DISABILITY INSURANCE. Some states require that employees be covered by disability or sick-pay insurance. The employer may be required to withhold a certain amount from the employee's salary to pay for this insurance.

References

Publication 334, Tax Guide for Small Business, 1980 Edition. Department of the Treasury, Internal Revenue Service.

Circular E and Supplement Reprint, 1980 Edition. Department of the Treasury, Internal Revenue Service.

Bibbero Systems, Inc.: Catalog for the Doctor's Office, 1978.

CHAPTER OUTLINE

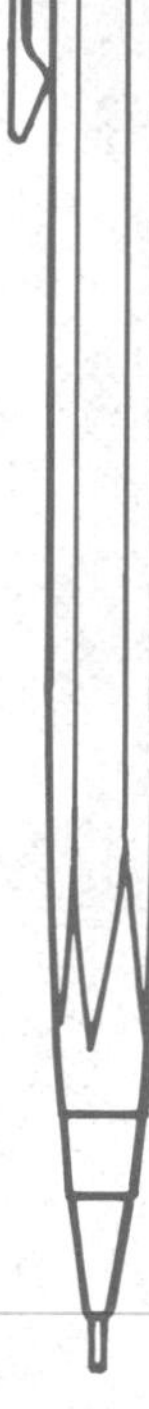

BEHAVIORAL OBJECTIVES

The medical office assistant should be able to:

- Describe the general types of private health insurance plans on the market.
- Compare the principles of group and individual policies.
- Compare the methods of payment under indemnity plans and service benefit plans.
- Describe the benefits and limitations of government-sponsored insurance plans.
- Identify and abstract from the patient record the necessary information for completing insurance claim forms.
- Minimize the rejection of insurance claims through correct completion of forms.
- Process insurance forms, checking for omissions or errors.
- Assist patient in completing insurance forms.
- Explain Medicare coverage and forms to beneficiaries.
- Maintain record of forms filed for easy reference.
- Contact insurance company concerning unpaid or incorrectly paid claims.
- Complete Worker's Compensation forms.
- Abstract medical records for insurance coverage applications.
- Define common insurance terms.

17

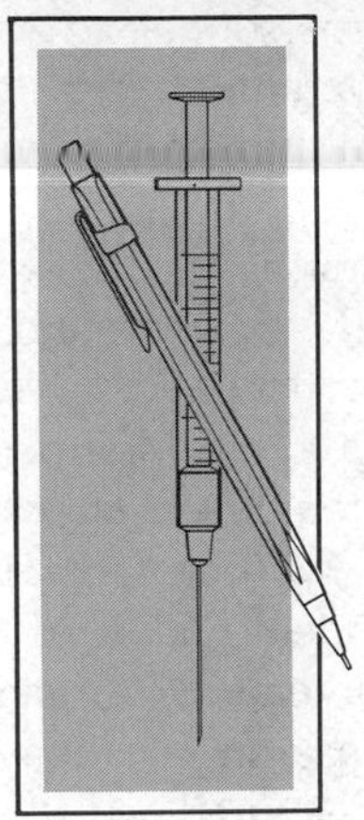

ACCIDENT AND HEALTH INSURANCE

The person without health insurance today is a rarity. Who can afford to be without it? — only the very wealthy or the very healthy! Since no one can be certain that either wealth or health will continue, practically everyone does have some kind of health insurance coverage, either privately or through government-sponsored programs. Just a few days of hospitalization with today's astronomical costs could cripple a family financially for years. Few would be able to keep up with even the daily cost of living were the breadwinner to be disabled for any length of time without the benefits of Worker's Compensation or disability insurance. Yet 50 years ago health insurance as we know it today was very uncommon. But, although the rapid growth of health insurance coverage is a recent phenomenon brought about somewhat by economic necessity, the concept of health insurance is not new.

A BRIEF HISTORY OF HEALTH INSURANCE

The first company organized specifically to write health insurance was founded in 1847. The nation's earliest accident insurance company came into being in 1850 in response to public demand for coverage against frequent rail and steamboat accidents of the mid-nineteenth century. By the turn of the twentieth century, 47 American companies were issuing accident insurance.

In its embryonic stage, the emphasis of health insurance was directed toward replacement of income rather than toward hospital or surgical benefits. The early insurance company policy protected the policyholder against loss of earned income due to a limited number of diseases, including typhus, typhoid, scarlet fever, smallpox, diphtheria, diabetes, and a few others. This policy contained a provision for a seven-day waiting period to take place before the start of benefit payments. The benefit period was limited to 26 consecutive weeks. Emphasis on the income aspects of the insurance continued until 1929, the start of the great Depression.

At this time a group of schoolteachers banded together to form an arrangement with Baylor Hospital in Dallas, Texas, to provide themselves with hospital care on a prepayment basis. This was the origin of the Blue Cross service concept for provision of hospital care.

A further major change occurred during World War II. The freezing of industrial wages made the fringe benefit a significant element of collective bargaining. Group health insurance became a large part of the fringe benefit package.

In 1956, government became a major insurer with passage of Law 569, which authorized dependents of military personnel to receive treatment by civilian physicians at the expense of the government. We know this today as CHAMPUS (Civilian Health and Medical Program of the Uniformed Services).

Title XIX of Public Law 89–97, under the Social Security Amendments of 1965, provided for agreements with states for assistance from the federal government in providing health care for the medically indigent, and is known as Medicaid.

Medicare under Social Security for the patient over 65 went into effect on July 1, 1966. The law was expanded in 1973 to disabled persons under 65 who had been receiving Social Security or railroad retirement checks for two or more years. This included disabled workers, persons who became incapacitated before age 22, disabled widows, and disabled dependent widowers.

The passage of the Health Maintenance Organization (HMO) Act in 1973 provided for federal aid to health insurance prepayment plans that met certain criteria. This brought about an accelerated growth of HMOs. An HMO is an organization that provides for comprehensive health care to an enrolled group for a fixed periodic payment. Available to HMO enrollees is a wide range of medical and hospital services, with emphasis on preventive care, early detection of disease, and ambulatory treatment. An outgrowth of this movement was the development of the Independent Practice Association (IPA), which is a prepaid group practice sponsored by independently practicing physicians who continue to practice in their own offices. By the end of 1978, five years after the passage of the HMO Act, 72 HMOs had qualified for federal aid and 22 of these were IPAs. There were also many more IPAs that had not applied for the federal aid. By 1980, 112 HMOs had qualified for federal aid.

The provision of medical and health care is the second largest industry in the United States. There are seven major forms of health insurance: hospitalization, surgical, regular medical, major medical, disability (loss of income), dental and vision care. The principal insurers may be classified as private insurance companies; Blue Cross, Blue Shield and medical society plans; and government-sponsored plans. Of the total amount spent on medical and health care in 1970, 37 per cent came from government sources.

PURPOSE OF HEALTH INSURANCE

Voluntary health insurance is designed primarily for those who can take care of the costs of routine illnesses but to whom a major illness may prove a real financial burden. Practicality dictates insuring against only those risks that would result in a considerable financial loss. It would be impractical, for example, to insure against minor bills for preventive injections, routine office calls, and treatment of ailments of short duration such as colds. These should be considered a predictable expense in a family budget. Covering such items in an insurance program boosts administrative costs of the insurance plan out of proportion to the small benefits received.

Few insurance policies pay all expenses resulting from accident or illness. However, in many families both husband and wife are wage earners, and frequently both are eligible for health insurance benefits through their own employment and that of their spouse. In order to prevent the available benefits from exceeding the covered expenses and also to hold down the cost of insurance, many groups have a "coordination of benefits" or "nonduplication of benefits" provision. Under such a provision the patient's plan is the primary carrier and will pay the full benefits of its policy. Any remaining covered expenses will be paid by the spouse's plan. In the case of a child, the father's insurance is usually considered the primary carrier.

Health insurance may be purchased under a group policy or an individual policy.

AVAILABILITY OF HEALTH INSURANCE

GROUP POLICIES. Insurance written under a group policy covers a group of people under a master contract, which is generally issued to an employer for the benefit of the employees. The individual employee may be given a certificate of insurance containing information regarding the master policy and indicating that the individual is covered thereunder. Group coverage usually provides greater benefits at lower premiums, and a physical examination is seldom required for the enrollees. Every person in a group contract has identical coverage. In many instances the employer pays the entire premium for the employee and family; in some instances the employee must pay for optional family coverage; and in even fewer instances the employee shares the cost of his own coverage.

INDIVIDUAL POLICIES. Some people who desire health insurance do not qualify for inclusion in a group policy. Most of the companies that write group insurance also offer individual policies. The applicant may be required to have a physical examination prior to acceptance and, if there is an unusual risk, may be denied insurance or may have to accept a rider or limitation on the policy. In any event, the individual premium will probably be greater and the benefits less than in a group policy.

TYPES OF PLANS

There are several hundred private insurance companies that offer both group and individual medical and hospital benefit coverage in this country today, as well as numerous local plans, including those sponsored by medical societies, rural cooperative societies, labor unions, industries, and other organizations. The insurance package is tailored to the needs of each group, and the combinations of benefits are limitless. A group or individual insurance package may contain any one or any combination of the following plans.

HOSPITALIZATION. Hospital coverage pays the cost of all or part of the insured's hospital room and board and special hospital services such as x-ray and the use of special rooms (for surgery, cystoscopic exam, intensive care, recovery, cast application, and so forth). Most plans cover in-hospital pharmacy charges, laboratory services, physical therapy, and blood transfusions. Hospital insurance policies frequently set a specific maximum amount payable per day and a maximum number of days of hospital care to which a patient is entitled under the contract. Some insurance companies require that the hospital be an accredited or a licensed hospital. Most hospital plans exclude admission for diagnostic studies.

SURGICAL. Surgical coverage pays all or part of the surgeon's fee. Some plans do not pay for the assisting surgeon. Surgery includes any incision or excision, removal of foreign bodies, aspiration, suturing, and reduction of fractures. The surgery may be accomplished in a hospital, doctor's office, or elsewhere. The insurer frequently provides the subscriber with a surgical fee schedule that sets forth the amount payable for commonly performed procedures.

REGULAR MEDICAL. Medical coverage pays the physician's fee for nonsurgical services, including hospital, home, and office visits, depending upon coverage. It may include provision for diagnostic and x-ray services, which would embrace special laboratory, x-ray, and pathology fees. It may pay for *detention time,* additional time the physician spends with a patient who is in critical condition. There may also be compensation for being called out at night or on a holiday, and for extra mileage traveled. Many medical plans do not cover a routine physical examination when the patient does not have a specific complaint or illness.

MAJOR MEDICAL (FORMERLY CALLED "CATASTROPHIC" COVERAGE). Major medical insurance provides protection against especially heavy medical bills resulting from catastrophic or prolonged illnesses, and is used as a supplement to basic medical care insurance or as a comprehensive, integrated program providing both basic and major medical protection, including charges for private duty nursing, drugs, and medical appliances. This kind of insurance grew out of the realization that it is not necessary to provide protection against small bills; it is the major medical expenses that constitute the real financial drain.

DISABILITY (LOSS OF INCOME) PROTECTION. This protection provides weekly or monthly cash benefits to employed policy holders who become unable to work owing to an accident or illness. Many policies do not start payment until after a specified number of days or until a certain number of sick leave days have been used. Payment is made directly to the patient and is intended to replace loss of income resulting from illness. It is not intended for payment of specific medical bills.

DENTAL CARE. Dental coverage plans have become more popular since 1965 and are now included in many fringe benefit packages. Some are based on a copayment and incentive program. For instance, the portion that the carrier will pay starts at 70 per cent of covered services during the first calendar year and increases to 80 per cent, 90 per cent, and 100 per cent, respectively, during the second, third, and subsequent calendar years of a patient's eligibility, provided he visits a dentist and has all prescribed dental care rendered during the preceding calendar year. After the initial investment of providing good oral health, the costs are kept down because the incentive program discourages dental neglect.

VISION CARE. Vision care insurance is the latest development in the total health package. It may include reimbursement for all or for a percentage of the cost for refraction, lenses, and frames.

SENIOR CITIZEN POLICIES. These are contracts insuring persons 65 years of age or over, and in most cases supplement the coverage afforded by the government under Medicare.

SPECIAL CLASS INSURANCE. Some applicants for health insurance cannot qualify for a standard policy by reason of health but may be issued special class insurance with limited coverage.

SPECIAL RISK INSURANCE. Some persons may purchase special risk insurance to protect themselves in the event of a certain type of accident, such as automobile or airplane crashes, or for certain diseases, such as tuberculosis or cancer. There is usually a maximum benefit.

LIABILITY INSURANCE. There are many types of liability insurance, including automobile, business, and residence policies. Such policies often include benefits for medical expenses payable to individuals who are injured in the insured person's home or car, without regard to the insured person's actual legal liability for the accident.

LIFE INSURANCE. Sometimes the proceeds from life insurance are used to meet the expenses of the insured person's last illness. Some policies provide additional monthly cash benefits if the policy holder becomes permanently and totally disabled.

OVERHEAD INSURANCE. Overhead insurance reimburses the insured for specific, fixed, monthly expenses, normal and customary, in the operation and conduct of his business or office.

PAYMENT OF BENEFITS

Insurance benefits may be determined and paid in one of several ways: by indemnity schedules, by service benefits, or by determination of the usual, customary, and reasonable fee.

INDEMNITY SCHEDULES. In indemnity plans, the insurer agrees to pay the subscriber a specific amount of money for a certain procedure or service. For example, the company agrees to pay an amount up to $500 for an appendectomy, with no consideration for the time or complications of the surgery. Indemnity plans do not agree to pay for the complete services rendered. Many times there is a difference in the amount paid by the insurance company and the amount of the physician's regular fee. This type of plan takes the major expense out of medical bills and helps to keep the premiums down. It also discourages overuse of a policy. Indemnity payments are usually paid to the insured unless the insured has authorized payment direct to the provider. When the insured purchases the policy, he is given a schedule of indemnities or fee schedule, that is, specified amounts payable for specified procedures. The amount of the premium often determines the schedule of benefits.

SERVICE BENEFIT PLANS. In service benefit plans, the insuring company agrees to pay for certain surgical or medical services without additional cost to the insured. There is no set fee schedule. Service benefit plans are usually sponsored by medical societies or groups. In a service plan, an appendectomy with complications would warrant a higher surgical fee than a routine procedure. Premiums are sometimes higher for this type of coverage, but often payments are larger. Frequently the payments are sent directly to the physician and are considered full payment for the services rendered.

USUAL, CUSTOMARY, AND REASONABLE FEE. Some insurance companies agree to pay on the basis of all or a percentage of the physician's usual, customary, and reasonable fee.

Usual Fee. The usual fee is that fee usually charged for a given service, by an individual physician, to his or her private patient — that is, his or her own usual fee.

Customary Fee. A fee is customary if it is in the range of the usual fees charged by physicians of similar training and experience, for the same service within the specific and limited geographic area (socioeconomic area of a metropolitan area or of a county).

Reasonable Fee. A fee is reasonable if it meets the two criteria given above or, in the opinion of a responsible review committee, is justifiable considering the special circumstances of the particular case in question.

THE BLUE PLANS AND MEDICAL SOCIETY FOUNDATIONS

BLUE CROSS AND BLUE SHIELD. In the early 1930s, hospitals introduced Blue Cross plans to provide protection against hospital costs. Today there are local Blue Cross plans operating in all states of the union, the District of Columbia, Canada, Puerto Rico, and Jamaica.

In 1939 state medical societies in California and Michigan began sponsoring health plans to provide medical and surgical services; these became known as Blue Shield plans. Other states soon followed, and today Blue Shield is the largest medical prepayment system in the country, covering 73 million Americans under private programs and serving 12 million others under government-financed programs.

Currently, more than 90 per cent of all Americans under 65 have some form of health coverage, and it is estimated that one of every three is served by Blue Shield. Blue Shield was founded on the concept of cooperation and active involvement of the medical profession. Physicians helped originate the plans, and early in its development, Blue Shield was often known as "the doctor's plan." Member physicians agree to bill Blue Shield for services to subscribers and adhere to other prearranged procedures. Under many Blue Shield contracts, physicians will accept Blue Shield's payment as payment in full for covered services. Unlike commercial insurance arrangements, Blue Shield and its participating physicians agree on methods of reimbursement in advance of the service performed.

In most areas, Blue Shield plans operate in cooperation with Blue Cross plans, which provide hospital coverage. However, in some areas Blue Cross plans write medical and surgical insurance as well as providing hospital coverage. Conversely, some Blue Shield plans offer hospital insurance as well as medical and surgical coverage.

Blue Cross benefits are normally paid to the provider of service. In some cases a check issued jointly to the provider and the insured is sent to the insured, who must then endorse and forward it to the provider.

Blue Shield makes direct payment to member physicians. For service of a nonmember physician, the payment is sent to the subscriber.

Both Blue Cross and Blue Shield have national headquarters located in Chicago.

BLUE SHIELD RECIPROCITY. Blue Shield reciprocity is an agreement among Blue Shield plans to provide benefits to subscribers who are away from home. It means the subscriber can receive benefits almost anywhere in the country. The identification card of subscribers having reciprocity has a double-end red arrow symbol with an "N" followed by three digits. When the reciprocity beneficiary receives covered care outside his own district, the physician bills the local Blue Shield plan using the local Blue Shield form. For those who do not have the double-end red arrow, the subscriber's home plan must be billed.

FOUNDATIONS FOR MEDICAL CARE. A Foundation for Medical Care is a management system for community health services. It takes the form of an organization created by local physicians through their medical society and it concerns itself with the quality and cost of medical care. Under the Foundation concept the following procedure occurs:

An insurance company sells and negotiates the policy. It collects the premiums, assumes all the risks, and reimburses the Foundation for the cost of the claims office;

The Foundation sets policy standards; receives, processes, reviews and pays claims to doctors; sets maximum fees based on current fees in the area; elects doctor-members yearly; and continually studies local medical-economic problems;

Member doctors agree to accept Foundation fees as full payment under Foundation-approved policies;

The local *medical society* legally controls the Foundation and selects Foundation trustees;

The *patient* selects the doctor of his own choice; the patient, his union or employer pays the premium directly to the insurance company.

The Foundation for Medical Care originated in San Joaquin County, California, in 1954. Foundations now exist in more than 40 states. The American Association of Foundations for Medical Care was organized in 1970 with the avowed purpose of helping individual Foundations provide a better health care system for the American people. Its headquarters are in Stockton, California.

PRIVATE INSURANCE COMPANIES

More than half of those covered by some form of health insurance are covered by private (commercial) insurance companies. Physicians and medical societies do not control either the premiums paid or the benefits received from these private policies. The procedures to be followed in claims completion may vary somewhat from the Blue plans. It will save time for the office assistant to use the Universal Claim Form. If the insurance company has its own form, complete the universal form and attach it to the company's form. Be sure to have the insured sign both forms. Then send it either to the insurance company if it is an individual plan or to the insured's employer if it is group insurance through an employer. The employer will then complete its portion and forward the forms to the insurance company.

GOVERNMENT-SPONSORED PLANS

CHAMPUS: MILITARY MEDICAL BENEFITS. The term *Medicare* first became an important word in the medical assistant's vocabulary in December 1956, with the passage of Law 569, which authorized dependents of military personnel to receive treatment by civilian physicians at the expense of the government. This program was first called Medicare, but was later changed to CHAMPUS (Civilian Health and Medical Program of the Uniformed Services).

On September 30, 1966, the Military Medical Benefits Amendment Act of 1966 became law. This act added outpatient care benefits, including prescription drugs, to the in-hospital benefits previously allowed. The patient pays an out-of-pocket deductible (now $50, not to exceed $100 per family) each fiscal year (October 1 to September 30), plus 20 per cent of the balance.

Military retirees and their dependents and dependents of deceased members became eligible for the same benefits in January 1967, except that their copayment amount is 25 per cent after the deductible.

CHAMPVA. In 1973 a program similar to CHAMPUS was established for the spouses and dependent children of veterans suffering total, permanent, service-connected disabilities and for the surviving spouses and dependent children of veterans who have died as a result of service-connected disabilities. This is called CHAMPVA (Civilian Health and Medical Program of the Veterans Administration). Eligibility is determined, and identification cards are issued, by the nearest VA Hospital. The insured then are free to choose their own private physicians. Benefits and cost-sharing features are the same as those for CHAMPUS beneficiaries who are military retirees or their dependents, and dependents of deceased members of the military.

Under both CHAMPUS and CHAMPVA the patient pays his share of the charges directly to the physician. This includes the deductible and the coinsurance portion. The physician collects the remainder from the government by filing Form 500 with the fiscal agent. The patient or sponsor must complete Items 1 through 18 of the form. The physician completes Items 19 through 33 and must sign the form personally. The form must be filed no later than December 31 of the year following that in which services were provided (Fig. 17–1).

Since details of government-sponsored programs are changed from time to time and are regulated by law, the medical assistant is urged to keep a copy of the latest official manual on hand and note any changes that occur. Write to CHAMPUS, Denver, Colorado 80240, for further instructions.

MEDICARE UNDER SOCIAL SECURITY. Medicare for the patient over 65 went into effect on July 1, 1966. There are two distinct parts (A and B) to the program.

Part A. Hospital insurance, Part A, is financed by special contributions paid by employed individuals as deductions from salary, with matching contributions from their employers. There is no additional premium required from the insured when he becomes eligible for benefits. These sums are collected, along with regular Social Security contributions, from wages and self-employment income earned during a person's working years.

Any person who is receiving monthly Social Security or railroad retirement checks is automatically enrolled for hospital insurance benefits. Some federal employees and former federal employees who are not eligible for Social Security benefits are also not eligible for hospital insurance, but may enroll in the Part B medical insurance program.

CHAMPUS/CHAMPVA CLAIM FORM

For services or supplies provided by civilian sources except Institutions

Read cover instructions and the back of this form before completing and signing!

Form Approved OMB No. 022-RO382

Patient/Sponsor Information (Items 1 through 18 to be completed by the beneficiary/patient or sponsor)

1. PATIENT'S NAME (Last name, First name, Middle initial): CARTER, ELAINE
2. PATIENT'S DATE OF BIRTH: MONTH 07 DAY 16 YEAR 53
3. PATIENT'S ADDRESS (Street, city, state, ZIP code): 337 Peppertree Drive, Baldwin, NY 11510 — PHONE NO. (Include area code) 516 323 0897
4. PATIENT'S SEX: ☐ MALE ☒ FEMALE
5. MILITARY/VA IDENTIFICATION CARD — CARD NO. S12345 — ISSUE DATE MONTH DAY YEAR; EFFECTIVE DATE MONTH 06 DAY 01 YEAR 80; EXPIRATION DATE MONTH 06 DAY 01 YEAR 85
6. PATIENT'S RELATIONSHIP TO SPONSOR: ☐ SELF ☒ SPOUSE ☐ NATURAL or ADOPTED CHILD ☐ STEPCHILD OTHER (Specify):
7. SPONSOR'S NAME (Last name, First name, Middle initial): CARTER, SCOTT W
8. SPONSOR'S SOCIAL SECURITY NO. OR VA FILE NO.: 123 45 6789
9. VA STATION NO.
10. SPONSOR'S DUTY STATION OR ADDRESS FOR RETIREES: HHC 2nd Batt., 24th Infantry, APO New York NY 10026 — PHONE NO. (Include area code)
11. SPONSOR'S BRANCH OF SERVICE: ☒ USA ☐ USAF ☐ USMC ☐ USN ☐ USCG ☐ USPHS ☐ NOAA ☐ VA
12. SPONSOR'S GRADE/RANK: SSG(6)
13. SPONSOR'S STATUS: ☒ ACTIVE DUTY ☐ RETIRED ☐ DECEASED
14. DO YOU HAVE OTHER HEALTH INSURANCE? ☐ YES ☒ NO — IF YES, ENTER NAME OF OTHER PLAN OR PROGRAM: — ADDRESS — CITY STATE ZIP
14a. TYPE OF COVERAGE: ☐ EMPLOYMENT (GROUP) ☐ MEDICAID ☐ STUDENT PLAN ☐ PRIVATE (NON-GROUP) ☐ MEDICARE ☐ OTHER:
14b. OTHER IDENTIFICATION NUMBER
14c. EFFECTIVE DATE MONTH DAY YEAR
14d. OTHER PROGRAM THROUGH EMPLOYMENT? EMPLOYER NAME:
15. IS CONDITION WORK RELATED? ☐ YES ☒ NO — MILITARY SERVICE RELATED? ☐ YES ☒ NO — AUTOMOBILE ACCIDENT RELATED? ☐ YES ☒ NO
16. INPATIENT/OUTPATIENT CARE: ☐ OUTPATIENT ☐ INPATIENT-EMERGENCY ☐ INPATIENT HOSPITAL-OUTSIDE 40 MILE RADIUS ☐ INPATIENT-SKILLED NURSING FACILITY ☐ INPATIENT-OTHER ☒ INPATIENT HOSPITAL-WITHIN 40 MILE RADIUS (ATTACH DD FORM 1251)
17. DESCRIBE CONDITION FOR WHICH YOU RECEIVED TREATMENT. IF AN INJURY, NOTE HOW IT HAPPENED: Gallbladder disease
18. SIGNATURE OF PATIENT OR AUTHORIZED PERSON, CERTIFIES CLAIM INFORMATION AND AUTHORIZES RELEASE OF MEDICAL OR OTHER INSURANCE INFORMATION. READ INSTRUCTIONS AND BACK OF THIS FORM BEFORE SIGNING. SIGNED *Elaine Carter* DATE 6/3/81 RELATIONSHIP TO PATIENT: *self*

Physician / Other Provider (Items 19 through 33 are to be completed by the physician or other provider.)

19. NAME, ADDRESS & PHONE NO. OF REFERRING PHYSICIAN: John E. Adams, M.D., 94 Kenmore Parkway, Garden City, NY 11530, 516 445 8394 — ☒ PRIVATE PRACTICE or ☐ UNIFORMED SERVICES
20. NAME & ADDRESS OF FACILITY WHERE SERVICES RENDERED (other than home or office): Island Hospital, 50 Kenmore Parkway, Garden City, NY 11530
21. PROVIDER OF SERVICES: ☒ ATTENDING PHYSICIAN ☐ OTHER:
22. HOSPITALIZATION INFORMATION: ADMITTED MO 05 DAY 28 YEAR 81 — DISCHARGED MO 06 DAY 03 YEAR 81
23. LAB WORK OUTSIDE YOUR OFFICE? ☐ YES ☐ NO CHARGES:
24. DIAGNOSIS, SYMPTOM OR NATURE OF ILLNESS OR INJURY, RELATE DIAGNOSIS TO PROCEDURE IN COLUMN "D" BY REFERENCE TO NUMBERS 1, 2, 3, or DX CODE
    1. Acute cholecystitis with cholelithiasis
    2.
    3.

25. A. DATES OF SERVICE MO/DAY/YEAR	B* PLACE OF SERVICE	C PROCEDURE CODE IDENTIFY:	D. DESCRIBE PROCEDURES/SUPPLIES FOR EACH DATE. SUBMIT REPORT EXPLAINING UNUSUAL SERVICES OR CIRCUMSTANCES	E DIAGNOSIS CODE	F CHARGES	LEAVE BLANK
05 28 81	1	47610	Cholecystectomy with open exploration of common duct	1	1200 00	

26. PATIENT'S ACCOUNT NO.: ---
27. PROVIDER'S SOCIAL SECURITY NO.: 000 00 0000
28. PROVIDER'S EMPLOYER I.D. NO.: 00 1111111
29. PHYSICIAN'S OR OTHER PROVIDER'S NAME ADDRESS, ZIP CODE & PHONE NO. (INCLUDING AREA CODE): Clifford Z. Turner, M.D., 94 Kenmore Parkway, Garden City, NY 11530 — PROVIDER NO. A 43550
G. TOTAL CHARGES: $ 1200 00
30. AMOUNT PAID BY BENEFICIARY: $
31. AMOUNT PAID BY OTHER INSURANCE: $
32. AGREEMENT TO PARTICIPATE (READ BACK OF THIS FORM): ☒ YES ☐ NO
33. SIGNATURE OF PHYSICIAN OR OTHER PROVIDER (READ BACK OF THIS FORM BEFORE SIGNING): SIGNED *C Z Turner* DATE: 06 30 81

*PLACE OF SERVICE CODES

1 — (IH) — INPATIENT HOSPITAL
2 — (OH) — OUTPATIENT HOSPITAL
3 — (O) — DOCTOR'S OFFICE
4 — (H) — PATIENT'S HOME
5 — (DCF) — DAY CARE FACILITY (PSY)
6 — (NCF) — NIGHT CARE FACILITY (PSY)
7 — (NH) — NURSING HOME
8 — (SNF) — SKILLED NURSING FACILITY
9 — (AMB) — AMBULANCE
0 — (OL) — OTHER LOCATIONS
A — (IL) — INDEPENDENT LABORATORY
B — (OF) — OTHER MEDICAL/SURGICAL FACILITY
C — (RTC) — RESIDENTIAL TREATMENT CENTER
D — (STF) — SPECIALIZED TREATMENT FACILITY

CHAMPUS FORM 500 JUNE 1978

FIGURE 17–1 CHAMPUS claim form.

Part B. Medical insurance, Part B, is voluntary. The insured must apply for coverage within a specified period and pay a monthly premium. This premium was initially $3 in 1966. By 1972 it had increased to $5.80, and in 1981 had reached $11.00. More than 70 per cent of the cost of medical insurance is paid by the federal government from general revenues. The law requires that the premium be reviewed every two years.

A new patient who says he is covered by Medicare should always be asked to show his identification card (Fig. 17–2). This card will show the name of the beneficiary, identification number, effective date, and type of coverage. Keep in mind that the older patient is frequently confused by the complexity of such programs, and the medical assistant can do much to assist this patient. The patient may be under the impression that he is fully covered under Medicare. Part B has a deductible ($75 in 1982). After the deductible is met, Medicare will pay 80 per cent of the covered benefits; the patient must pay the remaining 20 per cent plus any amount not allowed by Medicare.

Beginning July 1, 1973, *disabled* persons under 65 who had been receiving Social Security or railroad retirement checks for two years or more became eligible for Medicare. Persons able to receive disability coverage include disabled workers, persons who became incapacitated before age 22, disabled widows, and disabled dependent widowers. Insured workers and their dependents who need dialysis treatment or a kidney transplant because of permanent kidney failure also have Medicare protection.

At the same time the law was extended to persons 65 and over who had not worked long enough under Social Security to be eligible for the hospital insurance under Medicare, enabling them to buy this protection on a voluntary basis. Anyone who chooses to buy the hospital insurance protection must also enroll and pay the monthly premium for medical coverage.

17

Billing for Medicare Services. Billing for Medicare services may be accomplished easily in any one of these three ways:

1. If the doctor accepts assignment (which means that the doctor agrees to accept the charge determination of the Medicare carrier), ask the patient to sign Part I of the billing form on his first visit (Fig. 17–3). Itemize the services on Part II of the claim form, have the physician sign it, and submit it to the Medicare carrier. When the charge determination has been made, you then bill the patient for his 20 per cent plus the deductible if this has not already been met for the current year.

2. If the doctor does not accept assignment, you may bill the patient directly. The patient then must submit the billing form to the Medicare carrier (Fig. 17–4). In order to do this he will need from the doctor either an itemized bill, which he can attach to the claim form, or an itemization of services on Part II of the form.

3. If the doctor does not accept assignment, he can still submit the claim for Medicare for the patient, and check the box, ☐ *I do not accept assignment*, on

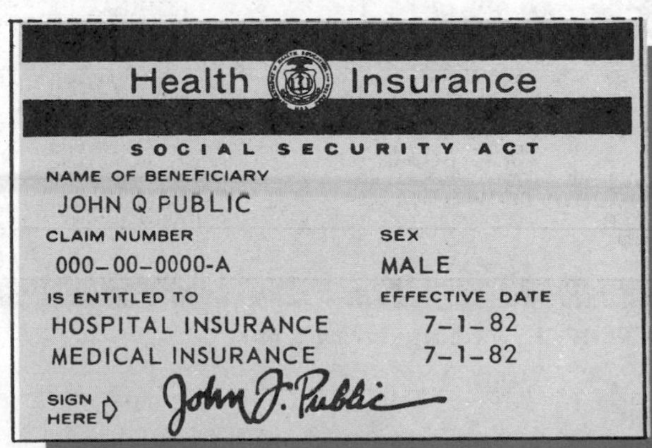
Health Insurance
SOCIAL SECURITY ACT
NAME OF BENEFICIARY
JOHN Q PUBLIC
CLAIM NUMBER
000–00–0000-A
SEX
MALE
IS ENTITLED TO
HOSPITAL INSURANCE
MEDICAL INSURANCE
EFFECTIVE DATE
7–1–82
7–1–82
SIGN HERE
John Q. Public

FIGURE 17–2 Identification card for a Medicare patient.

THIS FORM TO BE USED TO BILL **BLUE CROSS OF SOUTHERN CALIFORNIA** OR **BLUE SHIELD OF CALIFORNIA ONLY.**
PLEASE VERIFY WITH YOUR PATIENT THE CORRECT ORGANIZATION TO BILL.

READ INSTRUCTIONS BEFORE COMPLETING OR SIGNING THIS FORM

TYPE OR PRINT [X] MEDICARE [ ] MEDI-CAL [ ] STANDARD

PATIENT & INSURED (SUBSCRIBER) INFORMATION

1. PATIENT'S NAME (*First name, middle initial, last name*): Arthur O. Switzer
2. PATIENT'S DATE OF BIRTH: 06 06 14
3. INSURED'S NAME (*First name, middle initial, last name*): Arthur O. Switzer
4. PATIENT'S ADDRESS (*Street, city, state, ZIP code*): 4705 Waring Place, Los Angeles, CA 90033
5. PATIENT'S SEX: MALE M FEMALE
6. INSURED'S I.D. NO., MEDICARE NO. AND/OR MEDICAID NO. (*include any letters*): 066 11 7865 A
7. PATIENT'S RELATIONSHIP TO INSURED: SELF X SPOUSE CHILD OTHER
8. INSURED'S GROUP NO. (*Or Group Name*): ------
9. OTHER HEALTH INSURANCE COVERAGE - Enter Name of Policyholder and Plan Name and Address and Policy or Medical Assistance Number: -----
10. WAS CONDITION RELATED TO:
    A. PATIENT'S EMPLOYMENT: YES NO X
    B. AN AUTO ACCIDENT: YES NO X
11. INSURED'S ADDRESS (*Street, city, state, ZIP code*): 4705 Waring Place, Los Angeles, CA 90033
12. PATIENT'S OR AUTHORIZED PERSON'S SIGNATURE (*Read back before signing*) *I Authorize the Release of any Medical Information Necessary to Process this Claim and Request Payment of MEDICARE Benefits Either to Myself or to the Party Who Accepts Assignment Below*
    SIGNED *Arthur O Switzer* DATE 9/11/82
13. *I AUTHORIZE PAYMENT OF MEDICAL BENEFITS TO UNDERSIGNED PHYSICIAN OR SUPPLIER FOR SERVICE DESCRIBED BELOW*
    Arthur O Switzer
    SIGNED (*Insured or Authorized Person*)

PHYSICIAN OR SUPPLIER INFORMATION

14. DATE OF ILLNESS (FIRST SYMPTOM) OR INJURY (ACCIDENT) OR PREGNANCY (LMP): 07 21 82
15. DATE FIRST CONSULTED YOU FOR THIS CONDITION: 07 21 82
16. HAS PATIENT EVER HAD SAME OR SIMILAR SYMPTOMS? YES NO x
17. DATE PATIENT ABLE TO RETURN TO WORK: NA
18. DATES OF TOTAL DISABILITY: FROM NA THROUGH
    DATES OF PARTIAL DISABILITY: FROM NA THROUGH
19. NAME AND ADDRESS OF REFERRING PHYSICIAN OR OTHER SOURCE: -----
20. FOR SERVICES RELATED TO HOSPITALIZATION GIVE HOSPITALIZATION DATES: ADMITTED 07/21/82 DISCHARGED 09/11/82
21. NAME & ADDRESS OF FACILITY WHERE SERVICES RENDERED (*If other than home or office*): St. Vincent's Hospital, Los Angeles
22. WAS LABORATORY WORK PERFORMED OUTSIDE YOUR OFFICE? YES NO X CHARGES
23. DIAGNOSIS OR NATURE OF ILLNESS OR INJURY. RELATE DIAGNOSIS TO PROCEDURE IN COLUMN D BY REFERENCE TO NUMBERS 1, 2, 3, ETC. OR DX CODE
    1. Subacute bacterial endocarditis
    2.
    3.
    4.

    [ ] FAMILY PLANNING SERVICE

24. A DATE OF SERVICE	B * PLACE OF SERVICE	PROCEDURE NUMBER (RVS NUMBER / SMA NUMBER)	UNIT MODIFIER	C FULLY DESCRIBE PROCEDURES, MEDICAL SERVICES OR SUPPLIES FURNISHED FOR EACH DATE GIVEN (EXPLAIN UNUSUAL SERVICES OR CIRCUMSTANCES)	D DIAGNOSIS CODE	E CHARGES	F LEAVE BLANK
07 21 82	1	90220		Initial history and physical	1	100 00	
07/22 to 08/13/82	1	90250		Ex. visits (23) @ $35/visit	1	805 00	
08/14/82	1	90270		Complete cardiac re-evaluation	1	60 00	
08/15/82 to 09/11/82		90250		Ex.visits (27) @ $35/visit		945 00	

25. SIGNATURE OF PHYSICIAN OR SUPPLIER
    I certify under penalty of perjury that the foregoing is true and correct (read back before signing).
    SIGNED *R O Elam MD* DATE 9/15/82
26. ACCEPT ASSIGNMENT (*Government claims only*) SEE BACK: YES x NO
27. TOTAL CHARGE: 1910 00
28. AMOUNT PAID: -0-
29. BALANCE DUE: 1910.00
30. YOUR SOCIAL SECURITY NO.: 222-33-4444
31. PHYSICIAN'S OR SUPPLIER'S NAME, ADDRESS, PROVIDER NUMBER, ZIP CODE & TELEPHONE NO.:
    ROBERT O ELAM MD
    300 NORTH BROADWAY
    LOS ANGELES CA 90005
32. YOUR PATIENT'S ACCOUNT NO.: ------
33. YOUR EMPLOYER I.D. NO.: 00 0000000

PLACE OF SERVICE CODES

1 – (IH)	INPATIENT HOSPITAL	7 – (ICF)	INTERMEDIATE CARE FACILITY
2 – (OH)	OUTPATIENT HOSPITAL	8 – (SNF)	SKILLED NURSING FACILITY
3 – (O)	DOCTOR'S OFFICE	9 –	AMBULANCE
4 – (H)	PATIENT'S HOME	O – (OL)	OTHER LOCATIONS
5 –	DAY CARE FACILITY (PSY)	A – (IL)	INDEPENDENT LABORATORY
6 –	NIGHT CARE FACILITY (PSY)	B –	OTHER MEDICAL/SURGICAL FACILITY

C 4359

FIGURE 17–3 Medicare billing form.

MEDICARE STATEMENT

ROBERT O. ELAM, MD
300 NORTH BROADWAY
LOS ANGELES CA 90005

Mr. Arthur O. Switzer
4705 Waring Place
Los Angeles, CA 90033

DATE 9/15/82 HEALTH INSURANCE CLAIM NUMBER 066 11 7865 A

A DATE OF EACH SERVICE 1982	B PLACE OF SERVICE	C FULLY DESCRIBE SURGICAL OR MEDICAL PROCEDURES AND OTHER SERVICES OR SUPPLIES FURNISHED FOR EACH DATE GIVEN	D NATURE OF ILLNESS OR INJURY REQUIRING SERVICES OR SUPPLIES (DIAGNOSIS)	E CHARGES
07/21	IH	Initial History and Physical #90220	Subacute bacterial endocarditis	$ 100.00
07/22 to 08/13	IH	Ext. visits (23) @ $35/visit #90250		805.00
08/14	IH	Complete cardiac re-evaluation #90270		60.00
08/15 to 09/11	IH	Ext. visits (27) @ $35/visit #90250		945.00
			TOTAL	$1910.00

O - DOCTOR'S OFC.
IH - INPATIENT - HOSP.
OH - OUTPATIENT - HOSP.

H - PATIENT'S HOME
OL - OTHER LOCATION (SPECIFIED IN C)

NH - NURSING HOME
ECF - EXTENDED CARE FACILITY

PATIENT CLAIM COPY

FIGURE 17–4 Patient can submit his own claim to Medicare when billed on this form. (Courtesy of the Colwell Co., Champaign, Illinois.)

the form. In this situation Medicare sends its payment to the patient. The doctor bills the patient for the full amount of the fee.

Claims for Medicare must be filed by December 31 of the year following that in which services were rendered. Care received in 1980 must be billed no later than December 31, 1981. If the patient had his first covered services during the last three months of any year, the cost of these services may be applied to the deductible for the following year.

Medicare patients are particularly appreciative of your assistance in preparing claim forms. In addition to the public relations value, an advantage of submitting claims directly is that supportive documents, such as operation reports, x-ray reports, and so forth, may be attached.

MEDICAID. Some patients who qualify for Medicare will still be unable to pay the portion for which they are responsible. They may qualify for aid from a public welfare agency.

Title XIX of Public Law 89–97, under the Social Security Amendments of 1965, provides for agreements with states for assistance from the federal government in providing health care for the medically indigent. All states and the District of Columbia have Medicaid programs, but there may be wide variations among them.

Eligibility for benefits is determined by the respective states. The state also determines the type and extent of medical care that will be covered. A card showing proof of eligibility is usually issued to the beneficiary on a monthly basis. The dates of issuance will vary, but the medical assistant should always check the patient's current card or coupon to establish the fact of current coverage. This is sometimes referred to as proof of eligibility.

At the federal level the administration of the Medicaid program is handled by the Social and Rehabilitation Service of the Department of Health and Human Services. Direction at the state level is usually in the Department of Social Welfare.

Billing restrictions and requirements must be followed as directed in each individual state. The physician is free to accept or to refuse to treat a patient under Medicaid. However, if the physician does accept Medicaid patients, the office assistant must continually strive to keep current on Medicaid billing practices and the physician must accept the allowance as payment in full.

WORKER'S COMPENSATION. All state legislatures have passed Worker's Compensation laws to protect wage earners against the loss of wages and the cost of medical care resulting from occupational accident or disease. State laws differ as to the classes of employees included and the benefits provided. None of the states' Worker's Compensation laws cover all employees. However, if a patient says that he was injured during the course of his employment or is suffering from an illness associated with his work, the medical assistant should check with the patient's employer to verify the insurance coverage.

Compensation benefits include medical care benefits, weekly income replacement benefits for temporary disability, permanent disability settlements, and survivor benefits where applicable. The provider of service (doctor, hospital, therapist, and so forth) accepts the Worker's Compensation payment as payment in full and does not bill the patient.

Time limitations are set forth for the prompt reporting of Worker's Compensation cases. The employee is obligated to promptly notify the employer; the employer in turn must notify the insurance company and must refer the employee to a source of medical care. In some states the employer and the insurance company have the right to select the physician who will treat the patient. In essence, the purpose of Worker's Compensation laws is to provide prompt medical care to the injured or ill worker so that he may be restored to health and return to full earning capacity in as short a time as possible.

The physician who sees the injured worker first will complete what may be called the Doctor's First Report of Work Injury within the time limit imposed by state regulations (Fig. 17–5). The insurance company will usually require at least two copies, one copy will go to the state regulatory body, the employer may get a copy, and one file copy should remain with the physician. The assistant who types the report should make a minimum of five copies. This report must be personally signed by the physician and should contain the following information:

1. The history of the case as obtained from the patient, noting any preexisting injuries or diseases.
2. The patient's symptoms and physical complaints.
3. The complete physical findings, including laboratory and x-ray findings.
4. A tentative diagnosis of the condition.
5. An estimate of the type and extent of the disability. Where permanent disability has resulted, there should be a very careful survey, and the extent of disability given in detail.
6. Treatment that is indicated, including type, frequency, and duration. It may be necessary to attach a letter giving more detailed information to assist in making an evaluation of the case.
7. Whenever possible, the date the patient may be able to return to work, if he has been totally disabled.

In severe or prolonged cases, supplemental reports should be sent to the insurance carrier at least once a month (Fig. 17–6). At the termination of treatment, a final report and bill are sent to the insurance carrier. DO NOT BILL THE PATIENT.

Keep Separate Records. The records for Worker's Compensation cases, sometimes referred to as industrial cases, preferably should be separated from the physician's regular patient histories.

If the patient who is seen for an industrial injury has previously been treated as a private patient, a new chart and ledger should be started to be used only for the treatment rendered under conditions of the Worker's Compensation law. The insurance carrier may request and is entitled to receive copies of all records pertaining to the industrial injury but not the records of a private patient. There may be a lawsuit or a hearing before a referee or Appeals Board for which records are subpoenaed. If separate records are kept, there is no question of privilege involved.

LIFE INSURANCE

When an individual whom the physician is treating or has treated in the past makes application for life insurance, the insuring company naturally wants to know the current state of the applicant's health and any significant previous history.

In order to get an account of the applicant's current health, the insurance company authorizes one or more physicians in each community to perform physical examinations of prospective clients. The examining physician will make a report to the insurance company following the examination. The insurance agent arranges the applicant's appointment for the physical examination — and he will probably want the appointment as soon as possible so that his prospect doesn't get away! The insurance company, or its agent, will supply the necessary forms for completion. The company may require that the forms be completed in the doctor's own handwriting, but the assistant will make certain the forms are on hand at the time of the appointment. She may want to double check the form before mailing it, to be certain no details have been overlooked. The insurance company pays the physician a stipulated fee upon receipt of the report.

For a summary of the applicant's previous history, the agent asks the applicant to supply the names and addresses of any physicians consulted in the past. The company, in turn, will request reports from these physicians. Your employer may receive a request for such information concerning a previous patient. Before completing the form, make certain the applicant has signed an authorization for

DOCTOR'S FIRST REPORT OF WORK INJURY

STATE OF CALIFORNIA
DEPARTMENT OF INDUSTRIAL RELATIONS
DIVISION OF LABOR STATISTICS AND RESEARCH
P. O. Box 965, San Francisco, Calif. 94101

Immediately after first examination mail one copy **directly** to the Division of Labor Statistics and Research. Failure to file a report with the Division is a misdemeanor. (Labor Code, Sections 6407-6413.) Answer all questions fully.

A. INSURANCE CARRIER State Compensation Insurance Fund

Do not write in this space

1. **EMPLOYER** Jones Hardware
2. Address (No., St. & City) 750 Tenth Street, San Francisco, CA 94100
3. Business (Manufacturing shoes, building construction, retailing men's clothes, etc.) retail store
4. **EMPLOYEE** (First name, middle initial, last name) John J. Doe **Soc. Sec. No.** 000-00-0000
5. Address (No., St. & City) 234 -11th Street, San Francisco, CA 94100
6. Occupation clerk **Age** 40 **Sex** M
7. Date injured 10/13/82 **Hour** 3 P.M. **Date last worked** same
8. Injured at (No., St. & City) 750 Tenth Street, San Francisco **County** San Francisco
9. Date of your first examination 10/13/82 **Hour** 5 P.M. **Who engaged your services?** employer
10. Name other doctors who treated employee for this injury none
11. **ACCIDENT OR EXPOSURE:** Did employee notify employer of this injury? yes **Employee's statement** of cause of injury or illness:
    Fell from ladder a distance of four feet to the floor. Twisted right ankle.
12. **NATURE AND EXTENT OF INJURY OR DISEASE** (Include all objective findings, subjective complaints, and diagnoses. If occupational disease state date of onset, occupational history, and exposures.)
    Simple fracture lateral malleolus rt. ankle - undisplaced.
13. X-rays: By whom taken? (State if none) St. Martha's Hospital
    Findings: as above
14. Treatment:
    Short leg cast applied - no anesthesia
15. Kind of case (Office, home or hospital) office **If hospitalized, date** **Estimated stay**
    Name and address of hospital
16. Further treatment (Estimated frequency and duration) weekly
17. Estimated period of disability for: Regular work 3 months **Modified work** 6 weeks
18. Describe any permanent disability or disfigurement expected (State if none) none
19. If death ensued, give date
20. **REMARKS** (Note any pre-existing injuries or diseases, need for special examination or laboratory tests, other pertinent information.)

Name Friend Hunton (Type or print) Degree M.D. [PERSONAL SIGNATURE OF DOCTOR] Friend Hunton M.D.

Date of report 10/14/82 Address (No., St. & City) 450 Sutter Street, San Francisco, CA 94100

FORM 5021 *Use reverse side if more space required* 87938-607 10-65 600M OSP

FIGURE 17–5 First report of work injury.

DOCTOR'S FINAL (OR MONTHLY) REPORT AND BILL

Itemized bills, IN DUPLICATE, are to be submitted at the termination of the case.
Monthly statements are POSITIVELY required on cases under treatment.
Mail to State Compensation Insurance Fund Address 525 Golden Gate Avenue, San Francisco
Services beginning late in month and extending into succeeding month may be itemized on one statement.

EMPLOYER Jones Hardware, 750 Tenth Street, San Francisco, CA 94100
EMPLOYEE John J. Doe Social Security # 000-00-0000
DATE OF INJURY 10/13/82 SERVICES FOR MONTH OF October, 19 82

Patient refused treatment -- , 19
Patient stopped treatment without orders -- , 19
Patient entered hospital -- , 19
Patient able to return to work -- , 19
Patient discharged as cured -- , 19
Condition at time of last visit convalescent

Any other charges authorized such as Drugs? -- (Check) Hospital? -- (Check)

Code: O—Office; V—Home Visit; H—Hospital Visit; N—Night Visit; S—Operation; X—X-Ray.

Month	1	2	3	4	5	6	7	8	9	10	11	12	13	14	15	16	17	18	19	20	21	22	23	24	25	26	27	28	29	30	31
Oct													S														O				

Totals

First aid treatment (describe) $
Office Visits 10/27/82 CRVS #90060 $ 12.00
Home Visits $
Hospital Visits $
Operations 10/13/82 Short leg walking cast CRVS #29425 $ 40.00
MATERIAL (Itemized at cost) $

TOTAL $ 52.00

Any charges shown above which are in excess of the minimum fee must be explained below regarding nature of such services, indicating the date rendered.

Make check payable to:

Doctor Friend Hunton
Address 450 Sutter Street, San Francisco
Signature Friend Hunton MD
Date October 31, 1982

FIGURE 17–6 Monthly statement for Worker's Compensation.

release of information. The request form usually has a voucher check for a minimal fee attached. The physician may accept the proffered fee or, if he deems it inadequate, may bill the insurance company for "balance of fee." If it is reasonable, it will be paid without question.

THE PROCESSING OF INSURANCE CLAIMS

Understanding the correct procedures for the completion and filing of insurance claims is extremely important for the medical office assistant. A majority of patients will have some kind of insurance coverage, and many of them will have no idea how to make the claim. The office assistant who can handle this efficiently will have better collections as well as better public relations (Fig. 17–7). Since few policies will cover all medical charges, it may be necessary to bill the patient as well as the insurance company. Generally it will not be necessary to bill the patient who has a service-type policy or Medicaid or who is being treated under Worker's Compensation. Most others will have a deductible and/or copayment provision requiring some payment from the patient.

The required forms should be completed as soon as possible after service is rendered. Many times payment to an assisting surgeon, anesthesiologist, radiologist, or consultant is delayed until the attending physician's statement is received. A patient's loss of income protection payment is also delayed until the physician's statement is processed. This, in turn, could delay payment to the physician from the patient.

UNIVERSAL CLAIM FORM. The Universal Claim Form has now evolved from the Simplified Claim Forms that were developed by the Health Insurance Council (HIC) in cooperation with the American Medical Association (AMA) and gradually refined over the years. The Universal Claim Form is accepted by most commercial insurance companies, the Blue plans, and in many cases by government-sponsored insurance. It contains all essential information for processing a claim; it is simple to complete; and if the physician will give the patient a statement that includes the essential information, the claim form can be completed by most patients (Fig. 17–8).

SUPERBILL. One method of supplying insurance information to the patient is by use of what has become known as the superbill. This is a record that is generated at the time of service and includes all essential information for billing the patient or his insurance: date of services, description of services with treatment codes, fees for services, patient's personal data, and name, address, and identification number of the provider. If billing is done by the physician's office, a copy of the superbill can simply be attached to the insurance form. Many providers totally eliminate insurance billing by preparing the superbill in multiple copies that are either handed to the patient upon completion of service or mailed with instructions for the patient to use this form in billing for his insurance.

INSURANCE CARRIER Name & Address	Department and Individual to Contact	POLICYHOLDER Indiv to Contact	Group or Policy Number	SPECIAL NOTES
BLUE SHIELD P O BOX 12345 Anytown, USA	Tom Jones Professional Relations 123-456-7890	Aerospace Industries Joan Crawford 123-888-3030	AI-89037	Tom Jones will speak to groups or give personal assistance in office
		Bell Burgers Nancy Donovan 123-465-2210	BB-3415Z	Scheduled Benefits
OCCIDENTAL P O BOX 42873 Anytown, USA	Cathy Redding Claims Dept. 213-440-3131	Town School Dist. Mary Embers 312-055-3210	Group No. 4414	Does not pay for assistant surgeon

FIGURE 17–7 A page from the procedure manual. Insurance problems can be diminished by knowing who to contact at the insurance carrier and the policyholder.

THIS FORM TO BE USED TO BILL **BLUE CROSS OF SOUTHERN CALIFORNIA** OR **BLUE SHIELD OF CALIFORNIA ONLY.**
PLEASE VERIFY WITH YOUR PATIENT THE CORRECT ORGANIZATION TO BILL.

READ INSTRUCTIONS BEFORE COMPLETING OR SIGNING THIS FORM

TYPE OR PRINT ☐ MEDICARE ☐ MEDI-CAL ☒ STANDARD   Connecticut General

PATIENT & INSURED (SUBSCRIBER) INFORMATION

1. PATIENT'S NAME *(First name, middle initial, last name)*: Richard DeWitt
2. PATIENT'S DATE OF BIRTH: 01 23 18
3. INSURED'S NAME *(First name, middle initial, last name)*: same
4. PATIENT'S ADDRESS *(Street, city, state, ZIP code)*: 837 North Harbor Boulevard, Irvine, CA 92714
5. PATIENT'S SEX: MALE x FEMALE
6. INSURED'S I.D. NO., MEDICARE NO. AND/OR MEDICAID NO. *(include any letters)*: 333 22 4444
7. PATIENT'S RELATIONSHIP TO INSURED: SELF x SPOUSE CHILD OTHER
8. INSURED'S GROUP NO. *(Or Group Name)*: California Bean Growers
9. OTHER HEALTH INSURANCE COVERAGE - Enter Name of Policyholder and Plan Name and Address and Policy or Medical Assistance Number: ------
10. WAS CONDITION RELATED TO:
    A. PATIENT'S EMPLOYMENT: YES NO x
    B. AN AUTO ACCIDENT: YES NO x
11. INSURED'S ADDRESS *(Street, city, state, ZIP code)*: same
12. PATIENT'S OR AUTHORIZED PERSON'S SIGNATURE *(Read back before signing)*
    I Authorize the Release of any Medical Information Necessary to Process this Claim and Request Payment of MEDICARE Benefits Either to Myself or to the Party Who Accepts Assignment Below
    SIGNED DATE
13. *I AUTHORIZE PAYMENT OF MEDICAL BENEFITS TO UNDERSIGNED PHYSICIAN OR SUPPLIER FOR SERVICE DESCRIBED BELOW*
    SIGNED *(Insured or Authorized Person)*

PHYSICIAN OR SUPPLIER INFORMATION

14. DATE OF: 07 12 81 ◄ ILLNESS (FIRST SYMPTOM) OR INJURY (ACCIDENT) OR PREGNANCY (LMP)
15. DATE FIRST CONSULTED YOU FOR THIS CONDITION: 07 15 81
16. HAS PATIENT EVER HAD SAME OR SIMILAR SYMPTOMS? YES NO x
17. DATE PATIENT ABLE TO RETURN TO WORK: 07 26 81
18. DATES OF TOTAL DISABILITY: FROM 07 12 81 THROUGH 07 25 81
    DATES OF PARTIAL DISABILITY: FROM THROUGH
19. NAME AND ADDRESS OF REFERRING PHYSICIAN OR OTHER SOURCE
20. FOR SERVICES RELATED TO HOSPITALIZATION GIVE HOSPITALIZATION DATES: ADMITTED 07 15 81 DISCHARGED 07 17 81
21. NAME & ADDRESS OF FACILITY WHERE SERVICES RENDERED *(If other than home or office)*: St. John's Hospital, Santa Monica, California
22. WAS LABORATORY WORK PERFORMED OUTSIDE YOUR OFFICE? YES NO x CHARGES:
23. DIAGNOSIS OR NATURE OF ILLNESS OR INJURY, RELATE DIAGNOSIS TO PROCEDURE IN COLUMN D BY REFERENCE TO NUMBERS 1, 2, 3, ETC. OR DX CODE
    1. Leg pain
    2.
    3.
    4.

    ☐ FAMILY PLANNING SERVICE

24. A DATE OF SERVICE			B* PLACE OF SERVICE	PROCEDURE NUMBER (RVS NUMBER / SMA NUMBER)	UNIT MODIFIER	C FULLY DESCRIBE PROCEDURES, MEDICAL SERVICES OR SUPPLIES FURNISHED FOR EACH DATE GIVEN (EXPLAIN UNUSUAL SERVICES OR CIRCUMSTANCES)	D DIAGNOSIS CODE	E CHARGES	F LEAVE BLANK
07	15	81	3	90050		Office visit limited exam	1	20 00	
07	15	81	1	90220		Init hosp care compr HPX	1	100 00	
07	16	81	1	90215		Hosp visit intermed exam	1	30 00	
07	17	81	1	90275		Hosp visit w/discharge	1	35 00	

25. SIGNATURE OF PHYSICIAN OR SUPPLIER
    I certify under penalty of perjury that the foregoing is true and correct (read back before signing).
    SIGNED DATE
26. ACCEPT ASSIGNMENT *(Government claims only)* SEE BACK: YES NO
27. TOTAL CHARGE: 185 00
28. AMOUNT PAID
29. BALANCE DUE
30. YOUR SOCIAL SECURITY NO.: 111-22-3333
31. PHYSICIAN'S OR SUPPLIER'S NAME, ADDRESS, PROVIDER NUMBER, ZIP CODE & TELEPHONE NO.:
    ROBERT O ELAM MD
    300 NORTH BROADWAY
    LOS ANGELES CA 90005
32. YOUR PATIENT'S ACCOUNT NO.
33. YOUR EMPLOYER I.D. NO.: 95-1234567

*PLACE OF SERVICE CODES

1 – (IH) – INPATIENT HOSPITAL	7 – (ICF) – INTERMEDIATE CARE FACILITY
2 – (OH) – OUTPATIENT HOSPITAL	8 – (SNF) – SKILLED NURSING FACILITY
3 – (O) – DOCTOR'S OFFICE	9 – – AMBULANCE
4 – (H) – PATIENT'S HOME	O – (OL) – OTHER LOCATIONS
5 – – DAY CARE FACILITY (PSY)	A – (IL) – INDEPENDENT LABORATORY
6 – – NIGHT CARE FACILITY (PSY)	B – – OTHER MEDICAL/SURGICAL FACILITY

C 4359

FIGURE 17–8 Universal Claim Form, Standard Insurance.

1

SYSTEMATIZING CLAIM PREPARATION

Whenever you find medical assistants "talking shop," a frequent topic of discussion is insurance claims. It is not always just the volume of forms that causes problems. Failure to systematize the work, procrastination, failure to keep informed, and possibly an unconscious resentment contribute to the undesirable situation. Simplification of claim forms has eliminated much of the burden. With the right attitude and an efficient system, insurance billing need not be a cause for concern. It is certainly less troublesome than billing an account for several months, then writing a series of collection letters, and perhaps eventually having to resort to third-party collection procedures, with a considerable loss in income. If the volume of insurance is so great that the office assistant using efficient systematized procedures cannot keep up-to-date, then the practical physician will hire extra help for this purpose. The collection potential in most medical practices is increased in proportion to the proper handling of the patients' insurance. Therefore, it behooves the medical office assistant and the physician to give proper attention to the processing of the claims.

WHO IS RESPONSIBLE? The receptionist, the medical assistant, the bookkeeper, the insurance clerk, the nurse, the doctor — anyone who treats the patient, keeps records, or handles the telephone or appointments plays a role in insurance claims.

The processing of insurance claims begins with the receptionist. When the first appointment is made, she can ask the patient to bring along all insurance information and any special forms. If the patient has an identification card, the receptionist should first determine that the coverage is current, then photocopy the card for the office record. If more than one insurance is involved, get information for ALL companies.

It is important to obtain complete and accurate information on every new patient, including:

1. Full name, address, and telephone number
2. Date of birth
3. Occupation
4. Name, address, and telephone number of employer
5. Social Security number
6. Driver's license number
7. Name and address of insurance carrier
8. Group and member numbers, or policy number
9. Name and address of subscriber if other than patient
10. Other health insurance coverage, if any
11. Name and address of referring physician, if any
12. Photocopy of identification card, if any

Insurance information can change. For continuing patients, the receptionist should recheck insurance coverage every six months or so. Date-stamp forms as they are received, and keep a log of all insurance forms (Fig. 17–9). A log such as this will enable you to tell an inquiring patient immediately whether or not his claim form has been completed and mailed.

The doctor, office nurse, or medical assistant is responsible for the complete and accurate reporting of diagnosis and services performed. Unless the full information is on the chart, the insurance clerk cannot do her work well.

The person who does the bookkeeping must post the charges promptly and accurately.

COMPLETING THE FORMS. The importance of systematizing the processing of claims cannot be overemphasized. The work will be much easier if the following points are observed:

1. A definite time is set aside for this task.
2. There is a central location for all insurance forms.
3. The necessary manuals, code books, and other references are nearby.
4. The superbill or Universal Claim Form is used as often as possible.

INSURANCE CLAIM FORMS			
PATIENT	INSURANCE CO.	DATE IN	DATE OUT
James Bush	Continental Casualty	3-14	3-15
Virginia Ellis	Aetna Life	3-14	3-15
Robert Haskell	Occidental	3-15	3-15
Mary Blodgett	Travelers	"	3-15
Stan Wilson	Prudential	"	3-15
" "	[illegible]	"	3-15
Wm. Price	County Employees Group	3-16	3-18 returned to pt.
Earl Jacoby	Fireman's Fund	"	3-17
Mary Frederick	Aetna Casualty	"	3-17

FIGURE 17–9 Insurance log.

17

5. Forms are completed by category (all Blue Cross, all Medicare, and so forth).

6. Tabulator stops are set for the form being completed. (Make a note of where these stops are so they can be easily found when doing the same kind of form again.)

REASONS FOR CLAIM REJECTION. Many complaints made against insurance companies are not the fault of the companies but of the individuals completing the claim forms. The company processors are not mind readers; the claim form must be sufficiently detailed, complete, and accurate. Perhaps recounting some of the reasons for claim rejection will emphasize this point.

1. Diagnosis is missing, or incomplete, or does not correspond with treatment performed.
2. Charges are not itemized.
3. Patient's group, member, or policy number is missing or incorrect.
4. Patient's portion of form is incomplete or unsigned.
5. Birth date is missing.
6. Doctor's name or address is missing.
7. Dates are incorrect.
8. Claim form is not signed.

GUIDELINES FOR THE INSURANCE CLERK

When the patient brings in his insurance form, check to see that his portion has been completed and signed.

With the doctor's approval, have the patient sign *Assignment of Benefits* (Fig. 17–10) and *Authorization to Release Information* (Fig 17–11) on first visit.

Typewrite all claim forms and keep a copy (either carbon or photocopy).

If insured's statement is on a separate page from the physician's statement, photocopy the insured's completed page. Then use the reverse side of the photocopy for a carbon copy of the physician's statement. You then will have complete information and only one sheet of paper to add to your record.

Use standard nomenclature in diagnosis and procedure. If your state does not have a procedure code book, use *The Physician's Current Procedural Terminology*, published by the American Medical Association, or *International Classification of*

ASSIGNMENT OF INSURANCE BENEFITS

I, the undersigned represent that I have insurance coverage with and do hereby authorize __________ (NAME OF COMPANY) to pay and assign directly to __________ (NAME OF DOCTOR) all surgical and/or medical benefits, if any, otherwise payable to me for services as described on the attached forms hereof, but not to exceed the charges for those services. I understand that I am financially responsible for all charges whether or not paid by said insurance. I hereby authorize said assignee to release all information necessary to secure the payment of said benefits.

Date __________ Signed __________

FIGURE 17–10 Assignment of Benefits form.

RECORDS RELEASE

DATE __________

TO __________
DOCTOR

____
ADDRESS

I HEREBY AUTHORIZE AND REQUEST YOU TO RELEASE

TO __________
DOCTOR

____
ADDRESS

THE COMPLETE MEDICAL RECORDS IN YOUR POSSESSION, CONCERNING MY ILLNESS AND/OR TREATMENT DURING THE PERIOD FROM __________ TO __________

SIGNED __________
(PATIENT OR NEAREST RELATIVE)

____
WITNESS

RELATIONSHIP __________

FORM 122 - EASTMAN, INC.

FIGURE 17–11 Release of Medical Information form.

Diseases, 9th revision, Clinical Modification (ICD-9-CM), published by The Commission on Professional and Hospital Activities in the United States.

List ALL procedures performed — one procedure per line. Be specific. If a laceration is treated, give location, length and depth, number of sutures required, and time of treatment involved. If a sterile surgical tray was used for office surgery, itemize and bill as a separate fee. If a treatment injection was given, state injected material and amount given.

Attach a copy of x-ray report, hospital report, or consultant's report in complicated cases.

State usual and customary fee on all claim forms, regardless of what payment is expected.

Never alter a claim as to services performed, date of service, or fees established.

If more than one visit per day is required, state the times of day so that the claims processor will know they were separate procedures.

Fill in ALL blanks. Type "DNA" (does not apply) or "NA" (not applicable) or simple dash lines (----) rather than leave an item blank. This prevents possible tampering, and is an added assurance that the item was not overlooked.

Note on the copy the date and to whom the form was mailed.

Process all claims promptly and cheerfully.

ANSWERING PATIENTS' QUESTIONS ABOUT INSURANCE. Many times patients will ask questions about their policies and the extent of coverage. The assistant should be familiar with basic information about health insurance but should refrain from attempting to interpret specific contracts, since there may be many unknown factors that will have a bearing on benefits. Suggest that the patient take his policy or questions to his local insurance representative for detailed answers to his questions. If the policy is one held by an employees' group in a large company, the employer or the insurance clerk can probably answer the question.

Blue Cross and Blue Shield representatives may call at the office from time to time. In many areas, representatives hold special meetings for doctors' assistants in order to familiarize them with insurance forms and the types of coverage offered. The medical office assistant should attend such meetings in order to keep current on insurance practices.

Since she understands the need for health insurance, the medical assistant should be enthusiastic about its success. Today it is economically disastrous to be without medical insurance. Any patient who does not have insurance should be encouraged to purchase it. The medical assistant should be cautious about recommending a specific carrier, but can give general advice such as:

1. Purchasing from a recognized carrier
2. Reading the policy carefully or having a trusted friend or advisor read it
3. Not expecting "total" coverage
4. Knowing how claims will be handled
5. Understanding any deductibles or copayment clauses
6. Inquiring about cancellation or guaranteed renewable provisions
7. Checking policy limitations.

Cheap insurance is available, but it is no bargain since it gives limited coverage. Policies are available for moderate sums that may provide the coverage suitable for the individual's particular need.

AVOIDING INSURANCE ABUSE. When patients or physicians abuse health insurance, premiums for the insurance inevitably rise. No physician should send a patient to the hospital just for the patient's or the physician's convenience. Few plans cover diagnostic work. Furthermore, there are many procedures that can be done in the office with safety and efficiency, and at considerably lower cost than in the hospital. Procedures that would benefit from the additional safety of a hospital but do not require an overnight stay may be scheduled in the outpatient department. Inclusion of outpatient services in insurance coverage helps to eliminate overutilization of hospital services. Many hospitals have a utilization committee that guards against unnecessary admissions. The medical assistant who understands the regulations and can explain them to the patient can promote the compliance and goodwill of the patient.

INSURANCE TERMINOLOGY

Allocated Benefits. Payments provided in some policies for certain specified hospital services such as x-rays and drugs, up to a maximum amount.

Assignment of Insurance Benefits. To facilitate prompt payment of bills, a medical assistant should have the patient sign an assignment of insurance benefits form. This form is often provided by the insurance company, or a standard form from a printer may be used. Some offices use a rubber stamp. The assignment authorizes the insurance company to make direct payment of benefits to the physician. Most insurance companies honor these assignments.

Beneficiary. The person receiving the benefits of the policy is the beneficiary; the term usually refers to the policy owner, who may sometimes be called the subscribing member or the enrolled member, rather than to the dependents. (In a life insurance policy the beneficiary is one receiving the proceeds in the event of the death of the policy owner.)

Certificate of Insurance. A document containing information regarding the master policy of a group, indicating that the individual is covered thereunder.

Claim. This is a demand to the insurer by the insured person for the payment of benefits under a policy.

Coinsurance (Copayment). A policy provision, frequently found in major medical insurance, by which both the insured person and the insurer share in a specified ratio the hospital and medical expenses resulting from an illness or injury.

Coordination of Benefits. (see Nonduplication of Benefits).

Deductible. Many policies, especially major medical policies, carry a deductible clause, which states that the insuring company will pay the expenses incurred after the insured has paid a specified amount. This amount ranges from $50 to $500, depending on how the contract is written.

Disability. It is said that disability exists when illness or injury makes an individual unable to be employed, either partially or totally. Total disability is the inability of the insured to perform any duties of his occupation. Partial disability is the inability to perform a part of one's occupation; there may be a partial loss of income. The insured may do limited duties, with shortened hours or lighter work. Both total disability and partial disability may be considered "temporary" disability. Temporary disability exists when the insured expects to return to work and regain earning power. Permanent disability, on the other hand, is expected to continue for the person's lifetime. These disability terms are important when reporting Worker's Compensation cases or in the case of cash settlements.

Dismemberment. The loss of a limb or sight.

Effective Date. This is the date the coverage starts to take effect. There may be a probationary period; that is, a specific number of days during which no coverage will be available for any sickness commencing during this period. There may be a waiting period or a time limitation, during which a policyholder is not entitled to benefits for a year or some other specified length of time for certain preexisting conditions, such as hemorrhoids, hernia, varicose veins, tonsillitis, and adenoiditis.

Eligible Family Members. These include the spouse (husband or wife) and any unmarried children under 18 or 21 (or occasionally 23) years of age. There is usually a waiting period of 14 days to one month for a newborn dependent. A family policy covers all members of a family, as previously stated.

Exclusions (also called Exceptions). Exclusions are specific hazards or conditions listed in the policy for which the policy will not provide benefit payments. Common exclusions include the following: sickness or accident resulting from warfare, suicide or self-inflicted injury, air travel on nonscheduled flights, any sickness or injury covered by Worker's Compensation or cared for in a government hospital such as a VA Hospital, and the services of a dentist or oral surgeon. Some policies exclude any illness or injury connected with pregnancy, hernia, or cosmetic surgery; certain major diseases such as tuberculosis may also be excluded.

Fee Schedule. A list of services or procedures indemnified by the company and the specific dollars that will be paid for each service.

Health Maintenance Organization (HMO). An organization that provides for a wide range of comprehensive health care services for a specified group at a fixed periodic payment. The HMO can be sponsored by the government, medical schools, hospitals, employers, labor unions, consumer groups, insurance companies, physicians, and hospital-medical plans.

Indemnity. A benefit paid by an insurer for a loss insured under a policy.

Independent Practice Association (IPA). A prepaid group practice sponsored by independently practicing physicians who continue to practice in their own offices. Most IPA–HMOs operate on a fee-for-service basis, just like an ordinary private practice. Fees for members are billed directly to the IPA rather than to the patient, and a percentage may be discounted to meet the plan's contingencies. Fees for nonmembers are handled the same as any fee for service.

Insurance Clause. The clause that indicates the parties to a health insurance contract, sets forth the type of loss covered, and broadly defines the benefits to be paid.

Lapse. This is termination of a policy upon the policyholder's failure to pay the premium within the time required.

Loss of Income Benefits. Payments made to an insured person to help replace income lost through inability to work because of an insured disability.

Member Physician. A medical doctor who has joined a group or enrolled with the insurance company and has agreed to accept the contracts. He will meet certain obligations of the contract, such as accepting the insurance benefits as payment in full for care of persons receiving less than a certain income.

Nondisabling Injury. One that may require medical care but does not result in loss of working time or income.

Nonduplication of Benefits. Most group insurance plans have the nonduplication of benefits provision, which is also known as a coordination of benefits provision (double coverage). Its purposes are to prevent the available benefits from exceeding the covered medical expenses and also to prevent increase in insurance costs. It is important to identify the primary carrier, as it will be the first to pay benefits.

Other Benefits. These benefits are specified in each instance and often include x-ray, laboratory, anesthesiologist, and assistant surgeon. Some provide benefits for drugs, oxygen, and blood. The contract may read that the insurance company will pay the first $15 to $25 and then one-half of all additional charges, which are usually limited to drugs or other benefits supplied and used while in the hospital.

Patient Status. There are frequently stipulations of payment for procedures if a patient is an inpatient or outpatient. An inpatient is one who is registered as a bed patient in a hospital; he has been admitted to the hospital and is considered a resident of the institution. An outpatient is one who is receiving the services of the hospital but is not a registered bed patient; he does not stay overnight and is not considered a resident of the institution.

Preexisting Condition. A physical condition of an insured person that existed prior to the issuance of his policy.

Premium. The periodic payment required to keep a policy in force.

Prepaid Group Practice Plan (PGP). A plan under which specified health services are rendered by participating physicians to an enrolled group of persons, with fixed periodic payment in advance made by or on behalf of each person or family. If a health insurance carrier is involved, it contracts to pay in advance for the full range of health services to which the insured is entitled under the terms of the health insurance contract. Such a plan is one form of a Health Maintenance Organization (HMO).

Professional Standards Review Organization (PSRO). A group of physicians working with the government to review cases for hospital admission and discharge under government guidelines. This process is sometimes referred to as Peer Review.

Probationary Period. A specified number of days after the date of the issuance of the policy during which coverage is not afforded for sickness. The purpose of the period is to eliminate coverage for sickness actually contracted before the policy went into force.

Proration. The adjustment of benefits paid because of a mistake in the amount of the premiums paid or the existence of other insurance covering the same accident or disability.

Reinstatement. The resumption of coverage under a policy that has lapsed.

Release of Medical Information Form. A form that authorizes the release of medical information to the insurance company or allows the hospital to release information.

Rider. A legal document that modifies the protection of a policy, either expanding or decreasing its benefits, or adding or excluding certain conditions from the policy's coverage.

Service Benefit. An insurance benefit that fully pays for the specific hospital or medical care services rendered.

Termination Conversion. Most group policies stop coverage when an employee terminates his employment or association with the group. One of the most important benefits given to the person terminating from an insured group is the right to convert from the group plan to an individual plan. In some cases the insuring company agrees, subject to the desire of the individual, to continue coverage of the employee after he retires or is not employed, but usually with a change in benefits: either the premiums are increased or the benefits are decreased. The employee no longer has the protection of the group and is issued an individual policy.

Usual and Customary Fee. Some insurance plans do not publish a fee schedule but agree to pay all or a percentage of the usual and customary fee for any given procedure. The usual fee is the charge a physician makes to his private patients. The customary fee is one that is within the range of the usual fees charged by physicians in the same geographic and socioeconomic area and by physicians with similar training and experience.

CHAPTER OUTLINE

Editorial Duties
- The Physician's Library
  - Card Catalog of Books
  - Periodical File
- Preparation of an Abstract
  - Reprints
  - Other Reference Files
  - Diagnostic Files
  - Patients' Library
- Helping to Gather Information
  - Library Facilities
  - Preparing a Bibliography
- Manuscript Preparation
  - Rough Drafts
  - Final Drafts
  - Footnotes
  - Final Bibliography
  - Illustrations
  - Revision
  - Mailing the Manuscript
  - Proofreading
  - Indexing
  - Reprints
  - Speeches

Meeting and Travel Arrangements
- Meeting Calendars
- Transportation Arrangements
- Meeting Responsibilities
  - Agenda
  - Minutes

BEHAVIORAL OBJECTIVES

The medical office assistant should be able to:

- **Assist the physician in maintaining a personal library.**
- **Assist in the preparation of abstracts.**
- **Help gather information for lectures and manuscripts.**
- **Typewrite and proofread manuscripts suitable for publication.**
- **Prepare and maintain a meeting calendar.**
- **Assist with transportation arrangements.**
- **Prepare an agenda.**
- **Typewrite minutes of meetings.**

18

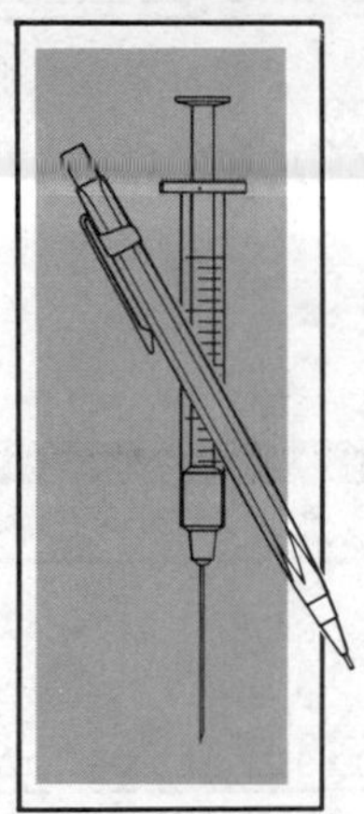

EDITORIAL DUTIES, MEETING AND TRAVEL ARRANGEMENTS

EDITORIAL DUTIES

The practicing medical assistant is well aware of the difficulties of keeping up with the changes in medicine. Medical progress is so rapid that the doctor must devise efficient ways of keeping abreast. The medical profession is unique in that the doctor traditionally shares with others, through writing and speaking, the discoveries, information, and observations gained in practice, research, and private study. You, the assistant, can be of immeasurable help if you become proficient in maintaining the doctor's personal library and in assisting with the preparation of articles and speeches.

The Physician's Library

The doctor just starting in practice has the basis of a personal library consisting of books acquired while in medical school. To this he will add new books relating to his special interests and to the inevitable changes that are occurring all the time. He may also accumulate a file of the *Journal of the American Medical Association* (JAMA), the journal of the state medical society, certain specialty journals in his field, trade journals, and even informative material provided by pharmaceutical companies. The individual physician's library may not be large; however, it must be systematically organized so that the contents are quickly accessible.

Libraries must have some plan of organization. In setting up or rearranging a small library, books should be classified by subject groupings that reflect medical specialties. Those dealing with related topics should be placed together. Journals and periodicals are usually arranged alphabetically.

Periodicals should be bound at regular intervals, generally by volume, in order to preserve the individual copies. The doctor's assistant should see to it that copies are bound in a consistent manner, as several different types of bindings present an untidy appearance. Most journals in the medical field publish indexes, either

Medical Office Assistant: Administrative and Clinical, The
5th Edition
Portia M. Frederick and Mary E. Kinn
Philadelphia, W. B. Saunders Company, 1981

Textbook and reference covering all
phases of medical assisting in the
physician's office

Title Card

Medical Assisting

The Medical Office Assistant: Administrative and
Clinical, 5th Edition, Philadelphia, W. B.
Saunders Company, 1981

Portia M. Frederick and Mary E. Kinn

Subject Card

Frederick, Portia M

The Medical Office Assistant: Administrative and
Clinical, 5th Edition, Philadelphia, W. B.
Saunders Company, 1981

1. Medical Assisting 2. Kinn, Mary E., joint author

Author Card

Kinn, Mary E

The Medical Office Assistant: Administrative and
Clinical, 5th Edition, Philadelphia, W. B.
Saunders Company, 1981

1. Medical Assisting 2. Frederick, Portia M., joint author

Author Card

FIGURE 18–1 Title, subject, and author cards for referencing a book in the personal library.

annually, semiannually, or quarterly. Make sure that the index for the copies is bound with them. In most cities the bindings of periodicals can be done locally. The hospital librarian is a good source of information for locating a bookbinder.

CARD CATALOG OF BOOKS. The books in the doctor's library should be indexed in a card catalog or book. A 3 by 5 card file is useful for this purpose. Generally, three or more cards should be prepared for each book: a title card, a subject card, and an author card. Here's how to index a book in this manner, using the book you are reading as an example.

A *title* card should be prepared with the heading *The Medical Office Assistant: Administrative and Clinical.* A *subject* card should be prepared with the heading "Medical Assisting." Two *author* cards should be prepared (Fig. 18–1). The four cards should then be filed either in a lexicographic file (all entries alphabetized together) or in a file divided into sections for title, subject, and author. With such a file and cross-reference system, books can be located very quickly.

PERIODICAL FILE. One of the doctor's greatest difficulties is in keeping up with medical literature. The problem becomes clear when it is pointed out that hundreds of medical and scientific journals are published in English in this country alone each year. The system that a physician uses for examining periodical literature will determine the method of filing periodicals.

It is unlikely that the individual doctor will want to maintain a complete index of all articles appearing in the periodicals he receives. This is a task for a skilled medical librarian. Most doctors do want to keep track of those articles that are of particular interest to them. Abstracts are of great value in the continuing task of keeping abreast of scientific developments.

Preparation of an Abstract

An **abstract** is a kind of summary or **epitome** of a book, paper, or case history. It is brief, indicating the nature of the article and summarizing the most important points and conclusions. The value of abstracts to busy doctors is indicated in this statement by Dr. Lewis J. Moorman:

> "It is obvious that both the general practitioner and the specialist need the help of those who read for the express purpose of sifting, culling, choosing, and epitomizing the pertinent facts for publication. Placing the kernel of medical knowledge stripped of all superfluous verbiage before the busy physician represents a great service."

Many doctors prepare abstracts of the articles that they find of particular value, and in some offices the secretary or medical office assistant is trained to do abstracting for the doctor. An assistant who can prepare a good abstract of an article can save the doctor from reading 10 to 20 pages of the original article and can help focus attention upon information of particular interest in the article.

Abstracts must clearly indicate the nature of the information contained in the article. Each should note any new procedures or revealed facts, as well as results of studies and experiments and conclusions noted. Naturally, the length and character of the article itself will determine the type and length of the abstract. In most scientific articles, the writer himself will summarize his conclusions at the end of the piece. This summary is of great help in preparing an abstract.

These abstracts are typed on cards, with the text of the abstract preceded by the title, surname and initials of the author, name of publication, volume, inclusive page numbers, month, and year. The cards are then filed. If abstract cards are kept, it is not necessary to clip and file the actual articles separately. The journals in which they appear can be kept in the usual alphabetical order.

REPRINTS. When doctors write articles or present papers before scientific meetings, their work is often published in a periodical and reprints of it made available to their colleagues. A portion of each doctor's library is usually composed of a collection of such reprints. In some cases the reprints come into the office unsolicited, owing to the doctor's interest in a particular person's writing in the past;

in other cases, the doctor may request his secretary to write for a particular reprint. Sometimes the doctor may have a special postcard made up for ordering reprints:

Please send me ______ copies of your article,
(title) ______________________________,
which appeared in ______ (publication) ______
______________________, 19______.

______ (Doctor's signature) ______

Other doctors prefer to write personal letters in which they compliment the author upon the excellence of the article and request copies of it for their files. Reprints often present a storage problem in the office, since they are not of uniform size. However, references to these reprints can be placed in the library card file and the reprints themselves placed in a separate drawer.

OTHER REFERENCE FILES. Doctors must have at their fingertips a variety of miscellaneous medical information. For this reason some doctors build up, in addition to periodical and book collections and indexes, a separate reference file of valuable information. Often this consists of pages photocopied from journals or reference books. The material is valuable only if it can be found when needed. The physician and the assistant together may set up a subject index for filing the material and a cross reference card file for locating the material easily. File dividers can be tabbed with the main topics and folders tabbed with subheadings. When an article or item is photocopied, a card is made up with the title of the article, its author, the periodical in which it appeared, and the date of publication placed on the card. The copy of the reference material is then filed in the appropriate folder and the card filed by subject for easy reference. As new developments occur, later articles may be filed and the outdated material discarded.

DIAGNOSTIC FILES. Physicians often draw material for their writing and speaking from the case histories of their own patients. For this reason, many doctors like to set up diagnostic files so that they can quickly pull out information on, for example, the incidence of certain side effects among patients treated with a particular medication. The assistant familiar with basic medical terminology will have no difficulty in maintaining such a file. The system used will vary from office to office, but subject cards generally will carry the name of the disease or surgical procedure, with subheadings for various aspects with the patient's name, diagnosis, and type of treatment listed below. For example, one subject entry might be "blood diseases" with subheadings for anemia, leukemia, toxemia, and so forth. Personal or patient cards will be headed with the patient's name and diagnosis, treatment, prognosis, and miscellaneous information below. By keeping such a file a doctor can readily obtain the charts from his case history file of all patients with a particular condition. This is particularly valuable to physicians who do a great deal of teaching, writing, or research.

PATIENTS' LIBRARY. Many doctors keep a small library of educational information for patients. This library generally contains some books written in language that the average patient can understand and a number of pamphlets and reprints that the patient can take home for his own file. This might include information on such subjects as diabetes, heart disease, skin conditions, danger signals of cancer, lung disease, first aid, and other subjects. This library service saves the doctor considerable time in repeating simple educational information and is generally welcomed by patients.

Helping to Gather Information

The secretary-assistant employed by a doctor who teaches, writes, or speaks frequently can increase her value as an employee by actually assisting him with the preparation of the paper. She may make up a list of references for a particular paper or talk or may even do actual research and preparation of abstracts. Any assistant who is called upon to assume such responsibility must know how to make the best use of the available library and reference facilities.

LIBRARY FACILITIES. Almost every doctor, even though he may be practicing in a rural area, has access to medical libraries. The doctor who practices in a metropolitan area or near a medical center such as a university is particularly fortunate, since these areas offer good library facilities. All general hospitals also maintain medical libraries comprising a basic collection of carefully selected, authoritative medical textbooks and reference works of the latest edition and files of current journals. The Medical Library Association sets standards for member libraries. A physician usually has access to a county society library or can utilize the package library services of his state society. In addition, extension library facilities can be used to obtain information from special supplemental collections. The American Medical Association, for example, and some other specialty societies, offer periodical lending services and package library services to their members. The facilities of the National Library of Medicine can also be used by doctors. The National Library of Medicine has established a system whereby doctors may get materials from a Regional Medical Library Program when information is not available locally. In those instances when the Regional Program cannot satisfy the need, the request is channeled to the National Library of Medicine.

How to Use a Library. All libraries systematically organize the books, periodicals, and other materials in a fairly uniform manner in order that the information be easily located and accessible. The doctor's assistant who finds it necessary to go to a library to do special work should introduce herself to the librarian or her assistant and get an idea of what the library has to offer in the way of materials. At this time she can also learn about the arrangement of materials, privileges, rules, and regulations for use of the library. After a brief discussion, the trained medical librarian usually can suggest shortcuts that are of great help in locating references or doing research.

Card Catalog of Books. All books, monographs, treatises, handbooks, dictionaries, and encyclopedias contained in a library are indexed by author and subject and sometimes by title in the card catalog. This catalog is really an index of the book contents of the library. Cards are arranged alphabetically, with subject, author, and title cards alphabetized in one series, or are alphabetized within separate sections for subject, author, or title.

There are a number of systems for classifying library books. In library procedure, classification means putting together materials on a given subject with related materials placed nearby.

Medical libraries use various classification systems. The Dewey decimal system, used not only in medical but all types of libraries, is sometimes used for arranging medical library collections. This system utilizes decimal numbers to indicate particular subjects and arranges the book collection in numerical sequence for easy location. For example, 616 indicates Pathology, Diseases, Treatment. Here's an example of how the Dewey decimal system works:

616.1	Diseases of the cardiovascular system
616.9	Communicable and other diseases
616.96	Parasitic diseases
616.99	Other general diseases
616.992	Neoplasms and neoplastic diseases

The Library of Congress classification system is also used. This consists of a number of separate, mutually exclusive classifications based upon combination of letters of the alphabet and numerals:

QR: Bacteriology
RD: Surgery
RC 321–431: Diseases of the nervous system

The National Library of Medicine classification system is replacing the Library of Congress system in many medical libraries.

There are some other systems, such as the Boston Medical Library Classification, the Cunningham Classification and the Barnard Classification, which are used by some medical libraries. However, a brief discussion with the librarian and a quick look at the card catalog will generally help acquaint you with the system used.

How the Card Catalog Can Help You Locate Books. No matter what system of classification is used, the main purpose is to help those who use the library to locate volumes quickly. The symbol for the particular book, whether it be a numeral, a letter, or a combination of numerals and letters, appears on the card for the book in the card file. This symbol is called a "classification mark." It also appears on the spine of the volume. To locate a volume, check the (classification) mark on the card and if an open shelf system is used, find that shelf in the library where corresponding symbols appear. If a closed shelf system is used in the library, give the number of the book and its title to the librarian and she will locate it for you.

Using Periodical Reference Books. The bulk of current medical literature appears in medical periodicals and journals. Some reference system for these hundreds of articles is necessary. In medical libraries at least three indexes are available to help researchers and others locate various periodical references: the *Cumulative Index Medicus,* the *Current List of Medical Literature,* and the *Cumulative Index to Hospital Literature.*

A monthly *Index Medicus* and the annual *Cumulative Index Medicus* are published by the National Library of Medicine. An author and subject index to periodicals in many languages is contained in the volumes, along with a list of new medical books published recently.

The National Library of Medicine has developed two bibliographic retrieval systems, MEDLARS and AIM-TWX. According to Wilhelm Moll, Director, Medical Center Library, University of Virginia, Charlottesville, in a letter appearing in *Library Journal,* March 1, 1972:

> . . . MEDLARS (or Medical Literature Analysis and Retrieval System) has been operating for eight years. It is a computer-based system in operation at the National Library of Medicine designed to achieve rapid bibliographical access to the library's store of information. Becoming operational in January 1964 with the publication of the first computer-produced issue of *Index Medicus,* the system has been turning out the monthly and annually cumulated indexes to the world's (approximately 2500) biomedical journals. It also makes possible retrospective demand bibliographical searches, recurring bibliographies on specialized subjects, and a host of other important bibliographical publications. These publications are used in practically every country of the world today.
>
> AIM-TWX, on the other hand, is an on-line, remote-access retrieval service used by some 65 hospital and medical libraries presently. It allows a librarian with access to a TWX (teletype) machine to search a five-year file of the 122 most commonly used clinical medical and nursing journals, including the 100 titles in *Abridged Index Medicus.*

The development of MEDLARS and AIM-TWX has provided an invaluable service to the profession by making possible easy access to references on an unlimited number of medical subjects. A library with a small staff could never provide this service to physicians without such electronic assistance.

Bibliographies for reference work can be prepared by referring to such volumes as the *Cumulative Index Medicus.* The *Current List of Medical Literature* is a similar volume listing by subject the contents of current medical journals. Each volume contains an author and subject index and an alphabetical listing of journals.

The *Cumulative Index to Hospital Literature* contains an author and subject index to more than 300 journals in the hospital and related fields, including references to hospital literature in medical, nursing, public health, business, architectural, and other periodicals. It is published quarterly with five-year cumulative indexes by the American Hospital Association in Chicago.

Also valuable in some instances is the index to the *Journal of the American Medical Association,* published three times a year.

Other Reference Sources. There are a number of other specialized reference volumes that a medical librarian may use to locate particular literature. The *Monthly Catalog of U.S. Government Publications,* for example, contains certain medical listings and is sometimes valuable in research work. Or, in securing biographical information about physicians or other professionals, it is often necessary to turn to such books as the *Directory of Medical Specialists, American Men of Science,* the *American Medical Directory,* or *Who's Who Among Physicians and Surgeons.* Encyclopedias such as *Encyclopedia Britannica* and the *Practical Medicine* series also are sometimes helpful in obtaining basic information.

PREPARING A BIBLIOGRAPHY. Utilizing the various reference sources of the medical library, a bibliography or list of references on a specific topic can be made up with comparatively little difficulty. It does take time, since the list of references must be accurate. Many researchers recommend listing each reference separately on a card or in a small loose-leaf notebook. This simplifies the actual preparation of the formal bibliography that always accompanies any published medical paper. Take down all this information: subject, author, title of book or article, publisher or periodical, volume, date of publication, and pages (Fig. 18–2). Sometimes card catalogs and other periodical references will list brief summaries of the specific

Author.. **Subject**............................
Title.. **Available at:**............................
.... **Call No.**............................
Publisher/Journal.. **Reference: Excellent, Good, Fair**
Copyright Date.............. **Volume:**.............. **Pages:**.............. **Illustrated:**..............
Student's Name:..

(Summary, including problem, source of data, method, results, quotations, references.)

Summary:..
....
....
....
....
....

FIGURE 18–2 Card for reporting bibliographic data.

reference cited; this information is also helpful in research and should be taken down.

Some libraries will prepare medical bibliographies free of charge or for a small fee. Some also will abstract or review literature, translate articles, and collect case reports. The American College of Surgeons library, for example, offers this service at a modest fee to its members. The American Medical Association also offers this service to its members. It is best to remember, however, that most hospital medical librarians do not have the time to perform such complete services, although they are ready and willing to help the doctor or his assistant make up individual bibliographies.

Manuscript Preparation

In most cases the secretary's tasks in connection with the preparation of a talk or a manuscript for publication are mainly mechanical; the doctor himself is responsible for the actual writing. However, since many physicians ask their assistants to serve in the capacity of editorial secretaries, smoothing out and actually editing their copy before submitting it for publication, a basic understanding of the style, format, and characteristics of medical papers is necessary.

A good medical paper must present established new facts, modes or practices, or principles of value, results of suitable original research, or a review of facts on a subject from which the reader can draw a legitimate conclusion. The subject should be limited to a definite area or problem before writing is begun and the purpose determined in advance.

The writing style for a scientific paper should be simple and straightforward. Excess words should be ruthlessly pared from the article. Grammatical construction should be correct in order to facilitate direct, clear expression. Slang, colloquialisms, personal allusions, and reminiscences should generally be avoided in papers for publication; they are often acceptable and add a friendly tone to a paper to be delivered in person before a medical meeting. The paper should be well organized and proceed smoothly from the beginning to end in a direct fashion.

Dr. Morris Fishbein, former editor of the *Journal of the American Medical Association,* stated in his book, *Medical Writing:* "A florid, roseate style, full of polysyllabic, metaphorical phraseology, distracts the reader's attention. Seldom is it necessary in scientific writing to employ other than simple English terms to express an idea or to state a fact."

Summing it up very simply, Selma DeBakey says, "Clarity, unity and coherence, with emphasis in the right direction, combine to make pleasing style."

Each medical periodical usually has its own style for publishing papers. The individual hoping to write for a journal should request a copy of the journal's guidelines for manuscripts in advance and then prepare the manuscript accordingly in order to minimize editorial changes. There are certain fairly uniform procedures, however, in the mechanical preparation of a manuscript to be submitted for publication.

ROUGH DRAFTS. Although most authorities still suggest triple-spacing for first drafts, very few modern typewriters have this feature. Double-space rough or first drafts of the article to provide plenty of space for corrections and revisions. Sometimes different colors of paper are used to distinguish between first, second, and final drafts of the article.

FINAL DRAFTS. Double-space the finished paper on 8-1/2 by 11 inch good quality, white paper. Double-spacing provides space for the editor who receives the manuscript to make corrections or insert instructions for the printer. Type on one side of the paper only and make at least one, preferably two, copies. The original is submitted to the editor; the author retains at least one copy for later checking of proofs. Allow a margin of at least one inch at each side and clearly indicate all paragraphs. Gauge bottom margins carefully.

In the center of the first page the title of the article should be typed in all capital letters. If there is a subtitle, this is typed on the second line below the main title, capitalizing the first letter of each important word. Then the author's name and identification are listed. If the paper was presented at a scientific meeting, this information should appear either below the author's name or at the bottom of page one with an asterisk.

Begin the text of the article on the third line below the title. No title page is necessary for manuscripts submitted for publication. Subsequent pages should be numbered, either in the center of the top or bottom margin or in the upper right- or upper left-hand corner. Generally, the author's name should also appear with the page number of each sheet for identification purposes.

The typical medical article begins with an introductory section outlining the nature of the material or problem to be covered, follows with actual discussion of the subject, and concludes with a summary in which conclusions are usually noted in numerical form. The format for case reports is somewhat similar. Case reports based on clinical information should be written clearly in smooth narrative style and should not read like a collection of telegraphic notes. There should be a clear presentation of sequence of events. A brief abstract may appear at the beginning or end of any article. This summary should be rigidly condensed and should contain the deductions as well as clearly reflect the author's viewpoint. Only the actual conclusions reached should be numbered.

FOOTNOTES. When a paper is based upon a study of the writing of others, it is necessary to acknowledge the sources used. In medical and scientific papers, footnotes usually provide exact references to sources of material. Forms of footnotes differ slightly, depending upon the style of the particular periodical, but in general a footnote contains the author's name, the title of the work cited, the facts of publication, and the exact page from which the citation was taken. Footnotes may be typed in the copy directly below the statement referred to and separated by two solid lines, or placed at the bottom of the page. Or, some editors prefer that footnotes be numbered in the paper and typed on a separate sheet of paper at the end of the article. An alternative referencing system recommended by the American Psychological Association's 1975 edition of its *Publication Manual* is the identification of references in the body of the manuscript at the appropriate place by enclosing in parentheses the author's surname, year of publication, and page reference. The complete reference is then listed at the end of the article. Here is how a footnote would appear if the first system were used:

Obesity is most apt to develop in infancy, the age of starting to school, puberty, and, for females, during pregnancy and menopause.[1]

---

1. Phyllis Sullivan Howe: *Basic Nutrition in Health and Disease,* 5th Ed. Philadelphia, W. B. Saunders Company, 1971, page 170.

The first time a book or article is mentioned in a footnote, all the information about publication should appear in the footnote; after that, references to the same source can be shortened to the author's last name and the page number cited. When a periodical is concerned, a later reference need contain only the author's name, the magazine, and the page number.

The abbreviation "ibid.," which means "in the same place," can be used with a page number to indicate subsequent reference to the same book or article already cited if it directly follows the first reference. For example, second reference to the Howe book coming right after the first one in the paper described would read:

Detailed information about footnote preparation can be obtained from the University of Chicago's *Manual of Style* or one of several published reference manuals for office workers.

FINAL BIBLIOGRAPHY. All scientific papers should carry a complete bibliography of source materials. Great care should be exercised in making up the final bibliography to make certain all references are correct. List only those sources that directly pertain to the paper and were used in its preparation. The form of bibliographies is fairly uniform. A periodical listing includes the author's name and initials, title of article, name of periodical (either in a commonly used abbreviated form or written in full), volume number, pages cited, and date of publication. A book reference includes the author's name and initials, title of book, edition, place of publication, name of publisher, year of publication, and volume number.

Book: Miller, B. F., and J. Burt, *Good Health: Personal and Community,* 2nd ed., Philadelphia, W. B. Saunders Co., 1966.

Periodical: Gerber, Paul C., New Consent Rules for Physicians Dealing with Minors, Physician's Management, Vol. 20, No. 10, 46–52, October, 1980.

Punctuation in bibliographies varies, depending upon the style of the particular publication. The main parts of the entry can be separated either by periods or by commas. The period at the end of the line is sometimes omitted.

Certain types of references present problems, since they do not fall into either the book or periodical categories. Government bulletins, for example, should be listed in this manner: author's name, title of article, number of the bulletin, name of the department, name of the bureau, and date of publication. Monographs and reports should be treated as books.

Bibliographies may be arranged alphabetically according to author's names or numerically as the references appear in the text. The main point to remember is that whatever punctuation and form is used, it should be consistent throughout the entire listing.

ILLUSTRATIONS. All drawings, photographs, and other illustrative material submitted with a manuscript should be placed on separate sheets. Never include such materials in the body of the manuscript. Illustrations add value to a paper but are expensive and should be used with restraint and judgment. The explanation of the drawing or illustration should appear in a legend. Glossy photographs reproduce best. Captions for photos should be typed on separate sheets or may be pasted with rubber cement below the photo. On the back of the photograph or drawing the author's name and the number of the illustration should be penciled lightly. Do not use pins or paper clips on photos. Credit lines should be given for copyrighted or commercial photos or illustrations. If x-ray films are submitted, make sure the prints are shiny; indicate on the back where they may be cropped, but leave localizing landmarks.

Charts and line drawings must be carefully prepared in order to get good reproduction. Such drawings preferably should be done with India or black ink on heavy white bond paper. The charts should be condensed and simplified as much as possible. Letters and identifying numerals can be placed on the face of the chart with the explanation in the legend below.

Tables should be typewritten on separate sheets in a uniform style, each numbered consecutively and with a descriptive heading.

All illustrative material should be keyed to the manuscript. In other words, illustrations should be numbered and indications placed in the manuscript as to where each illustration should be placed. The editor may not be able to place the illustration at exactly the spot indicated, but he must have this information in order to group the pictures and charts correctly.

REVISION. An important step in the preparation of any manuscript is a careful revision of copy. This is a duty often assigned to the secretary. Revisions should be made with these specific objectives in mind: (1) organization, (2) accuracy, (3) content, (4) conciseness, (5) correct sentence and grammatical construction, and (6) clarity and smoothness. The secretary should check for correct spelling, using a medical dictionary as well as a regular dictionary to aid her in this task.

MAILING THE MANUSCRIPT. Generally, manuscripts should not be folded but should be mailed flat in a large envelope. However, sometimes a paper of fewer than four pages can be folded twice and mailed in a regular business envelope. Or a manuscript running from four to eight pages is sometimes folded once and mailed in a 6 by 9 envelope. A letter stating that the manuscript is being submitted for publication should be enclosed. Photos and illustrations should be mailed flat with protective cardboards.

PROOFREADING. A paper accepted for publication will be set in type, and proofs of the article will usually be returned by the editor to the author for checking. Since changes in a manuscript once it is set in type are costly, revisions should be limited to correction of errors and minor changes. It is best to work in a team with someone when checking galley proofs, with one person holding the proofs and the other person reading from the original copy. Check for typographical errors, omitted lines and words, and so forth. Use a different-colored pencil for corrections on the proofs from the one used by the proofreader on the publication. Corrections should be entered in the margins of the proof, on a line with the error to be corrected.

The assistant whose employer does a great deal of writing for publication should become familiar with the proofreader's marks commonly used. A list of these appears in *A Manual of Style*, published by the University of Chicago Press, and in other books on writing for publication. Most of the common proofreader's marks are shown in Figure 18–3.

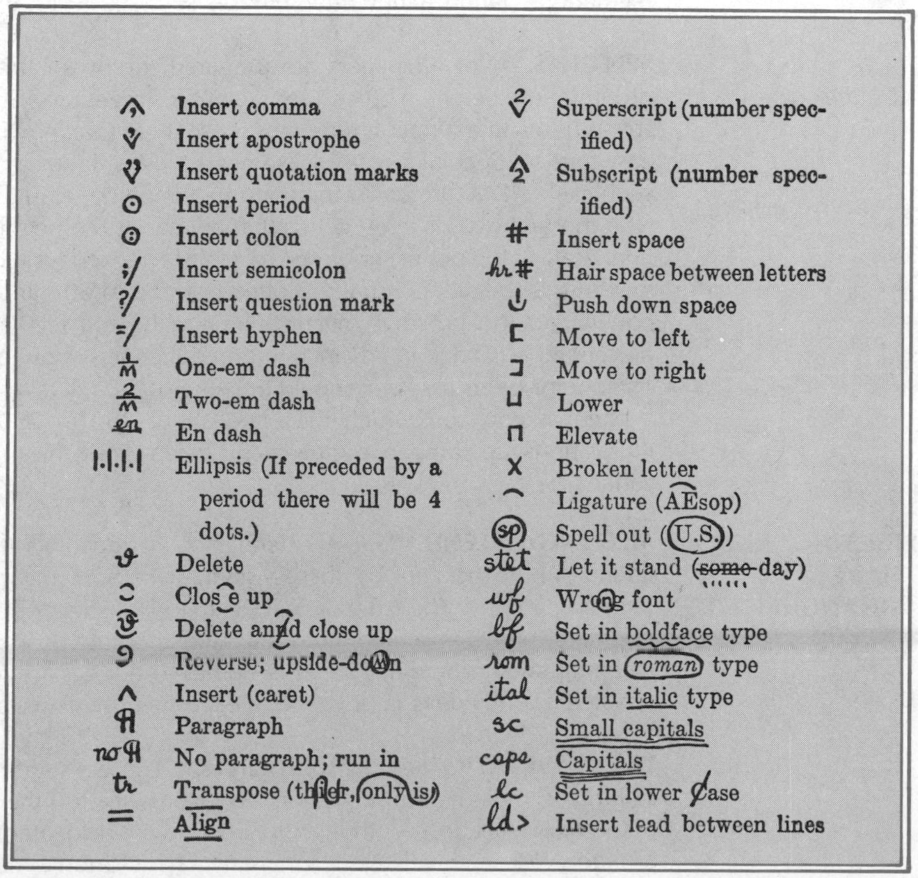

Mark	Meaning	Mark	Meaning
,̂	Insert comma	²∨	Superscript (number specified)
’∨	Insert apostrophe	∧₂	Subscript (number specified)
“ ”∨	Insert quotation marks	#	Insert space
⊙	Insert period	hr #	Hair space between letters
⦂	Insert colon	⊥	Push down space
;/	Insert semicolon	[	Move to left
?/	Insert question mark	]	Move to right
=/	Insert hyphen	⊔	Lower
1/m	One-em dash	⊓	Elevate
2/m	Two-em dash	X	Broken letter
en	En dash	⌒	Ligature (AEsop)
I.I.I.I	Ellipsis (If preceded by a period there will be 4 dots.)	(sp)	Spell out (U.S.)
₰	Delete	stet	Let it stand (~~some~~-day)
⁐	Close up	wf	Wrong font
₰̑	Delete and close up	bf	Set in boldface type
9	Reverse; upside-down	rom	Set in (roman) type
∧	Insert (caret)	ital	Set in italic type
¶	Paragraph	sc	Small capitals
no ¶	No paragraph; run in	caps	Capitals
tr	Transpose (thier, only is)	lc	Set in lower Case
=	Align	ld>	Insert lead between lines

FIGURE 18–3 **Proofreader's marks.**

One corrected galley should be returned to the editor and one set of proofs should be retained in the office. If a second set of proofs is sent later, check the first corrected set against the second set to make sure all corrections have been made.

INDEXING. Often it is necessary to provide an index for a long paper or a book. An author and subject index can be made from page proofs. One system for indexing is to use slips of paper or 3 by 5 cards. Each index entry is listed on a separate card or slip; this simplifies alphabetizing under major headings later. The whole index can then be typed from the alphabetized cards.

REPRINTS. At the time the article is set in type the doctor should order the quantity of reprints he feels he will need. Most doctors send copies of their articles to colleagues, to physicians who have evidenced an interest in their work, and to hospitals and teaching institutions with which they have had contact. The secretary will generally handle the ordering of the reprints; the doctor may request from 100 to 500 or more. Order enough to cover future needs, since type is often destroyed after the original press run. When the reprints arrive, it is best to count them to make sure the order is complete.

A list of those to whom reprints are to be sent should be made up. Some doctors maintain a separate card file in which the names and addresses of those to whom they want to send reprints are kept. Addresses should be checked from time to time in the *American Medical Directory* or by scanning membership and request lists. Some record of reprints should be kept and acknowledgments checked. A person who does not acknowledge two or three reprints should be taken from the mailing list.

An enclosure card, printed up in advance, is sent by some authors with a copy of the reprint. Others prefer to enclose a short letter stating that the reprint is a complimentary copy. Reprints usually are mailed as third class printed matter; postal regulations permit handwritten phrases such as "With the author's compliments."

SPEECHES. Not all papers are prepared for publication. Some are prepared for presentation before medical and scientific meetings. Speeches should be double spaced; in some offices a jumbo or magnatype machine is used so that the speech is easy to read. Special large-type elements are available for single element typewriters, such as the IBM Orator. At the bottom of each page, in the lower right-hand corner, type the first two or three words that appear at the beginning of the next page. The final draft of the paper should be carefully checked for typographical errors. At large meetings a speaker is usually allotted from 10 to 20 minutes to present his paper; at county society and small meetings he may have from 30 minutes to an hour for his presentation. Check in advance to find out exactly how much time will be allowed. The doctor or his assistant should time the speech. It takes about two minutes to read a page of copy on which there are about 200 to 250 words. If slides or other illustrations are planned, arrangements for showing this material must be made in advance.

MEETING AND TRAVEL ARRANGEMENTS

MEETING CALENDARS. A calendar of all meetings that the physician plans to attend should be kept by the assistant, with both the physician and the assistant retaining a copy. The calendar can be merely a sheet of paper listing name of meeting, date, place, and time, but it must be accurate. Any changes or additions to the calendar should be made on both copies as notices are received. A reminder to the physician a few days in advance of each meeting is usually appreciated.

TRANSPORTATION ARRANGEMENTS. The assistant may also have the responsibility of making transportation arrangements for the doctor when he attends out-of-town meetings. Although the doctor who is located in a metropolitan area will probably use a travel agent for many of his arrangements, the assistant may be charged with the responsibility of working with the agent and preparing the detailed itinerary. The assistant who does not deal with a travel agent may be expected to make hotel and transportation arrangements. For this reason she should keep a list of the telephone numbers of railroads, airlines, and buses in a special file. A folder with descriptions and telephone numbers of hotels is also useful. The doctor who is a member of an auto club can use membership privileges to obtain names of good hotels and motels, road maps, and other vital travel information.

Even though reservations are made in advance, recheck a day or two before the doctor is scheduled to leave, since slip-ups do sometimes occur. When all arrangements are final, typewrite the itinerary. Keep one copy in the office file. Give the doctor the original and several copies for distribution to members of his family or other individuals. Since it is sometimes necessary to reach the doctor during his absence, it is important that his itinerary be carefully prepared so that he can be reached at any point in his trip.

MEETING RESPONSIBILITIES. The progressive physician often accepts official responsibilities in his or her professional society or on the hospital board. The administrative assistant for this physician may be expected to assist in preparing an agenda or in typing minutes of the meeting dictated by the physician.

Agenda. Organizations whose bylaws specify *Robert's Rules of Order,* Newly Revised as parliamentary authority, and which have not adopted a special order of business, use the following prescribed order of business:

1. Reading and Approval of Minutes
2. Reports of Officers, Board, and Standing Committees
3. Reports of Special (Select or Ad Hoc) Committees
4. Special Orders
5. Unfinished Business and General Orders
6. New Business

Minutes. The record of the proceedings of a meeting is called the *minutes.* The minutes contain mainly a record of what was *done* at the meeting, not what was *said* by the members.

The first paragraph of the minutes should contain the following information: the kind of meeting (regular, special, and so forth); the name of the association; the date, time, and place of the meeting; the fact that the regular chairman and secretary were present or, in their absence, the names of the persons who substituted for them; and whether the minutes of the previous meeting were read and approved.

The body of the minutes should contain a separate paragraph for each subject matter. It should include all main motions; the wording in which each motion was adopted or otherwise disposed of; the disposition of the motion; and the name of the mover. The name of the seconder of the motion should not be entered in the minutes unless ordered by the assembly. The body of the minutes should also include any points of order and appeals, whether they were sustained or lost, and the reasons given by the chair for the ruling. The minutes may include the name and subject of a guest speaker, but no attempt should be made to summarize the speech.

The last paragraph should state the hour of adjournment.

The minutes should be signed by the secretary. In some organizations the president also signs the minutes. The practice of including the words *Respectfully submitted* is obsolete and rarely used today.

The assistant who might be expected to type the minutes of meetings should consult an authoritative book on the subject and prepare a model to follow in typing the minutes of each meeting so that every set of minutes will be in the same style.

References

Library Journal, October 1, 1971.
Library Journal, March 1, 1972.
Strunk, W. Jr., and White, E. B.: *The Elements of Style,* 2nd ed. New York, The Macmillan Company, 1972.

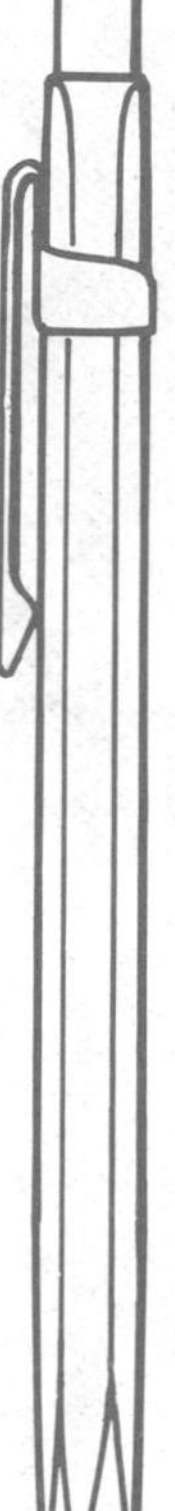

CHAPTER OUTLINE

Office Housekeeping Details
- Woodwork
- Floors
- Rugs
- Radiators, Vents, Furnaces
- Sinks
- Counter Surfaces
- Cabinets
- Boiler Sanitizers
- Autoclaves
- Linens
- Blankets

Removal of Stains
Reception Room Care
Assistant's Desk
Doctor's Office and Other Rooms
Office Security
Supplies
- Labels
- Ordering of Supplies
- Drug Samples
- Storage of Drugs

The Doctor's Bag

BEHAVIORAL OBJECTIVES

The medical office assistant should be able to:

- **Organize and plan the housekeeping details in a medical office.**
- **Apply proper methods of stain removal.**
- **Observe necessary precautions for office security.**
- **Correctly label and store drug supplies.**
- **Maintain a card system for supply inventory.**
- **Keep the doctor's bag ready for immediate use.**

19

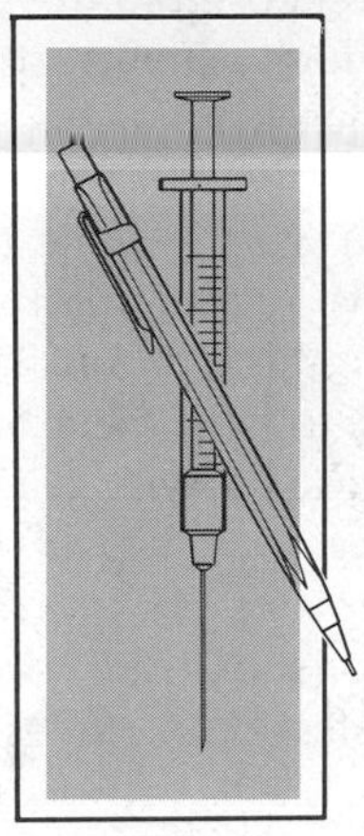

FACILITIES AND SUPPLIES: ORGANIZATION AND CARE

A harmonious, orderly office helps create a good working environment and lifts the morale of patients as well as office personnel. Supervision or the actual performance of certain housekeeping duties in the office often is a responsibility of the medical assistant. These duties may grow in proportion to the growth of the physician's practice as the medical office assistant becomes an experienced, loyal employee. She should be completely dependable and willing to assume the duties that will help keep the office running smoothly.

The same principles of organization and planning that guide the business management of an office are essential in the assistant's housekeeping duties. To maintain an atmosphere of organization and harmony, duties should be planned to avoid rushing and confusion. Here's a good housekeeping rule to follow: have a place for everything, and keep everything clean and *ready for use*. This saves time, conserves property, and eliminates incorrect use of materials. Adoption of sound housekeeping procedures also saves the assistant's personal energy. Furthermore, an office managed on a hit-or-miss basis holds potential dangers for patients, doctors, and assistants alike.

Medical equipment and supplies are expensive and sometimes hard to obtain. If properly cared for, they have a longer life and their use is increased. When you receive a piece of equipment in the office, read the instructions carefully. Do not attempt to assemble or use articles you have not first studied. File these instructions in a special folder and save them for future reference or for your successors. If there is a guarantee with the item, copy the code number, fill in the blank, and mail as instructed. Instructions and guarantees are enclosed for a definite purpose; do not misplace them. For income tax purposes it is necessary to keep a copy of the invoice for the date purchased and the amount. This is necessary for depreciation as well as for insurance. Keep a service file for equipment that needs regular servicing. This file should contain: guarantee dates, how often item should be serviced, when and by whom item was last serviced, and cost of servicing.

OFFICE HOUSEKEEPING DETAILS

Patients in a professional office are especially critical of the condition of the office and its contents. Anyone who visits a physician expects cleanliness and order to prevail. A patient does not want to be exposed to the diseases of other patients, nor should there be any evidence of previous patients in inner office rooms. Here are some suggestions for general office housekeeping.

Woodwork should be washed regularly with a mild cleanser and water solution. It is the assistant's job to see that such work is done and to make arrangements to have someone do it. Many offices have night janitor or custodial service; if not, a patient who is having difficulty paying his account may be glad to perform such services at the regular prevailing wage to help meet his obligations.

Floors should be scrubbed and waxed with a nonskid wax. Highly finished floors look beautiful but are very dangerous, especially for those who are ill and inclined to be unsteady on their feet.

Rugs should extend wall to wall or should be secured to prevent tripping. It is not advisable to use scatter rugs in professional offices; they are too likely to slip or be tripped on and cause falls.

Radiators or vents should be dusted with a dampened cloth; use a paint brush to clean the corners. Check the heater and pilot light for leaks. Furnaces should be oiled regularly and the filters cleaned or changed. A professional service may be best.

Sinks should be scrubbed daily or more often, if necessary, to prevent pitting and contamination. Frequent polishing with a mild cleanser will keep a smooth, glossy finish on porcelain, preventing acids from collecting. Hot water should be flushed through the tap and a drain cleaner used frequently. A sink is often the source of infection and odors; it needs constant care and disinfection. Any solid material should be removed from the sink, wrapped in paper, and placed in the waste container. Waste containers of the closed variety, especially those in the treatment or examining rooms, are lined with disposable bags.

Surfaces of counters, table tops, and so forth should be covered with a stain-resistant material that can be washed regularly. Stained surfaces are a sign of contamination. Use paper towels directly under any bottles. The newer equipment has a plastic-finish counter surface that is highly resistant to acids and medicine stains. These surfaces are heat resistant and do not scratch easily. They are easy to keep clean. They should be scrubbed daily, or after each patient, with a germicidal cleaner. The undersides of towel and tape dispensers are frequently overlooked in the daily cleaning. Tops of cabinets that are exposed should be dusted daily. These last two items are usually noticed by the patient.

Cabinets should be kept scrupulously clean and orderly (Fig. 19–1). Many of the modern medical offices are substituting closed cabinets for those that expose contents to view, since displays of instruments are disturbing to many patients. Even though they may not be visible, all instruments should be cleaned and organized for immediate use.

Do not begin cleaning cabinets unless you have time to complete the job. The doctor's afternoon off is a good opportunity for such jobs. Do one shelf at a time, starting at the top.

1. Remove the material from the shelf and place on a table in the same order as on the shelf.
2. Wash the shelf and rinse well. Dry.
3. Clean and polish the instruments and check for faults. Examine hinges and blades.
4. Check all labels to make certain of clarity. Retype and reglue labels, if necessary. Cleaning time is a good time to examine supplies for expiration dates, quantity, and deterioration. Make a list of those items that should be reordered.

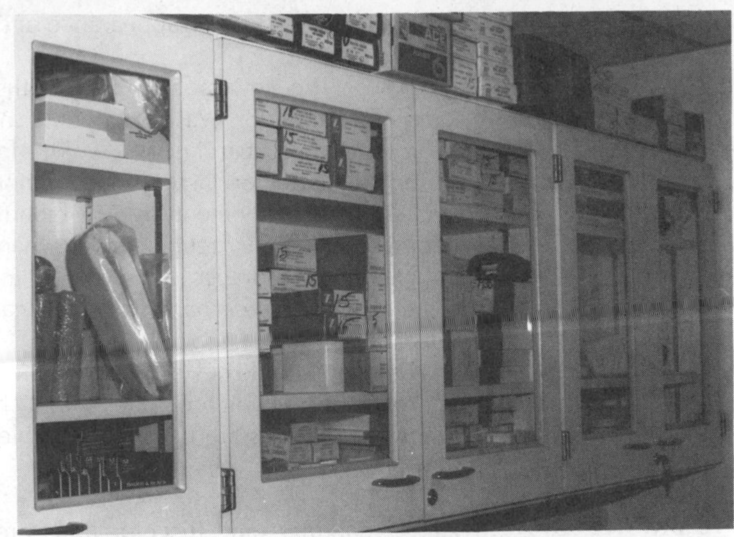

FIGURE 19–1 An example of a neat cabinet for orthopedic supplies.

5. Replace the supplies in their original places on the shelf. Two major dangers in the medical office are the changing of medications from their original locations and the incorrect reading of labels by the doctor or the staff. Even if a bottle has been in the same position for years, its location should never be taken for granted. When using a product, always read the label three times before proceeding and once again after administration.

Boiler sanitizers should be cleaned daily, especially if tap water is used in place of distilled or demineralized water. If there is no sediment from the water, the boiler can be cleaned less frequently. At the end of the day the boiler should be left open with the tray clearing the water level. Acquire the habit of turning off the boiler before opening it for the night and you will eliminate the after-hours fear that you left it on. Many an assistant has had to return to the office in the evening to check the boiler for that very reason.

In areas where water forms a heavy scum inside the boiler, it is necessary to boil it out with an 8 per cent hydrochloric acid (muriatic acid) solution each month. Fill the boiler completely with this solution, bring it to a boil, cool, and drain. Rinse the equipment well and it is again ready to use. Vinegar also is a good cleaning agent, but it is not advisable for office use because of its noticeable odor. Some boiler manufacturers advise the use of a 10 per cent solution of hydrochloric acid at room temperature for cleaning. Do not boil this solution; allow it to stand in the boiler until the scale becomes softened and can be scrubbed off with a stiff brush. When using acids for cleaning purposes, be careful not to spill them on the outside of the boiler, as they will remove the chrome finish. Also take care not to spill such substances on cabinet tops. The manufacturer's recommendations should be followed.

Sterilizer tablets are excellent for prevention of scale or rust. These tablets often are available from manufacturers of sterilizers and boilers, who distribute them with their own equipment. Sodium bicarbonate also can be used as a rust deterrent, but it does not do as thorough a job as tablets.

Autoclaves should be given special care, and instructions for proper use and cleaning should be followed closely. If you are new in an office and cannot find the proper instructions, write the manufacturer of the equipment for another copy. *Use only distilled or demineralized water in the autoclave.* Place instructions in a transparent plastic folder and tack inside a cupboard door near the autoclave.

Linens, if owned by the doctor, must be carefully marked with a special linen marker ink or linen pen. This ink will not smear or wash out. All laundry should be counted before it it sent and recounted when it is returned. Keep a copy of the laundry list in a special folder, for use in checking the returned laundry. Clean linen should be stored in a clean, dry place free from dust and insects. Provide a definite place for each type of linen. When storing, place folds on the outside toward the front; this gives a neater appearance and makes it easier to pick up one piece at a time.

Never use towels as scrub cloths, even though they are rented from a commercial laundry. Wash your hands immediately after handling dirty laundry and before handling clean linens. Avoid unnecessary waste of linens. If the linens are owned by the doctor, inspect pieces before putting them away and remove damaged pieces for discard or mending. The laundry will perform this checking service if your office uses a laundry rental service. Many offices are now using disposable towels and examination drapes, *so remember to separate them from the soiled linen going to the laundry. These paper products can cause no end of trouble in the washing processes.*

Blankets should never be allowed to touch a patient's body. The blankets should be protected from such contact with a sheet. Blankets should be cleaned regularly. Treatment blankets are usually washable; blanket sheets are also warm and washable.

REMOVAL OF STAINS

Stains, markings, and discolorations are frequent and inevitable eyesores in the professional office. Such blemishes on linens, furniture, supplies, clothing, or the skin often have a distressing effect on the morale of patients. Immediate action very often results in successful removal of such stains. Various agents for removal of stains should be kept on hand in a convenient place. General directions for stain removals should be memorized.

TABLE 19–1 Removal of Stains

Substance Causing Stain	How to Remove
Aniline dyes	Use lye solution or weak hydrochloric acid solution. Acid alcohol also may be used. Wash.
Silver nitrate	Remove fresh stains by soaking in salt water. Treat old stains with a warm solution of sodium thiosulfate, about 10 to 20%. Silver nitrate stains on the skin can be removed by painting the surface with iodine and then applying alcohol.
Coffee or cocoa	Wash in concentrated salt water and rinse well. It is sometimes necessary to soften the stain with glycerin before rinsing with cold water and borax.
Feces	Soak well in cold water and wash with soap and water.
Merthiolate	Remove with Dakin's solution (chlorinated soda).
Iron rust	Cover with lemon juice and salt and bleach in sunlight. There are also excellent commercial products for removal of rust.
Chlorophyll (grass stains)	Use warm alcohol to remove fresh stains. Kerosene can be used on older stains along with sodium perborate, diluted hydrogen peroxide, or diluted aromatic spirits of ammonia. Some commercial products are excellent.
Iodine (on hands or clothes)	Moisten with ammonia or sodium thiosulfate solution. Starch is sometimes a successful removal agent.
Mercurochrome	Immerse first in a 20% solution of potassium permanganate and then in a 5% solution of oxalic acid. Rinse well.
Petroleum jelly	Use ether, alcohol, or benzol (benzene) and wash with soda and hot water solution. An absorbent material placed under the stain will facilitate absorption while treating the stain.
Adhesive plaster	Use ether or benzol. There are special removers on the market that do not sting the tissues and are pleasant-smelling.
Ink	Remove ink stains from the skin with glycerin, acetic acid, or citric acid. To remove ink stains from fabric, immerse in tepid water and skim milk for a long time. It is sometimes necessary to cover the surface with lemon juice and salt and place in the sun.

THIS FORM TO BE USED TO BILL **BLUE CROSS OF SOUTHERN CALIFORNIA** OR **BLUE SHIELD OF CALIFORNIA ONLY.**
PLEASE VERIFY WITH YOUR PATIENT THE CORRECT ORGANIZATION TO BILL.

READ INSTRUCTIONS BEFORE COMPLETING OR SIGNING THIS FORM

TYPE OR PRINT ☐ MEDICARE ☐ MEDI-CAL ☒ STANDARD Connecticut General

PATIENT & INSURED (SUBSCRIBER) INFORMATION

1. PATIENT'S NAME (*First name, middle initial, last name*): Richard DeWitt
2. PATIENT'S DATE OF BIRTH: 01 23 18
3. INSURED'S NAME (*First name, middle initial, last name*): same
4. PATIENT'S ADDRESS (*Street, city, state, ZIP code*): 837 North Harbor Boulevard, Irvine, CA 92714
5. PATIENT'S SEX: MALE x FEMALE
6. INSURED'S I.D. NO., MEDICARE NO. AND/OR MEDICAID NO. (*include any letters*): 333 22 4444
7. PATIENT'S RELATIONSHIP TO INSURED: SELF x SPOUSE CHILD OTHER
8. INSURED'S GROUP NO. (*Or Group Name*): California Bean Growers
9. OTHER HEALTH INSURANCE COVERAGE - Enter Name of Policyholder and Plan Name and Address and Policy or Medical Assistance Number: ------
10. WAS CONDITION RELATED TO:
    A. PATIENT'S EMPLOYMENT YES NO x
    B. AN AUTO ACCIDENT YES NO x
11. INSURED'S ADDRESS (*Street, city, state, ZIP code*): same
12. PATIENT'S OR AUTHORIZED PERSON'S SIGNATURE (*Read back before signing*) *I Authorize the Release of Any Medical Information Necessary to Process this Claim and Request Payment of Medical Benefits Either to Myself or to the Party Who Accepts Assignment Below*
    SIGNED DATE
13. *I AUTHORIZE PAYMENT OF MEDICAL BENEFITS TO UNDERSIGNED PHYSICIAN OR SUPPLIER FOR SERVICE DESCRIBED BELOW*
    SIGNED (*Insured or Authorized Person*)

PHYSICIAN OR SUPPLIER INFORMATION

14. DATE OF: 07 12 81 ◄ ILLNESS (FIRST SYMPTOM) OR INJURY (ACCIDENT) OR PREGNANCY (LMP)
15. DATE FIRST CONSULTED YOU FOR THIS CONDITION: 07 15 81
16. HAS PATIENT EVER HAD SAME OR SIMILAR SYMPTOMS? YES NO x
17. DATE PATIENT ABLE TO RETURN TO WORK: 07 26 81
18. DATES OF TOTAL DISABILITY: FROM 07 12 81 THROUGH 07 25 81
    DATES OF PARTIAL DISABILITY: FROM THROUGH
19. NAME AND ADDRESS OF REFERRING PHYSICIAN OR OTHER SOURCE
20. FOR SERVICES RELATED TO HOSPITALIZATION GIVE HOSPITALIZATION DATES: ADMITTED 07 15 81 DISCHARGED 07 17 81
21. NAME & ADDRESS OF FACILITY WHERE SERVICES RENDERED (*If other than home or office*): St. John's Hospital, Santa Monica, California
22. WAS LABORATORY WORK PERFORMED OUTSIDE YOUR OFFICE? YES NO x CHARGES:
23. DIAGNOSIS OR NATURE OF ILLNESS OR INJURY. RELATE DIAGNOSIS TO PROCEDURE IN COLUMN D BY REFERENCE TO NUMBERS 1, 2, 3, ETC. OR DX CODE
    1. Leg pain
    2.
    3.
    4.

    ☐ FAMILY PLANNING SERVICE

LEAVE BLANK	24. A DATE OF SERVICE			B* PLACE OF SERVICE	PROCEDURE NUMBER (RVS NUMBER / SMA NUMBER)	UNIT MODIFIER	C FULLY DESCRIBE PROCEDURES, MEDICAL SERVICES OR SUPPLIES FURNISHED FOR EACH DATE GIVEN (EXPLAIN UNUSUAL SERVICES OR CIRCUMSTANCES)	D DIAGNOSIS CODE	E CHARGES	F LEAVE BLANK 1	2	3	4	5	6	7
	07	15	81	3	90050		Office visit limited exam	1	20 00							
	07	15	81	1	90220		Init hosp care compr HPX	1	100 00							
	07	16	81	1	90215		Hosp visit intermed exam	1	30 00							
	07	17	81	1	90275		Hosp visit w/discharge	1	35 00							

25. SIGNATURE OF PHYSICIAN OR SUPPLIER — I certify under penalty of perjury that the foregoing is true and correct (read back before signing).
    SIGNED DATE
26. ACCEPT ASSIGNMENT (*Government claims only*) *SEE BACK* YES NO
27. TOTAL CHARGE: 185 00
28. AMOUNT PAID
29. BALANCE DUE
30. YOUR SOCIAL SECURITY NO.: 111-22-3333
31. PHYSICIAN'S OR SUPPLIER'S NAME, ADDRESS, PROVIDER NUMBER, ZIP CODE & TELEPHONE NO.: ROBERT O ELAM MD, 300 NORTH BROADWAY, LOS ANGELES CA 90005
32. YOUR PATIENT'S ACCOUNT NO.
33. YOUR EMPLOYER I.D. NO.: 95-1234567

**PLACE OF SERVICE CODES*

1 – (IH) – INPATIENT HOSPITAL
2 – (OH) – OUTPATIENT HOSPITAL
3 – (O) – DOCTOR'S OFFICE
4 – (H) – PATIENT'S HOME
5 – – DAY CARE FACILITY (PSY)
6 – – NIGHT CARE FACILITY (PSY)
7 – (ICF) – INTERMEDIATE CARE FACILITY
8 – (SNF) – SKILLED NURSING FACILITY
9 – – AMBULANCE
O – (OL) – OTHER LOCATIONS
A – (IL) – INDEPENDENT LABORATORY
B – – OTHER MEDICAL/SURGICAL FACILITY

C 4359

FIGURE 17–8 Universal Claim Form, Standard Insurance.

1

SYSTEMATIZING CLAIM PREPARATION

Whenever you find medical assistants "talking shop," a frequent topic of discussion is insurance claims. It is not always just the volume of forms that causes problems. Failure to systematize the work, procrastination, failure to keep informed, and possibly an unconscious resentment contribute to the undesirable situation. Simplification of claim forms has eliminated much of the burden. With the right attitude and an efficient system, insurance billing need not be a cause for concern. It is certainly less troublesome than billing an account for several months, then writing a series of collection letters, and perhaps eventually having to resort to third-party collection procedures, with a considerable loss in income. If the volume of insurance is so great that the office assistant using efficient systematized procedures cannot keep up-to-date, then the practical physician will hire extra help for this purpose. The collection potential in most medical practices is increased in proportion to the proper handling of the patients' insurance. Therefore, it behooves the medical office assistant and the physician to give proper attention to the processing of the claims.

WHO IS RESPONSIBLE? The receptionist, the medical assistant, the bookkeeper, the insurance clerk, the nurse, the doctor — anyone who treats the patient, keeps records, or handles the telephone or appointments plays a role in insurance claims.

The processing of insurance claims begins with the receptionist. When the first appointment is made, she can ask the patient to bring along all insurance information and any special forms. If the patient has an identification card, the receptionist should first determine that the coverage is current, then photocopy the card for the office record. If more than one insurance is involved, get information for ALL companies.

It is important to obtain complete and accurate information on every new patient, including:

1. Full name, address, and telephone number
2. Date of birth
3. Occupation
4. Name, address, and telephone number of employer
5. Social Security number
6. Driver's license number
7. Name and address of insurance carrier
8. Group and member numbers, or policy number
9. Name and address of subscriber if other than patient
10. Other health insurance coverage, if any
11. Name and address of referring physician, if any
12. Photocopy of identification card, if any

Insurance information can change. For continuing patients, the receptionist should recheck insurance coverage every six months or so. Date-stamp forms as they are received, and keep a log of all insurance forms (Fig. 17–9). A log such as this will enable you to tell an inquiring patient immediately whether or not his claim form has been completed and mailed.

The doctor, office nurse, or medical assistant is responsible for the complete and accurate reporting of diagnosis and services performed. Unless the full information is on the chart, the insurance clerk cannot do her work well.

The person who does the bookkeeping must post the charges promptly and accurately.

COMPLETING THE FORMS. The importance of systematizing the processing of claims cannot be overemphasized. The work will be much easier if the following points are observed:

1. A definite time is set aside for this task.
2. There is a central location for all insurance forms.
3. The necessary manuals, code books, and other references are nearby.
4. The superbill or Universal Claim Form is used as often as possible.

Blood stains, common in the medical office, can be removed by soaking the article in cool, *not hot,* water and then washing it. To remove old blood stains, soak in hydrogen peroxide or ammonia, then wash. Naphtha or benzene should never be applied to blood; this sets the blood stain, making removal impossible. Hydrogen peroxide is best for removing blood stains from white materials.

Acids should be neutralized immediately with an alkaline substance such as ammonia or sodium bicarbonate, then washed thoroughly. Then test for neutrality with litmus paper. *Alkalis* should be treated with a mild acid, such as vinegar or a weak (10 per cent) solution of citric or acetic acid. Wash the article well and test for neutrality with litmus paper.

See Table 19–1 for directions for removing stains of various types.

RECEPTION ROOM

The importance of a neat, attractive reception room was pointed out in Chapter 7, *Your Role as Receptionist.* It is the room from which patients gain their first impression of the office. From a housekeeping standpoint, then, it is particularly vital that the reception room be kept clean, orderly, and in good condition. The assistant must see to it that cleaning duties such as dusting and vacuuming are performed regularly. Even if you have maintenance service in your office, morning dusting is advisable.

Provide plenty of fresh air but guard against drafts, since people who are ill are very susceptible to chills. There should be a constant change of air by means of open windows or air conditioners. If you have air conditioning, do not keep it too cool. The ideal temperature for a reception room is about 74° F. Room thermometers are a great help in maintaining the proper temperature. If your office does not have a thermometer, purchase one and place it in a location where you think the temperature is neither too hot nor too cold in the room.

Lighting should be balanced, and there should be no glare. Lamps are very decorative, but they are useful only if properly placed. Lamps should be at reading height; otherwise, they shine into the eyes of others in the waiting room or are so low patients have to slump to read by them.

The supply of accessories such as magazines and ash trays should be constantly checked. Smoking is usually discouraged in a professional office, since some people object to it. If a patient insists on smoking, have an ashtray ready if he asks for it. Then remove it immediately after the patient leaves.

Flower arrangements are a delight to see, but they should be attractively arranged and discarded immediately when they start to wilt. The water should be changed and kept fresh to prevent any odor. Because artificial plants are now so attractive, they are frequently used, but they too take care. Keep the leaves wiped free of dust to give a fresh appearance. These should also be rearranged and occasionally changed.

Toys present definite housekeeping problems. They are necessary in offices where children are visitors and have to wait any length of time. Such articles should be chosen for their cleanability and noiselessness. In some offices, the toys are kept in another room and are given to the children as needed, with an explanation to the mother that the article has been washed since the last child used it. Some offices have discontinued having toys and find that large animal pillows and plenty of good picture books satisfy the children and make a quieter waiting area. Television is good but should be mounted high enough to prevent the little patients from adjusting the channel and sound.

Draperies and upholstery should be cleaned regularly. This may be done at vacation time. Today much office furniture is plastic and washable; the dark, gloomy appearance of the reception room furniture of the past is being replaced with lighter colored furniture that is easier to clean.

Step into the reception room several times a day to check on the lighting and temperature and straighten the magazines. In more than one office patients have been left in the dark at the close of the day because the assistant was too busy to ...tion room duties properly.

...posed of by wrapping it in paper and ... Glassware should be immersed in a ... there for several hours. Autoclave any ...e. Sterility must be maintained in the ...nent rooms.

...d after contact with any contaminated ...ked for leaks; electric wires should be ...o leave the laboratory window open ...n you leave the office. There are many ...ceable to the office force but are very ... when using any volatile material,

...finite storage places away from too ... in brown bottles, since light causes ... be spotlessly clean and free from ... glassware that has been cracked or ...us.

...lean, and quiet. Provide facilities so ...; reading material will help the time ...nes to sleep, see that no one enters ...n the recovery room doubles as a

... in the inner office rooms. These ...quipment and supplies should be ... well as pleasant and comfortable. ...of the past. Treatment tables and ...soft pastels, and the general decor ...uipment are out of sight, but the

...ples lightens the assistant's tasks ...ways in working condition and

OFFICE SECURITY

...e say it is the small-time thief or ...Small time or not, this kind of ...e far too often making it easy, at ...ug addict is doubly dangerous ...asily if he breaks in and cannot

...n office before breaking in. The ... staff can be alert to certain ... possible "easy" target. Be on ...st, "glassy" eyes and a runny ...erested in the location of your ... too intently when you make ...us of anyone hanging around ...plex. If you notice such an

...dows as well as doors. Have ...ay be well worth the cost to ...advice. Check with the local ...e name of such an agency. ...y can be made difficult, and

...xtremely helpful. Leaving a ...e local police which lights

warning

WE HAVE JOINED
OPERATION IDENTIFICATION
ALL ITEMS OF VALUE
ON THESE PREMISES
HAVE BEEN INDELIBLY MARKED
FOR READY IDENTIFICATION
BY LAW ENFORCEMENT AGENCIES

FIGURE 19–3 Sign for office window indicating that valuables have been marked for purposes of identification.

will always be left on. If the inside of the office is visible to passersby, all small movable items that might be tempting should be put away out of sight before you leave the office at the end of the day.

Alarms can be helpful if they are reliable and are not easily disconnected by an expert. Loud local alarms are usually sufficient to frighten off a prowler. It is possible, though, to install an alarm that will ring in the local police station or at a special security office.

Police departments are urging that all valuables be protected by etching them with personal identification, such as the owner's name or social security number. This is easily done with an electric engraving tool that cuts into the equipment, and the marking is practically impossible to eradicate. Even if an attempt is made to scratch it off, a sufficient mark will be left so that the police, with the aid of a special chemical, can bring the engraved characters up again. Articles so marked are almost impossible to "fence." Place a sign in the office window (Fig. 19–3) showing that you have identified your valuables.

The most effective step in protecting your office is to remember to check carefully at the end of the day to make certain all doors and windows are doubly locked. Unless you make this an unvarying part of your routine, it is easy to leave a window unlatched. You may as well write an invitation on it or hand the thief the items through the window.

SUPPLIES

Although the care and ordering of supplies have been mentioned previously, there are some special notations that should be considered.

Follow good housekeeping rules in storing supplies. Supplies should be kept where they are most accessible yet protected from damage and exposure to moisture, heat, light, and air. Most drugs and solutions should be stored in a cool, dark cupboard because direct light and sunlight cause drug deterioration. Poisons should be stored separately from products used routinely. Have a *distinct label or cap* for these poisons. You might use a bright color, such as red, for their labels or caps. Narcotics must be stored in a secure place, out of sight. Acids and caustics should have special resistant lids; never use metal lids for these substances. Do not store strong acids next to alkalis. Inflammable items must be stored away from heat.

If drugs and solutions are to be stored for some time, the stoppers should be dipped in paraffin to seal them from the air. Do not fill these bottles to the very top; leave a little room for expansion.

desk is usually in view of the patients, and consequently it
imes. Everything should have its place and should be returned
nished. Provide desk trays for records and business papers
not leave such items lying around to be lost or to be read by
rsonal belongings out of sight. Never smoke, eat, or keep a
k. This does not lend to a professional-appearing office.
the assistant has a private corner that is separated from the
ass partition of some sort. She can see entering patients and
reception room but can also carry on private conversations
shot of those who are waiting.

ld always be kept neat and clean. Give this room a quick
tient departs, and remove any evidence of the preceding
changes without first consulting your doctor. Never throw
it of paper with a number on it. It may be important to the
fessional literature in convenient order and to his liking.
as batteries in the flashlight, tongue depressors, the cuff of
and so forth, daily. In offices where the doctor likes to keep
ent for his little patients, such as candy or pencils, the
to see that the supply of these items is adequate.
ping is a full-time job in many offices. Good system and
here. Consulting, examining, treatment, diagnostic, and
atories must be spotless. These rooms should be straight-
h patient (Fig. 19–2). All linen must be changed and medi-
t of sight. Frequently a patient may know who was in the
e a telltale bottle of medication in view. Watch the tem-
nce patients are usually asked to disrobe. These rooms
ner than other parts of the office. Deodorants are often
n rooms; these help remove the medical odor that many
d surgical supply companies carry nonperfumed room

uipment often. Reorder when supplies are low; do not
usted. If you are not familiar with the supplies in a new
u feel he may change brands, check with him on new
deterioration of materials must be watched constantly.
health by using outdated or spoiled medication.
he office catch-all. Even though it is out of sight, it
te work cannot be done in the midst of disorder. All

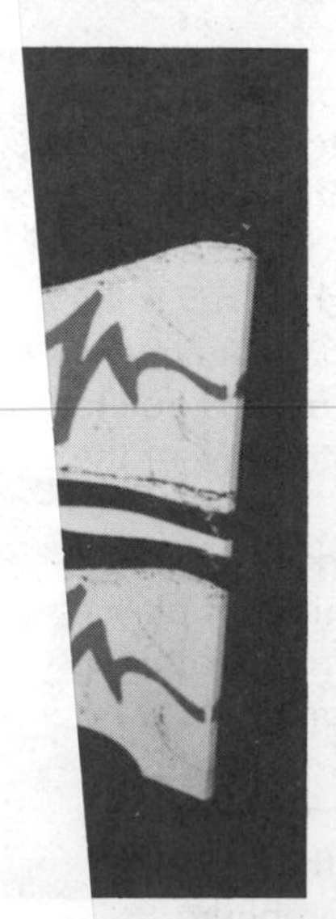

FIGURE 19–2 A clean, neat, and orderly patient examination room.

LABELS. If a bottle is to be used for a long time, the label should be indestructible. The original one is best and should be treated to preserve it when it is first received. If it has not been preserved, however, and shows signs of wear or mutilation, replace it with a neatly typed or printed fresh one.

When you are making new labels (and this cannot be overstressed!), make sure that the new label is an accurate, identical copy of the original. If there are varying strengths or dosages, make certain this information appears correctly. Never change a direction or a name on a label. These labels should be placed on the upper edge of the bottle and on the side opposite the pouring spout if there is one.

Careful use of the bottles will also protect the labels. Always pour away from the label side to prevent dripping over the label. Plastic screw caps are best because they protect the lip of the bottle and keep it clean. Glass stoppers are necessary for some solutions but are not very practical. They are individually ground and generally are not interchangeable. They break easily and often stick.

There are many different methods for securing a label. Use whatever is best for the particular bottle, but keep it neat and accurate.

Sprays. Plastic sprays are excellent and very easy to apply.

Transparent Tape. Although commonly used for securing labels, some transparent tapes are not very durable for solutions because they tend to curl on the edges and turn yellow. 3-M Magic Transparent Tape is good and does not curl or yellow.

Glass Ink or Lab-Ink. This is a superior method of labeling. The ink can be printed directly on the glass, and it is very resistant to all solutions. You can obtain inks in dark or light colors for various bottles.

Metal Tags. Tags are used in many cases, especially for flasks and bottles of stock solutions whose containers are constantly changing. They are durable and can be placed in the autoclave without damage.

Tape Writing. A hand-operated tape writer has solved many labeling problems. The self-adhering tape is available in many colors and several widths and is quite resistant to damage.

ORDERING. Ordering supplies is usually the duty of the medical assistant. Although not an easy task for a new assistant, it is an excellent way to learn about supplies and their storage. Never trust your memory to recall amounts, types, or styles to be ordered. Keep an established list or sort of running inventory where you can note dwindling supplies. Record exactly what has been previously used. Do not change brands when ordering unless you consult the doctor and get his consent.

It is advisable to establish good credit with certain reputable supply companies. Very seldom can you save money by purchasing from cut-rate or unknown supply houses. This does not mean that you cannot obtain estimates from competitive houses and purchase wisely. However, do not shift your purchases from company to company without good reason. If you are well known to a supply house, the people there will endeavor to please you and hasten your order. Also, the company will often give you the privilege of trying out a piece of equipment in the office before you actually purchase it. As a result, you will have a better guarantee of the quality of your purchases.

There should be an established method for ordering supplies. Set up a pattern for this task and do not vary it except in emergencies. Many representatives of supply houses will call at regular intervals. This facilitates ordering because you can ask questions and explain to them just what you want.

In some cases, you may save money by purchasing in larger quantities, but there are several factors which must be first considered.

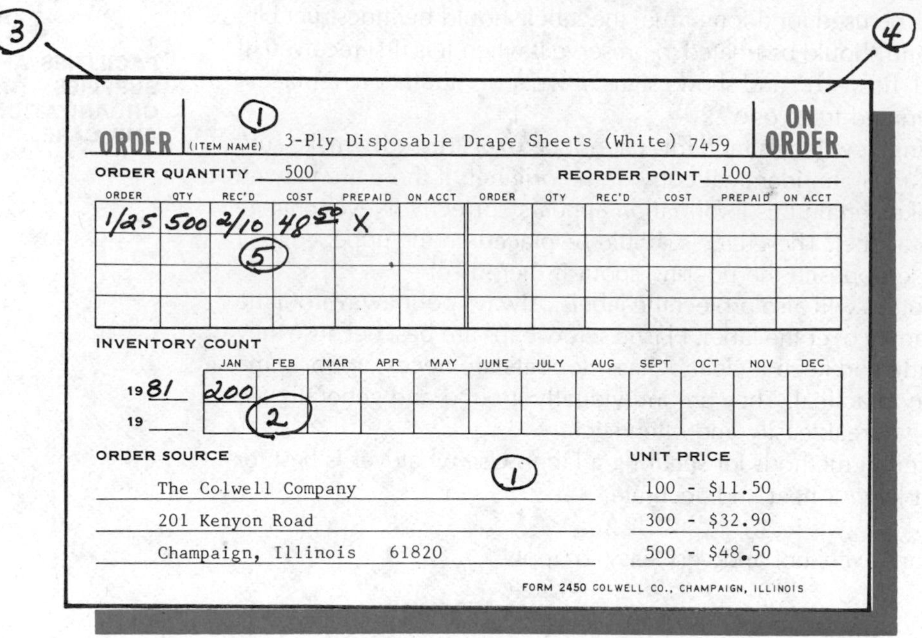
ORDER (ITEM NAME) 3-Ply Disposable Drape Sheets (White) 7459 ON ORDER

ORDER QUANTITY 500 REORDER POINT 100

ORDER	QTY	REC'D	COST	PREPAID	ON ACCT	ORDER	QTY	REC'D	COST	PREPAID	ON ACCT
1/25	500	2/10	48.50	X							

INVENTORY COUNT

	JAN	FEB	MAR	APR	MAY	JUNE	JULY	AUG	SEPT	OCT	NOV	DEC
1981	200											
19__												

ORDER SOURCE
The Colwell Company
201 Kenyon Road
Champaign, Illinois 61820

UNIT PRICE
100 - $11.50
300 - $32.90
500 - $48.50

FORM 2450 COLWELL CO., CHAMPAIGN, ILLINOIS

FIGURE 19–4 Inventory and order control card.

1. Will the supply be used in a reasonable length of time?
2. Will it spoil or deteriorate?
3. Is there proper space in the office?
4. Will the doctor continue to use the product?

Before you reorder, be sure you have the correct name of the item and any other identifying information needed. Attention to detail in ordering will be greatly appreciated by the supply houses. It will also speed delivery and assure you of obtaining exactly what you want.

A card system can be used for inventory control of all supplies. Start with 4″ × 6″ Inventory and Order Control Cards (Fig. 19–4).* These can be kept in a file box divided into two indexed sections: one for clinical materials and one for office supplies. Fill in the appropriate data on the cards (*1*),† using a separate card for each item. Next take inventory and write the amount of stock on hand in the space provided (*2*). Place a flag, such as the one shown in Figure 19–5, at the point where the supply should be replenished.

When an item needs to be ordered, place a metal tab over the "Order" section of the card (*3*). When the item is ordered, place the tab over to the right of the card in the "On Order" section (*4*). Note too the date and quantity ordered at this time.

When the order has been received, note the date and quantity in the correct column (*5*), remove the tab, and refile the card in your file box. If the order is only partially filled, let the tab remain until it is complete. The system is simple, it's accurate, and it can eliminate the problem of running out of needed supplies.

If you have any questions regarding various supplies or if you have a complaint to make, gather the following information before contacting the company: invoice number, date ordered, and name of the person who ordered it. List on paper your questions and the information you desire. If a catalog was used in making the order, open your copy to the correct page and secure additional information.

Even a reputable supply house can make mistakes, so check all the supplies you receive against your original order and the enclosed invoice. Check for correct items, sizes, and styles as well as the number or amount received. Keep all invoices and order forms for at least three years.

*Available from The Colwell Company, Champaign, Illinois
†Refer to corresponding numbers on Figure 19–4 for location of items on Inventory and Order Control Card.

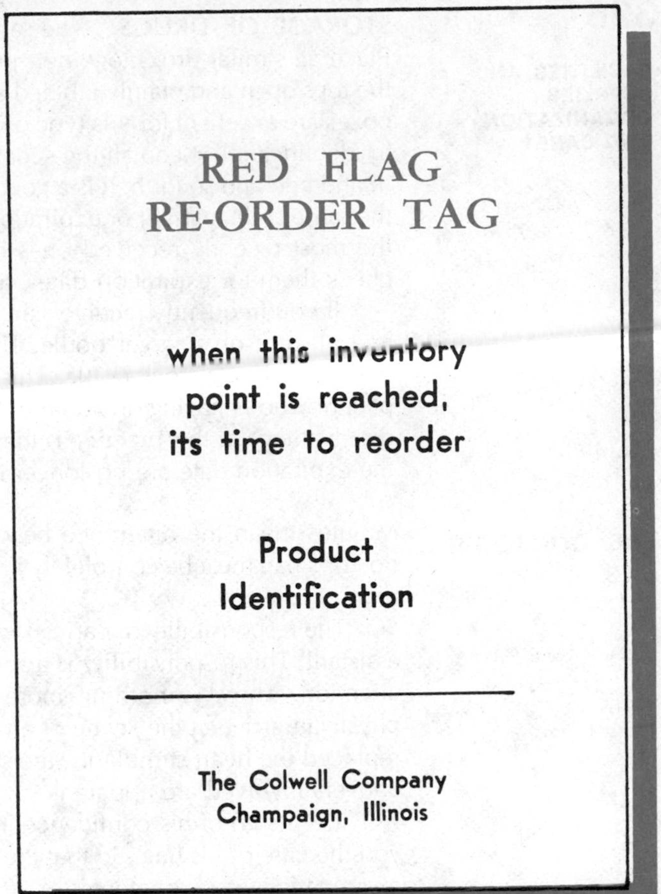

FIGURE 19–5 Red flag reorder tag.

Orders for supplies usually should be listed in a set style — that is, the actual title of the supply listed first, then the special name and size. Here are examples: "Scissors, Lister bandage, chrome, 5½ inch" or "pipette, Thoma blood diluting, for white corpuscles."

Your order should state whether payment is to be charged to the doctor's account, paid by check, or COD. Very few physicians use COD. Most doctors have established credit and prefer to pay their accounts by check at given times each month.

It is good business to inventory all equipment and supplies each year. First, list all capital purchases, such as furniture, sterilizers, and treatment machines. These items are expensive but permanent equipment. List date purchased and original price. Next, list the smaller items that are considered expendable but are less expensive, such as instruments, syringes, and thermometers. Last, estimate the usable supplies and drugs. Keep this inventory to check against the inventory for the coming year. It is also invaluable for income tax purposes.

DRUG SAMPLES. Samples of drugs and medications are continually arriving in the physician's office. These drugs should not be simply discarded. Separate those that are suitable to the doctor's practice and place them in the sample cupboard. The remainder can be saved for charitable agencies. There are many deserving medical missionaries who are very appreciative of medical supplies, but be sure to thoroughly examine the reliability of the drugs and the authenticity of the recipients before releasing the samples. The consent of the physician is, of course, also necessary. Under no circumstances should these samples be sold or given out randomly. The local medical society or the society auxiliary may be able to supply the name of a deserving charity for these samples. Sometimes they collect them and will handle the distribution.

STORAGE OF DRUGS. The sample cupboard should be organized categorically. Place all similar drugs together, preferably in boxes of similar size and shape, with the tops open and plainly labeled on the outside. Clear plastic shoe boxes or sweater boxes are excellent for this type of storage. Color-coded labels are an additional help in identification. Keep all the sedative samples in one box, all the stimulant samples in another, and so forth. It is a good practice to band together drug samples that have the same code number or expiration date. Do not forget to rotate the drugs by placing the most recently received ones in the back of the cupboard. At regular intervals check them for expiration dates, and properly discard those that have expired.

If you frequently receive samples of the same product, you can remove a label and place it on a larger bottle. Then each time this particular sample is received, empty it into the stock bottle. This may provide a good supply of the drug for some patient who is having financial difficulties and is unable to pay for his medicines. A disadvantage of this practice is that the manufacturer's drug batch code number and the expiration date are no longer known.

THE DOCTOR'S BAG

Minutes mean the difference between life or death in a medical emergency. The doctor's bag must be completely fitted and ready for his use at any hour of the day or night.

The responsibility of caring for the doctor's bag is often delegated to his medical assistant. This responsibility is a serious one and must be given close and continual attention. There is nothing more disconcerting or dangerous than to have the physician arrive at the scene of an emergency only to find that his assistant has not replaced the heart stimulants, the sedatives, or some other equally vital supply. The dangers involved are apparent.

It is a sign of his confidence in your reliability when your doctor turns over to you the care of his bag. So that the bag is always ready, establish a routine for daily examination of its contents. As a guide, keep an inventory of the bag's contents posted inside a cupboard above the place where you check and clean the bag.

If you have no time to check the bag routinely, do not fail to ask the doctor whether or not he made any house calls and find out what medications and equipment he used. You will need this information for your records and case histories.

When checking the bag, remove any specimens and see that they are properly labeled with the patient's full name, the date, and the type of test if the specimen is to be sent out for examination. If the doctor has used any instruments or gloves, remove them and replace with sterile ones. It is a wise idea to have a duplicate set of instruments and extra pairs of gloves handy so that they may be replaced immediately. Even if this equipment has not been used, it should be sterilized weekly. Keep the containers of alcohol, germicides, and other substances filled and check containers often for leaks. Do not fill fluid containers completely full to the stopper, but allow a small space for heat expansion.

If you have not received the information from the physician, you can tell what medications have been used by checking the contents of the bag against your inventory list. Medications should be routinely checked for deterioration and outdated material.

The physician usually carries only a small amount of narcotics in his bag. Whenever narcotics are dispensed from the bag, it is necessary to enter the patient's full name, the date, his address, the amount given, and the doctor's diagnosis in the office narcotic record book. This book will help you in your narcotic inventory.

You will find that the items your employer carries in his bag are determined by his personal preference, professional requirements, and the areas to be covered. When you clean the bag thoroughly each week, be careful to replace everything in its original position. The doctor organizes his bag to fit his individual needs. Often he is in a hurry, and this organization facilitates speed and accuracy. Do not substitute equipment or medications without the doctor's knowledge and consent. The many new disposable supplies make it much easier to care for the doctor's bag.

Here is a list of some items commonly found in a physician's bag:

Blood pressure set
Stethoscope
Thermometers (oral and rectal)
Flashlight and/or pen light
Sterile gloves and lubricating jelly
Wooden applicators
Assorted bandages
Adhesive tape (assorted widths)
Safety pins
Towel
Fountain pen
Prescription pads
Sterile suture set
Scalpel
Probe
Tourniquet
Percussion hammer
Illuminated diagnostic set (otoscope and ophthalmoscope)
Tissue forceps
Hemostatic forceps
Sterile syringes and needles (preferably disposable)
Sterile swabs
Sterile dressings
Tongue depressors
Scissors
Dressing forceps
Oral screw and airway
Microscopic slides and fixative
Culture tubes for throat cultures
Medications:
- Morphine
- Codeine
- Sedatives
- Adrenalin
- Digitalis
- Antibiotics (disposable type)
- Alcohol and/or skin disinfectant
- Sterilizing solution
- Spirits of ammonia

CHAPTER OUTLINE

BEHAVIORAL OBJECTIVES

The medical office assistant should be able to:

- **State the purpose of medical office management.**
- **List desirable qualities of a supervisor.**
- **Describe some of the duties of an office manager.**
- **Participate in the essentials of personnel recruitment.**
- **Plan and chair a staff meeting.**
- **Prepare an office policy manual.**
- **Prepare an office procedure manual.**
- **Supervise the selection and care of office equipment.**
- **Explain what is involved in financial management.**
- **Prepare a patient information folder.**
- **Prepare a financial policies folder.**
- **Prepare patient instruction sheets.**
- **Supervise arrangements for moving a practice.**
- **Assist in closing a practice**

20

MANAGEMENT RESPONSIBILITIES

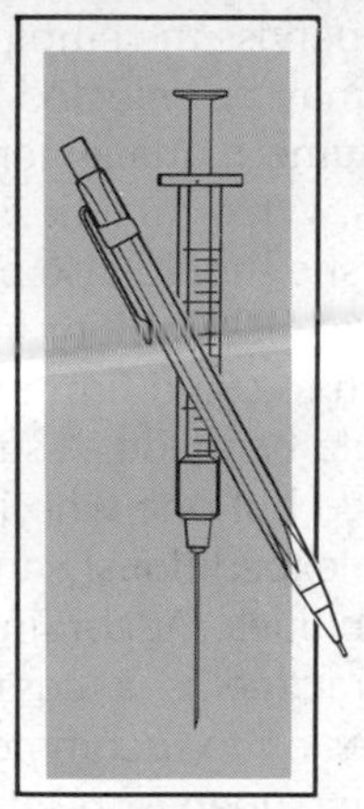

We have learned that the daily functioning of a medical office involves a multitude of details. Someone must supervise these details if there is to be harmony and not chaos.

PURPOSE OF MANAGEMENT

The purpose of medical office management is well expressed by Nourse and Marks.*

> The management of a medical office has a single purpose: to provide a quiet, functional environment in which the doctor can see and treat his patients as efficiently and effectively as possible. Everything else is secondary to this purpose. A medical office is the place where the doctor is *predictably available* to his patients for consultation, diagnosis and treatment at specified times. It is the place where he has on hand the facilities for examination and the treatment necessary for providing his patients with competent medical care. It is the place where medical records can be kept, charges for his services billed and his fees collected.

It is apparent that good management does not just happen. The lone assistant in a solo practice must be able to assume many of the management responsibilities with cooperation from the doctor. An office with three or more employees should have one person designated as supervisor or office manager. Other employees will answer to the supervisor; the supervisor will answer to the physician employer. This sets up an orderly way for the office staff to consult with the doctor regarding administrative or technical problems, complaints, or grievances; it provides an orderly way for the doctor to check on the operation of the office, disseminate information on policy changes, and correct errors or grievances. Many physicians say that friction between

*Alan E. Nourse and Geoffrey Marks, *The Management of a Medical Practice,* Philadelphia, J. B. Lippincott Company, 1963.

workers is their most common personnel problem. Management problems can often be avoided by carefully defining the areas of authority and responsibility of each employee. A definite chain of command must be established, and the physician should not undermine the supervisor's authority by circumvention. When employees know what is expected of them, they can plan both their daily and long-term work more effectively.

QUALITIES OF A SUPERVISOR

The selection of the right person to supervise the employees is critical. The supervisor may come from within the ranks or may be selected as a new member of the staff. Some employees do not wish to assume management responsibilities; others may not have the necessary qualifications. What qualities should a supervisor have? Job experience may be important, but he/she should also possess leadership ability, good judgment, good health, ability to organize, ability to learn and improve, original ideas, a sense of fairness, and strength to stand firm on policy but enough flexibility to recognize when an exception should be made. A supervisor should be one who is willing to work overtime when needed but one who isn't especially eager to do so. This person is likely to get work done expeditiously and to be intolerant of assistants who continually shirk their responsibilities. According to one writer, "running the administrative side of a medical practice is a complex job that's getting more complex every day."* The article goes on to recommend that physicians encourage and finance the attendance of their supervisors at management seminars. The American Medical Association's Department of Practice Management offers workshops designed to help medical assistants hone their office skills. One workshop called "Team Building — A Better Way to Supervise" is especially designed to sharpen the supervisory skills needed by the medical office manager to develop and manage the office team. Some practice management consultants also conduct seminars for medical office personnel. These are often arranged through a chapter of the American Association of Medical Assistants or the local medical society.

DESCRIPTION OF DUTIES

Office routines fall into three broad categories: patient scheduling, medical recordkeeping, and business management. It is the management processes that concern us here; we have dealt in detail with the first two categories in previous chapters. The duties of an office manager will of necessity vary with the practice. Management responsibilities may include any or all of the following: recruiting personnel, planning staff meetings, reducing staff friction, improving work flow, suggesting improved office efficiencies, supervising the purchase and repair of equipment, purchase and storage of supplies, office upkeep, supervising financial management and cost control, patient education, reducing physician strain, and eliminating time wasters for the physician. Some of the greatest time wasters are telephone interruptions, overscheduling, too many meetings, team conflict, too much paperwork, having to check employees' work, a cluttered desk, drop-in visitors, and fatigue.

STAFF MEETINGS

One of the most common complaints from office personnel is that of being unable to discuss problems with the doctor. There must be some formal mechanism for keeping the office manager and other key employees current on the daily business affairs of the practice. The answer may be in holding weekly staff meetings. Some of the best ideas for improvement come from the office staff, and this should be encouraged. The simplest technique is to set aside a specific time for meetings. The meetings need not be long or overly formal, but in order to be effective they must be planned and organized. Choose a chairperson (usually the physician) and a secretary to take notes. All members of the staff should be encouraged to submit ideas for discussion. Draw up a simple outline of the issues you want to discuss and prepare any supporting data needed for the meeting. The staff meeting should be a place to

---

*J. Wandres, "Seminars for staff home office efficiency," Physician's Management, October 1978.

discuss new ideas, any changes in office procedures, and resolution of any problems. It must not be allowed to deteriorate into a gripe session. Individual complaints should be handled privately. The agenda might be similar to that of any business meeting: (1) reading of the last meeting's minutes, (2) discussion of any old business, (3) discussion of any problems in the clinical area, (4) discussion of any problems in the administrative area, (5) discussion of any problems in common areas, and (6) adjournment. Some physicians like to combine the staff meeting with a breakfast or lunch. The time or place is not important so long as it suits the practice and the meetings are conducted regularly, democratically, and without interruption.

OFFICE POLICY MANUAL

An office policy manual serves as a training guide for the new employee, a ready reference for the temporary employee, and a reminder of policies for the regular employee. A policy manual accomplishes several goals: it solidifies what may have been vague thoughts into definite statements of policy, communicates these statements in exactly the same way to every employee, and provides a permanent record of these policies. This does not mean that they can never be changed, but a well-formulated policy may be the difference between order and chaos. The manual must be designed for a specific office, comprehensive but flexible, easy to read, and conform to professional ethics; it must be reviewed frequently and kept up to date as changes in policy occur.

What should an office policy manual contain? Because the manual is designed for the dissemination of information to all employees, it should probably start with a statement of the philosophy of the practice and any general office policies, followed by a personnel chart showing the line of authority and stating who has authority to enforce the policies.

Every employer has certain expectations regarding personal appearance of the employees. These should be set forth in the manual so that there is no misunderstanding. Dress code, the use of make-up and perfume, cleanliness, grooming, and hygiene are difficult topics to discuss on a personal basis but can be matter-of-fact in an office manual.

Describe the work week, listing the daily office hours and any days off, the doctor's daily schedule and where he can be reached with messages or emergencies. Specify the time allowed each day for lunch and breaks and whether they must be taken at a specific time. State the vacation policy, how much time the employee is

Name ______________________ Soc. Sec. No. ____________
Job Classification ______________________________
Employment Date ______________ Starting Salary ____________

Salary checks are issued every (week) (two weeks) (semi-monthly) (month) on ____________ (day or date).

Increase-in-pay review will be conducted six months after the completion of three-month probationary period and each six months thereafter.

Date of first pay review ______________
Current maximum salary for this job classification $____________
Revised ____________ $____________
Revised ____________ $____________

SALARY SCHEDULE

Date	Amount of Increase	Total Salary

FIGURE 20–1 Example of a page from an office policy manual.

allowed in working days, who authorizes it, and whether there are any restrictions.

What provision is there for sick leave, emergency leave, and any other absences? When is the employee eligible for benefits? Are medical services provided by the staff? What holidays does the office observe? What are the overtime policies?

Is there a policy for performance reviews, salary reviews, and merit increases? (Fig. 20–1). When is payday? Are there annual bonuses? If so, on what are they based? Are there other benefits for employees, such as professional dues, health insurance, uniform allowances, pension plan, profit sharing, free parking? How much notice should an employee give if she wants to quit? What are grounds for immediate dismissal?

To whom should employees go with problems or suggestions? Is time off given for education courses or for attending professional organization conventions or seminars? Is this paid time or vacation time? Does the office pay for courses, professional memberships, and expenses for professional conventions?

These are just suggestions. The policy manual must be tailored to the specific office for which it is designed.

OFFICE PROCEDURE MANUAL

The office procedure manual supplements the office policy manual. Sometimes the two are combined. Whereas the policy manual is informational, the procedure manual is a "how to" manual. It will contain a job description for each position in the practice and detailed steps for carrying out each task. Unfortunately, too few practices take the time to develop such a manual, and even those that do will often neglect to use it and keep it up to date.

A job description is a detailed account of the duties and the qualifications for a specific position (Fig. 20–2). In some cases it should state both primary and secondary duties, emphasizing that the employee must be flexible. Following the list of duties, there should be a procedure sheet for each task. A procedure sheet is a

POSITION: Office Manager
RESPONSIBLE TO: Physician

The office manager is responsible for the coordination of all office activities, including recruitment and training of personnel, accounting and financial procedures.

SPECIFIC TASKS:

1. Preparation of annual budget
2. Preparation of monthly profit and loss statement
3. Approval of all expenditures
4. Review and disposition of delinquent accounts
5. Approval of all write-offs
6. Liaison with accountant
7. Recruiting, hiring, and firing
8. Conducting performance appraisals and reporting to physician
9. Arrange personnal vacations and keep records of leave days
10. Assist in improving work flow and office efficiencies
11. Supervise purchase and repair of equipment
12. Purchase and storage of supplies
13. Arrange for practice insurance
14. Supervise regular staff meetings
15. Keep office policy manual current
16. Prepare patient education materials as needed

JOB QUALIFICATIONS: CMA-A or degree in business administration
Previous medical office experience
Supervisory experience helpful

FIGURE 20–2 Example of a job description.

verbal flow chart that lists step-by-step the logical sequence of activities involved in a given task. An employee should be able to perform the task by following the written instructions (Fig. 20–3). Procedure writing is sometimes difficult because we all tend to take for granted many of the simpler steps involved once we become proficient. After a task has been learned it is unnecessary to refer to the procedure sheet for instructions, but it is invaluable in training the new recruit and in assisting the temporary employee.

Job descriptions and procedure sheets help the employee achieve what is expected of him/her. Practice management specialists say that the most common remark from a discharged employee is "I didn't know I was supposed to. . ." A written job description may also help avoid legal problems with an employee who is dismissed for nonperformance.

A great deal of instruction can be incorporated into a procedure manual. Preferred office procedure, both administrative and clinical, should be spelled out in detail.

How are records prepared and filed? A description of the filing system may save the day if a temporary employee must find something in the file during the regular assistant's absence. How is the telephone to be answered? Which calls are put through to the doctor immediately, and which may the assistant handle? Include a list of the names and telephone numbers of persons you call often — for example, consulting physicians, hospitals, laboratories, and the physician's spouse. Explain the billing and collection procedures. Is billing done weekly, twice monthly, monthly? Are the statements prepared in the office? By what method? Is a collection agency used? Which one?

What kind of set-up does the doctor prefer for various office surgeries or treatments? Is there a card index showing these set-ups? If so, where is it kept? How much time is allotted for new patients? Established patients? Postoperative patients?

Have a page explaining where and how supplies are ordered and where they are stored. The name, address, and telephone number of each supplier should be included. List the major pieces of equipment with their serial numbers, where and when purchased, and a telephone number for servicing.

Note any special duties the doctor expects of the assistant, such as organizational activities or making travel arrangements. Professional information regarding the physician's education and specialty boards, hospital staff memberships, membership

PROCEDURE SHEET PROCESS INCOMING MAIL

1. Assemble all necessary tools and supplies: letter opener, paper clips, stapler, mending tape, date stamp.
2. Open all mail except letters marked *personal*.
3. Check to be sure writer's address is on letter before destroying envelope. Staple envelope to letter if address is missing.
4. Paper clip enclosures to letter (or note their absence if they are not enclosed).
5. Date stamp the letter or piece of mail.
6. Set aside cash receipts for processing.
7. Route insurance claim forms and inquiries to insurance clerk.
8. Arrange mail with second and third class on bottom, then first class, with any personal mail on top.
9. Place entire stack in mail tray on right side of doctor's desk.

FIGURE 20–3 Example of a procedure sheet.

in professional societies, state license number, and narcotic registry number belong in the manual.

A checklist of daily, weekly, monthly, quarterly, and yearly duties would be valuable. Completed samples of forms that need to be filled out and samples of correspondence provide excellent visual instruction.

Good management indicates that in the multiple-employee office, each position has an understudy who can substitute in an emergency. A well-documented procedure manual that is kept current ensures continuity where one employee must on occasion fill in for or assist another.

Development of a procedure manual is a good discussion item for staff meetings; the cooperation of the staff is essential if the project is to be successful. Keep it simple to update by using a three-ring binder. Be sure to destroy old pages when revisions are made. One master copy should remain in the custody of the office manager and one with the physician. Each employee should have a copy of the portion that affects him/her.

PERSONNEL RECRUITMENT

HIRING. Suggestions for interviewing and hiring were included in Chapter 2, Finding the Right Position. During the hiring proceedings, the interviewer may wish to invite the prospective employee to lunch with the staff, or for coffee in the more relaxed atmosphere of the employee lounge. This permits an opportunity to discover whether his/her personality will mesh with the atmosphere of the office.

Discuss the job description for the position being filled. This is essential if you are to be certain that the person being interviewed understands the required duties and responsibilities. Keep in mind, though, that job descriptions may change when personnel changes. No two people have the same capabilities and interests; and there's no need to try to mold a person to a job description when a simple shift in duties may accomplish a happier result. For instance, a clerical assistant might normally be expected to complete the computer sheets at the end of the day, but if a clinical assistant has a special aptitude for this and really enjoys the tasks, there's no reason this change in responsibility should not be made. Note it on the job description so that there's no confusion about who is responsible.

ORIENTATION AND TRAINING. Recruitment does not end with the hiring. The new employee must understand what is expected and should be given some preliminary training before she can develop her full potential. Show the new employee the physical environment in which she will work by giving her a tour of the office. Introduce her to the rest of the staff. Brief her on the nature of the practice and specialty, explain what type of patients will be dealt with, and how she will be

Dear___________:

Since your decision to leave our employ a few weeks ago, I have been concerned about your reasons for doing so. There may have been more than one reason—and one of them may have been dissatisifaction with the working conditions.

If there was in fact some reason for dissatisfaction that influenced your decision to leave our employ, I would appreciate your passing it along to me, so that I may avoid losing other valuable employees in the future.

Please drop me a note, telephone, or come in if you wish. I assure you that any comments you care to make will be treated with respect and appreciation.

Cordially yours,

FIGURE 20–4 Example of a letter from physician to an employee who resigns suddenly.

expected to interact with them. Explain office policies by having her read the office policy manual and then go over it with her. Be certain that the new employee understands your long-range expectations, but do not expect that she will handle all of them efficiently on her first day. Taking time to train the new member of the staff will lessen the chance of difficulties later.

PERFORMANCE AND SALARY REVIEW. The supervisor is responsible for an ongoing performance appraisal, complimenting whenever possible and appropriate, and offering helpful criticism when necessary. A formal performance appraisal at the end of the probationary period and at regular six-month intervals thereafter, with a report to the physician employer, is helpful in the employee's salary review.

The performance appraisal will include a judgment of both the quality and quantity of work, personal appearance, attitudes and team spirit, dependability, attendance, and any other qualities essential to satisfactory performance of the job in question.

DISMISSAL. The necessity of having to dismiss an employee is unpleasant at best, but if the ground rules are decided upon in advance, written into the policy manual, and explained to all employees, the problem is partially solved. The policies must be applied equally and impartially to all. The final decision for dismissal will probably be made by the physician but may be based on the recommendation of the office manager. The person who does the hiring should do the firing.

The probationary employee who does not prove satisfactory should be dismissed at the end of the probationary period with tact and a full explanation of the reasons for dismissal. It may be that some of the reasons for failure were present at the time of hiring, and the person who did the hiring must share the failure. It is important that the manager understand and profit from this experience.

An employee who has been in service for some time and is giving unsatisfactory performance should be warned and given an explanation of the specific improvements expected. If a second chance does not produce improvement in performance or attitude, then dismissal must follow. It should be done privately, with tact and consideration. Most practice consultants believe that firing should come close to the end of the day after all other employees have left and that the break should be clean and immediate. If the office policy provides for two weeks' notice, give two weeks' pay. A fired employee should not be allowed to train or influence a replacement. The exit meeting should be planned just as carefully as the employment interview. Be honest with the employee. Discuss the employee's assets as well as liabilities, and give the reasons for the termination before you announce the dismissal. There's no need to dwell upon the employee's deficiencies. These should have been thoroughly discussed at the warning interview, and the employee need only be told that the necessary improvements have not been made. Do listen to the employee's feedback, however. This may reveal some important administrative problems that need correction. And don't offer to give the employee a good reference unless you can do it sincerely.

Certain breaches of conduct, such as embezzlement, blatant insubordination, or violation of patient confidentiality, are grounds for immediate dismissal without warning.

Occasionally an employee will voluntarily terminate a job without giving a valid reason. The physician or office manager may wish to follow up with a letter to the former employee to seek out any problem that may have caused the resignation (Fig. 20–4).

OFFICE FACILITIES

Physicians are generally well aware of what is new in clinical and surgical equipment. Even those who want nothing but the best in surgical instruments may remain blissfully ignorant of what is new and improved in office equipment. The office manager must be the one who keeps informed of what is in the market place and how it can improve the efficiency of the administrative functions. It is up to her to know that the adding machine is on its way out, having been replaced with the multipurpose printing calculator; that the postage meter can expedite the mail; that an electric letter opener is inexpensive and may quickly pay for itself in time saved. Some doctors are now purchasing memory typewriters, whereas others still haven't heard that the electric typewriter was invented. Good equipment, strategically placed, can go a long way in boosting employee morale as well as efficiency. When you do purchase new equipment, make certain that it is in good working order, file the warranty in a safe place, and be sure that anyone using the equipment has first read the instruction manual. Keep the instruction manual near the equipment.

The office manager will oversee the purchase and storage of supplies. He/she will also coordinate office maintenance, safety, and security. These matters were discussed in the preceding chapter.

FINANCIAL MANAGEMENT

The degree to which an office manager is involved in the financial management of the practice will depend upon education, experience, and his/her willingness to accept responsibility. In all likelihood his/her duties will include supervising the cash receipts, banking, billing, and collections. The office manager will probably also write payroll checks, pay bills, and act as liaison with the accountant. The office manager who has accounting skills will probably prepare periodic profit and loss statements, and compute collection ratios and overhead percentage reports. Financial management also includes making provision for and seeing that premiums are paid on time for practice insurance such as professional liability, worker's compensation, employee's health coverage, and unemployment insurance.

PATIENT EDUCATION

One of the big time wasters in the medical office is having to explain the same details about office procedures over and over again to patients. The same principles discussed in personnel training apply here, namely, *put it in writing;* then a copy can be given to every new patient. Patients have many common concerns about the doctor's policies, such as office hours, the doctor's specialty, directions for reaching the office, parking facilities, emergency services, answering service, cancellations, house calls, prescription renewals, payment of fees, and so forth. Many management experts recommend that two separate folders or pamphlets be prepared — one devoted to general office information and another to financial policies.

PATIENT INFORMATION FOLDER. A patient information folder can be easily compiled by the doctor and office staff acting cooperatively in a staff meeting. Experience has shown that the patient information folder can reduce the number of incoming phone calls by an average of 20 to 30 per cent. It can also reduce misunderstanding and forgotten instructions. It must of necessity be tailored to the specific practice, but guidelines may be obtained free from the American Medical Association's Department of Practice Management.

The patient folder should be an introduction to your office, describing the services available, ancillary testing services provided, laboratory services if any, office hours, specialty information, what to do in case of emergency, night and weekend coverage, appointment and cancellation policies, telephone calls (office and answering service), hospitals used, prescription renewals, directions for reaching the office, parking facilities, house calls, and providing answers to any other questions frequently asked by the patients.

FINANCIAL POLICIES FOLDER. A small folder covering the financial policies of the office can eliminate many questions and possible misunderstanding. Keep it small enough to fit into the billing envelope and send it out with monthly statements.

1. State if office visits are payable at time of service.

2. State how payment can be made — for instance, are VISA and MasterCard acceptable? Can time payments be arranged?

3. Is there a charge for missed appointments?

4. Is there a charge for completing insurance and disability forms? How much? Are there any exceptions?

5. Are there charges for other services such as telephone prescriptions, year-end statements, returned checks?

6. Outline clearly that the ultimate responsibility for payment lies with the patient.

PATIENT INSTRUCTION SHEETS. In most medical offices there are patient procedures that occur over and over again. Instead of attempting to orally instruct a patient each time, why not develop clearly stated procedure sheets that you can review with the patient and then give the patient the written instructions to take along. Just be certain that the patient understands the instructions before he leaves the office. The instruction sheets can include such procedures as preparation for certain radiographic or laboratory tests, preoperative and postoperative instructions, diet sheets, taking an enema, dressing a wound — in fact, anything for which patients are repeatedly given instructions.

SPECIAL DUTIES

Before closing the chapter, we should mention certain events that do not occur with regularity but may confront the office manager at some time.

MOVING DAY. The thought of moving into a shiny new spacious office can be thrilling. Unless the move is planned in advance, however, moving day — and the weeks that follow — can be a nightmare. One way to handle the situation is for the doctor to plan a nice long vacation, giving the office manager full responsibility and authority to make the move. More often, though, the move takes place after hours or over the weekend, with all employees lending a hand, then reporting for work in the new facility, completely exhausted, on the next working day.

Do some careful measuring to see how the furniture and equipment you plan to move will fit into the new quarters. If possible, draw the rooms to scale and show where each item is to be placed by the mover. Include the location of available electrical outlets in your floor plan. If new furniture, carpets, or equipment will be needed, try to have them in place before moving day. Don't expect to have the new carpet installed the day of your move.

Decide what day you will move and whether you will close the office for one day or several. Select a mover and confirm the date. Patients must be notified of the move. As soon as the moving date is established, post a notice in the office and draw the patients' attention to it. You may want to send announcement cards to the active patients. Many doctors place a notice in the local newpapers.

At least 60 days in advance of the move, start a change of address notification campaign. Notify publishers of journals and suppliers of catalogs. Six weeks' notice is generally required on all subscriptions, and postage due on forwarded journals can be very expensive. Notify the telephone company and utility companies well in advance so that there will be no break in service. File a change of address card with the local post office. Order stationery and business cards with the new address.

The moving company will supply packing cartons for you to use. Have each employee be responsible for packing and labeling the items from his/her own work area. Tag each carton with a number and keep a master list of what is in each numbered carton. This will help you find items that you need. Also, if a carton should be lost or mislaid, you will have a record of what was in it. If time allows, just prior to moving is a good time to cull material from the files and discard old journals, supply catalogs, and any obsolete supplies or equipment.

Outline the moving day strategy showing each person's responsibility and give each one a copy. It may be wise to work in shifts to avoid confusion, but have one person at the new address to direct the movers when they arrive.

After the move, be sure to mention the new address when patients call for appointments.

CLOSING A PRACTICE. A doctor's practice may be closed because of retirement, death, a change in geographic location, or a change in profession.

If closing the practice is voluntary and can be planned in advance, the doctor may wish to consult an attorney or the local medical society for guidelines. Often, though, the closing is sudden and unexpected, and much of the burden falls on the office staff. The doctor who anticipates retirement can begin cutting back the practice months in advance. At this time he can notify patients as they come in that he will be closing the practice on a specified date and suggest that they begin arrangements for care from another physician. He can also ask that patients pay at the time of service to minimize accounts receivable at the time of retirement.

To avoid a charge of abandonment, the doctor should notify active patients by letter that he is discontinuing practice. The letter should be sent out at least three months in advance, if possible. If a patient has been discharged or has not been in to see the doctor for at least six years, there is no obligation to send the notice.

If another doctor is taking over the practice, tell the patient about the new doctor. However, be sure the patient understands that his records will be transferred to any doctor of his choice. The request for transfer of records must be in writing. For convenience, the doctor can have a form available that needs only the patient's signature. Remember that although the records belong to the physician they can legally be transferred to another physician only with the consent of the patient. Any records not transferred should be stored, either in bulk or on microfilm, until the statutes of limitations for malpractice and abandonment have run out.

Income tax returns and supporting documents should be kept for at least three years after the tax return was filed. Appoint someone to take care of any remaining outstanding accounts receivable.

Check with the Drug Enforcement Administration (DEA) of the U. S. Department of Justice for current regulations on disposal of controlled substances and the physician's certificate of registration. Do not simply toss them out. The certificate will have to be sent to the DEA for cancellation and then it will be returned. It may be necessary to produce an inventory of all controlled substances on hand when the practice is terminated along with duplicate copies of the official order forms that were used to obtain them. Return any unused order forms to the DEA. Don't use leftover prescription blanks for note pads. Burn them to avoid misuse.

The physician who is discontinuing active medical practice altogether can safely drop his professional liability insurance. However, do not destroy any of the previous policies. Most professional liability claims are covered by the policy that was in effect at the time the alleged act of negligence took place. The suit may be filed many years later and it is important that the old policy be available.

Some physicians reward loyal employees with severance pay. On the average this equals at least one month's salary plus prorated compensation for any unused vacation time.

Unfortunately, used office furniture and equipment do not bring much in the marketplace. If another physician is taking over the practice, the value of the furnishings and equipment can be negotiated. Many doctors donate their libraries to the local hospital and declare the gift as a deduction on their income tax. This is something to check with the accountant.

There are many details to take care of in closing a practice. Contact the local medical society for further guidance.

References

Hanna, J. M., Popham, E. L., and Tilton, R. S.: Secretarial Procedures and Administration, 6th Edition. Cincinnati, South-Western Publishing Company, 1973.

Horsley, J. E.: Don't close your practice until you read this. Medical Economics, June 14, 1976, pp. 187–193.

Johnson, H. W.: Selecting, Training, and Supervising Office Personnel. Menlo Park, California, Addison-Wesley Publishing Company, 1969.

Nourse, A. E., and Marks, G.: The Management of a Medical Practice. Philadelphia, J. B. Lippincott Company, 1963.

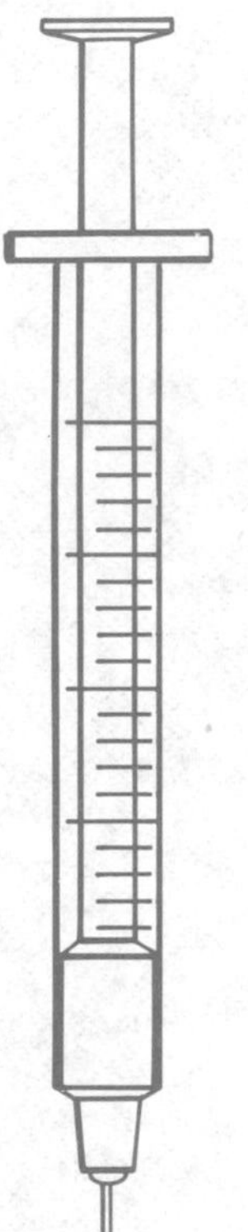

Chapter Outline

Normal Nutrition
- Nutrition and Dietetics
- Food
- Energy
- Dietary Evaluation
- Nutrients
  - Carbohydrates
  - Fats
  - Proteins
  - Vitamins
  - Minerals
  - Water
  - Fiber

Therapeutic Nutrition
- Modifying a Diet
  - Consistency
  - Calorie Level
  - Levels of One or More Nutrients
  - Bulk
  - Spiciness
  - Levels of Specific Foods
  - Feeding Intervals
- Prescribing a Diet

BEHAVIORAL OBJECTIVES

The medical assistant should be able to:

- **List the Four Basic Food Groups and know the major nutrients contributed by each group.**
- **Identify the Recommended Daily Allowances for a specific nutrient for a given individual by using the NRC table.**
- **Evaluate menus using either the Four Basic Food Groups or the NRC table.**
- **Describe the classic deficiency diseases, major food sources, and basic function in the body of the nutrients required for good health.**
- **Identify the seven basic methods of modifying the normal diet for therapeutic purposes.**
- **Name the general characteristics of a given therapeutic diet and describe its application in terms of the types of conditions for which it can be used.**
- **Describe the function of the medical assistant in teaching and interpreting the therapeutic diet for a patient.**

21

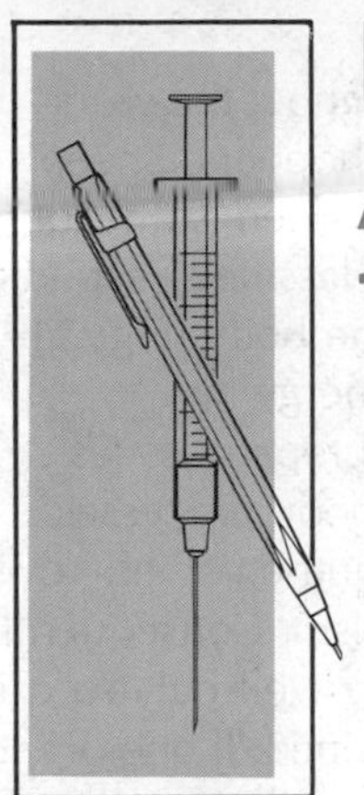

NUTRITION AND DIET THERAPY

LEE WELLER CALLAWAY, R.D., M.P.H., Ph.D.

NORMAL NUTRITION

Good health is a state of emotional and physical well-being which is determined to a large extent by a person's diet. We are, quite literally, what we eat, since the food we consume is used to build and repair every part of our bodies. Consequently, it is important that the food choices made are based on sound information and knowledge. A person who is well nourished will probably be more alert in every way and emotionally better balanced. He is also better able than the poorly nourished individual to ward off infections.

The physician, the nurse, and the **dietitian** are all closely involved in the nutritive care of a patient. The physician prescribes the diet, and, ideally, a dietitian instructs the patient on how to follow it. Frequently, however, such professional aid is not available. In this case, it is often necessary for the assistant to discuss the diet with the patient, answer questions, and explain certain aspects of the modifications involved. Many patients may hesitate to ask the physician details about the diet, or questions may arise after the patients leave the office. Such concerns are usually about methods of preparation, sources of information, interpretation of the label, and so forth, and the medical assistant is the one the patient turns to for answers. Consequently, the assistant should be able to answer basic questions on normal nutrition and have a fundamental knowledge of those diets which the doctor prescribes most often.

Nutrition and Dietetics

The definitions of these terms vary considerably throughout the literature. Basically, the science of **nutrition** is concerned with studying the nutritive materials taken into the body (food) and the **metabolic** processes that utilize them. Nutrition, as such, is defined in the *Handbook of Diet Therapy* as the "combination of processes by which the living organism receives and utilizes the materials necessary for the maintenance of its functions and for the growth and renewal of its components." In a slightly different context, nutrition is also used to indicate nutritional status or the condition of the body due to "the utilization of the essential nutrients available to the body."

Dietetics, on the other hand, is the practical application of nutritional science to individuals. It is "the combined science and art of feeding individuals or groups under different economic or health conditions according to the principles of nutrition and management."

Food

There are many materials eaten throughout the world that we in the United States do not consider acceptable food (grasshoppers, sheep's eyes, and so on). Similarly, many substances man can eat are forbidden, some for religious reasons or because of cultural custom. Nevertheless, to be classified as food a substance must perform one or more of three basic functions in the body (Fig. 21–1):

1. Provide a source of fuel or energy
2. Supply nutrients to build and repair tissues
3. Supply nutrients to regulate body processes

Most foods supply both fuel and nutrients; however, no one food supplies all nutrients required for proper metabolism. Consequently, a mixture of different foods is necessary. With a little planning, a well-balanced diet, one that supplies all the elements the body needs, can be obtained. If one or more of the required nutrients is inadequate, health suffers and the ability to function optimally is lowered. If prolonged **deficiencies** occur, specific diseases, even death, may follow.

Nutrients are substances from food that are utilized by the cells of the body. When food is consumed and broken down by the process of digestion, the nutrients derived are absorbed into the system.

Digestion is a series of reactions occurring in the mouth, the stomach, and the small intestine that result in reducing large food molecules into simple absorbable forms. Absorption is the process of assimilation of foods into the body when they are in their simpler forms. Most absorption occurs in the small intestines. The blood then carries the digested and absorbed nutrients to all parts of the body where they are **metabolized.**

Energy

Every bodily action, whether voluntary or involuntary, requires energy. Even when asleep the body still needs a source of energy for basal metabolism, to keep the heart beating, the lungs breathing, and other vital organs functioning. Voluntary action refers to muscular activities that are consciously carried out. The involuntary activities of digestion and respiration also require energy even though not consciously controlled.

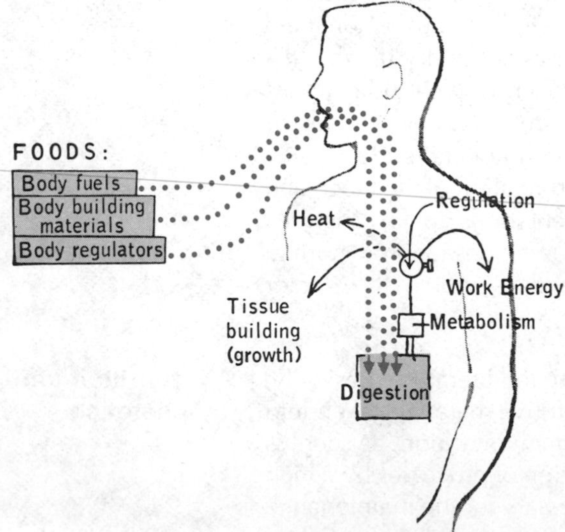

FIGURE 21–1 The functions of food. For an item to qualify as a food, it must offer substances that act as body fuel to provide energy, serve to build or maintain body tissues, or act as regulators of body processes. Many foods contain substances that serve all three purposes. (From Bogert, J. L., et al.: *Nutrition and Physical Fitness,* 9th Ed. Philadelphia, W. B. Saunders Co., 1973.)

There are basically two energy sources available to the body: **exogenous** and **endogenous.** If insufficient quantities of food (exogenous) are consumed to furnish the required fuel, the body will begin to break down its own fat reserves (endogenous) in an attempt to supply the necessary energy. Generally, it is desirable for the daily food intake to equal the total energy needs of the body (number of calories needed for both voluntary and involuntary activities).

Energy, or heat production, is measured in units called **calories.** In nutrition the "large calorie," or kilocalorie (kcal), is used to differentiate it from the smaller, more widely used calorie. One kilocalorie (or Calorie) is defined as the amount of heat required to raise the temperature of one kilogram of water one degree Centigrade.* Of the seven food constituents, carbohydrates, fats, and proteins are capable of furnishing the body with energy. One gram of either carbohydrate or protein yields 4 kcal/gm, whereas one gram of fat provides 9 kcal/gm. The amount of energy needed by a given individual varies considerably with his activity level and basal requirements; however, most adults require 1800 to 3600 kcal a day.

Dietary Evaluation

There are two basic methods commonly used for determining the nutritional adequacy of a given diet. The easier is a shorthand method and utilizes the Four Basic Groups. The other, using the recommended allowances, is more time consuming but more accurate.

THE FOUR BASIC FOOD GROUPS. Foods within a group supply similar nutrients, although the foods differ in caloric level and in nutrients supplied. If the Four Basic Food plan is followed and no other foods are included, the average diet will supply 1200 kcal. If the foods from each group are chosen wisely, a person can meet all of the nutrient requirements (with the possible exception of iron for women). Additional calories are easily obtained by either increasing the total quantity of food eaten from the Basic Four or adding sugars and fats to these foods (Table 21–1).

*Although the term calorie is currently being used, nomenclature is expected to change soon. The Joule is a unit of energy that is accepted by all scientists. Conversion: 1 Calorie = 4.184 Joules.

TABLE 21–1 The Four Basic Food Groups

Food Group	Average Amount/Serving	Average Servings/Day	Major Nutrients
Milk and dairy products	8 oz fluid milk ⅔ cup ice cream 1 oz cheddar cheese	children, 4 adults, 2	Calcium Phosphorus Protein Riboflavin
Meats (beef, lamb, poultry, fish, veal); eggs; and meat alternatives (dry beans, peas, lentils, nuts, or peanut butter)	3 oz cooked weight meat 1 cup dry beans or nuts 5 tsp peanut butter	2	Protein Iron Thiamine Niacin
Fruits and vegetables	½ cup	4 (1 citrus daily, 1 dark green leafy or deep yellow vegetable every other day)	Vitamin A Vitamin C
Breads and cereals	1 slice bread ½ cup cooked cereal ¾ cup dry cereal	4 (whole grain or enriched)	Thiamine Iron Protein Niacin Riboflavin

In planning daily menus a person should try to schedule regularly spaced meals. It is not an absolute necessity that three meals be consumed; however, it is extremely difficult to meet all of the nutrient and caloric requirements with fewer meals. Each meal should supply about one-third of the total daily requirements. This means that something from each group should be included at every meal.

RECOMMENDED DAILY ALLOWANCES. During World War II, the Food and Nutrition Board of the National Academy of Sciences–National Research Council was appointed to examine current research in the field of nutrition and to set up dietary standards. The first edition of the resulting dietary guide was published in 1943 and has been updated approximately every five years since then, as new research data have become available. The latest revision (1979) is shown in Table 21–2. The standards are known as the NRC's (National Research Council) or as the Recommended Dietary Allowances (RDA). These are suggested daily nutrient intakes that are "judged to be adequate for the maintenance of good nutrition in essentially all healthy persons in the United States under current conditions of living."* All nutrients, except for calories, allow a safety margin to cover individual physical or environmental variations. The allowances are not, however, meant to be adequate in cases of illness or injury. The allowances are grouped by both age and sex. Activity level is assumed to be moderate.

Nutrients

Nutrients are divided into seven classes: carbohydrates, fats, proteins, vitamins, minerals, water, and fiber. All of these must be supplied in sufficient quantities daily for good health.

*Recommended Dietary Allowances, Publication #1694, 8th Ed., Washington, D.C., National Academy of Science–National Research Council, 1973, adapted.

TABLE 21–2 Recommended Daily Dietary Allowances, Revised 1980, Food and Nutrition Board, National Academy of Sciences–National Research Council. Designed for the Maintenance of Good Nutrition of Practically All Healthy People in the U.S.A.*

		Weight		Height			Fat-Soluble Vitamins			Water-Soluble Vitamins	
	Age *(years)*	kg	lb	cm	in	**Protein** *(g)*	**Vitamin A** *(μg RE)*†	**Vitamin D** *(μg)*‡	**Vitamin E** *(mg α TE)*§	**Vitamin C** *(mg)*	**Thiamine** *(mg)*
Infants	0.0–0.5	6	13	60	24	kg × 2.2	420	10	3	35	0.3
	0.5–1.0	9	20	71	28	kg × 2.0	400	10	4	35	0.5
Children	1–3	13	29	90	35	23	400	10	5	45	0.7
	4–6	20	44	112	44	30	500	10	6	45	0.9
	7–10	28	62	132	52	34	700	10	7	45	1.2
Males	11–14	45	99	157	62	45	1000	10	8	50	1.4
	15–18	66	145	176	69	56	1000	10	10	60	1.4
	19–22	70	154	177	70	56	1000	7.5	10	60	1.5
	23–50	70	154	178	70	56	1000	5	10	60	1.4
	51+	70	154	178	70	56	1000	5	10	60	1.2
Females	11–14	46	101	157	62	46	800	10	8	50	1.1
	15–18	55	120	163	64	46	800	10	8	60	1.1
	19–22	55	120	163	64	44	800	7.5	8	60	1.1
	23–50	55	120	163	64	44	800	5	8	60	1.0
	51+	55	120	163	64	44	800	5	8	60	1.0
Pregnant						+30	+200	+5	+2	+20	+0.4
Lactating						+20	+400	+5	+3	+40	+0.5

*The allowances are intended to provide for individual variations among most normal persons as they live in the United States under usual environmental stresses. Diets should be based on a variety of common foods in order to provide other nutrients for which human requirements have been less well defined. See text for detailed discussion of allowances and of nutrients not tabulated.

†Retinol equivalents. 1 Retinol equivalent = 1 μg retinol or 6 μg βcarotene. See text for calculation of vitamin A activity of diets as retinol equivalents.

‡As cholecalciferol. 10 μg cholecalciferol = 400 IU vitamin D.

§α-tocopherol equivalents. 1 mg d-α-tocopherol = 1 α-TE. See text for variation in allowances and calculation of vitamin E activity of the diet as α-tocopherol equivalents.

Carbohydrates are chemical organic compounds composed of carbon, hydrogen, and oxygen. They are divided into three groups based on the complexity of the molecule: monosaccharides, disaccharides, and polysaccharides.

Carbohydrates

Monosaccharides and disaccharides are also called simple sugars, that is, they are made of one (mono) or two (di) units (saccharides). They are water soluble and sweet to the taste. The three most important monosaccharides in our diet are glucose, fructose, and galactose. Sucrose, lactose, and maltose are examples of disaccharides. Glucose (also called dextrose) and fructose (fruit sugar) are widely distributed in fruits and vegetables. During the process of digestion, disaccharides and the polysaccharide starch are broken down into monosaccharides and absorbed into the blood stream. Once absorbed they are transported to the liver where fructose and galactose are converted to glucose. Glucose, then, is an especially important sugar since it is the form of carbohydrate used by the body for energy and the only form of carbohydrate used in the brain and nervous system for fuel. Galactose is not present free in foods but is one of the two monosaccharides found in the disaccharide lactose.

Lactose is the major carbohydrate in milk and is the only common sugar not found in plant sources. It is not so sweet as many sugars and, therefore, is frequently used to sweeten formulas for tube feedings or to increase the caloric value of juices without appreciably changing the sweetness. Sucrose is granulated or table sugar obtained from either sugar cane or sugar beet. Maltose is produced mainly as an intermediate product of starch breakdown during the process of digestion. Some maltose is also found in cereal grains, malted drinks, and sprouting grains.

Polysaccharides are complex sugars, composed of many units of simple sugars. They are neither water soluble nor sweet to the taste. Sources of polysaccharides are starches, glycogen, and cellulose. Starches are found in grain products such as rice

TABLE 21–2 Recommended Daily Dietary Allowances, Revised 1980, Food and Nutrition Board, National Academy of Sciences—National Research Council. Designed for the Maintenance of Good Nutrition of Practically All Healthy People in the U.S.A. *(Continued)*

Water-Soluble Vitamins *(Continued)*					**Minerals**					
Riboflavin *(mg)*	**Niacin** *(mg NE)*‖	**Vitamin B_6** *(mg)*	**Folacin**¶ *(μg)*	**Vitamin B_{12}** *(μg)*	**Calcium** *(mg)*	**Phosphorus** *(mg)*	**Magnesium** *(mg)*	**Iron** *(mg)*	**Zinc** *(mg)*	**Iodine** *(μg)*
0.4	6	0.3	30	0.5**	360	240	50	10	3	40
0.6	8	0.6	45	1.5	540	360	70	15	5	50
0.8	9	0.9	100	2.0	800	800	150	15	10	70
1.0	11	1.3	200	2.5	800	800	200	10	10	90
1.4	16	1.6	300	3.0	800	800	250	10	10	120
1.6	18	1.8	400	3.0	1200	1200	350	18	15	150
1.7	18	2.0	400	3.0	1200	1200	400	18	15	150
1.7	19	2.2	400	3.0	800	800	350	10	15	150
1.6	18	2.2	400	3.0	800	800	350	10	15	150
1.4	16	2.2	400	3.0	800	800	350	10	15	150
1.3	15	1.8	400	3.0	1200	1200	300	18	15	150
1.3	14	2.0	400	3.0	1200	1200	300	18	15	150
1.3	14	2.0	400	3.0	800	800	300	18	15	150
1.2	13	2.0	400	3.0	800	800	300	18	15	150
1.2	13	2.0	400	3.0	800	800	300	10	15	150
+0.3	+2	+0.6	+400	+1.0	+400	+400	+150	††	+5	+25
+0.5	+5	+0.5	+100	+1.0	+400	+400	+150	††	+10	+50

¶The folacin allowances refer to dietary sources as determined by *Lactobacillus casei* assay after treatment with enzymes ("conjugases") to make polyglutamyl forms of the vitamin available to the test organism.

**The RDA for vitamin B_{12} in infants is based on average concentration of the vitamin in human milk. The allowances after weaning are based on energy intake (as recommended by the American Academy of Pediatrics) and consideration of other factors such as intestinal absorption; see text.

††The increased requirement during pregnancy cannot be met by the iron content of habitual American diets nor by the existing iron stores of many women; therefore the use of 30-60 mg of supplemental iron is recommended. Iron needs during lactation are not substantially different from those of nonpregnant women, but continued supplementation of the mother for 2-3 months after parturition is advisable in order to replenish stores depleted by pregnancy.

‖1 NE (niacin equivalent) is equal to 1 mg of niacin or 60 mg of dietary tryptophan.

and wheat, in vegetables, and in smaller amounts in fruits. **Glycogen** is not found in the food supply to any appreciable degree. Its importance is that it is formed during the metabolism of glucose and is the storage form of carbohydrate in the body. As such, it is stored in liver and muscle tissue and is used for energy by the body when broken down to glucose in the liver. **Cellulose** is the structural component of plants. Digestion of cellulose in the body is limited, so cellulose has little nutritive value. It is, however, important as a source of bulk or roughage, which aids in proper elimination. Cellulose and other indigestible carbohydrates will be discussed later in this chapter. (See pages 359 and 361.)

The major functions of carbohydrate in the body are to:

1. provide a source of energy supplying about 40 per cent of the calories in the American diet;
2. aid in **metabolism** of fat (without a source of carbohydrate, the metabolism of fat cannot go to completion); and
3. spare protein from being used as a source of energy (protein is needed for specific functions in the body which no other nutrient can replace).

Fats

Also composed of carbon, hydrogen, and oxygen, fats differ from carbohydrates in the proportions of each of these elements. Fats can be classified in several different ways: by their source, by their physical appearance, or by their chemical structure.

SOURCE: ANIMAL OR VEGETABLE. Animal fats are found in dairy products, meat, fish, and eggs. They are usually solid at room temperature. Vegetable fats are found in plants such as corn, olives, cottonseed, nuts, and beans. They are generally liquid at room temperature and are called oils.

PHYSICAL APPEARANCE: VISIBLE OR INVISIBLE. Visible fats are those that have a fatty appearance, such as butter or the fat around meat. Fats such as those in avocados or eggs are labeled invisible since they are not discernible.

CHEMICAL STRUCTURE: SATURATED OR UNSATURATED. Saturated fats are those fatty acids that contain all the hydrogen possible. They are usually from animal sources and are solid at room temperature. Examples of saturated fats are lard, butter, meat fat, and **hydrogenated** fats.

Unsaturated fatty acids can take on more hydrogen under the proper conditions. They are found in plants and are usually liquid at room temperature. Examples are oils from corn, cottonseed, peanuts, and safflower.

Some fats, such as some of the soft-type margarines, are partially hydrogenated. That is, an unsaturated fat is treated so that it takes up a predetermined quantity of hydrogen resulting in a product that exhibits properties of both a saturated and an unsaturated fat. These fats are usually soft at room temperature.

Cholesterol is a lipid commonly found with saturated fats. It is also made by the body. If abnormally high levels of cholesterol are in the blood (above 250 mg per 100 ml), the risk of deposition of this compound in the walls of blood vessels increases. Such a condition may increase the individual's chances of having a fatal heart attack. For such individuals a low cholesterol diet is usually prescribed. Foods such as egg yolk, organ meats, shellfish, whole dairy products, and meat fat are restricted since they are high in cholesterol and saturated fats.

Fats make up about 40 per cent of the total calories in the American diet. Since they supply 9 kcal per gm, they are the most concentrated source of energy in our diet. The major functions of fat in the body are to:

1. provide a source of energy;
2. carry fat-soluble vitamins A and D;
3. supply those fatty acids essential for growth and life; and
4. slow down emptying time of the stomach, thus increasing the satiety value of the diet.

When fat is stored in the body as adipose tissue, it acts as a reserve energy supply and as insulation and padding for the body and its vital organs.

Proteins

The word **protein** comes from a Greek word meaning "to take first place," and rightly so, for protein is necessary for all living cells. Chemically, proteins are made of carbon, hydrogen, and oxygen, similar to the composition of carbohydrates and fats. However, they also contain nitrogen and several other elements, such as sulfur, phosphorus, and iron. It is the nitrogen that distinguishes proteins from other molecules.

Proteins are very large, complex molecules. They are composed of units known as amino acids, which are the materials that our bodies use to build and repair tissues. They are the form in which proteins are absorbed into the system and metabolized. There are 22 amino acids, of which eight are essential in the adult (possibly ten in children) for normal growth and maintenance of tissues.

Proteins are classified according to whether or not they contain all essential amino acids in good proportions to one another. A complete protein is one that contains a well-balanced mixture of all eight essential **amino acids.** If it is the only source of protein in the diet it will support life and normal growth. A partially complete protein is one that supplies an imbalanced mixture of essential amino acids. If it is used as the sole protein source, it will maintain life but will not support normal growth. An incomplete protein will support neither life nor normal growth. It must not be the sole protein source, for it is missing or extremely low in one or more of the essential amino acids. Food sources of these proteins are:

Complete: meat, fish, poultry, eggs, dairy products.
Partially complete: grain and vegetable proteins.
Incomplete: corn, gelatin.

Fortunately, most foods have a mixture of proteins that supplement each other. Since there is little, if any, storage of amino acids in the body, it is important that a source of protein be included at each meal. If incomplete or partially complete proteins are used, attempts should be made to balance them. That is, a protein deficient in one amino acid should be eaten with one that is high in the same amino acid.

Vegetarianism has become increasingly popular recently. Many different forms exist: some vegetarians consume no red meats but will eat fish and poultry; some include eggs and/or dairy products; others (classified as vegans) consume no animal proteins at all, relying solely on vegetable foods for protein. Those who eat some animal protein in the form of fish, eggs, and milk are generally not at risk nutritionally. Vegans, on the other hand, must be sure to include a variety of foods to insure nutritional adequacy of their diets. To supply sufficient protein, vegetables that complement each other must be eaten together. As a guideline, vegetables belonging to the same general group (legumes such as beans and peas; grains and cereals; seeds and nuts) are usually deficient in similar amino acids. Consequently, mixing proteins from a variety of sources is required to produce a protein equivalent to that found in animal products.

The recommended intake of proteins is 0.8 gm per kilogram body weight (see Table 21–2). Of this, at least one-third should be obtained from complete proteins (one-half or more in children) unless the individual is a strict vegetarian, in which case, as already mentioned, care must be taken to balance the proteins consumed.

Proteins have numerous functions in the body, but the major ones are to:

1. build and repair body tissue (cannot be accomplished by any other nutrient);
2. aid in the body's defense mechanisms against disease;
3. regulate body secretions and fluids; and
4. provide energy.

Vitamins

Vitamins are defined in the *Handbook of Diet Therapy* as organic substances "occurring in minute quantities in plant and animal tissues; essential for specific

metabolic functions or reactions to proceed normally." They do not supply calories in our diet. Rather they function as **catalysts** and help or allow metabolic reactions to proceed. Originally they were lettered or numbered as they were discovered. However, as they have been identified chemically they have been given more specific names. In many cases their chemical names are as well known as their letter designations.

Vitamins are divided into two groups: fat soluble (A, D, E, and K) and water soluble (C and the B complex). Deficiencies of a vitamin cause illness. However, there is no good evidence that large intakes of vitamins are useful in the healthy individual since vitamins will not cure a disease or illness other than one caused by a lack of that nutrient. For example, vitamin C will not cure bleeding gums unless the condition is specifically caused by a lack of ascorbic acid, the chemical name for vitamin C. It should also be noted that toxic symptoms from excessive ingestion of vitamins A and D are proven clinical entities, and large intakes of some water-soluble vitamins may cause adverse effects.

FAT-SOLUBLE VITAMINS (Fig. 21–2)

Vitamin A, or Retinol. We can obtain vitamin A by two methods: (1) as vitamin A or (2) from a compound called **carotene,** which the body converts to vitamin A. Carotene is known as a precursor for vitamin A and is probably a more important source of the vitamin than the preformed compound, since vitamin A, as such, is present in very few foods.

Functions of Vitamin A	***Deficiency Symptoms***
1. Required for healthy skin and mucous membranes in the nose, throat, eyes, gastrointestinal tract, and genitourinary tract.	1. Tissues become dry, cracked, and unable to resist infection.
2. Necessary for proper vision.	2. Night blindness — ability to adapt to darkness is impaired. If deficiency progresses, the eye dries out, becomes infected, and **xerophthalmia** occurs, in which the patient goes blind.
3. Required for normal growth and body functions.	3. Skeletal retardation.

Human Requirements. The recommended daily allowance for the adult is 800 to 1000 RE* (4000 to 5000 International Units) per day (see Table 21–2). This could be supplied by many different foods, for example, ½ oz beef liver, half a large potato, ⅓ cup cooked, drained spinach, or 3 medium raw tomatoes.

Sources. The sources of vitamin A are limited to animal products. The best sources are liver, fish liver oils, egg yolk, butter, and cream. Carotene is much more widely distributed in nature and is found in foods that have a deep yellow or dark green color (the green pigment is much stronger and hides the yellow color of the carotene). Foods such as carrots, yellow squash, pumpkin, dark green leafy vegetables, sweet potatoes, apricots, peaches, and cantaloupes are excellent sources.

Stability. Vitamin A and carotene are not water soluble and are resistant to heat if not in prolonged contact with it. Consequently, they are not lost through most

---

*RE = retinol equivalents. This term was introduced in 1967 so that utilization of the different forms of vitamin A could be taken into account when suggesting individual vitamin A allowances. By definition, 1 RE = 1 gm retinol or an equivalent amount of other compounds, corrected for efficiency of utilization. Since most food composition tables do not presently distinguish sources of vitamin A, the International Unit requirement may be more useful until transition to use of this new unit is complete.

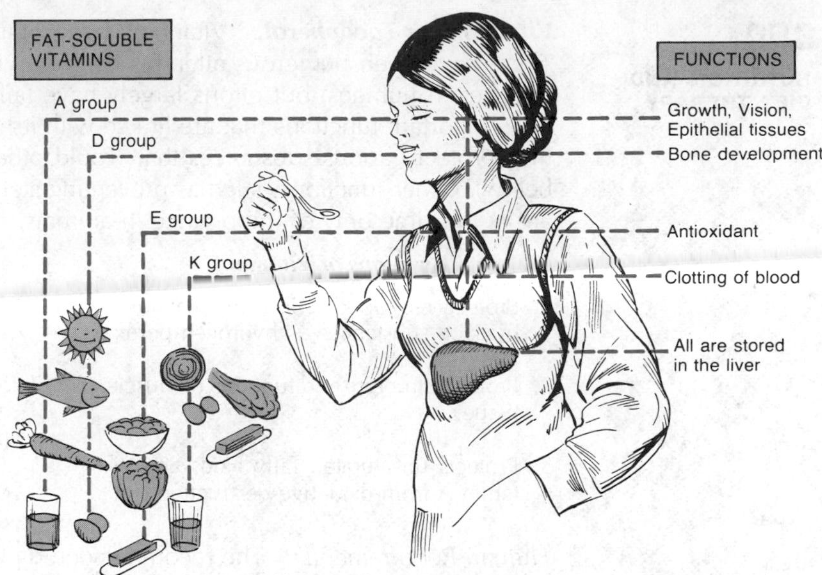

FIGURE 21–2 Fat-soluble vitamins and their functions. (From Bogert, J. L., et al.: *Nutrition and Physical Fitness,* 9th Ed. Philadelphia, W. B. Saunders Co., 1973.)

cooking methods. However, fats will become rancid when in contact with warm air, and once this occurs the major portion of vitamin A and carotene present is destroyed.

Toxicity. It is possible to get too much vitamin A. Toxic reactions are characterized by joint and bone pain, loss of appetite, loss of hair, and **jaundice.** The Council on Foods and Nutrition of the American Medical Association warns that 50,000 IU of this vitamin taken for a prolonged period of time can be dangerous.

Vitamin D, or Cholecalciferol. Vitamin D may be obtained from a few foods, but the most significant source is produced in the body upon exposure to sunlight. The preformed vitamin is not widely distributed. However, through enrichment processes it is added to a number of foods, mainly dairy products.

Functions of Vitamin D	***Deficiency Symptoms***
1. Required for absorption of calcium and facilitates absorption of phosphorus. Necessary for metabolism of calcium and phosphorus in normal nourishment and formation of bones and teeth.	1. Rickets: bones bend easily and do not form correctly since calcium is not absorbed adequately. Teeth are also malformed.

Human Requirements. The recommended daily allowance for the adult is 5 μg, which should be readily supplied by exposure to sunlight. The level for children and pregnant or lactating women is 10 μg per day (10 μg cholecalciferol = 400 IU vitamin D) (see Table 21–2). This latter could be supplied by ½ tsp. cod liver oil, 3½ oz tuna (water packed), or 2 cups fortified milk.

Sources. Fortified milk and milk products, egg yolk, liver, butter, cream, and fish liver oils. The best source is probably sunlight for most adults.

Stability. Vitamin D is stable to heat and is not affected by most cooking methods.

Toxicity. Excesses of this vitamin can cause toxicity symptomized by nausea, diarrhea, loss of appetite, and calcium deposits in tissues and joints. No exact figure can be given for an overdose since exposure to sunlight varies greatly among individuals.

21

Vitamin E, or Tocopherol. Vitamin E is the vitamin that is still looking for a disease. There have been numerous attempts over the years to link this vitamin with many illnesses in humans, but efforts largely have failed. It does, however, have several very important functions that are linked with its ability to combine with oxygen and thus protect various substances that would otherwise be subject to oxidation (see below). Other functions, such as preventing sterility or curing **muscular dystrophy,** are at this time only of importance in animals, not in man.

Functions of Vitamin E	***Deficiency Symptoms***
1. Protects red blood cells from breakdown by such substances as hydrogen peroxide.	1. Anemia, so far seen only in infants.
2. Protects structure and function of muscle tissue.	2. Some forms of muscle degeneration have been seen in patients with low plasma vitamin E levels.
3. Protects unsaturated fatty acids and vitamin A from oxidative destruction.	

Human Requirements. The recommended daily allowance for the adult is 8 to 10 mg TE* (see Table 21–2). This adult allowance could be met by 1 tbs safflower, corn, or soybean oil, or 3 oz wheat germ.

Sources. The best sources of this vitamin are vegetable oils and wheat germ. Other sources include milk, eggs, meats, grains, and leafy vegetables.

Toxicity. None identified as yet. This vitamin, unlike other fat-soluble vitamins, is stored in adipose tissue.

Vitamin K. The major function of this vitamin in the body is that it is required for the formation of **prothrombin,** which is a clotting agent in the blood. Consequently, the vitamin is often used to treat certain types of hemorrhages. Deficiency is rare and is usually due to absorption problems rather than inadequate supply of the vitamin.

Functions of Vitamin K	***Deficiency Symptoms***
1. Required for formation of the protein prothrombin by the liver.	1. Blood will not clot; hemorrhages will occur.

Human Requirements. There is no RDA for this vitamin. However, estimated safe and adequate daily intakes have been established (see Table 21–2) for adults at 70 to 140 mcg per day. Probably one-half to two-thirds of this would be supplied by bacterial synthesis in the intestine. The remainder could be supplied by ½ cup broccoli, 3 oz beef liver, or ⅛ head lettuce.

Sources. Good food sources include green leafy vegetables, egg yolk, and organ meats. A form of vitamin K is produced by intestinal bacteria.

Toxicity. In large doses, vitamin K can produce a hemolytic anemia and jaundice in infants.

WATER-SOLUBLE VITAMINS

Vitamin C, or Ascorbic Acid (Fig. 21–3). Vitamin C was first used to treat **scurvy** in British sailors during the eighteenth century. Of course, at the time the curative factor

---

*TE = alpha tocopherol equivalent. Alpha tocopherol is the chemical form of vitamin E that is the most common and the most biologically active. One mg of d-α-tocopherol has been designated as 1 α-tocopherol equivalent.

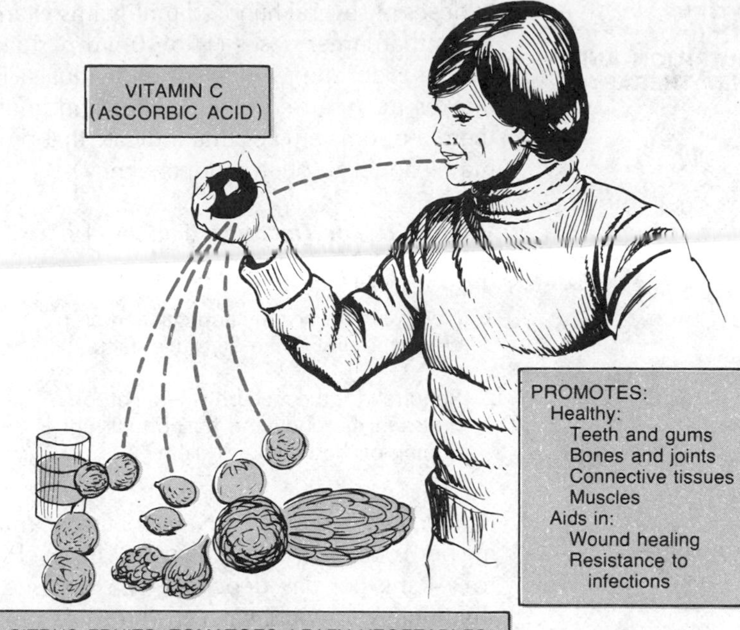

FIGURE 21–3 Vitamin C and its functions. (From Bogert, J. L., et al.: *Nutrition and Physicial Fitness.* 9th Ed. Philadelphia, W. B. Saunders Co., 1973.)

in the limes each sailor was required to consume daily while at sea was unknown. However, they did know that a lime daily seemed to prevent the dread disease. As a result, the British sailors were nicknamed "limeys," a term which is still used today.

Functions of Vitamin C	*Deficiency Symptoms*
1. Required for proper wound healing and helps in the body's resistance to bacterial infection.	1. Minor illnesses, general listlessness.
2. Necessary for the structure and maintenance of capillary walls.	2. Gums bleed, small pinpoint hemorrhages appear under the skin. If deficiency continues the disease scurvy develops. Patients with this disease have skeletal malformations that are irreversible.

Human Requirements. The recommended daily allowance for adults is 60 mg per day. This amount of ascorbic acid would be supplied by 6 oz orange or grapefruit juice, 1 cup strawberries, or 3 spears fresh or frozen broccoli, cooked.

Sources. Best sources of this nutrient are citrus fruits, cabbage, dark green leafy vegetables, and strawberries. Some sources are relatively low in vitamin C but are consumed in sufficient quantities so that they can be an important source as, for example, potatoes.

Stability. Vitamin C is very easily destroyed by both heat and exposure to air. Since it is water soluble, care must be used in cooking fruits and vegetables that contain vitamin C. Small amounts of water and short cooking times should be used. An alkaline medium will speed up the loss of vitamin C.

Toxicity. Because ascorbic acid is water soluble and easily excreted from the body, toxic effects of this vitamin were previously believed to be unlikely. Symptoms typical of gastrointestinal tract irritation (such as nausea and diarrhea) were observed at doses of several hundred milligrams vitamin C daily, but it has only been in recent years that larger doses (1 to 10 gm per day) have been shown to have potentially serious side effects in some individuals. For example, evidence shows that high intakes may cause kidney stones and gout in susceptible individuals. In addition, there are some studies that indicate that prolonged intake of high doses of vitamin C may lead to nutritional dependency.

Vitamin B_1, or Thiamine (Fig. 21–4)

Functions of Vitamin B_1	***Deficiency Symptoms***
1. Necessary for healthy appetite and proper functioning of the digestive tract.	1. Loss of appetite, diminished gastric secretions, fatigue, irritability.
2. Required for the metabolism of carbohydrates in the body and for normal functioning of the nervous system.	2. Edema, foot drop, **beri-beri.**

Human Requirements. Need for the vitamin depends on caloric intake; generally 0.5 mg per 1000 calories is adequate. The level set by the National Research Council is 1.0 to 1.4 mg per day depending on sex (see Table 21–2). To obtain this amount of thiamine, you could eat 1 tbs brewer's yeast, 4 oz lean pork, or 2 cups 40 per cent bran flakes.

Sources. Meats are not as good a source of thiamine as they are of most of the other B vitamins, although pork and organ meats, such as liver, can contribute good amounts if consumed in large enough quantities. Although not concentrated sources of thiamine, whole grain or enriched breads and cereals and potatoes are the most practical sources of vitamin B_1 because of the quantity of these products consumed. Legumes, wheat germ, and brewer's yeast are excellent sources, but the latter two are not included in the usual American diet.

Stability. Thiamine is destroyed by heat and alkaline mediums. Since it is water soluble, small amounts of water should be used in cooking in order to preserve this nutrient.

Toxicity. None.

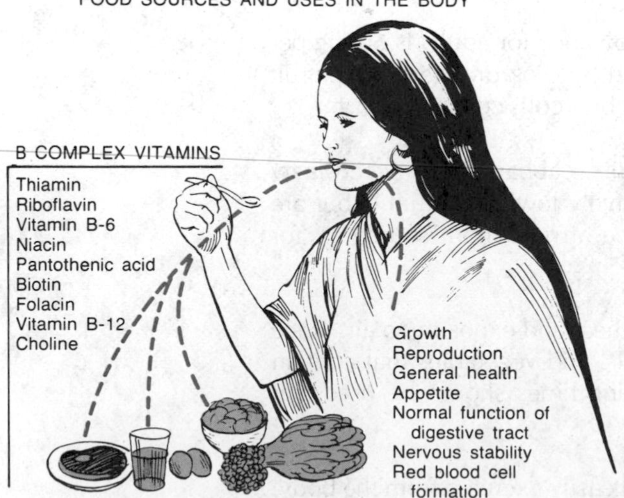

FIGURE 21–4 Food sources and uses in the body. (From Bogert, J. L., et al.: *Nutrition and Physical Fitness.* 9th Ed. Philadelphia, W. B. Saunders Co., 1973.)

Vitamin B_2, or Riboflavin

Functions of Vitamin B_2	*Deficiency Symptoms*
1. Necessary for all tissues, particularly for healthy skin and lips.	1. Cheilosis, cracking of the corners of the mouth.
2. Required for maintaining healthy eyes.	2. Itching and burning of eyes, sensitivity to light, headaches.
3. Essential for proper growth.	
4. Vital as a coenzyme in energy metabolism.	

Human Requirements. 1.2 to 1.6 mg per day as established by the National Research Council (see Table 21–2). Foods supplying this would be 1½ oz calf liver, cooked, 3 cups yogurt or milk, or 3 cups 40 per cent bran flakes.

Sources. The major source of this vitamin is milk, since one quart supplies 2 mg. Other sources include meats and enriched grains.

Stability. Riboflavin is very unstable in light. Consequently, milk should be stored in either dark glass or plasticized paper containers. Riboflavin from foods other than milk can also be lost in cooking water or drippings since it is water soluble.

Toxicity. None.

Niacin. Niacin is obtained from two sources: either from preformed niacin or from conversion of its precursor, **tryptophan**, in the body. Tryptophan is an essential amino acid, and the body converts it into niacin. About 1 mg of niacin is produced from approximately 60 mg of tryptophan.

Functions of Niacin	*Deficiency Symptoms*
1. Composes part of some enzymes and is required for proper growth and metabolism of carbohydrates.	1. **Pellagra:** characterized by the three D's (dermatitis, dementia, diarrhea).
2. Necessary for proper function of the gastrointestinal tract and the nervous system.	

Human Requirements. 13 to 18 mg per day is the recommended allowance (see Table 21–2). This amount of niacin would be found in 6 oz round steak or 1½ cups pinto beans.

Sources. Probably one-third to one-half of our niacin comes from tryptophan, which is obtained from meat and other complete sources of protein. Flour and cereal products are also good sources.

Stability. Niacin is fairly stable to heat and air, but it can be lost in the cooking water.

Toxicity. In large amounts niacin causes vasodilation, which is evidenced by facial flushing and tingling sensations in the extremities. Massive doses (3 gm or more daily) cause liver damage.

Vitamin B_6, or Pyridoxine

Functions of Vitamin B_6	*Deficiency Symptoms*
1. Many generalized functions in relation to muscle and nervous system function.	1. Microcytic anemia, muscle weakness, difficulty in walking. Generally produced experimentally by using an antagonist. Induced symptoms include nausea, skin rash, oral lesions. Convulsions have been reported in extreme cases of deficiency in infants.
2. Functions as a coenzyme in protein metabolism.	

Human Requirements. The National Research Council recommends 2 to 2.2 mg per day for adults (see Table 21–2). No single food is an outstanding source of vitamin B_6, but it is widely distributed in foods and eating a variety of foods easily supplies adequate amounts. The NRC allowance could be supplied by 4 bananas, 2 avocados, or 12 oz beef liver, fried.

Sources. Occurs in many foods, mainly meat and vegetables.

Toxicity. At doses of up to 150 mg, mild side effects and sleepiness have been reported. Over 200 mg, nutritional dependency has been shown and deficiency symptoms are seen when large intakes are discontinued. Toxic effects are seen at doses over 300 mg per day.

Folic Acid, or Folacin

Functions of Folic Acid	***Deficiency Symptoms***
1. Essential for all cells, particularly in the formation of red blood cells.	1. Smooth, red tongue; diarrhea; megaloblastic anemia; retarded growth.

Human Requirements. Allowance established at 400 μg per day for adults (see Table 21–2).

Sources. Best sources are green leafy vegetables, liver, and whole grains.

Stability. Folacin is destroyed by heat and frequently lost in cooking water. Storage and cooking losses are usually high irrespective of methods used.

Toxicity. No toxic effects are presently known, but excessive folacin may interfere with effectiveness of anticonvulsant drugs. Because folacin may mask early B_{12} deficiency symptoms, supplementation of folacin over the NRC allowance should not be taken unless the possibility of a B_{12} deficiency has been ruled out.

Vitamin B_{12}, or Cobalamin. Deficiency of this vitamin produces an anemia identical to that produced by a folic acid deficiency. However, if a deficiency of vitamin B_{12} is allowed to continue untreated, serious neurologic symptoms will result. (For this reason, folic acid cannot legally be added to multi-vitamin capsules except at very low levels so that it will not inadvertently mask the early symptoms of a vitamin B_{12} deficiency.)

Human Requirements. Three μg per day for adults (see Table 21–2). Easily supplied by ¼ oz beef liver, fried, ¼ cup frozen peas, cooked, or ¼ cup canned pineapple.

Sources. Liver and muscle meats are the best sources.

Stability. Stable under most conditions since it is attached to a protein in foods.

Toxicity. None.

Other B Vitamins. Other vitamins that belong to the B complex, but for which no requirements have as yet been established, are biotin, pantothenic acid, and choline. **Biotin** is synthesized by bacteria in the gastrointestinal tract and is important in several enzyme systems. Raw egg white contains a protein, avidin, which is capable of binding biotin, thus making it unavailable to the body. Avidin is changed by heating, so it will not function in this manner in cooked egg whites. The estimated safe and adequate intake of biotin is 100 to 200 mcg, which could be supplied by 4 oz beef liver or 2 cups cooked oatmeal. **Pantothenic acid** is involved in carbohydrate and fatty acid metabolism. It is present in almost all foods, and a deficiency should not be seen if a mixed diet is consumed. The Food and Nutrition Board suggests an intake of 4 to 7 mg per day. An equivalent of this amount would be found in 3 oz beef liver, 4 to 6 eggs, or 1 qt of milk. **Choline** is important in the body mainly as a constituent of compounds known as phospholipids (primary lecithin). Among other roles, it is involved in the transportation and metabolism of fats. Choline is found in whole grains, meats, egg yolks, and legumes. No deficiency has been demonstrated in humans.

Minerals

Minerals are inorganic chemical elements that make up about 4 per cent of body weight. Of the many that are used by the body only 13 are felt to be essential, and of those there are allowances established for only six. Most minerals are required in relatively small amounts, but even so they are absolutely essential for life.

Those minerals that are needed only in trace amounts seem either to behave as part of hormone or enzyme systems or to work with vitamins in various metabolic reactions throughout the body. For example, iodine is part of the thyroid hormone, thyroxine, and another hormone, insulin, has zinc as part of its structure. Cobalt, on the other hand, is an essential part of the B_{12} molecule.

Generally, if an individual consumes a well-balanced diet he will receive adequate amounts of most minerals. Those that may require special attention to insure that they are in sufficient quantities are calcium, phosphorus, iron, and, in some cases, iodine. During illness, of course, other minerals may also be of more concern.

MAJOR MINERALS

Calcium. Calcium is the mineral which, in the American diet, is most likely to be deficient. The body requires calcium at all ages, but the highest requirements are during pregnancy, lactation, and childhood.

Functions of Calcium	***Deficiency Symptoms***
1. Forms the body's skeleton and teeth.	1. Rickets: characterized by retarded growth and malformations of the bones.
2. Aids in forming blood clots.	2. Delayed blood clotting; hemorrhage.
3. Required for normal muscle activity, especially the heart muscle.	3. Tetany, abnormal twitching of the muscles.

Human Requirements. 800 mg per day (see Table 21–2). Supplied by 2 to 3 cups milk or yogurt, or 4 oz cheese.

Sources. Milk of any kind (skim, whole, low fat, buttermilk, chocolate milk, and so forth) or milk products, such as ice cream or cheese. Other sources include dark green leafy vegetables and shellfish (for instance, clams and oysters).

Phosphorus. Phosphorus is a constituent of every living cell and as such has numerous functions in the body. In many cases it works in very much the same manner as calcium. However, in addition it is required for protein, fat, and carbohydrate metabolism, in energy metabolism, and in various buffering systems in the body. It is also involved in a number of vitamin and enzyme reactions. No specific disease is associated with a deficiency of this nutrient, but excessive and prolonged use of antacids containing aluminum hydroxide can produce symptoms of phosphorus deficiency (weakness, anorexia, and bone demineralization).

Human Requirements. 800 mg per day for the adult (see Table 21–2). Occurring in many foods along with calcium, phosphorus is also supplied by 2 to 3 cups milk or yogurt, or 4 oz cheese or tuna fish.

Sources. Phosphorus is present in most foods, particularly in milk and meat products. Other good sources are cereals and legumes.

Magnesium. Most magnesium is found in combination with calcium and phosphorus in bone tissue. In addition to its role in bone metabolism, magnesium functions mainly in carbohydrate and amino acid reactions in the body. With other minerals it is also important in nervous activity and muscle contractions. A deficiency of this element results in nervous irritability and eventually in convulsions similar to those seen in cases of **tetany (hypocalcemia).**

Human Requirements. 300 to 350 mg per day for adults, depending on sex (see Table 21–2). No single food, eaten in normal amounts, is an outstanding source of magnesium, but a combination of ½ cup peanuts and 3 bananas would supply the NRC allowance.

Sources. Magnesium occurs in many foods, particularly dairy products, cereal grains, legumes, and dark green vegetables.

Sodium. This mineral is required mainly for control of fluid volume in the body; an increase in the level of sodium in the serum leads to water retention. One compartment expanded as a result of fluid retention is the vascular system. Sodium, then, is directly related to blood pressure. It also functions in acid-base balance and is involved in both carbohydrate and protein metabolism. Deficiencies of sodium can result from inadequate production of adrenocortical hormone or from excessive perspiration. Symptoms of deficiency include nausea, vomiting, and muscle cramps. Extreme cases may lead to heart failure.

Excess sodium may cause an effective increase in blood volume and hence an increase in blood pressure. Although many other factors besides sodium and water retention are involved in causing high blood pressure (hypertension), it would appear reasonable to suggest that sodium intake should be closely monitored. Estimates presently place sodium consumption at roughly ten times the level actually required. Therefore, at least those persons who are predisposed to hypertension probably should try to use the salt shaker less frequently and should avoid obviously salty foods such as potato chips and broth. Salt substitutes, however, should not be used without medical supervision.

Human Requirements. The Food and Nutrition Board set the safe and adequate intake for this mineral at 1100 to 3300 mg daily. One teaspoon of table salt supplies 2000 mg sodium, but 12 green olives or 4 oz ham could also supply over 1000 mg sodium.

Sources. Found naturally in a wide variety of foods, sodium is also added extensively to many foods during commercial production. Meats and dairy products are naturally high sources, but salt is added to foods like soups, butter, and potato chips for flavor.

Potassium. This mineral functions in much the same way sodium does except that potassium is concentrated within the body cells. In addition to its involvement with fluid volume, potassium plays a multitude of roles in carbohydrate and protein metabolism. Deficiencies of potassium are rare and are usually related to either severe vomiting or diarrhea or to use of **diuretics** (drugs that cause excretion of sodium and potassium, frequently used in treating hypertension). Symptoms of a potassium deficiency include nausea, vomiting, and muscle weakness. Severe losses of potassium result in rapid contractions of the heart and eventually death due to heart failure.

Too much potassium can also be dangerous. Usually hyperkalemia is due to kidney failure or to a combination of a reduced ability to excrete potassium along with overingestion of potassium, either from supplements or salt substitutes.

Human Requirements. The safe and adequate intake set at 1875 to 5625 mg per day. No single food source could supply this amount but many fruits and vegetables supply 300 to 400 mg per serving, so a variety of foods from these groups should adequately supply potassium in the American diet.

Sources. Bananas, oranges, and raisins are good sources of potassium as are most other fruits. Potatoes in the skin and avocados are excellent sources; milk and meat contain smaller amounts.

Chlorine. As the ion chloride, this mineral acts as a companion to sodium. It is primarily involved in acid-base and fluid balance, and is a component of hydrochloric acid in the stomach. Deficiencies are unusual and are generally related to sodium losses or to excessive vomiting and diarrhea. Toxicities of dietary chlorine are unknown since it is readily excreted by the kidney. Chlorine in its gaseous form, however, is lethal.

Human Requirements. Safe and adequate intake has been established to be 1700 to 5100 mg per day for adults. The amount of salt in the diet supplies more than enough of this nutrient.

Source. Table salt.

TRACE MINERALS

Iron. Although required in small amounts in comparison with nutrients like phosphorus and calcium, iron is a vitally important element. It is an essential part of hemoglobin, which is the protein that is the oxygen-carrying substance in the blood and is responsible for the color of red blood cells. The body is very conservative with iron, and it reuses it again and again. However, deficiencies do occur, particularly in premenopausal women or during pregnancy or hemorrhagic conditions. A deficiency of iron results in a microcytic anemia.

Human Requirements. The NRC allowance is 18 mg per day for adult women. Unless a woman eats liver and other rich sources of iron frequently, the ordinary diet may not supply a sufficient quantity of iron. In this case an iron supplement may be desirable. Ten mg per day is recommended for men (see Table 21–2). This lower amount for men can be supplied by 1 cup 40 per cent bran flakes or 4 oz beef liver.

Sources. Best sources are liver and other organ meats, egg yolks, whole grain products, and green leafy vegetables. Some other products, such as raisins, dried fruits, and molasses, are good sources of iron if eaten in sufficient quantities. Eating foods containing ascorbic acid along with iron-containing foods will increase the availability of iron to the body.

Toxicity. In some cases, overdoses of iron may be a problem. Although unusual to see in the United States except in instances of excessive use of supplements, iron accumulation can occur because the body has no mechanism for excreting excess iron. Consequently, iron is deposited in soft tissues (liver, pancreas, lungs) causing cell death, and may lead to complications such as diabetes and liver damage.

Iodine. Iodine's only function in the body is as a part of the thyroid gland hormone thyroxine. Although the requirement for iodine is small, the thyroid gland fails to function properly without it and the condition known as **goiter** occurs. Iodine deficiency in a pregnant woman can result in **cretinism** in the infant. This disease is characterized by dwarfing and retarded physical and mental growth.

Human Requirements. 150 mcg per day for adults (see Table 21–2). One tsp iodized salt supplies 420 mcg iodine, much more than the RDA. Three glasses of milk will supply 150 mcg of iodine.

Sources. The iodine content of plants is determined by the amount of iodine in the soil in which they are grown. Generally, vegetables grown in the Atlantic coastal area or regions around the Gulf of Mexico have the highest iodine content. Fish, seafood, and seaweed are excellent sources of iodine but are usually not eaten frequently enough to be considered dependable sources. The most reliable source of iodine is iodized table salt.

Zinc. Zinc is necessary for growth and **gonadal** development in man. Zinc is part of the hormone insulin, which regulates carbohydrate metabolism. It is also a component of several enzyme systems in the body. A deficiency of this nutrient retards skeletal growth and sexual maturation. Additional symptoms include decreased ability to taste and delayed wound healing.

Human Requirements. 15 mg per day for adults (see Table 21–2). This could be supplied by 1 oyster. One milligram of zinc is found in 1 oz of most meats.

Sources. The best sources of zinc are oysters, herring, whole grain, meats, milk, and egg yolk.

Fluoride. The major function of fluoride is in hardening bones and teeth. As a result it is beneficial in reducing the amount of dental decay in infancy and childhood. Some evidence indicates that fluoride may also benefit adults who take it throughout life in protecting them against osteoporosis. In areas of the country where water is naturally fluoridated in excess of 6 to 8 ppm, mottling (brown staining) of the tooth enamel is observed. However, at levels used in artificial fluoridation programs, no health hazard has been documented.

Human Requirements. The safe and adequate intake is set at 1.5 to 4 mg per day for adults. This would be supplied by 1.5 liters of fluoridated water.

Sources. Food sources of fluoride are unreliable. Soil content varies, so vegetables and grains are sometimes good sources. Seafood and seaweed are excellent sources. Water, when fluoridated, contains 1 ppm (1 mg per liter).

OTHER MINERALS. There are many other minerals that are required by the body. Slowly, as methods improve, deficiencies may be identified and allowances established as, for example, in the following minerals.

Copper. Contributes to iron absorption and metabolism and is involved in the formation of hemoglobin. Copper deficiencies are unusual and generally linked to genetic defects. The safe and adequate intake is established at 2 to 3 mg per day for adults. Richest sources of this mineral are shellfish, liver, legumes, and raisins.

Sulfur. Used in protein synthesis and in reactions in the liver. Normally adequate in diets where the complete protein content of the diet is adequate.

Water

Water is the most important nutrient, yet it is all too often overlooked when the average person considers nutritional status. It has a wide variety of functions in the body: (1) it regulates body temperature, (2) it acts as a solvent and a medium for most biochemical reactions in the body, and (3) it maintains electrolyte balance. Extensive water losses due to diarrhea, vomiting, burns, or perspiration lead to electrolyte losses and resultant life-threatening imbalances. Drinking too much water (water intoxication) can also be dangerous.

Human Requirements. None set but the Food and Nutrition Board recommends 1 ml per kcal per day.

Fiber

Fiber, or "roughage," is composed of many different substances. Three polysaccharides (cellulose, pectin, and hemicellulose) as well as the noncarbohydrate lignin contribute roughage to the diet. Fiber is not found in animal foods but comes only from plants. Dietary tables generally show "crude fiber" or dietary fiber, which is estimated to be 20 to 50 per cent lower than actual fiber content of the diet. Much work is needed to clarify this area of nutrition.

Fiber absorbs water easily and consequently functions to carry waste products from the gastrointestinal tract. Lack of sufficient fiber in the diet has been linked to many problems of the gut from hiatus hernia to diverticulosis to cancer of the colon. However, most of the data are based on epidemiologic surveys rather than on controlled laboratory studies, so conclusive proof is presently not available.

Human Requirements. No requirement has been established, but the average fiber content of the American diet (4 to 5 gm per day) is believed to be low. This may result in reduced movement of waste material through the colon, leading to increased irritation and eventual damage to the tissues. It is generally suggested that we increase the fiber content of the diet to 12 to 20 gm per day.

Sources. Whole grains, fruits, and vegetables. Bran is a concentrated source of fiber and, if added to the diet, should be added in small amounts. It can absorb up to 200 times its dry weight in water and so may cause blockage of the intestinal tract. Increased fiber content of the diet should always be accompanied by increased water consumption.

THERAPEUTIC NUTRITION

Although the majority of patients a physician sees will be treated medically without using a therapeutic diet, there are some illnesses and diseases that can be cured and patients whose recovery can be facilitated by the use of a special diet. In such cases, the normal (sometimes referred to as house or regular) diet is used as a basis of planning. This is used for two major reasons:

1. The closer the special diet is to a normal one, the fewer changes the assistant will be asking the person to accept, and the easier it will be for him to adhere to the diet.
2. It is easier to be certain that the patient's diet supplies adequate amounts of essential nutrients if a regular diet pattern is used as a baseline.

Modifying a Diet

The normal diet can be modified in the following ways (or any combination thereof) to supply a therapeutic diet:

1. Consistency
2. Caloric level
3. Levels of one or more nutrients
4. Bulk
5. Spiciness
6. Levels of specific foods
7. Feeding intervals

CONSISTENCY. Changes in consistency are sometimes ordered for individuals who have problems with their mouth, teeth, or esophagus. A texture restriction is also frequently called for in cases of illnesses of the gastrointestinal tract.

Soft or Light Diet. Foods with roughage are eliminated (no raw fruits or vegetables). No strongly flavored or gas-forming vegetables are allowed (onions, beans, broccoli, cauliflower, and so on). In many cases, spices are limited.

Mechanical Soft. A regular diet in which the food is either chopped, ground or **pureed**, depending upon the degree of texture change required. No foods or spices are restricted.

Liquid. There are two types of liquid diets. The clear liquid diet includes only broth soups, tea, coffee, and gelatin. In some cases, apple juice and cranberry juice may be allowed. The full liquid diet includes all foods allowed on a clear liquid diet plus milk, custards, strained cream soups, refined cereals, eggnogs, milkshakes, and all juices.

Adequacy. The soft and mechanical soft diets should supply all nutrients required by an individual. The clear liquid diet is not adequate and should be used for very brief periods of time. Full liquid diets can be made adequate, but they are usually not and so should also be used only for short periods.

CALORIE LEVEL. Calories may be either increased or decreased. Increased calories are ordered in cases of chronic underweight, following an illness, for malnutrition and hyperthyroidism, during times of growth, such as infancy and childhood, and during pregnancy and lactation. In such circumstances the total amounts of foods on the regular diet are increased, and the diet is usually higher in fats (since fat supplies more calories per gram than either carbohydrates or proteins). The number of meals eaten may also be increased from three to six or more.

Calories are restricted in cases of **obesity** and **diabetes.** Quantities of food consumed should be decreased, but no one food group should be eliminated. For diabetes, foods containing carbohydrates, particularly the simple sugars, are controlled. Lists of foods that enable the diabetic to plan his diet more easily have been prepared by the American Diabetic Association. (The lists are known as Exchange Lists, and various modifications of them are frequently used for calorie-restricted diets in general.)

Adequacy. High calorie diets should be adequate in all nutrients. Low calorie diets can usually be made adequate. However, diets supplying less than 1800 kcal per day become monotonous, and it becomes progressively difficult to meet nutritional requirements as calories decrease. At caloric intakes below 1000 kcal, the diet will probably be inadequate.

LEVELS OF ONE OR MORE NUTRIENTS. A large number of therapeutic diets fall into this category. This type of diet is used to treat specific deficiency diseases (for example, high iron) or in cases where a patient has had a toxic reaction to a specific vitamin or mineral (for example, low vitamin A). Many inborn errors of metabolism are treated by eliminating or limiting the ingestion of a nutrient (for instance, **phenylketonuria** is treated by limiting the quantities of the essential amino acid, phenylalanine). In cases of hypertensive heart disease, sodium is restricted. For patients with **atherosclerosis,** a low fat or low cholesterol diet may be prescribed. Protein levels are changed for kidney and liver disease therapy. Fat is also restricted for gallbladder or liver disease.

In any case, the normal diet is modified by restricting foods that are sources of the nutrient involved.

Adequacy. Except for the nutrient in question, the NRC allowances can usually be met, although if several restrictions are ordered for the same patient, a nutrient supplement may be necessary.

BULK. Bulk or residue is changed when treating problems of the colon or large bowel. In some cases high residue diets are ordered; in others, low residue diets. In either case, foods high in cellulose are considered to be high in residue because the body does not digest this carbohydrate well and a residue is left in the colon. In some instances, a low residue diet is distinguished from a low **fiber** diet. In this case a low fiber diet eliminates those foods with a high cellulose content, and a low residue diet restricts milk, in addition to fiber content.

Adequacy. Either diet should supply all nutrients needed, although if milk is restricted drastically the calcium level must be watched carefully.

SPICINESS. A bland diet restricts those dietary components that are classified as gastrointestinal irritants. A bland diet restricts any foods that are chemically (for instance, caffeine, pepper, chili, nutmeg, and alcohol) or mechanically (high fiber) irritating. No fried foods or highly concentrated sweets are included. Gas-forming vegetables belonging to the onion and cabbage family are also eliminated. The diet is usually used for problems occurring in the gastrointestinal tract (such as ulcers).

Adequacy. The bland diet should supply sufficient nutrients for the individual to meet the NRC allowances, unless fruits and vegetables are eliminated (in which case, a supplement may be necessary).

LEVELS OF SPECIFIC FOODS. Diets that fall into this category are most frequently used to treat allergies of various kinds. There are two basic elimination-type regimens. A simple elimination diet removes only one or two foods that are suspected of causing the allergy. The Rowe elimination diet involves a more extensive program. Using this method, the basic diet consists of a few hypoallergenic foods such as rice cereal, apples, pears, carrots, sweet potatoes, lamb, and milk substitutes. If no allergic reaction is observed, single food-family groups are added slowly in periods of about ten days. In children the most common allergies are to chocolate, wheat, eggs, and milk. A disease known as **celiac** disease is treated by eliminating those foods that contain a protein called **gliadin** (found in wheat, oats, and barley products).

Adequacy. In some cases it may be difficult to meet the NRC allowances for all nutrients. When this situation occurs, supplements should be ordered.

FEEDING INTERVALS. Feeding intervals can be changed. Usually more meals are ordered rather than fewer. Generally the increase is from three meals to six or eight meals. Feeding intervals are shortened for treating problems dealing with the gastrointestinal tract, malnutrition, or underweight. An individual who has had part or all of his stomach removed surgically requires more meals. In some cases, the total food consumed per day is the same, but it is fed in smaller quantities at any given time. In other cases more food is added at the extra meals.

Adequacy. Unless the number of meals is reduced severely, the NRC allowances should be met.

There are, of course, many other diets that have not been mentioned. If further information is required, a text on diet therapy should be consulted (see list at end of this chapter).

Prescribing a Diet

Since there are so many different types of therapeutic diets, it is frequently impossible for the physician to stay abreast of all the restrictions and other considerations involved. For this reason he will often rely on either a local dietitian or a nutrition consultant *to plan the therapeutic diet and instruct his patients* on the modifications they should follow.

Basically, diet therapy involves a problem-solving process. First, data concerning the nutritional status of the patient must be collected. This information is generally accumulated by a variety of health professionals (headed by the physician), including in some cases medical assistants, and is expanded and coordinated by the registered dietitian. The second step is the planning phase, during which the collected data are analyzed, the nutrition-related problems are delineated, and the possible solutions are outlined. The proposed dietary measures are then implemented as a planned dietary program. (Some of the most common nutrition-related problems and the dietary modifications used to treat them are shown in Table 21–3). Lastly, the program or diet being used is evaluated in terms of the medical problem to see if the nutrition-related disorder is being or has been corrected. If necessary, the entire process is repeated over again. At all times it is preferable to involve the client as much as possible in order to maximize results and maintain long-term dietary modifications.

If it is not feasible to use professional dietetic assistance, the physician may wish to use a service offered by some firms which develop diets, printed with the physician's name on them, if desired, that can be handed to the patient. Numerous pharmaceutical or medical suppliers also supply diet lists, which usually are used as additional advertising for the products of that manufacturer. If such diets are used, remember that one list is frequently used for more than one type of diet (for example, several different calorie levels may be listed in chart form), and it is left to the patient to decipher the information. Diets of this nature must be as clear and concise as possible so that the patient is not unduly confused or frightened.

In any event, it is important that the patient return home with something he can read after leaving the office. All questions will not occur to him at the time the diet is first introduced. He must have some method of finding out information, and a written diet list is the easiest method of accomplishing this.

If, as a medical assistant, it is your duty to discuss the diet with the patient, be sure that you understand it well enough to talk with the patient in a convincing manner. There may be some questions you cannot answer. If so, have the patient ask the physician or contact a person more versed in diet therapy. It is important that the patient understand the diet and the rationale behind its use. If he feels uneasy or has a lot of unanswered questions, he will be far less motivated to follow the diet.

TABLE 21–3 Common Diet-Related Disorders

Disorder	Major Dietary Components	Corrective Dietary Measures
Allergies	Wide variety of foods as possible allergens: wheat, milk, eggs, chocolate are most common.	Eliminate or restrict food sources of allergen.
Anemia	Deficiency of iron, B_{12}, or folacin.	Increase amount of deficient nutrient.
Atherosclerosis	High cholesterol, high saturated fat, excessive calories.	Control calories, decrease total fat in diet to 30 to 35 per cent of calories, change to more unsaturated fats, lower cholesterol content of diet, stress complex carbohydrates rather than simple sugars.
Cancer of the Colon	Low fiber.	Increase dietary fiber, increase fluids.
Cirrhosis of the Liver	Excessive ingestion of alcohol or nutrients such as iron, lead, vitamin A or D.	Reduce dietary level of excessive nutrient or substance.
Constipation/ Diverticulosis	Poor fiber intake, poor fluid intake.	Increase dietary fiber and fluids.
Diabetes Mellitus	Obesity, excessive sugar consumption.	Control calories and carbohydrates.
Hypertension	Obesity, high salt intake.	Control calories, decrease sodium intake.
Obesity	Excessive calorie intake, inadequate physical activity.	Decrease calories, increase activity.

You, as the medical assistant, can be a very valuable asset to the physician, the dietitian, and particularly, the patient. A sound understanding of nutrition and especially of diet therapy will enable you to function in your role in the most effective manner possible.

References

Briggs, J. L., and Calloway, D. H.: *Bogert's Nutrition and Physical Fitness.* 10th ed. Philadelphia, W. B. Saunders Co., 1979.

Goodhart, R. S., and Shils, M. E.: *Modern Nutrition in Health and Disease.* 5th ed. Philadelphia, Lea &. Febiger, 1973.

Krause, M. V., and Mahan, L. K.: *Food, Nutrition and Diet Therapy.* 6th ed. Philadelphia, W. B. Saunders Co., 1979.

Turner, D.: *Handbook of Diet Therapy.* 5th ed. Chicago, University of Chicago Press, 1970.

Williams, S. R.: *Nutrition and Diet Therapy.* 3rd ed. St. Louis, C.V. Mosby Co., 1977.

CHAPTER OUTLINE

BEHAVIORAL OBJECTIVES

The medical office assistant should be able to:

- **Name the different major types of microbial pathogens that cause disease in humans.**
- **List at least three different diseases caused by each major type of microbial pathogen listed in objective one.**
- **Describe how each of the major types of microbial pathogen can be cultured and identified.**
- **Distinguish between and define: infection and disease; signs and symptoms of disease.**
- **Indicate the value of serology in the diagnosis of infectious disease.**
- **List and describe some pitfalls or problems that might be encountered in doing diagnostic office microbiology.**
- **Suggest some useful office microbiologic procedures that may be initiated or routinely done.**
- **Define and compare specific and nonspecific host defenses.**
- **Name the cellular components of blood and their function.**
- **Define B-cell, T-cell, antibody, inflammatory response, active immunity, passive immunity, artificial immunity, natural immunity, delayed hypersensitivity, immediate hypersensitivity.**
- **Name at least five different diseases of the specific or nonspecific immune system.**
- **Indicate why diagnostic protozoology and helminthology are sometimes considered as important studies of clinicodiagnostic microbiology laboratories. Name five diseases caused by protozoa and five diseases caused by helminths.**

22

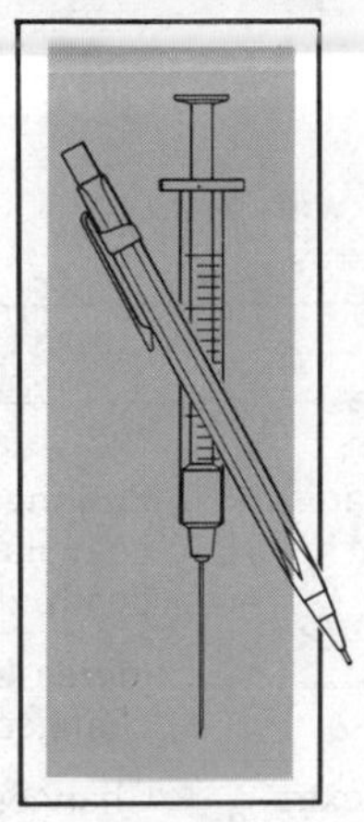

BASIC MEDICAL MICROBIOLOGY

DONALD J. REINHARDT, Ph.D.

In this chapter **infectious** diseases will be discussed. *Disease* may be defined as any sustained, harmful alteration of the normal structure, function, or metabolism (biochemistry) of an organism or cell. We recognize and categorize many different types of diseases: hereditary (genetic), drug-induced, structural, degenerative, and infectious, to name a few. Sometimes a specific disease may fit two or more categories. Table 22-1 lists some examples of the different kinds of diseases and explains the abnormality. Infectious diseases are caused by infection, which is the entrance of a living **microbe** onto or into a cell or organism.

Infection itself is not disease, for until the infected cell or organism shows a continuing harmful alteration of its structure, physiology, or biochemistry, disease is either not detected or not considered present. A living microbe may be ingested, injected, or inhaled and may never cause an infectious disease, as when the infected host organism or cell expels or destroys the microbe.

The study of microbes (microbiology) and of their effects on the defense systems of the body (immunology) is complex. Many factors determine the role of microbes in disease, the identification of microbes in the laboratory, and the ability of the body to maintain or recover health. This chapter is necessarily technical; its contents will become more familiar in practice and should serve as a comprehensive reference for your work.

MICROBIOLOGY

Types of Microbes

Microbes (or microorganisms) are generally microscopic organisms. Some microbes may cause infectious disease and are termed pathogens. The first observations of microbes were made in the 1600s by Anton van Leeuwenhoek, who observed bacteria, protozoa, and fungi with microscopes that he had made. Leeuwenhoek's microscopes were the first ever constructed. After many subsequent years of research, scientists now recognize the following kinds of microorganisms: **protozoa, fungi** (including yeasts and molds), **bacteria** (including **rickettsiae, chlamydiae,** and **mycoplasma**), and **viruses**.

TABLE 22–1 Simplified Explanation of Selected Diseases with the Abnormality and Consequences

Category and Disease	Abnormality	Consequences
Hereditary		
Hemophilia	Defective blood-clotting mechanism; one or more chemical factors missing or defective.	Prolonged bleeding without coagulation factor; bleeding to death, if not corrected.
Baldness	Loss of hair.	Increased heat loss via scalp and changed appearance of head.
Down's Syndrome	Affected individuals have one extra chromosome (47 instead of 46).	Changes in metabolism and function lead to distorted physical features (mongoloidism) and lowered mental processes (IQ)
Metabolic		
Diabetes	Inability to use glucose effectively inside the body.	High levels of sugar in blood and urine. If uncorrected, formation of ketone bodies, acidosis, followed by coma and death.
Hyperthyroidism	Excessive secretion of thyroxine and thyronine, two hormones of the thyroid.	Nervousness, irritability, muscle weakness, weight loss despite good appetite.
Addison's Disease	Adrenocortical hormone insufficiency.	Fatigue, weakness, pigmentation of skin in pressure areas and sometimes face; postural hypotension. Delayed excretion of water, loss of sodium via urine.
Infectious		
Trichomoniasis	Growth and multiplication of the flagellate, *Trichomonas vaginalis,* in urinary tract of females or males.	Itching, burning of urethra.
Gonorrhea	Growth and multiplication of the bacterium *Neisseria gonorrhoeae* in the genitourinary tract of males and females.	Inflammation, pus; in males, burning on urination with release of pus; females may be asymptomatic.
Infective Osteomyelitis	Growth and multiplication usually of the bacterium *Staphylococcus aureus* in bone marrow.	Bone pain and ache; bone destruction; fever.

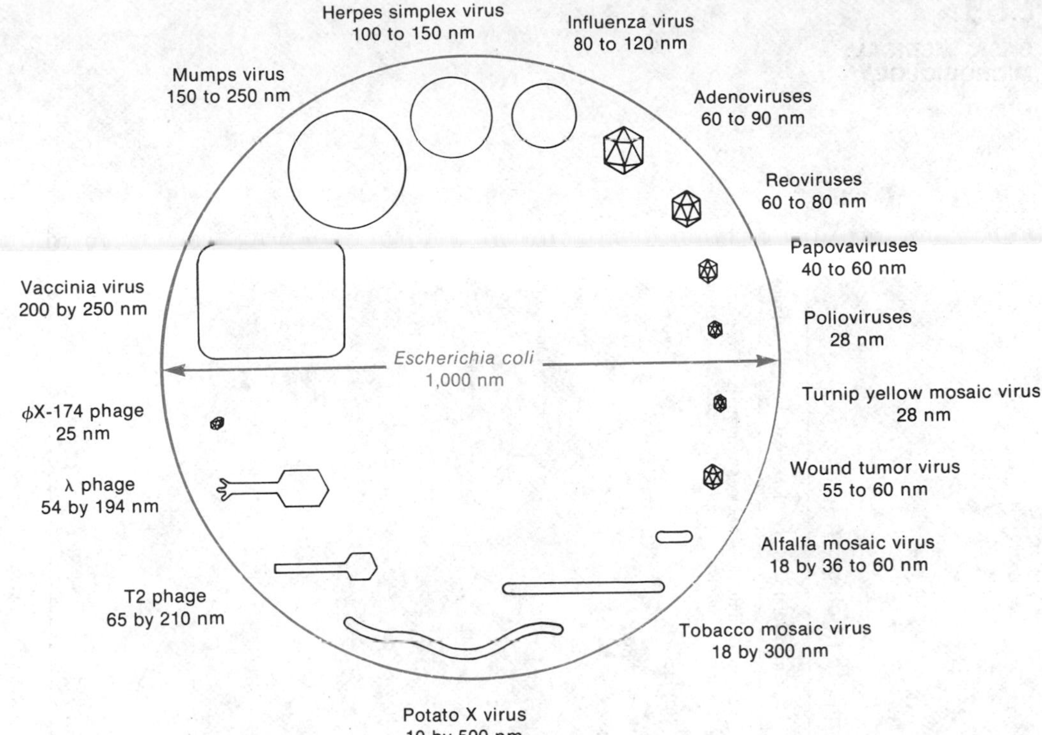

FIGURE 22–1 Diagrammatic comparison of sizes of viruses and related structures. The largest circle, enclosing the whole, represents the diameter of *Escherichia coli,* a small cylindrical bacterium about 1 μm (1,000 nm) in diameter. The other organisms are drawn to approximately the same scale. (From Frobisher, M., et al.: *Fundamentals of Microbiology*. 9th edition. Philadelphia, W. B. Saunders Company, 1974; reprinted with permission.)

Size of Microbes

One of the largest microbes that can cause infectious disease in humans is the protozoan *Balantidium coli*, an intestinal **ciliate** that is responsible for diarrhea and ulceration of the colon. The virus group contains some of the smallest pathogens, for example, polio and hepatitis viruses. Figure 22–1 compares and contrasts the sizes of several different kinds of microbes. Because of the small size of microbes and because of the preciseness and universality of the metric system, microorganisms are regularly measured in micrometers (μm; one millionth of a meter). Many bacteria are about 1 μm, approximately 1/25,000 of an inch.

Diseases

Microorganisms cause many different kinds of infectious diseases. Some of the infectious diseases are mild and usually not life-threatening: acne, warts, the common cold, septic sore throat. Other infectious diseases are more serious and life-threatening: hepatitis, malaria, infectious endocarditis, rheumatic fever, infectious meningitis. Table 22–2 presents different infectious diseases caused by bacteria, rickettsiae, fungi, viruses, mycoplasma, chlamydiae, protozoa, and **helminths** (worms, sometimes included in microbiology because diagnosis and identification frequently requires microscopy).

Signs and Symptoms

How does the physician know that a patient has an infectious disease? The patient's **signs** (objective criteria observable by the physician) and **symptoms** (the patient's subjective description of the disease) frequently suggest that an infectious disease is present. Sometimes the signs and symptoms are so distinctive that the disease can be accurately diagnosed by physical examination (as in measles, chickenpox, acne, boils, and abscesses). In many other instances, laboratory tests and further examinations are needed to confirm or reject the possibilities. A simple example of this is the sore throat. Sore throats are frequently caused by viruses, or bacteria, or both.

TABLE 22–2 Selected Types of Infectious Diseases Classified According to Etiologic Agent*

Bacterial	Viral	Mycotic	Protozoan	Mycoplasmal	Chlamydial	Rickettsial	Helminthic
Anthrax	Chickenpox	Candidiasis	Amebic dysentery (amebiasis)	Nongonococcal urethritis	Lymphogranuloma venereum	Rocky Mountain spotted fever	Creeping eruption
Boils	Common cold	Coccidioidomycosis	Balantidiasis	Primary atypical pneumonia	Psittacosis	Typhus fever	Hookworm
Botulism	Equine encephalitis	Cryptococcosis	Giardiasis		Trachoma		Pinworm
Brucellosis	Hepatitis	Histoplasmosis	Leishmaniasis				Roundworm
Diphtheria	Herpes (fever blisters)	Ringworm (Athlete's foot, jock itch, etc.)	Malaria				Tapeworm
Gonorrhea	Measles	Thrush (Candidiasis)	African sleeping sickness				Trichinosis
Meningitis	Mumps		Trichomoniasis				Whipworm
Rheumatic fever	Polio						
Septic thrombophlebitis	Smallpox						
Shigellosis							
Subacute infectious endocarditis							
Syphilis							
Tetanus							
Tuberculosis							
Typhoid fever							
Urinary tract infections							
Whooping cough							

*Mycoplasma, chlamydia, and rickettsia are specialized types of bacteria.

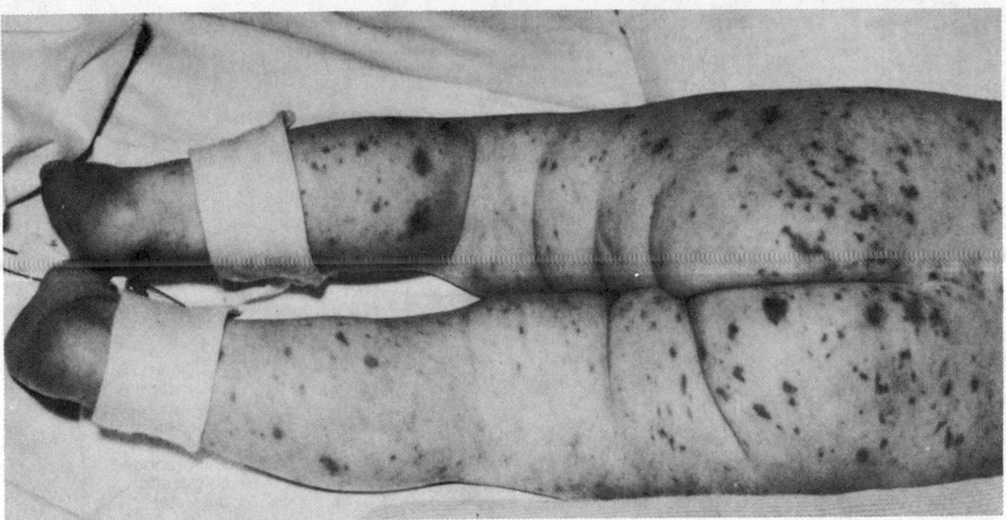

FIGURE 22–2 Representative cutaneous eruption of acute meningococcemia in a young child with meningococcal meningitis. (From Bell, W. E., and McCormick, W. F.: *Neurologic Infections in Children*. Philadelphia, W. B. Saunders Co., 1975.)

Classic sore throat is caused by *Streptococcus pyogenes*, a bacterium susceptible to **antibiotics** like penicillin or erythromycin. However, it has been shown that only about 50 per cent of all sore throats are caused by this bacterium. Some viruses cause the same signs and symptoms as evident with a typical bacterial septic sore throat, and antibiotic therapy is not helpful. Therefore, a throat culture (done by streaking swab specimens on **blood agar plates**) must be performed to identify *Streptococcus pyogenes*. This will suggest that the bacterium is the etiologic agent and antibiotic therapy is warranted.

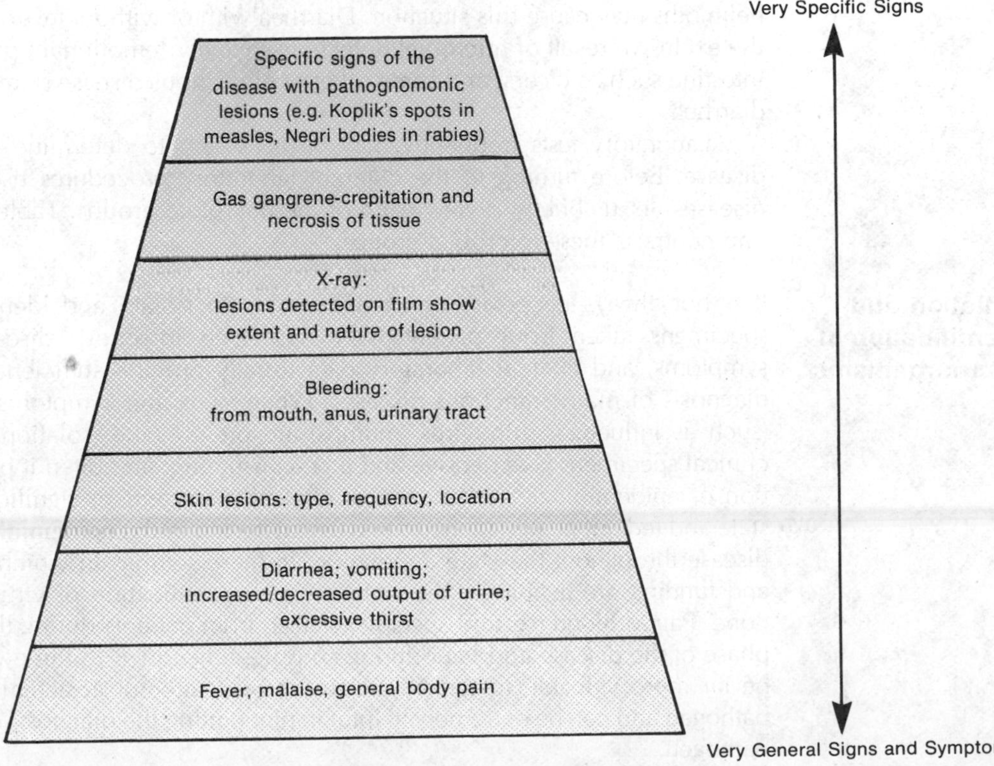

FIGURE 22–3 A pyramid illustrating increased specificity of some signs or symptoms encountered in some infectious diseases.

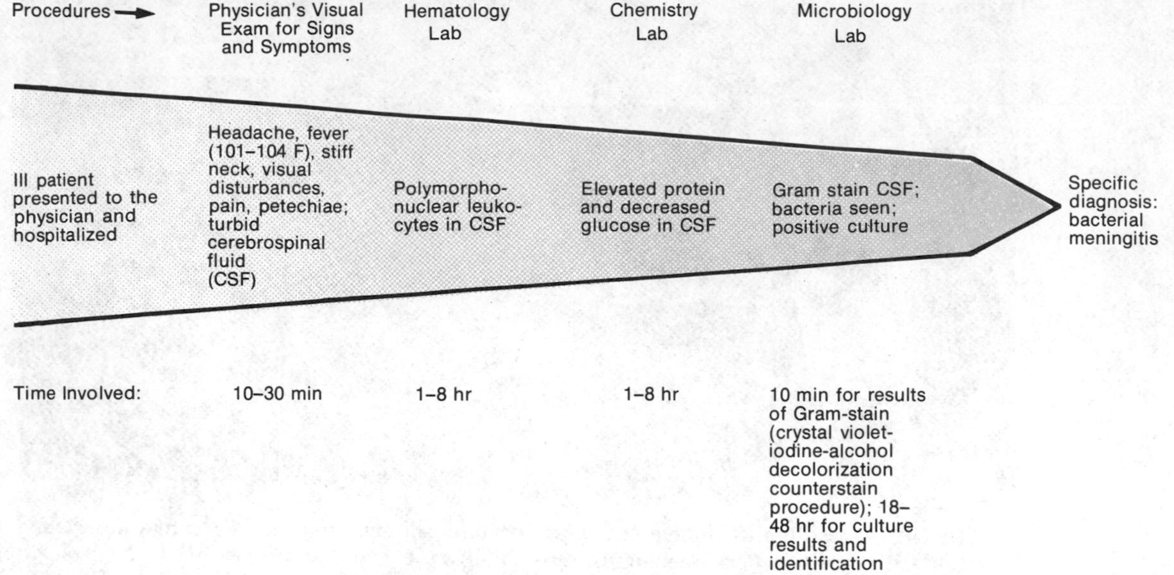

FIGURE 22–4 Example of steps in the diagnosis of a disease such as bacterial meningitis.

Figure 22–3 presents a brief overview of some signs and symptoms of infectious diseases. Fever and **malaise** are common, general signs of most infectious diseases. The figure illustrates signs that show increasing diagnostic value to the physician. Figure 22–4 illustrates steps in the diagnosis of one infectious disease.

The signs and symptoms of disease provide the initial clues that assist the physician in arriving at a tentative or specific diagnosis. *Sometimes the presentations by the patient are so general that the possible diagnoses are many*. A simple example of a typical presentation of an infectious disease is *diarrhea with fever*. At least five different genera of bacteria as well as several viruses and some protozoa and helminths may cause this situation. Diarrhea with or without fever, moreover, is not the exclusive result of microbial (infectious) activity: emotional upset, lesions in the intestine such as ulcers, and some other noninfectious disease states may also cause diarrhea.

Laboratory tests frequently may be necessary to determine the identity of a disease. Before turning to the different laboratory procedures used for infectious diseases, let us briefly review each of the microbial groups. Table 22–3 compares and contrasts these microbial groups.

Isolation and Identification of Microorganisms

It is not always necessary or even desirable to isolate and identify microbes in specimens taken from patients with suspected infectious diseases. The signs, symptoms, and clinical laboratory data usually provide sufficient information for diagnosis of many infectious diseases. When signs and symptoms of *viral* disease (such as influenza, rhinovirus, mumps) are present, the isolation of viruses from clinical specimens is expensive and time-consuming, and often it provides information of epidemiologic rather than of clinical management significance. However, state and federal health agencies may be interested in the **epidemiology** of infectious disease throughout the state and nation. In these settings in which time, expertise, and funding are available, the isolation and identification of viruses is frequently done. Paired blood (**serum**) specimens taken from patients during the acute or early phase of the disease and later during convalescence (two to three weeks later) may be far more valuable to the physician than the attempt at actual isolation of the pathogen and can be extremely helpful in pinpointing the diagnosis or suggesting the pathogen.

Serologic studies are applicable to almost any infectious disease state, whether bacterial, viral, protozoan, rickettsial, or fungal. The episodes of Legionnaire's

TABLE 22–3 Comparison of Different Types of Infectious Disease Agents

	Viruses	Rickettsiae	Chlamydiae	Mycoplasmas	Bacteria	Fungi	Protozoa	Helminths
Size (μm) Range	0.02–0.3	0.3–0.6	0.3–1.0	0.05–0.3	0.2–50	2–60	2–60	10–20 to several meters
DNA and RNA	0	+	+	+	+	+	+	+
Cultivable on Media	0*	0*	0*	+	+	+	some	some
Serological Tests	Available for all of the above, using specific antisera or antigens							
Main Types of Disease	many	systemic fevers	trachoma; lymphogranuloma venereum; conjunctivitis; psittacosis	atypical pneumonia; Nongonococcal urethritis	many	dermatologic, pulmonary; disseminated	intestinal; blood	intestinal; blood
Arthropod Vector Required	some	most	no	no	some	no	some	few

* = Some viruses and all chlamydiae and rickettsiae are usually cultivable in embryonated eggs. None of these organisms can be grown on nonliving media.
0 = Absent
† = Present

22

disease are relevant in this respect. Samples of serum obtained from patients with some atypical pneumonias over the years and kept frozen for later analysis clearly showed that in the past some pneumonia was due to *Legionella* (the Legionnaire's bacterium). A short time after the outbreak in Philadelphia, the Center for Disease Control in Atlanta, Georgia, mobilized its resources, isolated and characterized this bacterial pathogen, and developed varied and useful serologic tests. These tests are now available for analysis of any serum, whenever Legionnaire's disease is suspected.

Protozoa and Helminths

In parasitology, identifications frequently can be made by microscopic examination of the appropriate specimens. Eggs of roundworms, tapeworms, and flukes frequently may be seen in feces of patients with these parasites (Fig. 22–5). Sometimes whole or segments of worms or larvae may be passed in feces (Fig. 22–6). **Cysts** or

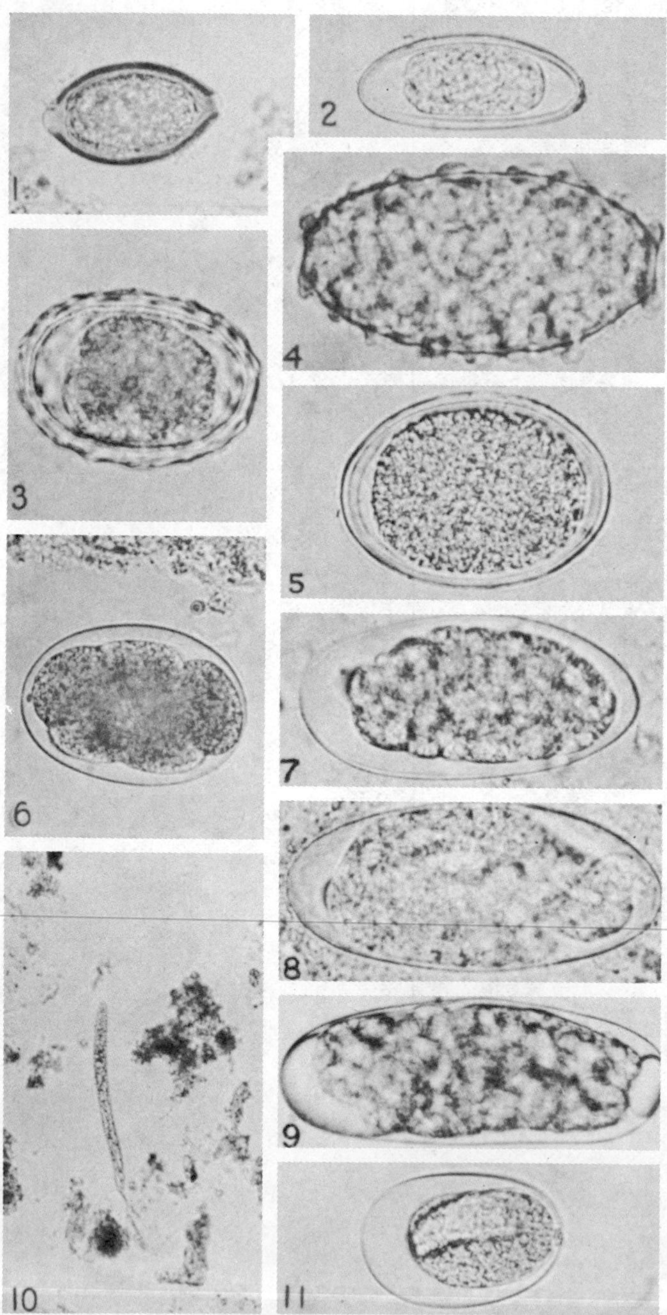

FIGURE 22–5 Nematode eggs: 1, *Trichuris trichiura;* 2, *Enterobius vermicularis;* 3, *Ascaris lumbricoides,* fertilized egg; 4, *Ascaris,* unfertilized egg; 5, *Ascaris,* decorticated egg; 6, hookworm; 7, *Trichostrongylus orientalis,* immature egg; 8, *Trichostrongylus,* embryonated egg; 9, *Heterodera marioni;* 10, *Strongyloides stercoralis,* rhabditiform larva; 11, *Strongyloides* egg (rarely seen in stool). All figures 500 × except 10 (75 ×).

Illustration continued on opposite page

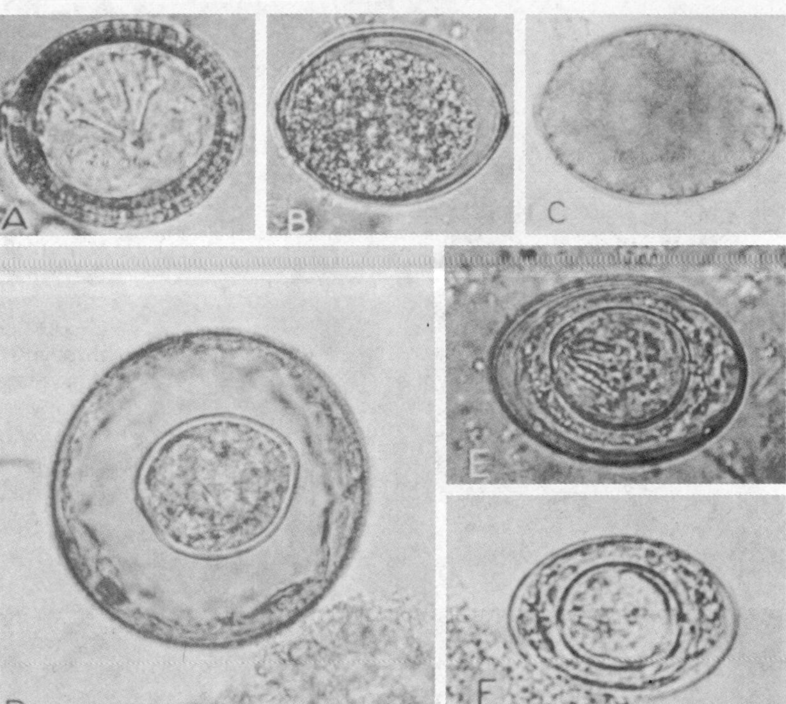

FIGURE 22–5 *Continued* Cestode eggs: *A, Taenia* sp.; *B, C, Diphyllobothrium latum; D, Hymenolepis diminuta; E, F, H. nana. A, E and F,* 750 ×; *D,* 650 ×; *C,* 500 ×. (Figure parts 1–11 and A–F from Hunter, G. W., Swartzwelder, J. C., and Clyde, D. F.: *Tropical Medicine*. 5th edition. Philadelphia, W. B. Saunders Company, 1976; reprinted with permission.)

trophozoites (feeding cells) of parasitic **amebae, flagellates,** or ciliates may also be noted in stools from patients infected with these protozoa. *Trichomonas vaginalis*, a flagellate, may cause vaginitis or urethritis in some patients and can be seen in urine specimens (Fig. 22–7).

Stool and urine specimens can be examined for protozoan and helminth pathogens in a physician's office by a qualified assistant or technologist. The best procedure is to submit these specimens to diagnostic laboratories that are equipped to do this work routinely. Concentration procedures are available to increase the chances of detecting certain diagnostic stages of parasites in feces or blood. The

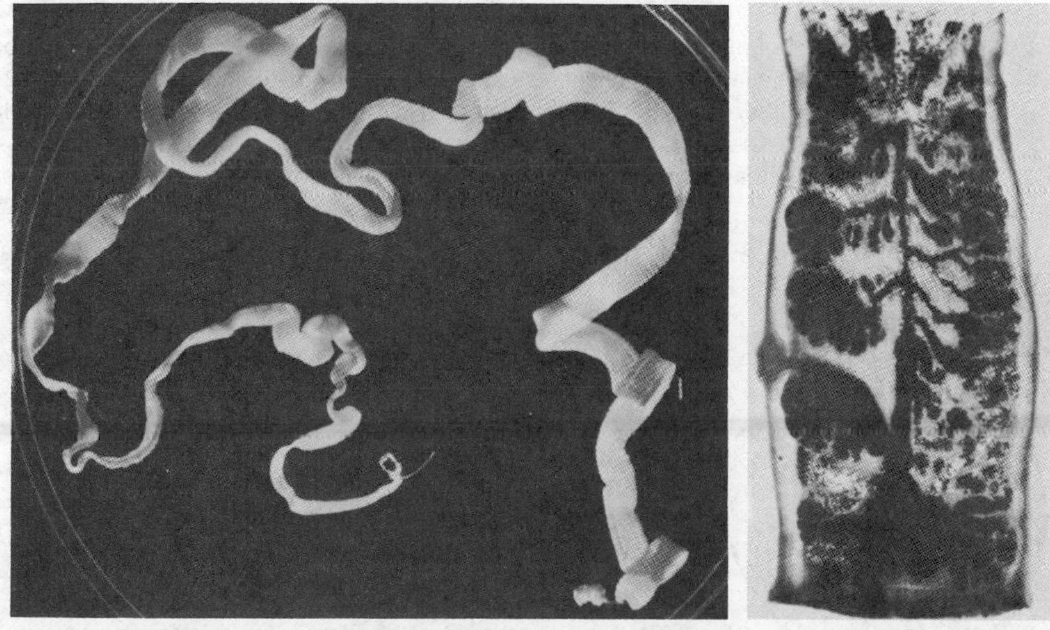

FIGURE 22–6 *A,* Entire tapeworm — *Hymenolepis diminuta.* (Photograph by Zane Price.) *B, Taenia solium,* gravid proglottid. (Photomicrograph by Zane Price.)

Illustration continued on following page

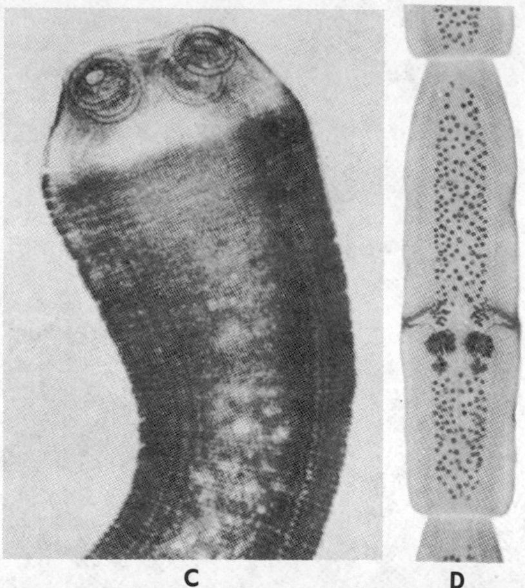

FIGURE 22–6 *Continued* C, *Taenia saginata*, scolex. (Photomicrograph by Zane Price.) D, *Dipylidium caninum*, mature proglottid. (Photomicrograph by Zane Price.) E, *Ascaris lumbricoides*, female worm passed spontaneously (natural size). F, *Enterobius vermicularis* adult female worms. Note shapes and the clear, attenuated and pointed posterior end. (*A* through *E* by Zane Price; *F* courtesy of Louisiana State University School of Medicine; all from Markell, E. K., and Voge, M.: *Medical Parasitology*, 5th edition. Philadelphia, W. B. Saunders Company, 1981; reprinted with permission.)

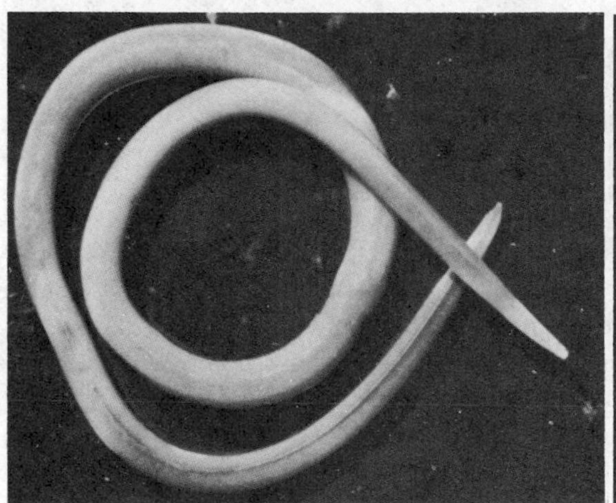

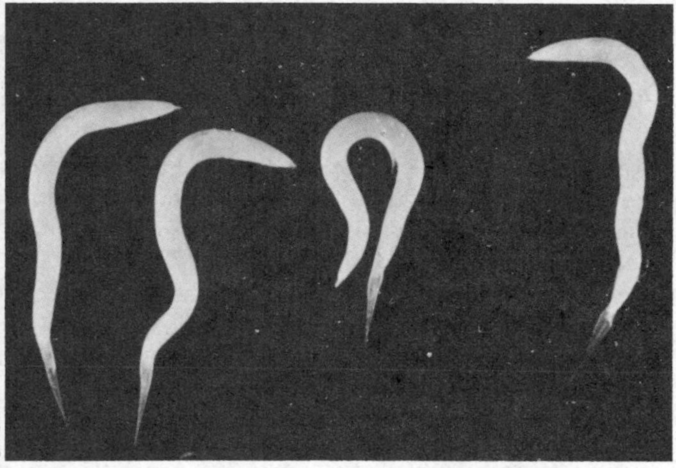

helminthic disease trichinosis is unusual in that it requires a muscle **biopsy** to detect the larvae of *Trichinella spiralis* in certain striated muscle cells (Fig. 22–8). Blood and tissue parasites may be detected with Giemsa or Wright stains of blood and other tissues. Malaria, leishmaniasis, trypanosomiasis (sleeping sickness and Chagas disease), toxoplasmosis, and interstitial plasma cell pneumonia (*Pneumocystis carinii*)

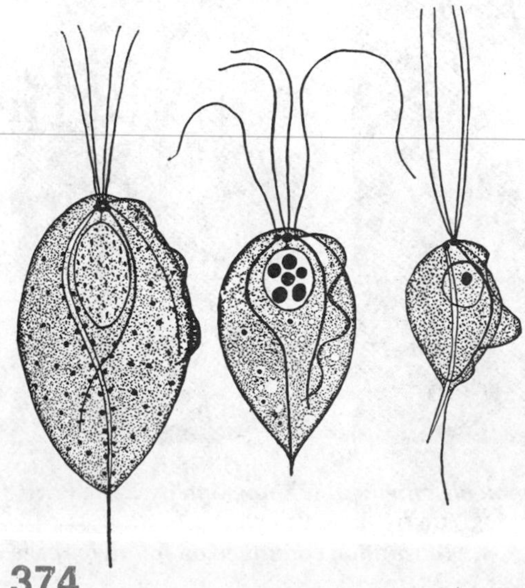

FIGURE 22–7 Three species of *Trichomonas* found in humans: (left to right) *T. vaginalis, T. buccalis* (or *T. tenax?*), *T. hominis*. The size differences shown are not very constant. *T. buccalis* is not known to be pathogenic, but its continuous presence in the mouth in considerable numbers indicates bad oral hygiene. (2,000 ×) (Courtesy of Dr. S. J. Powell, Institute for Parasitology, Durban; from Frobisher, M., et al.: *Fundamentals of Microbiology*. 9th edition. Philadelphia, W. B. Saunders Company, 1974; reprinted with permission.)

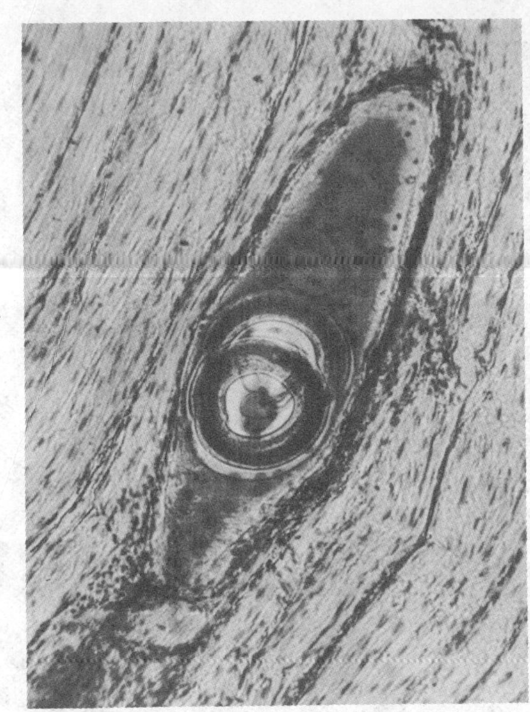

FIGURE 22–8 *Trichinella spiralis,* larva in muscle. (Photomicrograph by Zane Price; from Markell, E. K., and Voge, M.: *Medical Parasitology,* 5th edition. Philadelphia, W. B. Saunders Company, 1981; reprinted with permission.)

are important diseases caused by blood and tissue parasites (Fig. 22–9). When results of microscopic tests are equivocal or when additional confirmation is desired, serologic tests may be used.

Fungi

22

Fungal (mycotic) diseases of man range from relatively **benign** diseases such as vaginitis or dermatophytoses (ringworm) to life-threatening situations such as candidal endocarditis or **disseminated** disease (coccidioidomycosis, cryptococcosis, or histoplasmosis). In practice, physicians most often encounter ringworms [dermatophytoses or tineas (Fig. 22–10)] of the hands, feet, nails, face, scalp, groin (jock itch) or general body and vaginitis or urethritis due to *Candida albicans*. Skin manifestations may also occur with disseminated or lymphatic fungal diseases, which are frequently difficult to diagnose. *Coccidioides, Histoplasma, Blastomyces,* and *Sporothrix* are a few of the pathogenic fungi that cause such cutaneous lesions when disseminated (Fig. 22–11). Fungi may cause pneumonia, mycetomas, fever, endocarditis, and meningitis (*Cryptococcus neoformans*) and are sometimes overlooked or missed in clinical diagnostic settings. Patients who are **immunocompromised** (such as those with leukemia or immune deficiency diseases, or those

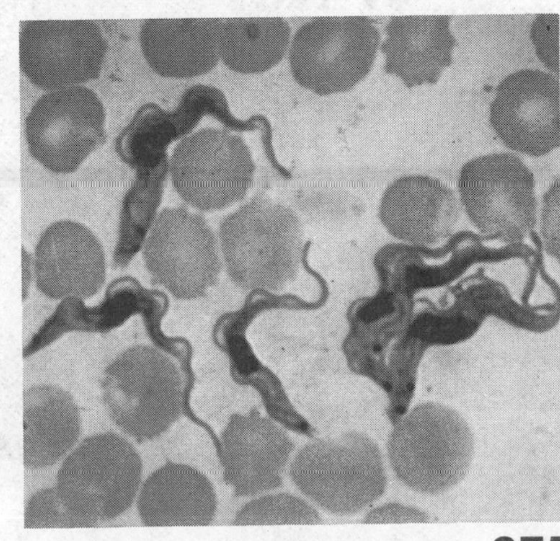

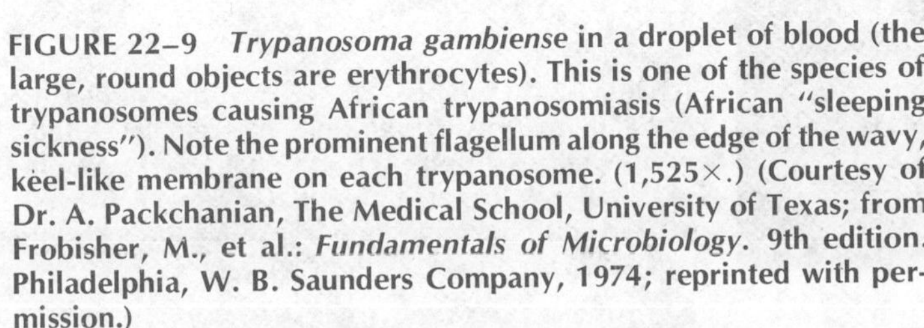

FIGURE 22–9 *Trypanosoma gambiense* in a droplet of blood (the large, round objects are erythrocytes). This is one of the species of trypanosomes causing African trypanosomiasis (African "sleeping sickness"). Note the prominent flagellum along the edge of the wavy, keel-like membrane on each trypanosome. (1,525×.) (Courtesy of Dr. A. Packchanian, The Medical School, University of Texas; from Frobisher, M., et al.: *Fundamentals of Microbiology*. 9th edition. Philadelphia, W. B. Saunders Company, 1974; reprinted with permission.)

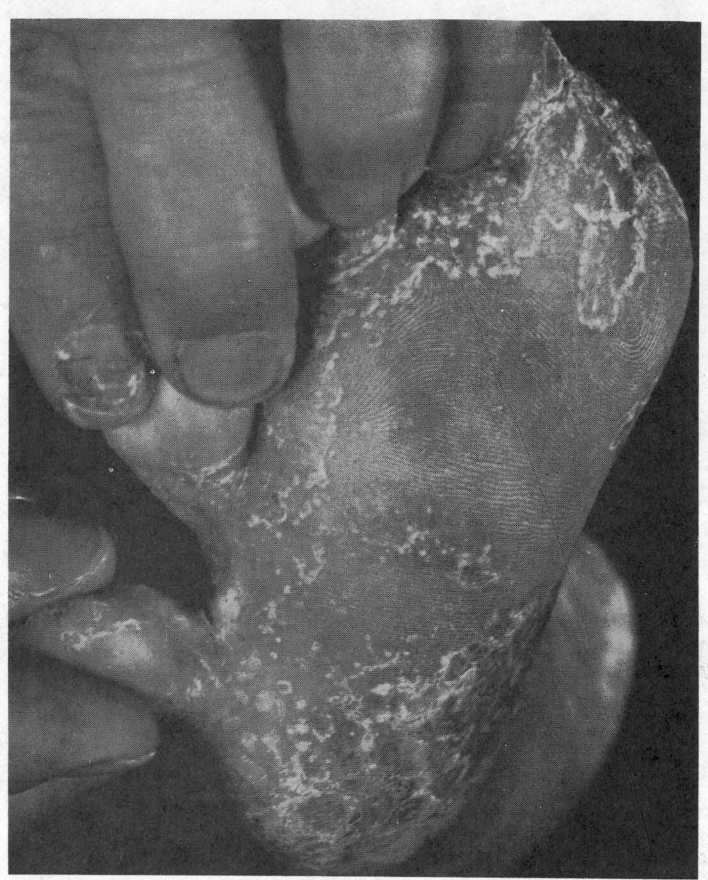

FIGURE 22–10 Chronic intertriginous type of tinea pedis, showing maceration and fissure between fourth and fifth toes. (From Conant, N. F., Smith, D. T., Baker, R. D., et al.: *Manual of Clinical Mycology*. 3rd edition. Philadelphia, W. B. Saunders Company, 1971; reprinted with permission.)

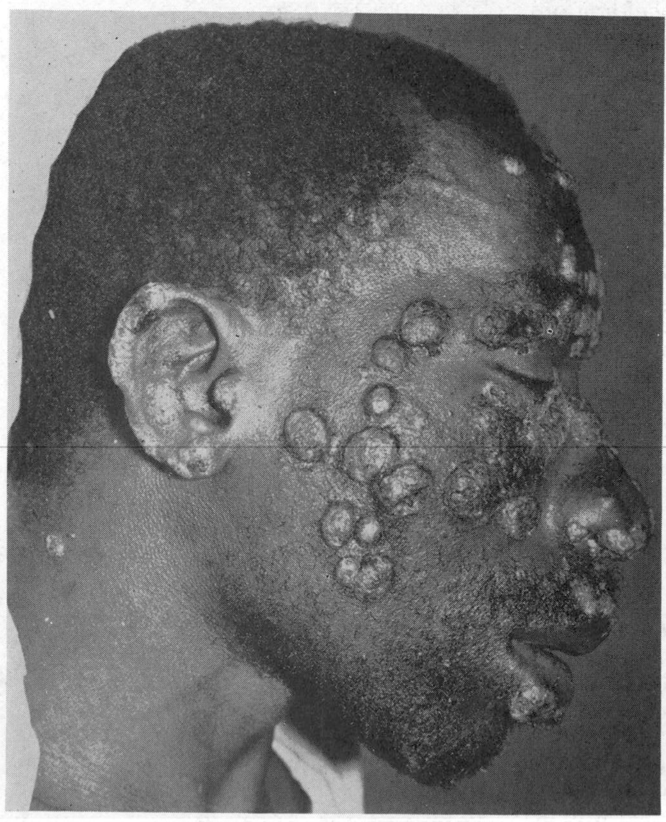

FIGURE 22–11 North American blastomycosis of the skin, showing multiple discrete, elevated, granulomatous lesions. (From Conant, N. F., Smith, D. T., Baker, R. D., et al.: *Manual of Clinical Mycology*. 3rd edition. Philadelphia, W. B. Saunders Company, 1971; reprinted with permission.)

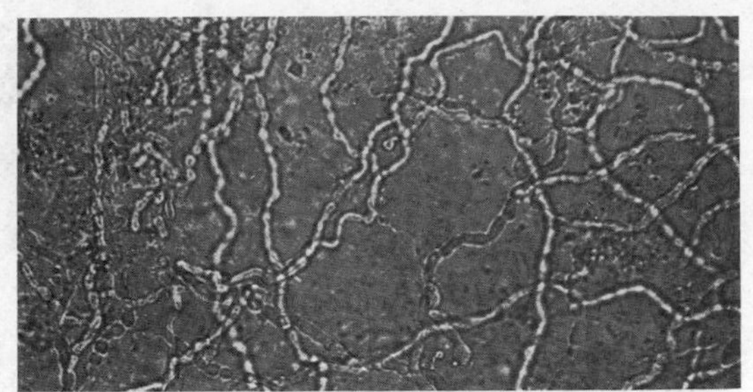

FIGURE 22–12 A mold *(Trichophyton)* causing "ringworm" of feet or "athlete's foot," sometimes contracted in swimming pools and gymnasiums. This slide shows material scraped from superficial lesions on the foot and treated with 10 per cent KOH (× 350). (Courtesy of Miss Rhoda W. Benham; from Fuerst, R.: *Frobisher and Fuerst's Microbiology in Health and Disease*. 14th edition. Philadelphia, W. B. Saunders Company, 1978; reprinted with permission.)

maintained on corticosteroids, immunosuppressive drugs or antibiotics) are particularly at risk.

In the diagnosis of dermatophytoses, samples of diseased skin scrapings or hairs are taken. Culture of those specimens on dermatophyte test medium (DTM) and microscopic observation of the specimens, cleared in 10 per cent potassium hydroxide, for **hyphae** (fungal filaments) and **arthrospores**, can help establish a preliminary diagnosis (Fig. 22–12).

Cultures and microscopy of dermatophytes may be done routinely in the general practitioner's office. In disseminated, tissue, and pulmonary mycoses, special stains such as Giemsa, Gomori, Gridley and periodic acid-Schiff reagent can help detect the pathogens in clinical specimens (Fig. 22–13). Most fungi are relatively easy to cultivate on simple **media** such as brain-heart infusion, Sabouraud's agar, and blood agar (Fig. 22–14). Antibacterial antibiotics are usually incorporated into the medium to preclude or minimize bacterial contamination. Excellent serologic tests are available to assist the physician with the diagnosis of mycotic diseases. Skin tests are also available to assist in the differential diagnoses of those diseases (such as coccidioidomycosis, histoplasmosis, and blastomycosis) that may mimic pulmonary tuberculosis.

The antibiotics available for the treatment of mycotic diseases are limited in number but are usually effective. Tolnaftate is available for topical application to certain dermatomycoses, and griseofulvin may be taken orally to cure more difficult situations. Candidal vaginitis is controllable by mycostatin. Many systemic and pulmonary diseases are usually treated with the drug amphotericin B, which may be damaging to the kidneys. Cryptococcosis and some other diseases caused by yeasts may be treated with 5-fluorocytosine. Sporothrixosis can be treated with iodine orally administered in carefully measured doses.

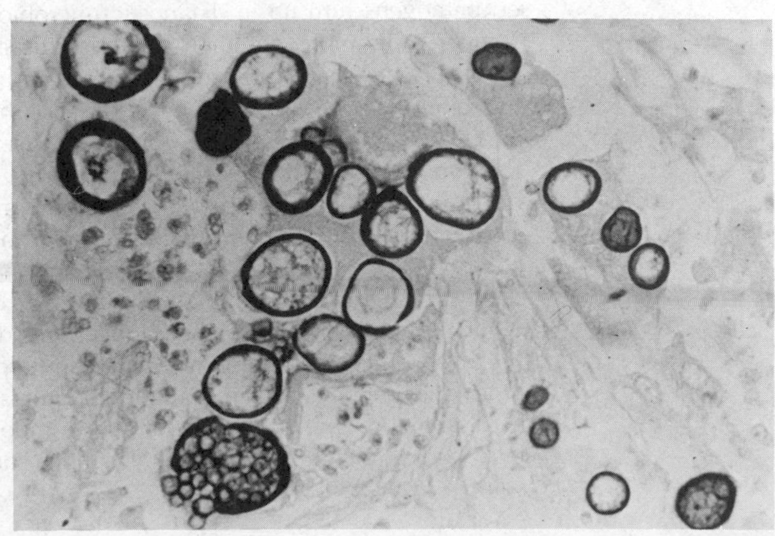

FIGURE 22–13 Coccidioidomycosis. Tissue section showing developing and mature spherules, some containing endospores. (From J. W. Rippon, *in* Burrows, W.: *Textbook of Microbiology*. Philadelphia, W. B. Saunders Co., 1973; reprinted with permission.)

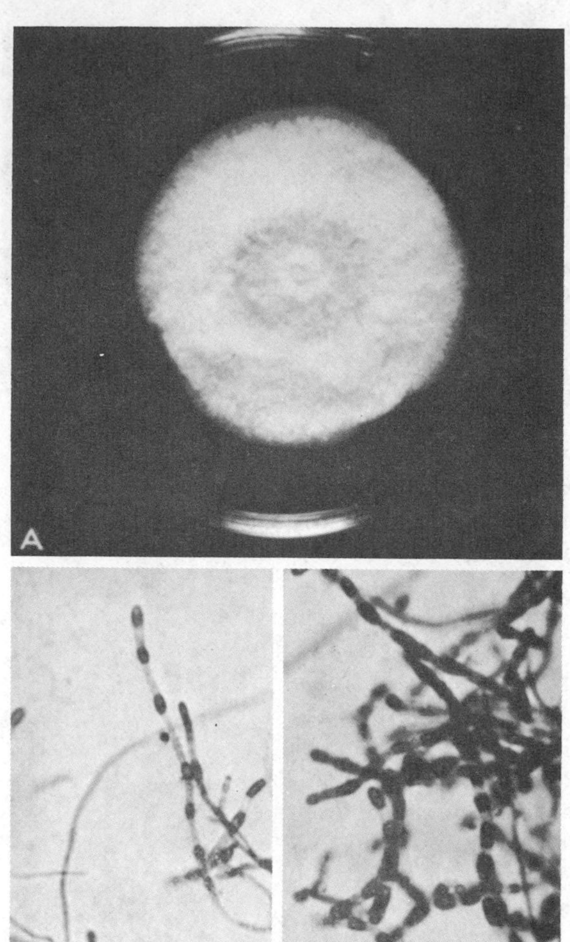

FIGURE 22–14 *Coccidioides immitis. A,* Culture on Sabouraud's glucose agar, 19 days, at room temperature. *B,* Arthrospore formation in young culture. (× 580) *C,* Arthrospore formation of old culture. (× 700) (From Conant, N. F., Smith, D. T., Baker, R. D., et al.: *Manual of Clinical Mycology.* 3rd ed. Philadelphia, W. B. Saunders Co., 1971.)

Bacteria

The identification of bacteria accounts for the great majority of diagnostic microbiology done in office and clinical laboratories. The usual pathogens sought or expected to be found in clinical specimens are shown in Table 22–4. Occasionally, unexpected pathogens turn up in diagnostic microbiology. In this chapter we present only some of the more common bacterial diseases. There are many rarer bacterial diseases (such as plague, anthrax, tularemia, cholera) that are beyond the scope of this brief introduction.

Caution — Some simple, rapid, and useful microbiologic procedures may be done in physician's offices that are properly equipped. However, novices should be reminded that microbiology is a complex and detailed discipline. Care must be exercised by all who attempt clinical microbiology. If some office microbiology is attempted, it would be appropriate and beneficial to have the actual set-up, procedures, and media initially supervised by a qualified medical technologist or clinical microbiologist. The additional, limited payment of a consultant-teaching fee for this individual's pertinent advice can help eliminate future errors and waste of time and money. When handling cultures or specimens, the use of aseptic (contamination-preventing) technique is important. Cultures or specimens accidentally contaminated can waste time and resources and will lead to erroneous results.

TABLE 22–4 Some Important Bacterial Diseases and Common Etiologic Agents

Disease	Some Possible Organisms
Sore Throat	*Streptococcus pyogenes* (Group A Streptococci)
Urinary Tract Infections	*Escherichia coli* and other members of the Enterobacteriaceae; occasionally gram-positive bacteria.
Meningitis	*Haemophilus influenzae, Neisseria meningitidis, Streptococcus pneumoniae.* In infants, *E. coli* and occasionally other enterics.
Pneumonia	*Staphylococcus aureus, Streptococcus pneumoniae, Haemophilus influenzae, Klebsiella pneumoniae, Mycobacterium tuberculosis.*
Skin Lesions	*S. aureus, Streptococcus pyogenes.*
Conjunctivitis	*S. aureus, Haemophilus aegypticus, Pseudomonas aeruginosa.*
Otitis (inflammation of the ear)	*S. aureus, Pseudomonas aeruginosa.*
Sexually transmitted	*Neisseria gonorrhoeae, Treponema pallidum.*
Diarrhea (usual pathogen)	*Salmonella* spp., *Shigella* spp.
Diarrhea (special pathogens)	*Vibrio parahaemolyticus, Vibrio cholerae.*
Pharyngitis	*Haemophilus influenzae, Streptococcus pyogenes, S. pneumoniae, Staphylococcus aureus.*

Sterile and Nonsterile Specimens

When doing clinical microbiology it is important to keep in mind that some specimens are normally sterile (have no viable microbes) and that others are normally contaminated (that is, they contain viable microbes). All specimens from *mucocutaneous sites* such as mouth, respiratory tract, urethra, anus, and gastrointestinal tract, *are contaminated with normal flora.* Specimens that are *expected to be sterile* in *healthy individuals* include blood, cerebrospinal fluid, **aspirates**, aspirated and **catheterized** urine, biopsies, and **pleural** and **peritoneal** fluids. Therefore, the detection of microorganisms, by stain, culture, or both, in clinical specimens expected to be sterile is significant. Accidental contamination of the specimen may occur, occasionally, during collection or processing or both.

22

Aseptic, Sterilization, Disinfection, and Discard Procedures

Aseptic procedures are all those techniques that are used to preclude microbial contamination of specimens, surfaces, and the environment.

The caps or plugs on tubes must be carefully handled to avoid contamination. Unscrewed caps may be temporarily set down on a clean, *disinfected* (antiseptic-treated) surface, with the inside of the cap facing upward. There is more chance of contamination if the caps are placed downward on the surface. Cotton plugs from tubes may be held at the end of the plug, between the fingers, when transfers of **inoculum** from one tube to another are being made. The plug should never be touched or held where the plug contacts the inside of the tube. The mouths of all glass specimen tubes should be flamed for two to three seconds right after the cap or plug is removed and just before recapping. This procedure will kill microbes that are occasionally deposited at this site.

A quiet, clean, low-traffic area is ideal for office microbiology. Minimization of air currents is important to keep the accidental air contaminations as low as possible. Benchtops where bacteriology is done should be disinfected before and after working at the site. The disinfectant is swabbed over the surface with a clean paper towel and allowed to dry for a few minutes. Disinfection kills most but not all microbes. Alcohol (either isopropanol or ethanol) is a good disinfectant. Tincture of iodine (a mixture of alcohol and iodine) is even more effective; organic iodides (iodophors) are excellent disinfectants.

In microbiology, sterilization is defined as any procedure that kills all viable (living) microbes in or on something. The flaming of inoculating needles or loops to redness prior to dipping them into a specimen for plating or subculture is a sterilization procedure. To avoid killing viable pathogens in the specimen, the loop is allowed to cool in the air for 15 to 20 seconds prior to placement in the sample or specimen. Media are usually sterilized in an autoclave (pressure cooker) for 15 minutes at 15 lbs of pressure at 121° C (250° F) (see Chapter twenty-six). **Heat-labile** media (those that are easily decomposed by heat) are frequently sterilized by passing them through filters that retain bacteria, thereby rendering the media free of bacteria. Dry heat (in an oven set at 160 to 170° C for 1½ to 2 hours) is an effective sterilization procedure for glass and metal objects. Sterile plastic materials are usually sterilized by ethylene oxide, a potent sterilizing gas. Sterilized media or items are packaged or wrapped in a manner that protects the contents. Opening a package or container that is sterile exposes it to potential and actual contaminants. The goal for effective clinicodiagnostic microbiologic asepsis is to prevent and prohibit microbial contamination whenever and wherever possible. Additional details on sterilization procedures are given in Chapter 26.

Used plates, tubes, and pipettes that are contaminated are usually autoclaved or incinerated prior to discarding. It is important to have an adequate procedure for decontamination of clinical materials prior to discarding them in the municipal waste system.

Specimens and Media

The acquisition of clinical specimens from the patient for microbiologic analysis is one of the most important clinical procedures. Improperly collected specimens, which can easily lead to an incorrect diagnosis, are worthless and waste time and money. Some guidelines for specimen collection and processing are reviewed in Table 22–5. All specimens acquired from **mucocutaneous** surfaces (gastrointestinal, throat, vaginal, urethral, nasal, nasopharyngeal) will be contaminated with normal flora. In these clinical settings usually a particular pathogen is being sought among the organisms that comprise the normal flora.

Special selective differential media are available to facilitate the isolation and identification of suspect pathogens. These media contain a nutritious substrate with or without additional supplements such as inhibitors, indicators for acid production,

TABLE 22–5 Synopsis of Specimen Containment and Processing in Microbiology

Type of Specimen	Commentary
Cerebrospinal Fluid	Sterile vial or tube used. Gram stain, streak loopfuls onto blood agar and chocolate agars (always incubate chocolate agar in CO_2 incubator). Inoculate 0.1 ml into thioglycollate for anaerobes.
Blood	Collect blood directly into blood culture bottles with anticoagulant (preferably with SPS, Liquoid). One vented and one unvented bottle are used. Check bottles by aspiration, followed by plating onto blood, chocolate and EMB agars, and Gram stains on days 1, 3, 5, 7, and 14.
Aspirates, Pus, Wound, Biopsy; Ocular, Otic, and Nasopharyngeal Discharges	Use sterile vials or tubes for the specimens. Transport medium should be used to prevent drying of specimens on synthetic fiber swabs (preferable to cotton). Gram stain, inoculate blood, chocolate, EMB and anaerobic blood plates. Swab may be added to thioglycollate medium aseptically, by carefully bending and breaking the swab at the tip against the inner wall and lip of vial or tube and permitting it to drop into the thioglycollate.
Throat	Inoculate blood plates directly with swab, previously applied to fauces or tonsils. Swab one quadrant and then streak for isolation. Swab that cannot be processed immediately may be placed in transport medium.
Feces	Usually collected in coffee container or sterile "bucket." Bloody and mucoid areas should be selected. Swab specimens should be in transport medium. Streak XLD, Hektoen, and brilliant green agars. Enrich a portion of the specimen in gram-negative or tetrathionate broths. Plate onto selective agars above at 1, 3, and 7 days.

supplemental vitamins, and amino acids. These media may be purchased in sterile, packaged plates or tubes from major scientific companies (such as Scientific Products and Fisher). Blood agar is a very good basic medium to use for most sterile specimens (aspirates, biopsies, catheterized and aspirated urines, cerebrospinal fluids, and blood). Specimens such as midstream (clean-catch) urines, pus and material from wounds should be streaked on blood agar and a medium that is selective for gram-negative bacteria (MacConkey agar or eosin-methylene blue agar). Thayer-Martin medium and Trans-Grow are useful for the isolation of *Neisseria gonorrhoeae*. Whenever bacteria with fastidious nutritional characteristics are suspected, such as *Haemophilus* spp. or *Neisseria meningitidis*, **chocolated blood agar** should be used and the streaked cultures incubated in a CO_2 jar (candle or Brewer jar). Cerebrospinal fluid specimens, in particular, should be processed in this fashion. XLD (xylose, lysine deoxycholate) and Hektoen agars are useful media for some fecal pathogens such as *Salmonella* and *Shigella*. Blood agar is a good differential medium for detecting *Streptococcus pyogenes* from throat specimens and *Staphylococcus aureus* from nasal specimens.

ANAEROBES. **Anaerobic** bacteria will grow only when incubated under conditions where oxygen is deficient or absent, or where the solution is highly reduced [has a low oxidation-reduction (O-R) potential, that is, electrons move easily from one compound to another]. Low oxidation-reduction potentials indicate good growth conditions for anaerobes. Thioglycollate tubes and blood agar plates supplemented with menadione (vitamin K) and incubated in a Brewer anaerobic jar with a Gas-Pak set-up are useful for the isolation of anaerobes (Fig. 22–15). Material from wounds, pus, blood, and pleural and peritoneal fluids are particularly important specimens that may contain anaerobic pathogens. It is important to remember that anaerobic specimens are part of the normal **flora** of the mouth, small and large intestines, feces, vagina, and urethra and that the same caution that applies to facultative anaerobic bacteria from normally-contaminated mucocutaneous areas applies to anaerobes from these sites.

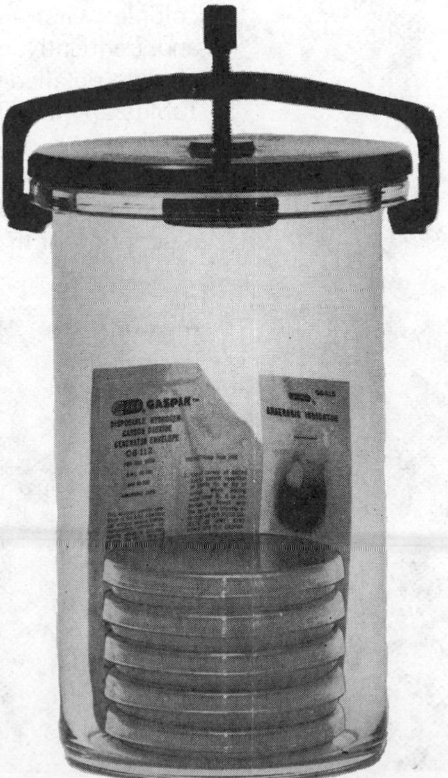

FIGURE 22–15 Simplified form of anaerobe jar utilizing hydrogen and carbon dioxide from the "Gaspak" envelope. Combination of hydrogen and oxygen in the jar is catalyzed at room temperature. (Courtesy of Baltimore Biological Laboratories, Division of Becton-Dickinson Laboratories, Baltimore, Md; from Frobisher, M., et al.: *Fundamental of Microbiology*. 9th edition. Philadelphia, W. B. Saunders Company, 1974; reprinted with permission.)

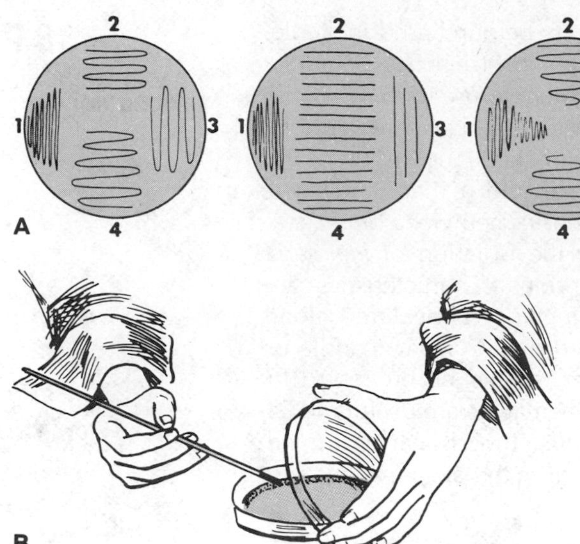

FIGURE 22–16 *A* and *B*, Correct technique for streaking a Petri plate of nutrient agar for isolated colonies. Note the comfortable position of the right hand and the protective angle of the lid held by the left hand. When one sector is completed, the loop is withdrawn and the lid closed. The plate is rotated 90°, and the next sector streaked. (From Bradshaw, L. J.: *Laboratory Microbiology*. 2nd Edition. Philadelphia, W. B. Saunders Co., 1973; reprinted with permission.)

PURE CULTURE TECHNIQUES

Streak Plates. The streaked agar plate is the most useful procedure in clinical microbiology for obtaining well-isolated bacterial or fungal colonies. A loopful of specimen is spread over each quadrant of the plate. After the first quadrant has been streaked and before a new quadrant is started, the loop is stabbed into the agar at the periphery to clean it off; streaking is then continued to the next gradient by running the loop three or four times across the previously-streaked quadrant (Fig. 22–16). The purposes of this streaking procedure are to determine the *number* and *types* of microorganisms that may be isolated from the clinical specimen and to obtain *well-isolated* colonies for subsequent staining or biochemical testing. Different bacteria will frequently vary in the appearance of their colonies. Streptococci and diphtheroids (*Corynebacterium*) form small colonies; *Staphylococcus* forms larger colonies. Gram-negative bacteria form medium to large-sized colonies that are *gray* and frequently mucoid or gummy in character. Books on clinical microbiology provide detailed descriptions of the typical colonies of most microorganisms. (See Table 22–4 for a list of some bacteria that are commonly expected in certain clinical specimens).

Gram Stain and Other Tests. Biochemical tests should be considered after description of th colonies and a Gram stain of each *significant* and different type

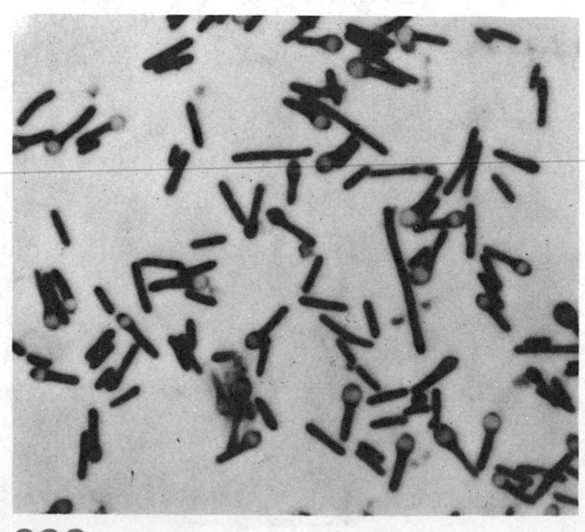

FIGURE 22–17 *Clostridium tetani,* a gram-stained smear showing terminal spores that swell the rods and produce the typical drumstick appearance. Cells of this species range in size from 0.3 to 0.8 by 2.0 to 5.0 μm. (Courtesy of General Biological Supply House, Chicago, Ill. From Frobisher, M., et al.: *Fundamentals of Microbiology*. 9th edition. Philadelphia, W. B. Saunders Company, 1974; reprinted with permission.)

colony have been done. Regardless of the organism to be studied only pure, well-isolated colonies should be tested. A colony containing two or more organisms is not that uncommon when the culture is very contaminated. Tests done with mixed organisms are confusing and useless.

Gram stains of pus, wound material, biopsy specimens, cerebrospinal fluid, sputum, aspirates, and pleural and peritoneal fluids are very informative. The chemical reagents used in the Gram stain enable us to determine biochemical and morphologic characteristics of bacteria. **Gram-positive bacteria** have a large amount of **mucopeptide** and stain blue-purple; **Gram-negative bacteria** have little mucopeptide and stain pink. The shapes (such as round or rod) and sizes of bacteria are clearly evident in a Gram stain that is properly done (Fig. 22–17). The specimen to be stained is spread over about half of a clean slide, which is air-dried and heat-fixed over a Bunsen flame for three to five seconds (Fig. 22–18). Colonies from agar plates

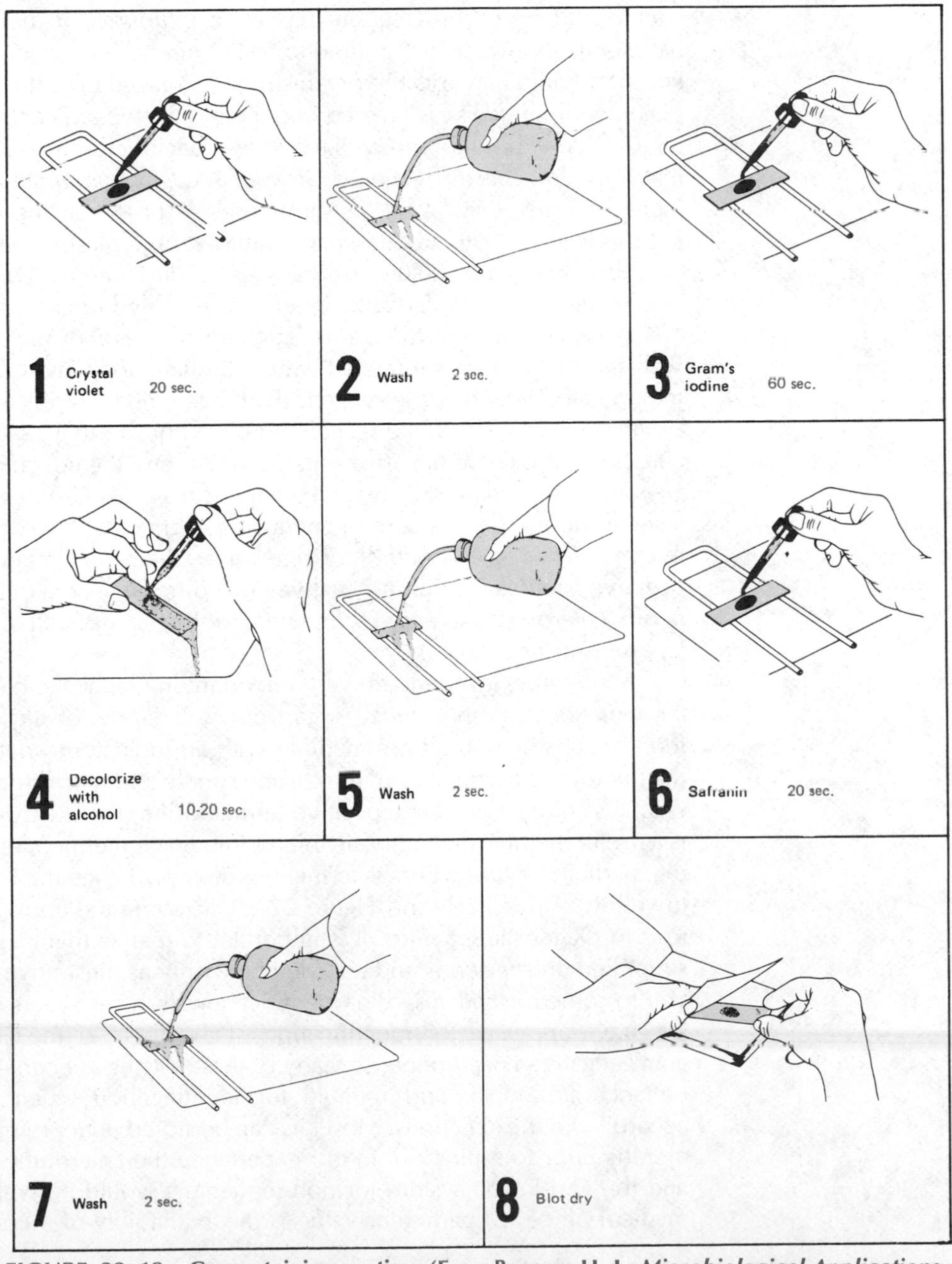

FIGURE 22–18 Gram-staining routine. (From Benson, H. J.: *Microbiological Applications.* Dubuque, Iowa, Wm. C. Brown Co., 1973; reprinted with permission.)

may also be Gram-stained by mixing a very small portion in a drop of tap water, followed by spreading, drying, and heat fixation. The reagents are then added, each followed by a brief wash in tap water; crystal violet (10 seconds), wash, iodine (10 seconds), wash, 95 per cent alcohol decolorization (three to five seconds with constant running alcohol), wash immediately, safranin (20 seconds), wash, blot dry, air dry, and observe under the oil immersion lens of a microscope for color reactions and morphology. Bacterial preparations that are too dense or too light may be under- or over-decolorized and give false Gram reactions. Most clinical microbiologists can determine the general type of organism and its expected Gram reaction by the appearance of the colonies on clinical plates. Organisms stained directly from clinical specimens may or may not be typical. However, all things considered, the Gram stain is one of the most valuable diagnostic procedures in clinical microbiology and has a place in a physician's emergency or quick-check approach to clinical diagnosis.

There are various kinds of tests useful for the presumptive identification of bacteria. Some of the tests are based on *inhibition of the organism with certain biochemicals* such as the antibiotic bacitracin or the surface-active agent optochin. For these inhibition tests the organisms are streaked onto the surface of a blood agar plate and the test disk is pressed into the inoculated area and incubated overnight at 35° C. A zone of inhibition with the *A disk* (bacitracin) suggests group A *streptococci*, that is, *Streptococcus pyogenes. Streptococcus pneumoniae* are inhibited by P or O (optochin) disks (Fig. 22–19). Another test is based on the reaction obtained after gram-positive cocci are inoculated into rabbit plasma with EDTA, a chemical compound added to ensure accurate test results. *Staphylococcus aureus* **coagulates** (gels) the plasma; *Staphylococcus epidermidis* and *Micrococcus* spp. do not.

A very useful test for gram-negative bacilli is the oxidase test. A portion of a well-isolated colony is removed with a sterilized loop and rubbed onto a paper strip impregnated with oxidase reagent (Pathotec oxidase strips are excellent). Oxidase-positive organisms turn the reagent purple within 15 to 30 seconds; there is no color change with oxidase-negative organisms. Among the cocci, only the gram-negative *Neisseria* are oxidase-positive; all other cocci are oxidase-negative. Oxidase-positive tests are found among some genera of the gram-negative bacilli such as *Pseudomonas, Alcaligenes, Achromobacter, Flavobacterium,* and *Vibrio.* Most gram-negative bacilli are oxidase-negative, including all genera of the large and important family *Enterobacteriaceae: Escherichia, Klebsiella, Serratia, Enterobacter, Salmonella, Shigella,* and *Proteus*.

Some other tests that are very important in diagnostic clinical microbiology are *fermentation tests* that utilize sugar, polysaccharide, or alcohol carbon sources as food or substrates in a base medium with an indicator to detect acid production. If the microbe is a fermenter of the carbon source and if acid is produced, the indicator changes color to indicate a positive **fermentation** (Fig. 22–20). *Triple sugar iron* (TSI) is a useful medium in diagnostic microbiology. Nonfermenting organisms do not turn the medium yellow, whereas fermenters always change the butt of the tube from red to yellow. Table 22–6 and Figure 22–21 illustrate the application of TSI and other tests in diagnostic schemes. It is important to realize that these are abbreviated and simplified presentations and are used here only as illustrative examples to introduce you to some methods used for identification. In recent years commercial diagnostic kits have appeared for identification of members of the Enterobacteriaceae and gram-negative nonfermenters. Many of these kits have been evaluated and found to be accurate, rapid, and reliable for identification when used judiciously and according to the directions. Most kits can be stored under refrigeration for three to six months prior to expiration. In our experience the Enterotube II* system for enterics and the Oxi-Ferm* system for non-fermenters would be well suited for use in the medical office. Of particular value is the availability of numerical code books that

*Roche Diagnostic Laboratories, Nutley, New Jersey.

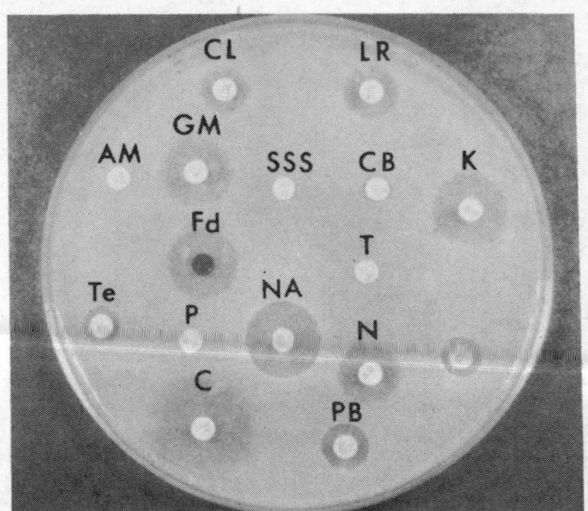

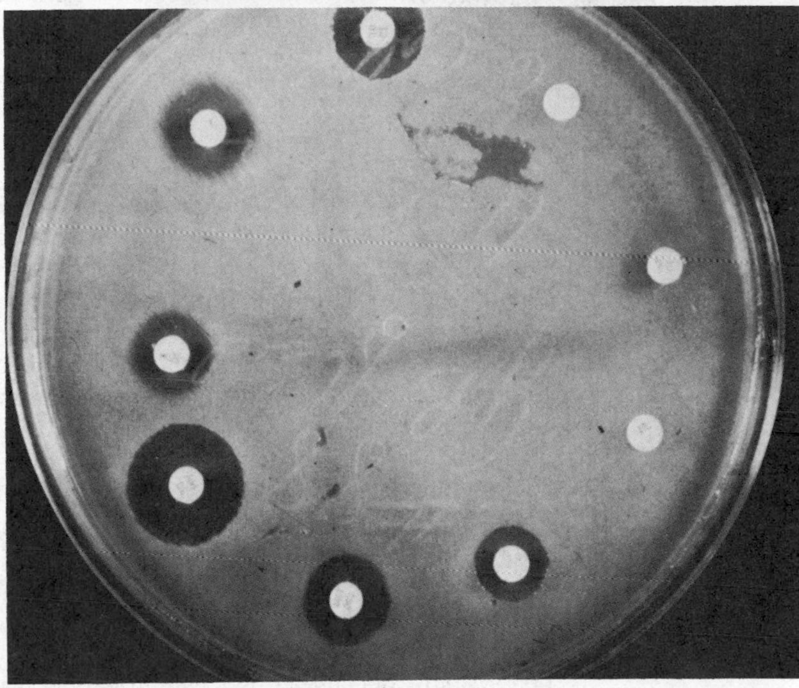

FIGURE 22–19 *A,* Chemotherapy and antibiotics. Testing sensitivity of a bacterium to antibiotics or other chemotherapeutic agents by the "disk method." (Courtesty of Linda Kaye Hickey; from Frobisher, M., and Fuerst, R.: *Microbiology in Health and Disease*. 13th edition. Philadelphia, W. B. Saunders Co., 1973; reprinted with permission.)

CL-Coly-Mycin
AM-Ampicillin
TE-Terramycin
P-Penicillin
C-Chloramphenicol
PB-Polymyxin B
N-Neomycin
Fd-Nitrofurantoin
T-Tetracycline
K-Kanamycin
LR-Cephaloridine
GM-Garamycin
SSS-Triple Sulfa
CB-Carbenicillin
NA-Nalidixic Acid

B, An agar plate inoculated with *Escherichia coli* shows a series of paper disks containing different antimicrobial agents. The size of the zone of growth inhibition is measured and the susceptibility of the microorganism is determined by reference to an interpretive chart. (From Youmans, G. P., Paterson, P. Y., and Sommers, H. M.: *The Biologic and Clinical Basis of Infectious Disease*. 2nd edition. Philadelphia, W. B. Saunders Company, 1980; reprinted with permission.)

utilize numerical values obtained from positive and negative tests to logically and systematically assist in identification of the bacterium.

ANTIBIOTIC SUSCEPTIBILITY TESTS. Physicians often initially prescribe antibiotics for patients with infectious diseases on the basis of the antibiotic most likely to control the probable pathogens. This practice is important because early and effective therapy prohibits further growth and multiplication of the pathogen and leads to an earlier resolution of the disease. Penicillin, for example, is frequently prescribed for sore throats because 50 per cent of all sore throats are caused by *Streptococcus pyogenes*, which is routinely susceptible to that antibiotic or its derivatives. Urinary tract infections are frequently caused by *Escherichia coli*, and antibiotic treatment is directed at this potential pathogen. However, despite the usefulness of this method of prescribing antibiotics, the patient may not respond well to the antibiotic administered. A **strain** (isolate) of the usual or common pathogen *may be resistant* to an antibiotic that kills or inhibits most other isolates of the same species. Or, the pathogen may be a completely different species, representative of a less common bacterium. In urinary tract infections a species of *Klebsiella, Enterobacter, Proteus* or *Pseudomonas* may be the **etiologic** agent. Each of these species may have different antibiotic susceptibility patterns. *The Kirby-Bauer antibiotic susceptibility test* is one of the most

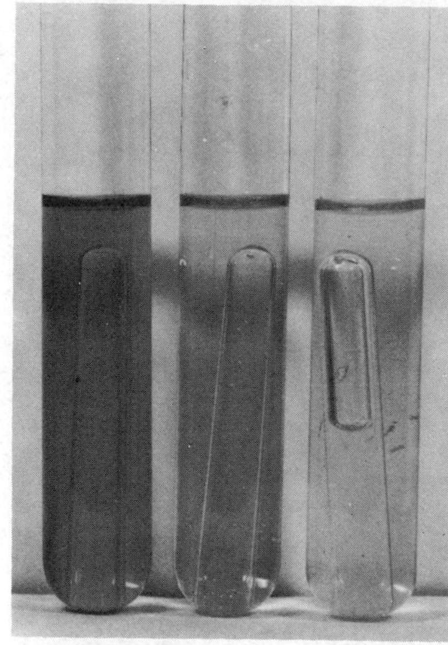

FIGURE 22–20 Carbohydrate fermentation reactions in glucose broth. The bacteria did not ferment the sugar in the left tube. The liquid is still red and no displacement of the medium in the tube (inverted to catch gas produced) has occurred. Acid produced in the tube in the center changed the indicator color of the broth from red to yellow. The tube on the right shows acid (the broth also turned yellow) and gas production. (From Fuerst, R.: *Frobisher and Fuerst's Microbiology in Health and Disease.* 14th edition. Philadelphia, W. B. Saunders Company, 1978; reprinted with permission.)

useful and widely used antibiotic susceptibility tests. In this test a suspension of the etiologic agent is obtained by using well isolated colonies of the organisms added to enriched broth medium. The organisms are permitted to grow for a few hours and diluted with sterile broth to give a density comparable to a standard McFarland tube, which contains barium chloride of a known density that mimics bacterial turbidity. The suspension of cells is then uniformly swabbed in three overlapping directions over the entire surface of the plate. High potency antibiotic disks are added to the plate and overnight incubation follows. The next day zone sizes are measured in millimeters, and a standardized chart is read to determine whether that size correlates with susceptibility or resistance. For details on this method, consult the selected references at the end of the chapter or obtain directions from a local hospital microbiology laboratory.

Viruses

Viruses, the smallest microbes known, *will grow only inside living cells.* Therefore, in clinical and research laboratories they are isolated and grown in tissue culture or cell systems. Because viruses will grow only inside other living organisms, they are

TABLE 22–6 Characteristics of Selected Common Gram-Positive Cocci Useful for Presumptive Identification

Gram-positive cocci, small colonies

1. *Beta-hemolytic* (clear hemolysis around the colony), A or bacitracin disk sensitive. *Streptococcus pyogenes.*
2. *Alpha-hemolytic* on blood agar (green hemolysis around the colony) O or optochin disk sensitive. *Streptococcus pneumoniae.* Alpha-hemolytic colonies that are not O disk sensitive are usually *Streptococcus* of the viridans group. The latter are typically nonpathogens of the normal mouth flora.

Gram-positive cocci, medium to large colonies after 24 to 48 hours incubation

Ferment in butt of TSI (Triple Sugar Iron Agar) tubes.

1. *Uniform-sized cocci,* may or may not be beta-hemolytic or yellow in color. Coagulase positive. *Staphylococcus aureus.*
2. *Uniform-sized* cocci, usually nonhemolytic, cream white colonies. Coagulase negative. *Staphylococcus epidermidis.*

Growth on slant of TSI, no acid in butt of TSI.

1. Cocci in packets of four or irregular-sized cocci or uniformly sized cocci. *Micrococcus* spp. (common skin contaminants).

Gram-negative cocci, usually in pairs, oxidase positive

Ferments glucose only. *Neisseria gonorrhoeae.*

Ferments glucose and maltose. *Neisseria meningitidis.*

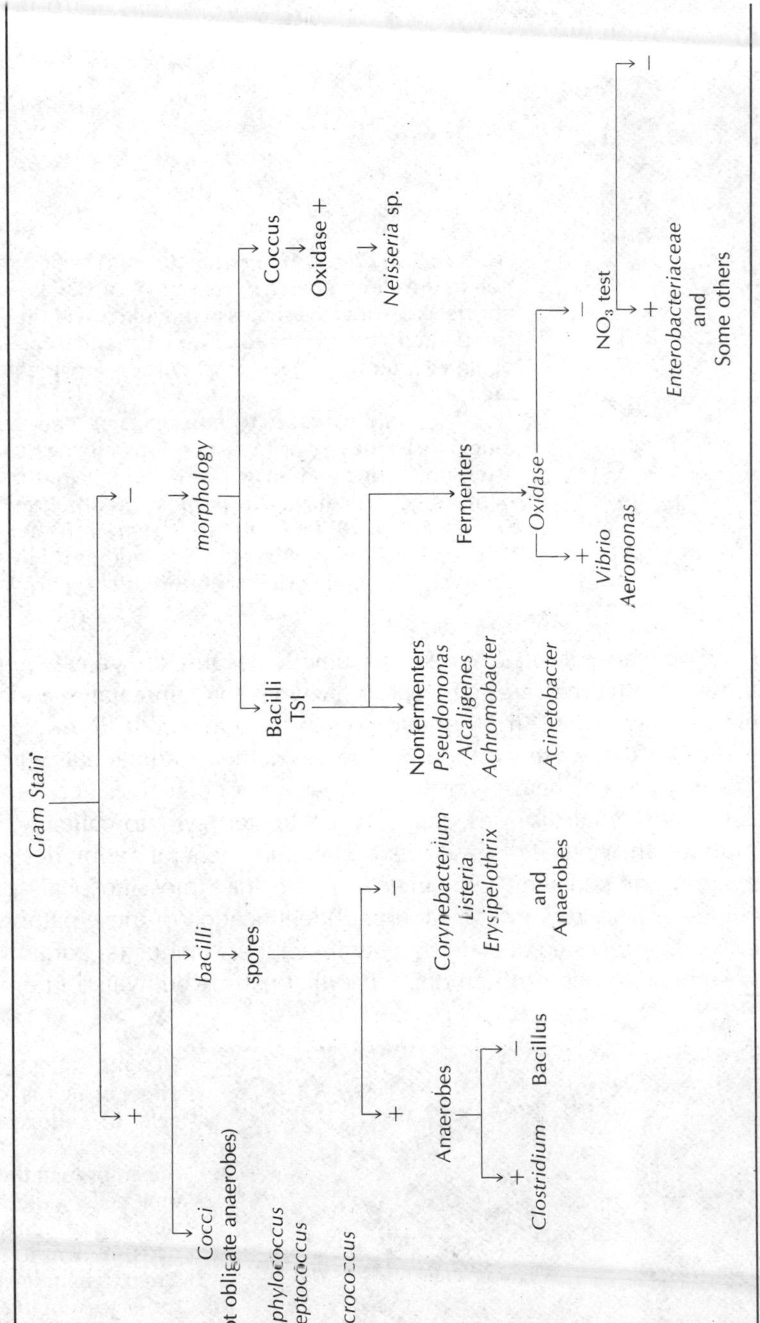

KEY: + = positive reaction
− = negative reaction

FIGURE 22–21 Simplified dichotomous scheme of microbial identification.

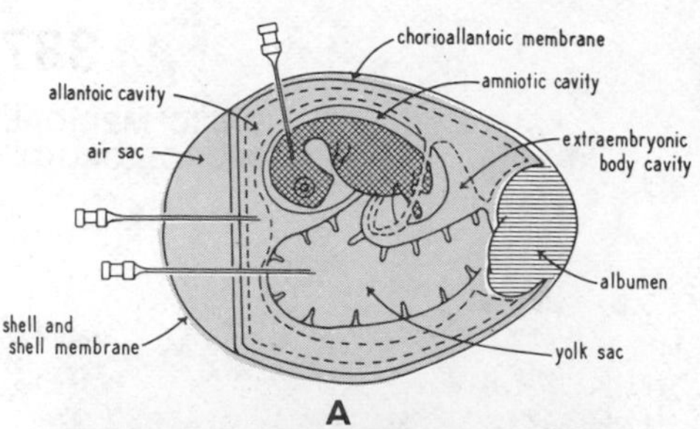

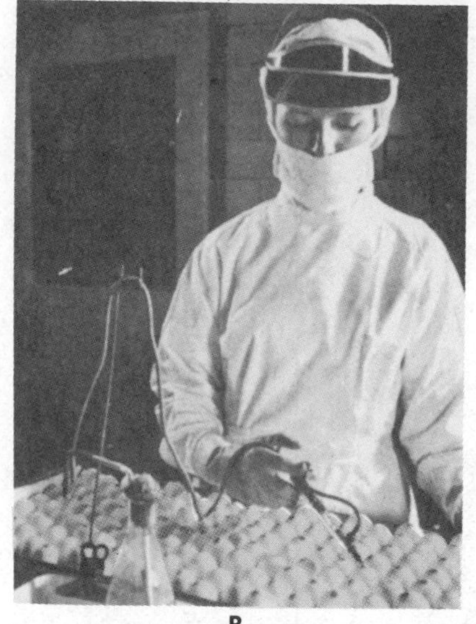

FIGURE 22–22 *A,* Diagrammatic representation in sagittal section of the embryonated hen's egg 10 to 12 days old. The hypodermic needles show the routes of inoculation of the yolk sac, allantoic cavity, and embryo (head). The chorioallantoic membrane is inoculated after it has been dropped by removing the air from the air sac.

B, Carefully dressed technician using a pressure-fed syringe to inoculate fertile eggs with suspension of living rickettsiae. The eggs, after suitable incubation, will be used in the preparation of vaccines or of antigens for diagnostic purposes. (Photograph courtesy of E. R. Squibb & Sons, Princeton, N.J.; from Frobisher, M., et al.: *Fundamentals of Microbiology.* 9th edition. Philadelphia, W. B. Saunders Company, 1974; reprinted with permission.)

termed *obligate parasites*. Viruses are unique because they have either RNA *or* DNA but never both. They are deficient in **enzymes** (protein catalysts) that would enable them to grow alone. All other microorganisms have both RNA and DNA.

Viruses cause many important diseases of man, and patients with viral infections frequently present themselves to the physician for diagnosis and treatment. Unfortunately, most viral diseases can only be treated symptomatically, that is, for the symptoms and not the disease agent. Therefore, general antibiotics are ineffective in preventing or curtailing viral infections. Because most hospitals do not have the facilities or resources for isolation and identification of these pathogens, specimens are usually processed at state or federal facilities. Influenza, parainfluenza, mumps, and smallpox viruses are among those that can be cultivated in embryonated fowl

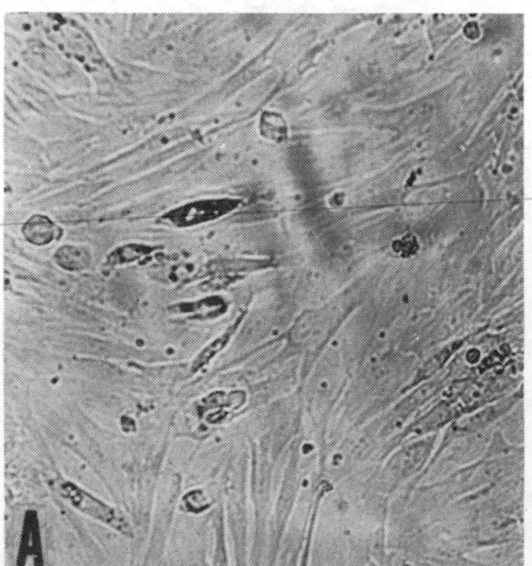

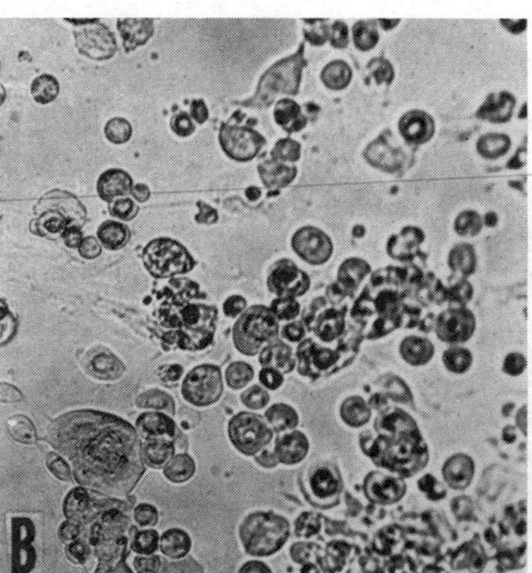

FIGURE 22–23 The cytopathic effect of a virus on human chorion cells in culture. (The chorion is one of the membranes protecting the embryo in the uterus.) *A,* Normal cells: culture five days old showing a fairly regular, organized network of uniformly elongated, spindle-shaped cells of rather distinctive appearance. *B,* The same sort of cells 72 hours after being inoculated with the virus of herpes simplex ("fever blister"). The cells have lost their distinctive form and arrangement and have become mere shapeless, disconnected, disorganized blobs of dead protoplasm. (1,500 ×.) (From Frobisher, M., et al.: *Fundamentals of Microbiology.* 9th edition. Philadelphia, W. B. Saunders Company, 1974; reprinted with permission.)

eggs (Fig. 22–22). Blood, cerebrospinal fluid, aspirates, and throat and nasal washings (mixed with appropriate antibiotics to inhibit or kill bacteria) may be added to tissue or cell cultures, enabling observations for **cytopathogenic effect** (CPE) or growth interference to be done (Fig. 22–23). Viruses that grow in these cell systems may be tested to detect typical **antigens** using one or more of the following tests: neutralization, complement fixation, gel filtration, gel diffusion, counter immuno-electrophoresis, radioimmunoassay, and passive hemagglutination, among others. The last three tests are of particular value for detection of the viruses of infectious hepatitis (hepatitis A) and serum hepatitis (hepatitis B). A list of viruses encountered in medical practice follows. The DNA viruses will be discussed first.

DNA Viruses

POXVIRUSES. Poxviruses are the largest viruses known. Smallpox virus is the most important virus in this group. In 1977, smallpox was declared an eradicated disease, meaning that smallpox immunizations are no longer necessary because no human case of smallpox has been detected in the world since the announcement date for eradication. The vaccination strain for smallpox will be maintained in laboratories; should smallpox ever appear again, it would be necessary to vaccinate (immunize) potentially susceptible persons to protect them. Smallpox virus invades the host through the upper respiratory tract, where it first lodges on the mucocutaneous membrane and then invades the lymph nodes, lymphatics, and bloodstream. The virus ultimately causes obvious skin damage (pox lesions). Smallpox lesions may cover the entire body, including the soles of the feet and the palms. The lesions are initially red (macules), then watery and raised (vesicles), and finally pustular and crusty. Extensive scarring remains after the scabs fall off. Smallpox was once a dreaded disease, killing 5 to 50 per cent or more of the people it parasitized. It remains to be seen if smallpox may one day reappear. Two possible sources of the smallpox virus that have not been eliminated are wild monkeys that sometimes harbor the virus and some research laboratories. No other poxviruses are significant disease agents.

HERPESVIRUSES. There are four main kinds of herpesviruses: Herpes 1 and 2, Varicella-Zoster, Epstein-Barr, and cytomegaloviruses. Herpes 1 virus is responsible for fever blisters and cold sores, acute gingivostomatitis, and occasionally cases of eczema, conjunctivitis, and meningitis. By far the most common ailment is recurrent fever blisters or cold sores, which occur about the mouth, lips, and nose and may spread to the face. The virus seems to be activated by sunlight, temperature changes, and in females, by the menstrual period. The lesions are clustered, somewhat painful, and may disappear for weeks or months, only to recur. There is no known cure. Herpes 2 virus is different from Herpes 1 because it attacks tissue in the urogenital tract. The virus is frequently transmitted during sexual intercourse and may, therefore, be classified as a **venereal** disease agent. Evidence obtained in recent years shows that the virus is frequently *associated* with cervical cancer in women, but the virus is not yet the proven agent of that disease.

Varicella-Zoster virus causes chickenpox and shingles. The virus that causes chickenpox is *not* a member of the poxviruses. Chickenpox is a relatively mild disease that infects in a fashion similar to smallpox, predominantly in children but may afflict adults as in shingles, a painful attack on the sensory nerves. Chickenpox virus causes fever and skin lesions that are distributed in a centripetal rather than a centrifugal fashion, that is, lesions are more common on the trunk of the body than on the extremities. Chickenpox lesions do not form on the palms or the soles of the feet. Adults who are immunocompromised (that is, have weakened body defenses) may be particularly susceptible to the virus that causes chickenpox.

The Epstein-Barr virus causes infectious mononucleosis, sometimes called "kissing" or "lover's" disease, which is a debilitating condition that frequently occurs in young adults. Infectious mononucleosis does not result in skin lesions like chickenpox or herpes. Instead, the signs and symptoms are swollen lymphatic glands, fever, and extreme lassitude (fatigue). Effects of the disease may last for several months to a year or more.

Cytomegaloviruses cause upper respiratory tract and systemic infections. At risk are immunocompromised hosts — frequently those with malignancy or immunologic deficiencies or who are immunosuppressed. This virus may cause infections of the fetus in utero and lead to microencephaly and mental retardation.

ADENOVIRUSES. Adenoviruses cause disease that resembles influenza. Some of the possible signs of the disease include fever, cough, pharyngitis, laryngitis, tracheobronchitis, and otitis. These viruses also cause acute conjunctivitis (eye infections involving the conjunctiva). People become infected when they contact water or fluids contaminated with these viruses. Typical hazards include swimming pools, ophthalmic solutions, and secretions from diseased people. The virus commonly causes epidemic flu-like disease in military populations.

PAPOVAVIRUSES. The papillomavirus, a member of the papova viruses, is responsible for human warts. Warts may spread from one body site to another. Frequently, the soles of the feet and hand are infected. Warts are usually treated by surgical removal or direct destruction with harsh chemical treatment.

RNA Viruses

These are very important viruses that cause a variety of diseases involving cells of one or more of the following organ systems: respiratory, gastrointestinal, nervous, or circulatory. Some of the most significant viral diseases are caused by RNA viruses: rabies, influenza, parainfluenza, polio, rubella (German measles), rubeola (measles), respiratory syncytial disease, the common cold, enteroviral disease, mumps, and encephalitis.

INFLUENZA VIRUSES. These viruses cause severe respiratory tract infections in epidemic proportions throughout the world. The disease is characterized by fever (101 to 103° F for two to three days), body ache (muscle, joints, or generalized), and cough. The disease lasts for approximately one week, after which a permanent immunity to that particular influenza is acquired. Very young and very old individuals are at the greatest risk. Epidemics of bacterial pneumonia frequently occur in conjunction with influenza. The influenza viruses destroy epithelial tissue and predispose the host to infections with bacteria such as *Streptococcus pneumoniae, Klebsiella pneumoniae,* and *Staphylococcus aureus.*

PARAMYXOVIRUSES. The mumps, measles (rubeola), parainfluenza, and respiratory syncytial viruses are in this group. Vaccines prepared from live but weakened viruses are available for mumps and measles. All these viruses infect and cause disease in the upper respiratory tract. Most often the diseases are mild but, occasionally, they are serious and life-threatening. Mumps produces fever and enlargement of one or both parotid salivary glands. When mumps occurs in adult males, there may be testicular involvement with subsequent sterility. The virus may invade the central nervous system (causing viral meningitis) or other organ sites such as the pancreas or ovaries. Fever, coughing, and runny nose are classic signs of measles, and in about 95 per cent of patients **Koplik's spots** (vesicular lesions on the buccal area of the mouth) are seen. A rare and late manifestation of measles is subacute sclerosing panencephalitis, a disease that causes extensive damage of brain tissue.

The parainfluenza viruses cause coryza, croup, pharyngitis, bronchitis, and pneumonia. Infants and children are most susceptible. In hospitalized children, about 20 per cent of acute, nonbacterial respiratory distress is caused by this virus; another 25 per cent is due to the respiratory syncytial virus responsible for the significant epidemic among infants in Italy in 1978–1979. The respiratory syncytial virus causes bronchiolitis and pneumonia. Older children and adults seldom present with serious signs and symptoms when infected with the virus; however, infants are very susceptible. All of the paramyxoviruses are readily identified by standard virologic procedures.

RUBELLA VIRUS. The rubella virus causes German measles, a relatively benign disease in children and young adults. German measles is frequently called "3-day measles" to distinguish it from the rubeola type. When German measles affects women in the first three months of pregnancy, the rubella virus is able to attack and destroy portions of the developing fetus. This situation can lead to mortality of up to 20 per cent of the infected babies. When the disease is acquired by the mother in the first month of her pregnancy, there is up to an 80 per cent chance that her infant will have one or more birth defects. Should infection occur in the third month, only 15 per cent of infants will be affected. Therefore, the virus is most damaging in the early development of the embryo. Viral effects on the neonate include deafness, **encephalitis**, anomalies of the heart and blood vessels, and eye defects (cataracts, glaucoma, and chorioretinitis). In congenital rubella the viruses may persist for months or weeks in the infected infant and be released in large numbers from urine, feces, saliva, and the nasopharynx. This is a serious and important source of viral dissemination to new, susceptible (nonresistant) individuals.

In children and adults the viral disease is manifested as an acute, febrile illness. The rash starts on the face and spreads over the trunk and extremities. Rubella is usually self-limiting and benign, with a mild upper respiratory tract infection. Arthralgia, arthritis, and encephalitis may occur rarely in infected persons.

PICORNAVIRUSES. Picornaviruses include the *enteroviruses* (the polio, Coxsackie, and ECHO viruses) and the *rhinoviruses*. The rhinoviruses, which number over 100, cause the common cold with its typical stuffy and runny nose. Enteroviruses cause summer and fall epidemics.

There are three types of polio viruses: 1, 2, and 3. These viruses infect the lymphatics of cervical lymph nodes and also the Peyer's patches of small intestine. Viremia (viruses in the blood) occurs; the nervous system may be invaded. Flaccid paralysis occurs in some individuals but not in others. Cerebrospinal fluid analysis shows an early granulocyte (white cell) response followed by an increase in lymphocytes. The original vaccine was the killed Salk strain. The oral polio vaccine of Sabin is now used routinely.

There are 24 types of Coxsackie A and six types of Coxsackie B viruses. These cause fever, sore throat, and vesicular lesions in the throat and pharynx, herpangia, a syndrome similar to the common cold, and occasionally aseptic meningitis. The virus may also cause vomiting. Analyses of throat and stool specimens are best for diagnosis. This virus inoculated into suckling mice causes paralysis and death.

ECHO (enteric cytopathic human orphan) viruses cause febrile and common cold-like illnesses, and occasionally *aseptic meningitis*.

Hepatitis Viruses

These cause damage to the liver, with jaundice an important manifestation. Hepatitis viruses may be either RNA or DNA viruses.

Hepatitis-A virus, the RNA virus, causes the infectious form of the disease and is usually acquired by ingestion of contaminated food or water. Hepatitis-B, a DNA virus, causes serum hepatitis and is usually obtained parenterally by injection of contaminated blood or serum into the body. There is also a new hepatitis virus that is neither A nor B.

All hepatitis viruses have a characteristically long incubation period of several weeks prior to the manifestation of overt disease. There are excellent serologic tests for determining the type of hepatitis virus infecting the patient.

Rickettsiae

Rickettsiae are microorganisms that are usually transmitted by wood or dog ticks, mites, or lice and cause spotted fever diseases. Only Q-fever (*Coxiella burnetii*) does not have an insect vector (carrier and transmitter). Physicians are most apt to encounter Rocky Mountain spotted fever which, besides being prevalent in the region of its namesake, is also fairly common to the South and along the Eastern seaboard. Rickettsioses are treated effectively with tetracyclines.

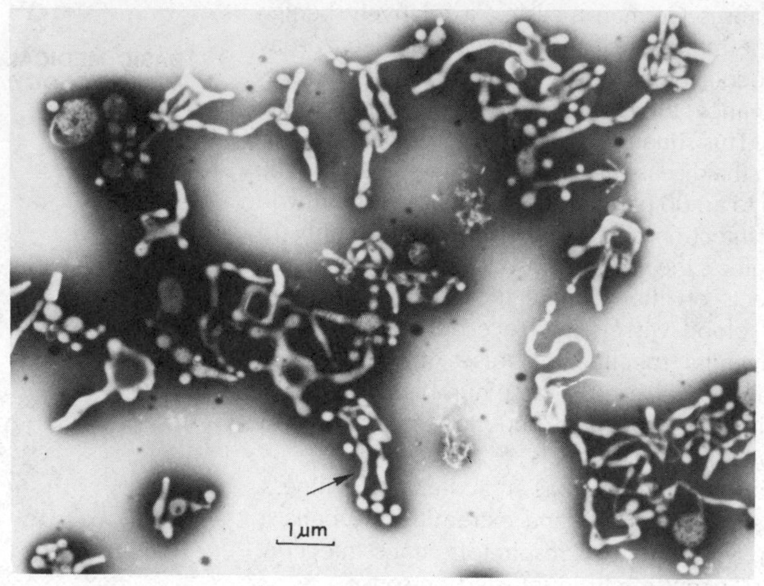

FIGURE 22–24 *M. pneumoniae,* negatively stained. The electron micrograph shows numerous forms of variable morphology, some of which are clearly ring-shaped with lobes and some which have beaded filaments (arrow). (Courtesy of E. S. Boatman; from Frobisher, M., et al.: *Fundamentals of Microbiology*. 9th edition. Philadelphia, W. B. Saunders Company, 1974; reprinted with permission.)

Chlamydiae and Mycoplasmas

These microorganisms are less exacting in their nutritional requirements than rickettsiae and viruses. Some hospital labs have the media and facilities to isolate and identify chlamydiae and mycoplasmas. Mycoplasmas but not chlamydiae may be grown on artificial, nonliving media, usually with added serum. The mycoplasmas cause nongonococcal urethritis (T-strain mycoplasma or *Ureoplasma ureae*) and atypical pneumonia (*Mycoplasma pneumoniae*). *Ureoplasma ureae* form tiny colonies and decompose urea (positive test). *Mycoplasma pneumoniae* usually causes a rise in cold agglutinins, a type of antibody found in serum (Fig. 22–24).

The diseases caused by chlamydiae include lymphogranuloma venereum (a venereal-like disease causing granuloma and swelling in the lymphatics of the groin), conjunctivitis, trachoma, and psittacosis (parrot-fever). Both chlamydiae and mycoplasmas are not common pathogens and are, therefore, sometimes omitted in the differential diagnosis by some physicians.

HOST DEFENSES AND IMMUNOLOGY

Despite the fact that microbes exist in many diverse environments — air, soil, water, food, skin, and throughout the gastrointestinal tract from the mouth to the anus in large numbers — the human body seldom becomes diseased. How can we account for the fact that we are not destroyed by these ubiquitous organisms? It is known that shortly after death organisms on the mucocutaneous membranes of the body begin to invade the deeper tissues of the body. Therefore, it is the *living* body that affords protection. These protective factors may be grouped into two main categories: specific and nonspecific defenses.

BRIEF HISTORY. In the 1890s and early 1900s scientists such as Von Behring and Kitasato argued that the blood fluids (sera) possessed powerful antibacterial factors that destroyed or controlled microbes. Metchnikoff, on the other hand, observed the engulfment of microbes by white blood cells and he believed the cells in the blood were the most important factors. As scientists studied the blood fluid and the blood cells over the years, they began to realize that both the fluids *and* the cells were important.

Host Defenses

NONSPECIFIC DEFENSES. The nonspecific defenses are all those protective elements of the body that are not mediated by lymphocytes or antibody. Skin, hair, tears, lysozyme, saliva, stomach acid, peristalsis, the normal microbial flora, sneeze and cough reflexes, cilia, mucus, complement, and granulocytes and the inflammatory response are among the most important of the nonspecific defenses.

The skin protects the internal body tissues and organs by forming a physical barrier to microbes that is basically impenetrable. Most microbes cannot readily penetrate intact, living skin. Cuts, abrasions, and puncture wounds expose deeper tissues sites to infection. Evaporated perspiration of the skin leaves a salt residue that is tolerated by only a few gram-positive bacteria such as *Staphylococcus* and *Corynebacterium*. Species of *Corynebacterium* utilize the oils in the skin and produce fatty acids that are inhibitory to many other bacteria that happen to land on the skin. The skin thus is biochemically inhospitable to the growth of most microorganisms and generally is difficult to penetrate.

Hair is nonliving and composed of protein. It prohibits microbes from landing directly on the skin, attracts and traps dirt, dust, pollen, spores, and microbes, and prohibits microbes from contacting the skin. When the hair is washed, much of this debris is removed.

Tears are protective in that their washing effect removes debris from the eye. Lysozyme in tears lyses (breaks down) some bacteria.

Lysozyme is an enzyme produced by the body and found in tears and tissue fluids. This enzyme weakens the cell wall of the gram-positive bacteria and causes them to explode and die.

Saliva, produced by the salivary glands, washes nonattached microbes and epithelial tissue from the mouth into the stomach acid. Saliva, therefore, has a cleansing effect.

Stomach acid is extremely harmful to many microbes. Most microbes are inactivated or killed in the stomach by hydrochloric acid, which often lowers the pH in this portion of the gastrointestinal tract to 2.0 to 3.0.

Peristalsis is the involuntary undulating motion of the gastrointestinal tract that moves and propels masses of dead and living microbes along it. Peristalsis prohibits the localized accumulation of metabolic wastes and toxins that might be harmful to the mucocutaneous tissues.

The role of *normal microbial flora* as a protective element of the skin has already been discussed. In the human intestine there are over 100 different species of commensal bacteria. These bacteria are numerous; as many as 10- to 100-billion viable bacteria per gram of feces are found when quantitative studies are done. These different commensal bacteria compete with one another for food, and their byproduct wastes either encourage or inhibit the growth of other microbes. The fact that so many different species grow and multiply in our intestines is amazing and informative. An important consideration is that these bacteria often inhibit or kill certain intestinal bacteria such as *Salmonella* that are pathogenic to humans. It is also important to note that it is difficult to render the bowel microbe-free with antibiotics, as some surgeons have attempted to do prior to gastrointestinal tract surgery. Furthermore, the prolonged use of antibiotics kills off only the sensitive microorganisms, leaving many antibiotic-resistant types that may sometimes infect other tissues of the patient or be released into the environment.

Sneeze and cough reflexes expel irritants such as dust, pollen, mucus, and microbes before they reach deeper lung sites, where they would pose serious disease hazards. Patients with repressed cough responses may acquire lobar or general pneumonia.

Cilia line the nose and upper respiratory tract. These beating hairs whip trapped dust, debris, microbes, and mucus upward and outward through the nose and mouth.

Mucus is a complex polysaccharide produced by glands in mucocutaneous sites of the body. The material traps particulates and facilitates their removal during breathing, sneezing, coughing, and swallowing.

Complement is a complex of 11 protein factors that acts in conjunction with antibodies to destroy microorganisms and foreign antigens. Complement is a serum factor that assists some antibodies in their protective role.

Granulocytes and the inflammatory response are evident in many infections (Fig. 22–25). The inflammatory response is characterized by redness, swelling, pain,

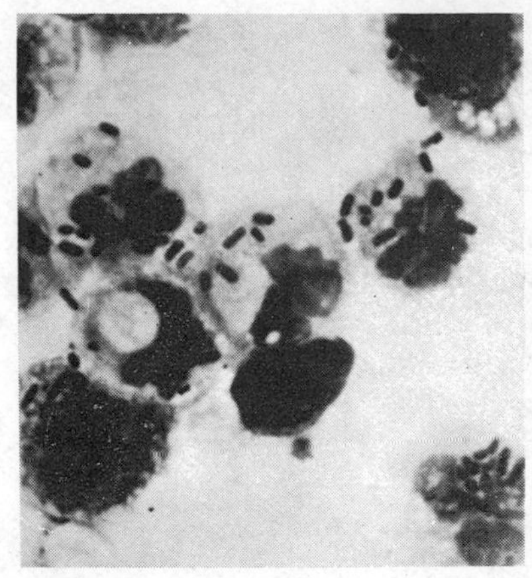

FIGURE 22–25 Stained smear of pus from lung of mouse inoculated with a species of pathogenic bacilli. The bacilli are seen to have been engulfed by the leukocytes (phagocytized) in large numbers. This is an excellent illustration of one of the most important defensive measures. (From Frobisher, M., et al.: *Fundamentals of Microbiology*. 9th edition. Philadelphia, W. B. Saunders Company, 1974; reprinted with permission.)

and heat. An abscess caused by *Staphylococcus aureus* is an example of a classic inflammatory response. A foreign antigen usually incites the inflammatory response. The capillaries contract initially, then dilate; blood flow is increased and the number of cells passing the site is increased. Granulocytes stick to the wall of the capillaries and pass through to get at the antigen. The antigens are frequently ingested and destroyed inside **vacuoles** of the granulocytes.

SPECIFIC IMMUNE DEFENSES. For the purpose of our discussion, specific host defenses may be defined as those protective features that reside in the immunoglobulins and in the lymphocytes (white blood cells). To understand this more clearly, refer to Table 22–7 on the composition and features of human blood. Regardless of the origin or source of the lymphocyte, it should be remembered that the function of lymphocytes is to destroy or neutralize foreign antigens. An antigen is any substance that can induce the formation of antibody. Most commonly, antigens are proteins, glycoproteins, lipoproteins, polysaccharides, and lipopolysaccharides. Each living thing forms its own special kind of antigens. Each human body can usually recognize its own antigens (self-antigens), and it does not attack and seek to destroy self. However, when foreign antigens are introduced, certain body cells can determine that these antigens are foreign (nonself) and they attempt to neutralize and destroy them in an immunologic attack. Table 22–8 shows some important types of immunity.

These specific immune defenses of the body include (1) production of **immunoglobulin** by B **(bursal)** lymphocytes and (2) the protective activities of T **(thymus)** lymphocytes and associated **macrophages.** Figure 22–27 illustrates the origin of the two main types of lymphocytes, B- and T-cells, both of which are found in the **reticuloendothelial system.** They arise from a type of bone cell termed **stem cells.** Stem cells that move to the thymus and develop there and finally move to the lymph node and other reticuloendothelial sites are known as T-cells. The stem cells that move to the intestine and develop in the bursal equivalent are termed B-cells. When

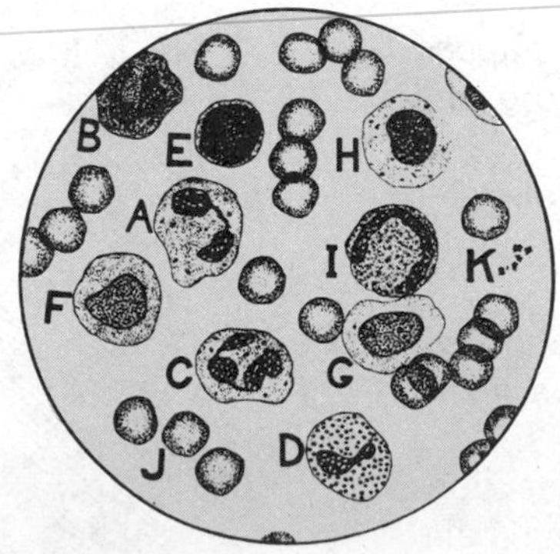

FIGURE 22–26 Drawing of a smear of blood stained with Jenner's stain, showing common forms of blood cells. *A, B, C,* Polymorphonuclear leukocytes with two-, three-, and four-lobed nuclei, respectively. *D,* Eosinophil showing lobular nucleus and prominent, eosinophilic (red-staining) granules. *E,* Lymphocyte. *F, G,* and *H,* Various forms of monocytes. *I,* Lymphocyte with horseshoe-shaped nucleus ("transitional cell"). *J,* Erythrocytes (red blood cells); note biconcave-disk shape, thin at center. *K,* Platelets. (About 1,000 ×.) (From Frobisher, M., et al.: *Fundamentals of Microbiology*. 9th edition. Philadelphia, W. B. Saunders Company, 1974; reprinted with permission.)

TABLE 22–7 Type and Amount of Cellular Components of Normal, Adult Human Blood

Cell Type	Average Amount (No /mm³)	Leukocytes (%)	Nature and Function
Erythrocytes (red cells)	5×10^6	*	Contain hemoglobin; Carry O_2 to cells and CO_2 away from cells to lungs for exchange with O_2.
Leukocytes (white cells)	7000	100	Multiple functions listed below include surveillance, recognition and destruction of nonself antigen, protection, homeostasis.
Granulocytes			
Neutrophils	4500	40–70	Ingest and destroy large particles.
Eosinophils	150	0–5	Involved in allergic cell responses.
Basophils	30	<1	Release histamine and other factors to mobilize body defenses.
Lymphocytes (large and small types)	2000	20–45	Can differentiate into antibody-producing cells (immunocytes).
B-cells (bursal)			Antibody production
T-cells (thymic)			Cell-mediated immunity
Monocytes (macrophages)	450	2–10	Ingest and destroy antigens.

*Does not apply.

stimulated by appropriate antigen, these B-cells can become plasma cells that manufacture antibodies (immunoglobulins) (Table 22–9). Why are two types of lymphocytes necessary? The answer is not absolutely clear. The control of bacterial infection seems to be mediated predominantly by the nonspecific neutrophil defense system and immunoglobulins. The control of viral, fungal, and protozoal infections seems to be orchestrated predominantly by the T-lymphocytes and macrophages, with immunoglobulins also playing some role in the defense system.

ANTIBODIES AND B-LYMPHOCYTES. A lymphocyte B-cell becomes a protein-synthesizing factory that manufactures large amounts of a protein called immunoglobulin. Immunoglobulins made by B-cells are termed antibodies. Antibodies are relatively large protein molecules that can unite with or tie up antigens. In one

TABLE 22–8 Types of Immunity

Natural	Obtained from the environment by unintentional ingestion, injection, or inhalation of antigens, or receipt of antibodies by infant from mother.
Active	Person becomes infected from environmental sources: food, water, air, arthropods. Antibodies are produced in response to infection.
Passive	Antibodies passed from mother to child via colostrum postpartum or in utero via placenta.
Artificial	Obtained by injection or immunization. Man-mediated introduction of antigens or antibodies.
Active	Antigen intentionally administered to stimulate the production of antibodies (for example, diphtheria, pertussis, tetanus—DPT immunization).
Passive	Antibody (gamma globulins) intentionally administered by injection to provide protection for actual, suspected or threatened infection (for example, tetanus or botulism antitoxins).

TABLE 22–9 Characteristics of Immunoglobulins

Class Immunoglobulin and Function	Molecular Weight	Mg/100 ml	Site of Synthesis	Crosses Placenta?	Fixes Complement?
IgG – precipitin reaction	160,000	800–1600	lymph nodes and spleen	yes	yes
IgM – involved in intravascular agglutination reactions	900,000	50–190	lymph nodes and spleen	no	yes
IgA – functions on tissue surfaces to inactivate and neutralize microbes contacted	160,000, 320,000, 400,000, (3 types)	140–400	mucous membranes of gut, lung, lymph nodes	no	no
IgD – role not defined	160,000	0.3–40	lymph nodes and spleen	no	no
IgE – involved in allergic responses of the host	200,000	0.2	mucous membranes	no	no

manner of speaking, antibodies serve to neutralize, tie up, or inactivate the foreign antigen. Each B-cell makes only one type of antibody, usually an antibody specific for one type of antigen. There are thousands of different nonself antigens that each human encounters in a lifetime, and thousands of different B-cells, each making one type of antibody for one specific antigen. After the specific antibody has reacted with the antigen and formed an antigen-antibody complex, the complex is ingested by phagocytic cells and destroyed. The analogy of a magnet and vacuum cleaner may be used. Each B-cell produces a special biochemical magnet (antibody) that reacts with only one type of antigen. After the antibody has complexed with the antigen, the phagocytes (vacuum cleaner) take in the complex and destroy it.

Agglutination Tests. Antibodies that have reacted with antigens can form large cellular complexes (agglutinations — commonly mediated by IgM) or macromolecular complexes (precipitations — mediated by IgG) (Fig. 22–28). These antigen-antibody reactions are useful in certain diagnostic tests when screening for antibody in a patient's serum. We can take the serum of the patient and react it with a known antigen (such as *Streptococcus* or *Salmonella* cells or extract). In positive agglutination tests, a visible flocculation (clumping) is seen on the test slides. In positive precipitation tests, a **precipitin band** of antigen-antibody is seen. The molecular complexes that form are the result of the immunoglobulin molecule tying one antigenic site to another. This resembles a bridge spanning a void and joining two

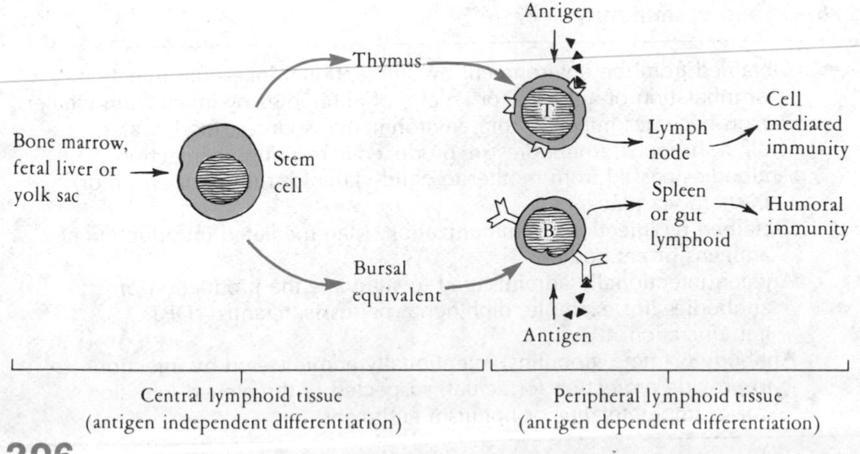

FIGURE 22–27 Development of the lymphoid system. (From Bellanti, J. A.: *Immunology II*. Philadelphia, W. B. Saunders Company, 1978; reprinted with permission.)

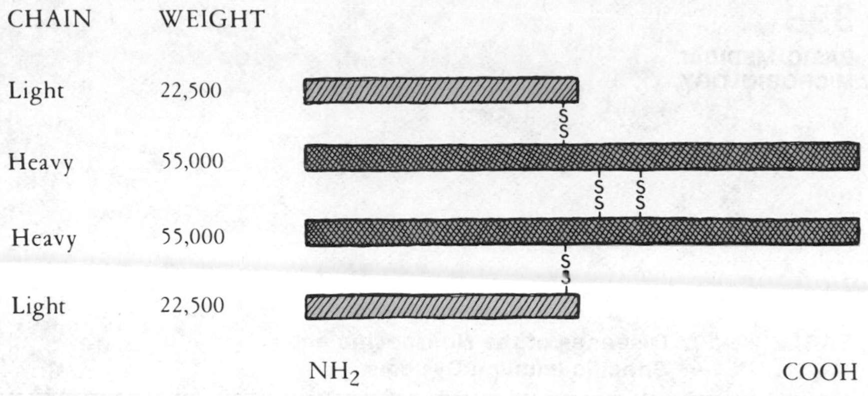

FIGURE 22–28 Schematic diagram of human IgG1 showing the location of interchain disulfide bonds. The molecule consists of two light chains and two heavy chains. The amino-terminal end is at the left and the carboxyl-terminal end is at the right. The structure depicted here is also applicable to other immunoglobulins with varying heavy-chain composition and polymerization. (From Bellanti, J. A.: *Immunology II*. Philadelphia, W. B. Saunders Company, 1978; reprinted with permission.)

portions of land (antigenic or determinant sites). Antibodies are like fingerprints in the serum of blood. The immunoglobulins signify that a nonself antigen has encountered the body immune system and caused it to respond. These agglutination reactions enable physicians and research scientists to determine recent and past infections.

T-LYMPHOCYTES, DELAYED HYPERSENSITIVITY, AND ALLERGY. Cellular, immune reactions are mediated by T-lymphocytes. For example, the tuberculin or tine test involves the introduction of test antigen derived from *Mycobacterium* into the skin. If a person has been infected with *Mycobacterium* some weeks, months, or years in the past, he usually has developed a good cellular immune response to the antigens of the *Mycobacterium*. When this antigen is introduced into the skin of these individuals, the T-cell–mediated immune response results in an accumulation of T-lymphocytes, macrophages, and serum at the injected site. The reddened and edematous (swollen) site is measured. A predetermined size (millimeters) of swelling determines a positive (that is, previously infected) result. Skin tests are valuable as screening tests in diseases such as tuberculosis, trichinosis, coccidioidomycosis, and histoplasmosis. This type of reaction is termed **delayed hypersensitivity** and usually occurs 36 to 72 hours after the antigen has been introduced. For this reason, skin test reactions based on T-lymphocyte (delayed hypersensitivity) are routinely read at 48 to 72 hours by the physician.

Immediate Hypersensitivity and Allergy. Delayed hypersensitivity reactions should be contrasted with **immediate hypersensitivity** reactions (**anaphylaxis**). Immediate hypersensitivity reactions occur with insect stings or bites or hypersensitivity to drugs such as penicillin. In these settings, the patient has been previously sensitized with a chemical compound (such as penicillin or venom from an insect) and antibodies have been produced. The antibodies are attached to certain cells in the body and when the sensitizing antigen is introduced into the blood stream, it contacts the antibodies, reacts with them, and stimulates the cells possessing the attached antibodies to release vasoactive substances (histamines). When severe, immediate hypersensitivity reactions are called anaphylactic shock reactions. These reactions are life-threatening. Not infrequently, individuals who have received penicillin in the past become sensitized to the antibiotic. When they receive the antibiotic next time there is a binding of penicillin to antibodies, and an immediate hypersensitivity reaction occurs with shock, rapid heart beat, and stasis (pooling and stagnation) of body fluids. Extremely sensitized (allergic) individuals have been known to die within a few minutes after receiving penicillin or a bee sting. Adrenalin and antihistamines are among the drugs administered to reverse allergic shock reactions. Accurate information must be obtained and kept on each patient's allergies and drug sensitivities.

TABLE 22–10 Diseases of the Nonspecific and Specific Immune Systems

Disease	Signs and Symptoms
Phagocytes/Complement	
Neutropenia acquired or inherited	Low numbers of neutrophils, frequent bacterial infections especially of skin and respiratory tract.
Chronic granulomatous	Granuloma lesions form in different body sites with multinucleated giant cells, plasma cells, lymphocytes, and histiocytes. Recurrent infections with catalase-positive bacteria.
Defective Complement	Ineffective phagocytosis and lytic activity. Frequent infections with gram-positive and gram-negative bacteria.
Gamma Globulins	
Agammaglobulinemia	Low levels of gamma globulins. Susceptibility to encapsulated pyogenic organisms: *Streptococcus pyogenes, S. pneumoniae, Haemophilus influenzae,* and *Staphylococcus aureus.*
Dysgammaglobulinemias	Deficiencies in amounts of gamma globulins, but not all classes. Recurrent infections such as pneumonia and sepsis, resembling agammaglobulinemia in character.
Wiscott-Aldrich Syndrome	Defect in destroying/inactivating polysaccharide antigens. Eczematoid and purpuric lesions, thrombocytopenia, and recurrent infections. Susceptibility to bacteria, fungi, protozoa, and viruses.
Cellular	Sporadic birth defect.
Di George Syndrome	Absence of thymus and parathyroid glands. Frequent fungal and viral infections due to absence of T-cells (T-cells are necessary for cellular mediated immunity).
Nezelof Syndrome	Faulty development of thymus gland. Severe, recurrent mycotic, viral and bacterial infections.
Combined: Cellular and Gamma globulins	Very severe and dangerous with very low survival rate. Several instances of successful bone marrow transplants. Graft vs. host reaction common form of rejection by bone marrow of host.
Autoimmune Disease	Antibody made against self tissue results in destruction of host tissue. Lupus erythematosus, rheumatoid arthritis, scleroderma, polyarteritis nodosa, and polymyositis are examples of different autoimmune diseases.

Diseases of the Immune and Other Systems

Diseases of the immune system are many and varied. Some of these diseases are congenital (occurring at birth) and are the result of genetic abnormalities. Table 22–10 presents an overview of different diseases of the nonspecific and specific immune systems. It is important to remember that immunoglobulin deficiencies (B-cell diseases) are often characterized by frequent, recurrent, severe infections with bacteria, and cellular immune deficiencies (T-cell disease) are characterized by frequent, recurrent, and severe infections with viruses, fungi, or protozoa and, occasionally, bacteria.

On occasion the body's defense system may go awry in another fashion, as when it makes antibody that reacts with self. Among these **autoimmune diseases** are systemic lupus erythematosus, rheumatoid arthritis, scleroderma, polyarteritis nodosa, and polymyositis.

References

Freeman, B. A.: *Burrows' Textbook of Microbiology*. 21st ed. Philadelphia, W. B. Saunders Co., 1979.

Youmans, G. P., Paterson, P. Y., and Sommers, H. M.: *Biologic and Clinical Basis of Infectious Diseases*. 2nd ed. Philadelphia, W. B. Saunders Co., 1980.

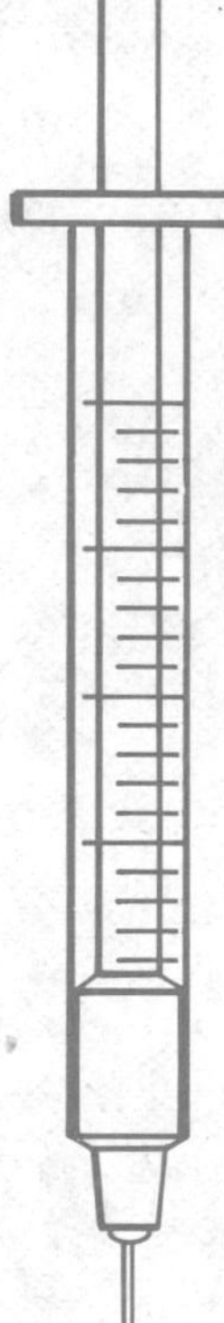

CHAPTER OUTLINE

Sources of Drugs
Drug Names
Uses of Drugs
Drug Standardization
Legal Regulations
    Narcotics
Forms of Drugs
Prescriptions
Terminology
Drug Actions
Solutions
Practical Problems in
    Preparing Medications
Poison Control Centers
Burn Centers

BEHAVIORAL OBJECTIVES

The medical office assistant should be able to:

- **Read a prescription.**
- **Make out a prescription under the physician's direction.**
- **Order Federal Narcotic Order Blanks and make them out properly for the physician to sign.**
- **Order State Narcotic Prescription Blanks.**
- **Make up a solution by either the per cent or the ratio method of calculation, according to the strength and the type of the solution.**
- **Prepare a part of a drop.**
- **Prepare a dose of a given strength from a tablet of another strength.**
- **Prepare a dose of a given strength from a solution of a specific strength.**
- **Assist the physician to quickly secure information relative to a poison and its antidote.**

23

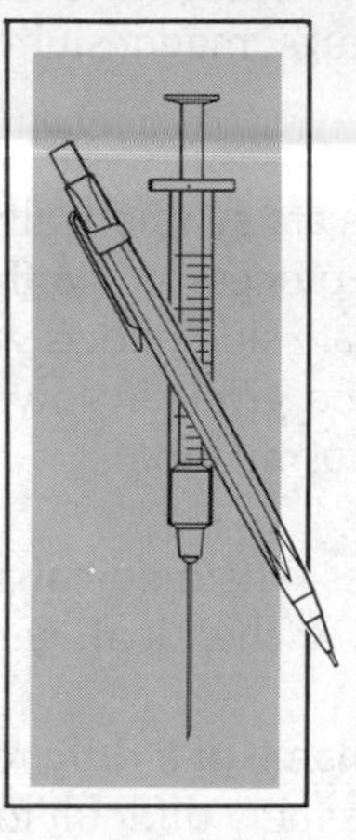

PHARMACOLOGY AND PREPARATION OF MEDICATIONS

MARY W. FALCONER, R.N., M.A.

Revised by Edward A. Gustafson, B.S., Pharm.D.

Drugs are weapons in the doctor's **armamentarium** for fighting sickness and disease. A drug is defined as a medicinal substance used in the treatment of a disease. The science and study of the effect of drugs is called "pharmacology." Records of pharmacology date back to ancient Egypt.

There are over one thousand drug manufacturers today, and it is estimated that it costs about four million dollars to develop a drug ready for market. Few people fully realize the cost and time involved in the research and manufacture of a drug. About eight out of ten drugs prescribed today were not even on the market ten years ago.

The purchase of a modern drug may save a patient's life; it may be the deciding factor in restoring his health; it will probably help him to return to work much sooner, or he may not need to miss work at all. The consumer must share in the cost of drug research. Although many drugs may at times seem very expensive, if they reduce hospitalization, shorten the illness, and return the individual to health and productivity, they may actually result in monetary savings. Their value in terms of human suffering and loss of health, or life itself, cannot be measured.

It is important that every doctor's assistant have a basic understanding of the common drugs used in the professional office. The assistant not only maintains the supply of drugs but often prepares drugs for use or administers them to patients on the physician's directions.

SOURCES OF DRUGS

Drugs are obtained from four principal sources: animal, vegetable, mineral (natural sources), and the chemist's laboratory (synthetic sources).

NATURAL SOURCES. Drugs are obtained from the leaf, seed, sap, stem, or root of certain plants. Digitalis is an extract from the leaf of the foxglove, opium comes from the poppy, and quinine is derived from the bark of the cinchona tree.

Animals have been the source of therapeutic hormones. Insulin is the hormone extracted from the islet cells of the pancreas; thyroid is obtained from the thyroid gland. Antibiotics are substances secreted or excreted by living organisms (bacteria, yeasts, and molds). Animal fats give us bases for ointments.

Minerals are another source of drugs: magnesium sulfate as Epsom salts or sulfur is derived from wells.

SYNTHETIC SOURCES. Most drugs are synthetically produced today by laboratory processes that duplicate a natural process or **synthesize** a new formula. Often a synthetic process can virtually eliminate side effects while increasing the potency of a drug. Synthetic drugs can usually be given in lower dosage than similar natural drugs since they contain no extraneous material.

DRUG NAMES

A drug may bear many different names. The medical assistant should understand the three types of names a drug may have: chemical, **generic**, and trade.

CHEMICAL NAME. The chemical name of a drug represents its exact formula and is frequently long, unwieldy, and extremely difficult to understand. For example, the chemical name of Chlor-Trimeton is

2-[p-Chloro-ax-(2-dimethylaminoethyl) benzyl] pyridine maleate.

This name is of no value to the medical assistant.

GENERIC NAME. The generic name is the common name of the chemical or drug. This name is not owned by any particular company; it is **nonproprietary.** A generic name refers to a single substance. "Chlorpheniramine maleate" is the generic name for Chlor-Trimeton.

TRADE NAME. The trade name is the name by which the manufacturer identifies the drug. It is a copyrighted name and cannot be used by another company. The same formula may have several different trade names from several different pharmaceutical companies. Chlor-Trimeton is a trade name of the Schering Corporation; the same product manufactured by Smith, Kline & French is called Teldrin.

There are certain types of preparations of drugs, usually taken by mouth, which have varying rates of releasing the medication within the body. These are also identified by registered trade names — for example, Repetabs by Schering Corporation, Spansules by Smith, Kline & French, Gradumets by Abbott, Extentabs by Robbins. There are many more names used, as there are many more pharmaceutical houses, and each has its own name for time-release action medications.

USES OF DRUGS

Many people think that drugs are used for therapeutic purposes only — that is, for the treatment of disease or for their curative value. However, drugs are also used for many other purposes. Some of the more important reasons include:

1. Relief of undesirable symptoms of the disease — morphine to relieve pain.
2. Immunizations to prevent disease — vaccine for typhoid fever, toxoid for diphtheria.
3. To aid in the diagnosis of the disease — dyes used as opaque media in radiographic examinations, antigens used for skin testing in allergy.
4. To hasten recovery from illness — usually vitamins, minerals, and supplementary food substances, such as amino acids.
5. To give the patient substances his body is not producing (at all or in insufficient amounts) — thyroid extract for hypothyroidism, insulin for diabetes mellitus.

DRUG STANDARDIZATION

Drugs are standardized in the United States, and two books are recognized as authoritative treatises. These are the *United States Pharmacopeia* (USP) and the *National Formulary* (NF). These two books are being combined into one book, and the United States will have only one official book for drug standards, the *United States Pharmacopeia* (USP). This book will be revised every five years.

The Council on Drugs of the American Medical Association (AMA) at intervals publishes books that give up-to-date information on drugs. Originally, these books were called *New and Non-Official Remedies,* but later were entitled *New Drugs.* They were published yearly. The present book is *Drug Evaluation.* It is not published yearly but as conditions dictate. There are innumerable publications available to the physician for quick reference. Among these are *Model's Drugs in Current Use, Falconer's Current Drug Handbook,* and *Physician's Desk Reference.* All these publications, and others of the same type, give "thumbnail" information about drugs that are in general use at the time. The first two books listed cover a large number of drugs without respect to their manufacturers. The last gives information on the main drugs manufactured by those pharmaceutical houses supporting the publication. The *Current Drug Handbook* is revised every other year; *Drugs in Current Use* at irregular intervals; and *Physician's Desk Reference,* yearly, with supplements during the year.

Additionally, each box of medications has in it a brochure giving all pertinent information about that particular drug. The assistant will do well to keep an index file of these brochures. It should be kept up to date and be where she and the doctor can reach it easily. This will be the very latest information possible.

LEGAL REGULATIONS

Drug standards are established and enforced by the United States Food and Drug Administration (FDA), a part of the Department of Health & Human Services, by authority of the Federal Food, Drug, and Cosmetic Act enacted in 1938. The purpose of the act, as far as drugs are concerned, is to ensure the identity, strength, purity, and quality of drugs shipped in interstate commerce. The first law regulating the sale of foods and drugs was enacted in 1906 and was aimed primarily at the prevention of adulteration of products (the substitution of one product for another — usually a cheaper for a better, more expensive one). This was a rather weak law with many loopholes. The jurisdiction of the FDA is limited to products that have been involved in interstate commerce. However, this includes practically all drugs with which the doctor's assistant is concerned.

The AMA has had a history of active support of laws that protect the public through pure food and drugs. It is constantly working toward effective controls of quack medicines and devices, cosmetic and food faddism, and quackery in vitamin preparations and dietary foods. The AMA has never hesitated to sponsor or endorse legislation in the health field when it has been indicated.

In 1951 Congress passed the Durham-Humphrey amendment to the Federal Food, Drug, and Cosmetic Act. The main purpose of this amendment was stricter control of the dispensing of dangerous drugs.

Narcotics

The Harrison Narcotic Act was passed in 1915 to regulate the manufacture, sale, dispensing, and prescribing of narcotics. This was a federal law under the supervision of the Bureau of Narcotics, United States Treasury Department, making it necessary for every person who prescribed narcotics to register with the Collector of Internal Revenue on or before July 1 of each year and pay a special tax. The renewals are now made during an assigned month based on the first letter of the last name of the doctor. This enables the agency to handle the paper work in an even flow throughout the year. The possession of narcotics by unauthorized persons is a federal offense and subject to a severe penalty.

In 1970 a new law was enacted covering medications, including narcotics. This was called the Controlled Substance Act of 1970. It became effective in May, 1971; with a few drugs the effective date was January 1, 1972. By this law the Bureau of

Narcotics became the Bureau of Narcotics and Dangerous Drugs (BNDD), under the Department of Justice. The Food and Drug Administration, under the Department of Health, Education and Welfare, retained jurisdiction of all foods and those medicinal substances that were not included under the BNDD. As of 1973 the name of this bureau was changed to the Drug Enforcement Administration (DEA) but was still under the Department of Justice. Narcotics and various other drugs are covered by this agency. The substances that are included in this category are mainly those that tend to be or have been "abused." The drugs are listed in five schedules. A complete list of all drugs included in each schedule can be obtained from the Regional Office of the DEA. The assistant should secure this list for the physician's office and ask that the doctor's name be placed on their mailing list so that as drugs are added, deleted, or moved from one schedule to another, the office list can be kept up to date. Briefly the drug schedules are:

SCHEDULE I. This schedule includes substances that have no accepted medicinal use. The manufacture, importation, and sale of these chemicals is prohibited. Some state laws vary as to the use and possession of marihuana.

EXAMPLES: Heroin, marihuana, lysergic acid diethylamide (LSD), mescaline, and peyote.

SCHEDULE II. This schedule includes drugs previously known as Class A Narcotics and some nonnarcotic medicines. The prescription for these drugs must be entirely handwritten by the physician, usually on special prescription blanks. The states vary from one to another in this matter. Some require only one copy, some duplicates, and some triplicate copies. Where special blanks are required they are obtained from the State Department of Health. The assistant should be sure that there are ample blanks on hand at all times. In any case the physician's narcotic license number must appear on the blank. The nonnarcotic drugs listed in Schedule II may be written on the physician's regular blank, but the doctor must write the prescription himself. Preprinted blanks given out by the pharmaceutical houses may not be used.

EXAMPLES: Narcotics: opium and opium **derivatives** (morphine, codeine, Percodan, Pantopon, Dilaudid, methadone [Dolophine]) and cocaine (not technically a narcotic, but treated here as are the narcotics).

Nonnarcotics: amphetamine (Benzedrine and other trade names), methamphetamine (Methedrine and other trade names), methylphenidate (Ritalin), and phenmetrazine (Preludin), the barbiturates, amobarbital (Amytal), pentobarbital (Nembutal), secobarbital (Seconal), and the nonbarbiturate sedative glutethimide (Doriden), and methaqualone (Quāalude).

SCHEDULE III. This schedule includes the narcotics previously classified as Class B narcotics and some nonnarcotic drugs. The physician must write the prescription for these as in Schedule II, but his regular prescription form may be used. Preprinted forms from pharmaceutical companies may not be used. Refills, up to five in any six-month period, may be allowed. This must be indicated on the prescription. Telephone requests must be handled by the physician himself.

EXAMPLES: Narcotics: various combinations of drugs containing codeine, dihydrocodeinone, hydrocodone, and camphorated tincture of opium (Paregoric), previously an "exempt narcotic".

Nonnarcotics: Amphetamine-like compounds not listed in Schedule II and aprobarbital, butabarbital (Butisol), and methyprylon (Noludar).

SCHEDULES IV AND V. These two schedules are handled in much the same manner. The prescription may be made out by the assistant, but must be signed by the physician. Refills are the same as for Schedule III, except that requests for refills over the phone may be handled by the assistant under the direction of the doctor.

EXAMPLES: Schedule IV: Barbiturates not previously listed, some hypnotics, such as chloral hydrate and similar drugs; some muscle relaxants, such as meprobamate (Equanil and other names); the benzodiazepine tranquilizers, such as chlordiazepoxide (Librium), diazepam (Valium), flurazepam (Dalmane), etc. The nonnarcotic analgesic propoxyphene (Darvon) is also in Schedule IV.

EXAMPLES: Schedule V: This schedule includes most cough medications containing codeine and some drugs used for gastrointestinal disorders, such as Donnagel and diphenoxylate (Lomotil).

Canadian assistants will find that Canada has had a similar law for some time. Information as to the schedules there can be obtained from the Provincial or the Dominion Office of the Department of Health and Welfare.

Specific narcotic laws are lengthy, and it is not important that the medical assistant be familiar with them in detail. It is, however, her responsibility to know the provisions of the laws for handling narcotics.

Regulations of the Drug Enforcement Administration governing the purchase and inventory of controlled substances by medical practitioners were outlined in Chapter 5, Medicine and the Law.

PRESCRIPTIONS FOR CONTROLLED SUBSTANCES. Although the federal government does not furnish triplicate prescription blanks, many states do require and provide them. These prescription blanks must be used for narcotic prescriptions only. Do not confuse them with the Federal Triplicate Order Forms, which are used to order Schedule II drugs for the office or the doctor's bag.

All prescriptions for controlled substances must be dated and signed on the day when issued and must bear the full name and address of the patient, and the name, address, and registration number of the physician. The prescription must be written in ink or indelible pencil or typewritten and must be signed by hand by the practitioner. The prescription may be prepared by a nurse or secretary for the signature of the physician, but the prescribing physician is responsible in case the prescription does not conform in all essential respects to the law and regulations.

A written prescription is required for drugs in Schedule II and must be signed by the physician. *The refilling of Schedule II prescriptions is prohibited.* In the case of a bona fide emergency (as defined by the DEA), a physician may telephone a prescription to a pharmacist for a drug in Schedule II. In such a case, the drug prescribed must be limited to the amount needed to treat the patient during the emergency period. The physician must furnish, within 72 hours, a written, signed prescription to the pharmacy for the drug prescribed. The pharmacist is required by law to notify the DEA if he has not received the prescription within 72 hours.

A prescription for drugs in Schedules III, IV, and V may be issued either orally or in writing and may be refilled *if so authorized* on the prescription up to five times within six months after the date of issue. After five refills or after six months, a new prescription is required in either oral or written form from the physician.

CONTROLLED SUBSTANCES RECORDS. As set forth in Chapter 5, the physician must keep an accurate record of certain narcotic and nonnarcotic drugs that he dispenses to his patients. A special book, kept in a definite place, should be maintained for this purpose. An example of one type of record is shown in Figure 23–1. The record should show

1. Full name and address of the patient to whom the drug was given
2. Date drug was given
3. Character and quantity of drug
4. Method of dispensing (prescription, dispensing, or injection)

NARCOTIC, STIMULANT AND DEPRESSANT RECORD

DATE	NAME	ADDRESS	DRUG AND QUANTITY	RX	DISP	INJ

FORM 3301 COLWELL CO., CHAMPAIGN, ILLINOIS

FIGURE 23–1 Page from Narcotic, Stimulant and Depressant Record.

The patient's record will show the condition and purpose for which the drug was given.

CONTROL OF DRUG ABUSE. In February 1966, Congress passed the Federal Drug Abuse Control Act, also known as the Harris Bill (HR 2). The purpose of this bill was to stop the flow of illicit drugs, such as **stimulants** and **depressants,** as well as certain **tranquilizers** and **hallucinogenic** drugs. Most of these drugs are listed in the various schedules given under the Controlled Substances Act.

The laws governing the prescribing of drugs differ somewhat from state to state, but in all states prescriptions may be legally written or telephoned only by the physician; in most states they may be filled only by a registered pharmacist.

The future will bring tighter control of drugs sold over the counter, known as OTC products. The Department of Health and Human Services has already shown this by the removal of antibiotics from throat lozenges. Pharmacists are becoming more cautious because they are sharing in the legal responsibility of prescriptions. They are pointing out precautions, exposing quackery, and are cautious in recommending OTC items. Pharmacists often ask the patients what other medications they are taking in an attempt to avoid interactions that can prove serious, and even fatal. Many pharmacies keep personal and family records so as to be able to better advise people concerning the use of the numerous OTC products. This is especially applicable for the family using one pharmacy regularly. So often patients fail to tell the physician of the OTC drugs they are taking. The pharmacist, if he notes a possible interaction or other problem, can consult with the physician before he fills the prescription.

FORMS OF DRUGS

There are many different ways to classify drugs. One of the most common methods is by their source, as mentioned earlier in this chapter. Another way is by their reaction on the body or by the part or system of the body they affect. Drugs may also be classified by form.

Drugs are produced in a variety of forms, but they are mainly solids and liquids. The solids are found in powder, capsule, tablet, and pill forms.

Tablets vary greatly in size, shape, color, and coating. An *enteric-coated* tablet does not dissolve until it has reached the intestinal tract, thereby delaying its action from two to four hours. The coating is insoluble in the stomach. *Sugar-coated* and *chocolate-covered* tablets dissolve in the mouth and have a flavor. *Compressed* tablets have a filler or binding ingredient in them with the medication and have no coating. A *triturate* tablet is a powder that has been moistened with a volatile liquid and then molded into shape; the liquid evaporates and leaves the shaped powder. These tablets dissolve readily in the mouth and are usually mild. Antacid tablets are an example of a triturate tablet. *Hypodermic* tablets are to be dissolved and injected. The diluent is usually sterile distilled water or injectable normal saline. Hypodermic tablets are rarely used anymore for injection as their sterility cannot be assured, but they can be given sublingually.

The following terms will acquaint the assistant with some other forms of drugs:

Pure Drug. Any unadulterated powder, crystal, or gum employed as a medicine in the treatment of disease. A pure drug appears in its highest possible concentration. It is chemically pure.

Saturation. A solution is saturated when it is impregnated to the greatest possible degree. This saturation is reached when no more of the substance can be dissolved and remain in solution.

Stock Solution. Any solution in concentrated form or highly saturated that is kept on hand for the convenience of making up lesser strengths of the same solution at a desired time.

Tincture. An alcoholic preparation of a soluble drug or chemical substance, such as iodine.

Mixture. A liquid preparation of one or more drugs that unite without chemical action and retain their individual physical properties. A mixture may or may not contain a dissolved substance.

Elixir. An aromatic, alcoholic, sweetened preparation usually employed as a vehicle for an active medicine, i.e., elixir of phenobarbital. Elixirs differ from tinctures in that they are sweetened.

Emulsion. An oily or resinous substance held in suspension in some liquid such as water or gum acacia. Cod liver oil is usually in emulsion form.

Syrup. A solution of sugar and water, usually containing flavoring and medicinal substances, often used as a vehicle. Cough syrups are the most common.

Diluent. A substance added to a solid or viscid substance which reduces the strength of the solution or mixture. It is the substance that dilutes. Many injectable medications come in dried or crystalline forms and have a diluent with them to be added prior to administration.

Suspension. The diffusion of fine particles of a solid through a liquid. A suspension differs from a solution in that particles do not dissolve but retain their solid form; eventually these particles may sink to the bottom. Such preparations are labeled "Shake well before using."

Extract. A preparation obtained by dissolving the medicinal substance in alcohol, ether, or water and evaporating to a prescribed consistency. Extracts are prepared from plant- or animal-derived drugs. Liver extract is an example.

Suppository. Mixture of drugs formed into a small mass that is shaped to introduce into a body orifice. Such suppositories are usually formed of a material that melts at body temperature. There are rectal, vaginal, or urethral suppositories.

Ointment. A semisolid preparation of a drug in a base, to be applied externally. The base may be wool fat, petroleum, lard, or cholesterol. Creams are similar to ointments but are water soluble.

Spirits. Alcoholic solutions of a volatile substance, easily vaporized. They are also known as essences. An example is aromatic spirits of ammonia.

Inhalant. A drug that can be placed in a volatile substance and is capable of being absorbed through the epithelial tissue of the lungs. It has rapid effects. Examples are anesthetics, oxygen, aerosols, ephedrine, and penicillin.

Vehicle. A substance, usually medicinally inactive, that is used to carry a medication. Wild cherry syrup is a common vehicle for cough medications. Many pediatric medications, such as penicillin, are in sweet, flavored syrups.

PRESCRIPTIONS

What is a prescription? A prescription is a written order to a pharmacist, by a licensed physician, to supply a particular patient with certain drugs of specific quantity and prepared according to the doctor's direction. These directions may be written in English or Latin. A prescription is a legal document. The prescription will contain

1. Full name and address of the patient
2. Date written
3. Rx symbol, meaning recipe or "take thou"
4. Name and amount of the drug
5. Instructions to the pharmacist regarding compounding
6. Instructions to the patient
7. Signature of the physician
8. The doctor's name, full address, telephone number, and narcotic registry number

The formal parts of a prescription are as follows:

A. *Superscription:* Patient's name, address, and the Rx symbol
B. *Inscription:* Name and quantities of the ingredients
C. *Subscription:* Directions for compounding
D. *Signatura:* (or "S" for signa) Directions for the patient

Prescription writing today is not as complicated as in earlier times, because pharmaceutical manufacturers now prepare most medications ready for administration. It is comparatively rare for a pharmacist to have to compound or mix a medication. A typical prescription is shown in Figure 23–2.

A medical assistant does not write prescriptions, but she will find a knowledge of prescription terms and abbreviations of great value in medical transcription, in taking telephone messages from the pharmacist, and in understanding instructions for administration of medications. Prescription writing is faster and will enable the assistant to take messages more rapidly and more accurately. It is much easier to write "one tab t.i.d.p.c./c aq or p.r.n." than "one tablet three times a day after meals with water or whenever necessary."

Guard all prescription pads well, especially the narcotic forms, lest they be appropriated and used by addicts who may enter the office. It is best to keep prescription forms, both regular and narcotic, in the doctor's desk drawer. If the prescription pad is left on a desk or table top, it is easy for an addict to tear a few pages from the back of the pad while the desk is unattended. In states where the narcotic prescription forms are numbered serially, the medical assistant should regularly check the numbers to see that they are all in sequence. If a number is missing, report this to the physician immediately.

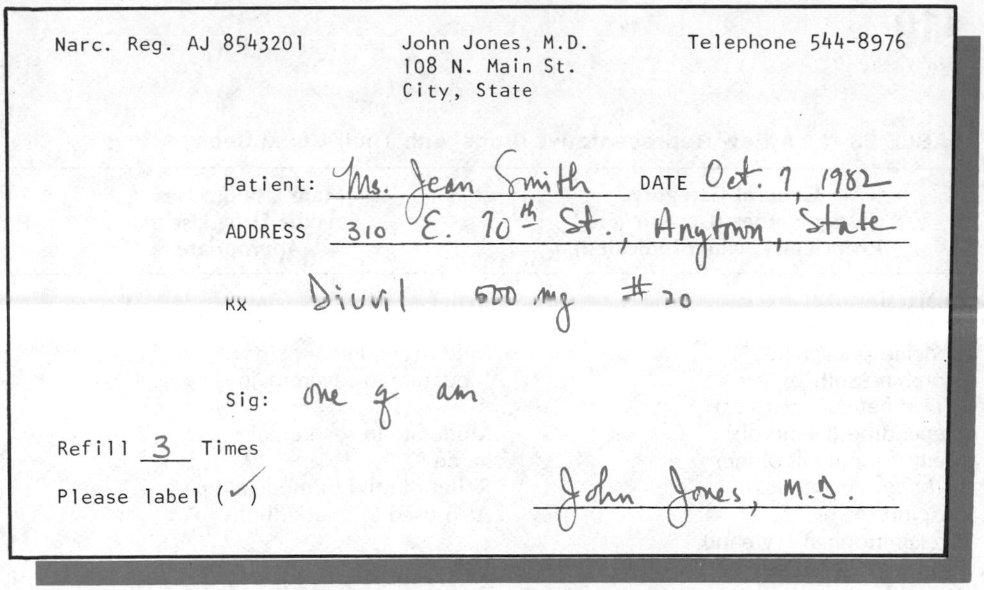

Narc. Reg. AJ 8543201 — John Jones, M.D. — Telephone 544-8976
108 N. Main St.
City, State

Patient: Ms. Jean Smith DATE Oct. 7, 1982

ADDRESS 310 E. 70th St., Anytown, State

RX Diuril 500 mg #20

Sig: One q am

Refill 3 Times

Please label (✓)

John Jones, M.D.

FIGURE 23–2 A sample prescription.

In an article that appeared in Medical Economics on "The Law and Your Prescriptions," Dr. William MacDonald told of a doctor who used prescription blanks for bridge score pads. "He said he got them free from a local pharmacy," said Dr. MacDonald, "and, from his viewpoint, the blanks could be used as freely as scrap paper." Dr. MacDonald wisely advises doctors and medical assistants to use prescription forms only for the purpose for which they are intended.

Dr. MacDonald also warns doctors to follow narcotic laws to the letter. "Last year, as you know, I moved my office across the street," he writes. "Believe it or not, I got a call from the Collector of Internal Revenue. He said my dollar-a-year stamp authorized me to prescribe narcotics from 28 Maple Street and not from 25 Maple Street. He said I should have notified him *before* I actually moved so that he could amend the tax stamp." Such notifications are the responsibility of the medical assistant.

PRESCRIPTION ABBREVIATIONS. The assistant often prepares medications under the doctor's supervision. For this reason she must be familiar with the measuring systems and terminology associated with pharmacology. Symbols and abbreviations widely used in prescription writing and drug dispensing are shown on page 412.

SOME FREQUENTLY PRESCRIBED DRUGS AND THEIR USES. Table 23–1 shows but a very few common drugs that are prescribed by physicians, drugs that patients will be asking about or reporting about to the physician. The medical assistant should remember that her knowledge of drugs is to aid the physician and help the patient, *not* to advise or prescribe.

SYSTEMS OF MEASUREMENT. The metric system of weights and measures is now used throughout the world as the primary system for weight, capacity, and length. In the United States, it is used for scientific work, including most pharmaceuticals, and it may soon be in use for all purposes. However, some physicians still use the apothecaries' system. This necessitates learning both systems and the relationships between the two. A few hints may aid in understanding the system: The metric system is based on the decimal (10); each higher or lower measure is ten times or one-tenth of the measure at hand. The fraction is always written as a decimal and the number precedes the letters designating the actual measure; thus, one and one-half

TABLE 23–1 A Few Representative Drugs with Their Usual Uses

General Category Drug Names (Generic and Proprietary, when Indicated)	Main Use or Uses Specific Drug Use as Appropriate
Analgesics	**Relief of pain**
(Opium alkaloids)	
Codeine phosphate	Mild to moderate pain
Morphine sulfate	Moderate to severe pain
(Synthetic Analgesics)	
Meperidine (Demerol)	Moderate to severe pain
Methadone (Dolophine)	Same
(Minor Analgesics)	Relief of mild to moderate pain
*Aspirin (ASA)	Also used to treat arthritis
Acetaminophen (Tylenol)	
Propoxyphene (Darvon)	
Antacids	**Reduce gastric acidity**
Compounds of aluminum, bismuth, magnesium	Many preparations often combined Many proprietary names
Anti-infectives	**Destroy microorganisms**
(Antibiotics)	
Penicillin (many forms)	"Narrow spectrum," active against a relatively few organisms
Streptomycin	As above
Tetracyclines (many forms)	"Broad spectrum," active against many organisms
(Nonantibiotics – specifics)	Effective against one or a limited number of diseases
Dapsone (Avlosulfon)	Leprosy
Isoniazid (INH)	Tuberculosis
Quinacrine hydrochloride (Atabrine)	Malaria
Quinine sulfate	Malaria
Anticoagulants	**Delay bleeding time (clotting time)**
*Heparin sodium (Liquaemin)	Action rapid, but relatively short
Bishydroxycoumarin (Dicumarol)	Action slower, but more prolonged
Warfarin sodium (Coumadin, Panwarfin)	As above
Cathartics and laxatives	**Cause evacuation of intestinal contents**
Agar (from seaweed)	{Hydrophylic – increases content
**Psyllium (Betajel, Metamucil)	{Bulk laxatives
Bisacodyl (Dulcolax)	Mucosal stimulant
Cascara sagrada	Mild intestinal irritant
Magnesium sulfate (Epsom salts)	{Saline cathartics – withdraw fluid
Magnesium magma (Milk of Magnesia)	{ from the circulation – help in edema
Monosodium phosphate (Sal Hepatica)	
Dioctyl sodium sulfosuccinate (Colace, Doxinate)	Wetting agent
Diuretics	**Increase the flow of urine**
Ethacrynic acid (Edecrin)	
Furosemide (Lasix)	
Mercurial compounds	
Thiazide compounds	
Heart (Cardiac) Depressants	**Decrease the rate of heartbeat and aid in overcoming cardiac arrhythmias**
Procainamide hydrochloride (Pronestyl)	
Propranolol (Inderal)	
Quinidine (several salts)	
Heart (other important drugs)	**Varied**
Digitalis (many forms)	Strengthens beat and lengthens rest period

TABLE 23–1 A Few Representative Drugs with Their Usual Uses *(Continued)*

General Category Drug Names (Generic and Proprietary, when Indicated)	Main Use or Uses Specific Drug Use as Appropriate
Nitroglycerin Papavarine	Relax spasms of the coronary arteries
Iron Compounds	**Iron deficiency anemia**
Ferrous gluconate (Fergon)	
Ferrous sulfate (Feosol)	
Muscle Relaxants	**Relax skeletal muscles**
(Strong)	
Dimethyl tubocuracrine chloride (Mecostrin) Succinylcholine chloride (Anectine, Sucostrin)	Used mainly in surgery
(Mild)	
Mephenesin (Tolserol) Meprobamate (Equanil, Miltown)	Mild relief of tension
(Anticonvulsants)	
Diphenylhydantoin (Dilantin) Paramethadione (Paradione) Phensuximide (Milontin)	Used mainly in epilepsy
Respiratory Stimulants	**Used for shock and depressant drug poisoning**
Doxapram (Dopram)	
Sedatives – Hypnotics	**Light doses produce sedation, heavier doses cause sleep**
(Barbiturates)	
Pentobarbital (Nembutal)	
Phenobarbital (Luminal)	
Secobarbital (Seconal)	
(Nonbarbiturates)	As above
Chloral hydrate	
Ethinamate (Valmid)	
Flurazepam (Dalmane)	
Glutethemide (Doriden)	
Sympathomimetics	**Stimulate the sympathetic portion of the autonomic nervous system**
Ephedrine sulfate Epinephrine hydrochloride (Adrenalin) Isoproterenol hydrochloride (Isuprel)	Used for the relief of bronchial spasms and to treat allergy. The drugs increase rate and strength of heart beat and raise blood pressure. (Ephedrine is used more for maintenance, epinephrine in emergencies, and isoproterenol according to dosage in both situations)
Tranquilizers	**Treatment of tension, anxiety, neuroses and psychoses**
Chlordiazepoxide (Librium)	
Prochlorperazine (Compazine)	
Promazine hydrochloride (Sparine)	
Dimenhydrinate (Dramamine)	Used for motion sickness
Uterine Stimulants	**Increase the strength of uterine muscle contraction – initiate labor**
Ergonovine maleate (Ergotrate)	
Oxytocin injection (Pitocin, Syntocinon)	Also control uterine bleeding

*Most important drug listed in category.
**Placed here owing to nature of its action.

Common Prescription Abbreviations

$\overline{aa}$	of each	inj.	injection, to be injected
a.c.	before meals	kg.	kilogram
ad	up to	M.	mix
adde	add, let it be added	mcgm.	microgram
ad lib.	as much as needed	M. et sig.	mix and label
agit.	shake, stir	M. et f. pil.	mix and make into pill
alt. dieb.	alternate days		
alt. hor.	alternate hours	M. et f. pulv.	mix and make into powder
alt. noc.	alternate nights		
a.m.	morning	mg. (mgm.)	milligram
ante	before	noct.	night
aq.	water	o.h.	every hour
aq. bull.	boiling water	o.m.	every morning
aq. com.	common water, tap water	o.n.	every night
aq. dest.	distilled water	p.c.	after meals
aq. ferv.	hot water	pil.	pill
aq. frig.	cold water	p.r.n.	whenever necessary
aq. susp.	water suspension	pulv.	powder
b.i.d.	two times a day	q.h.	every hour
/c	with	q.i.d.	four times a day (not at night)
caps.	capsule		
comp.	compound	q.2 h.	every two hours
contra	against	q.4 h.	every four hours
coq.	boil	q.n.s.	quantity not sufficient
dil.	dilute	q.s.	quantity sufficient
div.	to be divided	℞	take (recipe)
dos.	doses	rep.	let it be repeated
elix.	elixir	/s	without
emul.	emulsion	sat.	saturated
et	and	sig.	write on label, give directions
ext.	extract		
f. (ft.)	make (let there be made)	sol.	solution
		ss	one-half
fl.	fluid	stat.	immediately
garg.	gargle	suppos.	suppository
gm.	gram	syr.	syrup
gr.	grain	tab.	tablet
gt.	drop	t.i.d.	three times a day
gtt.	drops	tr. (tinct.)	tincture
guttat	drop by drop	troc.	lozenge
h.	hour	u.	unit
h.s.	bedtime (hour of sleep)	ung.	ointment

Abbreviations and Symbols

Apothecaries' System

Symbol	Abbreviation	Meaning
♏	min. (m.)	minim.
℈	scr.	scruple
ʒ	dr.	dram
fl. ʒ	f. dr.	fluid dram
℥	oz.	ounce
fl. ℥	fl. oz.	fluid ounce
O	pt.	pint
C	gal.	gallon
	gr.	grain

Metric System

gm.	gram
L.	liter
cc.	cubic centimeter
ml.	millimeter

Table of Weights and Measures

Apothecaries' System	Metric System
Weights	*Weights*
20 grains = 1 scruple	1000 milligrams = 1 gram
60 grains = 1 dram	1000 grams = 1 kilogram
8 drams = 1 ounce	
12 ounces = 1 pound*	
Liquids	*Liquids*
60 minims = 1 dram	1000 milliliters = 1 liter
8 drams = 1 ounce	(1 milliliter = 1 cubic centimeter)
16 ounces = 1 pint	
2 pints = 1 quart	
4 quarts = 1 gallon	

*Avoirdupois weight: 16 ounces = 1 pound.

liter would be written 1.5 L. The letters cc and ml are used interchangeably. The term ml is more accurate, since it is 1/1000 of a liter. Cc refers to cubic centimeters and is a measure of capacity. Under specific conditions of temperature and barometric pressure, a ml of water will just fill a cubic centimeter (cc) of space. Arabic numerals are used.

With the apothecaries' system either Roman or Arabic numerals are used (although Roman numerals were used exclusively at one time), but not properly in the same prescription. Symbols or abbreviations may be used. One and one-half ounces might be written ℥iss *or* oz1½. The number follows the symbol or abbreviation. The letters ss mean semesis (one-half). Some persons dot the i, but no other letter should be dotted.

TERMINOLOGY

Aerosol. A solution that can be finely atomized and inhaled for producing local respiratory or systemic action. Epinephrine (adrenalin) is used in an aerosol.

Analgesic. A drug to relieve pain by lessening the sensory functions of the brain. It may be taken internally or used topically. Analgesics vary greatly in their ability to quiet pain, from aspirins to the opium derivatives.

Anesthetic. A drug used to produce insensibility to pain or the sensation of pain, local or general. *Topical* anesthetics are surface applied and have local action. Other *local* anesthetics are *infiltration* (injected into a nerve), *intraspinal* (spinal fluid withdrawn and an equal amount of anesthetic injected into the spinal canal), and *caudal* (drug injected into base of the spine, used in obstetrics).

Antibiotic. An agent that is produced by a living organism and is effective against bacteria. There are many antibiotics on the market today, including penicillin, streptomycin, erythromycin, and tetracycline.

Conversion From One System to Another

Liquids		Weights	
Metric	*Apothecaries'*	*Metric*	*Apothecaries'*
0.06 cc. =	1 minim	0.1 gram =	1½ grains
1 cc. =	15 minims	0.2 gram =	3 grains
4 cc. =	1 dram	0.3 gram =	5 grains
30 cc. =	1 fluid ounce	0.06 gram =	1 grain
500 cc. =	1 pint	0.5 gram =	7½ grains
1000 cc. =	1 quart	1 gram =	15 grains
4000 cc. =	1 gallon	1 kilogram =	2.2 pounds

23

Approximate Equivalents Within Systems

Metric	Apothecaries'
0.06 gram = 0.06 cc.	1 grain = 1 minim
1 gram = 1 cc.	15 grains = 15 minims
4 grams = 4 cc.	60 grains = 60 minims
30 grams = 30 cc.	480 grains = 480 minims (1 oz.)

Antidote. A substance used to counteract a poison or the effects of a poison.

Carminative. A medication which relieves flatulence and aids in the expulsion of gas from the stomach and intestines. Usually contains volatile oils or carbonated beverage.

Cathartic. An agent that increases and hastens bowel evacuation (defecation). Commonly called a laxative. Types range from mild laxatives and purgatives to drastic cathartics. Some increase the bulk in the bowel; others irritate the intestinal mucosa.

Chemotherapeutic Agents (Anti-infective). Chemical substances that are used to inhibit or kill microorganisms that cause disease. Sulfonamides are chemotherapeutic.

Decongestant. A drug that relieves local congestion. The most popular of this group are the nasal decongestants, such as ephedrine or phenylephrine (Neo-Synephrine).

Diaphoretic. A drug used to induce and increase the secretion of perspiration.

Digestant. A drug that promotes the progress of digestion. Enzymes, acids, and bile salts are included in this group.

Diuretic. An agent that increases the function of the kidneys and stimulates the flow of urine. Increases the water content of the blood through osmosis or salt action, freeing water from the tissues, reducing edema.

Emetic. A drug used to induce vomiting. Mild mustard and plain tepid water are home remedies used as emetics. Ipecac syrup is commonly used.

Household Measurements and Equivalents*

1 minim = 1 drop
1 teaspoon = 5 ml or 75 drops
4 teaspoons = 1 tablespoon (15 cc)
1 dessert spoon = 2 drams
1 tablespoon = 4 drams
4 tablespoons = 1 wineglass
16 tablespoons = 1 cup
(liquid)
12 tablespoons = 1 cup
(dry)
1 cup = 8 fluid ounces (1/2 pint)
1 glass = 8 fluid ounces
1 wineglass = 2 fluid ounces
1 pint = 1 pound
1 tablespoon = 16 cc
1 ounce = 1 whiskey glass

*These measurements and equivalents are approximate because of the great variation in household measuring devices.

Mathematical Equivalents

Percentage	Decimal	Fraction	Ratio
25%	.25	1/4	1:4
50%	.5	1/2	1:2
60%	.6	3/5 (6/10)	3:5
1/2% (.5%)	.005	1/200	1:200
1/10% (0.1%)	.001	1/1000	1:1000
85%	.85	17/20	17:20
1%	.01	1/100	1:100

Expectorant. A drug used to increase the secretions and mucus from the bronchial tubes. Makes a cough more productive and breaks up congestion. Some cough medicines are expectorants; some are a combination of antihistamines and expectorants; others are used to decrease flow of mucus.

Hemostatic. Drug used to check bleeding; blood coagulants. Absorbable hemostatics are applied directly to the oozing surface, and an artificial clot is formed, which gradually absorbs. Gelfoam and Surgicel are examples.

Hypnotic. A drug that produces sleep and lessens the activity of the brain. A hypnotic has a sedative action when used in smaller doses. The barbiturates are the most common hypnotics, both oral and injectable: pentobarbital (Nembutal), amobarbital (Amytal), secobarbital and amobarbital (Tuinal).

Miotic. Any agent that causes the pupil of the eye to contract, by contraction of the ciliary muscles.

Mydriatic. An agent used to dilate the pupil of the eye. Used by ophthalmologists in eye examinations. (Cycloplegics cause loss of accommodation by paralyzing the ciliary muscle of the eye.) Mydriatics have little or no effect on the muscles of accommodation.

Nutrient. A substance that supplies nourishment or affects the metabolic rate of the body; a food supplement. Vitamins are considered nutrients.

Opiate. Any drug that is derived from or contains opium. It is the oldest known remedy and was used long before the time of Christ. It comes from the opium poppy. There are more than 20 alkaloids from the opium plant, but morphine, codeine, and papaverine are the most common. The synthetic narcotics are similar in action but are not opiates. These synthetics are meperidine (Demerol), methadone (Dolophine), levorphanol tartrate (Levo-Dromoran), and pentazocine (Talwin). They are usually less habit-forming than the opiates.

Parenteral. A sterile solution of a medication prepared for injection. A medication given parenterally is given by injection into the body. The various types are intravenous, intramuscular, subcutaneous, intraspinal, intradermal, intraperitoneal.

Relaxant. An antispasmodic; a drug used to reduce or relax muscular spasm, usually skeletal muscle. They are often used with a general anesthetic, as in eye or rectal surgery. Curare (South American arrow poison) produces good muscular relaxation. Uterine relaxants for the nongravid uterus are used to relieve painful menstruation.

Sedative. A drug that reduces excitement; a quieting agent, but does not produce sleep as a hypnotic drug does. They are often the same drug, a smaller dose acting as a sedative while a larger dose acts as a hypnotic.

Stomachic. An agent used to increase the secretory activity of the stomach and aid in digestion. Not to be confused with a *stomatic,* which pertains to the mouth.

Tranquilizer. A calming agent that reduces anxiety and tension without acting as a depressant. Tranquilizers are called "psychotherapeutic" drugs. This group of drugs has increased in large numbers during recent years. The phenothiazine derivatives are often given. These include chlorpromazine (Thorazine), perphenazine (Trilifon), thioridiazine (Mellaril), and several others.

Vasoconstrictor. A drug that causes a blood vessel to constrict, narrows the lumen of a vessel, raises blood pressure, and causes the heart to beat more forcefully. Used to stop superficial bleeding, raise and sustain blood pressure, relieve nasal congestion.

Vasodilator. The opposite of a vasoconstrictor, a drug that dilates blood vessels, lowers blood pressure by making blood vessels larger, causing the heart to pump less forcefully. Used in the treatment of hypertension, angina pectoris, and peripheral vascular diseases. Nitroglycerine placed sublingually gives prompt vasodilator action. Aminophylline dilates coronary vessels and bronchial tubes and is used in asthmatic cases.

DRUG ACTIONS

There are many different methods, or channels, for administering a medication, either on the body surface in a local area (topical action) or into the body (systemic action).

TOPICAL ACTION. A topical drug is one applied locally to the skin or mucous membrane, sometimes to the ear or eye. These drugs are usually in the form of a liquid, lotion, emulsion, ointment, or foam. They are used for the treatment of infection, irritation, or an allergic reaction or are given to produce local anesthesia.

Topical anesthetics would be applied to produce a lack of feeling or sensation. Cocaine is an example; it paralyzes sensory nerve endings and produces a surface anesthesia. Other topical anesthetics can be in the form of an ointment, such as Surfacaine, Nupercaine, and Tronothane. Some eye medications like Butacaine have a topical anesthetic action. These are used in the eye prior to testing with the tonometer.

Astringents are used to harden or contract tissues. An example of this is witch hazel when applied locally.

Antiseptics are the best example of local action. When we have a skin abrasion we apply a local antiseptic, such as alcohol, tincture of iodine, Merthiolate, and Zephiran.

A local medication can also act as a *counterirritant.* This is an agent that is applied locally to reduce inflammatory reaction in some other part, usually underlying the area where the counterirritant is applied. It relieves a congested organ or an inflamed muscle. Grandmother's mustard plaster is an excellent example.

Anodynes, such as oil of clove for toothache or oil of wintergreen for rheumatism, relieve pain but are milder than analgesics. *Irritants* are often applied to produce warmth of the skin. They dilate the blood vessels and usually produce a reddening where applied. *Emollients* have a soothing effect on the skin. They are usually a fatty or oily substance, such as cocoa butter or anhydrous lanolin. Demulcents are similar to emollients but do not contain oil or fat. *Styptics* are applied to a small bleeding area to check the flow of blood. Protective medications, such as colloidin and silicone, form a coating on the skin ("new skin"). *Keratolytics* are agents that aid in the loosening of the dry horny layer of skin such as in dandruff or some fungal infections. Selenium sulfide and Whitefield's ointment are keratolytics.

SYSTEMIC ACTION. Systemic actions are also called *general actions*. They occur after absorption of a substance into the circulation, and they may affect the entire body. Effectiveness of a systemic drug depends on how it is introduced into the body. In order to be most effective, it must be able to be absorbed — that is, have the ability to permeate the cells. The drug must be utilized by the specific organ or part of the body for which it is intended, and it must be utilized or be excreted, either unchanged or with other body wastes such as through urine, the lungs, or the skin.

There are many types of systemic actions. When it is intended to increase the activity of a tissue, a *stimulant* is used. Caffeine is a stimulant. In some cases an overdose of a stimulant can give a reverse action and cause depression. *Depressants* cause a decreased activity of the tissues. Bromides and sleeping capsules can be depressants. There are several types of depressants, such as cardiac, cerebral, and respiratory.

Systemic drugs may also cause *irritation* or *stimulation*. These two words are often confused, and understandably so. An irritation causes a slight temporary damage, such as the action of castor oil on the mucous membrane of the intestines. A mild irritation can result in a stimulation, while a prolonged stimulation can produce an irritation.

The words *cumulative action* appear in pharmacologic writings. This means that a drug accumulates in the body; it is eliminated more slowly than it is absorbed. Digitalis, a heart stimulant, is cumulative.

Frequently a physician will say a patient has an *"idiosyncrasy"* to a certain drug. He is referring to the fact that the patient has an unusual response to the drug. An idiosyncrasy may show itself in many different ways, such as a sleeping capsule keeping a person awake, acting as a stimulant to this person. These are abnormal symptoms that cannot always be explained.

Tolerance is of major concern to the physician. This is the ability to withstand a quantity of a drug. Often a physician must progressively increase a dosage in order to maintain the desired therapeutic effect. Substances to which people usually develop a tolerance are narcotics, alcohol, and tobacco.

If the patient is taking more than one drug at a time, *interaction* between the drugs may take place. This may or may not be desirable. There are many types of interaction. One drug may enhance the action of another; one may negate another or decrease its action. In some cases, the interaction may produce toxicity. This is one reason why the physician must be aware of *all* drugs being used by the patient, including simple OTC drugs.

SOLUTIONS

A solution is made up of two parts called the *solute* and the *solvent*. The solute is the substance dissolved, and the solvent is the dispersing fluid or the liquid in which the solute is dissolved. The solute may be a solid, gas, or liquid. Most solutions are made of a solid or liquid dissolved or mixed into the solvent. The strength of the solution is the amount of the pure drug or solute in a definite quantity of the solvent. Solute plus solvent equals a solution.

If water is used as a solvent, the result is called an aqueous solution. There are many solvents — for example, alcohol, ether, acids, or oils.

Solutions are spoken of in percentages or ratios. A 5 per cent solution is 5 parts of the solute in 100 parts of solution, or a ratio of 1:20. Many crystals do not displace

Table for Making Weight in Volume Percentage Solutions*

The following table gives the proportion of material to be used with solvent q.s. to make the volume at top of the column. Multiples or fractions of these volumes may be calculated from these figures.

Strength of Solution	Dissolve the weight specified below in distilled water q.s. to make 100 cc.	Dissolve the weight specified below in distilled water q.s. to make 500 cc.	Dissolve the weight specified below in distilled water q.s. to make 1 fl. oz.	Dissolve the weight specified below in distilled water q.s. to make 1 pint
0.25 per cent	0.25 gm.	1.25 gm.	1.14 gr.	18¼ gr.
0.5 per cent	0.5 gm.	2.5 gm.	2.28 gr.	36½ gr.
1 per cent	1 gm.	5 gm.	4.56 gr.	73 gr.
2 per cent	2 gm.	10 gm.	9.13 gr.	146 gr.
3 per cent	3 gm.	15 gm.	13.7 gr.	219 gr.
4 per cent	4 gm.	20 gm.	18.26 gr.	292 gr.
5 per cent	5 gm.	25 gm.	22.8 gr.	365 gr.
6 per cent	6 gm.	30 gm.	27.38 gr.	437 gr.
8 per cent	8 gm.	40 gm.	36.5 gr.	583 gr.
10 per cent	10 gm.	50 gm.	45.6 gr.	729 gr.
12.5 per cent	12.5 gm.	62.5 gm.	57 gr.	913 gr.
15 per cent	15 gm.	75 gm.	68.5 gr.	1095 gr.
16⅔ per cent	16.6 gm.	83.3 gm.	76 gr.	1217 gr.
20 per cent	20 gm.	100 gm.	91.28 gr.	1460 gr.
25 per cent	25 gm.	125 gm.	114 gr.	1825 gr.
30 per cent	30 gm.	150 gm.	137 gr.	2187 gr.
33⅓ per cent	33.3 gm.	166.6 gm.	152 gr.	2433 gr.
50 per cent	50 gm.	250 gm.	228 gr.	3500 gr.

437.5 grains = 1 Avoirdupois ounce; 480 grains = Apothecaries' ounce.

*Reprinted from Conn, H. (ed.): *Current Therapy 1973*. Philadelphia, W. B. Saunders Co., 1973.

any appreciable volume, so the volume of the solution is practially the same as the quantity of the solvent. Strong solutions are usually given as per cent and weak solution as ratios.

To make a 5 per cent solution of acetic acid you would measure 5 ml acetic acid 100 per cent (solute) and add sufficient water (solvent) to make up a total of 100 ml. In other words, you would add 95 ml water.

The USP XIV specifies: "When *per cent* is used in prescriptions without qualification, it means for mixtures of solids, per cent weight in weight; for solutions of solids in liquids, per cent weight in volume; for solutions of liquids, per cent volume in volume; and for solutions of gases in liquid, per cent weight in volume." (See table above.)

PRACTICAL PROBLEMS IN PREPARING MEDICATIONS

HOW TO GIVE A FRACTION OF A DROP

RULE: To one drop of the given solution add sufficient number of drops of water (or solvent) to equal the denominator of your desired fraction, then use the number of drops in the numerator. DILUTE TO THE DENOMINATOR, ADMINISTER THE NUMERATOR.

EXAMPLES: (1) Give ⅓ of a drop.

To the one drop add 2 drops, thus making three drops. Then give one drop, or one-third of the original drop.

(2) Give ¾ of a drop.

To the one drop add 3 more drops, making a total of four drops. Then give three drops, or three-fourths of the original drop.

HOW TO CALCULATE A FRACTION OF AN AMPULE OR VIAL

Sometimes a portion of a drug must be withdrawn from a vial or ampule. Markings on the container give the concentration of the solution, usually as the amount of the drug per milliliter or cubic centimeter. Given the amount of drug needed, the amount of fluid to be withdrawn must be determined. This is best done by setting up a proportion with the three known quantities: the amount of the drug per unit, that unit, and the amount of drug needed.

EXAMPLE: An order is received for 0.5 mg of a drug. The vial is marked 0.25 mg per ml.

$$\frac{0.25}{1} = \frac{0.5}{\times}$$ (0.25 mg is to 1 ml as 0.5 mg is to how many milliliters (×)?)

$$0.25 \times = 0.50$$

$$\times = 2$$ 2 ml will be required

Some drugs are measured in units that signify the amount of the drug required to obtain a specific reaction, instead of in weight or volume. Again, a proportion is used to determine the proper amount as in the following example.

EXAMPLE: A vial is marked "1 ml (cc) contains 20,000 units." The order is for 30,000 units.

$$\frac{20{,}000}{1} = \frac{30{,}000}{\times}$$

$$20{,}000 \times = 30{,}000$$

$$\times = 1.5 \text{ ml}$$

POISON CONTROL CENTERS

Within the last few years over 300 poison control centers have been established around the nation to provide quick and handy sources of information on many chemical products containing potentially injurious substances. These are usually located in major community hospitals or in medical colleges and are often cooperatively set up with local and state health departments, hospitals, and physicians. The medical assistant should post the telephone number of the nearest poison control center in a prominent place in the office so that it will be readily available should the doctor need to secure information fast to help treat a poisoned person.

BURN CENTERS

The same information should be available for the nearest burn center. So much expensive equipment is used and such specialized personnel needed that the average community hospital is not prepared to care for the severely burned patient. The nearest center should be known and the address and telephone readily available.

Reference

Falconer, M. W., Sheridan, E., Patterson, H. R., and Gustafson, E. A.: *The Drug, the Nurse, the Patient.* 6th ed. Philadelphia, W. B. Saunders Co., 1978.

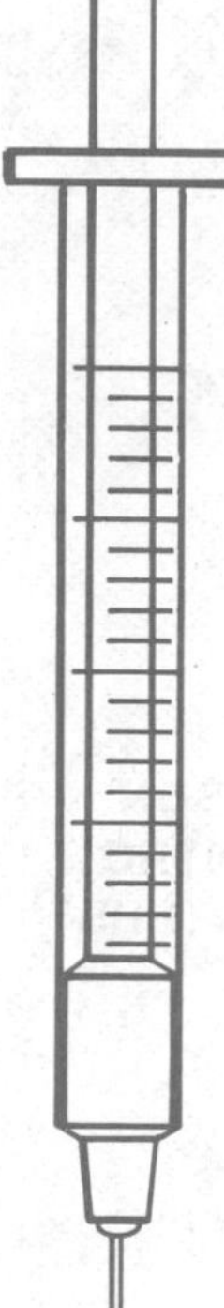

CHAPTER OUTLINE

Factors Influencing Dosage
Channels of Administration
- Topical Drugs (Applied to the Skin)
- Topical Drugs (Used in Cavities that Connect with the Exterior)
- Systemic Drugs

Parenteral Administration
- Types of Injections
  - Intramuscular
  - Subcutaneous
  - Intradermal

Children and Infants
Preparing for an Injection
Giving an Injection
Dangers of Incorrect Injecting Technique
Avoiding Dangers of Incorrect Injecting Technique

BEHAVIORAL OBJECTIVES

The medical office assistant should be able to:

- **Give medications by any of the methods usually used by paramedical personnel, such as sublingually, orally, subcutaneously, intramuscularly, and intradermally.**
- **Instruct the patient or a relative how to give medications as directed by the physician.**
- **Answer most of the patient's questions concerning the taking of medications prescribed by the physician.**
- **Prepare for, assist with, and clean up after the physician gives a medication intravenously.**
- **Properly care for all office medicines and the equipment used to administer them.**

24

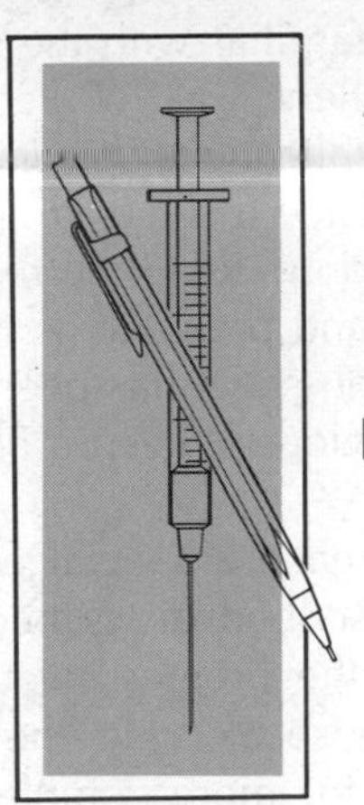

ADMINISTRATION OF MEDICATIONS

MARY W. FALCONER, R.N., M.A.

The administration of medications has become one of the most significant functions of the medical world. One of the most important responsibilities that a physician may delegate to a well trained and reliable assistant is the administration of certain medications to his patients. It cannot be said often enough in this book that the doctor relies upon the accuracy and dependability of his assistant far more than the businessman does upon his secretary, for example. Dollars and cents are at stake in the business world — but health and lives are at stake in the medical world. Accuracy is essential! Carelessness is intolerable!

The assistant who is asked to administer medications must have a thorough understanding of the scientific principles of diagnosis and therapy to be able to give them with assurance. She must have certain skills to administer the medications correctly at the doctor's request. She must understand the time element in relation to absorption, tolerance, and so forth of medications. She first should acquaint herself thoroughly with the medications used by her doctor. She should, for example, read all literature enclosed with medications, *not* so that she can treat or diagnose but so that she understands the specific uses, values, limitations, side effects, interaction with other drugs, and dangers of these medications. Additional information about drugs can also be obtained from local pharmacists or drug company representatives.

No assistant should ever give medications except on the instructions of the doctor or on the basis of his acknowledgement. If a patient is coming into the office for medication while the doctor is not present, consent should be secured from the doctor beforehand, *not after* the medication has been given.

It is important to observe the patient closely during the administration of any medications. If the assistant has any question, no matter how insignificant, in her mind about administering the medication or the patient's condition, she should immediately check with the doctor. Under no circumstances should she go beyond the doctor's instructions.

PRECAUTIONS. The administration of medicine must be done with the utmost care. It cannot be said enough: BE CAREFUL . . . BE ACCURATE. If there is ever any doubt, do not give the medication but check with the physician. Always check the patient's chart, making certain it is the correct patient and not just the "patient in the second room." Never use medication from a bottle with a damaged label. Know the medications you are giving.

No medical assistant needs to learn all the drugs used or prescribed by her physician, but she should become familiar with the medications that are frequently prescribed and used. An excellent way of acquainting yourself with these medications is to read medical publications, paying particular attention to drug advertisements. Every physician's office receives drug samples. Read the manufacturer's literature enclosed with the drug. Read the recommended dosage carefully, the contraindications, side effects, and precautions. Know the actions and uses of the drug. If this enclosed information sheet has been destroyed, consult the office reference books. As mentioned previously, keep a file of the brochures that come with the drugs.

The medical assistant should make a special effort to know the side effects and precautions of commonly prescribed drugs because patients will frequently telephone the office to report on the progress of their illnesses. Since it is not always possible for the patient to speak with the physician, an alert medical assistant may question the patient for more complete information. If she has an understanding of drugs she will know what information should be brought to the physician's attention immediately. This knowledge may aid in preventing a patient from having a drug reaction.

A knowledge of drugs can save many hours in transcribing medical records for the medical assistant who has the name of the drug and the correct spelling at her fingertips. Many drug names sound similar to the untrained ear, and considerable damage can be done through misinterpretation.

The trend toward labeling prescriptions with the name of the drug is helpful in discussing a patient's medication. In case of an emergency, considerable time may be saved by having the name of the drug rather than just a prescription number and a description of the drug's appearance. This also offers a double-check on a medication, because patients can transpose a number when giving it to you over the telephone. There may also be a financial saving to a patient when a similar illness proceeds through several children in a family and the physician prescribes the same medication. However, there is a danger here that must be stressed. The parent must not give a medication ordered for one child to another without the doctor's express order. The assistant must warn the parent if he or she asks and must confer with the physician before telling the parent that the drug may be used for the second child. Symptoms of various diseases are often very similar, but the cause may be entirely different. As an example, gastroenteritis (plain old "stomach ache") due to dietary indiscretion and acute appendicitis often have the same symptoms: nausea, vomiting, and abdominal pain. The drug given for the former would be contraindicated for the latter. Occasionally a physician does not want a patient to know the name of the medication; in this case, the medical assistant must be careful not to give the name of the drug to the patient. If the patient asks for this information, he should be referred to the physician.

POINTS TO REMEMBER. Read each label carefully before administration — not merely the name of the drug but also its strength. Medications are prepared in various strengths; this is especially true with injectables. For example, a chorionic gonadotropin hormone comes in three different strengths: 500 I U per cc, 1000 I U per cc, and 2000 I U per cc. The last one is four times the strength of the first.

When recording a medication on a patient's chart, make certain the strength is recorded as well as the amount, how it was given, and where. To write 1 cc does not tell whether it was 500 or 2000 I U. Also, was it given intramuscularly in the deltoid, buttocks, or thigh, on the right or left side?

Check the patient's name again with the physician's orders. Know your patient as well as the medication.

Never use a medication from an unmarked bottle or when the label is not clear and easy to read.

Measure the exact amount. Don't measure air bubbles.

When pouring a solution or medication, pour away from the label. This keeps the solution from running down over the label and damaging it.

If a medication has changed color or has a precipitation, do not use it. The assistant should examine the label to see if there is an expiration date and be sure that the drug is still usable.

Do not mix medications unless you have been instructed to do so. Some medications are incompatible.

Remain with a patient if there is any question of a possible reaction, or if he feels ill. If there is any doubt, call the physician immediately.

Do not hesitate to admit a mistake! If you have given a patient the wrong medication, tell the physician immediately. This is no time for you to hide your errors; a patient's life may be at stake.

Occasionally newspapers carry stories of tragic accidents that occur when a doctor's assistant, a nurse, or even a physician mistakenly administers the wrong drug to someone. To avoid mistakes, get in the habit of reading every label twice before you administer the medication and once after administration.

FACTORS INFLUENCING DOSAGE

Insofar as the patient is concerned, there are certain factors to be considered when giving medications. These factors make it necessary on occasion to vary the standard dose: age, weight, sex, previous habits and tolerances, idiosyncrasies and susceptibility, temperament and occupation, condition of the patient, object of medication, time of administration, and channel of administration.

The age of the patient determines the strength of the dose of a medicine to be given. A child or a very aged person may take a smaller dose. Weight is important, too; the lighter the person, the smaller the dose. In some cases, the physician will order the dose on the basis of the patient's optimal weight rather than his actual weight. This is especially true if the patient is very much overweight or underweight.

The average female may be given a smaller dose of a medicine than a male. Concerning previous habits and tolerances, you must consider the patient's medical history. What medicines has he been taking? Does he need more of the drug now than when he started taking it? A "Yes" here indicates tolerance. Remember, to many nonprofessional individuals, medicines or medications are substances prescribed by the physician, drugs are illicit agents used by drug addicts, and remedies are things you buy in a drug store without a prescription that make life a little easier. They do not realize that many of these over-the-counter drugs are actually potent medications. Many patients are allergic to certain drugs. Respect any statement they may make as to previous reactions.

Temperament and occupation also influence the amount of a given medicine that can be administered. A nervous person often should take a smaller dose, and a phlegmatic type sometimes will require a heavier dose of certain drugs, such as the antidepressants. Physically active persons may take a larger dose.

The patient's condition is an extremely important factor to consider. What is the intensity of the pain to be stilled, for example? Or, what is the cumulation of the drug in the patient's body? Dyspnea (shortness of breath or labored respiration) may call for smaller, more frequent doses.

It is also necessary to consider what the object of the medication is. For example, in sedation is a deep sleep or rest required? Time of administration also affects the strength of the dose. Is the drug being administered with meals, on an empty stomach, or at bedtime?

Finally,what is the channel of administration?

CHANNELS OF ADMINISTRATION

It seems unnecessary to say that medications are administered to people for their benefit. However, medical personnel often become so imbued with the scientific actions of drugs that they overlook this very basic fact. Never forget that it is the patient who is of paramount importance; it is his health that is being restored or maintained. Also remember that it is far better to prevent disease and to keep people healthy than to have to cure them of illnesses.

Medicines are given to patients in a variety of ways. Medical substances may have their main action at the point of contact with the body or in an organ or tissue far removed from the entry area. The former types, as stated in the previous chapter, are called local or topical drugs. These act on the skin and the mucous membranes lining cavities that connect directly with the exterior. The latter kinds are systemic drugs, which must first enter the blood and the lymph circulation in order to be carried to the target area.

Topical Drugs (Applied to the Skin)

The average patient will understand the use of many of the topical drugs perfectly. However, it is important that the physician or his assistant make sure this is true. It is surprising how many patients need a detailed explanation of even the simplest procedure.

The more common forms of topical drugs are ointments, creams (water-soluble preparations similar to ointments), lotions, solutions (wet dressings), sprays, and preparations to be "painted" on. These substances were defined in the previous chapter.

OINTMENTS AND CREAMS. These are well understood by most people and will usually require no specific instructions, except perhaps to know whether or not a dressing or other covering should be applied. If the assistant does not know and the prescription does not state the information, the doctor should be consulted to ascertain his wishes in the matter. If the area is to be covered, the type of covering should be explained to the patient.

Though this may not be required information for the assistant, a word of caution concerning ointments may help in an emergency. "Burn ointments" may be used on small, superficial burns. For these injuries they are useful and beneficial. However, *never* put any ointment, cream, or other oily or greasy substance on a deep or extensive burn. Such cases should be taken immediately to the nearest hospital emergency room, burn center, or doctor's office. If any ointment or other oily material has been put on the burn, it will have to be removed before the burn can be treated, and this is often a very painful process. If it is essential to cover the burned area while transporting the patient, a clean cloth may be put over the wound. The inside of folded linen that has been ironed is relatively sterile (it is free from microorganisms, or at least nearly so).

A wet dressing may be used. Water from the hot water heater is also relatively free of bacteria. The dressing should be of saline or drinking water and should be as close in temperature to the surface of the body as possible. The wet dressing should be covered with an impervious material.

LOTIONS. Lotions are often used to control itching. Calamine, with or without phenol, is one such preparation. It should be dabbed on, using a soft cloth or cotton. It should not be rubbed in as this will increase the itching. With this type of medication the area is left uncovered. Lotions are also used to relieve the congestion and pain in muscles and joints — called rheumatism by many individuals. In these cases, the lotion may be rubbed in and is often covered with a thick cloth (wool or other heavy cloth) to retain heat. These lotions dilate the superficial blood vessels, thus drawing the blood to the surface and away from the congested parts below.

SOLUTION AND WET DRESSINGS. These can be a real problem, especially if they are to be applied to body parts other than the feet and hands. It is easy to immerse the extremities into a solution or wrap them in a cloth wet with the solution. If the area to be treated can be covered, plastic wrap can be put over the wet dressing and adhesive put around the edges, thus containing the solution. If this is not practical, plastic may be put under the part and the top left open to the air. If the medication in the solution is a dye, the patient should know about this and be advised to use old bedding and clothing so that if they are stained, it will not be too great a loss.

DRUGS TO BE PAINTED ON THE SKIN. These drugs are frequently used by most individuals. They are common household articles. Included in this category are tinctures (tr. of iodine) and nonalcoholic compounds, such as Merbromin (mercurochrome). The alcoholic solutions are thought by many to be superior to the nonalcoholic types, but they do sting. Tincture of iodine should not be put on wet skin or into a deep (punctured) wound, nor should it be covered. Some of the new iodine products, such as Betadine (which is not a tincture), may be covered.

SPRAYS. Sprays are used more for cavities that connect with the exterior than they are for the skin. But they are sometimes used to apply antiseptics to large surfaces. Generally, the same types of drugs are used for sprays as are used for painting on the skin.

Topical Drugs (Used in Cavities That Connect with the Exterior)

The cavities that communicate with the exterior that will be considered here are the ears, eyes, nose, mouth and throat, vagina, and rectum. The bladder, through the urethral opening, also communicates with the exterior, but the patient rarely, if ever, applies medication to the bladder.

EARS. Ears are usually treated with ear drops or ointments. If ear drops are ordered, the patient should lie on the unaffected side. The medication is usually supplied in small bottles, with a dropper attached to the cork or cap. The bottle should be held closely in the hand for a few minutes before using, to warm the solution. If any agitation is required, the bottle should be rolled in the hand, never vigorously shaken. The drops should be as close to body surface temperature as possible. Drops too hot or too cold should not be used, as they will increase pain and may cause dizziness. The ear lobe should be pulled slightly downward and backward in the infant and small child, slightly backward in the child, and slightly upward and backward in the adult. This procedure straightens the ear canal. The drops should be allowed to flow by gravity down the side of the canal. The patient should lie still for 15 to 30 minutes to allow the medicine to work — to spread over the area and at least partially dry. No ear plug should be used unless specifically ordered. Ointments and creams are often applied by the doctor, but the assistant may do this under the doctor's direction. The ointment is applied on a cotton applicator to the side of the canal. Be careful not to go too deep as the tympanic membrane must not be touched. An otoscope will help in locating the portions of the canal needing treatment.

EYES. The eyes are treated with the same types of medications as the ears, namely, drops and ointments. In giving eye drops, the patient is asked to look up, and the lower lid is gently pulled outward a very little. This makes a cup into which the designated number of drops are placed. Eye solutions also come in dropper bottles. The solution may be at room temperature but should not be very cold. *Never* drop the medication directly on the sensitive cornea, the covering over the iris (colored portion), or the pupil. Ointments are applied in the same way. Eye ointments come in very small tubes with a minute opening through which the ointment is applied. Be extremely careful never to let the tip of the dropper or the tube touch any portion of the eye or eyelids. A patient can be taught to give himself eye drops and can become very adept at the procedure. The patient is told to hold the head back, open the eyes widely, and let the drops fall into the lower portion of the eye. The assistant can lighten the procedure a bit, if necessary, by telling the patient that his first try may result in a face wash with the drops, but no harm is done except for a small loss of solution.

Tears flow from the upper outer canthus to the inner lower canthus and then drain into the upper portion of the nasal cavity. It may be wise after putting drops into the eyes to place light pressure on the inner canthus for a few minutes to avoid having the drops excrete too rapidly.

NOSE. In the nose, drops and sprays are the most commonly used forms. To apply nose drops, the patient should be lying down, with the head lower than the body, for instance, over the head of the bed, examining table, or couch. This is to allow the drops to reach the upper nasal cavity, where they are usually needed. Short, rapid breaths (like those of a rabbit) will help spread the solution. With the use of sprays, only one precaution needs to be taken — be sure that the tip of the apparatus is free in the nasal cavity and not against the side of the cavity. For both drops and sprays, one thing must be impressed on the patient: "Do not exceed the amount or frequency for the medication ordered." Usually, these drugs contain a vasoconstrictor, a decongestant. If used too often, the medicine can cause blanching and drying of the mucosa and this can make the condition worse.

Cold sores and other small sores and infections in the openings of the nares are common. They are treated as any skin condition of a similar nature, since there is a small bit of skin lining the outer end of the nares.

MOUTH. The care of oral disorders may be the province of the dentist or the physician. Usually, the patient needs few or no directions for mouth care. However, if the throat is affected, instruction may be important. The three most commonly used methods of getting medicines to the throat are painting, spraying, and gargling. Most patients understand the latter process without discussion. If they do not, the directions are simple: the patient takes the medicinal solution into the mouth (not too much at one time); takes a deep, but not a forced breath; holds the head back; opens the mouth and exhales through the fluid. The solution is not swallowed. The procedure is repeated until the prescribed amount has been used.

For painting and spraying it is *absolutely essential* that the person doing the procedure (patient, friend, assistant, or doctor) first look into the mouth and the throat to see where the inflammation is. Many people, professional as well as laymen, fail to do this. They take the applicator or atomizer and blindly dab around in the back of the mouth, frequently touching the posterior pharynx, which is rarely involved in the infection. Often, in this type of procedure, the part most needing treatment is missed entirely. The parts most commonly infected are the tonsils and the pillars at the side of the oropharynx (where the mouth and throat meet). Incidentally, touching the posterior pharynx will cause gagging. One means of producing vomiting is to fluff out the cotton on the tip of an applicator and "tickle" the posterior pharynx.

VAGINA. The vagina is treated with many kinds of medicines in many different ways. Some of these are tampons (cotton or other absorbent material, with a string attached for removal), douches, capsules, ointments, and suppositories.

Tampons are used to apply fluid medications, as well as ointments. They are inserted well into the vaginal canal, left in the prescribed amount of time, and then removed. Capsules are usually relatively large. They are lubricated slightly and inserted well into the vaginal canal. If not contraindicated, a plain tampon may be placed at the orifice to aid in the retention of the capsule. Sometimes the capsules are to be inserted at bedtime and remain in place while the patient is asleep. They gradually dissolve and release the medication. Suppositories act in much the same way and are treated like capsules. Douches require little, if any, instruction for the adult female, for whom they are usually ordered. Here a bit of feminine hygiene can be taught. The vaginal secretions are antiseptic in nature, and too frequent douching can remove too much of the secretion, with infection following. The occasional douche is quite all right, but it should not be used too much.

RECTUM. Rectal applications are much the same as those for the vagina. However, by far the most commonly used form is the suppository. The patient must be instructed to insert the suppository well into the rectum. There are two sphincters (a muscle that closes an opening) in the rectum. The suppository must be placed about two inches beyond the second sphincter.

A word of caution here that may seem superfluous, but really is not. Be sure that the patient knows the relationship of the three openings in the vulva (perineal) area. Many patients have inserted a rectal suppository into the vagina and vice versa, or have irrigated the rectum or the bladder when a douche was ordered. This latter mistake could cause a severe infection of the bladder and even of the kidneys.

Another precaution which is essential: be sure that the patient understands that the aluminum foil is removed from the suppository before it is inserted. Many patients have lubricated the foil and inserted the suppository, covering and all. The doctor cannot understand why no results are obtained until a bit of detective work reveals what happened. Suppositories are usually oil based and need little, if any, lubrication, but a little petroleum jelly or a few drops of oil (salad oil is acceptable) may help with the insertion.

Systemic Drugs

The external cavities can be used for giving medications for systemic, as well as for topical, action. This is usually limited to the mouth and rectum.

SUBLINGUAL AND BUCCAL. Medications given by these methods are usually small, readily soluble tablets. Buccal medications are placed in the lower portion of the mouth, at the sides, but outside the teeth. Sublingual (under the tongue) drugs are placed as the name indicates, under the tongue. These areas are richly supplied with blood vessels, and the dissolved medication is taken directly into the blood stream. The patient is warned not to eat or drink anything or swallow saliva until the tablet is dissolved and the medicine has disappeared. Of course, the number of drugs that can be given this way is limited. There are several reasons for using this method: the drug would be destroyed by the digestive juices; there is no one to give the patient an injection (which is the case in most homes); and the effect of the medicine is needed quickly. The oral route (swallowing) is much slower. Nitroglycerin, a drug used for certain types of heart diseases, is usually given sublingually. It can be given orally, but its action is much slower by that route. Certain enzymes used for biologic debridement are given buccally. The digestive juices destroy these enzymes. Drugs given by these methods act almost as quickly as those given subcutaneously (by hypodermic).

RECTAL. Rectally, systemic drugs are given by suppository. The drug is absorbed by the rectal mucosa, which is likewise richly supplied with blood vessels. Unlike the oral route, the rectal route is slow. This may be an advantage, if the physician wants a delayed action. Like the sublingual and buccal procedures just discussed, the rectal method can be used for drugs that the digestive juices destroy. It can also be used when the patient cannot take anything by mouth owing to such conditions as nausea and vomiting.

ORAL ROUTE. By far the majority of medications are given by the oral route. Usually no directions other than amount and times of medication need to be given. However, a few hints may be useful.

Cough medications should not be diluted or followed by water. They should be allowed to trickle down, as part of their action is on the throat.

Fluid iron preparations, acids, and certain other minerals should be taken through a straw as they tend to stain the teeth. Rinsing of the mouth following these medications is often advisable.

Capsules are usually easier to swallow than are tablets. Both of these, and pills as well, should be placed on the back of the tongue and swallowed with a little water. Most are best followed with water, but this should be checked, as some are not to be followed by water or any other fluid. Large tablets, especially those that disintegrate quickly, can cause choking. To avoid this, unless contraindicated, tablets can be crushed and put into capsules. This method cannot be used for the various "time-release" medicines, as that would defeat their purpose. However, these tablets are rarely large. The large tablet also may be swallowed with a bolus of soft food, unless contraindicated.

Fluid drugs given to increase the appetite are "bitter." Nothing should be done to disguise the taste, as it is the bitter taste that is wanted. This stimulates the digestive juices and not only makes the patient want to eat more but also assures that the food will be better digested.

INHALATION. Drugs may be given by inhalation, again either for local or systemic effect. Most drugs given this way are administered by means of a special apparatus. Various inhalators, vaporizers, atomizers, nebulizers, intermittent positive pressure machines, and respirators are used. Each machine has its own rules, and the patient must be instructed in the proper way of using the specific equipment ordered. No general rules can be given. The assistant must consult the brochure for each apparatus. Some are for the nose, some for the mouth, and some for both. The entire procedure must be carefully explained to the patient. The drug used may be in the form of a fine powder, a fluid, or a gas. If the latter, it is often oxygen or given with oxygen. Usually this is reserved for hospitalized patients, but this is by no means always true. The patient with severe, long-term asthma or heart disease may need oxygen, with or without other medicinal gaseous substances, for months. This would require medication administration in the home. The amount of medicine to be used, in any form, must be carefully measured if it does not come premeasured, as is often the case. If the assistant studies the brochure that comes with the equipment and checks the drug to be used, she should have no difficulty explaining the process to the patient or the member of his family who will be preparing and administering the drug.

It is becoming more and more common for medications to come premeasured and ready for dispensing to the patient. This practice has greatly reduced medication errors. A word here that bears repeating: left-over drugs in the home should be destroyed! They should never be taken by anyone other than the patient, nor should the patient himself take the drugs later for "the same condition," which may or may not in fact be the same. Drugs should never be given to a neighbor when she or he has the "same" disorder. This is not only a highly dangerous practice, it is actually illegal. It constitutes practicing medicine without a license and can be punished by law. Many patients have been made worse and there have been deaths owing to such practices.

An increasing number of drugs are being given by injection. There are many reasons for this trend: topical drugs, applied to the skin, allow very little, if any, absorption, making them very unpredictable; some medicines cannot be given orally; the drug is needed for immediate action, and the oral route would be too slow; and many other reasons. The injection method of administration will be elaborated upon in the next few pages.

PARENTERAL ADMINISTRATION

The term **"parenteral"** covers all methods of giving medication (and also fluids, **electrolytes** and nutrients) by means of a needle or **cannula** introduced through the skin. The term "hypodermic" is derived from "hypo" meaning "under" and "derma" meaning "skin". Therefore, a hypodermic needle administers a medication beneath the skin. The term hypodermic has been used to designate all parenteral channels but is now mainly used in the same manner as subcutaneous ("sub" below and "cutis" skin). The term parenteral is, therefore, preferred since it refers more correctly to the introduction of medication into the body tissues or fluids through the use of a needle and is not confined to a specific level of tissue. This method of administration is used because a greater reaction to the medication may be produced.

Some medications cannot be given by way of the digestive tract because they may be rendered inactive, their action may be changed, or they may be incompatible with digestive juices. The patient may not be able to take the medication orally. Absorption of medication by parenteral methods will vary somewhat, depending upon the type of solution, the condition of the circulation in the area, and the pressure of the injection. Parenteral administration may also be used when local action is desired as in a local anesthetic or when the medication is designated to remain in a local area such as occurs with steroid implants or hormone implants.

Types of Injections

The more important forms of parenteral administration with which the medical assistant will deal are the intramuscular, subcutaneous (hypodermic), intradermal,

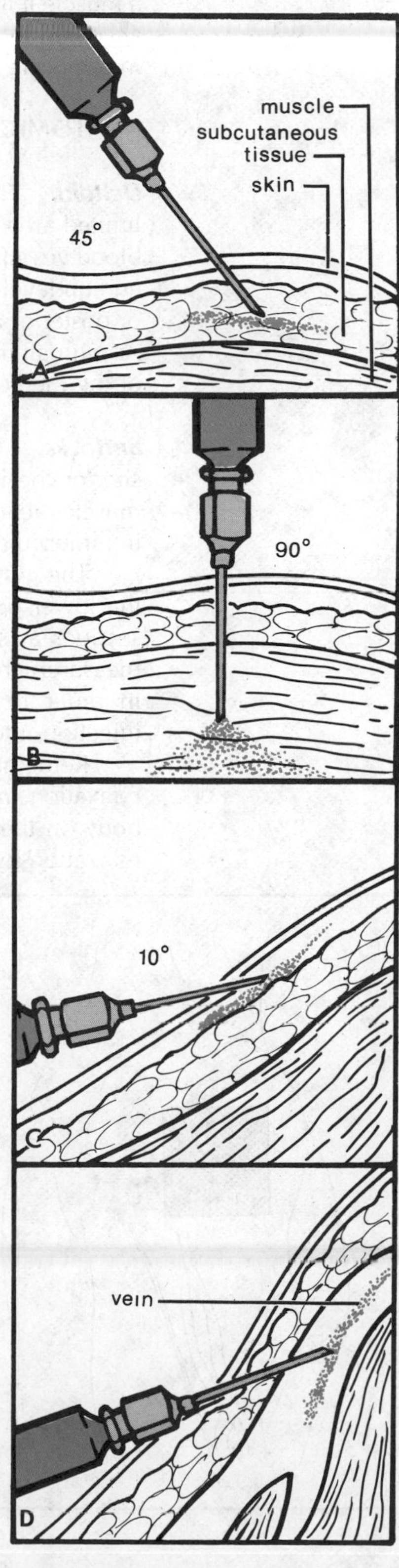

FIGURE 24–1 Needle insertion for types of injections. *A*, Subcutaneous; *B*, intramuscular; *C*, intradermal; and *D*, intravenous.

and intravenous methods (Fig. 24–1). The first three may be administered by the medical assistant under the supervision and instructions of the physician. Intravenous injections are administered by the physician with the medical assistant assisting, but some medical assistants are taught to withdraw blood intravenously for diagnostic purposes under the supervision of a physician.

Intramuscular

"Intra" means "within" and "muscular" signifies "muscle." Therefore, intramuscular injections are administered into a muscle. A medication may be administered into a muscle if it is irritating to the areolar tissue (connective tissue). Larger doses may be accepted by a muscle than by other tissues. Medications are more rapidly absorbed in a muscle than in the upper tissues.

ANATOMICAL SITES FOR INTRAMUSCULAR INJECTIONS

Deltoid. The upper outer arm in the middeltoid muscle is used. This is a somewhat limited area and will not accept large amounts of medication. The major nerve and blood vessels are in the posterior portion. It will have some limited use if it is a small and undeveloped muscle, as in small children. Only the lateral area, not the anterior or posterior areas, is used. The brachial nerve and blood vessels are major hazards. As with all intramuscular injections, the muscle must be relaxed for proper injection of the medication (Fig. 24–2).

Buttocks. The gluteus medius muscle of the buttocks is probably the most common site for the intramuscular (IM) injection, especially in the ambulatory patient. This muscle accepts moderately large amounts of medication, more than the other intramuscular sites.

The gluteal area is measured from the crest of the ilium (top of the hip bone) to the lower portion of the cheek of the buttocks. This area is then divided into four sections as shown in Figure 24–3. Note the insert in this figure showing incorrect measurement. Injections must be restricted to the upper outer quadrant as indicated in order to prevent serious damage to the sciatic nerve and an **intravascular** injection into a major blood vessel.

Remember that the muscle must be relaxed for a proper injection. This relaxation may be obtained by having the standing patient bear the weight of the body on the opposite side of the injection. The standing patient may also contain relaxation by placing the toes inward as far as possible in an exaggerated "pigeon–

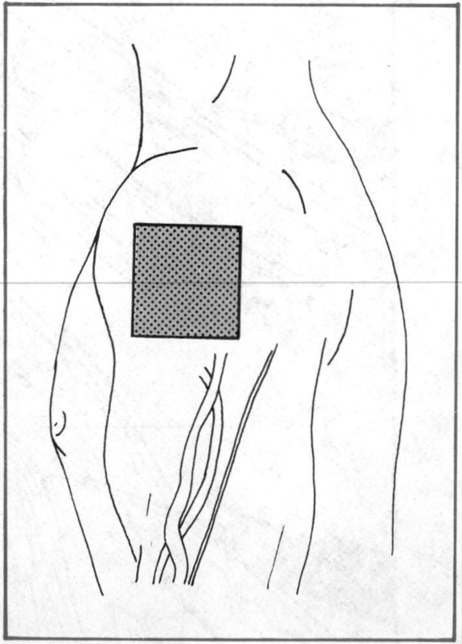

FIGURE 24–2 Injection site in the mid-deltoid muscle.

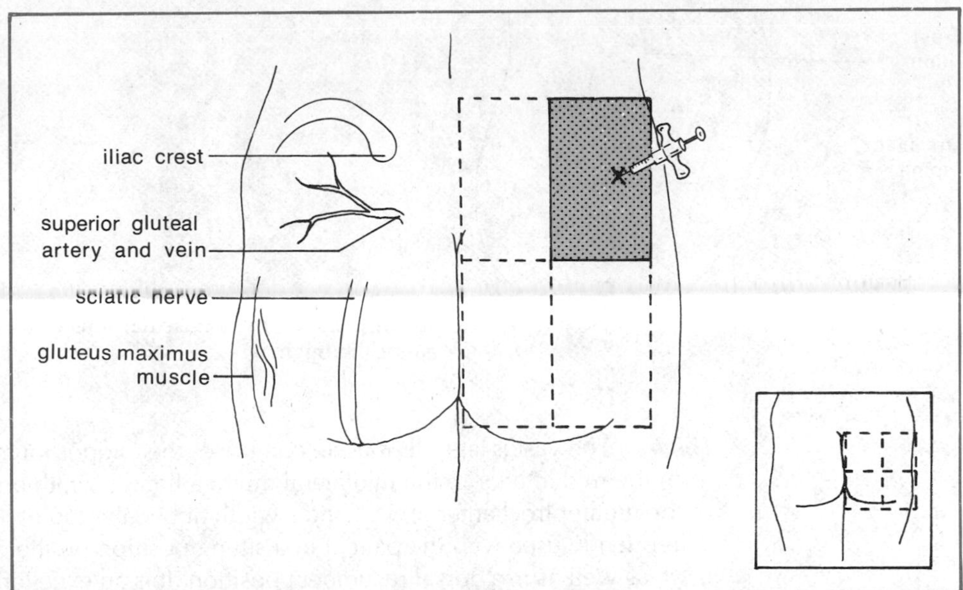

FIGURE 24–3 Injection site in the upper outer quadrant of the gluteus. Inset shows a common *incorrect* marking of the site. Remember to consider the whole buttock, not just the lower, fleshier area.

toed" posture. The patient may lean only slightly forward and have the support of the examining table. It is not advisable to bend too far because this will extend the muscle and diminish its ability to accept the medication easily. If the patient is in a prone position, the toes should be turned inward while the heels are allowed to fall out in a relaxed position. The site of the quadrant does not change whether the patient is standing or prone.

The prone position is recommended in the following situations:

1. administration of the medication is painful.
2. administration of a medication that must be given very slowly.
3. the "Z" tract method of injection is used (Fig. 24–14).
4. the patient feels faint or is weak.
5. the patient does not appear to be able to hold still in the standing position.
6. the medication is of a large quantity and has a rapid seepage into the lower tissues.

Remember — It is believed that some injections into the buttocks are not given deep enough, thus depositing the medication into adipose tissue rather than into the muscle. This fatty tissue does not absorb medication well, and the medication may remain at the site of injection. There is less discomfort to the patient if the medication is properly placed in the muscle and not in fatty tissue. You should be certain to select long enough needles for obese patients.

Hip. The ventrogluteal muscle is gaining use as a site for intramuscular injections. It has been used for the bedridden patient for some time but only recently has this site been used for the **ambulatory** patient. One of the advantages is it may have less fatty tissue overlying the muscle. This, of course, depends on the patient's distribution of fat. This muscle is also thicker than the gluteal medius.

The patient is best placed in the Sims's position but may lie dorsally or prone, if necessary. To locate the site, place your right palm on the patient's left greater trochanter, put your index finger on the anterior iliac spine, and spread your middle finger posteriorly as far as possible from your index finger, trying to touch the crest of the ilium. The center of the triangle formed by the index and middle fingers is the site for the injection (Fig. 24–4). The opposite hand is used on the patient's other side, that is, your left hand is used to select the site on the patient's right hip.

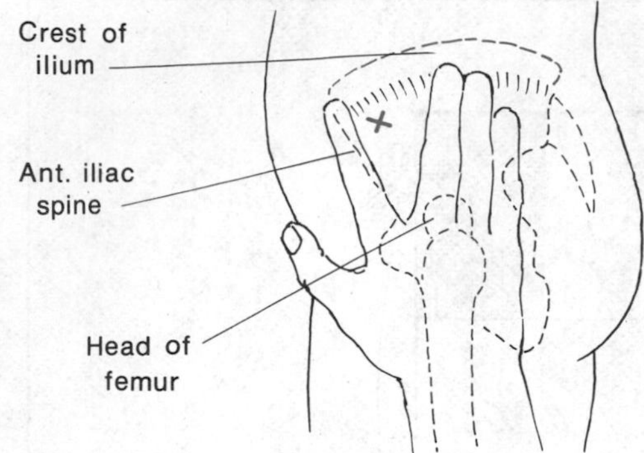

FIGURE 24–4 **Intramuscular injection in the ventrogluteal muscle of the thigh.**

Thigh. The vastus lateralis muscle comprises the midportion of the thigh, extending from the midanterior to the midlateral thigh, a hand's width below the proximal end of the greater trochanter and a hand's width above the top of the knee cap. The area is frequently used with the patient in a sitting position on the edge of the examining table as well as in a dorsal recumbent position. It is an excellent site for patients who have to administer their own injections and is used for both adults and children (Fig. 24–5).

EQUIPMENT USED FOR INTRAMUSCULAR INJECTIONS. Intramuscular injections use a wider range of needle lengths and gauge than any other injection. The selection will depend upon the **viscosity** (thickness) of the medication and the depth of the muscle to be reached. A deltoid may use a 25 gauge, ⅝ in. for a small arm to a 23 gauge, 1 in. for an average arm. If there is considerable adipose tissue over the site, this must be taken into consideration. Remember to consider the depth of the adipose *plus* the depth into the muscle. The buttocks will take a greater range of needle sizes because of the wide variation of the overlying fatty tissue. A child may take a 1 in. needle, whereas an obese adult patient may take one 2½ in. or longer. The average buttocks needle is from 1¼ to 1½ in. Remember that **adipose** tissue does not absorb medication. It should also be remembered that there is less discomfort with a medication given deep in a muscle than one given more shallowly.

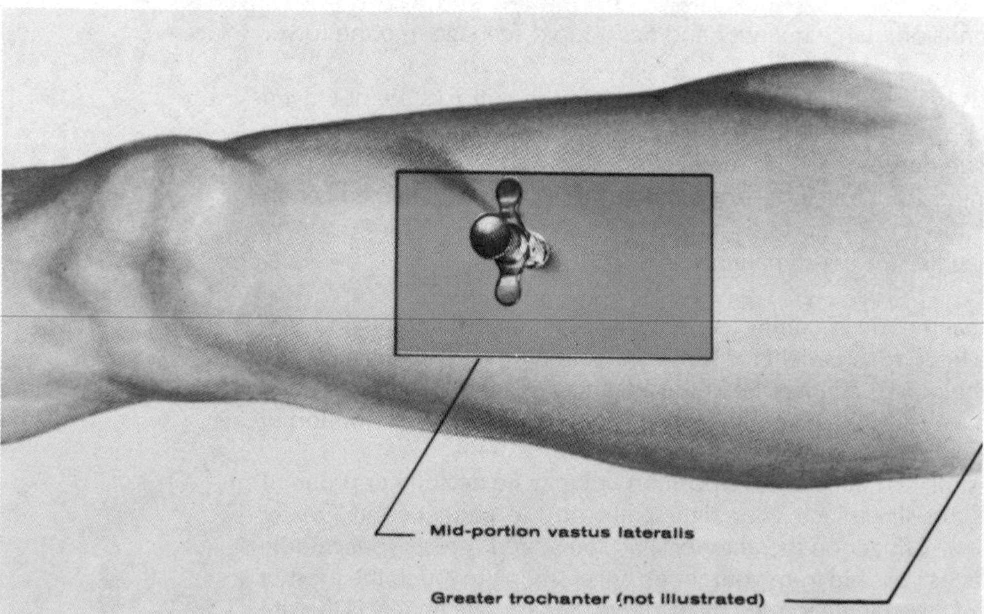

FIGURE 24–5 **Vastus lateralis muscle of the thigh for intramuscular injection (Courtesy of Wyeth Laboratories, Philadelphia, Pa.)**

The gauge of the needle is dictated by the medication and the needle's length. A patient cannot feel the difference between a 22 gauge and a 20 gauge needle, but the medication is forced into the tissue with less force when a 20 gauge is used. A longer needle should be of a larger gauge to prevent too much flexibility.

Subcutaneous

As mentioned before, this method is sometimes called "hypodermic injection." Medications administered by this method are given when the rate of absorption is moderate. It takes about 30 minutes for the maximal effect. The subcutaneous tissue does not accept as large a dose as does a large muscle. Because the skin is the largest organ of the body there are numerous sites for "subq" injections. The upper outer arm is probably the most common site. Another is the anterior and lateral aspects of the thigh. Patients who are taught to administer their own injections often find that the thigh and lower abdomen are easily reached. Patients receiving frequent injections, as is often the case with subcutaneous medications, should alternate the sites of injection.

The subcutaneous layer contains the connective tissue that binds the skin to the deeper tissues. There is some degree of elasticity in these tissues, but the sensitivity is greater and larger doses give more discomfort. Doses are usually less than 1 cc or 1 ml and are usually never more than 2 cc. The thickness of the skin does vary somewhat over the body, so there are slight variations in length of the needles used. Most subq needles are ⅜ to ½ in. long. Gauges range from 27 to 25; the larger gauges are not often used because heavier medications are not usually given into the subcutaneous areas. The length of the needle is not selected because of the depth. Whether a shorter or longer needle is used, the depth is approximately the same since the injecting needle is held at an angle of about 45°, and the needle is slipped under the skin into the connective tissue layer (see Figure 24–1B).

Intradermal

The majority of intradermal (Id) injections are done for diagnostic purposes, such as testing for allergic reactions, sensitivities to drugs, and the presence of or resistance to disease. Examples of these are the tuberculin skin test, the Schick test for susceptibility to diphtheria, and the Dick test for susceptibility to scarlet fever. This method of injection also has a longer period of absorption than the intramuscular and subcutaneous methods.

Because the solution is injected into the upper layer of the skin, there is sometimes a slight stinging or burning sensation relative to the amount of the substance injected.

As with the subcutaneous injection, the sites are as great as the area of skin. The preferred sites are the **dorsal** (inner) surface of the lower arm and the **lateral** portion of the upper arm. Since it is essential that the skin be pulled taut, these sites allow for an easy, proper injection. Skin reactions are also easy to observe in these locations. The anterior portion of the thighs are also used when many intradermal tests are done, especially in allergy testing. The upper and lower limbs are usually preferred to the back since a tourniquet may be applied to localize the absorption in the appendage, preventing a possible **systemic** reaction.

The amount of fluid injected in an Id injection is very small. It will range from 0.01 to 0.2 cc. The lesser amount is usually sufficient to give a reaction for allergy testing. When an Id injection is correctly performed, a small **wheal** will be formed, lasting only a few moments (Fig. 24–6). The site is not massaged after the injection, only blotted gently.

The tuberculin syringe is usually used for an intradermal injection because the smaller calibrations of this syringe are necessary for accurate measurement. The needle used is a small 27 gauge ⅜ in. or 26 gauge ½ in. Often these needles have an intradermal bevel that is shorter than the regular bevel. The shorter bevel makes it unnecessary to go as far into the skin as would be necessary with a regular bevel (Fig. 25–18B).

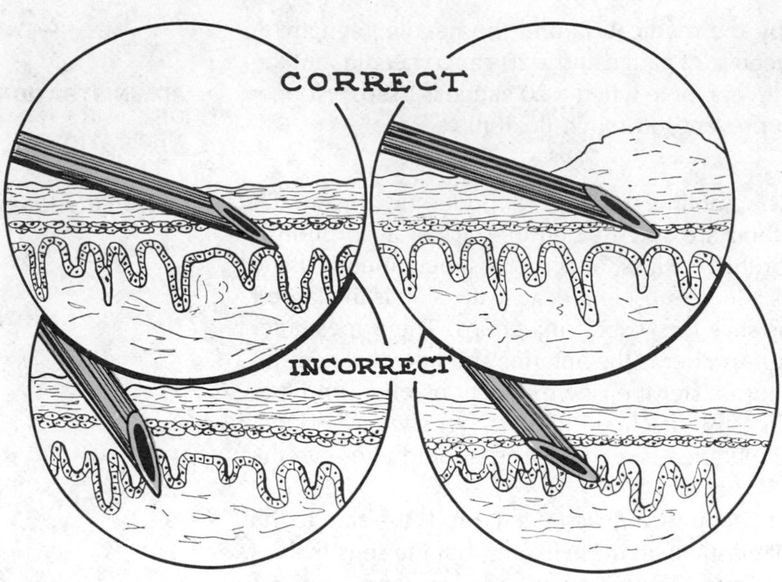

FIGURE 24–6 Angle of needle insertion for intradermal injection. (From Halsted, J. A.: *The Laboratory in Clinical Medicine*. Philadelphia, W. B. Saunders Company, 1976.)

METHOD OF INTRADERMAL INJECTIONS. There are several methods for holding a needle and syringe unit for an intradermal injection. Individuals doing many Id injections each day work out the best method for themselves. Whichever method is preferred, it is advisable to pull the skin as taut as possible, being careful not to pinch or give the patient any discomfort. With the bevel facing up the needle will slide easily into tightly pulled skin. A sudden insertion usually goes too deep for an intradermal injection. Remember that only the bevel of the needle should slide under the skin. When the bevel is within the skin's upper layer, press the plunger in very carefully until a small wheal is formed. There will be some resistance in the plunger if you are in the correct layer of the skin.

The usual method of injection, especially for the patient's anterior forearm, is to grasp the patient's arm from the underside so the skin may be pulled tight (Fig. 24–7). The skin also may be spread tightly from above. Use the long flat surface of the thumb to prevent a gouging pressure that only causes discomfort for the patient and does little to tighten the skin. The syringe unit is held between the index and great fingers, allowing the thumb to push the plunger in. Another technique that is

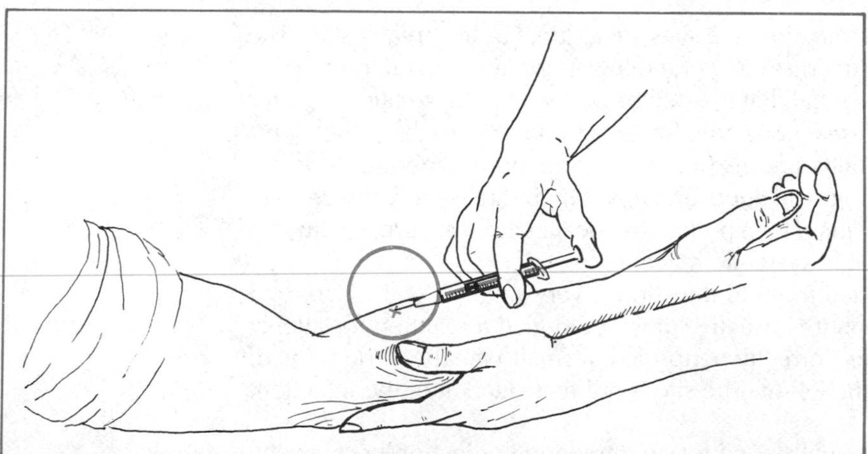

FIGURE 24–7 Intradermal injection on the lower inner arm. The site is located about 2 in. below the antecubital area (bend) on the inner arm. The patient is seated with the arm resting on a table top. The medical assistant stands directly in front, facing the patient. The patient's skin may be pulled taut by grasping under the arm as shown, or by pulling the skin taut from directly above the injection site with the medical assistant's hand over the arm.

useful for the upper arm is to grasp the upper arm the same way as you would the lower arm. The syringe is held in the palm of the hand as an artist holds a brush. The unit is positioned so the plunger may be pushed in with the **proximal** area of the little finger. It is very difficult to push the plunger in if you have positioned the plunger near the distal joint of the little finger. The needle is gently eased into the skin as if you were taking out a very small splinter in the skin. If a wheal does not appear as you are injecting the solution, you are probably too deep. You can also tell if you are too deep if the plunger is pushed in easily.

This type of injection of medication has a longer period of absorption compared to the intramuscular and subcutaneous routes. If allergy skin testing is done, any reaction usually appears locally within 20 to 30 minutes.

Children and Infants

Administering injections to small children and infants may present special problems. There are three sites used for intramuscular injections: midanterior portion of the rectus femoris muscle of the thigh, the midlateral portion of the vastus lateralis muscle of the thigh, and the deltoid muscle of the lateral portion of the upper arm. The gluteus medius muscle in the buttocks is not usually used because it is less developed in the very young patient. For the same reason, the deltoid may be used only for smaller doses (Fig. 24–8).

Any site that is selected on an infant or small child for a injection has a greater margin of error because of the limited surface area, as compared to an adult, and the smallness of the underlying muscle used. Safety restraints are sometimes in order to avoid injury to the infant or child. If the child is old enough to understand, then be

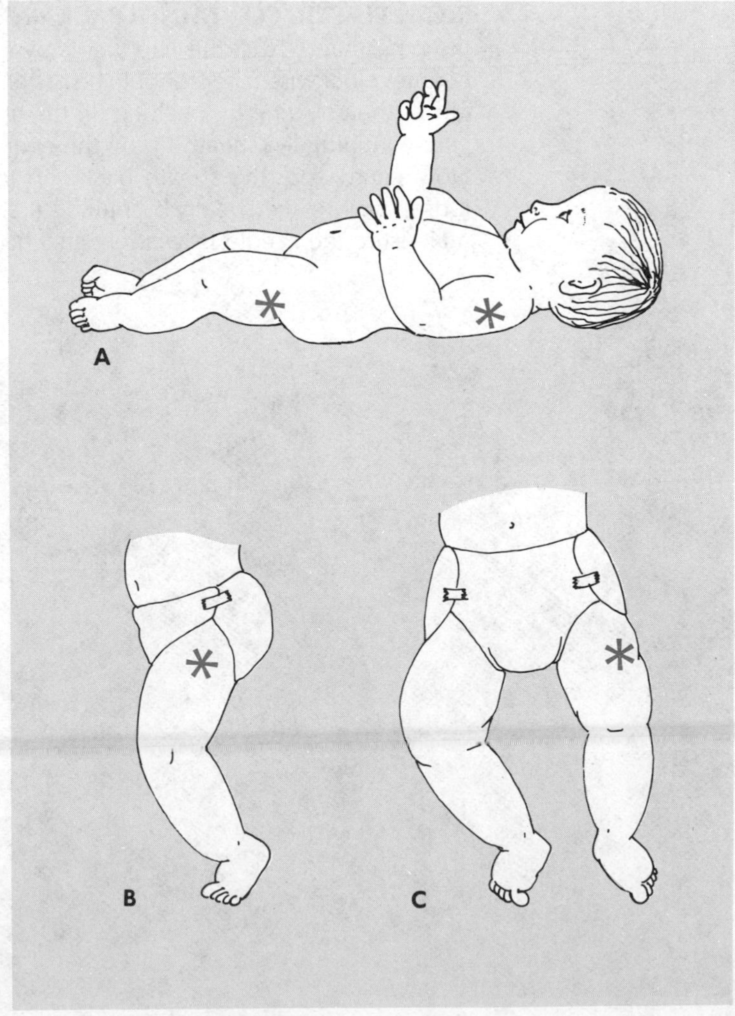

FIGURE 24–8 Injection sites on infants. *A*, upper arm (deltoid muscle) or lateral thigh (vastus lateralis muscle). *B*, lateral thigh (vastus lateralis muscle). *C*, anterior thigh (rectus femoris muscle).

honest and tell the child it may hurt for a moment but that it is important to hold very still. After the injection, remain with the child, giving assurance and affection that will aid in decreasing the fear and hurt. Always have the physician show you where to give the injection and then make certain you follow all the instructions carefully.

Preparing for an Injection

1. Wash your hands.
2. Check the patient's name and medical record. It is a double check to call the patient by name when greeting him.
3. Select the correct syringe and needle unit and assemble the necessary disinfecting materials for the medication container and the patient's skin.
4. Check the medication again.

PEEL-APART PAPER PACKAGE UNIT. This type of packaging is designed so the contents may be dropped on to a sterile area without being touched (Fig. 24–9). The syringe is exposed but the needle sheath (needle covering) remains on the needle. Remove the sheath by grasping the syringe with one hand and, with the other hand, grasp the portion of the sheath over the hub of the needle and gently rock. Do not twist because this will loosen the needle from the syringe tip. Then pull the sheath *straight* off slowly in order to prevent jerking back and contaminating the needle as well as possibly injuring yourself. The thumbnail of the hand holding the syringe may be placed on the small flange at the base of the needle hub in order to help secure the needle while removing the sheath. Now grasp the hub of the needle to check that it is securely attached to the syringe tip.

RIGID PLASTIC CONTAINER PACKAGING. Grasp the unit in your hand and, with the other hand, twist the cap that is over the plunger end of the syringe by turning counter clockwise. There should be a slight snap as the seal is broken. Slide the syringe out of the covering by pushing on the tip of the needle sheath with your thumb or gently tapping the sheath tip on the counter. The sheath will remain on the needle. Now gently rock the sheath back and forth by grasping over the hub end. When loose, remove the sheath by pulling it straight off. Grasp the hub of the needle to make sure the needle is securely attached to the syringe (Fig. 24–10).

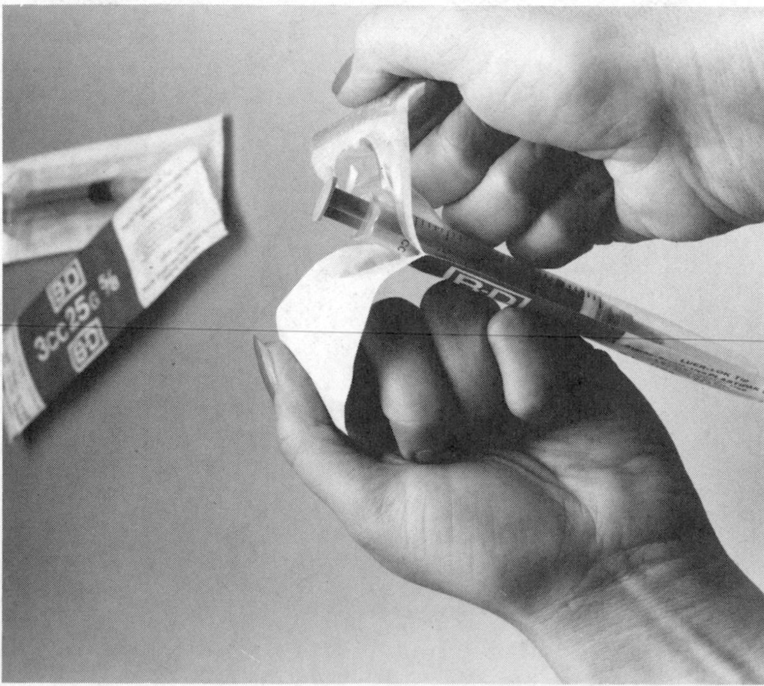

FIGURE 24–9 Peel-apart package for disposable syringe and needle unit. (Courtesy of Becton, Dickinson and Co.)

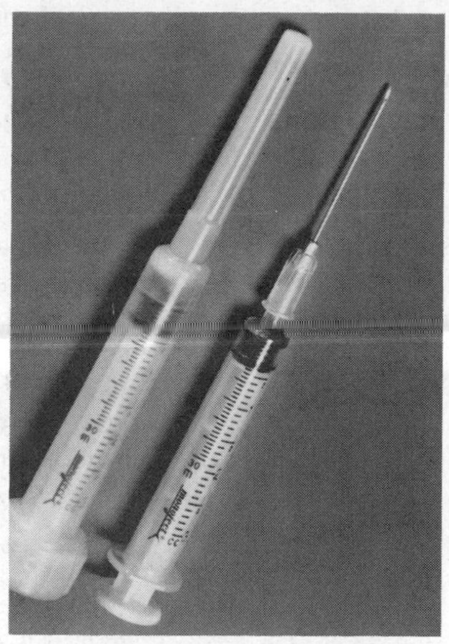

FIGURE 24–10 Rigid plastic package for disposable syringe and needle unit. (Courtesy of Wyeth Co.)

MULTIPLE SYRINGE PACKAGING. Multiple packaging is convenient for the medical office that uses a considerable number of a single type of syringe each day. An allergist's office is one likely example. These packages may be referred to as an "Allergy Tray" (Fig. 24–11). A single opening will expose 25 syringes with individual needle sheaths to maintain sterility. The trays are of lightweight plastic and are easily stored. There is considerable time saved with this type of multiple packaging.

FILLING A SYRINGE FROM A MULTIPLE DOSE VIAL. A vial is usually a multiple dose container that has a rubber stopper to facilitate multiple entries. Vials vary greatly in size, from 1 or 2 cc to 50 or more doses. Because they are entered more than once, extreme caution must be taken every time a needle is inserted into the medication. Contamination of the contents could be very serious. If at any time an error is made and there is danger of possible contamination, the medication should be discarded. Never return unused medication to the vial. Avoid danger of an infection; no medication is more valuable than a patient's health.

Read the Label Three Times

1. Read the label carefully when removing it from the storage place.
2. Read the label again when you are preparing the medication.

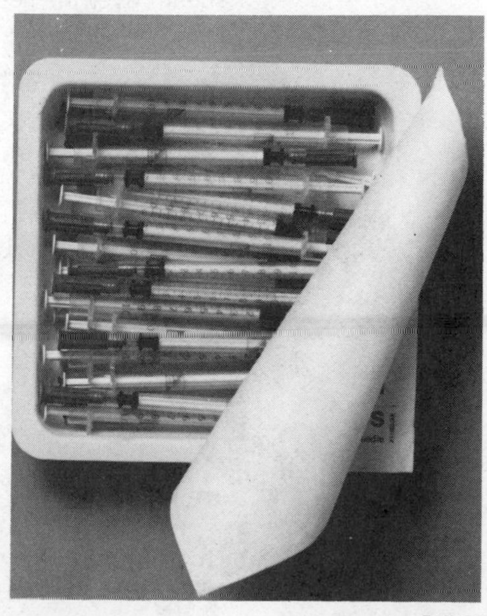

FIGURE 24–11 An allergy tray, opened to reveal syringes. (Courtesy of Becton, Dickinson and Co.)

3. Read it again when you return the medication to the storage place. Make certain it is the correct patient by repeating the patient's name. Check the patient's medical record again to see that you have the correct medication, the correct dose, and you understand the physician's instructions.

Preparation

1. Cleanse the rubber stopper of the vial thoroughly. Many manufacturers package vials with a "dust cap" to guarantee sterility and to show it has not previously been entered. This cap is easily torn off and sometimes may be replaced after use as an added precaution.

2. Pull the plunger of the syringe back to draw into the syringe enough air to equal the amount of medication that will be withdrawn from the vial. This air-medication exchange prevents a vacuum from forming in the vial and thus permits easy withdrawal of the medication and utilization of the entire amount of the contents. A very slight pressure maintained in the vial will make withdrawal easier.

3. Insert the needle into the cleansed rubber stopper with the bevel of the needle facing upward, and put slight pressure on the back of the needle so the needle enters the stopper at a slight angle. This method of entering a vial prevents the possibility of a rubber plug cut, which would then be injected into the medication. Be careful not to use so much pressure that the needle bends. Push the needle in so the tip of the needle is through the stopper.

4. The air in the syringe is now injected into the vial. It is best to inject the air into the space in the vial and not through the medication.

5. Now invert the vial directly above the syringe and, with the tip of the needle in the medication, gently pull the plunger back and fill the syringe with the correct dosage of medication (Fig. 24–12). Some air bubbles may be removed by gently tapping on the syringe and pushing the plunger back a little. Since it is not good procedure to "play" medicine and air back and forth, it may be best to withdraw the amount of medication needed and then withdraw the unit from the vial. Return vial to counter. Pull the plunger back, creating one large bubble in the tip of the syringe. Tap the syringe with your finger, then slowly push the plunger into the barrel. The unit must be held straight up in order to expel all the air. Stop when the correct dosage is measured and a drop of medication appears in the tip of the needle. Then withdraw the plunger very slightly in order to clear the medication from the lumen of the needle.

If the medication is not administered immediately, replace the sterile needle sheath over the needle to protect it from contamination.

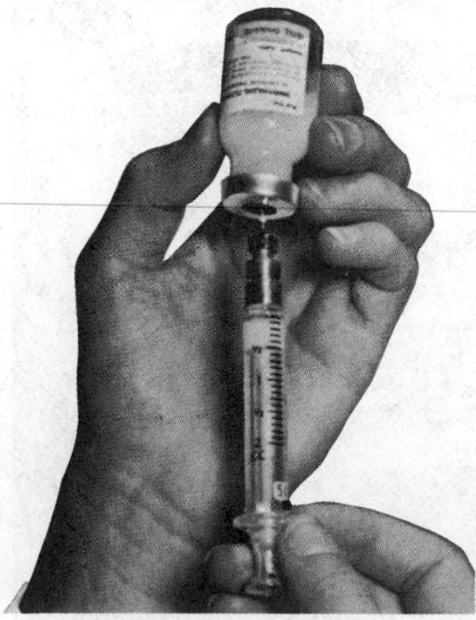

FIGURE 24–12 Filling a syringe from a multiple-dose vial.

FILLING A SYRINGE FROM A SINGLE DOSE AMPULE. Many medications are prepared in single dose glass ampules. Remember to check the label carefully for the correct content and strength of the desired medication.

1. Gently tap the top of the ampule to remove any contents that may be in the top. Do not shake or tap too hard because some medications foam easily.

2. Cleanse the ampule at the breaking point with an antiseptic. This area is usually marked by a line or there is a depression in the neck of the ampule. It may be necessary to use a small file provided by the manufacturer and found in the box. Score the ampule at the breaking point to facilitate easier breaking.

3. The ampule may be opened by giving the top a sharp tap so the top will break away from you. If the ampule is large or does not snap off easily, it may be necessary to break off the top by carefully "bending" it at the weakened breaking point. This is done by folding a sterile gauze around the area. Do not squeeze because this may shatter the glass. Ampules are manufactured with a slight pressure within the ampule so as to "blow out" any minute pieces of glass.

4. Do not put any air in the syringe.

5. Insert the needle into the distal portion of the ampule, being careful not to touch the opening of the ampule.

6. Withdraw the medication slowly.

7. Hold the syringe unit straight up and withdraw the plunger slightly in order to collect all the air bubbles in the tip of the syringe. Slowly push the plunger into the barrel until the air has been expelled and the medicine appears in the tip of the needle. Withdraw the plunger very slightly in order to clear the lumen of the needle of medication (Fig. 24–13).

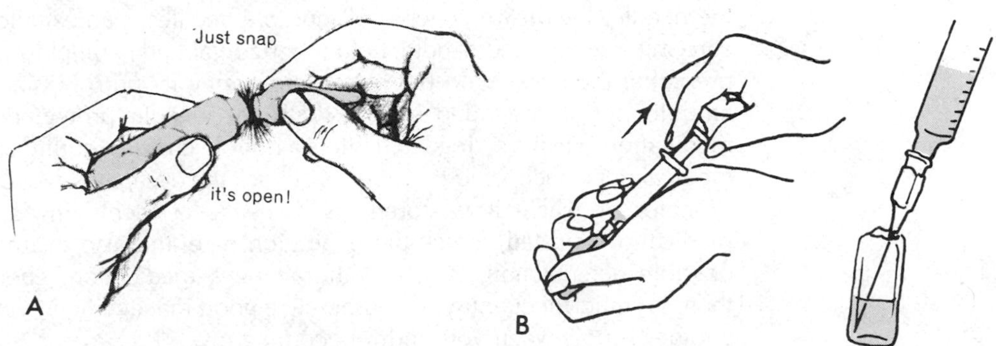

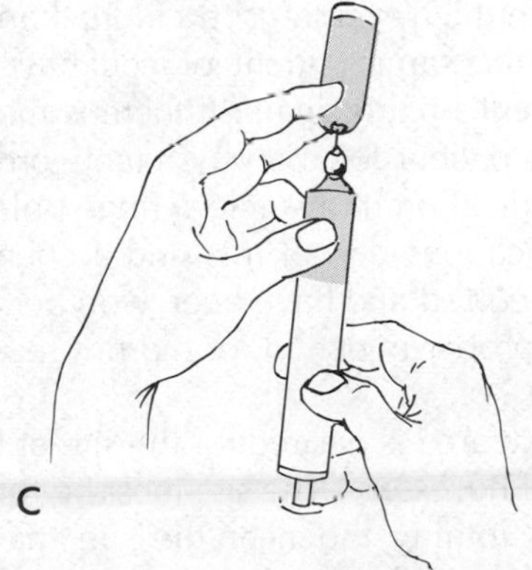

FIGURE 24–13 **Filling a syringe from a single-dose ampule. *A,* Snap it open. *B,* Holding syringe in a downward position. (From Wood, L. A., and Rambo, B. J.: *Nursing Skills for Allied Health Sciences.* 2nd ed., vol. 3. Philadelphia, W. B. Saunders Co., 1980.) *C,* Holding the syringe in an upright vertical position. The needle tip is only slightly entered into the ampule opening and the plunger withdrawn immediately. Surface tension of the liquid prevents the medication from running out. You must keep a steady suction on the plunger if this method is used.**

To facilitate more rapid withdrawal of a viscid medication, it is sometimes advisable to withdraw it from the container with a shorter needle of larger gauge, such as an 18 gauge, 1 in. than will be used for the injection. This is also recommended if the medication is irritating to the tissues nearer the body surface as with medications administered by the "Z" tract method. The injecting needle is then free of any medication.

Needles are changed by grasping the sheath over the hub and giving a slight turn to loosen. The replacing needle is then secured to the syringe top, holding the needle in the same place and with pressure, forcing the needle onto the syringe tip with a slight turn. Check to make sure that the needle is secured with the syringe tip. Remove the needle sheath with a gentle rocking motion.

Read the manufacturer's package insert before administering a medication by injection. Some medications have special precautions. Heavy oil-based medications recommend that 0.5 cc of air be injected following the medication. This will clear the needle and prevent a leakage along the injection tract. This is especially important with medications that irritate the upper tissues.

Giving an Injection

When giving a medication by injection great care should be taken. The procedure may become easy and even automatic, but as stated before and stressed often, always use the correct technique, follow the physician's orders, recheck the patient's name, and read the label carefully again. Do not vary from your instructions.

Make certain that all the materials needed are ready for use. Many offices have a central room where medications are prepared and then taken to the waiting patient in another room. This has many advantages, but care must be taken that the syringe and needle unit are transported to the other area with sterile technique. Always cover the needle; the **sheath** covering disposable needles is an excellent protector. When carrying a syringe and needle, hold it horizontal and parallel to your body. If you are preparing the medication but not administering it yourself, place the vial or empty ampule beside the filled syringe with the needle protected. This shows what medication is in the syringe and offers a double check. Acquire the habit taught to all medical personnel: *Read the label . . . check the dosage.* Never depend on the shape or color or where it is stored, as a means of identifying a medication. If the medication is dated, check the expiration date and also examine the contents for possible deterioration. Before withdrawing a medication, check to make certain there is sufficient quantity. If you practice good management, you will have ordered another supply when you find it becoming low.

If the medication is prepared in a central room, great care must be taken to ensure that the medication is given to the right patient. Do *not* wrap the needle with a piece of gauze or cotton to keep it sterile. Never transport more than one injection at a time unless two or more are for the same patient or you have a special medication injection tray. Check the patient's name again. If there is more than one physician, make certain it is the correct patient for the physician's orders you are following. Never put more than one medication in a single syringe unless specifically ordered by the physician. Some medications do not mix and a chemical change may take place. Many lawsuits have occurred and have been won because a patient received the wrong medication, an improper injection, or did not receive a drug ordered for him.

Explain to the patient what area is desired for the site of the injection. Assist the patient in exposing the area, if necessary. The site must be fully exposed to facilitate correct anatomic selection. Clothing too near the site may also be a source of contamination or may act as a possible tourniquet, increase the depth of fatty tissue, or slip during the injection and interfere with the procedure.

Cleanse the site of the injection thoroughly with a sterile sponge saturated with a skin disinfectant. Keep the sponge between the index and middle fingers of the hand that does not give the injection. This still allows the hand to grasp the patient's skin and also to have the sponge ready immediately after the injecting needle is removed.

Hold the syringe and needle with your injecting hand. With the other hand, which has cleansed the skin, draw the skin to make it taut. When the skin is spread, make certain your fingers have not rubbed over the site that was cleansed for the injection. If the skin is not pulled tightly at the point of injection, the needle will not penetrate readily and some pain may be felt. Also, the gentle tautening of the skin will distract the patient from the actual injection. Sometimes the skin is squeezed up at the site of the injection. This depends on the type of skin, the area used, and the position of the patient relative to the medical assistant. Its appropriateness is learned mostly through experience. The technique may, however, change the distribution of fatty tissue and prevent the administration of the medication at the correct depth.

Hold the syringe unit between the thumb and the fingers and, with the wrist relaxed, insert the needle with a short, quick darting motion. In intramuscular injections, the needle is inserted to about ⅛ in. from the hub of the needle. It is best never to insert the needle completely to the hub; in case it breaks off, the small amount exposed makes removal comparatively easy. (A broken needle is *extremely* rare and practically never happens if proper technique has been used.)

All intramuscular and subcutaneous injections should be aspirated. To **aspirate** is to create a suction by pulling the plunger of the syringe back slightly. This precaution must not be omitted. Although it is extremely rare, there is always danger that the tip of the needle has been introduced into a blood vessel and an intravascular injection would inadvertently be given. This is especially dangerous with a medication that reads "for intramuscular administration only."

Aspiration may be done by holding the syringe between the thumb and the ring finger and pulling the plunger up between the index and great fingers. This technique is helpful when the hand that is holding the skin taut cannot be moved. The plungers of some syringes are difficult to pull, and it is necessary to use the noninjecting hand to pull the plunger back. If the tip of the needle is in a blood vessel, blood will appear in the tip of the syringe. Only a gentle pull is necessary, enough to slightly move the plunger outward. **Take care that the position of the needle does not change during the aspiration or after the aspiration,** because the change of location of the needle tip may place it in a blood vessel. *If* blood is aspirated *do not inject into this area*; withdraw the needle and inject about an inch from the original site. It is preferred that another complete unit of medication be prepared and administered. If you are not in a blood vessel, about 0.2 cc of air may appear in the syringe tip. This will do no harm and will aid in the diffusion of the medication, minimize pain, and prevent leakage of the medication along the puncture site.

As you start injecting the medication, release the hand that is holding the tissue slightly to facilitate entrance of the medication at a moderately slow speed to allow for distention of the tissue and to avoid pain from the pressure of the medication entering the tissue. Most medications can be injected by placing the index finger on the plunger of the syringe and gently pressing. Take extreme care not to move the syringe about while aspirating and injecting, because there is equal amount of movement of the needle within the tissue and it will cause pain as well as destroy tissue or may cause the needle tip to slip into a blood vessel.

After all the medication has been injected, withdraw the needle quickly in the same path as it was injected. If a slight clicking sound is heard on removal, it may mean that the syringe was not brought out along the same line on which it was inserted. This will cause pain to the patient as well as increase the size of the canal through which the needle passed into the tissue.

Immediately upon removal of the needle place the sterile sponge over the site of the injection. Do not push in with one finger, but use a broad flat surface of several fingers. Massage the site gently but firmly. Most beginners tend to rub the skin surface rather than massage. If the instructions are "Do not massage site of injection," hold the sterile sponge firmly over the site for a few moments. If the injected area shows signs of bleeding, keep pressure on it for a few more moments. Cover with a small dressing or Band-Aid if necessary.

Assist the patient from the examining table. Some patients may appreciate assistance in dressing; if not, respect the patient's privacy. If the medication was painful or the patient was apprehensive of the injection, it may be best to allow the patient to rest for a few minutes. Never leave a patient unattended immediately after an injection but wait for a few minutes and chat.

If the syringe and needle are reusable, rinse immediately in running tap water. If a disposable unit was used, make certain the needle is broken and the syringe destroyed. Manufacturers of disposable syringes and needles are now marketing small units that destroy these items and make them safe for the trash (see Figs. 25–20 and 25–21).

Record the medication given, the strength and the site of the injection, the date, and by whom it was administered, if there are several persons giving injections.

"Z-TRACT" METHOD OF INTRAMUSCULAR INJECTION. Some medications are absorbed more rapidly into the muscle than in the subcutaneous tissue. Because of poor absorption and possible irritation in the subcutaneous tissue, the injection must be given in such a method as to prevent any leakage back from the deep muscle into the upper subcutaneous tissue. These medications are always given into the gluteal muscle of the buttocks and never given into the deltoid or other less deep areas. For these medications the "Z-tract" method is used for injection and a longer needle than usual is employed (Fig. 24–14). This method of injection displaces the upper tissue laterally before the needle is inserted.

1. Prepare the skin for injection as previously instructed.

2. Before the needle is inserted, pull skin to one side and hold firmly in place. If the skin is slippery from the cleansing solution, the cleansing gauze will aid in holding the skin in place.

3. Insert the needle, making certain you are deep in the muscle and not in adipose or cutaneous tissue. DO NOT RELEASE THE SKIN.

4. You may aspirate by using the first and second fingers of the syringe hand to pull upwards on the plunger.

5. If the needle tip is in the correct area, inject the medication slowly. Some medications will carry the instruction to inject 0.5 cc of air following injection of the medication. This air will clear the needle of the medication and prevent it from following along the tract of injection. This air can be pulled into the syringe after the medication has been drawn in. Because the patient is in a prone position the air will be the last to enter the tissue.

6. Wait a few seconds before withdrawing the needle. Immediately upon withdrawal of the needle release the skin.

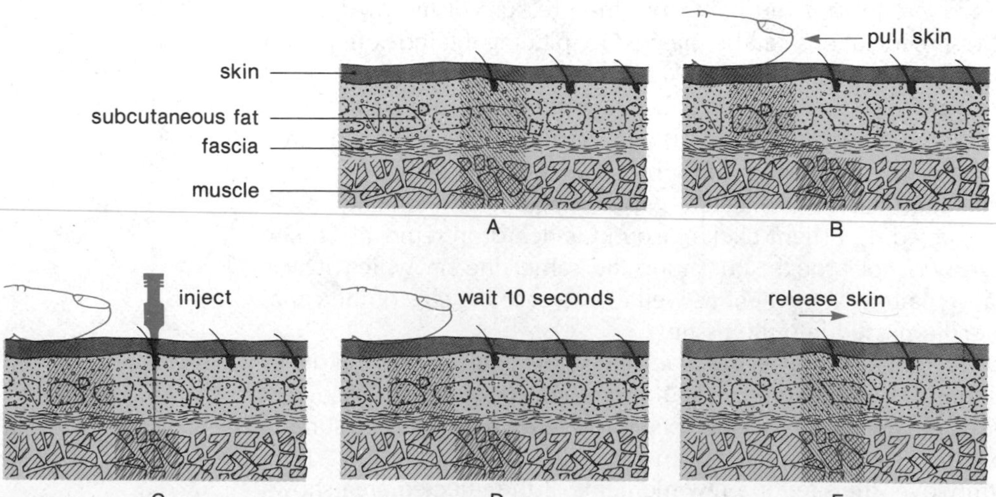

FIGURE 24–14 "Z–tract" method of lateral skin displacement prior to insertion of hypodermic needle. The injection channel is sealed off after release.

7. Check the instructions accompanying the medication. Many medications that require the "Z-tract" method of injection should not be massaged after injection; just hold a sterile sponge over the area for a few moments.

8. Walking will not hurt but will help in the absorption. Avoid pulling a tight girdle over the site of injection. Use alternate buttocks for injections.

Dangers of Incorrect Injecting Technique

1. One of the greatest dangers is the introduction of an infection through the hole made in the skin by a contaminated needle, syringe, or medication.

2. There may be irreparable damage to a major nerve or other structure due to incorrect selection of the injection site or needle.

3. Medication deposited into the wrong tissue may result in tissue damage, resulting in a health hazard to the patient.

4. There may be tissue damage due to the selection of the wrong needle, a dull needle, or excessive movement of the needle while it is within the tissue.

5. The introduction of a foreign particle into the tissue could result in a sterile or nonsterile abscess. This may be the result of a piece of lint from cotton caught on a needle or left on the skin from the disinfectant pledget, or it may be a minute particle in the lumen of the needle.

Avoiding Dangers of Incorrect Injecting Technique

1. Never inject into anything but normal tissue. Avoid lesions, scars, pigment changes, moles, freckles, and changes in the texture of the skin. Do not inject into an area covered with hair.

2. Always aspirate on all intramuscular and subcutaneous injections to make certain the tip of the needle is not in a blood vessel. Start over again if blood is aspirated.

3. Use only the strictest sterile technique at all times. If there is any doubt about a possible contamination, start over again with sterile equipment. Don't use a disposable unit if the seal has been previously broken.

4. Select the injection site very carefully to avoid major blood vessels and nerves. Know the anatomy of the site and the depth of the injection site for the various types of injection.

5. Never inject into an arm that has had surgery resulting in the removal of the lymph nodes, such as after a **radical mastectomy.**

6. Rotate injection sites for patients receiving frequent injections.

7. Carefully select the correct length and gauge of needle to be used. Consider the overlying fatty tissue or the smallness of a child's muscle.

8. Obtain assistance as needed when giving an injection to an uncooperative child or adult.

9. If indicated, massage the site after the injection with a sterile dressing and apply a Band-Aid if necessary. Children like bright colored Band-Aids as a badge of bravery.

10. Do not allow a patient to hold up a sleeve or other tight clothing that may slip and interfere with the injection, act as a tourniquet, contaminate the site, or increase the depth of the overlying fatty tissue. This is frequently an error when a tight undergarment is pulled only half way down for a buttocks injection or a tight sleeve is held up for a deltoid intramuscular. The adipose tissue can be increased to twice the usual depth, and the medication is deposited into fatty tissue and not into the muscle as indicated.

11. Keep the gauze skin disinfectant pledget in the minor hand ready for immediate use when giving an injection.

12. Destroy the needle and syringe of a disposable unit immediately so that it cannot be reused.

13. Do not give the injection unit to a child as a reward or as a toy. DESTROY IT IMMEDIATELY.

CHAPTER OUTLINE

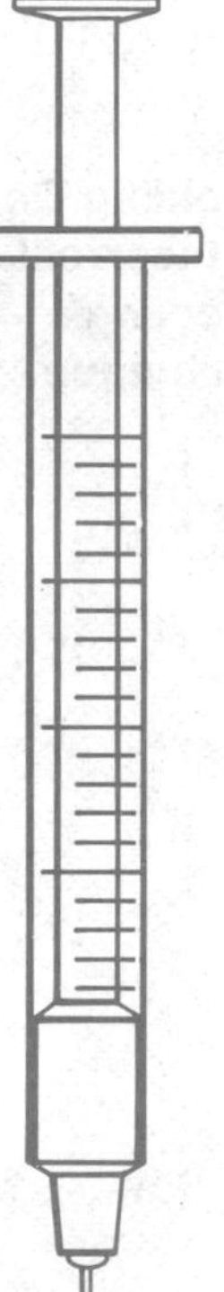

BEHAVIORAL OBJECTIVES

The medical office assistant should be able to:

- **Identify the most commonly used instruments and explain their basic use.**
- **Protect instruments through correct usage and storage.**
- **Correctly sterilize instruments.**
- **Correctly identify the various syringes and hypodermic needles.**
- **Clean, sharpen, and sterilize the various syringes and needles.**

25

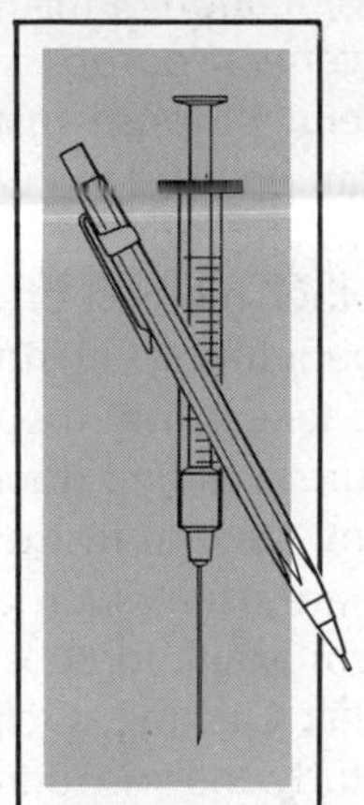

INSTRUMENTS, SYRINGES, AND NEEDLES

The identification and care of surgical instruments are often the core of clinical procedures in the physician's office. A clinical assistant must have a knowledge of instruments, how they are used, and their specific place in a setup. She must know how to care for them and how to sterilize them correctly. An administrative assistant must recognize the names of instruments so as to aid in transcribing the physician's dictation. This knowledge is also necessary for the correct purchasing and inventory of instruments.

George D. Wolf, M.D. says, "The artist and the surgeon alike require special tools for the delicate techniques they have developed." Medical instruments are precision instruments and are very expensive. For this reason a chapter has been devoted to their identification, use, and care. Special instrument setups are covered in the chapters on Physical Examinations and Office Surgery. This chapter will cover briefly those instruments found in the physician's office. Since this is not a book on surgical instruments, the most frequently used nomenclature will be used to identify the instrument and its purpose. There are thousands of surgical instruments cataloged in books, and there are great variations in names. The same instruments may carry two or three different names depending on the physician, hospital, or geographic location in which they are found.

LEARNING SURGICAL INSTRUMENTS

If you have looked through a surgical or medical catalog, you have seen many strange and confusing names. The medical assistant is not confronted with the instruments a hospital central supply person would encounter or those the operating room nurse must know, but she must know the basic instruments. Train yourself to look at each instrument carefully and recognize the distinctive parts. For example, compare the mosquito **hemostatic** forceps and the physician's splinter forceps. They are both the same size and, at first glance, may appear to be identical. More careful inspection reveals that the hemostatic forceps has **ratchets** and that the splinter forceps does not. Both have **serrations**, but the splinter forceps has a much sharper tip, as is common with all splinter forceps. Another example is the 6 in. dressing forceps and the 6 in. tissue forceps. They are both thumb forceps, also known as "spring handle" forceps, but the tissue forceps has teeth.

There are many methods of classification of instruments, but basically, there are those instruments that are used for *general purposes* and those that have only one *specific* use. An example of a general purpose instrument would be the general operating, or surgical, scissors that can be used to cut tissue, soft sutures, or delicate fabrics. An example of the second classification would be the ophthalmoscope, used to view the interior of the eye. Another method of naming an instrument is by its use — cutting, draining, scraping, puncturing, or holding. Along with these usage names there may be a specific name taken from the surgeon who designed it or the hospital or clinic where the procedure was first done. Sometimes a manufacturer's name is given to an instrument. Many general instruments will be further identified by the part of the body where they are used, such as a rectal speculum, a vaginal speculum, and a nasal speculum. Hemostatic forceps often carry the proper name of some renowned surgeon such as **Allis, Cushing, Ochsner,** or **Sims.**

To start learning instruments, study the instrument catalogs. Look carefully at each instrument, identify its length, handle, serrations, ratchets, and movable parts. Then look at the instruments in your office and handle them, visualizing how they are used. As you study instruments you will be able to pick up an instrument that you have never seen before and at least identify its purpose. For example, the many different retractors all have one thing in common — they hold back tissue and retract or pull away from the area in order to facilitate better vision. Often the length of an instrument will aid in its identification. The uterine vulsellum and the Bozeman uterine dressing forceps are designed with long handles to reach through the vaginal speculum to the uterine cervical area. Apply these observations to the identification of all instruments, both therapeutic and diagnostic.

Identifying Parts of Instruments

Most instruments have either a ring handle (Fig. 25–1*A*) or a spring handle, called "thumb handle," as shown in Figure 25–1*B*. Forceps of the ring handle type are usually made with a ratchet catch (Fig. 25–1*C*) and a box lock (Fig. 25–1*D*). The ratchets may be closed at any one of three or more positions; the more teeth engaged, the tighter the grip of the instrument. The box lock is composed of two parts that are riveted together, giving the instrument permanent strength.

The inner surfaces of the jaws on some instruments have sawlike teeth called serrations. Both ring-handled and thumb-type instruments may have serrations. These serrations may be crisscross, horizontal, or lengthwise (Fig. 25–1*E*). They may be on plain-tipped or mouse-toothed instruments. Serrations prevent small blood vessels and tissue from slipping out of the jaws of the instrument.

The tooth ends on instrument jaws are called mouse-toothed, and sometimes rat-toothed (Fig. 25–1*F*). They are found on ring-handled and thumb-type instruments, on plain and serrated jaws. Usually one jaw has one more tooth than its partner to prevent a sharp edge from being exposed. Toothed instruments are usually called tissue forceps and are identified by the number of intermeshing teeth — 1×2, 2×3, 3×4, and so forth. Similar to the mouse-toothed is the soft tissue forceps, which also has teeth of less depth and sharpness, as shown in the Allis forceps (Fig. 25–1*G*). These teeth are finer and slightly rounder, and there is usually a greater number of them. Their grip is also closed by ratchets, as on the hemostat, but they are used for a delicate grip that provides a secure hold with a minimum of injury to the tissue.

Other teeth that may be seen are the rather long single or double teeth of the tenaculum and vulsellum. Usually the tenaculum has a single sharp tooth on each jaw (see Fig. 25–7*D*), whereas the vulsellum (see Fig. 25–7*C*) has a double tooth that

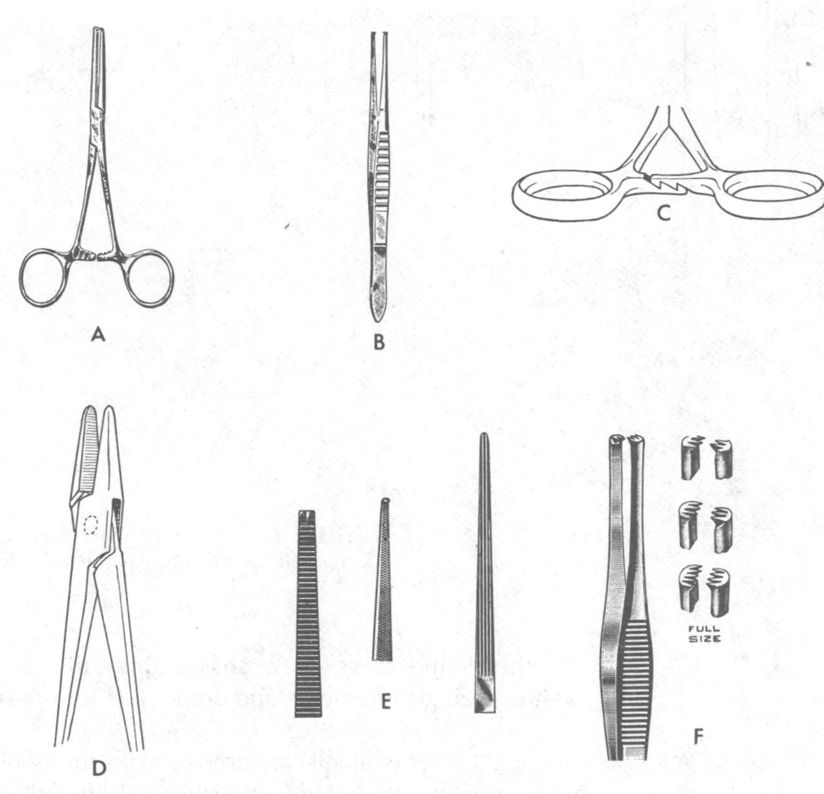

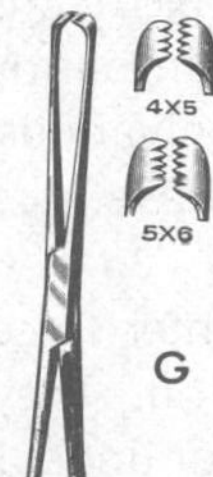

FIGURE 25–1 Identifying parts of an instrument. *A,* Ring handle. *B,* Thumb-type or spring-type handle. *C,* Ratchets. *D,* Box-lock. *E,* Serrations (horizontal, crisscross, longitudinal). *F,* Mouse-toothed. *G,* Allis tissue forceps.

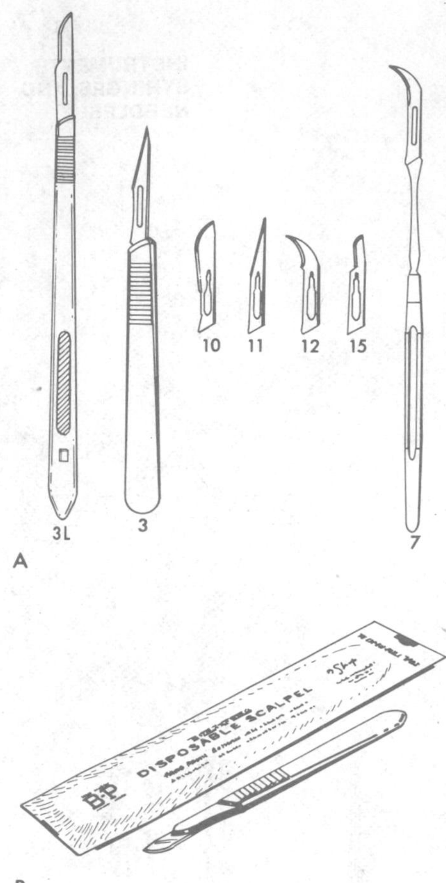

FIGURE 25–2 *A,* **Bard-Parker operating knives (handles with various disposable blades).** *B,* **Disposable sterile blade and handle.**

resembles the fangs of a snake. Both the tenaculum and the vulsellum are tissue-seizing instruments and are locked into position by ratchets.

Surgical Knives

Surgical knives (scalpels) are used to make incisions. Most knives are now disposable or have disposable blades furnished in different shapes and sizes (Fig. 25–2). The three standard handles are No. 3, No. 3L (long), and No. 7. The No. 3 is the most commonly used, and No. 3L is the same except for its increased length; No. 7 is more delicate for use in narrower places. Combinations of disposable blades and handles are available in various blade sizes. Some of the reusable handles now have a "flip-off" spring for ease in removing the blade.

Splinter Forceps

The four types of splinter forceps shown in Figure 25–3 (*A* through *D*) are quite different in construction. They are all used, however, to grasp foreign bodies embedded in the skin or under fingernails. The fine tips lend themselves particularly to the retrieval of splinters and other foreign objects.

Towel Clamps

The two popular styles of towel clamps, or towel forceps, are shown in Figure 25–3 (*E* and *F*) and are used to place sterile drapes around the site of the operation. In office surgery the towel clamp holds various layers of drapings or towels in place. All towel clamps have sharp points, which are used occasionally to hold the drape to the edge of the incision. The curved tips allow them to hang freely without interfering with the line of vision. Towel clamps come in various lengths from 3 to 6½ in.

Hemostatic Forceps

Figure 25–4 (*A* through *C*) shows the three most commonly used hemostats. These instruments are employed to clamp off small blood vessels and hold tissue. In

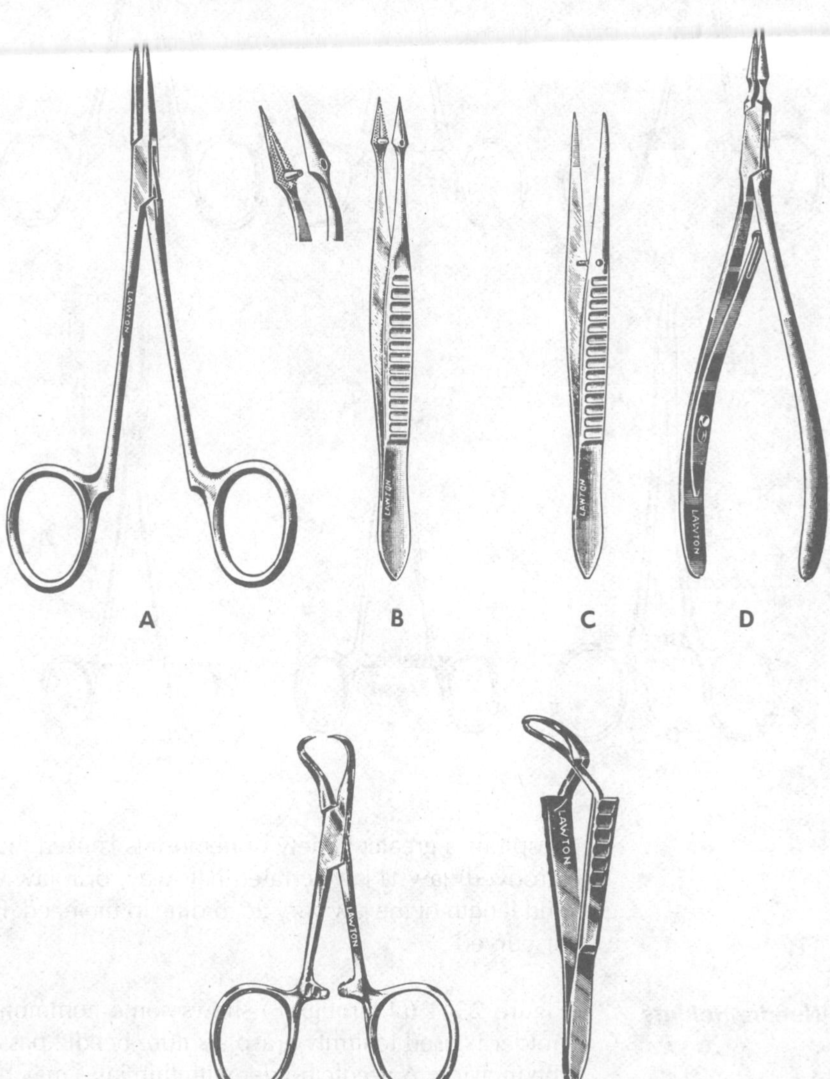

FIGURE 25–3 *A,* Physician's splinter forceps (ring handle). *B,* Hunter splinter forceps (thumb or spring handle), straight or curved. *C,* Plain splinter forceps. *D,* Virtus splinter forceps. *E,* Backhaus towel clamp. *F,* Jones towel clamp (spring handle).

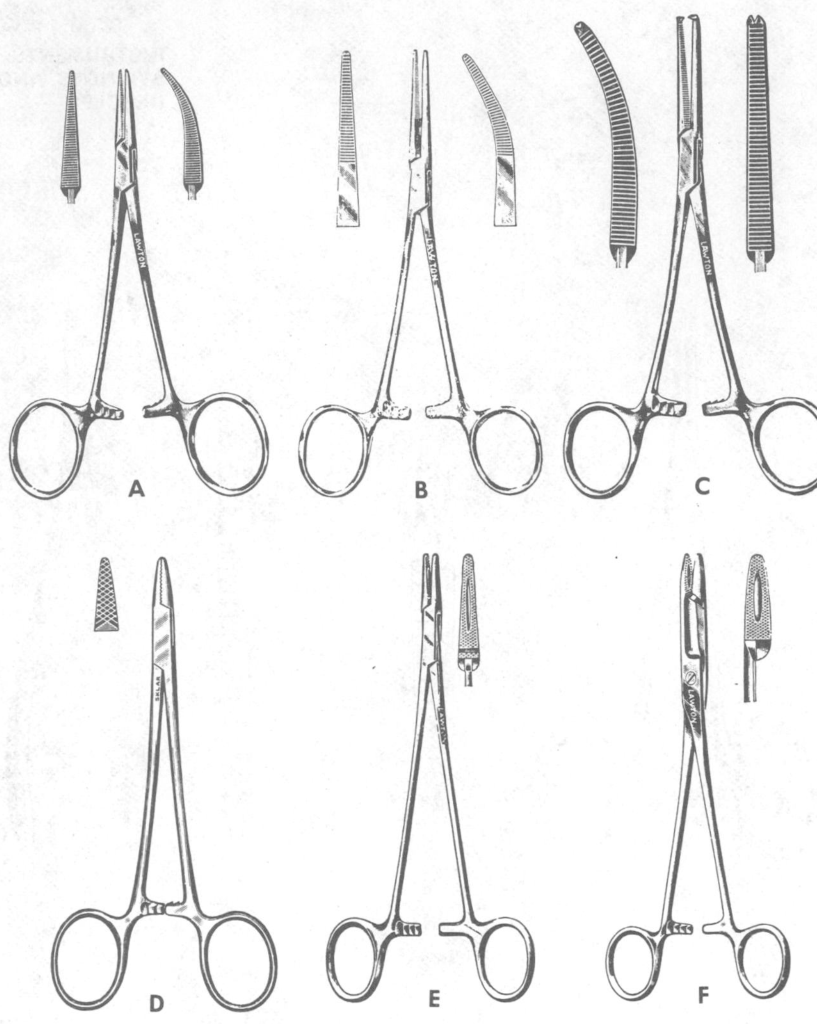

FIGURE 25–4 *A,* Halstad mosquito hemostat, straight or curved, 5 in. *B,* Kelly hemostat, straight or curved, 5½ in. *C,* Rochester-Ochsner hemostat, straight or curved (toothed 1×2), 6¼ in. *D,* Plain needle holder without grooved jaw, 6, 7 or 8 in. *E,* Plain needle holder with grooved jaw, 6 in. *F,* Needle holder with grooved jaw and scissors, 5½ in.

hospitals a greater variety of hemostats is used, but most have either a fully serrated (grooved) jaw, a jaw serrated half-way, or a jaw with serrations and teeth. The size and length of the jaw vary according to the need. Hemostatic forceps may be straight or curved.

Needle Holders

Figure 25–4 (*D* through *F*) shows some commonly used needle holders. A needle holder is used to firmly grasp a suture needle passed through the skin flap adjoining the incision. A needle holder with thin jaws may be advantageous for fine needles as used in plastic surgery or eye surgery. In addition to having a needle-grasping surface, a needle holder (*F*) may also have a scissors feature. This type of combination instrument can only be used for more delicate suturing since the screw joint does not lend strength to the instrument. The jaws of needle holders are usually shorter and look stronger than those of hemostats. Since needle holders wear smooth at the jaws after continued use, most now are available with a jaw insert of carbide to ensure that the needle will not twist.

Other Instruments

Figure 25–5 (*A* through *J*) shows a number of instruments one is likely to see in most physicians' offices.

STERILIZER FORCEPS. The two illustrated types of sterilizer forceps (tongs) are used to retrieve sterilized items such as instruments, syringes and needles from a boiler or autoclave. Both types shown have curved jaw surfaces, which facilitate holding the item (*A* and *B*).

TUNING FORK. The tuning fork (C) is used to test the perception of sound. The forks come in a variety of frequencies (wave lengths). It is held by the single stem end and gently tapped on the examiner's knuckle, or it may be plucked between the thumb and index finger. It is not advisable to rap it on a hard surface since this will damage the instrument.

FINGERNAIL DRILLS. Fingernail drills (*D*) are used to perforate a nail under which blood or exudates have formed. The drilled hole allows the fluid to escape, thus relieving the pain.

COMEDO EXTRACTOR. These extractors (*E*) come in various sizes and styles. The Saalfeld type shown here has a lance end that is used to incise small **abscesses** and a blunt end with a small hole in the center to press out foreign matter such as is found in a blackhead or whitehead.

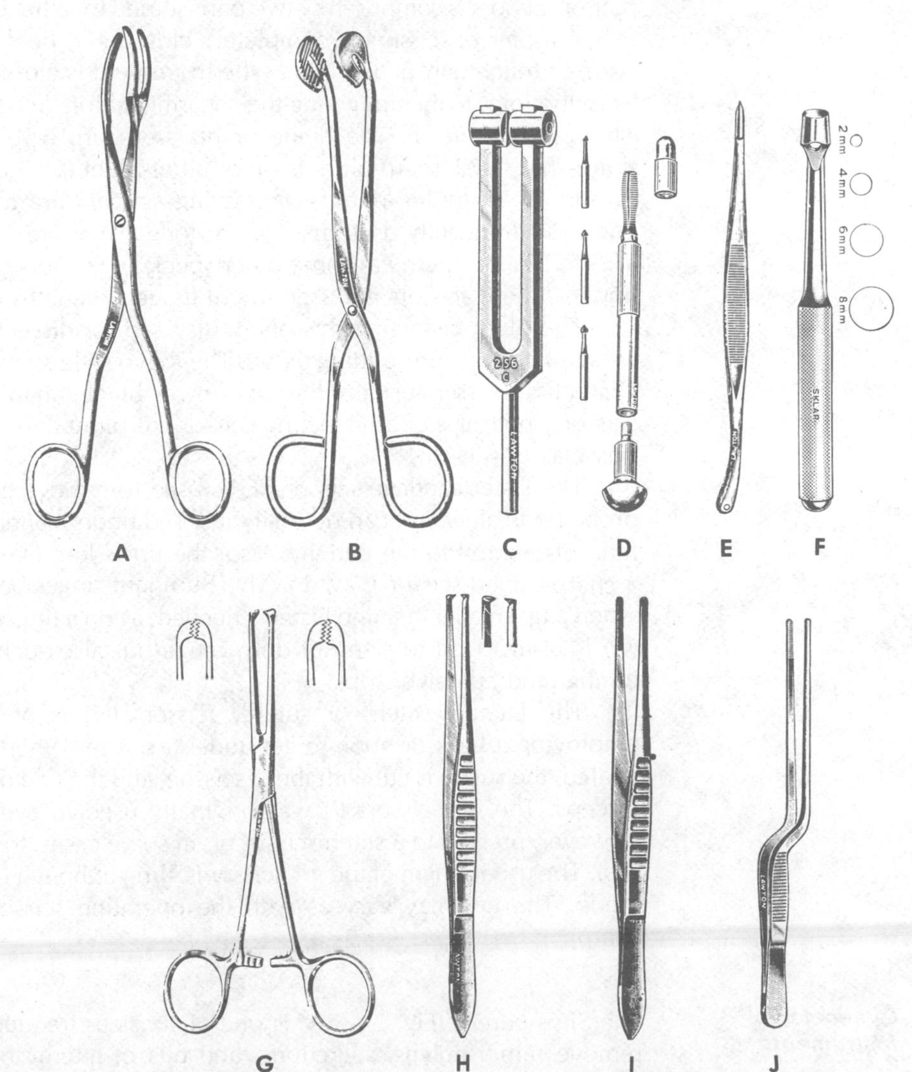

FIGURE 25–5 ***A,*** **Sterilizer forceps (tongs), 3-pronged, 8 in.** ***B,*** **Sterilizer forceps, 8 in. C, Tuning fork.** ***D,*** **Fingernail drill with attachments.** ***E,*** **Comedo extractor, double-ended.** ***F,*** **Cutaneous punch (skin biopsy punch).** ***G,*** **Allis tissue forceps.** ***H,*** **Plain tissue forceps, 5½ in.** ***I,*** **Plain thumb forceps, 5½ in.** ***J,*** **Lucae bayonet dressing forceps, 5½ in.**

CUTANEOUS PUNCH. Sometimes called a dermal punch (*F*), this is used for obtaining a small piece of skin for a biopsy. The cutting end comes in various sizes as shown.

FORCEPS. There are several hundred different types of forceps. It is an extremely broad term and does not really identify any particular instrument. The Allis tissue forceps (*G*) shown is used to grasp tissue such as muscle or epithelium. The same function is served by the plain tissue forceps (*H*), but the Allis forceps has a much more gentle grip because the teeth are less sharp. The number of teeth vary (1×2, 2×3, 3×4), depending on preference.

Thumb forceps (*I*) is primarily a dressing instrument designed to handle with a "no-touch technique" surgical dressings. It is made in lengths of 4 to 12 in. with varying serrated jaws and does not have teeth.

Lucae bayonet forceps (*J*) is a simple angled thumb forceps. It is used to best advantage in the nose and ear. The bayonet shape provides better vision. These are made in lengths up to 8½ in. Occasionally they are toothed.

Scissors

Figure 25–6 shows the many different types of scissors found in a medical office. A pair of scissors is composed of two parts joined together by a screw and a screw joint. When a pair of scissors is completely closed and held to the light, the two blades seem to touch only at the tips; as the instrument is closed, this meeting place travels from the joint to the tip, giving the shearing action. Scissors are identified as straight (str) or curved (cvd). The blade points are sharp or blunt. They are described as sharp-sharp (s/s), sharp-blunt (s/b), or blunt-blunt (b/b) as shown in Figures 25–6 (*A, B,* and *C*). These all-purpose operating scissors are also called surgical scissors. The most frequently used are 5½-in. long. They are made in ½-in. lengths, from 4½ to 5½ in. There are some other specialty scissors that are longer. As the name implies, these scissors are used to cut tissue or lengths of fine suture.

The blunt dissecting scissors (*D*) is used for **dissecting** or exposing growths or vessels from the surrounding tissue. The Mayo style shown here has a beveled blade. Dissecting scissors usually have narrower blades than do the blunt-blunt surgical scissors; both tips of a dissecting scissor are blunt and they appear to be a stronger scissors.

The Lister bandage scissors (*E*) is used to remove bandages and dressings. The probe tip is blunt and can be easily inserted under bandages with relative safety and little discomfort to the patient. Also, the tip is less likely to probe into the skin as a sharp-tipped scissor may do. The Burnham finger bandage scissors (*F*) is useful when a tip smaller than the Lister is needed, as on a finger bandage. The gauze shears (*G*) is used to cut to size not only gauze but also such things as rubber sheeting, tubing, and adhesive strips.

The Littauer stitch, or suture, scissors (*H*) is one of several popular types employing a beak or hook to get under a suture. When an incision has sufficiently healed, the suture is cut with these scissors and the end pulled with a thumb dressing forceps. The iris scissors (*I*) was originally used in eye surgery. Many physicians, however, prefer it to a stitch scissor or, in some cases, to a general operating scissors (s/s). The usual length of the iris scissor is 4 in., although longer or shorter patterns are made. The tips may vary as with the operating scissors (for example, blunt and sharp).

Gynecologic Instruments

The Sims curette (Fig. 25–7*A*) is one of six sizes frequently used. They are used to remove minor **polyps,** secretions, and bits of afterbirth (placental matter), and to obtain specimens from the uterine cavity. Identical sizes are also made with dull blades. The Bozeman dressing forceps (*B*) is used to reach the cervix, uterus, and vagina. Employed to hold sponges or dressings, it can also be handy in the application of a medication. The curved handle allows for better visibility. The

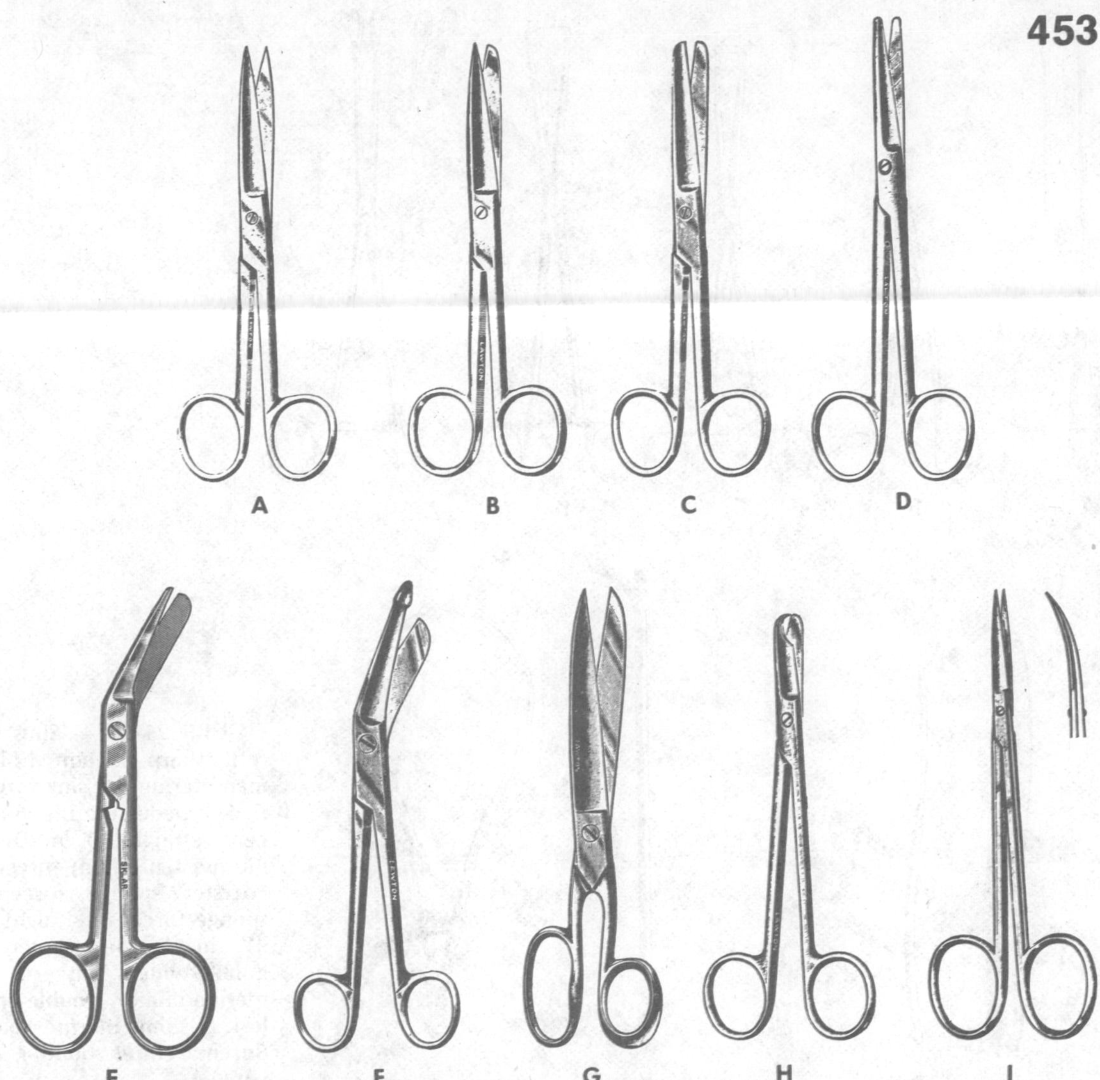

FIGURE 25–6 ***A,*** **Operating scissors, straight or curved, sharp-sharp;** ***B,*** **Blunt-sharp; and** ***C,*** **blunt-blunt.** ***D,*** **Mayo dissecting scissors, straight or curved, 6¾ in.** ***E,*** **Lister bandage scissors, 5½ in.** ***F,*** **Burnham finger bandage scissors.** ***G,*** **Gauze shears, Army type, 7½ in.** ***H,*** **Littauer stitch scissors or suture scissors, 5½ in.** ***I,*** **Iris (eye) scissors, straight or curved, 4⅛ in.**

Schroeder vulsellum (*C*) and the tenaculum (*D*) are used to hold tissue, such as the cervix, during the obtaining of a specimen or for lifting the cervix to view the **fornix.** The uterine sponge forceps (*E*) may be used in lieu of the Bozeman for dressing purposes.

The Hegar dilators, of which the largest (*F*) and the smallest (*G*) are shown here, come in sets of eight sizes. These are double-ended so that there are actually 16 different sizes. These are used to dilate the cervix for examination purposes and also prior to dilatation and curettage (D & C).

The Sims uterine sound (*H*) is graduated in centimeters and is used to check the **patency** of the cervical os. The Van Buren *urethral* sound (*I*), which also comes in graduated sizes, is used to dilate the urethra. The Martin pelvimeter (*J*) is used to measure the female pelvis and allows the physician to determine whether it is possible to deliver the fetus through the normal birth route.

Eye, Ear, Nose, and Throat Instruments

The Krause nasal snare (Fig. 25–8*A*) has a wire loop which, when tightened, may be used to remove polyps from the nasal cavity. A similar snare, smaller in size, is available for use in the ear. The Hartmann "alligator" forceps (*B*) has a 3½ in. shaft. It

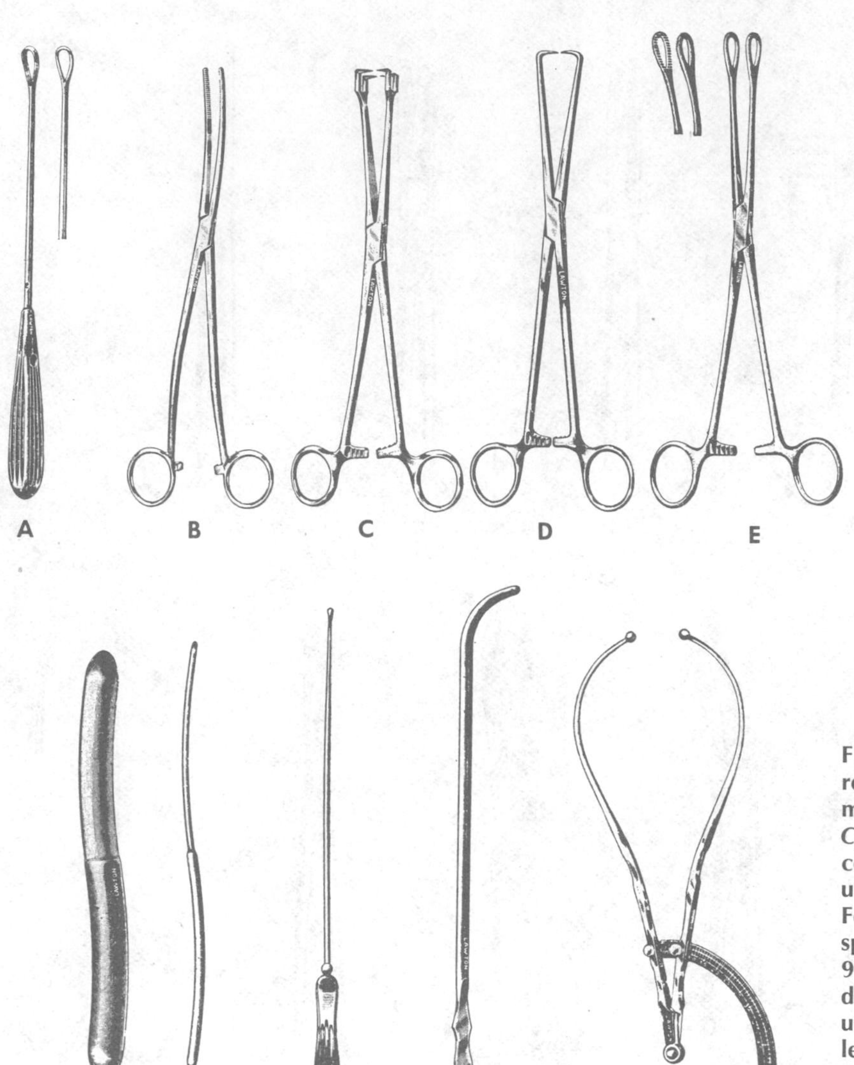

FIGURE 25–7 *A,* Sims uterine curette, sharp or blunt, 12 in. *B,* Bozeman uterine dressing forceps, 10 in. *C,* Schroeder uterine vulsellum forceps, straight, 9 in. *D,* Schroeder uterine tenaculum forceps, 9 in. *E,* Foerster sponge forceps (uterine sponge forceps), straight or curved, 9½ in. *F,* Hegar uterine dilator, double-ended, largest. *G,* Hegar uterine dilator, double-ended, smallest. *H,* Sims *uterine* sound. *I,* Van Buren *urethral* sound. *J,* Martin pelvimeter.

is so called because the jaw moves in an alligator-type action. It is employed through either a nasal or ear speculum for grasping and removing foreign objects. The alligator jaw is made in a variety of styles (for example, cup jaw or with teeth) so that it can be used on foreign bodies or polyps with different shapes.

The Weider tongue depressor (metal tongue depressor) (C) fits comfortably in the physician's hand during throat, postnasal, and oral examinations (*insert* shows serrations on the under side of the blade to minimize slipping).

The physician is frequently called upon to remove foreign bodies from the eye. Deeply embedded foreign objects are, of course, handled by a specialist; however, the Dix spud (flat end; *D*) is helpful in office procedures, as is the LaForce eye spud (golf club-shaped end; *E*).

Buck ear curettes (*F*) are used to remove foreign matter (usually wax) from the ear canals. They are made with sharp scraper ends or blunt rings and can be obtained in various sizes.

The Freer dissector and elevator (*G*), one end of which is sharp and the other dull, aids in separating tissue from bone or cartilage. This is its dissecting function. As an elevator, it is used to lift tissue away, either to permit improved examination or to facilitate dissection.

The Hartmann eustachian catheter (*H*) is used to blow air into the eustachian canal, which connects the nasopharynx to the cavity of the middle ear. The Senn (*I*) is a double-ended instrument with a skin hook and a retractor. The three-pronged end is used as the skin hook; the flat end is a retractor, which is used to hold open small incisions or lacerations for viewing or to secure a skin edge for suturing.

A trocar (*J*), such as the nested set of three sizes illustrated, is used to withdraw fluids from cavities. It consists of a **cannula** (outer tube) and a sharp pointed **stylet (obturator).** Once the trocar is inserted, the stylet is withdrawn. Another variety is the Ochsner trocar (*K*) with a drain. This also comes in various sizes and is used for draining and irrigating with a catheter inserted, as shown.

The Reiner irrigating syringe (*L*) illustrated happens to be all metal, but similar

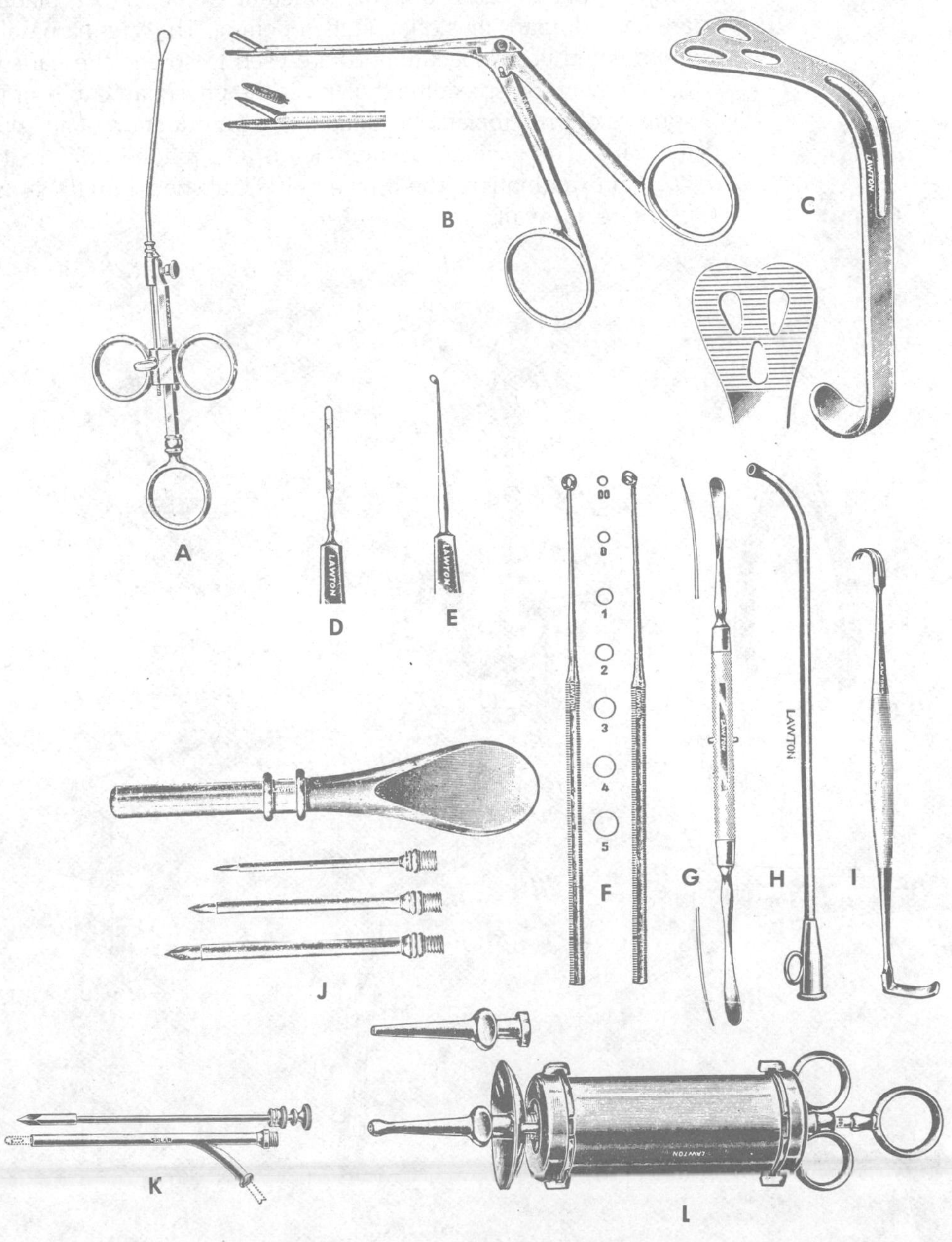

FIGURE 25–8 *A,* Krause nasal snare. *B,* Hartmann "alligator" ear forceps, plain or toothed. *C,* Weider "metal" tongue depressor. *D,* Dix eye foreign body spud, flat end. *E,* La Force eye foreign body spud, "golf-club eye spud." *F,* Buck ear curette. *G,* Freer dissector and elevator. *H,* Hartmann eustachian tube catheter. *I,* Senn double-ended retractor and skin hook. *J,* Nested trocar, three sizes. *K,* Ochsner trocar with obturator and drain. *L,* Reiner ear syringe with shield and control handle, plain tip and bulbous tip.

models are available in glass or disposable plastic. All types are fitted with a piston, by means of which a stream of fluid is forcibly injected into the ear or cavity, for removal of **cerumen** and for irrigations. A small splash shield has been mounted behind the tip to help collect the wash-back in a basin usually used during the procedure. The three-ringed control–type handle facilitates a firm grip. It is supplied with a plain catheter or a bulbous tip.

Specula

Among the important aids to the visual examination of the body orifices are the instruments known as specula (Fig. 25–9). A speculum is an instrument for opening or distending a body orifice or cavity to permit visual inspection. A bivalve speculum is one with two valves or parts, sometimes referred to as blades or bills. These valves are spread apart, thus dilating the opening. The Vienna nasal speculum (*A*) and the illuminated nasal speculum (*B*) are used to spread the naris for examination of the nasal cavity. By spreading the valves the physician can examine for nasal polyps or sources of irritation and be aided in the introduction of an applicator and snares into the naris. The vaginal speculum (C) is also made in different sizes and is used in a vaginal examination. The Brinkerhoff rectal speculum (*D*) is used in the examination of the rectal wall.

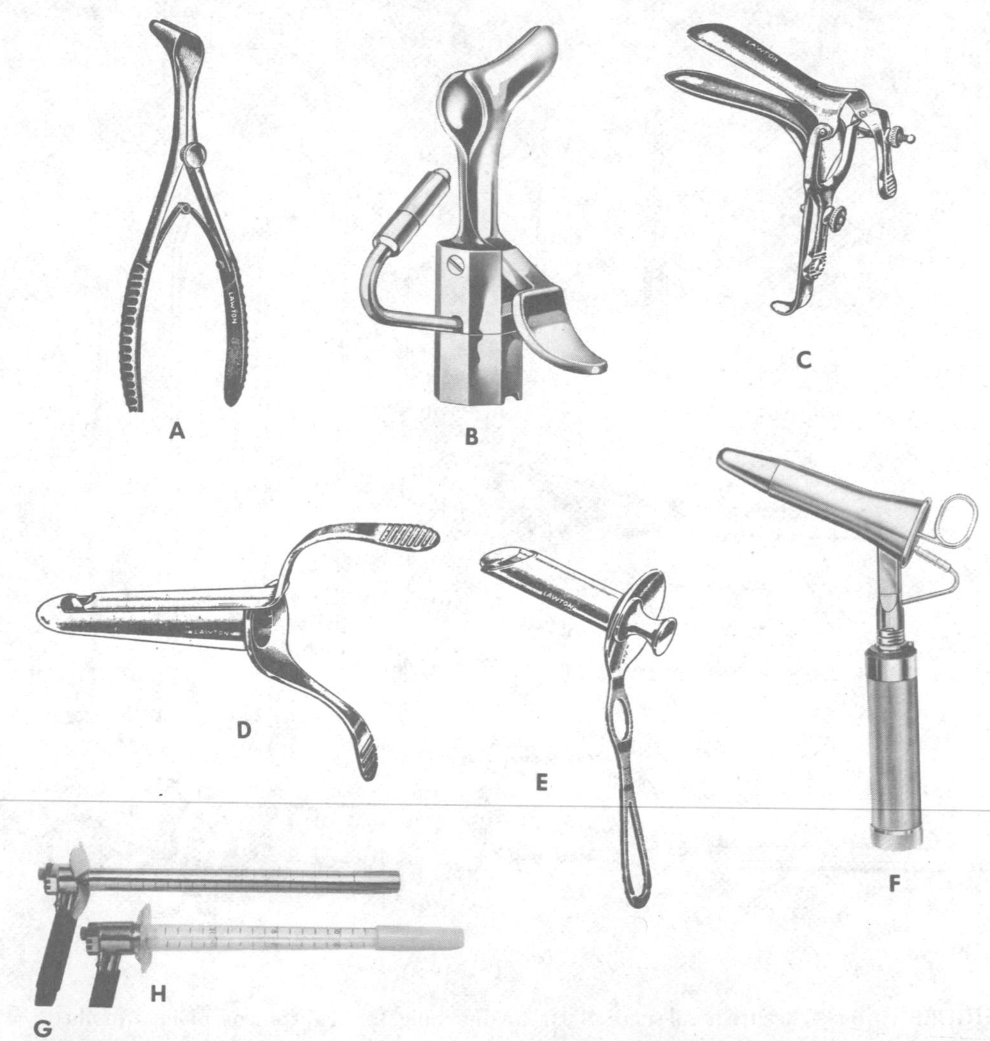

FIGURE 25–9 ***A,* Vienna nasal speculum. *B,* Nasal speculum, bi-valve, illuminated. *C,* Graves vaginal speculum. *D,* Brinkerhoff rectal speculum. *E,* Hirschmann anoscope. *F,* Illuminated anoscope with removable obturator. *G,* Sigmoidoscope, reusable, illuminated, 25 cm (obturator not shown). *H,* Sigmoidoscope, disposable, fiberoptic.**

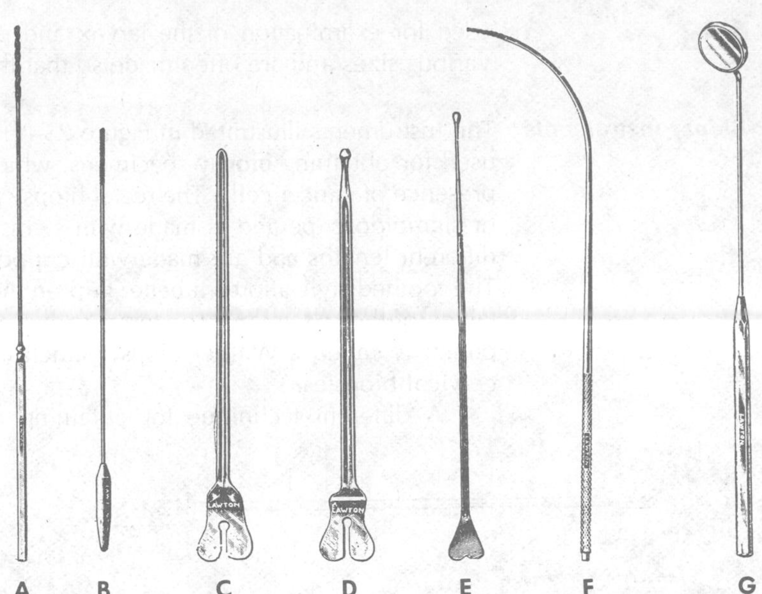

FIGURE 25–10 *A,* **Buck metal applicator, 8 in.** *B,* **Brown metal applicator, 6 in.** *C,* **Grooved director, plain tip.** *D,* **Grooved director, probe tip.** *E,* **Larry probe, bulbous tip.** *F,* **Ivan laryngeal metal applicator, curved.** *G,* **Laryngeal mirror.**

Scopes

The term "scope" is usually applied to a viewing instrument that is equipped with a light source. Generally a scope does not have movable parts that would increase **dilation** after the instrument has been inserted, as found in the Graves vaginal speculum or the Vienna nasal speculum.

The anoscope (*E* and *F*) is approximately 3½ in. (8.9 cm) in length and enables examination of the anal area and lower rectum. Because of their limited length, anoscopes are not always illuminated. A proctoscope, not shown, is approximately 6 in. (15 cm) in length and facilitates examination of the rectum above the limits of the anoscope. The sigmoidoscope (*G* and *H*) is approximately 10 in. (25 cm) in length and permits examination of the sigmoid bowel area. Both the proctoscope and the sigmoidoscope must be illuminated.

Obturators

An obturator is the part of an instrument that closes a lumen (opening) of the instrument in order to facilitate the insertion of the instrument into a body cavity. These obturators are usually removed after the initial insertion of the instrument has been made. The obturators for the rectal scopes are smooth and rounded to ease the insertion of the instrument through the anal sphincter muscle (Fig. 25–9*E* and *F*). Some obturators are sharp to aid in puncturing tissue. An example of this is the sharp-tipped obturator of the trocar that must be inserted through the skin. This type of obturator is sometimes called a stylet (Fig. 25–8*K*).

Applicators, Probes, and Directors

The ear and/or nose applicators shown all have the same function (Fig. 25–10). Cotton is twisted around the end, to which medication is then applied. The style with the six-sided handle (*A*) is called the Buck applicator and measures 7½ in. It is made with either a triangular, twisted, or roughened end to aid in securing cotton to the tip. The Brown applicator (*B*) with the oval handle is 6 in. in length and is frequently made of copper or nickeloid materials that aid in its flexibility.

The grooved director (*C* and *D*) is employed to guide a cutting instrument such as a surgical knife. Notice that the director may have a probe tip (*D*), which makes it easier to explore the direction of the hole or **fistula.** Probes and directors come in lengths ranging from 4 to 12 in. and with or without bulbous tips. The slender construction of the Larry probe (*E*) makes it suitable for rectal examinations. The probe is useful for exploring subcutaneous foreign bodies.

The long, curved applicator (*F*) is called an Ivan laryngeal applicator. It has a length of 9 in., and the curve lends itself to use in the throat and postnasal areas. The scored or roughened end aids in holding cotton in place. The laryngeal mirror (*G*) is used for examination of the larynx and postnasal areas. These also are made in various sizes and are often made so that the mirror surfaces will not fog.

Biopsy Instruments The instruments illustrated in Figure 25–11 (*A* through *D*) show a number of styles used for obtaining **biopsy** specimens, which is most usually done to ascertain the presence of cancer cells. The rectal biopsy punch (*A*) is used through a proctoscope or sigmoidoscope and is made with stems that may be interchanged. These have different lengths and are made with cupped, basket-type, straight, or angled jaws. The toothed style affords a better grip on the tissue and prevents slipping during the taking of the specimen. (The *insert* shows a different jaw). The ring-handled biopsy punch is called a Wittner biopsy punch (*B*) and is one of several styles used for cervical biopsies.

A different technique for obtaining cells for examination, such as for the

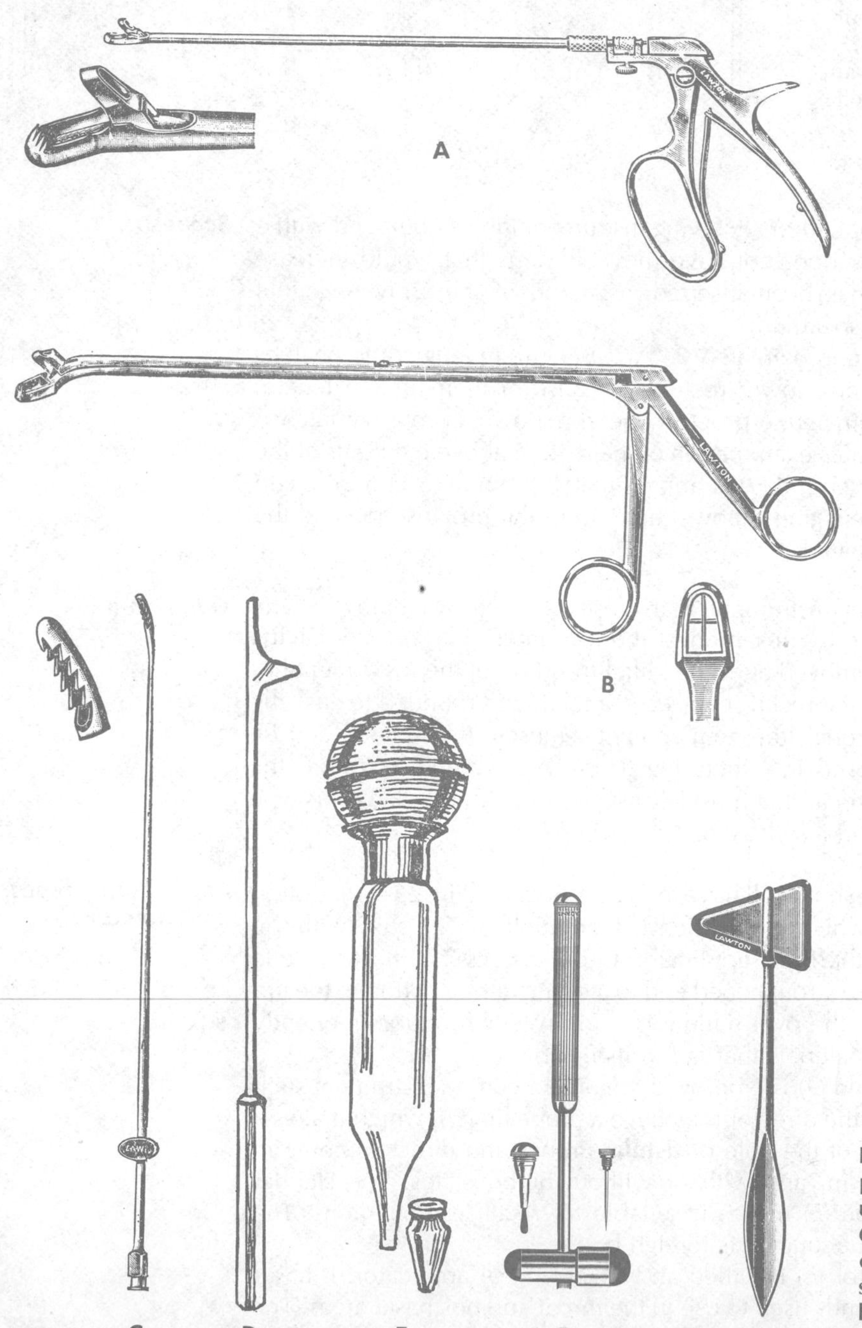

FIGURE 25–11 *A*, Rectal biopsy punch (forceps). *B*, Wittner uterine (cervical) biopsy forceps. *C*, Novak biopsy curette. *D*, Cervical spatula. *E*, Asepto irrigation syringe with tip. *F*, Neurologic hammer with pin and brush. *G*, Taylor percussion hammer.

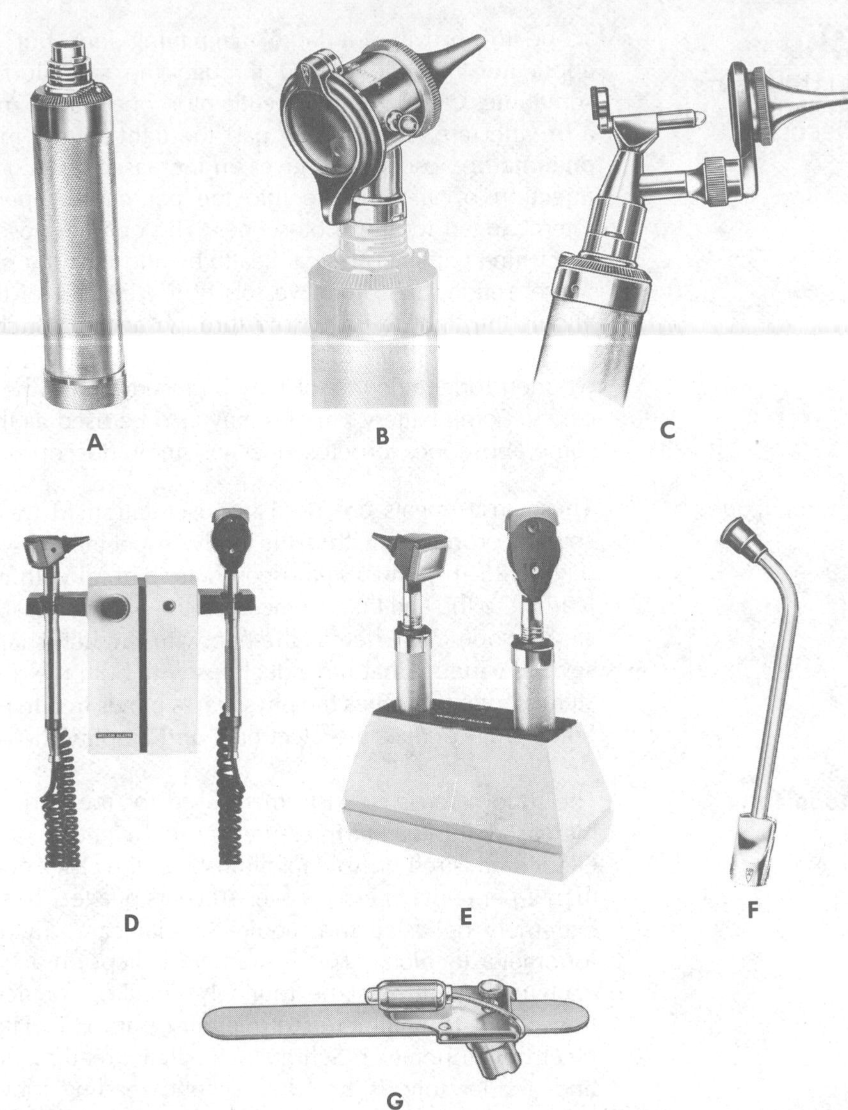

FIGURE 25–*12* Illuminating instruments. *A,* Battery handle for attachments. *B,* Diagnostic otoscope (removable speculum). *C,* Operating otoscope (removable speculum). *D,* Wall-hung transformer unit and handles for fiberoptic pneumatic otoscope and ophthalmoscope. *E,* Desk model with rechargeable handles for otoscope and ophthalmoscope. *F,* Transilluminator, curved. *G,* Tongue depressor holder, illuminating. (*D, E,* and *G,* Courtesy of Welch Allyn, Inc., Skaneateles Falls, New York.)

Papanicolaou test, involves the use of a curette. To the Novak biopsy curette (*C*), a suction machine is attached which collects the cells as they are dislodged by the curette. Much of this technique is now done with disposable kits such as the Gravlee Jet Washer or the Vabra endometrial aspirators. Another system to gather cells uses a long scraping instrument similar to a spatula. The type pictured here is known as the Eisenstein cervical spatula (*D*). These are now usually disposable items made of either wood or plastic.

Irrigating Syringes

The glass Asepto irrigating syringe (Fig. 25–11 *E*) varies in capacity from 1 to 4 oz and has a blunt cone tip, a fine pipette tip, or a catheter tip. It is also supplied with a detachable soft rubber tip. These are also supplied in disposable plastic.

Hammers

Number (Fig. 25–11 *F*) shows a neurologic hammer with pin and brush. The sharp pin and the brush are for testing the quality of nerve reflexes. The Taylor percussion hammer (*G*) is used to test muscular reflexes.

Illuminated Diagnostic Sets

The set illustrated in Figure 25–12 consists of several different attachments for the battery handle (*A*) that is the source of power for the light. These attachments may also be interchangeable with other light source attachments. The diagnostic otoscope (*B*) provides a large magnifying lens but restricts the area in which an applicator may be passed through the speculum. The operating otoscope (*C*), sometimes called the therapeutic otoscope, has a smaller magnifying lens but affords a broader area for working past the light source into the ear canal. The fiberoptic **pneumatic** otoscope (*D*) gives an increased level of illumination and allows for the injection of air pressure into the ear canal. Specula of different sizes may be interchanged for these otoscopes. The ophthalmoscopes in (*D*) and (*E*) are used to determine general physical health by allowing the physical examination of the optic nerve, retina, and blood vessels of the interior of the eye. The transilluminator (*F*) allows the light to be passed through an area such as the sinuses or breasts. The flexible rotating or curved transilluminator is adjustable for viewing the throat. A wooden tongue depressor may be inserted into the holder (*G*) for viewing the oral cavity. Some battery handles may also be used as the power source for the light on some anoscopes, proctoscopes, or sigmoidoscopes.

Stethoscopes

These instruments are used in auscultation to transmit to the examiner's ear the sounds produced within the body, especially the sounds of the heart and lungs (Figure 25–13). Most stethoscopes are biaural with two earpieces and a flexible tube leading to the end that is placed on the patient. The flat disc-shaped tip is the Bowles stethoscope (*A*), whereas the one with the bell-shaped end is a Ford (*B*). There are several varieties that have dual tips with both the disc and bell ends. The obstetrical stethoscope (C) leaves the physician's hands free to palpate and manipulate the fetus. Some stethoscopes are electronic and amplify the sounds.

Tonometer

The tonometer is an instrument used for measuring intraocular tension (pressure). Increased intraocular pressure causes a group of diseases known as **glaucoma.** Glaucoma is responsible for almost half the cases of adult blindness and strikes more than 2 per cent of persons over 40 years of age. These instruments are expensive and extremely delicate, and require special care. Figure 25–14*A* shows the standard tonometer (Schiötz). This instrument is kept on a special stand and is sterilized for each patient. It must be routinely checked for accuracy. The scale readings are transposed to millimeters of mercury (mm Hg). Figure 25–14*B* shows the Digiton electronic tonometer (Schiötz). The digital reading (in mm Hg) is automatically taken and a brief tone is heard; a second reading may be taken. These readings are displayed by pressing a recall button.

CARE OF INSTRUMENTS

Since instruments are expensive and a physician's skill is somewhat dependent on these "tools of the trade," the medical assistant must not only be able to identify

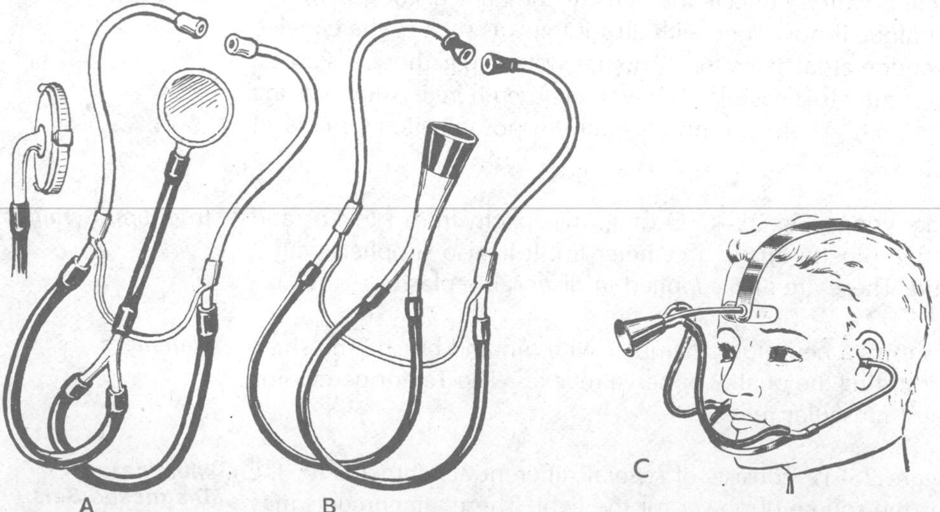

FIGURE 25–13 Stethoscopes. *A*, Bowles stethoscope with disk-shaped chest endpiece. *B*, Ford stethoscope with bell-shaped endpiece. *C*, Obstetric stethoscope with headpiece.

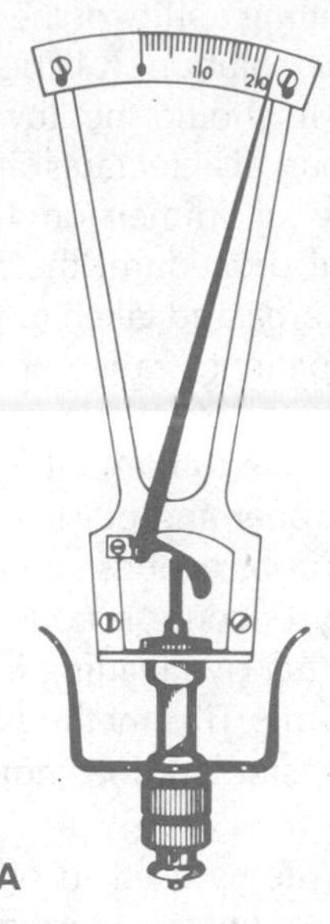

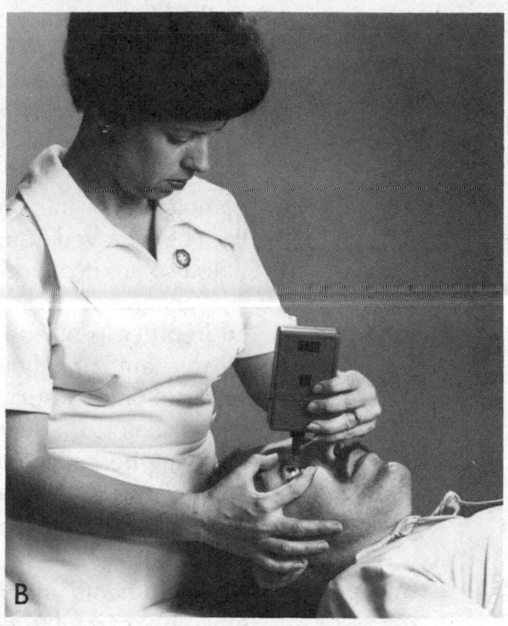

FIGURE 25–14 Tonometers. *A*, Standard tonometer, Schiötz. *B*, Electronic Digiton tonometer, Schiötz.

them and know their uses but must also be able to care for them properly in order to extend the lives of the instruments and enable them to be used as they were intended.

Most instruments are made of fine grade stainless steel. The term "stainless" is usually taken too literally. Even the best of stainless steel may water spot and stain, especially if water with a high mineral content is used, but it does resist rust and keeps a fine edge and tip longer. The proper hardness and flexibility is important. Inexpensive instruments may be too brittle, easily stained, and unable to function properly. Mistreatment of a chrome-plated instrument can cause minute breaks in the finish, which may become a source of contamination and may also tear the surgeon's glove.

Instruments should be carefully examined when they are first received from the supplier. Scissors should be tested to see if they shear the full length of the blades, clear to the tip. This can be checked by cutting a piece of cotton. If the scissors cut cleanly and do not chew at any point, even at the tip, then they are functioning correctly. Teeth and serrations are checked to see if they intermesh completely and if the jaws are even on the sides and tip. Each instrument should be felt over its entire surface for any rough areas that may tear or snag the surgeon's glove. Box locks and hinges must work freely but not be too loose. Thumb- and spring-handled instruments must have the correct tension and meet evenly at the tips.

Under no circumstances should instruments ever be bunched together or be allowed to become entangled. Avoid mixing stainless steel instruments with ones of aluminum, copper, or brass. This may cause electrolysis and may result in etching. Even mixing stainless steel with chrome-plated instruments is best avoided. If an instrument is accidentally dropped, it may be permanently damaged. If scissors are dropped while the blades are partially open there will be a nick at the point the blades are crossed. Do not leave ratchets tightly closed or leave a hemostat clamped onto thick material such as a drape or gauze. Use a towel clamp or dressing forceps for this.

Reserve a special place during a surgical procedure to receive contaminated instruments. This is usually a basin of disinfectant solution placed in the sink or within reach of the assistant. If a metal basin is used, it is advisable to place a small towel in the bottom of the basin in order to prevent damage to the instruments as they are dropped into the solution. Never allow blood or other **coagulable** substances to dry on an instrument. If immediate cleaning is not possible, they should be rinsed well and placed in a cold water solution of a blood solvent and a mild detergent. The detergent increases the wetting ability of the water, allowing the instrument's surface to be better exposed to the solution. It is best to use a detergent that is as nearly to neutral pH as possible. It should be low-sudsing and easy to rinse off. Each manufacturer of the various disinfectants and blood solvents will recommend the correct dilution and time of immersion for its product. Read the label. Upon completion of the surgical procedure, the receiving basin for the instruments can then be removed from the area and taken to the cleaning and sterilization room. This will also get it out of the patient's range of view.

Separate the various types of instruments. Sharp instruments should be separated in order to prevent damage to the cutting edges as well as possible injury to the person sanitizing them. Rubber and plastic items puncture easily and often discolor metals. Some plastic and rubber goods should not be soaked too long because they will discolor. Plastics may become porous and lose their glossy surface. Many of these are best sanitized either by cleaning in the usual way without soaking or with alcohol and by wiping/drying. This method is not sufficient for instruments that will penetrate the body tissues, since it does not sterilize them.

Sanitization

All instruments and other items used in office surgery, examination, or treatment must be carefully cleaned *before* **sterilization** or **disinfection. Sanitization** is sometimes incorrectly called disinfection, but sanitization comes before disinfection as well as before sterilization. It is a very important step and cannot be overlooked or done carelessly. Stainless steel instruments that are not cleaned immediately after use may acquire a tarnish that is difficult to remove. Plated instruments may rust in minute breaks in the plating and thus be a source of bacterial deposits.

If instruments were not rinsed thoroughly immediately after use but were received in a solution basin, then the solution should be drained off after the desired time of immersion and the instruments rinsed well in running water. Open all hinges and scrub serrations and ratchets with a small scrub brush or toothbrush. This step must not be skipped, because sterilization cannot penetrate to the instrument's surface through coagulable substances. At this time check the instruments carefully for proper workability.

Assembled instruments must be disassembled before they can be thoroughly cleaned. When finished, dry *completely* before reassembling. Trapped moisture will cause corrosion.

Boiled instruments should not be considered sterile, because boiling only eliminates the organisms that are killed at 212° F or less. Boiling is used to disinfect the instruments after they have been sanitized. The boiling water cannot reach the instrument's surface unless all foreign substances have been removed. The boiling method of disinfection is sometimes used for instruments that do not penetrate the body tissues and need not be sterile, such as nasal and ear specula. The efficiency of boiling water may be increased by the addition of enough sodium carbonate to make a 2 per cent solution. This increases the disinfecting power of the boiling water and decreases the corrosive action on metals. John J. Perkins states, "Bacterial spores in water resisted boiling for about 10 hours, but they are destroyed in a 2 per cent soda solution at 208°F (98° C) in 10 to 30 minutes. Other workers employing a similar technic demonstrated that when contaminated and oiled instruments were boiled in a 2 per cent soda solution, a period of 10 minutes' boiling was necessary to produce sterilization. Boiling water to which alkali has been added in the above-mentioned concentrations is adequate for destruction of most spores in an exposure period of 15 minutes."*

Remember that excessive exposure to any wide range of pH change from neutral is not recommended.

---

*Perkins, J. J.: *Principles and Methods of Sterilization in Health Sciences.* 2nd ed. Springfield, Ill., Charles C Thomas, 1970.

If instruments are to be disinfected by boiling they should have all the surfaces exposed by opening hinges and ratchets and then be placed on the tray of the boiler and protected from hitting each other. The water should be of sufficient level to completely cover the instruments when the tray is immersed. Instruments are usually boiled for 15 to 20 minutes. Do not start the timing until the water is at a rolling boil. Then lower to a gentle boil.

Chemical sterilization is recommended for instruments that are not thermally stable or that may be dulled by heat sterilization methods. Read the manufacturer's instructions on the bottle carefully. Many of these chemicals are disinfectants and *not* sterilizing agents. Gas is a new accepted method of sterilization but may have limitations in an individual physician's office. (See the chapter on Sterilization for further information on gas sterilization.) Both chemical and gas sterilization methods may require that an instrument be rinsed with sterile distilled water before use in order to remove any residual chemical that is not compatible with body tissue.

Handling Sterile Instruments

If instruments have been chemically sterilized by immersion in a chemical or boiled for the correct length of time, they are removed by sterile forceps from the container or boiler. If the sterilizing chemical is strong enough to damage contacted tissue, the instrument must be rinsed with sterile distilled water. The instruments are then placed on a sterile field that has a barrier drape to prevent moisture from drawing any contamination from the surface below the drape. Do not touch the instrument with your hands or allow any contaminated materials to come in contact with the field. This method of handling instruments is not satisfactory unless the instruments are used immediately. It is very difficult to dry, wrap, and label them for storage and still maintain sterility.

Instruments that need not be stored sterile should be removed from the solution with sterile forceps, but they can be rinsed under hot running water to remove the solution that could damage the instrument during storage. Dry it very carefully, since moisture is the main enemy of an instrument. Instruments may be wiped with an oiled cloth if they are to be placed in storage for any length of time, but remember, this oil must be removed before they are sterilized at a later date. Only water-soluble lubricants are recommended. These are non-oily and usually do not become sticky, are easier to remove, and do not interfere with steam sterilization.

Loading the Sterilizer

Here is an important rule to remember which applies to use of the autoclave. When loading the autoclave, prepare all packs and arrange the load in such a manner to present the least amount of resistance to the flow of steam and heat. Articles should be placed so that they rest on their edges rather than on their flat sides in order to permit proper permeation of the materials with moisture and heat. Tiers should be placed alternately. Under no conditions permit crowding of packs into tight masses. Jars and containers should be placed on their sides. When the container is right side up, even with the cover removed, air is trapped within the container and there is no flow. The perforated trays supplied with many autoclaves serve ideally for routine sterilization of instruments. Place a layer of muslin under and over the instrument to facilitate drying and prevent contamination when removing from the autoclave (Fig. 25–15). Because steam will not penetrate oil, all oil should be removed from the materials and instruments to be sterilized.

Sterilization in an Emergency

It is occasionally necessary to sterilize instruments in a great hurry or in places where there are no facilities for proper sterilization. In such cases, the instrument may be dipped in alcohol or gasoline and then ignited. As soon as the object is dry, it is considered sterile. These are emergency methods only, though sometimes necessary, and are not recommended, as the process is very hard on good instruments. The tip of an instrument may be dipped into tincture of iodine, Zephiran, or Merthiolate for a few minutes for emergency use, but these solutions are hard on the metal surfaces of the instrument.

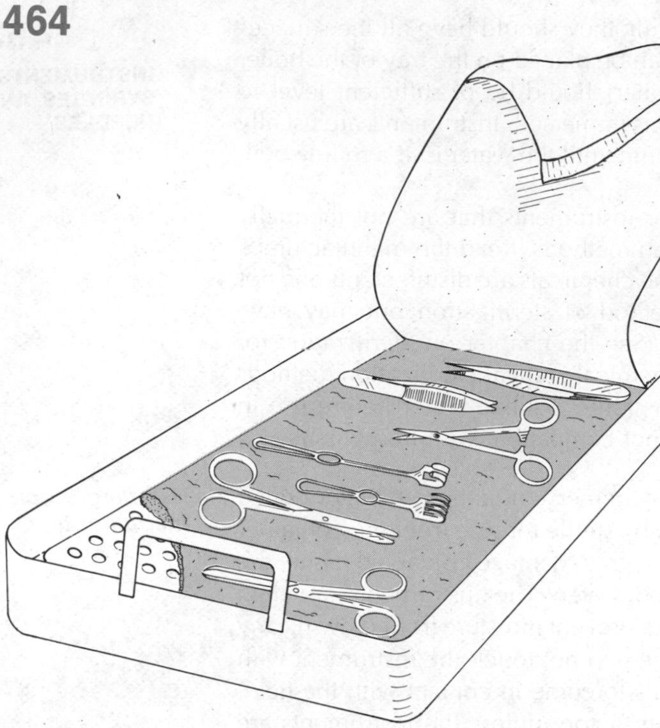

FIGURE 25–15 Instruments placed on soft fabric on an autoclave perforated tray and covered with fabric. A perforated bottom tray is necessary for effective steam flow. The cover is to protect against contamination after removal from the autoclave and to increase drying speed.

If an instrument is in need of oiling in order to make it work properly, use a small amount of water-soluble grinding or lapping (polishing) compound, and work the compound into the area by opening and closing the instrument several times until it moves freely. Rinse well and sterilize.

Because most knife blades in use today are disposable, it is seldom necessary to sharpen instruments. However, many scissors are reusable and may need sharpening and adjusting. It is advisable to send the scissors to a competent instrument repair service. Your surgical supply representative may be able to suggest where you can get this repair service.

CARE OF SYRINGES AND NEEDLES

It is necessary for the medical assistant to understand the construction of hypodermic syringes in order to care for them and to administer medication accurately. Figure 25–16 illustrates the construction of a 10 cc and 2 cc syringe. These parts (needle, tip, barrel, scale calibration, and plunger) are found in both the reusable and the disposable syringes. The value of the scale markings on a syringe must be noted. Are these scale calibrations in tenths or hundredths of a cubic centimeter, or in minims?

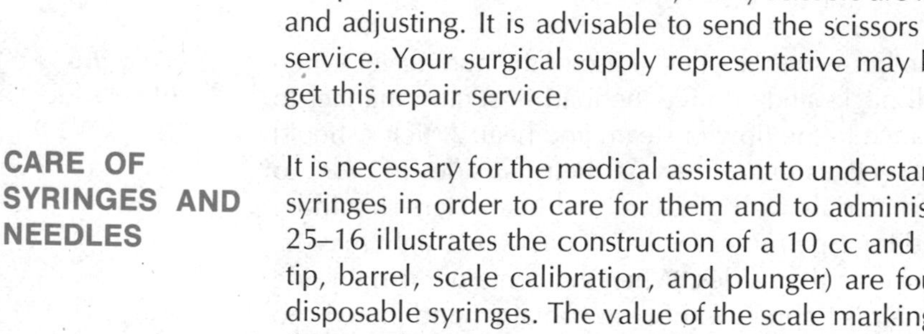

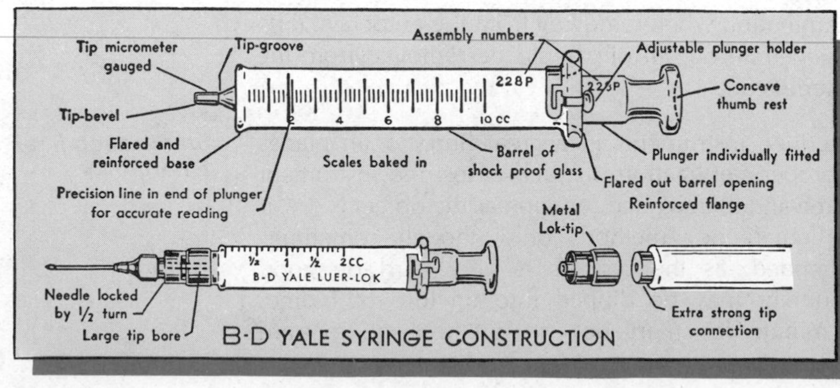

FIGURE 25–16 Syringe construction. (Courtesy of Becton-Dickinson and Co.)

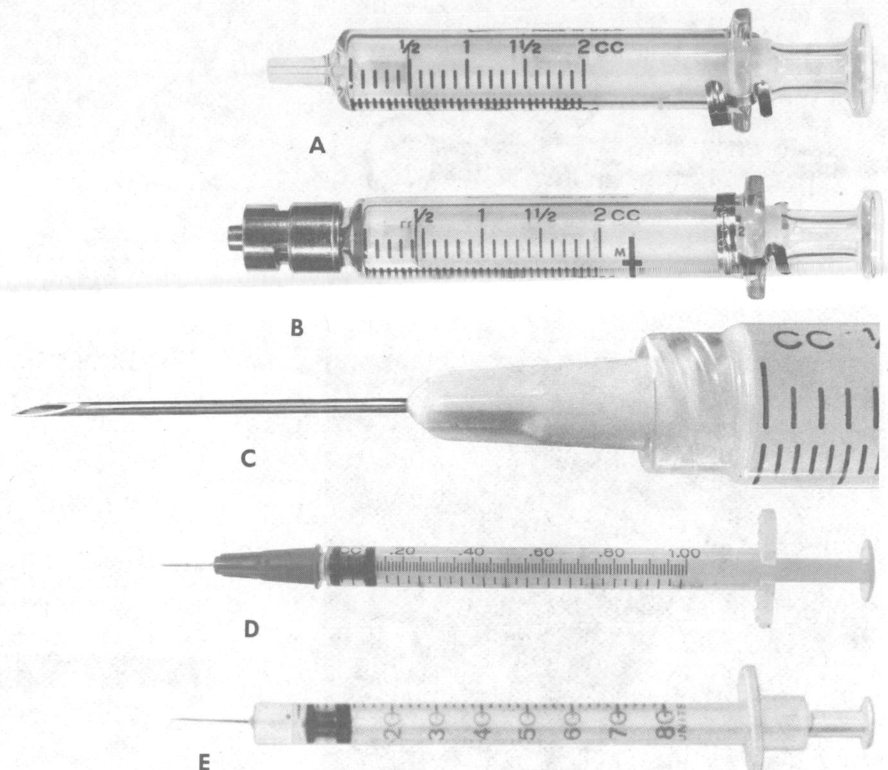

FIGURE 25–17 Types of syringe tips. *A,* Reusable glass syringe, 2 cc with regular tip (plain tip). *B,* Reusable glass syringe with metal Luer-Lok tip. *C,* Luer-Lok tip on disposable plastic syringe. *D,* Disposable tuberculin syringe with detachable needle. *E,* Disposable tuberculin syringe with hubless needle permanently attached.

For example, the smallest division of the 10 cc syringe in Figure 25–16 is 0.2 of a cubic centimeter (or milliliter), and that of the 2 cc syringe is 0.1 of a cubic centimeter. What is the total capacity of the syringe? Capacities range from ¼ cc (very small) to 100 cc (the largest).

Syringes may also be characterized by their tips (Fig. 25–17). Different tips allow for different modes of needle attachment. Some needles are permanently affixed to their barrels.

Some specialty syringe and needle units are designed for particular uses. Some have a control handle for smooth injection (Fig. 25–18*A*). Others are preloaded with medication and ready for immediate use (Fig. 25–18*B*). Another specialty syringe is an insulin syringe, where the calibration is not according to volume, but to the concentration of insulin, in insulin units (Fig. 25–18C).

It is important to learn the parts of a syringe that may be handled while preparing a medication and those parts that must remain sterile. When inserting the plunger into the barrel or attaching the needle, be sure that the fingers do not come into contact with the parts indicated in Figure 25–19. Also, when the plunger is fully extended after medication has been drawn into the syringe, remember to avoid contacting the plunger.

A majority of syringes and needles used in the modern medical office are disposable. The greatest advantage is the prevention of cross-infection. Disposable needles are siliconized and are extremely smooth and sharp; they have not been dulled by frequent use. Color coding makes easy identification. After a syringe has been filled with medication and not immediately used, the sterile needle sheath may be replaced. This also makes safer transportation of the unit to another room. Disposable syringes are easier to read, as the scales have not been worn away. This provides for fast, accurate measurement of the medication. Manufacturers of disposable items must meet extremely rigid standards. The sterilization methods for these items are carefully controlled, and constant inspection includes the use of biologic sterilizer indicators.

Although reusable syringes and needles are not used as frequently as in the past, there are some specialty syringes and needles that require special care. Often these

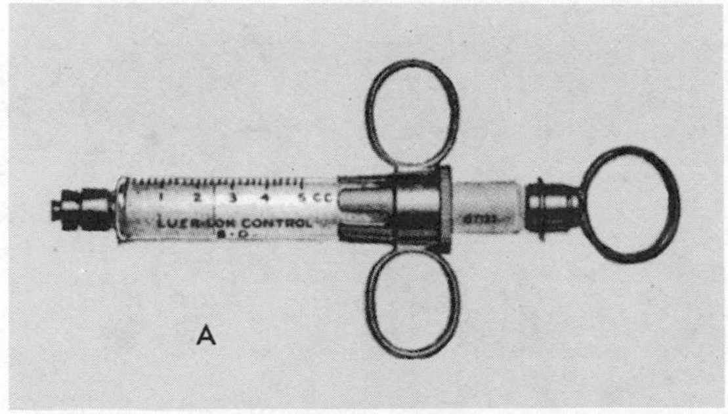

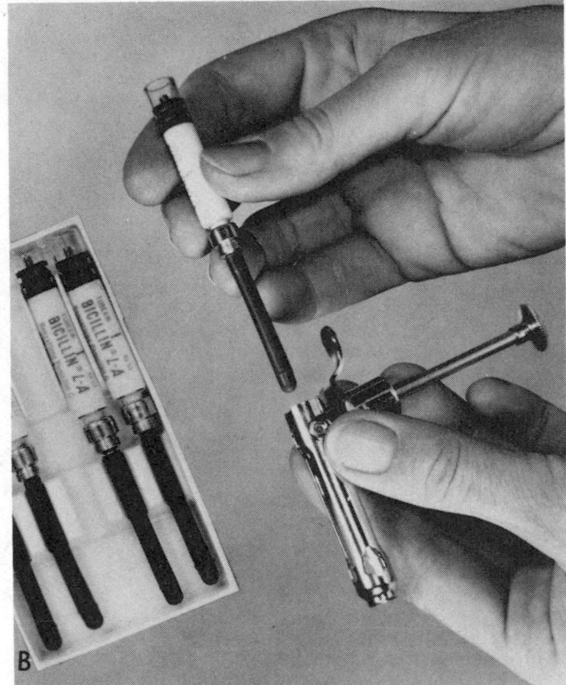

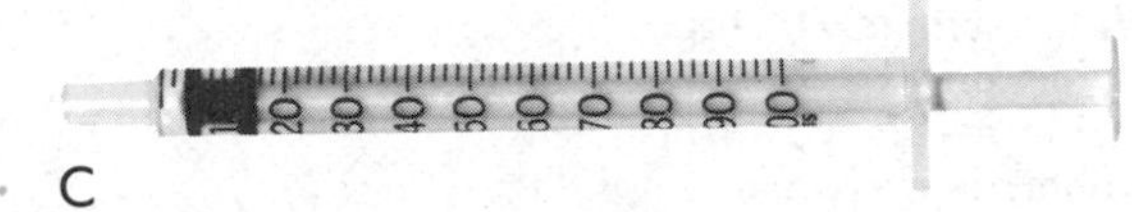

FIGURE 25–18 **Special syringes.** ***A,*** **Syringe with control handle. This type of three-ring handle provides for a secure grip, especially when used with one hand or for a slow, steady depression of the plunger. Control handles are found on both reusable (above) and on disposable syringes, as well as on other syringe-type instruments.** ***B,*** **Tubex syringe with cartridge-needle unit. (Courtesy of Wyeth Co.)** ***C,*** **An insulin syringe, 100 units per cc.**

specialty items are expensive, and extra care will extend the life of the syringe or needle. The most important rule to remember in caring for a syringe and needle is to rinse the unit under cool running water immediately after use. This practice is especially important if the syringe has been used for any blood work or for a medication that can form a film on the inside of the syringe and needle.

Rinse the syringe well by first separating the unit and allowing the water to run over both parts. Then reassemble the unit, draw the water into the barrel, and force it gently through. Repeat this process several times. If a reusable needle was used, attach the needle to the tip of the syringe and force the water through. Grip the unit well with your hand, and place your forefinger on the hub of the needle in order to prevent the needle's being forced off.

REMOVING SUBSTANCES FROM SYRINGES. If the syringe has sediment in it, scrub it with a small bottle brush. There are special brushes for syringe cleaning that have a smaller brush attached for cleaning the hub of a needle and a stiff plastic stylus that is used to clear out the syringe tip. An oily substance can be cleaned from a syringe by rinsing with ether, acetone, or alcohol. Then, wash the unit well with a detergent and rinse with distilled or demineralized water. Syringe barrels and

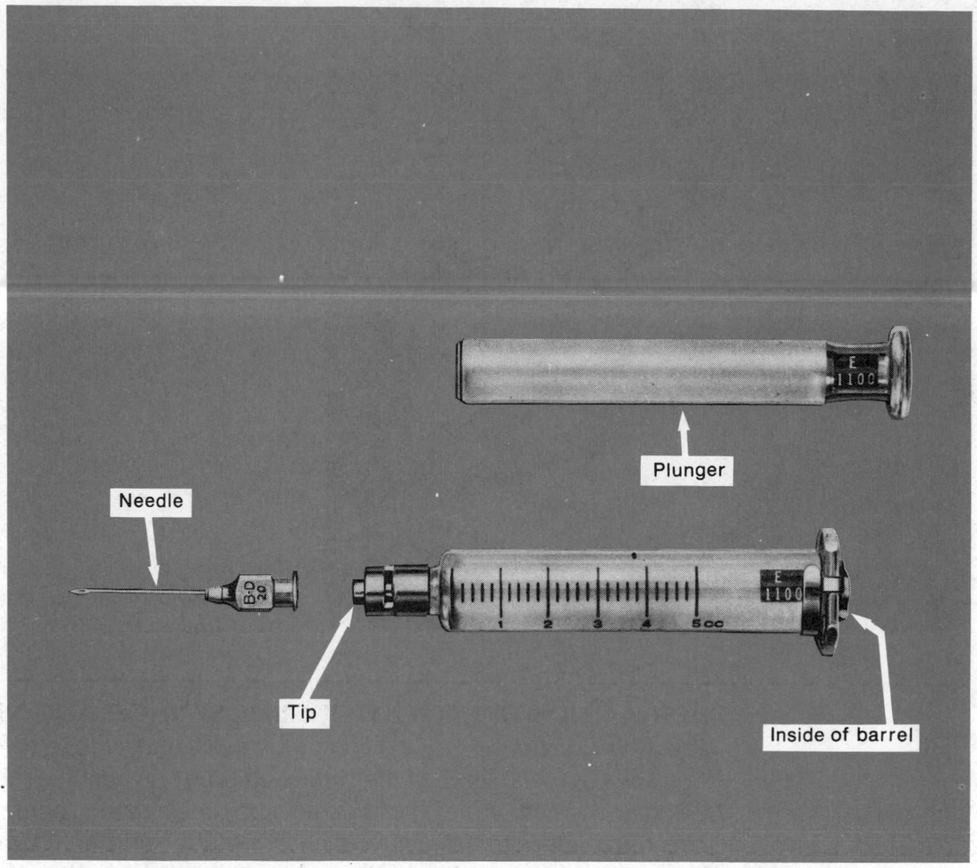

FIGURE 25–19 Parts of a syringe to be kept free of contamination.

plungers should remain separated until they are ready for use again. Alkali deposits may be removed with 10 per cent nitric acid solution. This solution will also remove some dyes and blood stains. Iron stains may be removed by a 10 per cent hydrochloric acid solution. It is not advisable to soak the syringe in an acid solution, because it will remove the markings and will erode any metal such as Luer-lok tip. It is best to saturate a cotton applicator and swab out the syringe, rinsing well afterwards. Take care that the acid solution does not come in contact with the metal. There are also excellent commercial cleaning products on the market.

Because reusable syringes are individually made by expert glass blowers, the surfaces must not be allowed to collect deposits. Some syringes are made with matching barrel and plunger. These units will bear a matching number on the barrel and plunger, and the numbers must match in order for the unit to be usable. The parts of these numbered units are not interchangeable with other syringes. Many reusable syringes are now Multifit* syringes. These plungers and barrels are interchangeable with other units. In case of breakage, unbroken parts may be used with other remaining parts.

Disposable syringes are made of plastic or other synthetic materials. These syringes are unbreakable and very sturdy. Disposable syringes are individually packaged and are color coded for easy identification. The use of disposable units absolutely prevents cross-infection of patients. It also eliminates the time lost in cleaning and sterilizing reusables. Disposable units are supplied in a wide range of types and sizes. Sterile disposable needles are used almost exclusively, with the exception of some special needles. These are also color coded by the hub for easy identification.

*Becton-Dickinson Company

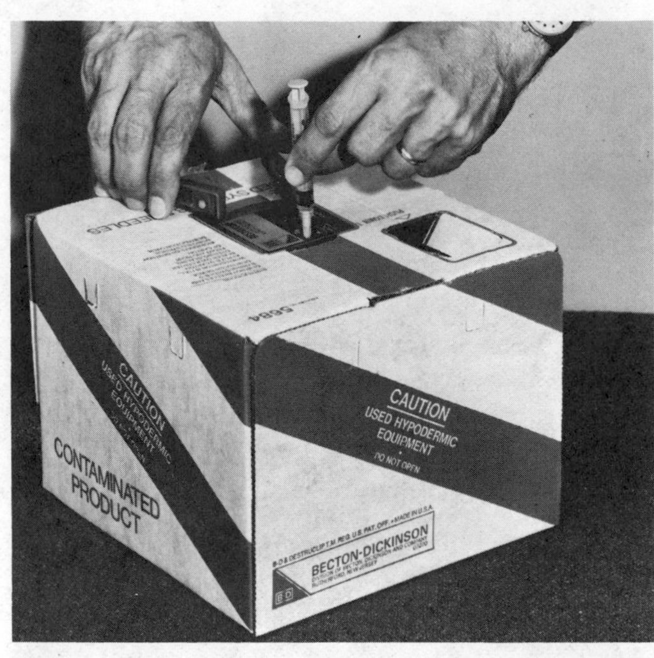

FIGURE 25–20 Disposable carton for destruction of syringes and needles. (Courtesy of Becton-Dickinson and Co.)

DESTRUCTION OF USED HYPODERMIC SYRINGES AND NEEDLES. Remember, *always break and destroy a disposable needle and syringe before discarding.* This is safe and easy with some of the cutting units now available. This method prevents the medical assistant and the physician from accidentally being injured and possibly becoming infected. Never give a child a syringe unit as a toy or reward. The unit in Figure 25–20 cuts off the needle and syringe tip and provides a place for storage of the destroyed unit. In Figure 25–21 the unit is smaller, and it destroys the needle and the syringe tip. It is of vital importance to destroy needles and syringes before discarding them. If a large quantity of disposable units is used, it may be advisable to have a small trash compactor, which would eliminate these syringes and needles going out of the office intact. Some areas have rather severe fines and/or penalties for discarding needles that have not been rendered unusable.

HOW TO OPEN A STUCK SYRINGE. Sometimes, even with careful handling, a syringe becomes stuck. If this happens, fill the air space of the stuck syringe with warm water by using another syringe and needle and injecting water through the tip.

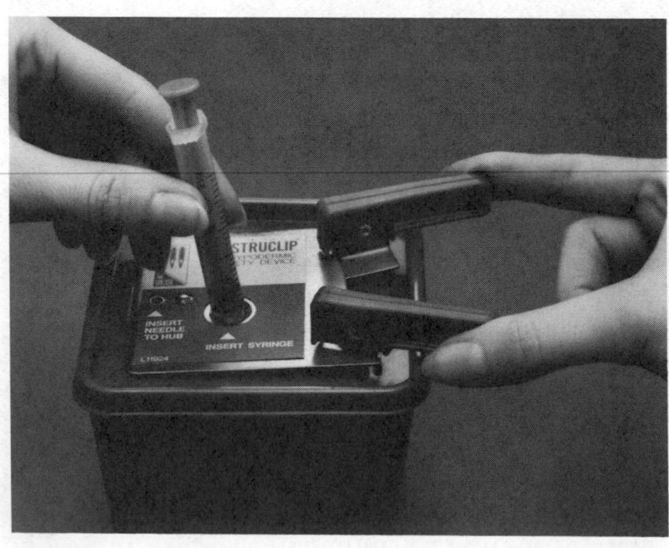

FIGURE 25–21 Cutting device for disposable syringes and needles. (Courtesy of Becton-Dickinson and Co.)

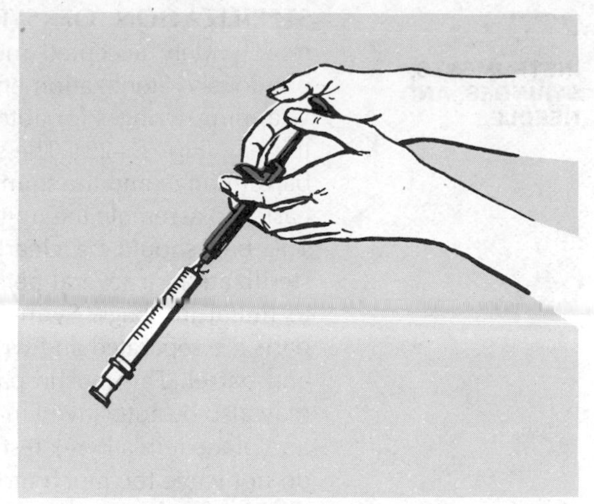

FIGURE 25–22 Opening a stuck syringe with the syringe opener. (Courtesy of Becton-Dickinson and Co.)

Then, allow the syringe to soak for some time. This, however, will not loosen a tightly stuck syringe.

Boiling the syringe in a 25 per cent aqueous solution of glycerine is sometimes successful in separating stuck syringes. This method often makes it possible to remove the plunger by rotating it with a circular motion while it is hot. It may help to immerse the syringe in cold water for ten minutes and then plunge it into boiling water for a few seconds. This heats the barrel and causes it to expand, while the plunger remains cool and contracted.

The most satisfactory method is the use of the B-D Syringe Opener No. 26, as shown in Figure 25–22.

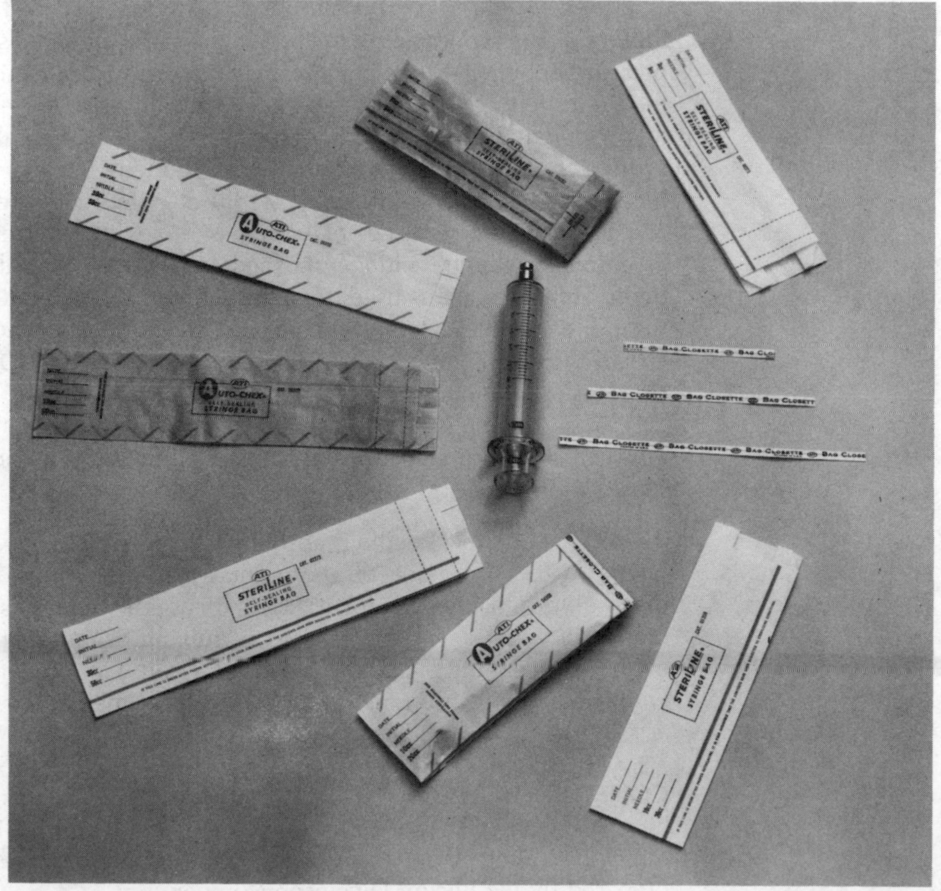

FIGURE 25–23 Envelopes for sterilization and storage of instruments and syringes. (Courtesy of Aseptic-Thermo Indicator Co.)

STERILIZATION OF SYRINGES. Sterilization by autoclaving or dry heat is the most widely accepted method. To prepare the syringe, sanitize it as mentioned previously. Sterilization envelopes or small bags are the most satisfactory method of wrapping syringes for autoclaving. These syringe bags have a sterilizer indicator on the bag (Fig. 25–23). The syringe parts are separated and placed in the bag with the barrel flange and the thumb rest of the plunger toward the open end. This makes it easier to assemble the unit without contamination when the sealed end is torn open. The bag should be clearly labeled with the size of the syringe and the date of sterilization. If several persons are cleaning and autoclaving syringes, it is advisable to initial the bags. Syringes may also be autoclaved in muslin wraps. The syringe parts are separated and wrapped together with a piece of gauze between the plunger and barrel. This muslin pack may be secured with string or sterilizer tape. Syringes may also be autoclaved in test tubes. Assemble the syringe after a thorough sanitizing and place it in a Pyrex test tube. The syringe does not have to be completely dry, but do not leave too much moisture on it. The tube is of large enough diameter to allow the syringe, but not the flange of the syringe, to drop in. This prevents the tip of the needle from touching the butt of the test tube. Cover the exposed plunger with muslin or sterilizer paper and secure with a string or rubber band. When sterilizing by this method, there is no need to label. The date of sterilization is sufficient. This method is useful if the unit may receive a little rough handling, as in a physician's bag. These units are autoclaved for 20 minutes at 250° F.

Dry Heat. This method of sterilizing glass reusable syringes is used, because all the moisture is eliminated and the sterilizing can be done in a regular oven, if necessary. The syringe is prepared in the same manner as for autoclaving. The exposure time is one hour at 320° F (160° C.). The oven should not be overloaded, as this would prevent circulation of air.

Boiling. The syringes are sanitized in the same manner as for sterilization by steam pressure or hot air. There are advantages to using distilled or demineralized water in the boiler, although using such water does increase the expense and is sometimes inconvenient. Hard water erodes the glass and leaves an alkali deposit that causes a syringe to stick. Boiling in hard water shortens the life of a syringe. The use of bicarbonate of soda or alkalizing sterilizer tablets is not recommended.

If hard water is used for boiling syringes, the barrel and plunger should be assembled with the plunger pushed completely into the barrel. If distilled or demineralized water is used, then the syringes are separated. Arrange all syringes in the boiler parallel to one another and all pointing in the same direction; do not crowd them. Boil for 15 to 20 minutes at a rolling boil. Do not overboil, since this shortens the life of the syringe.

Since boiling is effective against some organisms but not against all spores or viruses, like that of infectious hepatitis, boiling is not recommended as a method of sterilization.

CARE OF HYPODERMIC NEEDLES

A good hypodermic needle is absolutely essential. No one likes to use a dull needle or one with a fish hook on the point. Most needles used for injections today are disposable. Do not attempt to cut expenses by purchasing inferior or unknown brands of needles or syringes. This is truly an example of false economy and may even lead to injury of a patient and a lawsuit. Good disposable needles are made with exacting precision and are appreciated by the patient as well as by the medical assistant.

CONSTRUCTION OF NEEDLES. Figure 25–24 shows the construction of the hypodermic needle and four common needle points. There are some facts to remember about the construction of a hypodermic needle. This statement was prepared by the Becton-Dickinson Company.

The size of the needle is governed by four factors: safety, rate of flow, comfort of the patient, and depth of penetration. There are three standard dimensions: length, outside diameter of

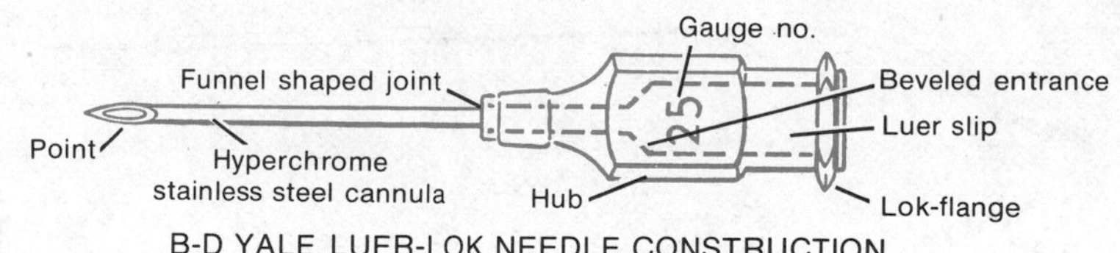

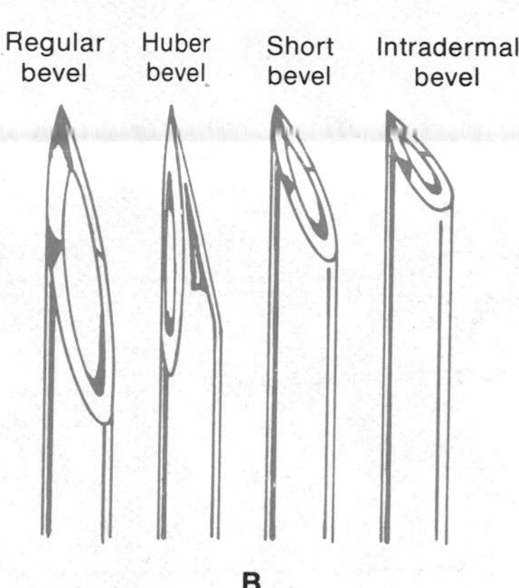

FIGURE 25–24 *A*, **Construction of a hypodermic needle.** *B*, **Types of bevels. (Courtesy of Becton-Dickinson Co.)**

the cannula, and wall thickness. Regular needles are measured for length from where the cannula joins the hub to the tip of the point (hub not included). The outside diameter or "gauge" of a needle is measured by a Stubb's English wire gauge, standard throughout the United States. The diameter sizes are indicated by gauge numbers running from 13 to 27. The larger the gauge number, the smaller the needle. Gauge numbers are often stamped on the flat surface of the hub for ready use.

As you can see in Figure 25–24*B*, the Huber point has a "closed" point. This is to prevent tissue plugs from forming when the needle is inserted. The Huber point gives a smooth sliding action through the tissues, thus reducing the danger of such plugs. The short and intradermal bevels are preferred when medication is injected into the outer layer of the skin and only the bevel of the needle needs to be inserted.

Figure 25–25 illustrates some specialty needles. The Silverman biopsy needle (Fig. 25–25*D*) has a 14 gauge cannula with a fitted stylus, shown inserted. The biopsy needle is used to obtain a specimen from an internal organ or underlying soft tissue. With the stylus in place, the needle is inserted through the body wall to the depth desired. The stylus is then removed, and the split cannula is inserted. The tissue specimen is picked up by the inner cannula. A needle biopsy is frequently preferred to an incisional biopsy for soft tissue. The abscess cannula (Fig. 25–25*E*) is 18 gauge, 1¼ in. with a bulbous tip and flexible cannula. The abscess needle is attached to a syringe and is used to withdraw fluids or pus from an abscess or cyst. These special needles are reusable and must be carefully cleaned and sterilized. The points should be protected when they are in storage.

HOW TO CLEAN NEEDLES. Although most of the needles used in physicians' offices are disposable, an occasional reusable needle must be cleaned and sterilized.

Clean the needle immediately after use, while it is still attached to the syringe, by forcing water through it several times. Then remove the needle from the syringe and rinse it under running water. Push a stylet through the needle to make certain the cannula is clean. *Always insert the stylet from the hub end,* not from the point. Clean the inside of the hub with a cotton applicator. Take care never to touch the point of the needle to anything. Needles become dull or have fish hooks only through misuse or abuse.

HOW TO REMOVE A STUCK NEEDLE. Sometimes a hypodermic needle becomes stuck on a syringe. If this happens, grasp the hub of the needle with a

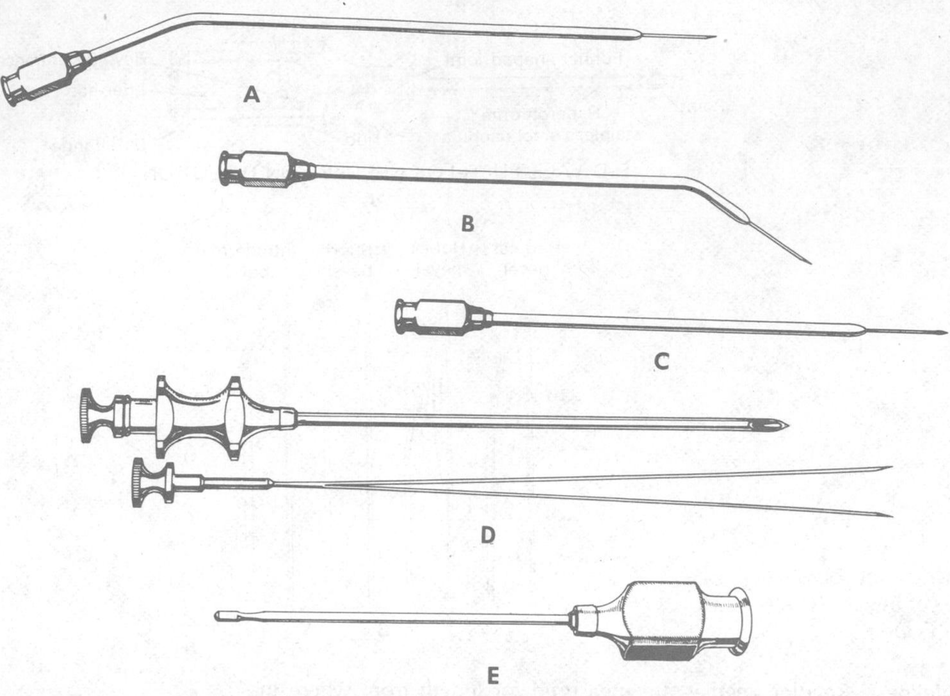

FIGURE 25–25 Specialty needles. ***A,*** **Hemorrhoid needle.** ***B,*** **Tonsil needle, curved.** ***C,*** **Tonsil needle, straight.** ***D,*** **Silverman biopsy needle with stylus (inserted) and biopsy cannula.** ***E,*** **Abscess needle. (Courtesy of Becton-Dickinson and Co.)**

forceps (Fig. 25–26) and turn the syringe counterclockwise. This should loosen the needle. Do not twist the needle or wiggle the syringe, since breakage may occur.

HOW TO SHARPEN A HYPODERMIC NEEDLE. Reusable needles should be kept sharp and smooth. Trauma, pain, and seepage are greatly reduced by eliminating burrs and fish hooks. Needles should always be inspected prior to each sterilization, and those needles requiring sharpening should be placed aside.

Instructions for sharpening hypodermic needles are given by the Becton-Dickinson Company as follows:

Use a magnifying glass to detect burrs, fishhooks, and dull, broken, and misshapen points. To remove burrs from the inside edges use a pointed stylet, trocar, or discarded needle. Use a smooth (Arkansas Stone) oil stone. A light mineral oil on the stone hastens sharpening and gives a smoother finish. To hold the needle more rigidly, attach a small syringe if desired. Use the index finger of the other hand for gentle pressure. Place the needle bevel flush on the

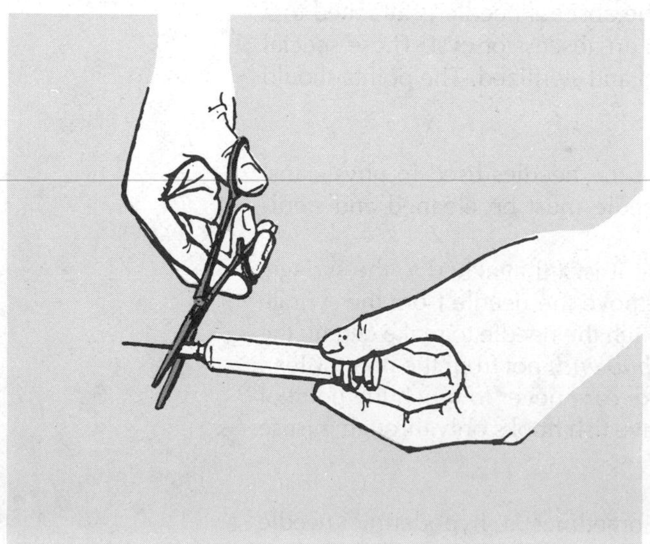

FIGURE 25–26 Removing a stuck hypodermic needle from a syringe.

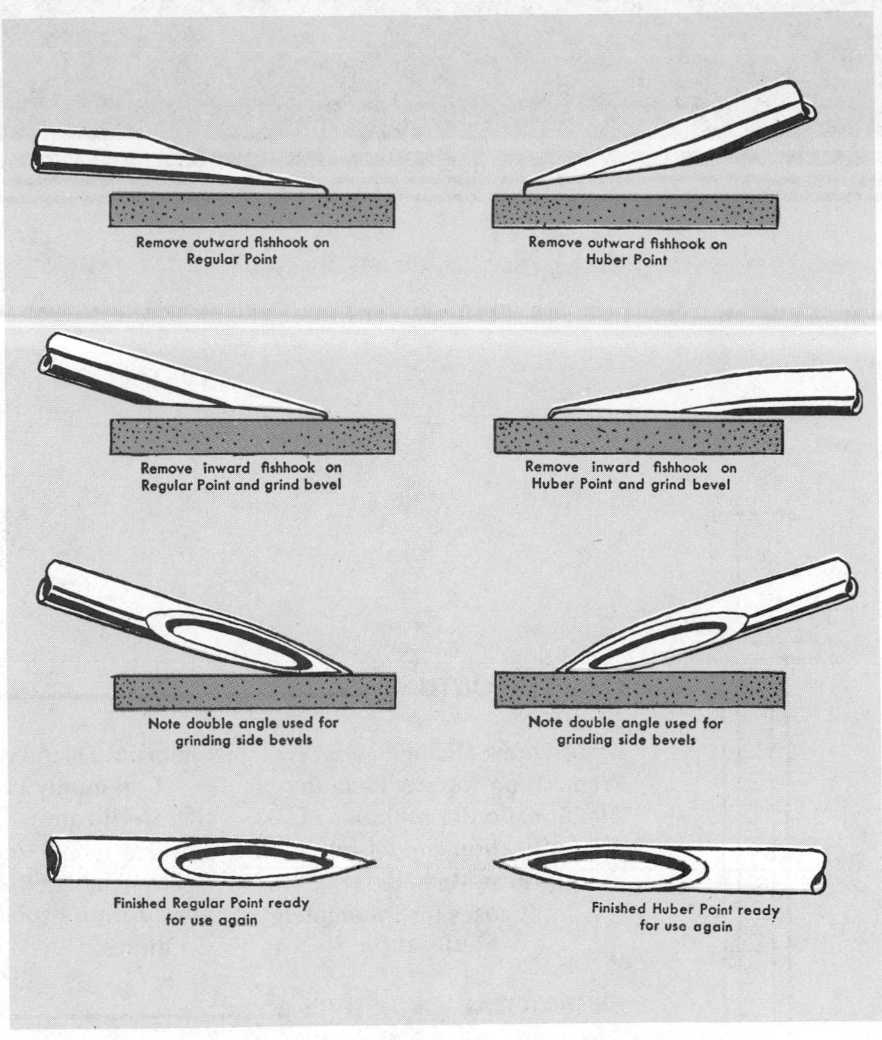

FIGURE 25–27 **Sharpening a hypodermic needle. (Courtesy of Becton-Dickinson and Co.)**

stone at the proper angle [see Figure 25–27] and sharpen by sliding forwards and backwards, and also by moving laterally across the stone to prevent wearing grooves in the stone. In sharpening a needle with a fitted stylet, keep the stylet in place so that perfectly matched bevels are maintained.

STERILIZATION OF HYPODERMIC NEEDLES. Like syringes, hypodermic needles are sterilized by autoclaving or hot air methods. Boiling is not recommended because sterilization is not assured. Chemical sterilization may be used, but it is unsatisfactory because the sterilizing chemical must be rinsed off with sterile distilled water before use. This extra step is often a source of contamination. Autoclaving is the most satisfactory and convenient method. Extra long needles, such as tonsil and hemorrhoid needles, may be placed in glass tubes for autoclaving. About one-half inch of cotton should be placed in the butt of the tube; then insert the needle into the tube, point first. Cover the end of the tube with gauze or sterilizer paper and date the package.

Constriction tubes are excellent for sterilizing regular needles because they prevent the point of the needle from touching anything by means of the constricture in the tube that holds the needle by the hub. Use a cotton plug (not too tight) or gauze or paper over the end. Do not use a rubber stopper because steam cannot penetrate it. It is a good idea to insert a sterilizer indicator, such as Diack, in one tube of each batch to be sterilized. There are also paper holders that protect the point of the needle and permit a needle to be placed in an envelope with a syringe without the danger of the needle puncturing the envelope.

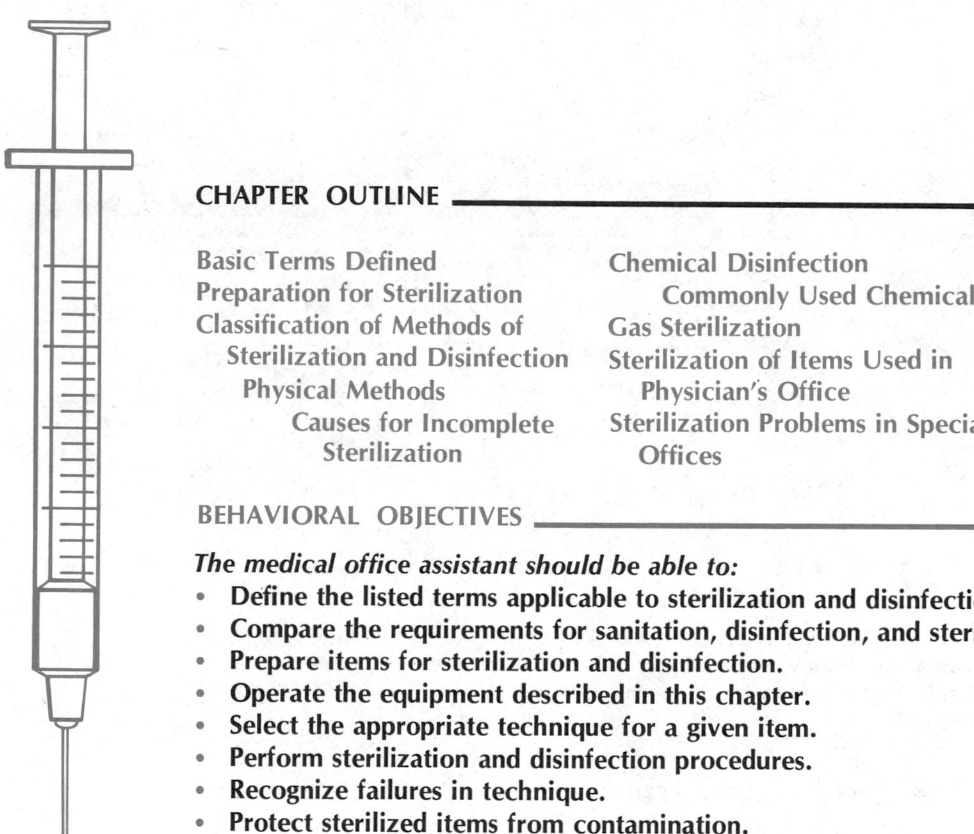

CHAPTER OUTLINE

Basic Terms Defined
Preparation for Sterilization
Classification of Methods of Sterilization and Disinfection
  Physical Methods
    Causes for Incomplete Sterilization
Chemical Disinfection
  Commonly Used Chemicals
Gas Sterilization
Sterilization of Items Used in Physician's Office
Sterilization Problems in Specialty Offices

BEHAVIORAL OBJECTIVES

The medical office assistant should be able to:

- **Define the listed terms applicable to sterilization and disinfection.**
- **Compare the requirements for sanitation, disinfection, and sterilization.**
- **Prepare items for sterilization and disinfection.**
- **Operate the equipment described in this chapter.**
- **Select the appropriate technique for a given item.**
- **Perform sterilization and disinfection procedures.**
- **Recognize failures in technique.**
- **Protect sterilized items from contamination.**

26

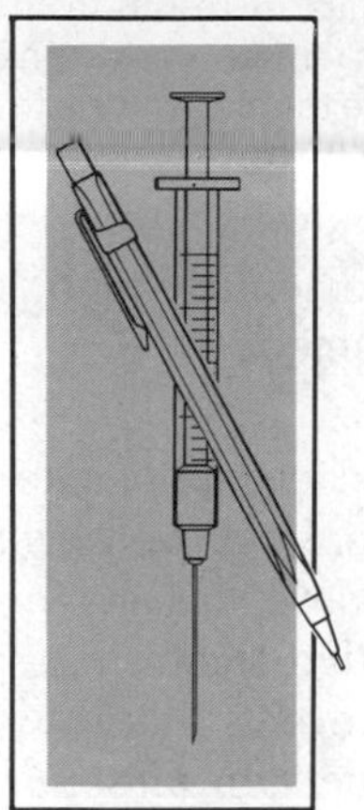

STERILIZATION TECHNIQUES

Sterilization and the attempts to reach and understand sterility are as old as recorded history. Many practices and theories have been tried and then discarded, but with each something has been added to the total knowledge.

Cremation was known to man centuries ago. Man has also known that desiccation sometimes preserves body tissue, and prevents the spread of sepsis. Moses, in about 1250 BC, gave the ancient Hebrews the first recorded sanitation laws. In a sense, Moses was our first "public health officer." The ancient Greeks used forms of fumigation to combat epidemics. Hippocrates (460–370 BC), who separated philosophy and medicine, realized the value of boiling water, washing hands, and using certain medications while dressing an infected wound. The next contribution of significance was the discovery of bacteria in 1683, chiefly by Anton van Leeuwenhoek. Then Joseph Lister (1827–1912), Louis Pasteur (1822–1895), and others started the world on the miraculous path of sterilization. Pasteur said on April 30, 1878, in a lecture to the Académie de Médecin:

> If I had the honor of being a surgeon, convinced as I am of the dangers caused by germs of microbes scattered on the surface of every object, particularly in hospitals, not only would I use absolutely clean instruments, but, after cleansing my hands with great care and putting them quickly through a flame (an easy thing to do with a little practice), I would only make use of charpie, bandages, and sponges which had previously been raised to a heat of 130° C to 150° C; I would only employ water which had been heated to a temperature of 110° C to 120° C. All that is easy in practice, and, in that way, I would still have to fear the germ suspended in the atmosphere surrounding the bed of the patient; but observation shows us every day that the number of those germs is almost insignificant compared to that of those which lie scattered on the surface of objects, or in the clearest ordinary water.

Joseph Lister was the first surgeon to use chemical disinfection. One of his principles, which was the basis for antisepsis, was that "all instruments, dressings and everything else in contact with operations, including the hands of the surgeon and the assistant, should be rendered antiseptic." Lord Lister has been given full honor for introducing the sterile instruments, dressings, and glassware used in the operating room. He gave this advice to his fellow surgeons:

> In order, gentlemen, that you may get satisfactory results from this sort of treatment, you must be able to see with your mental eye the septic ferments as distinctly as we see flies or other insects with the **corporeal** eye. If you can really see them in this distinct way with your intellectual eye, you can be properly on your guard against them; if you do not see them you will be constantly liable to relax in your precautions.

We all give thanks to these gentlemen and many others who contributed to the knowledge of sterility and sterile technique.

BASIC TERMS DEFINED

ANTISEPTICS. Substances which, when applied to microorganisms, will render them harmless either by killing them or by preventing their growth, according to the agent or the method of application. Antiseptics are agents made to prevent sepsis by inhibition or destruction of the **causative** organism, especially for application to the living tissue. If the substance only prevents the growth of bacteria it may then be referred to as a *bacteriostatic agent*. The term *antiseptic* is sometimes used to include disinfectants, although disinfectants are usually too strong to be applied to living tissue. Antiseptics are used in the treatment of wounds and infections and are applied to the skin before surgery. Antibiotics are not classified as antiseptics because they are taken internally.

ASEPSIS. The absence or prevention of access of microorganisms to materials. *Medical asepsis* refers to destruction of organisms after they leave the body. This technique is used in the care of patients with infectious diseases by preventing the transference of pathogenic organisms from person to person, but not all equipment is sterile. This is achieved by the isolation technique. *Surgical asepsis* refers to the destruction of organisms before they enter the body. In surgical asepsis an object is either sterile or nonsterile. Measures that can be taken to provide surgical asepsis include absolute sterilization of all instruments, linens, and other inanimate objects that come in contact with the surgical wound.

ASEPTIC TECHNIQUE. The process designed to exclude or avoid all germs. This technique is used in the operating area and in handling infectious diseases and contaminated material.

CONCURRENT DISINFECTION. Immediate disinfection and disposal of body discharges and infective matter through which a disease may be passed during the course of its progression. This process is being carried on constantly in professional offices and hospitals.

CONTAMINATION. The state of an article or surface that may have become soiled through contact with nonsterile material, especially with the introduction of disease-producing or infectious organisms. If an object is not sterile it is then considered to be contaminated.

DISINFECTION. The destruction of pathogenic organisms by chemical or physical means, but commonly reserved for use only with chemical agents. A disinfectant is an agent that destroys infectious organisms. As ordinarily employed, the disinfection process may or may not be adequate for the destruction of all pathogens, such as the tubercle bacilli, spores, or certain viruses. Disinfectants should be used only on inanimate objects and should not be confused with antiseptics that are applied to living tissue.

FUMIGATION. The process by which microorganisms or insects and vectors of infection are destroyed, usually by the use of gaseous agents; also defined as exposure to disinfecting fumes.

FUNGICIDE. An agent that destroys fungi (has fungicidal action).

GERMICIDE. An agent that destroys pathogenic organisms. Common usage involves the application of chemical agents to kill disease-producing germs, but not necessarily bacterial spores. Germicides are applied to living tissues, as well as to inanimate objects. Another commonly used term, with similar definition, is *bacteriocide*.

SANITIZATION. The act of making sanitary, an important step toward sterilization and disinfection. Sanitizing agents are usually water and detergents, utilized by scrubbing and soaking. Under no circumstances does sanitizing replace or substitute for sterilization. Sanitizing only reduces the number of bacteria on an item and removes certain protein substances so sterilization may be obtained. *Sanitization* is a less precise term than *disinfection* since it is more of a cleaning process.

STERILIZATION. The complete destruction of *all* forms of microbial life. An object that is free of all living organisms may be called *sterile*. Technically, there is no such thing as nearly sterile or partially sterile. An object is either sterile or it is contaminated.

VERMICIDE. An agent that destroys parasitic worms or intestinal animal parasites.

PREPARATION FOR STERILIZATION

In the physician's office cleanliness takes the extreme form of sterilization. Sterilization reduces the perpetual threat of contamination to patients, to the physician, and to the medical assistant.

To assure proper sterilization, a definite area should be set aside in each office for just this purpose. This area should be divided into two sections. One section is used for receiving contaminated materials. This area should have a sink, as well as receiving basins, proper cleaning agents, brushes, sterilizer wrapping paper and envelopes, and indicators. The other section should be reserved for receiving the sterile items after they are removed from the sterilizer. Clear, clean plastic bags in which to store sterile packs may be kept in the sterile area.

Both areas should be spotlessly clean and well organized. If highly contaminated materials are to be handled, or if the medical assistant has an open cut or wound on her hands, she should wear disposable gloves in handling the contaminated items.

CLASSIFICATION OF METHODS OF STERILIZATION AND DISINFECTION

There are many methods of sterilization and disinfection with varying degrees of value. It is extremely important to understand these methods, their advantages and disadvantages, the possible sources of error, and the proper technique of application.

Physical Methods

RADIATION

Ultraviolet. These rays, found in sunlight and ultraviolet lamps, are used to prevent airborne bacteria from spreading in operating rooms, classrooms, and bacteriologic laboratories. Beauty salons and barber shops use ultraviolet rays in their cabinets. These rays are sometimes used in the preparation of certain vaccines. The destructiveness of the ultraviolet ray varies greatly with the distance from the source, the air it passes through, and the surface of the article it hits. This form of radiation is not considered a method of sterilization because of its limitations and its lack of penetrating power.

X-rays. The x-ray, or roentgen ray, is known to have lethal power. These rays penetrate deeply and rapidly. Many authorities feel that the rays will be used for sterilization in the near future, but techniques must still be perfected. Their uses in a medical office are limited.

ULTRASONICS. Ultrasonics are vibratory sound waves of such high frequency that they cannot be heard by the human ear. To date, these sound waves have been used mainly for sanitization of instruments prior to their sterilization by placing the instruments in a bath and then passing the sound waves through it. This forms microscopic bubbles that create a terrific suction and pulling action on the materials attached to the instrument but do not damage even the most delicate of instruments.

REFRIGERATION. A few species of bacteria are killed by freezing temperatures, but a large majority of them survive even subzero temperatures. This method is not used for sterilization but rather for the preservation of foods. It prevents the growth of bacteria. Upon thawing, growth and multiplication can resume, and often foods spoil more quickly.

FILTRATION. When fluid substances cannot be subjected to heat without causing injury to them, they are filtered through unglazed porcelain with pores so minute that most of the bacteria are held back while the fluid passes through. This method is used for the sterilization of some drugs, bacterial toxins, antitoxins and certain culture media. Viruses and rickettsiae that pass through these filters are known as filterable organisms. The most commonly used laboratory filter for this is the Berkefeld filter. The water supply of some cities is purified by the filtration method.

DESICCATION. Desiccation, or drying, is used to inhibit or preserve, especially bacterial cultures and foods. Often freezing and drying are performed rapidly for preservation. Spores are extremely resistant to this method. Desiccation is extremely limited for sterilization.

HEAT. Heat is the most widely used method of sterilization and disinfection in medical offices (Table 26–1). The average organism is killed by heat of 145° F (65° C). The temperature at which an organism is killed is known as the *thermal death point*. This point of death is not a fixed temperature because of some variables, such as the time involved to reach this temperature, and the exposure time, as well as the surrounding environment. This is evident in the fact that if the temperature is increased the time may be decreased, or the reverse. In other words, the thermal death point is reached by a temperature and time formula. Other factors are also considered in this formula, such as toxins that are formed by the organism and pH changes.

Dry Heat. Dry heat can be produced by direct flame or ovens.

Incineration or burning by direct flame destroys an organism immediately. Bacteriologic loops are flamed until the wire glows. For years, mothers have flamed needles for the removal of splinters. Incineration is used to destroy disposable items, as well as contaminated dressings, swabs, sputum cups, and so on. Ironing is a form of burning and is used in the home by ironing dressings just to the scorching point.

The use of dry heat ovens is a preferred method when direct contact with saturated steam is impractical. Dry heat penetrates slowly and unevenly, so longer exposure time is required. Most dry heat sterilizers are electrically heated and

TABLE 26–1 Sterilization Chart

Article	*Method*	*Temperature*	*Time*
Gauze, small, loosely packed	Autoclave	250°F	30 minutes
Gauze, large, loosely packed	Autoclave	270°F	30 minutes
Gauze, small, tightly packed	Autoclave	250°F	40 minutes
Gauze, large, lightly packed	Autoclave	270°F	10 minutes
Gauze, tightly packed	Dry heat	320°F	3 hours
Gauze, loosely packed	Dry heat	320°F	2 hours
Glass syringes in tubes	Autoclave	250°F	30 minutes
Glass syringe and needle in muslin	Autoclave	250°F	30 minutes
Glass syringe in muslin	Dry heat	320°F	1 hour
Hypodermic needle in muslin	Dry heat	320°F	2 hours
Instruments on tray, muslin under and over	Dry heat	320°F	1 hour
Instruments on tray, muslin under and over	Autoclave	250°F	15 minutes
Rubber gloves in glove envelopes	Autoclave	250°F	15 minutes
Solutions in flasks with gauze plug	Autoclave	250°F	30 minutes
Glassware unwrapped	Dry heat	320°F	1 hour
Glassware wrapped	Autoclave	250°F	30 minutes
Petroleum jel, 1 oz. jar	Dry heat	340°F	1 hour
Petroleum jel, 1 oz. jar	Dry heat	320°F	2 hours
Petroleum gauze in instrument tray	Dry heat	320°F	150 minutes
Powder, 1 oz. jar	Dry heat	320°F	2 hours
Powder, small glove packs	Autoclave	250°F	15 minutes

Remember to always place an indicator in areas where there is doubt that the steam will penetrate.

DO NOT MEASURE BY CHAMBER POUNDS. A THERMOMETER AND INDICATOR ARE THE RELIABLE METHODS OF JUDGING A KILLING TEMPERATURE.

heavily insulated ovens with blowers to force air for even distribution of heat. The thermometer should be properly located in the top of the chamber. These ovens should not be overloaded. Glassware should not touch other objects. Items should be kept away from the sides of the oven so air can circulate freely. It is advisable to heat the oven and cool it slowly. Do not open the door during sterilization. There are many variations of temperature and time, depending on the load, but the following are suggested:

340° F (170° C) for one hour
320° F (160° C) for two hours
250° F (121° C) for six hours

The great variance found in temperature and time is influenced by the type of substances being sterilized. For example, the destruction of some spores in anhydrous oil requires 320° F for 160 minutes, but with a very small amount of water added, less than 0.5 per cent, sterilization can be reached in 20 minutes at 320° F.

Remember that organisms, both in **viable** and spore forms, are more resistant to heat when in a dry state. This is a major reason why dry sterilization is not as efficient as steam under pressure. Dry sterilization has definite use for the sterilization of petroleum oil (for petroleum jelly and mineral oil), certain powders, wax, and glassware. Indicators should be used on every item since there can be a variation of 40° to 60° in a chamber (Fig. 26–1). Overheating can cause damage to sharp instruments. Wrapping items in fabrics is not satisfactory since the wrap may become brittle through desiccation. Aluminum foil is an excellent wrap and also has a long shelf life.

Some offices have attempted to use the autoclave as a dry heat oven, but it is not the most satisfactory method of sterilization. An autoclave equipped with a steam jacket and manual controls must be used in order to prevent the steam from automatically being transferred to the chamber. If jacket pressure is maintained around 15 to 18 pounds, the chamber walls are heated to about 250° F. This is very difficult to gauge, however, because the chamber thermometer gives an accurate reading only when steam is in the chamber. Sterilization by this method would require six hours, and this would be very difficult to accomplish. It is best to use this as a heating and drying source and NOT as a method of sterilization.

Moist Heat. The forms of moist heat are boiling water, free-flowing steam, and steam under pressure.

Boiling water (212° F or 100° C) kills most vegetative forms of pathogenic bacteria, but bacterial spores and some viruses associated with infectious hepatitis are resistant to boiling. Because of these limitations, boiling is discouraged as a means of sterilization and is used for disinfection only.

No matter how much heat is applied or how vigorous the boil, water will reach only 212° F at sea level. The higher the elevation, the lower the temperature required to obtain a boil. For example, in Denver, Colorado, water boils at 202° F. Water in a boiler should first be taken to a brisk boil and then the heat turned down to produce a mild roll. Whenever bubbles are regularly formed, the water has reached the boiling temperature. Objects must be completely immersed and the timing started only after the water shows a rolling boil. All a violent boil does is to increase the amount of steam and the loss of water through evaporation. Boiling water is a very poor substitute for steam under pressure.

The addition of 2 per cent soda solution greatly increases the killing power of boiling water, as well as dissolves dried blood and other coagulable substances, but it is harmful to glass and rubber goods.

Free-flowing steam reaches the same temperature as boiling water. It is used for materials that would be harmed by higher temperatures and for those that cannot be immersed in water or subjected to dry heat. The fractional or intermittent method is used, that is, materials are exposed to flowing steam for 30 minutes on three successive days. The Arnold Sterilizer is used for this purpose. This fractional method is seldom employed in a medical office because of the time involved, but it is used in laboratories.

Steam under pressure as represented by the autoclave (Fig. 26–2) is the best and most accepted method of sterilization used to date in the medical office. It is fast,

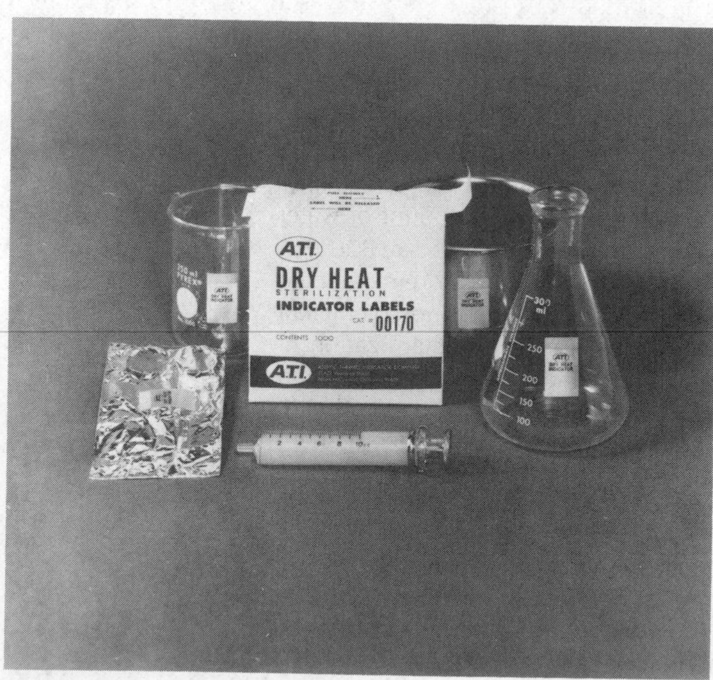

FIGURE 26–1 Dry Heat Indicator. (Courtesy of Aseptic-Thermo Indicator Co.)

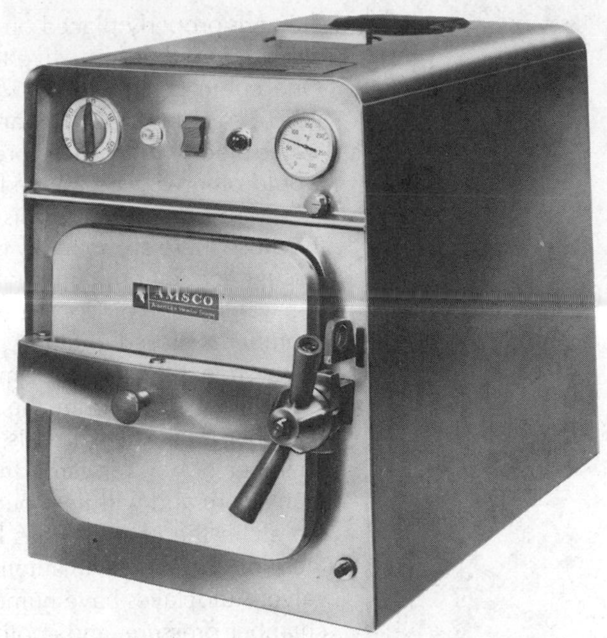

FIGURE 26–2 Medical office autoclave. (Courtesy of AMSCO, American Sterilizer Company, Erie, Pennsylvania.)

convenient, and dependable if certain rules of technique are followed. *Steam under pressure is used for the sole purpose of obtaining a higher moist heat*. The increased pressure alone offers no advantage. It is the higher heat plus the moisture of the steam that is more effective, with the moisture playing a very important part. The two factors of heat *and* moisture must be present to be effective. When steam is admitted into the autoclave chamber it condenses on the cold objects, simultaneously heating and wetting the object, coagulating proteins, and destroying all living organisms. *All* surfaces must be contacted by this moisture. Steam under pressure is capable of much faster penetration of fabrics and textiles than dry heat *but* it has definite limitations if the rules are not followed.

Incorrect operation of an autoclave may result in superheated steam. When the steam is brought to a higher temperature, it is literally dried out and the advantage of a higher heat is diminished. It then acts more as hot air, with less penetrative ability, and possibly is as ineffective as sterilization. Wet steam is another cause of incomplete sterilization. This presents a particularly difficult problem with fabric packs because the packs are soaked with moisture and the steam becomes ineffective. Moreover, it is extremely difficult to dry the packs during the drying cycle. A wet pack literally sucks up bacteria from the air and any surface it is placed upon.

Wet steam may result from failing to preheat the chamber, resulting in excessive condensation in the interior of the chamber. It can be compared to taking a hot shower in a cold bathroom, which results in heavily steamed mirrors and tile walls. Cold instruments placed in a hot chamber will also increase condensation. A little condensation is helpful, but excessive moisture is not. Other causes of a wet load are opening the door too wide during the drying cycle and allowing a rush of cold air into the chamber; also, overfilling the water reservoir may produce a wet load.

The main cause for incomplete sterilization in the autoclave is the presence of residual air. Without the complete elimination of air, an adequately high temperature cannot be reached. *Air and steam do not mix*. Since air is heavier than steam it will pool wherever possible. One-tenth of 1 per cent residual air trapped in the chamber will prevent complete sterilization. This is especially dangerous in older autoclaves that do not have a chamber thermometer separate from the temperature marks on the same gauge as the pounds pressure. *Fifteen pounds pressure does not guarantee 250° F.*

All escape valves and discharge lines must be kept clean and free from dirt and lint. Air will flow out of jars, cans, bottles, and containers, as water would flow out, if they are properly placed on their sides. If the operator mentally visualizes water for air, she can then visualize this air flowing out as water would flow out by gravity. One cubic centimeter of water will provide 865 cubic centimeters of steam (Fig. 26–3), so containers that cannot be placed on their sides should have a few drops of water placed in them before loading; the steam forming will force out the air that would otherwise be trapped in the container.

Many autoclaves consist of a sterilizing chamber surrounded by an outer jacket. (Because there are so many different models used in medical offices, the authors will discuss general principles only.) Steam is admitted in the bottom of the jacket from the water reservoir as the water boils and forms steam. The connection into the chamber is closed until the jacket pressure is sufficient to transfer into the chamber. This connection is opened manually or automatically, depending on the model. The steam then flows from the jacket into the chamber from the upper rear of the chamber (Fig. 26–4*A*). This flow of steam from the upper rear drives the air in the chamber down, forward, and out the air exhaust valve. Remember, air is heavier than steam and will flow out, if not trapped, like water flowing out of a sink. When the air in the chamber has been driven out and the temperature starts to rise, the thermostatic valve will automatically close, sealing off the chamber at the air exhaust valve. Autoclaves have numerous gauges: one indicates the jacket pressure, one the chamber pressure, and another the chamber temperature. Some of the older models have the temperature marking on the same gauge as the chamber pressure. As stated before, pressure gives no guarantee of temperature. When the pressure in the chamber starts to rise, you then should watch the chamber temperature gauge. You *do not* start your timing of the load until the desired temperature in the chamber has been reached. Then adjust the heat control to maintain the desired temperature and set the time clock.

The autoclave chamber must be cleaned before each loading. If there has been any ebullition of solutions, the water reservoir must be drained and thoroughly cleaned and rinsed. On many models there is no access to the reservoir and it must be cleaned by a professional serviceman. Check the manufacturer's instructions carefully and do not use a commercial cleaner unless advised by the manufacturer. A mild detergent may be used in the chamber, but make certain it is very thoroughly rinsed after any type of cleaner has been used. Many manufacturers will not honor a guarantee if anything other than distilled water is used or if any type of cleaner has been put through the reservoir tank.

The trays must also be kept clean and free of lint. Do not remove the bottom tray except to clean. It must be in place for proper steam circulation. The air exhaust valve is one of the most important parts of the autoclave and must be clean and free of lint, otherwise the air will not exhaust from the chamber. Unless proper care is taken of the autoclave, the dressings and instruments will have been *well heated but not sterilized.*

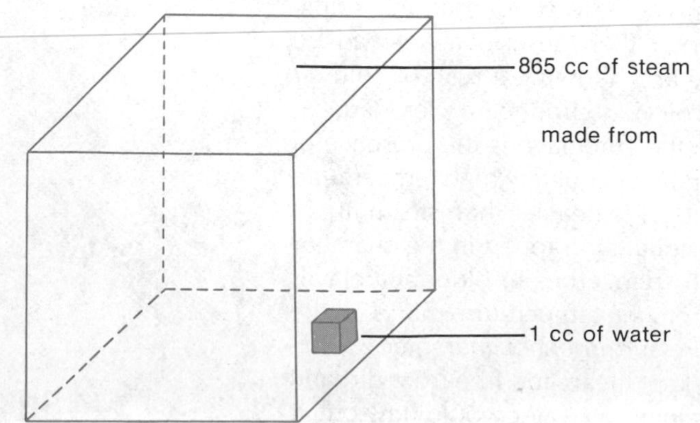

FIGURE 26–3 Quantitative aspects of water and steam.

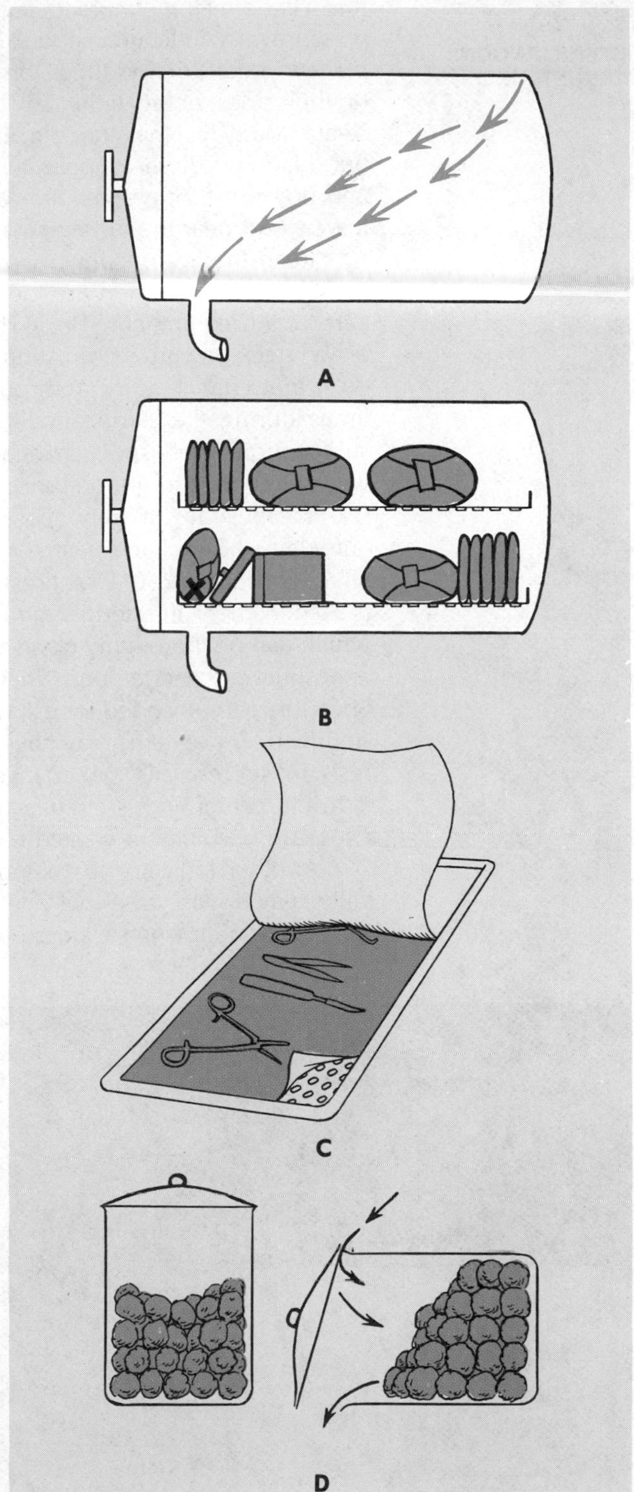

FIGURE 26–4 *A,* Cross section of a cylinder type autoclave. Arrows indicate the direction of the flow of steam and air elimination. *B,* The X marks the placement of an indicator near the exhaust outlet. Note the jar is placed on the side with the lid opened and the glove envelopes are on end. The packs are not crowded, and there is space between top and bottom shelf. *C,* Instruments are placed on a thin towel on a tray and covered with a layer of towel. All jointed instruments are opened to permit steam to all surfaces. All trays used should be perforated. *D,* Steam flows into the right container but not into the left one. An indicator should be placed in the lower back of the container on the right.

INDICATORS. In 1881 Robert Koch tried using anthrax spores to see if the items had been sterilized, but this method was difficult to use and gave unreliable results. Also in the 19th century, a British physician used raw eggs in a load. If the eggs were hard at the end of exposure, he considered the load to be sterile. Even with these extremely poor and unreliable methods, it was realized that there was a need to determine sterility. To eliminate the constant doubt of complete sterilization, *indicators* should be used. These indicators show, by melting or by changing color, that a certain temperature for a given period of time has been reached, irrespective of pressure. An indicator should be placed with each load, buried deep in packs, placed in constriction tubes, put in the bottoms of containers that cannot be turned on their sides, or located in any other places that might be inaccessible to the flow of steam. Many feel that an indicator is not necessary if the chamber has a thermometer, but this tells you the temperature only where the tip of the thermometer is located and not in the above-mentioned places. An indicator should also be placed in the lower front near the air exhaust valve.

Read the accompanying instructions for the indicator you use. The dangers of incomplete sterilization are too great for you to be lax in your technique or in the care of the equipment. The ATI Steam-Clox indicator (Fig. 26–5) will give you an extra check on your sterilization. It consists of a small piece of paper with four spots on it that change color from purple to green. The different spots indicate different times during the sterilization procedure and show the operator the progress of sterilization. These spots change color only in the presence of heat AND steam; they will not change in the presence of heat alone.

To illustrate: If only spot 1 changes color, there is a definite failure of the autoclave in supplying steam or eliminating air from the chamber. This spot changes after exposure of 250° F for two minutes, which is not enough for sterilization. Spot 2 is used to check the sterility of rubber goods, instruments, and other nonporous items which can be thoroughly cleaned before sterilization. This spot allows the minimum exposure time and temperature (250° F in 10 minutes) for such hard-surfaced items. Spot 3 is recommended for use when packs of gauze sponges and dressings are to be sterilized. These items may have bacteria embedded in the fibers that revert to more resistant spores. This spot changes color after 15 minutes exposure at 250° F. Spot 4 is in the center and is circular. If this spot turns green, it indicates needlessly long exposure, resulting in wasted time and unnecessary deterioration of materials.

Another indicator that is popular and has proved useful is the small, hermetically sealed glass tube that contains a tiny pellet which requires only five to eight minutes to melt when exposed to 250° F. At a slightly lower temperature (245° F) it

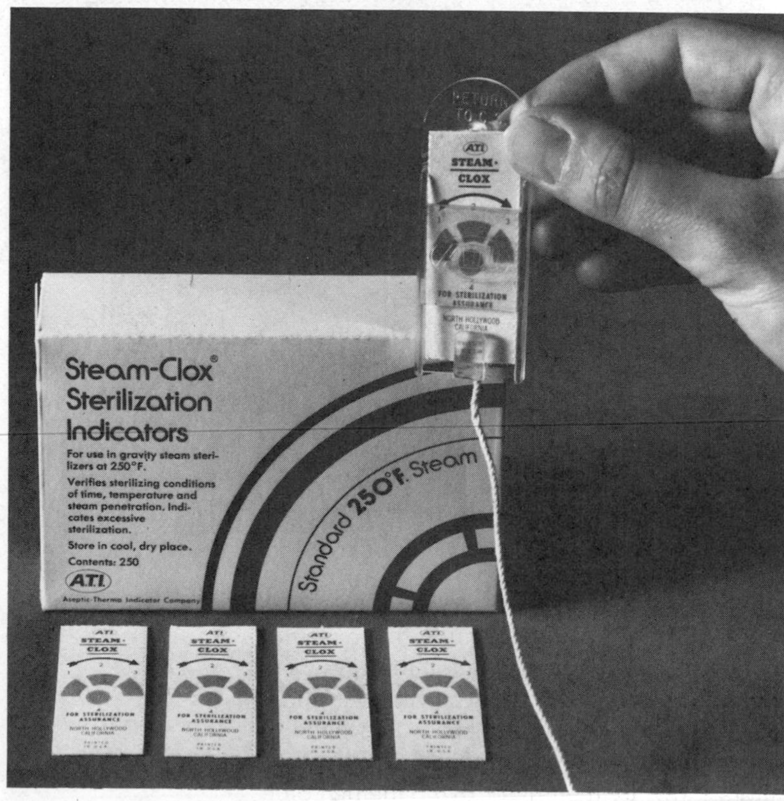

FIGURE 26–5 Steam-Clox autoclave indicator. (Courtesy of Aseptic-Thermo Indicator Co.)

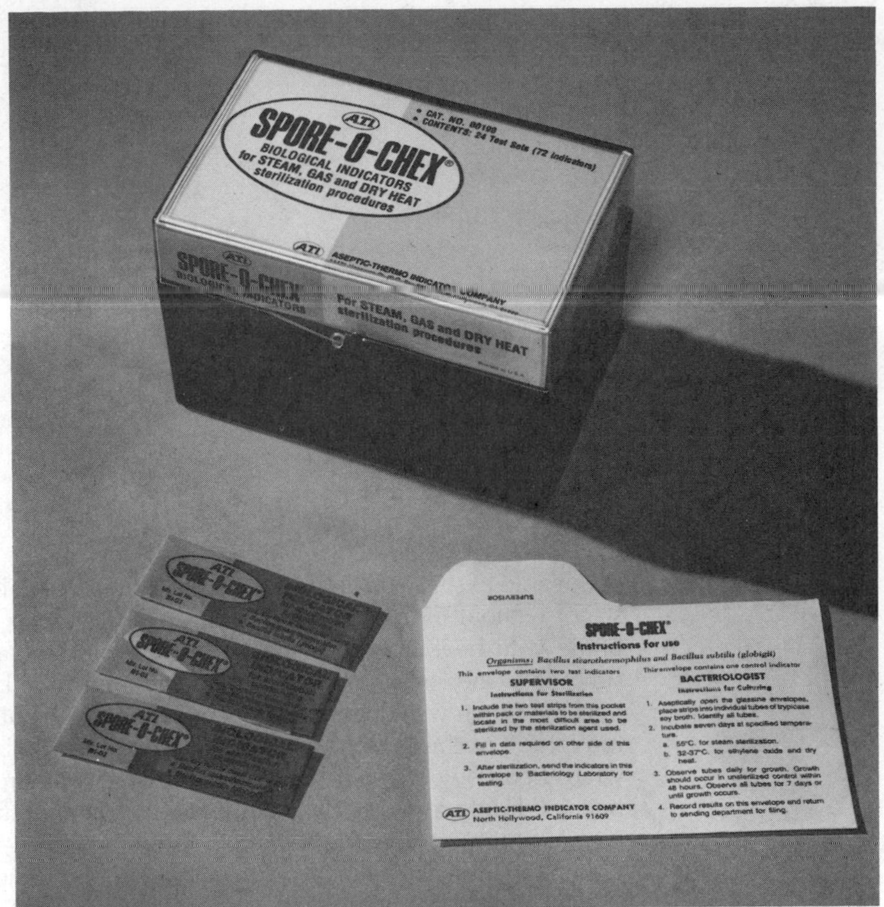

FIGURE 26–6 Spore-O-Chex biological indicator containing bacilli spores. (Courtesy of Aseptic-Thermo Indicator Co.)

requires 20 to 30 minutes to melt. These sealed glass indicators may be placed in a fluid without damage to themselves or to the fluid.

The most accepted means of determining the efficiency of sterilization processes is the indicator that contains dried bacterial spores of established, heat-resistant organisms (Fig. 26–6). These bacterial spore strips are available commercially from reliable suppliers, but the indicators are not always practical for a physician's office because the strip, after autoclaving, must be sent to a bacteriology laboratory for sterility testing.

Autoclave or sterilizer tapes frequently have some form of indicator on them that changes after exposure to sterilization procedures. These tapes are excellent for securing packages and bags, but they are not to be used as sterilizer indicators. They never were intended for this purpose; they only indicate that the package has been processed, not that sterility has been reached.

Sterilization indicator bags are also very convenient. They are made of disposable paper or thermostable plastic in which syringes, tubing and many other items can be sterilized and stored. The paper or transparent material is permeable to steam and provides a barrier against airborne bacteria during storage. Each bag has an indicator printed on it, similar to the sterilizer tape, which shows that the bag has been autoclaved but does not prove it is sterile (Fig. 26–7).

WRAPPING MATERIALS. The maintenance of sterility is completely dependent upon the wrapper and its porosity, as well as on the method of wrapping. The wrapping material must be permeable to steam but impervious to contaminants such as dust and insects. Muslin should be of 140-thread count and a double thickness used. Canvas or duck fabric is not advisable because steam cannot penetrate it properly. Paper is the most popular wrap in the physician's office. It should be

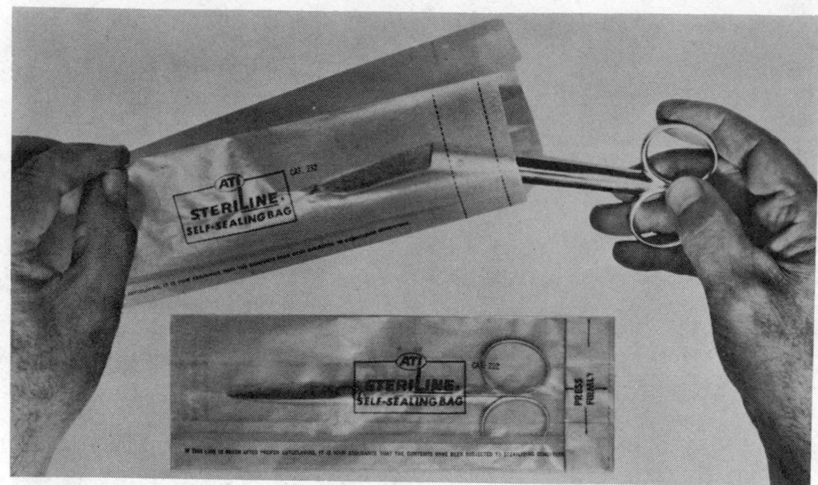

FIGURE 26–7 Instruments are autoclaved individually in transparent envelopes for easy identification and storage. (Courtesy of Aseptic-Thermo Indicator Co.)

permeable to steam, resistant to contamination, but able to withstand the moisture of steam without disintegrating. The paper must be of a quality that will not become brittle with heat or storage. There are several manufacturers of "sterilizer paper," such as Dennison and Kraft. Paper lends itself well to autoclaving but tends to become brittle with dry heat. This can happen with autoclaving if the drying cycle is too long. For this reason, it is not advisable to autoclave muslin wraps with paper wraps because of the difference in the drying cycle time. Glassine bags also tend to become brittle and may stick to a metal surface, but they are transparent and allow easy visibility of contents. Aluminum foil is used only for dry heat sterilization. Cellophane may be autoclaved but should not be subjected to dry heat sterilization. Plastics should not be used as wrappers unless specifically recommended. Regardless of which wrapping material is used, it should be folded in such a way that it may

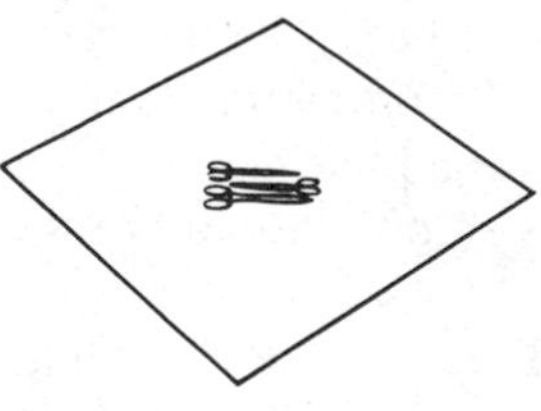

All items are placed in the center and

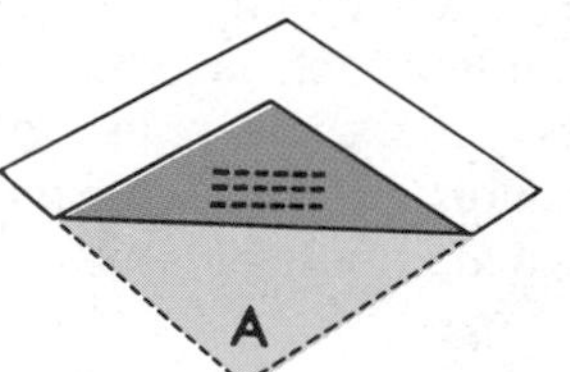

the material folded up from the bottom,

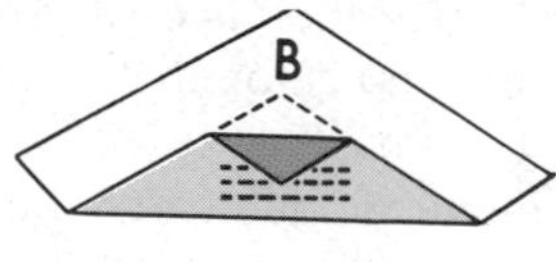

doubling back a small corner.

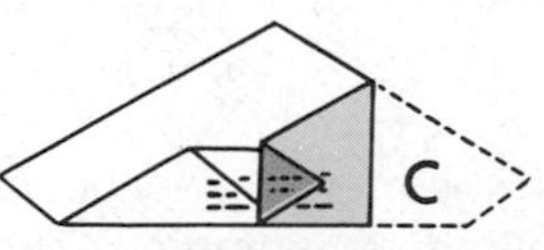

The right,

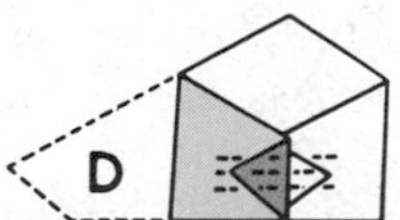

then left, edges are folded over, again leaving corners doubled back.

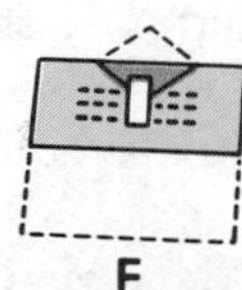

The pack is folded up from the bottom and secured with pressure-sensitive tape.

FIGURE 26–8 Steps in wrapping dressings for sterilizing.

be opened without contaminating the contents. Figure 26–8 illustrates the folded flaps that permit the pack to be opened without reaching in and under the fold.

There is great diversity in the length of time supplies may be considered to remain sterile. If the storage area is dust free and has very limited air circulation, if the packs are not handled and are covered with clean plastic bags, then it is generally felt they will remain sterile for at least 30 days. When an item is resterilized it must be completely reprocessed with a new wrapper. Any time a package seal is broken or damaged in any way, it is considered contaminated (Table 26–2).

Causes of Incomplete Sterilization

1. Inadequate sanitation
2. Incorrect loading of autoclave chamber
   a. overloading

TABLE 26–2 Tips for Improving Your Autoclaving Techniques

Probable Cause	Correction
LINENS	
Too Damp	
Clogged chamber drain.	Remove strainer; free openings of lint.
Goods removed from chamber too soon following cycle.	Allow goods to remain in sterilizer an additional 15 minutes with door slightly open.
Improper loading.	Place packs on edge; arrange for least possible resistance to flow of steam and air.
Stained	
Dirty chamber.	Clean chamber with Calgonite solution. Never use strong abrasives, steel wool, and so forth.
	Rinse thoroughly after cleaning.
INSTRUMENTS	
Corroded	
Poor cleaning; residual soil.	Improve cleaning. Do not allow soil to dry on instruments. Sanitize first.
Exposure to hard chemicals (iodine, salt, acids, and so on).	Do not expose instruments to these chemicals. If exposure occurs, rinse immediately.
Inferior instruments.	Use only top quality instruments.
Spotted or Stained	
Mineral deposits on instruments.	Wash with soft soap and detergent with good wetting properties.
Residual detergents from cleaning.	Rinse instruments thoroughly.
Mineral deposits from tap water.	Rinse with distilled water.
Stiff Hinges or Joints	
Corrosion or soil in joint.	Clean with warm, weak acid solution (10% nitric acid solution). Rinse thoroughly after.
Jaws and shanks out of alignment.	Realignment by qualified instrument repairman.
SOLUTIONS	
Ebullition or Caps Blow Off	
Exhausting chamber too rapidly.	Use slow exhaust, cool liquids, or turn autoclave off and let cool at its own speed. That is, let the pressure decrease at its own rate.
MECHANICAL	
Steam Leakage	
Worn gasket.	Replace
Door closes improperly.	Re-open door and shut carefully. Have serviced if unable to close door properly.
Chamber Door Will Not Open	
Vacuum in chamber (check chamber pressure gauge).	Turn on controls to starting steam pressure and wait until equalized, then vent and open door.

   b. placing jars in upright position
   c. allowing small trays to act as barriers
   d. placing articles horizontally and not vertically
   e. removing bottom tray and placing items on autoclave floor
3. Dirty or clogged discharge air exhaust line
4. Reading pressure rather than temperature
5. Improper placement of indicators
6. Inadequate drying during drying cycle
7. Incorrect wrapping
8. Using nonpermeable wrapping material
9. Failure to maintain full correct temperature during entire cycle
10. Starting timing before correct temperature is reached
11. Failure to preheat chamber for first load

Chemical Disinfection

Remember the term "sterilization" means the complete destruction of all living organisms. This is an absolute term and cannot be used with such words as "almost" or "partially." The Council on Pharmacology and Chemistry of the American Medical Association has reported:

> The Council on Pharmacology and Chemistry has formally gone on record as disapproving of the use of the terms "sterilize," "sterile" and "sterilization" in a bacteriological sense other than in their correct scientific significance; i.e., meaning the absence or destruction of all microorganisms. These terms are not relative and to permit their use in a relative sense not only is incorrect but opens the way to abuse and misunderstanding.

The term "disinfection" is therefore preferred when discussing chemical means of killing organisms. Chemical disinfection has certain limitations and is very difficult to verify since there are no convenient indicators such as those used for steam pressure sterilization. Most commercial promotions of disinfectants are directed toward the killing of staphylococci. Some claim lethal powers on tubercle bacilli, fungi, and even spores and viruses. Because physicians and medical assistants are not familiar with chemical disinfectants, they can only rely upon established, ethical manufacturers who have rigid tests and standardization of their products and do not make false advertising claims.

Disinfectants are used because they are convenient and are often the agent of choice because some materials are damaged by heat; e.g., fine cutting edges, lensed instruments, and synthetics that are not thermostable.

A good disinfectant and antiseptic should be effective in a moderately low concentration; it should not irritate tissue (this applies to antiseptics more than to disinfectants); it should retain its potency in the presence of some dead organic matter; it should not be too volatile with a high evaporation; and it should be effective within a reasonable length of time. Often a disinfectant solution is not effective because (1) it is left in an open container where evaporation changes its consistency; (2) sanitized instruments are not dried, and the wet instruments, when placed in the solution, dilute it beyond the manufacturer's recommendation; or (3) items are not thoroughly sanitized before being placed in the solution, and the attached organic matter changes the action of the disinfectant.

Fabrics placed in the bottom of a container or instrument tray are often the cause of weakening a solution because chemicals are trapped in the fibers and are not in solution. The solution in containers with fabric in the bottom should be changed more frequently than should the solution in containers without fabric pads.

Destruction of organisms by chemical means varies greatly, depending upon the type of chemical used. No chemical can kill unless it reaches the instrument's surface; therefore, complete sanitization is absolutely necessary. Very strong agents will kill in a short time but they are usually very hard on an instrument. Time and strength cannot be separated. Temperature is somewhat of a factor, although most agents are used at room temperature. The effectiveness of some agents is increased by adding to boiling water; others are less effective if chilled. Reliable manufacturers will state the organisms that can be expected to be killed by the solution in a specified dilution, for a specified time. They will also state which organisms will not be killed.

SOAP. For many years soap was considered the "all-purpose" disinfectant, but studies have shown that soap has very limited killing power. It is the scrubbing action and the running water that have real value, as in handwashing and sanitizing. The average household soap has limited effect, but since soap is not a single chemical there are additives that do have lethal power. Although there is considerable controversy on "germicidal" or "surgical" soaps, there are some germicidal soaps that do kill organisms, mainly staphylococci, which are the greatest offenders on our skin. These germicidal soaps leave a film of disinfectant on the skin that will last for several hours. Hexachlorophene is virtually insoluble in water but soluble in alcohol, so it will remain on the skin and not be removed by a routine handwash, but it is removed if the hands are rinsed in alcohol.

DETERGENTS. These are mainly wetting agents to increase penetrating and wetting power; they are sometimes called "soapless" soap. Because of their ability to emulsify fats and oils, they aid in the mechanical removal of bacteria, especially from the skin. Detergents that are very alkaline are corrosive to aluminum and will also attack ground glass surfaces, such as syringes. Strong alkaline detergents are also harmful to rubber. Most detergents are slightly alkaline and may be used for general purposes but it is best to use detergents that are manufactured for cleaning glassware and rubber goods.

ALCOHOL. Alcohol is the most widely used disinfectant. Ethyl alcohol had been widely used in the past, but isopropyl alcohol has become more frequently used. It exhibits slightly greater germicidal action than ethyl alcohol. It is an excellent fat solvent and therefore good for cleansing the skin, but continued use is hard on the hands. Iodine and other chemicals are sometimes added to alcohol to increase its lethal powers. Alcohol may be used to disinfect delicate instruments but it tends to rust them. Care should be used in cleansing lensed instruments with alcohol because it may dissolve the cement around the lenses. It is a good cleanser but any excess should be wiped off or allowed to evaporate before using the instruments.

ACIDS. Acids in concentrated form are excellent germicides but are corrosive. The more they are diluted to decrease these hazards, the less valuable they are as disinfectants. Boric acid is a very weak antiseptic, even in saturated solutions. On the other hand, nitric acid is extremely caustic.

Phenol. Phenol (carbolic acid) was first used as an antiseptic in 1865 by Joseph Lister. It is toxic to tissues in strong dilutions but is often added to other agents. Phenol is used as a standard for testing disinfectants. This standardization is the lethal quality of an agent as compared to phenol acting for the same length of time, on the same organisms and at the same dilutions. This procedure is useful but has limitations because of the various requirements an antiseptic should meet. These comparisons are carefully set according to the specifications of the United States Food and Drug Administration. Hexachlorophene is a phenolic derivative.

ALKALIES. These include lye and quicklime. They are extremely corrosive and are used mainly for sanitation of barns, chicken houses, and so on. A pasty mixture is called "milk of lime" and a thin dilution is known as "whitewash."

FORMALDEHYDE. Formaldehyde (formalin) has strong disinfectant properties and is used as a preservative of tissue (10 per cent solution). A 5 per cent solution is actively germicidal and sporicidal in the presence of organic matter. It is irritating to tissue, and any instrument disinfected with it must be thoroughly rinsed with sterile water before use. It should be used at room temperature because cooling reduces its effectiveness.

METALS. Certain metals are used in antiseptics and are very effective. Silver is used as silver nitrate ($AgNO_3$) in many different percentages, and as argyrol in 5 to 20 per cent aqueous solutions. Mercury is used as bichloride of mercury, mercurochrome, and merthiolate. Arsenic and zinc are also used.

OXIDIZING AGENTS. Oxidizing agents such as hydrogen peroxide (H_2O_2) are used for bacteria that are anaerobic — that is, they cannot exist in the presence of free oxygen. These agents are usually not stable and are considered only mildly antiseptic but are used to irrigate cuts and minor wounds.

DYES. Dyes are sometimes used as germicides, but they are considered mild. With the discovery of sulfonamides, dyes are not used as much today. Dyes are more bacteriostatic and fungicidal than antiseptic. Some of the dyes used are crystal violet, carbolfuchsin, and brilliant green.

OILS. Oils have a weak germicidal effect. They are used more for their pleasant odor and mild astringent effect than for antisepsis. Some of the oils used are clove, pine, wintergreen, thyme, and peppermint.

IODINE. Tincture of iodine and other iodine compounds are traditional agents for cuts and abrasions and for preoperative preparation of the skin. A 1 or 2 per cent solution dissolved in 70 per cent alcohol is an excellent skin antiseptic, but may be irritating to the tissues. A 2 per cent aqueous iodine solution is often used as an instrument disinfectant in emergency situations. However, because some iodine is a tincture, it tends to evaporate and become stronger, burning the skin and having less antiseptic power. There are many commercial iodine compounds that are less dangerous to use and are stable. It is generally considered to be more of an antiseptic than a disinfectant.

QUATERNARY AMMONIUM COMPOUNDS. These are very popular. Zephiran is an example. They are highly stable and nonirritating when used as directed. They are in tincture solutions for skin antisepsis and in aqueous solutions for instrument disinfection.

Remember with all chemical solutions that it is extremely important that you read the labels carefully and follow the manufacturer's instructions. Many times an anxious salesperson may mislead you or try to save you a few pennies. You can always check with your local hospital to see what they use for chemical disinfection.

Gas Sterilization

The use of gas as a sterilizing agent was known in ancient times. History tells us of the use of fumigation: formaldehyde was used over 60 years ago to fumigate a sickroom. Gases were used for killing insects by the ancient Greeks and Romans. In about 850 BC, Homer referred to the use of sulfur for this purpose. In 473 BC the Athenians attempted to use this method to stop a plague. Chaucer, in 1384, used the term "fumigacioun" in English. This early fumigation was adequate for some areas but effective only on the exposed areas and then required considerable airing afterwards before the site was tolerable. Even some of the modern methods require airing, which can present a problem. After World War II the Army Chemical Corps started a search for a new sterilizing agent that would be bactericidal and sporicidal at a moderately low temperature, would penetrate porous substances, and would not damage metals, plastics, rubber, leather, wood, or wool. It should be easily removed by aeration, be low in toxicity, noninflammable, and easy to store and use. Ethylene oxide answered all these qualifications except that it was explosively inflammable.

By mixing ethylene oxide with carbon dioxide, this problem has been overcome to some degree since 1949.

There are some variables with the use of gas sterilization as there are with steam under pressure sterilization. The major problem is the time of exposure, but this has been shortened by the slight increases of temperature. Moisture is also a variable factor. There is considerable difference in the various gas sterilizers on the market, and each manufacturer has its own set of conditions necessary to achieve sterilization.

Many researchers report that gas sterilization could possibly be used exclusively, eliminating both the steam pressure and the dry heat methods. The major disadvantage is the extended time needed for exposure and the time required for aeration after.

There is no doubt that gas sterilization is superior to the use of chemical disinfection methods. The United States Public Health Services (USPHS) does not recommend the use of disinfecting solutions as a method of sterilization.

PREPARATION AND WRAPPING OF ITEMS FOR GAS STERILIZATION. Items to be sterilized by gas are sanitized as carefully as for any type of sterilization. Excessive moisture is removed and all surfaces are exposed. There is not the great concern of having to position items as there is in the autoclave since gas flows in all directions and contacts all exposed surfaces. Almost all forms of sterilizer wraps are acceptable for gas sterilization, but the new transparent plastics made specifically for sterilization are preferred because the contents are visible. The manufacturer of the sterilizer will probably have suggestions. Do not use aluminum foil, nylon films, Saran wrap, or cellophane.

INDICATORS FOR GAS STERILIZATION. As with all forms of sterilization, indicators should be used. There are several excellent indicators on the market and, as with steam sterilization, bacterial cultures are the superior method of checking sterilization. The spores of *Bacillus subtilis,* var. *globiggi* are more resistant to ethylene oxide so it is the organism that is used. Ethylene oxide indicator labels, strips, and bags also are used and are reliable because they can be buried deep within a pack. Some gas indicator tape is useful, but, as with steam indicator tape, it indicates only that the item has been exposed to the gas on the outside of the package. It does not and never was intended by the manufacturer to be an indicator of complete sterilization (Fig. 26–9).

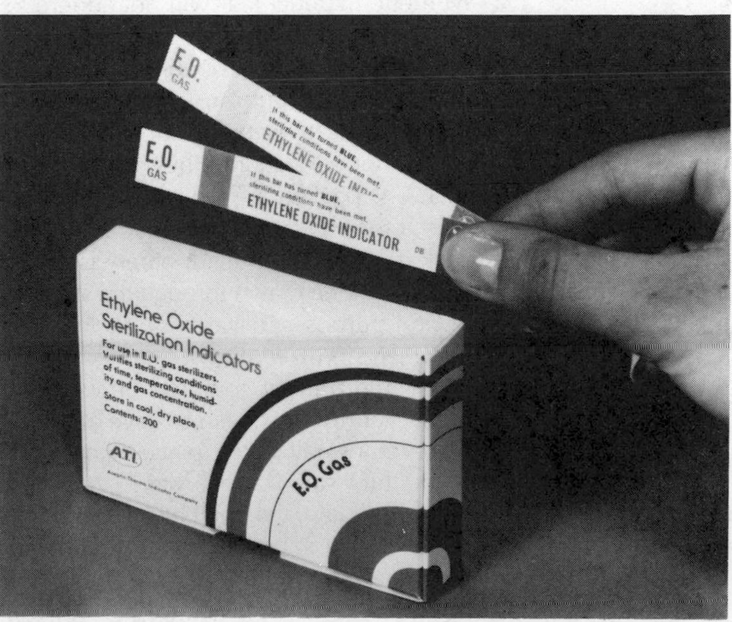

FIGURE 26–9 Ethylene oxide indicators for gas sterilizers. (Courtesy of Aseptic-Thermo Indicator Co.)

LOADING A GAS STERILIZER. The chamber is loaded in the same way as for the autoclave, allowing space between items for the gas to circulate. It is not as critical as in the autoclave because air pockets do not form in containers. Gas circulates in all directions.

Heat damage is not a problem because the heat is only slightly higher than room temperature. Wrapping materials that have a low ethylene oxide permeability also have a low air permeability and therefore may tend to burst when used in a sterilizer that has a vacuum cycle. To reduce this possibility, it is essential that as much air as possible be removed from the bag before sealing. A wrap material that is suitable for one type of gas sterilizer may not be suitable for another. Check the manufacturer's instructions.

EXPOSURE TIMES. Since there are several variables such as the type of sterilizer, gas concentration, temperature, and moisture, the following are not to be followed but are shown as examples only:

35 to 45 minutes at 130° F *or* 2¼ to 2½ hours at 75° F

AERATION TIME. Ethylene oxide gas diffuses fairly rapidly in the open air, but many porous materials will absorb the gas and therefore will require longer periods of aeration. There are so many variations that the manufacturer's instructions must be followed. These times will vary from 150 hours aeration for natural methods to only 5 to 8 hours for mechanical methods of aeration. The storage life of an item sterilized by gas will depend upon the type of wrap and the place of storage. The supplier of the wrapping material should supply this information.

Sterilization of Items Used in the Physician's Office

DRESSINGS. There are as many different designs of surgical dressings as there are surgical techniques. The American Medical Association has found about 5000 different styles in use. Frequently the same dressing has several different names.

Some medical offices make their own dressings, but usually the machine-made dressings are less expensive, are more uniform in size and shape, and save considerable time for the medical assistant as well. These dressings may be purchased in large bulk nonsterile packages and rewrapped in smaller packs for autoclaving. Presterilized individual packaging increases the cost considerably for materials that are used in quantity.

Most dressings and gauze sponges are made of cotton, but some are made of silk, wool, or wood fibers (cellulose). They are folded in various sizes and shapes, with all raw edges carefully placed inside the folds. Ravelings from raw edges could cling to a wound and act as a foreign body. Some dressings have a thin layer of synthetic material that will not adhere to a wound.

Dressings should be sterilized in the autoclave or by dry heat. Wrap them in small packets with a double layer of muslin or with sterilizer paper. Muslin wraps may be reused but must be washed, and checked for holes and lint. Muslin will discolor with repeated heating. Each packet should be firm enough to hold together during normal handling but not too tightly packed to permit the flow of steam and heat. The packets are sealed with sterilizer tape, labeled, and dated. Pins are not too satisfactory because they leave holes. Pins should be completely embedded in the pack except for the head; otherwise, when the pin is removed the unsterile areas of the pin will be drawn through the sterile dressing. The use of sterilizer tape can serve several purposes: to fasten a package, identify the contents, and indicate the pack has been sterilized. Do not crowd the packs too closely together in the chamber, as this would prevent complete circulation of steam and heat.

If your office does not have an autoclave and you need sterile dressings, make up several small packs, place them in a pillow case and send them to your doctor's hospital for sterilization. Make certain the package is well marked with the doctor's name, the date, the contents, and the manner in which you wish the dressings to be sterilized. Most hospitals are very cooperative, but they should be allowed ample time to complete the work. These extra packs are put into the autoclaves at odd hours whenever time permits.

Remember that a 6 in. pack takes twice as long to penetrate as a 3 in. pack. An indicator should be placed in the thickest part of a pack. It is inadvisable to mix dressings and instruments in the same load because the timing must be set for the longest time that is required for the dressings, and this increased time is hard on the instruments.

JARS, BOTTLES, AND TRAYS. Jars, bottles, and trays must be wrapped and placed on their sides to be autoclaved. The wraps should be secured with string and not with rubber bands if sterilized by dry heat. If these items are not to be stored sterile they need not be wrapped. Covers on jars and containers should never be in place, but put to one side or slightly ajar, otherwise steam cannot circulate inside to drive out trapped air. These caps and lids are replaced before being removed from the chamber, taking care not to contaminate them.

OILS AND OINTMENTS. The sterilization of oils and ointments presents a different problem. Because steam cannot penetrate oils, it is best to sterilize oily substances by dry heat, usually for one hour at 320° F for a 1 oz jar. A 4 oz jar would require 100 minutes for sterilization by dry heat.

The most common item in this group would be gauze dressings impregnated with petroleum jelly (Vaseline). These are sterilized in glass jars or metal instrument boats. Once the container has been opened and some contents removed, it is considered to be contaminated. For this reason, it is best to sterilize small amounts at a time. Use heat resistant glassware and metals, and do not place the cover directly over the top but tilt it slightly. Autoclave these items the same as you would a fluid (petroleum jelly is the same as mineral oil when heated). Be very careful not to decrease the pressure rapidly or there will be ebullition, which could possibly require a professional service cleaning of the autoclave. Read the manufacturer's instructions. Some guarantees are void if oils and solutions have been processed in the autoclave. The use of dry heat is suggested for these substances.

SOLUTIONS. Some medical offices wish to keep bottles of sterile distilled water or normal saline on hand for rinsing and irrigating purposes. (These solutions are not to be used as injectables.) Sterilization of irrigating and rinsing solutions may be done in an autoclave that has a "Fluids Vent" cycle; otherwise, there will be an ebullition of the solution.

To prepare these solutions for autoclaving, use a Pyrex container. Fill the container about two-thirds full, no more, and place a **hermetically** sealed glass tube indicator such as a Diack in the solution. Make a plug by covering a couple of cotton balls with gauze and securing with a rubber band. Do not make the plug too large or too tight in the neck of the container, because steam must circulate through. Do not use cotton alone because it will leave lint on the inside neck of the container. Next, cover the top of the container with a double layer of muslin or paper wrap and secure with a rubber band. This will keep the lips of the container sterile for pouring purposes. Now date and label the contents (see Fig. 26–10).

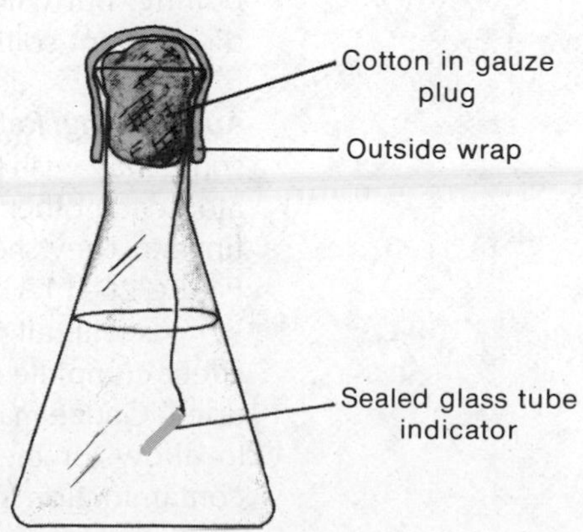

FIGURE 26–10 Preparation of solution for autoclaving.

POWDERS. Powders are best sterilized by dry heat. They are prepared the same as oils. The timing is two hours for a 1 oz jar at 320° F or one hour at 430° F. Some powders, such as sulfonamides, should be run at a lower temperature of 285° F for three hours. Talcum to be used with gloves may be run at 320° F for 55 minutes in small packets of about two tablespoons each. Always check first to make certain a powder may be sterilized by a heat method.

TUBING. Wash and clean well and rinse with distilled water. Shake out the excess water, leaving a small amount of moisture, which will form steam and drive out the trapped air. Steam pressure sterilization is best for tubing that can withstand the heat; therefore, follow the manufacturer's recommendations. If chemical disinfection is indicated, use 70 per cent isopropyl alcohol for 15 minutes, or other recommended agents. Then rinse again with sterile water before use. Nylons have excellent chemical resistance, except some may be soluble in alcohol and/or phenols. Also, some synthetics absorb chemicals if they are soaked too long.

RUBBER GOODS. Too much heat, light, moisture, or exposure to certain chemicals destroys many rubbers. These items are sterilized separately, not only because they require a different sterilization time but also because they discolor metals and may stick to them. Improper handling of rubber can destroy it.

Here are general instructions for handling rubber goods. Always rinse rubber in cool running water immediately after use. If necessary, such items should be placed in a basin of disinfectant, then washed well in warm water and cleansing agents, such as soap. Do not use detergents, scouring powders, ammonia compounds, or bleaches on rubber. Open all pockets and folds while cleaning and remove metal clips. Rinse well in warm water and towel dry as thoroughly as possible. Powder with a glove talcum to prevent sticking. Hot water bottles and ice bags should be drained by hanging upside down. When they are dry, they should be inflated and capped. The inside surfaces of rubber should not be allowed to touch. Tubing should be hung over two pegs to prevent sharp turns in rubber, which may crack. Do not soak rubber too long. All rubber goods should be dusted with powder and wrapped if placed in storage.

Methods of sterilization of rubber goods include autoclaving and some chemicals. Boiling and other chemicals are used for disinfection. Rubber goods that are to be boiled should be sanitized as previously described and wrapped lightly in gauze before being placed in the boiler, to prevent them from contacting the metal tray and sides of the boiler. Make certain all air pockets are eliminated. It is sometimes necessary to place a weight on the articles to keep them completely immersed. Boil about 15 to 20 minutes but do not overboil. Remove them with sterile tongs and place them on a clean or sterile field that has a barrier back to prevent contamination from the under side. They may be dusted with sterile powder, wrapped, and labeled. Rubber goods should be considered disinfected but not sterile.

Rubber goods are prepared for chemical disinfection in the same manner as for boiling, but will have to be rinsed with sterile water after being removed from the disinfectant solution.

Autoclaving Rubber Gloves. Although most offices now use disposable gloves, some may wish to have reusable gloves on hand. Gloves should never be autoclaved atop each other because the pressure will prevent the proper flow of steam into the fingers. They should be placed in glove envelopes with the thumbs up, as shown in Figure 26–11*A*.

As with all rubber goods, steam must contact all surfaces of the glove in order to effect complete sterilization. After the glove has been carefully sanitized it is towel dried. Gauze may be placed in the palm of the glove, but this should be large enough to allow for the flow of steam into the fingers and permit easy removal without contamination to the outside of the glove. The cuff is then folded down over another

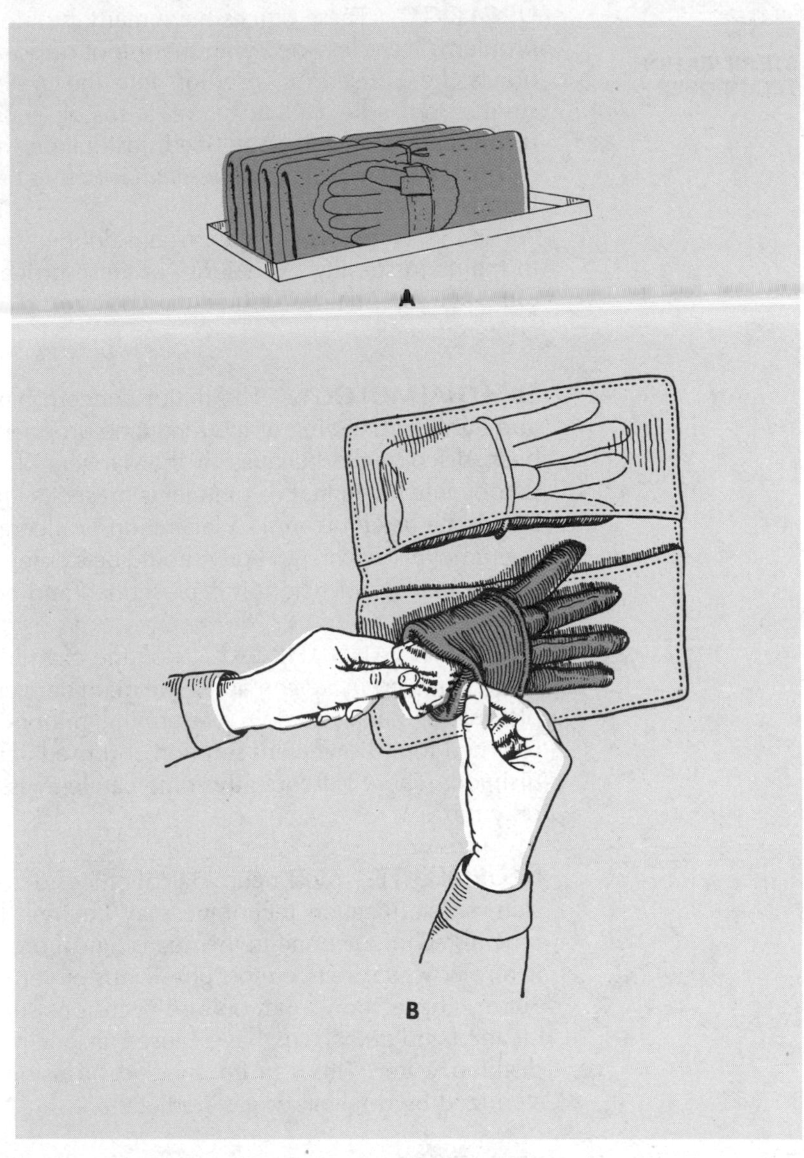

FIGURE 26–11 *A,* Packs of glove envelopes. *B,* Method of preparing gloves for autoclaving.

layer of gauze (Fig. 26–11*B*). Place in the glove envelope with the thumbs toward the outside folds. Load the packs in the autoclave with the thumbs up to allow the air to flow out. The usual grade of good rubber cannot withstand autoclaving of more than 15 to 20 minutes.

Remember that all wrapped and autoclaved items must be properly labeled and dated.

Sterilization Problems in Specialty Offices

OBSTETRICS AND GYNECOLOGY. Routine examination equipment, such as vaginal specula and uterine dressing forceps, is sometimes carelessly cleaned and "rushed through" chemical disinfectants. More offices are now autoclaving these instruments and storing them in clean toweling. Any instrument that penetrates the tissue MUST BE STERILIZED and stored sterile. Some examples include the uterine biopsy punch, uterine tenaculum, cervical dilators and sounds, and any item used for the insertion of an intrauterine device.

The common infections in the Ob/Gyn office are **venereal** disease, **Monilia, E. coli, Trichomonas,** and **Staphylococcus** from the perineal area and from vaginal discharges. Be very careful while handling contaminated items, especially from a gonorrhea infection, which could result in gonorrheal conjunctivitis and possible blindness.

UROLOGY. These offices have many problems that are unique to urology. Such problems have lessened with the use of disposable syringes, catheters, and solution bowls. Items used for insertion into the urethra and bladder instillation must be sterile. Reusable catheters are a major source of contamination and are not recommended. Office-sterilized instillation medications may contain pyogenic substances even if they are sterile. It is best to use reliable commercially prepared solutions.

If cystoscopic examinations are done in the office, extreme care must be taken to maintain sterility. A majority of these procedures are now done in the hospital. Office vasectomies must be done with sterile operating room techniques to prevent contamination.

OPHTHALMOLOGY. The major concern here is in the careless use of eyedrops and careless handling of the medicine dropper. The use of stock solutions has long been discouraged because of the dangers of the solution becoming a culture for pathogenic bacteria. Eye ointments present a similar problem. Only sterile solutions should be used if there is a laceration or ulceration in the eye. Instruments used for the removal of a foreign body should be sterile. It is advisable to reserve a medication for the patient for whom it is prescribed and not use it on other patients.

EAR, NOSE, AND THROAT. Routine examination instruments are sterilized after use and stored in a clean area. The main danger here is in the changing of dressings, placing of packs, and in performing minor surgery. Dressing forceps are often returned to a disinfectant solution and used again before the time lapse required to disinfect. There is frequently some carelessness in handling such items as tracheotomy tubes.

NEUROLOGY. Most neurological offices do not use many items that puncture the skin, so sterilization technique may become lax or is never practiced. The most crucial technique done in the neurological office may be a spinal puncture, but this is rare nowadays since most physicians prefer to use the hospital for this procedure. Surveys have shown that on rare occasions spinal needles that have been carefully cleaned and autoclaved have caused aseptic meningitis as a result of pyogens in the distilled water. This can be avoided by using disposable needles that have been sterilized by dry heat or gas sterilization.

PEDIATRICS. It has been known for many years that the main source of cross-infection in pediatrics has been the fever thermometer. Because it is used so frequently, the thermometer does not have time to disinfect between uses. Often there is some carelessness in rinsing and wiping the thermometer before returning it to the disinfectant. The disinfecting solution may not be changed or the container sterilized as frequently as it should be. Usually alcohol is used in the container and this solution is not a tuberculocide or virucide, especially for hepatitis virus. Thermometers used by patients with hepatitis should be discarded and not used again. Disposable thermometers will prevent cross-infection. Single-use thermometer sheaths are available in both oral and rectal types and are easy to use.

There is also carelessness involved in removing small foreign objects from the skin, such as splinters. Sterile procedure and sterile instruments must always be used when entering the skin, regardless of how uncooperative the patient may be.

THORACIC MEDICINE. The most common source of contamination here is in the use of the pulmonary function test equipment. These machines are difficult to sterilize, and asepsis is frequently ignored. The interior of the apparatus is not accessible and cannot be sterilized except by gas sterilization. The parts that are nearest the patient should be autoclaved or carefully disinfected. Disposable parts such as mouthpieces and tubes are available.

Aseptic-Thermo Indicator Co.: *Principles and Practices of Ethylene Oxide Sterilization.* North Hollywood, Cal., Aseptic-Thermo Indicator Co.

Perkins, J. J.: *Principles and Methods of Sterilization in Health Sciences.* 2nd ed. Springfield, Ill., Charles C Thomas Publishers, 1970.

Seedor, M. M.: *Introduction to Asepsis: A Programmed Unit in Fundamentals of Nursing.* Revised ed. New York, Bureau of Publications, Teachers College, Columbia University.

References

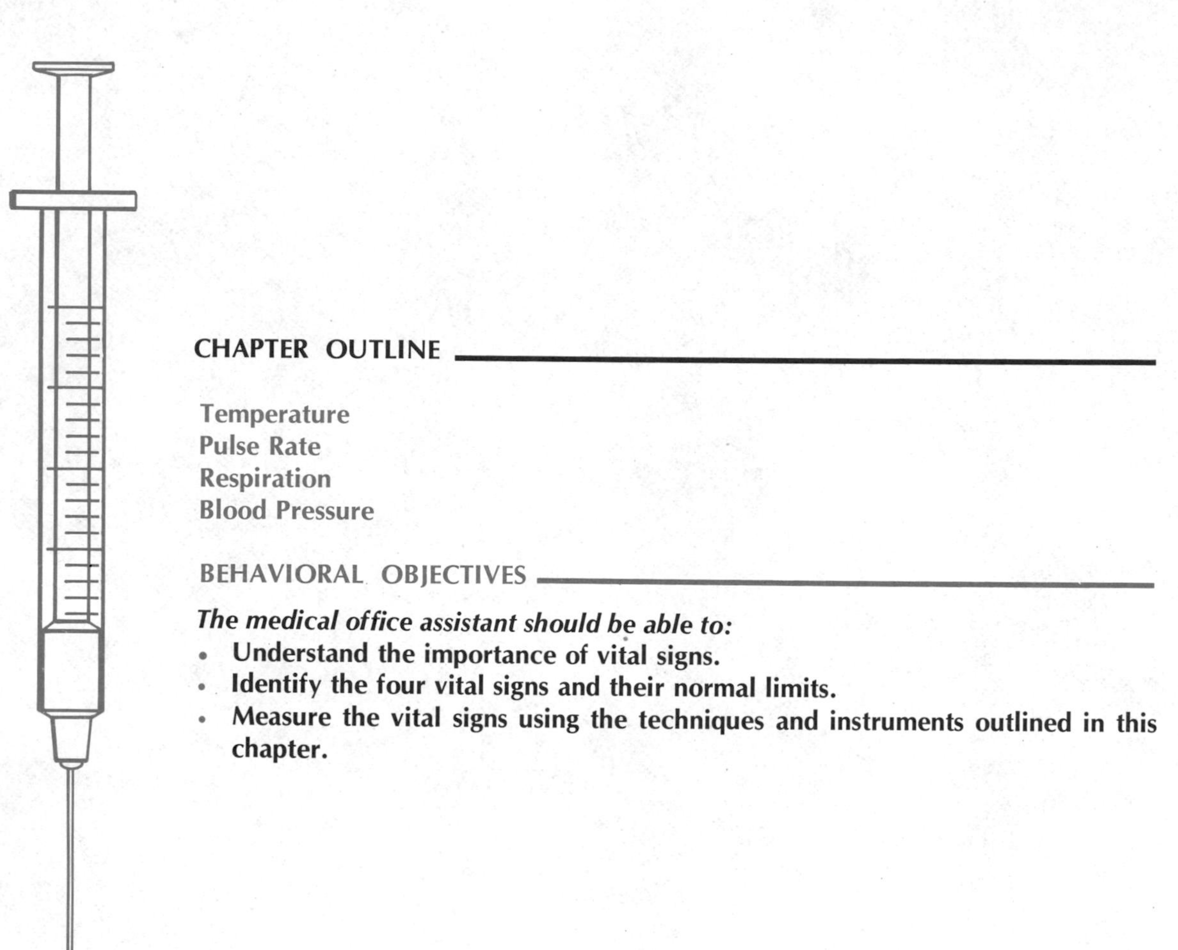

CHAPTER OUTLINE

Temperature
Pulse Rate
Respiration
Blood Pressure

BEHAVIORAL OBJECTIVES

The medical office assistant should be able to:

- **Understand the importance of vital signs.**
- **Identify the four vital signs and their normal limits.**
- **Measure the vital signs using the techniques and instruments outlined in this chapter.**

27

VITAL SIGNS

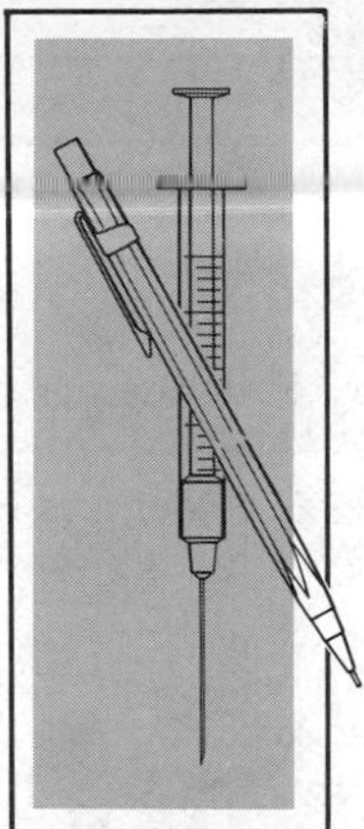

An important part of every physical examination is the determination and recording of the patient's **vital** signs, sometimes called **cardinal** signs. These vital signs include the patient's temperature, pulse, respiration, and blood pressure. It is essential the medical assistant have an understanding of these signs as well as the ability to determine and record them accurately. These signs are influenced by many factors, both physical and emotional. Since patients are often apprehensive during an office visit, it is necessary for the medical assistant not only to perform these diagnostic aids accurately but to create an atmosphere that is relaxing and comfortable. It is sometimes necessary to retake a vital sign a second time after a patient is more relaxed.

ACCURACY IS ESSENTIAL. A change in a patient's vital sign may indicate a departure from a normal condition. Variations may indicate that a disease is in progress and, therefore, indicate a change in treatment. It may show a change in the stage of a disease.

TEMPERATURE

A patient's temperature is an important part of the physical diagnosis. The Fahrenheit (F) scale has been used most frequently in the United States, but many doctors and hospitals are now using the Centigrade (or Celsius) scale (Fig. 27–1). Since most temperatures are taken orally, the quotes are assumed to be the oral temperature unless otherwise specified. If the patient is unable to cooperate, the temperature is taken rectally and registers one degree higher than the oral temperature. Rectal temperature is generally considered more accurate than oral temperature but is not as convenient to obtain. Occasionally it may be necessary to place the thermometer under the arm. This reading is called the axillary temperature and will record one degree lower than

Fahrenheit	Celsius
32°F	0°C
95.0	35
95.9	35.5
96.8	36
97.7	36.5
98.6	37
99.5	37.5
100.4	38
101.3	38.5
102.2	39
103.1	39.5
104.0	40
104.9	40.5
105.8	41
106.7	41.5

A

FAHRENHEIT

98.6°

NORMAL

37°

CELSIUS

To convert degrees F. to degrees C.
Subtract 32, then multiply by 5/9

To convert degrees C. to degrees F.
Multiply by 9/5, then add 32

B

FIGURE 27–1 *A,* **Comparison of Fahrenheit and Celsius temperatures.** *B,* **Comparison of Fahrenheit and Celsius thermometers. (From Brunner, L. S., and Suddarth, D. S.:** ***Lippincott Manual of Nursing Practice.*** **2nd ed. Philadelphia, J. B. Lippincott Co., 1978.)**

the oral temperature. A patient's oral temperature should not be taken within 30 minutes after his having taken anything by mouth, even smoking.

The body temperature will vary during a 24-hour period. It is influenced by many things, especially the body metabolism and the presence of infection. Lower temperatures are found in the early morning hours. Shock, congestive heart failure, and exposure to extreme cold will lower the body temperature.

The so-called normal temperature is 98.6° F (37.0° C). When the body's temperature is elevated, it is frequently said that the person "has a temperature," but this figurative expression should be avoided since the person always has a temperature, whether normal, subnormal, or elevated. The 98.6° F temperature is called the *normal* temperature, but it should be called the *average* temperature. There are some individuals with a normal temperature of 97° F, whereas others have a normal of 99.6° F. A persistently elevated temperature, called a *fever,* warrants a thorough investigation. There are several types of fevers.

In a *continuous* fever (Fig. 27–2*A*) the temperature is elevated and remains

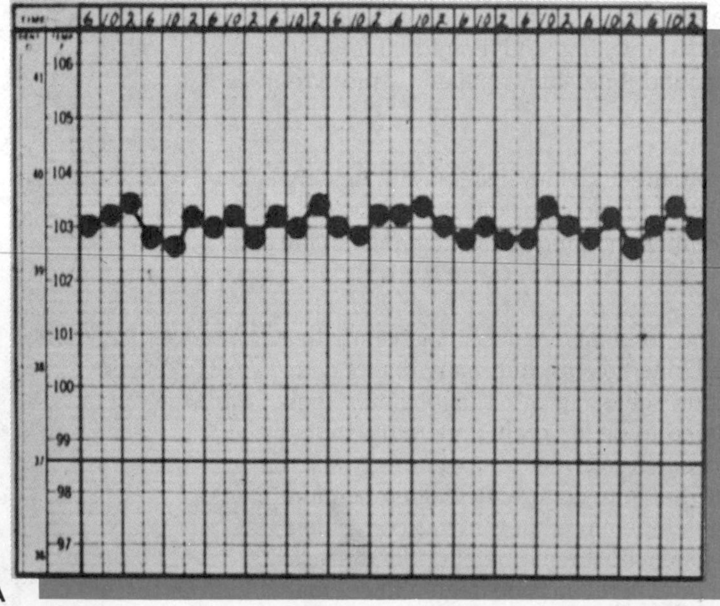

A

FIGURE 27–2 Types of temperature charts. ***A,*** **Continuous fever.**

Illustration continued on opposite page

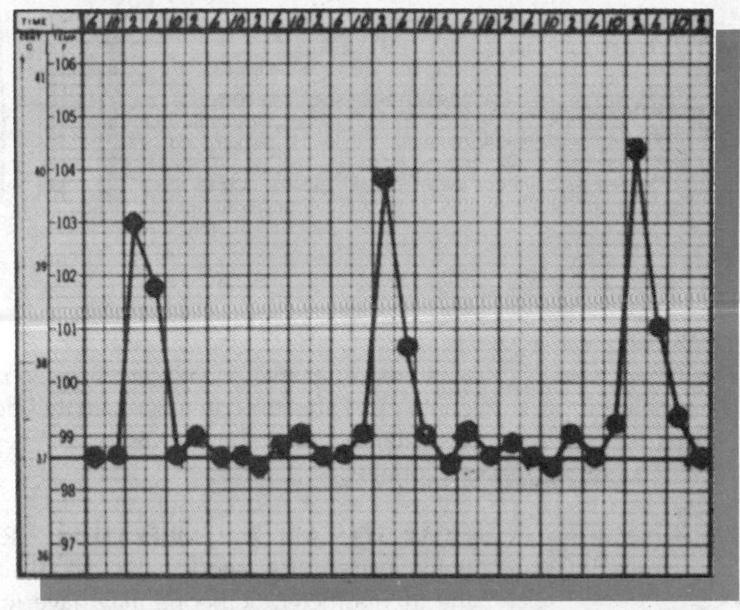

B

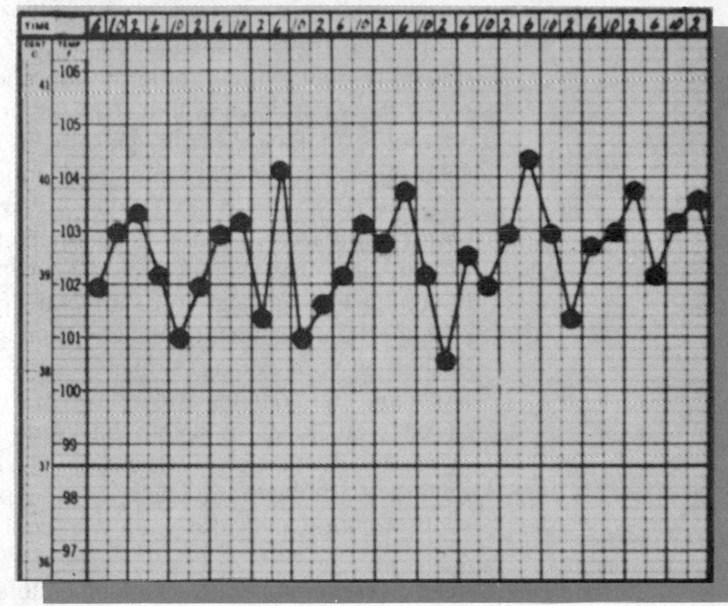

C

FIGURE 27–2 *Continued B,* Intermittent fever. *C,* Remittent fever. (From Hopkins, H.A.: *Leopold's Physical Diagnosis*. Philadelphia, W. B. Saunders Co., 1965.)

consistently elevated with no, or very little, fluctuation during a 24-hour period. In an *intermittent* fever (Fig. 27–2*B*) the temperature is elevated at times during the 24-hour period but falls to normal or even subnormal during this time. A *remittent* fever (Fig. 27–2C) shows a continuous temperature elevation with a rise and fall but never a drop to the normal level. A remittent fever differs from the continuous fever in that there is a greater variance in the rise and fall of the remittent fever.

A fever is said to be *relapsing* when it recurs after one or more days of normal temperature. Fevers resolve or disappear by lysis or crisis. *Lysis* occurs when a fever gradually falls over a period of several days. If a fever abruptly falls within a 36-hour period it does so by *crisis*. Frequently a fever crisis is accompanied by profuse sweating (**diaphoresis**). Diaphoresis also occurs in night sweats, extreme weakness, and nervousness. Chills and rigor (shivering) are frequently found in patients who are having a fever crisis.

THERMOMETERS. There are three types of fever thermometers used in a physician's office: oral, rectal, and security tipped (Fig. 27–3). Each thermometer should

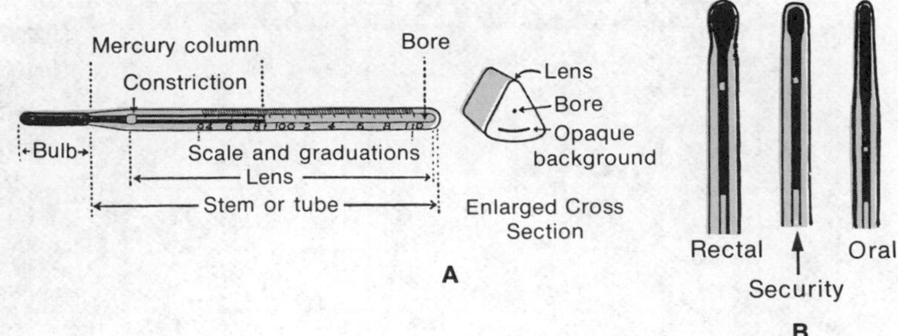

FIGURE 27–3 *A,* Construction of the clinical thermometer. *B,* Types of tips: rectal, security, and oral.

be stored in its individual container. *Do not* keep several thermometers in the same container. Label the container as to thermometer type, e.g., oral or rectal. Patients are very alert and apprehensive as to the type of thermometer, where it was used, and its cleanliness.

HOW TO TAKE A TEMPERATURE. Rinse the thermometer well with cool water before using it. It is a good habit to hold your finger under the water tap before rinsing the thermometer. Someone may have just finished washing in hot water, and the warm water in the tap could cause difficulties. After rinsing the thermometer with cool water, check to see that the mercury is below 95° F. If not, shake the mercury down. To shake down, hold the top end between the thumb and first finger and swing the wrist down with a snap, as though shaking water off the fingers. Do not attempt to shake it down by grasping in the fingers and striking the hand against a solid object, as this will injure the thermometer.

Oral Temperature. Place the thermometer in the patient's mouth under the tongue to one side. The patient should keep the mouth closed and the tongue down, breathing through the nose. An oral tip thermometer is kept in place for three minutes. Remove the thermometer from the patient's mouth and wipe the saliva and lipstick off with a rotary stroke over the bulb. Never touch the mercury bulb end. Hold the thermometer at eye level with the right hand so the calibrated scale is toward you. Rotate it slightly back and forth with the thumb and finger until the mercury column is clearly seen between the scale lines and the numbers. Read and record. Wash the thermometer with soap and cool water. Disinfect it with an antiseptic solution and rinse again with cool water before returning it to the container.

Rectal Temperature. Rectal temperatures are taken on the very young patient, the patient with breathing difficulty, the uncooperative patient, and the unconscious patient. The rectal thermometer has a stubby bulb for safety purposes. NEVER use an oral thermometer in the rectum. Rectal thermometers should be carefully labeled and stored in a separate container. The procedure is the same as for the oral temperature, except the tip of the rectal thermometer is lubricated with petroleum or lubricating jelly and then gently inserted into the rectum past the constricting muscle of the anus, about one and one-half inches. The rectal thermometer is held in place for five minutes. Do not leave a patient alone while the thermometer is in the rectum. Remove, wipe, read, and record. The normal rectal temperature is usually one degree higher than the oral temperature.

The rectal temperature is most frequently done on the infant. The infant is placed on his back with the buttocks exposed. With the index finger between the ankles, grasp the legs and flex the knees over the infant's abdomen, exposing the anus; with the other hand insert the lubricated rectal thermometer into the anus about one inch. Keep a gentle but firm hold on the legs. Hold the thermometer in place between your index and great finger while the palm of the hand and thumb grasp the infant's buttocks. This hold will steady the infant and will also hold the thermometer secure. Be very careful not to let go of your holds on the legs and the

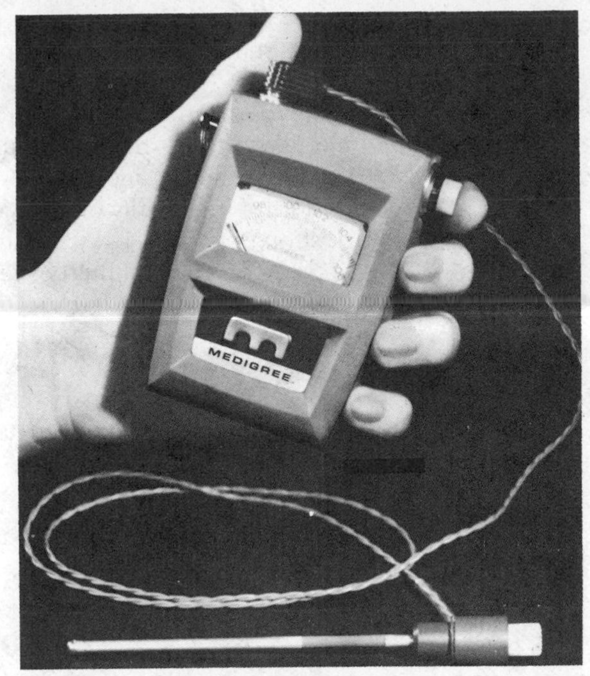

FIGURE 27–4 Electronic thermometer. (Courtesy of Chesebrough-Ponds, Inc.)

buttocks while the thermometer is in place. After five minutes, remove, wipe, read, and record.

Axillary Temperature. Use a rectal or security tipped thermometer. Rinse thermometer and shake down. Wipe the area dry before putting the thermometer in place. Allow it to remain in place ten minutes. Instruct the patient to remain quiet during this time. Remove and record. When recording this reading remember to place an "A" next to the numbers to indicate an axillary temperature. The normal axillary temperature will be 97.6° F (A). This is the least accurate method of taking a patient's temperature because it is difficult to hold the arm firmly in place for the needed time.

USING THE ELECTRONIC THERMOMETER. The electronic thermometers record very rapidly, usually within five seconds, and claim an accuracy of within ± 0.2° F. They have disposable tips for both oral and rectal use, which are color coded. The temperature reading on the dial remains in position until released, permitting an accurate recording on the patient's chart (Fig. 27–4).

These electronic thermometers require adjustment, and care must be taken to have the dial directly in front of you at eye level while adjusting it; otherwise, it will be inaccurately adjusted if you are viewing it from an oblique angle.

PULSE RATE

This is such a routine part of the physical examination that it is often taken in a mechanical way, and some of the finer aspects are neglected. It is a method of counting the heartbeat through the walls of an artery. What is felt is a shock wave that travels along the fibers of the arteries as the heart contracts, similar to the sound of hammering as it travels through a pipe. The pulse rate varies from person to person. It is affected by the individual's activities and illnesses. The average adult pulse rate is from 60 to 90 beats per minute. During resting periods the rate is usually 60 to 70 beats per minute, whereas during normal activity it may be from 70 to 90. The pulse rate of a young athlete may be as slow as 50 beats per minute. Infants and children usually have a slightly faster pulse rate of 90 to 120.

A pulse rate may be taken any place where an artery is near the surface of the body. This **rhythmical** throbbing may be felt several places in the body, such as the radial, brachial, carotid, temporal, femoral, popliteal, and dorsalis pedis arteries. The *radial artery* is by far most frequently used to take a pulse rate.

The patient should be in a comfortable position with the wrist preferably near the same level as the heart (Fig. 27–5*A*). The arm should be well supported and relaxed. The patient may be lying down or sitting. As with all pulse readings, the pads of your first three fingers are placed over the artery area with a slight pressure. The radial artery is best found just above the wrist bones and slightly outside of the cords on the thumb side (Fig. 27–5*B*). Now count the pulse for one minute. Making any note of irregularity or variations of the normal quality of the beat such as **arrhythmia**, strong or weak, jerky, or unequal.

The brachial pulse is felt at the inner (antecubital) aspect of the elbow. It is the artery heard and felt when taking a blood pressure. It is also felt in the groove between the biceps and triceps muscles just above the elbow on the inner surface of the arm.

The carotid artery is located between the larynx and sternocleidomastoid muscle in the front and to the side of the neck. It is most frequently used in

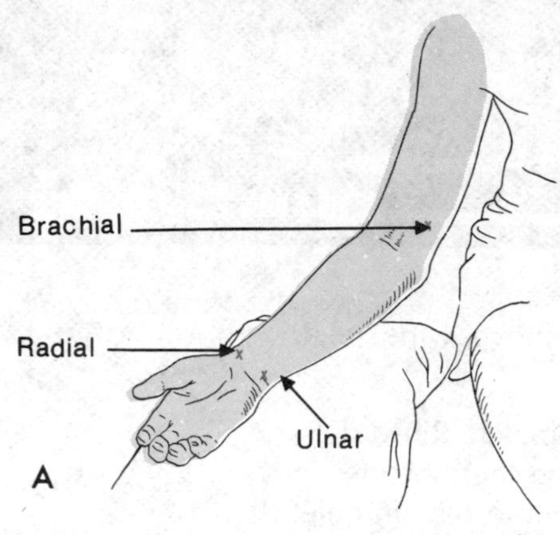

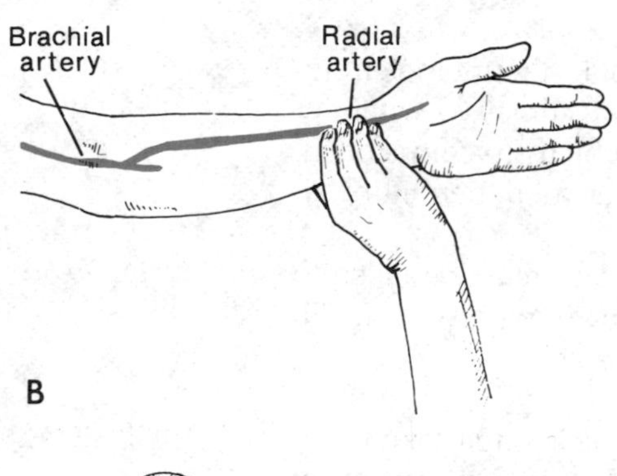

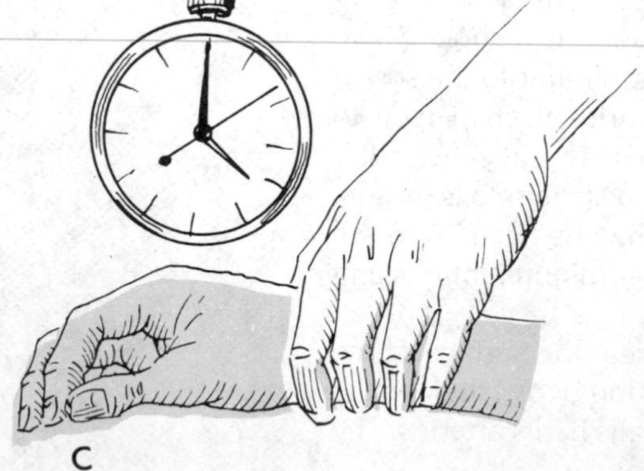

FIGURE 27–5 **Location of pulses on the arm. *A,* Sites of palpation of the brachial, radial, and ulnar pulses. *B,* Sites of the brachial and radial pulses. *C,* Taking the radial pulse with the patient's arm well supported. (From Wood, L. A., and Rambo, B. J., *Nursing Skills for Allied Health Services*. 2nd ed, vol. 1. Philadelphia, W. B. Saunders Co., 1977.)**

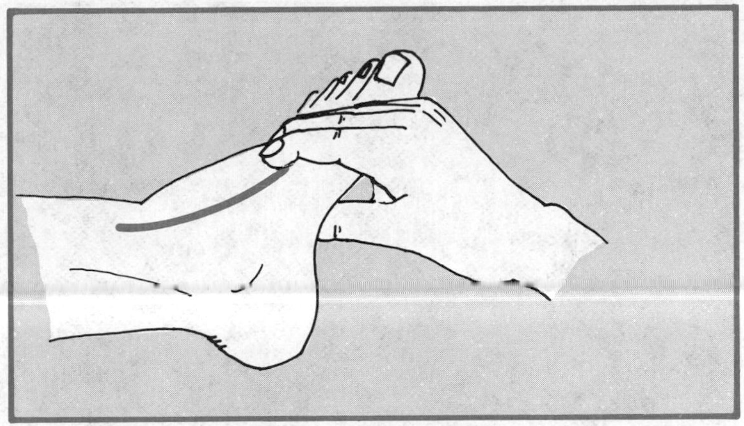

FIGURE 27–6 Taking the pedal pulse.

emergencies and during cardiopulmonary resuscitation (CPR). It can best be felt by pushing the muscle to the side and pressing against the larynx.

The origin of the temporal pulse is the carotid artery and is felt in the slight depression at the side of the head immediately off the side of the eye and above the zygomatic arch. This pulse is not often used.

The femoral pulse is located at the site of the femoral artery where it passes through the groin. One must press deeply below the inguinal ligament.

The popliteal pulse is found at the back of the knee. This is done with the patient in a recumbent position and the knee slightly flexed. This is difficult to feel since this artery is deeper than the others. This artery is also used when taking the blood pressure on the leg.

The dorsalis pedis pulse is felt on the top of the foot just slightly lateral to the midline by the extensor tendon of the great toe (Fig. 27–6). This pulse may be congenitally absent in some patients. It is frequently used by physicians in checking a patient's lower limb circulation and for arterial insufficiency.

Some pulses are more difficult to feel than others, and the medical assistant should remember to always have the patient in a comfortable relaxed position. The sensitivity of the fingers is greatly decreased if the medical assistant is in an awkward position. Remember that too much pressure will obliterate the patient's pulse and too little pressure will make it difficult to feel. The correct pressure requires practice.

Record the number of beats per minute. If the pulse rate is taken at any site other than the radial artery, the site should also be recorded.

RESPIRATION

The normal respiration rate is 16 to 20 per minute, somewhat slower in older persons and faster in infants and small children. The respiration rate generally increases as the body's temperature rises. An example of the respiration, pulse and temperature ratio is:

Respiration	*Pulse*	*Temperature*
18	80	99°F
21	96	101°F
23	104	102°F
28	126	105°F

Variations occur in the respiratory rate (fast or slow), volume (deep or shallow), and rhythm (regular or irregular). There are specific medical terms used in describing the alterations in breathing. **Dyspnea,** meaning difficult breathing, occurs in patients with pneumonia or asthma; it also occurs after physical exertion or at very high altitudes. Other alterations in breathing are **bradypnea** (abnormally slow respiration), **apnea** (temporary cessation of respiration), **tachypnea** (excessively rapid breathing), and **hyperpnea** (increased depth of breathing). Hyperpnea is usually accompanied by **hyperventilation** and is frequently found in emotional conditions. **Orthopnea**

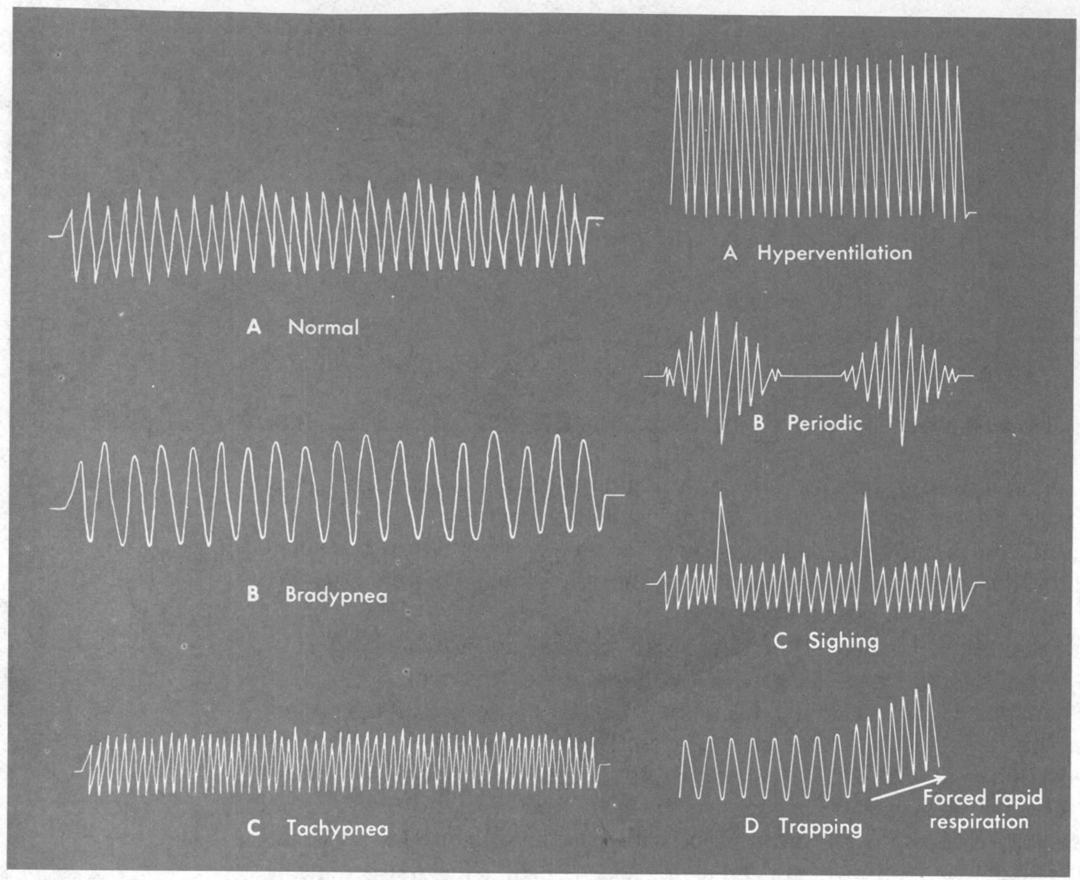

FIGURE 27–7 Spirograms demonstrating various respiratory patterns. (From Prior, J. A., and Silberstein, J. S.: *Physical Diagnosis*. 3rd ed. St. Louis, The C. V. Mosby Co., 1973.)

means a patient has difficulty breathing while in a supine position, as found in patients with congestive heart failure (see Fig. 27–7).

HOW TO TAKE THE RESPIRATION RATE. Because the respiration rate is easily controlled, and since a patient who is conscious of his breathing's being watched will control it to some extent, it is advisable to count the rate while appearing to be interested in something else, such as the pulse rate.

The medical assistant may keep her eyes alternately on the patient's chest and her watch while she is counting the pulse rate, and then, without taking her fingers from the pulse, she can count the respiration rate. If the patient is lying down, his arm can be crossed over his chest so the respirations can be felt with the rise and fall of the chest. Count the respirations for a minute and record. Also note any variations or irregularities in the rate.

BLOOD PRESSURE

Blood pressure is the pressure of the blood against the walls of the arteries. This pressure is determined by the pumping action of the heart, the resistance of the blood's flow through the arteries, the elasticity of the arterial walls, the amount of blood in the vessels, and the blood's viscosity (thickness). Because of these influencing factors, there are actually two blood pressures within the blood vessels. The *systolic* pressure is the highest pressure when the heart is contracting and when the pulse beat is felt. The *diastolic* pressure is the lowest pressure when the heart is relaxed and there is no pulse beat felt. The difference between the systolic and the diastolic is called the *pulse pressure*.

Blood pressure is recorded as a fraction, with the systolic reading on top and the diastolic reading on the bottom. The normal average blood pressure of an adult is between 90 and 140 mm Hg (millimeters of mercury) systolic reading, and 60 to 90 mm Hg for the diastolic reading, with an average of 120/80 mm Hg. The male adult has a slightly higher reading than the female. A child's reading is usually lower than an adult's. Older persons may have a slightly higher reading. A person of 60 years of age may have a normal reading of 140/90 mm Hg. For routine frequent blood pressure checks the readings should be taken at about the same time of day and by the same person.

A person is said to have **hypertension** if his blood pressure is consistently above the normal pressure. It is not diagnostic of any one disease but can be found in various renal diseases, during pregnancy, in certain endocrine disturbances, and in obesity. Blood pressure is increased in arteriosclerosis, atherosclerosis, and brain injury. It is also influenced by pain, fear, and exercise.

Low blood pressure is referred to as **hypotension** and is found in a wide variety of conditions such as hemorrhage, chronic wasting diseases, and shock, both emotional and traumatic. **Orthostatic hypotension** is a form of low blood pressure that occurs when a person changes from a supine position to an upright position rather rapidly or when standing for a long period of time.

The instrument used to take blood pressure is called the *sphygmomanometer* and is aided by the *stethoscope*. A manometer is an instrument used to measure pressure of a liquid or gas. By adding *sphygmo-* (pulse) it means an instrument used to measure the arterial blood pressure; that is, the pulse pressure. There are two types of sphygmomanometers used, the mercury (Fig. 27–8*A*) and the aneroid manometers (Fig. 27–8*B*). Both should be handled carefully; they are delicate and expensive instruments. The aneroid is easy to transport but should be frequently calibrated by the manufacturer. The recording needle on the aneroid dial should rest within the small square at the bottom of the dial. It should not have a stop pin at this point. The mercury column is considered to be more accurate, as long as the meniscus of the mercury is at zero (0).

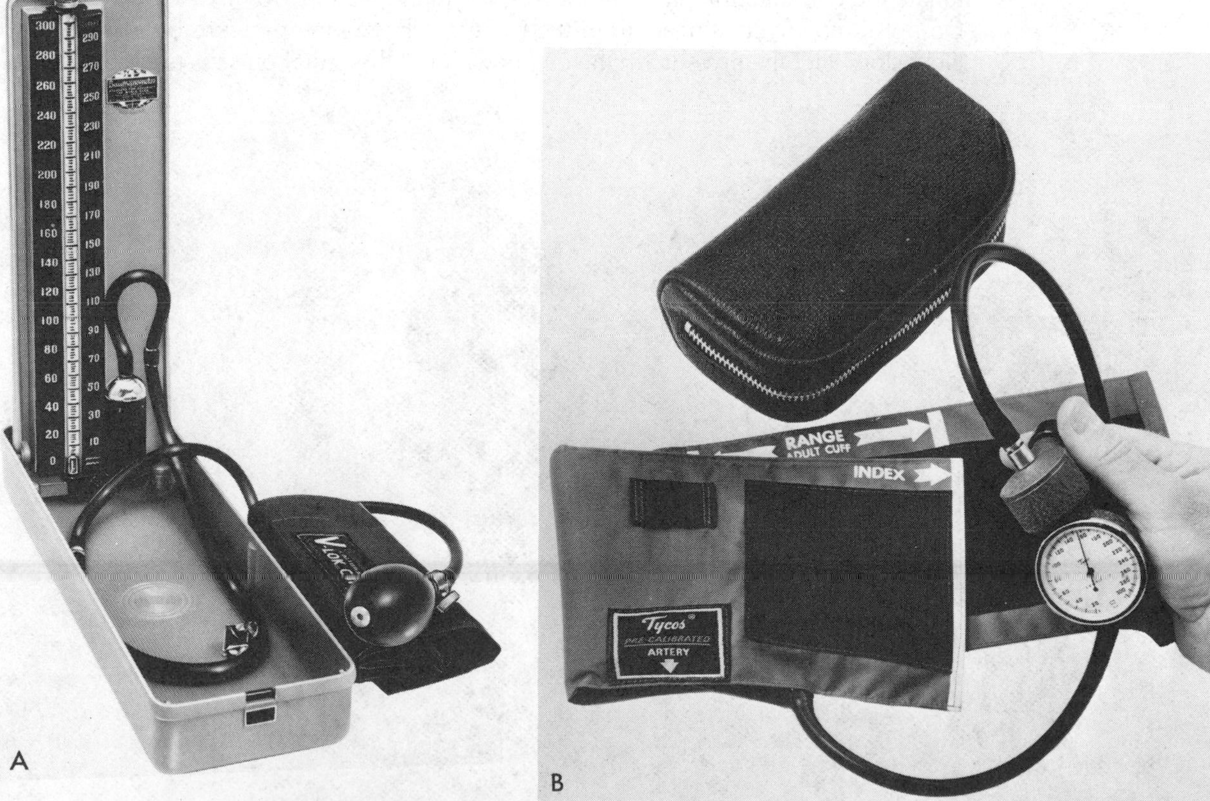

FIGURE 27–8 *A*, Baum mercury manometer. (Courtesy of Baum Co.) *B*, Tycos aneroid manometer. (Courtesy of Tycos Co.)

HOW TO TAKE A BLOOD PRESSURE. The patient may be lying down with his arm resting beside him and the palm turned upward, or he may be sitting with the arm resting on a firm surface, palm upward and on the same level as his heart. Explain to the patient that the arm must be relaxed. Roll his sleeve about five inches above the bend of the elbow. Be careful the sleeve does not constrict the arm. Apply the completely deflated cuff around the arm about two inches above the bend. The cuff should be high enough to place the stethoscope without touching the cuff. The cuff is applied evenly and should be slightly snug. Place the stethoscope in your ears (the earpieces of the stethoscope should be pointing away from the face). Palpate the brachial artery and place the stethoscope over this point. Listen for the pulse. Hold the stethoscope over this point gently but firmly. Gently tighten the screw on the rubber bulb to close the air escape valve. By pumping the bulb, inflate the cuff until the pulse ceases, then inflate to 20 mm higher. Now open the valve on the bulb slightly and listen for the return of the pulse beat, watching the mercury column or the aneroid dial. Slowly let the air escape from the bulb while watching the column and listening for the pulse beat. The first beat you hear is the systolic pressure. Continue to let the air escape slowly. The beat will become clearer and louder. Then suddenly the sound of the heart beat will be very dull and soft. This change in the beat is the diastolic pressure. Some physicians record the last sound heard as the diastolic pressure. It is advisable to check with your physician as to his preference (Fig. 27–9).

Clear all the air from the cuff and wait a few minutes; then repeat the procedure. Do not take one reading immediately after another and never take more than three successive readings on the same arm. Change arms. Record immediately. If others are using the stethoscope, be sure to wipe the earpieces off with alcohol.

Palpatory Method. The systolic pressure may be checked by feeling the radial pulse rather than using the stethoscope to hear the brachial pulse. Place the cuff in the usual position and palpate the radial pulse, noting the rate and rhythm. Now inflate the cuff until the pulse disappears and then go about 30 mm above this point. Do not remove your fingers from the pulse or change the pressure of your fingers. Now slowly let the pressure in the cuff down until the radial pulse is felt again. Note

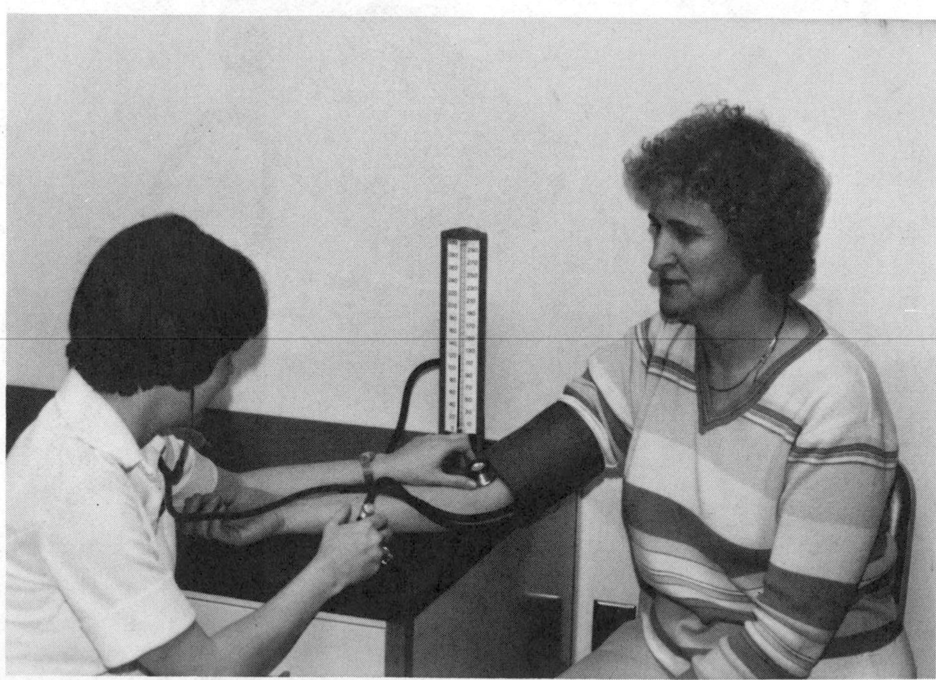

FIGURE 27–9 Taking a blood pressure reading.

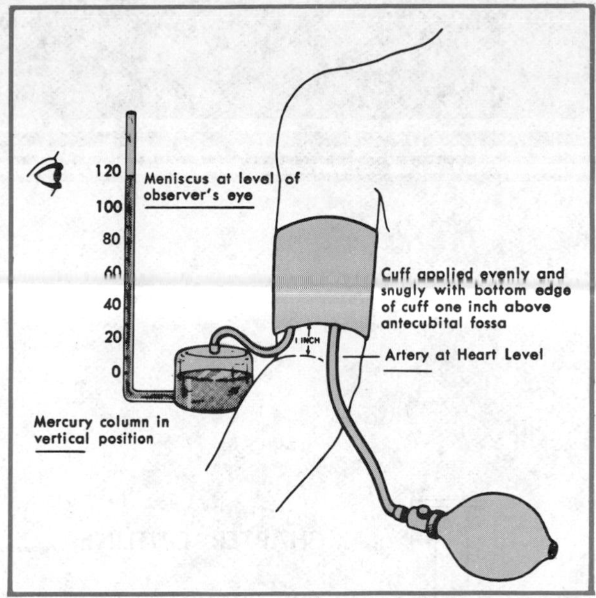

FIGURE 27–10 Important "rules" for accurate reading of arterial blood pressure. (From Burch, G. E.: *The Clinical Measurement of Blood Pressure*. Copiague, New York, W. A. Baum Co., Inc., 1969.)

the mercury reading and record as the systolic pressure. The diastolic pressure is difficult to measure by this method and is not determined by the palpatory method.

COMMON CAUSES OF ERROR

1. The patient's arm is not at the same level as the heart. (It is not necessary for the manometer to be at the level of the heart.)
2. The rubber bladder in the cuff has not been deflated before starting or retaking a reading.
3. The mercury column is allowed to drop too rapidly, resulting in inaccurate readings.
4. The patient is nervous, uncomfortable, or too anxious. This may cause a higher reading than the patient's actual blood pressure.
5. The cuff is improperly applied:
   a. Rubber bladder bulging out from the cover.
   b. Cuff not around arm smoothly.
   c. Cuff too tight or too loose.
6. Failing to wait a few minutes between retakes and not deflating the cuff completely between readings.
7. Defective apparatus:
   a. Air leak in a valve, especially the release valve.
   b. Leak in the rubber bladder.
   c. Mercury column is dirty.
   d. Mercury column is not at zero, although a zero reading on the aneroid manometer does not guarantee accuracy. It should be checked by the manufacturer.
8. On extremely obese patients it may be necessary to apply the cuff on the forearm and place the stethoscope over the radial artery.
9. Study Figure 27–10 for some important rules.

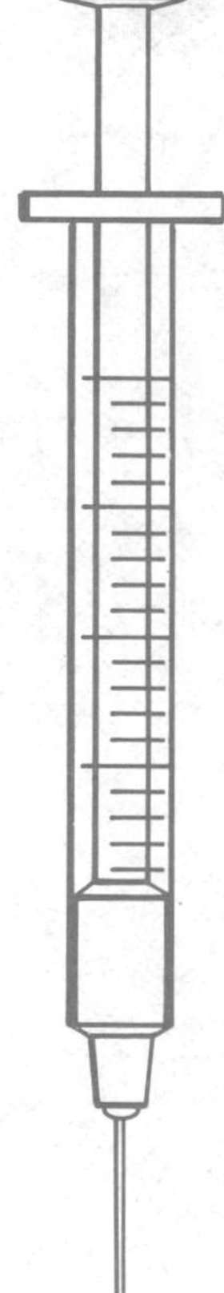

CHAPTER OUTLINE

BEHAVIORAL OBJECTIVES

The medical office assistant should be able to:

- **Prepare the patient for history-taking and physical examination.**
- **Record the patient's basic medical history, using the correct terminology and abbreviations.**
- **Define the principal methodologies of the physical examination, including the various methods used.**
- **Correctly position and appropriately drape the patient, preparatory to various forms of physical examinations.**
- **Assist the physician in conducting the complete physical examination with the correct instruments discussed in this chapter to facilitate the physician's handling of the examination.**
- **Define the terminology, pathology, and special tests performed in the specialties as discussed in this chapter.**

28

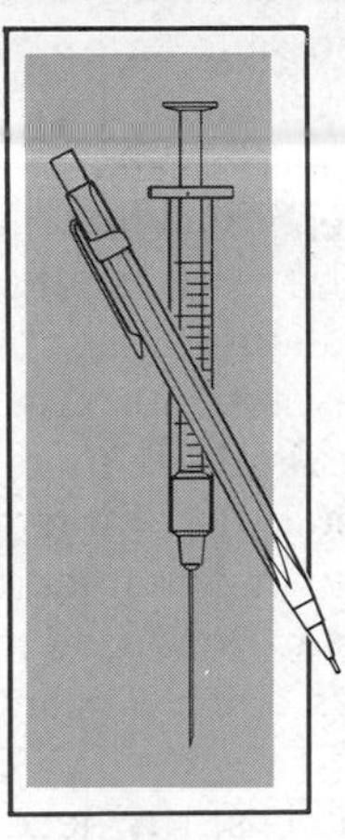

ASSISTING WITH PHYSICAL EXAMINATIONS

The clinical responsibilities of the medical assistant vary widely, depending upon the physician's specialty and the extent of his reliance upon auxiliary personnel. Some physicians are reluctant to delegate clinical duties. However, the physician who does utilize competent help appreciates how his own time is saved and his professional skills are amplified by the use of a well-trained medical assistant. The clinical assistant can ease the role of both the physician and the patient in many office procedures.

The medical assistant must have the ability to: (1) communicate with the patient and the physician, (2) evaluate their needs and respond to these needs, and (3) follow instructions quickly and accurately. She must also be able to relay the physician's instructions to the patient accurately and clearly. There is much the medical assistant can do to save the physician's time in physical examinations. She must maintain continuity between the patient and the physician as well as with the other office personnel and services. A good medical assistant follows an organized routine but is flexible enough to adjust to each individual problem.

ATTITUDE TOWARD THE PATIENT

These days everyone talks about environment, communications, reactions, and interactions. These are all essential when providing good patient care. Patient care does not start with the physical examination but when the patient first contacts the physician's office. As the care progresses through the various stages, the entire medical team utilizes special skills to enhance this care. These skills are not all technical and medical in nature but also entail the caring for one human being by another. Because medical care is of extremely personal nature, the medical assistant must always remember that each patient is an individual with anxieties. These anxieties often cause people to act and react in various ways. Because these anxieties do exist it is essential to remember to be effective in communicating with the patient, both verbally *and* nonverbally.

The clinical assistant can do much to put a patient at ease: the tone of her voice, the ease and confidence of her movements, and showing a sincere interest in the patient. In other words, give that patient your undivided attention. The patient is not concerned with the problems of the office, nor is the medical assistant there to impress the patient with her medical knowledge. She is there for one purpose only — to give that patient the best possible care.

If the medical assistant has been delegated the responsibility of taking a portion of the medical history, it should be done in an area free from outside interference and out of range of other patients. Patients will not talk freely when they may be overheard or frequently interrupted. The room should be physically comfortable and conducive to confidential communications.

Listen to the patient. Do not express surprise or displeasure at a patient's statement. Remember the medical assistant is there not to pass judgment but to gather medical data. Expressions should be of interest and concern. The medical assistant should not judge what is or is not of importance. The information gained should be reported to the physician in an organized manner, exactly as given by the patient, without the medical assistant's opinion or interpretation.

THE MEDICAL RECORD

In order to understand the patient's needs it is necessary for the physician first to interview and obtain a medical history. This permits the physician to correlate later the physical findings with information acquired in the history. Questioning the patient, or interrogating, is the usual method of obtaining this vital information. The interrogation and the physical examination cannot be separated and are the first basic skills of the medical profession.

TERMS AND ABBREVIATIONS. Here are some terms and abbreviations used in writing a patient's medical history:

Chief Complaint (CC). This is usually the reason for the patient's seeking medical care. Often it is recorded in the patient's own words. It is a list of the patient's symptoms.

Present Illness (PI). This is an amplification of the chief complaint. It is usually written in chronologic sequence with dates of onset.

Systems Review (SR) or ***Review of Systems (ROS).*** This serves as a guide to general health and tends to detect conditions other than those covered in the present illness. It is obtained by a logical sequence of questions, beginning with the head and proceeding downward.

Past History (PH) or ***Past Medical History (PMH).*** Questions regarding the patient's *Usual Childhood Diseases (UCHD)* are asked — major illnesses and operations, allergies, accidents, and immunizations with the date of onset.

Family History (FH). Details regarding the patient's mother and father are obtained — their health and, if deceased, the cause and age of death. Hereditary tendencies are recorded here.

The physician may wish to inquire about the patient's *Occupational History (OH)* and *Social History (SH).* Social history includes his eating and drinking habits, hobbies, and interests.

SYMPTOMS AND SIGNS. Many times you will hear that certain findings and conclusions in a medical history are either **subjective** or **objective.** These two terms are sometimes confused, as are the terms **symptoms** and **signs** which are often used interchangeably with subjective and objective.

Subjective findings are the *symptoms* that are perceptible only to the patient; they pertain to the individual only. They are the subjective conclusions or symptoms that often bring the patient to the physician. An ache, pain, or **vertigo** is felt only by the patient. The patient tells the physician about these symptoms and the physician records them as subjective findings. *Cardinal symptoms* are the most significant of the patient's complaints, the ones that are used to establish a diagnosis.

Objective findings are perceptible to a person other than the patient. They are the *signs* that a physician detects when he examines a patient. A physician feels, sees, or hears the signs that are often associated with a certain disease or abnormal condition. These objective findings are dependent on another's senses. A mass that a physician feels in the patient's abdomen is an *objective* finding. It is a *sign* of an abnormal condition.

Other terms used that require understanding are the words **functional** and **physical,** or organic. When a condition or disease is functional it means the disease is without discoverable lesion or organic cause. That is, the organ may appear "normal" but its function is not normal. A functional disease is any disease that alters the body functions but is not associated with any apparent organic or physical lesion. A physical disease or condition is one in which the abnormality or lesion can be seen or felt.

Some physicians may, at this time, make a summary of the history. Others may prefer to dictate it after the physical examination has been completed.

PROBLEM-ORIENTED MEDICAL RECORD (POMR). This method of medical record taking and keeping was designed to bring logical sequence to recording the information obtained from the patient. It is based on a scientific method and was designed to solve a problem. The medical history and the physical examination fit well into a format designed to clarify the reasons for the history and the physical examination. These are data that make sense and aid in solving the problem. Because the POMR is organized it makes it easier for anyone who deals with the patient to use the record. It lends to better audit of the medical record. It is said to be the tool for communication among the members of the health team caring for the patient.

Dr. Lawrence L. Weed is credited with bringing this logical system of recording a patient's record to the medical profession. Dr. Weed's system includes four basic parts for the POMR:

Data Base. The record of the patient's history, physical examination, and initial laboratory findings. As new information develops it becomes part of this data base.

Problem List. A list of the identified patient's problems kept in the front of the patient's chart. It is the "Table of Contents" or the "Index" of the patient's problems. Each problem entered here is supported by the data base. Each is numerically listed and dated.

Initial Plan. A written plan for each major problem identified, outlining further studies, treatment, and patient education. There are three sections — diagnostic, therapeutic, and patient education — for each problem.

Progress Notes. Structured notes that correspond to each defined problem in the problem list including subjective data, objective data, assessment of the problem, and further plans (diagnostic studies, treatments and patient education), each identified and in an organized "diary" form.

Further information on POMR may be found in Chapter 11, The Patient Record.

METHODS OF EXAMINATION

INSPECTION. This is the art of observation, the ability to detect significant physical features. This method of examination ranges from a patient's general appearance — the general state of health, including posture, mannerisms, and grooming — to the more detailed observations that may include contour, **symmetry,** visual injuries and deformities, tremors, rashes, and color changes.

PALPATION. This method uses the sense of touch. A part of the body is felt with the hand for the purpose of ascertaining its condition or that of an underlying organ. It may include touching the skin or a more firm feeling of the abdomen for underlying masses. This technique involves a wide range of perceptions: temperature, vibrations, consistency, form, size, rigidity, elasticity, moisture, texture, position, and contour. Palpation is performed with one hand, both hands (bimanually), one finger (digitally), fingertips, or the palmar aspects of the hand. A pelvic examination is done bimanually, whereas an anal examination is performed digitally. Do not confuse this with *palpitation*, which is a throbbing pulsation.

PERCUSSION. This tapping or striking of the body with fingers or a small hammer to elicit sounds or vibratory sensations aids in the determination of the position, size, or density of an underlying structure. The effect of percussion is both heard and felt by the examiner. It is helpful in determining the amount of air or solid matter in an underlying organ or cavity. The two basic methods of percussion are direct and indirect. Direct (immediate) is performed by striking the body with a finger. The indirect (mediate) is used more frequently and is done by the examiner placing his own finger on the area and then striking that placed finger with a finger of the other hand. Both a sound *and* a sense of vibration are evident here. The examiner will speak of sounds in terms of pitch, quality, duration, and resonance.

AUSCULTATION. This is the process of listening to sounds arising from the body — not the sound produced by the examiner such as in percussion but sounds that originate within the patient's body. This is a difficult method of examination because the examiner must distinguish between a normal and an abnormal sound. A stethoscope is usually employed to amplify these sounds. Auscultation is particularly useful in appraising sounds arising from the lungs, heart, and abdomen, distinguishing bruits and murmurs, rhythms, durations, and quality. Indirect listening is done with the stethoscope, whereas direct auscultation is done by the examiner placing his ear directly over the area.

MENSURATION. This is the process of measuring. (It should be remembered that a patient's weight and height are measurements.) Measuring is also an essential part of an orthopedic and neurologic examination. Measurements are taken of the length and diameter of an extremity, the extent of a flexion or extension, or the pressure of a grip. The expansion of the chest is also frequently measured. Even ophthalmologists and gynecologists employ measurements. These measurements are usually reported in centimeters determined by the use of a centimeter tape or a small, clear plastic centimeter ruler. Conversions are 1 cm = 0.3937 in., and 1 in. = 2.54 cm.

MANIPULATION. This is the forceful passive movement of a joint to determine the range of extension or flexion. Manipulation may or may not be grouped with palpation. It is usually considered separate from the four standard methods of examination (inspection, palpation, percussion, and auscultation) and is grouped with mensuration, especially by the orthopedist and the neurologist. Insurance and industrial reports will often request this information in detail.

EXAMINATION POSITIONS

There are various positions in which a patient may be placed to facilitate a physical examination. It is the obligation of the medical assistant to know these positions, to know how to instruct and assist the patient in obtaining these positions with as much ease as possible, and to assist the patient in retaining the position for as long as necessary with as little discomfort as possible. The medical assistant should also know how the various positions are draped in order to protect the patient from embarrassment, to facilitate the best visibility possible for the examiner, and not to have the drape interfere with the examination.

Figure 28–1 (*A* through *J*) illustrates the various positions most frequently used in a physician's office.

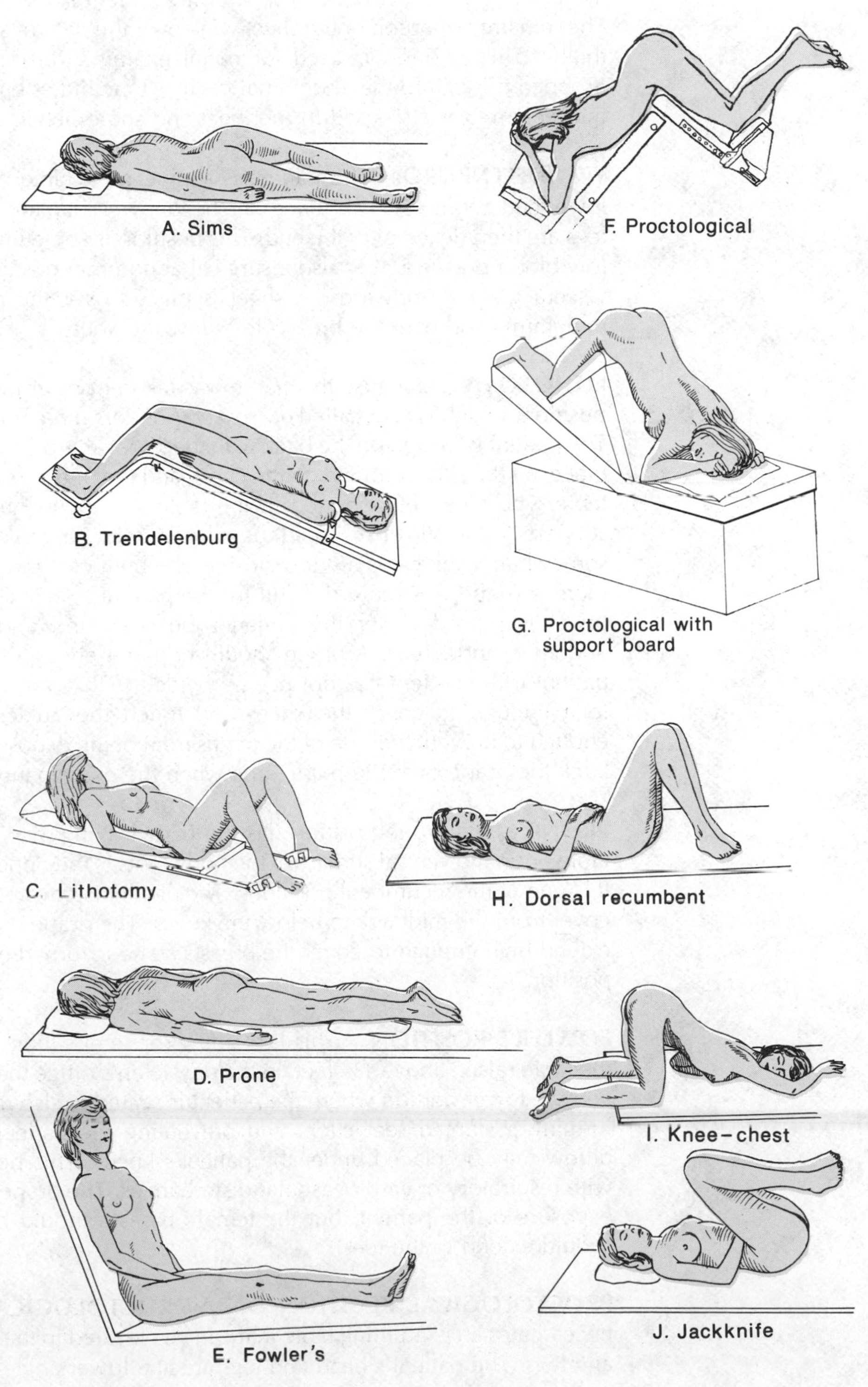

FIGURE 28–1

SIMS' POSITION. This position is sometimes called the "lateral" position, but since lateral only means "side" this does not clearly illustrate the complete position. The patient is placed on the left side with a towel or small pillow under the left cheek. The left arm and shoulder are drawn back behind the body so the body's weight is predominately on the chest. The right arm is flexed upward for support. The left leg is only slightly flexed and the buttocks are pulled to the edge of the table. The right leg is sharply flexed upwards. A towel is placed on the upper left thigh just below the perineal area. The patient is covered with a drape, preferably an aperture drape. If an aperture drape is not used, then a sheet is placed over the patient extending from under the arms to below the knees. The physician will raise a small portion of the sheet from the back of the patient sufficiently to expose the rectum. The remaining portion of the sheet will cover the patient's chest area and be over the thighs. This position is used for rectal examinations since the rectal ampulla is dropped down into the abdominal cavity; it facilitates entrance and examination of the rectum. It is also used for perineal and some pelvic examinations.

TRENDELENBURG. The patient is supine on a table that has been raised at the lower end about 45°. This places the head lower than the patient's legs. The patient's legs are then flexed over the end. This position is sometimes used in case of shock or low blood pressure. It is also a surgical abdominal position because the abdominal viscera gravitate upwards. A sheet is placed over the patient, covering from the underarms and over the breasts to below the knees.

LITHOTOMY. Because this name was taken from history, it does not describe the position, which is also called *dorsosacral* or *dorsal recumbent with the knees flexed.* The patient is placed on the back with the knees sharply flexed high, the arms may be placed at the side or folded on the chest, and the buttocks are at the lower edge of the table. The feet are supported in the table stirrups or hung in knee hammock-like supports. The stirrups should be placed wide apart and away from the table somewhat. If the heels are too close to the buttocks, the possibility of leg cramps is increased and it is more difficult for the patient to relax the abdominal muscles. A towel is placed under the patient's buttocks and a drape covers the patient's abdomen and knees. A drape should be large enough to cover the breasts of the patient if the patient has not been provided with a gown. The drape must then be long enough to cover the knees and touch the ankles. It should also be wide enough to prevent the side of the thighs from being exposed. The physician will push back the drape over the pubic area when the examination is performed.

PRONE. The prone position has the patient lying face down horizontally on the table or on the ventral surface of the body. This is the opposite of the supine position. It is one of the recumbent positions. The patient is covered with a drape sufficient to cover from the midback to below the knees. The drape on the female patient should extend high enough to cover the breasts if she is turned over to a dorsal recumbent position.

FOWLER'S POSITION. This is a sitting, or semi-sitting, position with the head of the table raised above 1½ feet. In the physician's office the head of the table is raised and the lower portion where the patient is seated is also raised about 3 to 4 in., thus forming a slanted seat effect and preventing the patient from possible sliding; a pillow may be placed under the patient's knees. This position is used for patients with respiratory or cardiovascular disturbances. The drape will vary according to the exposure of the patient, but the female breasts should be covered and the drape should extend to the feet.

PROCTOLOGICAL POSITION ON A PROCTOLOGICAL TABLE. This position necessitates an examining table that can be elevated in the center and lower the head and legs. The patient's head and legs are at a lower angle from the buttocks. It must be stressed that the patient's body is flexed at the hip joint and not at the waist. If this flexion is not correct the patient will experience considerable discomfort and the bowel will not be correctly displaced forward. A fenestrated or aperture drape is best, but a single sheet may be draped in a "U" around the anal area. Do not bind the patient's legs together with the drape because it may be necessary to separate the legs somewhat for adequate examination. This position is the superior choice for a sigmoidoscopic examination since the lower bowel is displaced forward into the abdominal cavity and somewhat straightens out the rectosigmoid area. It is also a convenient position for checking the perineal area and the anus, and for hemorrhoids.

PROCTOLOGICAL POSITION USING A SUPPORT BOARD OR PROCTO-REST*. Since many physicians' offices do not have a regular proctological table a support board may be used with great success. This is similar to the proctological table position. The rule that the patient's body is flexed at the hips and not the waist is equally important. The drape is similar. The support board may be placed on the examining table in either of two different directions: with the patient's head directed toward the head of the table or with the head toward the foot of the table. With the patient's head directed toward the foot of the table, higher elevation of the buttocks is permitted since the head of the table is elevated 8 to 10 in., creating more tilt to the board and downward slant of the patient's torso. A more conventional method is placing the support board on the flat surface of the examining table with the patient's head directed toward the top of the table.

DORSAL. This is also known as the *dorsal recumbent* position. The patient is lying on his back. The legs may or may not be slightly flexed. This position is used for examination of the abdomen and for resting. In the *dorsal elevated* position the patient is on the back with the head and shoulders slightly elevated, in a somewhat modified Fowler's position. The *supine* or *horizontal* positions have the patient on his back. These terms are used more frequently in x-ray positioning.

KNEE-CHEST. As the term implies, the patient rests on the knees and the chest. The head is turned to one side with one arm flexed under the abdomen and the other hanging over the side of the table. The thighs are perpendicular to the table and slightly separated. The patient's back should not be rounded but curved inward somewhat to an anterior convexity. The patient will need assistance and instructions from the medical assistant in order to obtain this position correctly. It is a difficult position for most patients to obtain and to sustain for a period of time. If the correct knee-chest position cannot be obtained, the patient may have to be placed in the knee-elbow position. This position makes for considerably less strain on the patient and is easier to maintain. The knee-chest is also known as the *genupectoral;* the knee-elbow is also called the *genucubital*. The drape for both positions is similar to the drape for the proctological positions, and the positions are used for the same types of examinations. An aperture drape is used or a single sheet may be draped in a "U" and pinned over the patient's sacral area. Two smaller sheets may be used, with one sheet over the patient's back and the other from the curve of the buttocks down over the thighs. It will be necessary to join the two sheets together on each side of the examination area with towel clamps. The knee-chest position is sometimes used as therapy for a postpartum prolapsed uterus.

JACKKNIFE. The patient is placed on the back with the shoulders slightly elevated and the legs flexed sharply up over the abdomen. This places the thighs at right angles to the abdomen and the lower leg at right angles to the thighs. This position, also called the *reclining* position, is used for the passing of a urethral sound. The drape is similar to that of the lithotomy position. (The proctological position has been incorrectly called a jackknife position.)

---

*Hamilton Manufacturing Co., Two Rivers, Wisconsin.

PREPARING AND DISMISSING THE PATIENT

After the physician has talked with the patient he may ask the medical assistant to prepare the patient for the physical examination. Frequently, the assistant may take the patient's weight and height at this time. If the patient is to be weighed at each subsequent visit it may be best to take the weight before the patient disrobes so the gain and loss will be consistent with the usual amount of clothing the patient will wear to the office. Ask the patient to remove his shoes. Place a paper towel on the scale's step for the patient to stand on. For accurate height, raise the height bar above the patient's head and ask the patient to face forward. Lower the bar until it touches the top of the scalp. It may be necessary to push down a little in rather thick hair. Remember to lower the bar immediately after the patient steps off the scale. A piece of brightly colored tape or ribbon on the tip of the bar may prevent a serious accident.

Direct the patient to the lavatory to empty the bladder before the examination. Have the patient save the specimen for a urinalysis. Remember to check the lavatory several times during the day to make certain there are sufficient supplies for a "clean-catch" urine specimen. It is helpful to post written instructions for the patients who are not familiar with the clean-catch method. Be certain to label the specimen immediately.

The medical assistant may wish to give the patient a brief explanation of the examination to be done. Patients are far more likely to cooperate and disrobe properly if they understand the necessity for it. If a patient appears to object to disrobing, then the medical assistant must tactfully explain the necessity of adequate exposure in order to facilitate a good examination. Failure to be properly prepared will often lead to unnecessary delays and difficulties for the physician. Do not ask a patient to disrobe in an area that does not afford privacy or a place to leave one's personal belongings. If a gown is used, tell the patient whether the gown is to be opened in the front or back. If the physician prefers that the belt not be used, it should be removed from the gown before it is given to the patient. Many gowns do not have a closure at the neck, so the medical assistant may apply a small piece of tape to close. This may be easily removed by the physician if necessary.

Rapport is often accomplished by conversation, but as soon as the physician starts the examination the medical assistant should keep her conversation to a minimum and should remain inconspicuous. When the patient is properly positioned and draped, the medical assistant may notify the physician that the patient is ready. She may remain in the room to assist the physician if she is needed or if the physician requests it.

After the examination is finished, assist the patient off the table. Remember to always raise or lower the foot board or leg rest when a patient is changed from a sitting to a **recumbent** position, otherwise there may be considerable strain on the back and abdominal muscles, as well as the back of the thighs.

The patient may now be permitted to dress. If it is not necessary to assist the patient, then respect his privacy while dressing. Never leave the room without giving the patient directions. Too often patients are left in a room not knowing if they should dress or not, or they dress and leave without further instructions on treatment, return visits, or a prescription.

Clean the room immediately. Put fresh paper on the table; change the towel on the pillow. Disinfect any surfaces that may have been contaminated. Remove all used instruments, medications used, or any evidence of the previous patient. Return all items to their proper places. Check labels on all specimens. Check the patient's medical history to see if all entries have been made, or direct the history to the proper person. Do not leave a patient's history where others may read it. A history is a legal confidential record, and a lawsuit may occur if it is mishandled. The room should now be ready for the next patient.

BASICS OF A ROUTINE PHYSICAL EXAMINATION

It has been said that there is no such thing as a really complete physical examination, nor would there always be a need for it. Examinations vary greatly, depending on the physician's specialty and the reason for the examination. There may also be a variance in the sequence of an examination as the needs for different areas are stressed. This book will follow only the average routine that an examiner may follow. There will be an overview with some terminology and description of pathology that may be used and seen. Only basic instruments will be described since each physician has individual preferences.

The physical examination really starts as soon as the patient appears before the examiner. The term "presenting appearance" may be used on the medical record. It is noted whether the patient appears well and in good health. The patient may appear disheveled, dull, or even in distress. Even a patient's responses to the opening remarks or questions may show an alertness or a dullness.

GAIT. The patient's gait, that is, the manner or style of walking, will often give some information by his limping, for example, walking with the feet wide apart, or having difficulty keeping balanced. This analysis of gait is usually done with the patient walking a straight line and may be without the patient knowing he is being observed. Some of the terms used are **ataxic,** which describes an unsteady, uncoordinated walk that employs a wide base; **slapping** or **steppage,** in which the advancing leg is lifted high enough for the toe to clear the ground; or **drag-to,** when the feet are dragged, rather than lifted, toward the goal. Other descriptions may be **scissors or spastic,** in which the legs are held together and move in a stiff manner, the toes seeming to drag and catch.

STATURE. This refers to the patient's height and is used as a criterion in identifying the genetically tall or short person and the abnormally large (as in gigantism) or small individual (dwarf). Gigantism may be **acromegaly** from the hypersecretion of the anterior pituitary gland growth hormone. Dwarfism can be seen in cretins, who have a congenital thyroid deficiency. Midgets are frequently classed with dwarfs; midgets, however, are perfectly proportioned in all respects, whereas dwarfs usually have normal-sized or large heads and short limbs.

POSTURE. A patient's posture may reveal significant information. This may be displayed in a rigid posture from a fixed spine; an extremity that has limited motion will alter a posture frequently. The patient may say that he cannot sleep unless in a sitting position (this is seen in some heart diseases). There may be a condition called **torticollis** (wryneck) that is the result of a shortening of the sternomastoid muscle. Examinations relating to the spine may show an abnormal curve as found in **kyphosis** (humpback), **scoliosis** (curvature of the spine), or **lordosis** (abnormal or exaggerated curve of the lumbosacral area, which causes the buttocks to protrude excessively). A patient's posture may indicate an area of pain.

BODY MOVEMENTS. These may be classed as *voluntary* or *involuntary*. The voluntary movements are usually the patient's normal habits and are sometimes limited in clinical value unless they are the result of an abnormal condition. Involuntary movements are frequently tics that may also be habit spasms and are usually found in the eyes, neck, or face, they may also be the result of various conditions. Tics are rhythmic involuntary movements of various rates under different conditions. A hand tremor may be the beating of the thumb against a flexing finger or there may be a rhythmic oscillation of the head as may occur in **senescence** (old age).

SPEECH. Patterns of speech may denote social history and the character of the patient, or they may reveal an abnormal condition. Some basic speech defects are

aphonia, the inability to speak because of a loss of the voice for various reasons as in severe laryngitis or overuse of the voice; **aphasia,** the loss of the power of expression through speech, writing, or sign due to an injury to the brain centers; and **dysphasia,** an impairment of speech or voice.

BREATH ODORS. These may or may not be diagnostic, although they often are associated with poor oral hygiene or dental care. Acidosis from diabetes mellitus will give the strong odor of acetone on the breath as a sweet, fruity odor. A musty odor is associated with liver disease, and the odor of ammonia may be found in cases of **uremia.**

NUTRITION. A patient is generally thought of as being overweight or underweight. Obesity may be of either of two origins: **exogenous** involves simply excessive caloric intake in ratio to the expenditure of calories, and **endogenous** is that found in certain endocrine disturbances such as Cushing's syndrome. **Edema** is the accumulation of fluid in the intracellular spaces of the body. It must be differentiated from fat by the simple test of pressing a finger on the skin over a bony area, like the ankle, and seeing if a pit or depression remains. Edema leaves a pit for a few moments and may be called *pitting edema.* Fat does not pit but returns to skin level immediately after the finger is removed.

SKIN. The skin is considered part of the general appearance, except in special complaints. Concerns would be an abnormal coloring such as redness, **cyanosis, pallor,** or excessive brown patches. **Jaundice** may indicate an increase in the level of **bilirubin** in the blood. A decreased pigmentation would be found in **vitiligo,** the acquired loss of **melanin** characterized by white patches. Lesions, ulcers, and bruises can be the result of pathologic conditions. Skin texture refers to smoothness, roughness, and scaling. Loss of elasticity is when the skin does not return immediately to normal when it has been pulled or stretched. This can occur when there has been chronic actinic damage, such as in excessive suntanning.

HAIR DISTRIBUTION. Distribution and the lack of hair as well as the texture of hair are important. Patchy baldness is seen in **alopecia areata.** Excessive hair on the body, especially facial hair on the female, indicates some bodily change. Heavy abdominal or thigh hair is diagnostic. Fingernails often give some indication of a person's health, especially if they are brittle, grooved, or lined. Clubbing of the fingertips is associated with some congenital heart diseases. Spooning of the nail is seen in some severe iron deficiency **anemias.** Beau's lines appear after a severe acute illness. These transverse depressions in the nail appear several weeks after the illness but will grow out with normal nail growth.

SEQUENCE OF A ROUTINE PHYSICAL EXAMINATION

The examination usually starts with the patient seated on the examining table. If the physician uses reflected light, then the light source should be behind the patient's right shoulder. If illuminated instruments are used, then the standard overhead lights are sufficient. Always be very careful never to shine a light directly into the patient's eyes. Turn lights on while they are directed away from the patient, and then carefully move the light toward the area to be examined.

Materials needed:

- Stethoscope
- Pencil flashlight
- Ophthalmoscope
- Otoscope
- Tongue depressor
- Gauze square
- Finger cot or disposable glove
- Lubricating gel
- Tape measure
- Percussion hammer
- Nasal speculum
- Tuning fork

HEAD. The patient's head and face are usually the starting place for the examination. The face reflects the patient's state and will tell the physician a great deal. It may appear puffy, especially the eyelids, giving the appearance that the patient has just awakened. This puffiness may be due to **myxedema** from a long-standing thyroid deficiency. A smoothening of the forehead and cheek could be the result of a paralysis of the seventh cranial (facial) nerve. With **scleroderma** the facial skin is characteristically tight and **atrophied.** Lipid or fatty patches that collect in the eyelids usually near the center are called **xanthelasma.** These appear as yellowish-white, slightly elevated small patches and may or may not be associated with a disease.

NECK. The neck is checked for range of motion (ROM) by having the patient voluntarily move his head in various directions. One limitation that may appear is **torticollis,** the shortening of the sternomastoid muscle. *Bounding* is an involuntary slight nodding of the head synchronized with the pulsation of the heart. The *thyroid gland* is always given special attention for asymmetry, enlargement, and texture. The patient is asked to swallow several times. The medical assistant may help by giving a small amount of water in a paper cup. The physician may palpate the thyroid gland anteriorly and posteriorly. The carotid artery is palpated and auscultated for possible *bruit,* that is, an abnormal sound or murmur. The cervical, submandibular, and supraclavicular lymph nodes are palpated.

EYES. Eyes are usually checked first for reaction to light into the pupils; this is known as "light and accommodation" (L&A). The color of the sclera may be abnormally red or yellow. The movements of the eyes are tested by having the patient follow the examiner's finger. **Exophthalmos** is an important observation that is seen in some cases of hyperthyroidism or of a tumor or fat pad behind the eyeballs. Intraocular pressure is checked with the tonometer in most individuals past the age of 35. Pressure within the eyeball could denote the presence of glaucoma, which results in pathologic changes in the optic disc, visual defects, and eventual blindness.

EARS. The ears are examined with the aid of the otoscope. Symptoms referable to the ears may be deafness, pain, discharge, **vertigo,** and **tinnitus.** The external ear is first checked for redness of the ear canal or the presence of ear wax **(cerumen).** The **tympanic membrane** (eardum) may be seen in most patients with the aid of the otoscope and appears pearly gray. The patient may be asked to swallow again in order to observe any movement of the tympanic membrane by the change of pressure through the eustachian tube. This tube is also called the auditory tube and serves as an equalizer between the middle ear and the throat. Scars appearing on the membrane are frequently the result of earlier ear infections and perforations. The color of the membrane is diagnostic since it may indicate fluids such as blood or pus in the middle ear.

MOUTH and THROAT. The mouth, or oral cavity, is usually thought of in terms of oral hygiene and dental care. A history of sore throats, bleeding gums, tooth extractions, and voice changes calls for a careful examination. The status of dental hygiene includes the condition of the teeth, whether the patient takes care of his teeth, and whether there is good occlusion, that is, whether the teeth of the upper and lower jaws meet properly for good chewing. Normal gums are a pale pink and glossy smooth and do not bleed upon slight pressure from a tongue depressor. **Pyorrhea** is the discharge of pus from the dental periosteum and is a progressive condition. It may also be called **periodontitis.** The palatine tonsils are usually visible, but it is sometimes difficult for a physician to tell the difference between a tonsillectomized throat and very small tonsils. Tonsils may be enlarged and cryptic. The pharyngeal tonsils (adenoids) in the nasopharynx area and the lingual tonsils at the base of the tongue are not easily accessible. The physician will use a tongue depressor and a piece of gauze to grasp the tongue. The floor of the mouth is examined by both inspection and palpation for enlarged lymph nodes and ulcerations.

The nasal cavity and the nasopharynx may reveal the presence of a discharge from the sinuses known as a postnasal drip (PND), which is a common complaint. Other abnormalities may be obstructions, a deviated septum, polyps, and ulcerations. The nasal cavity basically requires an examination of the color and texture of the mucosa. When a patient has a nosebleed it is correctly called **epistaxis.** The sinus meatus cannot be seen, but the frontal and maxillary sinuses may be examined by radiography or by the application of pressure over the area and transillumination.

CHEST. While the patient is still in the sitting position, the chest, heart, and breasts will be examined. The chest is noted for symmetric expansion. A tape measure may be used, especially if there is a variation between upper and lower chest expansion. A patient with a history of **emphysema** may display a chest that is barrel-like rather than the usual elliptical shape as viewed laterally. It is necessary to know the landmarks, or **topography,** of the chest in order to communicate effectively in locating the underlying structures (Fig. 28–2).

The types of respiration are noted. Some of the variations are **dyspnea** (labored or difficult breathing), **tachypnea** (very rapid breathing), **orthopnea** (the ability to breathe easier when in an upright position), hyperventilation, or irregular rhythm as noted in **Cheyne-Stokes** breathing. Chest sounds heard by the physician may be described as various types of **rales,** which are abnormal sounds that vary from coarse

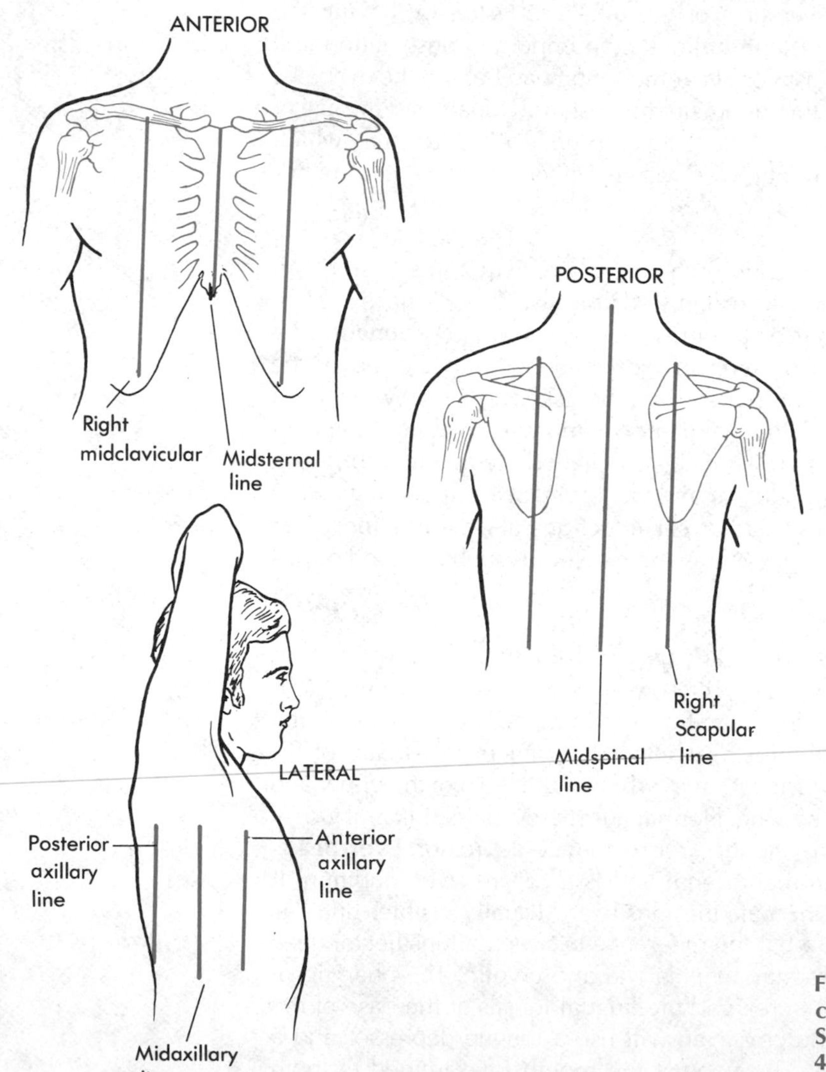

FIGURE 28–2 Topography of the chest. (Adapted from Prior, J. A., and Silberstein, J. S.: *Physical Diagnosis.* 4th ed. St. Louis, The C. V. Mosby Co., 1972.)

musical sounds to whistling or squeaking as heard in asthma or bronchitis. The term **stridor** describes a wheezing sound or a shrill, harsh, or crowing sound. **Fremitus** describes vibrations that may be both felt and heard by the examiner, as when a person is speaking.

Usually a patient is asked to take deep and regular breaths during a chest examination. This may produce a slight dizziness, sometimes erroneously called vertigo. This dizziness is not abnormal at this time, and the patient may be assured that it is only the result of the deep regular respirations and will rapidly pass.

Syncope and chest pains warrant careful examination. Much of the examination of the cardiovascular system comprises data gained from the vital signs and the electrocardiogram. (See Chapters 27 and 32.) Because it takes considerable concentration to interpret what is heard, it is necessary to have complete silence when the physician is listening to the patient's heart. The heart is examined from both the anterior and posterior approaches to the patient. The physician may at this time mark the patient's chest where special leads are to be placed if an electrocardiogram is to be done following the examination.

BREASTS. A careful breast examination is part of the examination of every female, whether the patient is symptomatic or not. Breast cancer is the most common malignancy occurring in women, and early detection is the key to successful treatment. Women should be instructed to examine their own breasts at regular intervals. The American Cancer Society has excellent pamphlets and films to supplement the physician's instructions.

The patient's gown is lowered to the waist. With the patient in the sitting position the breasts are inspected for symmetry, skin texture, and skin changes. An orange-peel or pigskin texture would indicate possible edema, which would cause the hair follicles to indent. Skin retractions may be the result of an underlying growth pulling the skin inward. Frequently the patient is asked to do several calisthenics in order to activate various muscles involved with the breasts. The patient may be asked to place her arms at her side while sitting for general inspection, raise her arms over her head in order to increase dimpling or skin retractions, press her palms together to tighten the pectoral muscles that will also exaggerate dimpling and retractions, or lean forward with her arms supported by the examiner (especially for examination of extra large or very pendulous breasts).

The breast examination may be continued when the patient is in the supine (dorsal recumbent) position. It will be helpful if a small pillow or rolled towel is placed under the shoulder of the side to be examined. This allows the breast to rest more evenly on the chest wall. The consistency of the breast tissue depends on the patient's age, obesity, stage of the menstrual cycle, and pregnancy.

REFLEXES. **Reflexes** are checked with the patient in the sitting and supine positions. While the patient is sitting, the biceps are checked with the patient's arm flexed and supported by the examiner; the knee-jerk (patellar) and the ankle-jerk (Achilles) are also checked with the patient sitting. The plantar reflexes (Babinski and Chaddock) may be examined with the patient in either the sitting or the supine position.

ABDOMEN. The patient is now lowered to the supine, or dorsal recumbent, position and the drape is lowered to the pubic hair line. The gown is raised to just under the breasts. A towel should be placed over the female breasts if a gown is not used. Whether he is right- or left-handed, the physician usually stands on the patient's right side. The patient's arms may be placed at the side or the hands may be crossed on the chest. If the table is narrow and the patient cannot relax completely, it may help to have the patient tuck his thumbs under his buttocks in order to relax the shoulders. Relaxation of the abdominal muscles is absolutely essential for an abdominal examination. It sometimes helps to place a small pillow under the

TABLE 28–1 Structures Underlying the Abdominal Quadrants

Right Upper Quadrant	Left Upper Quadrant
Liver	Stomach
Gallbladder	Spleen
Pylorus	Body of pancreas
Duodenum	Left kidney
Head of pancreas	Splenic flexure of colon
Right kidney	
Hepatic flexure of colon	
Right Lower Quadrant	**Left Lower Quadrant**
Cecum	Sigmoid colon
Appendix	Left ovary and tube
Right ovary and tube	
Portion of ascending colon	
Midline	
Bladder	
Uterus	

patient's head or to flex the knees. If the patient exhibits ticklishness it is best to disregard it and try to continue the examination by changing the routine somewhat.

First, it is important to know the topography of the abdomen and the underlying organs (Figure 28–3 and Table 28–1). For general location of the underlying organs, the abdomen is divided into quadrants. The vertical line extends from the xiphoid process of the sternum to the pubic symphysis; the horizontal line crosses the abdomen at the level of the umbilicus. Another method of dividing the abdomen is by regions or sections (Fig. 28–3*B*). Note the right and left hypochondriac regions are composed almost entirely of the costal margins. This is because the abdomen extends up under the rib cage to the diaphragm dome. The liver and spleen are located in these regions.

Some abdominal symptoms a patient may give during the history could be **dyspepsia** (indigestion), **dysphagia** (difficult swallowing), a change in bowel habits, excessive **flatulence** (gas), nausea, and vomiting. General abdominal discomfort is common since abdominal pain is frequently referred pain and not always located directly over the involved organ.

The inspection of the abdomen would start with noting any change in color such as jaundice. **Striae** (silver stretch marks), **petechiae** (small purple hemorrhagic spots), **cutaneous angiomas** (spider nevi), scars, and visible masses are all among what may be observed. The contour of the abdomen may be flat, rounded, or bulging in local areas. A bulging in the right and left lumbar regions (the flanks) may be the result of the presence of free abdominal fluid **(ascites).** Abdominal hernias are examined with the patient in the supine and standing positions. To complete the abdominal examination the patient may be placed in a knee-elbow position to better determine the presence of free abdominal fluid. The Sims' position is also used for this purpose.

RECTUM. The rectal examination usually follows the abdominal examination or may be part of the male and female examinations. A patient's comfort and dignity are vital since most people dislike this part of the physical examination most. The examiner will need a finger cot or examining glove and lubricating jelly. A good light is directed at the perineal area.

The rectum of the male is usually checked when the patient is in a standing position bending over the end of the examining table to have the prostate gland examined. The anus and perineal area are inspected for inflammation, rashes, excoriation, or external hemorrhoids. The buttocks are spread to facilitate visualization of the anus. If a **fissure** (an abnormal crack or cleft) or **fistula** (an abnormal

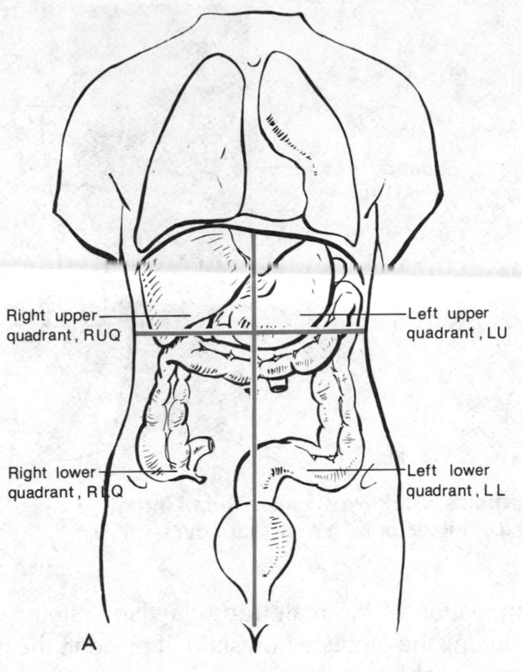

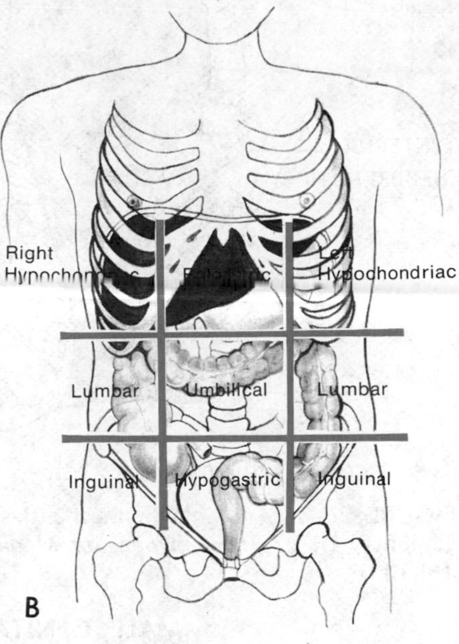

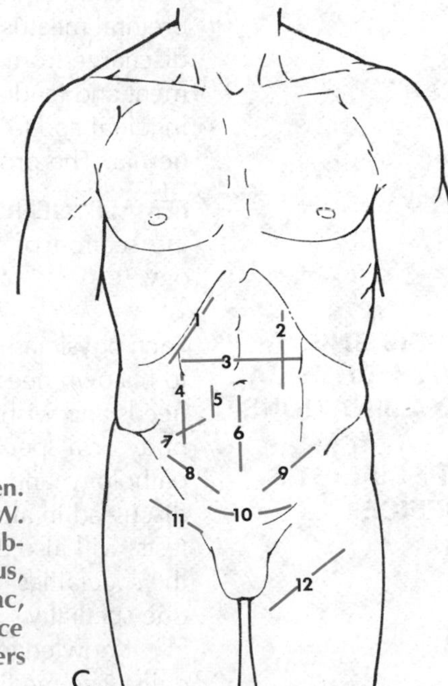

FIGURE 28–3 *A,* **Quadrants of the abdomen.** *B,* **Regions of the abdomen. (From Chabner, D. E.:** ***The Language of Medicine.*** **2nd ed. Philadelphia, W. B. Saunders Co., 1981.)** *C,* **Incisions of the abdomen, anterior view. (1) subcostal, (2) paramedial, (3) transverse, (4) upper right rectus, (5) midrectus, (6) midline, (7) lower right rectus, (8) McBurney's or right iliac, (9) left iliac, (10) suprapubic, (11) hernia, (12) femoral. (From Fordney, M. T.:** ***Insurance Handbook for the Medical Office.*** **2nd ed. Philadelphia, W. B. Saunders Co., 1981.)**

tubelike passage) is present, the patient will feel considerable pain (Fig. 28–4). These abnormalities make the digital examination of the rectum difficult to perform. The anal sphincter muscle is palpated; in the male, the prostate is checked for size, shape, and consistency. Internal hemorrhoids are difficult to palpate unless they are thrombosed.

The rectum of the female may be examined while the patient is in the lithotomy position for the pelvic examination. The posterior vaginal wall and the anterior rectal wall are palpated by the examiner by placing the index finger in the vaginal canal and the middle finger in the rectum. Since the digital examination limits the examination to an area of within 6 to 8 cm (2.5 to 3.5 in.), the physician may wish to further examine the bowel by sigmoidoscopy.

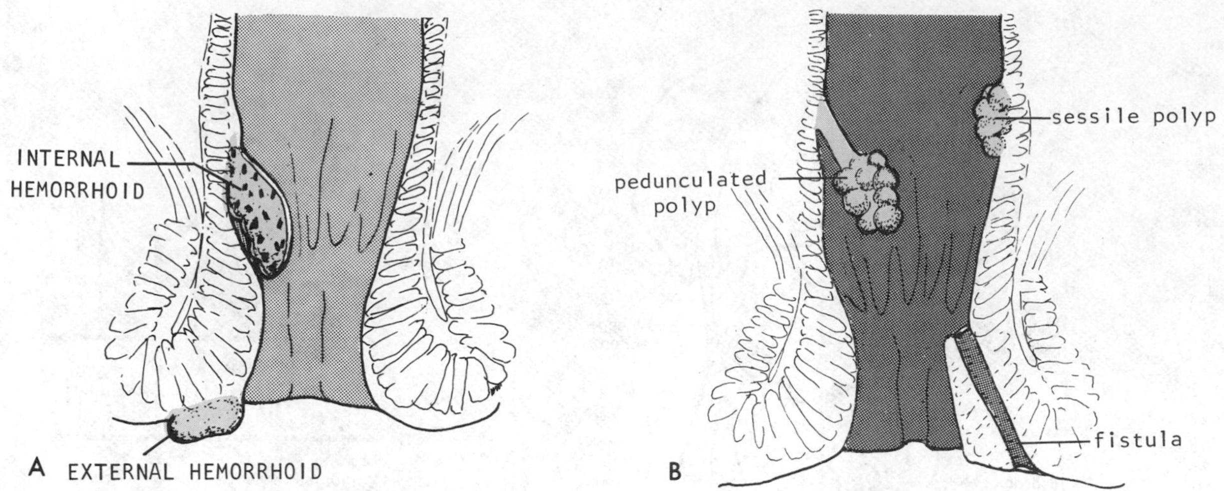

FIGURE 28–4 Anorectal abnormalities. *A,* Hemorrhoids. *B,* Polyps and fistula. (From Chabner, D. E.: *The Language of Medicine*. 2nd ed. Philadelphia, W. B. Saunders Co., 1981.)

MALE GENITALIA. Examination of the male reproductive system will consist of inspection of the penis including the prepuce (foreskin), if present, the glans, and the urethral meatus. The presence or absence of any ulcers, scars, or nodules as well as a discharge from the urethra should be noted. The scrotum is examined for enlargement and tenderness, which may be the result of a **hydrocele,** edema, or tumor. The inguinal and femoral areas are inspected and palpated for bulges denoting a possible hernia. The prostate gland is palpated as mentioned earlier.

FEMALE GENITALIA. This portion of the examination is covered in its entirety in the section of this chapter on specialty examinations, "Obstetrics and Gynecology."

ASSISTING WITH PHYSICAL EXAMINATIONS IN A SPECIALIST'S OFFICE

Each physician has a particular method of examination and treatment that lends itself to his own needs and habits. The medical assistant must be alert to these individual needs and wishes. In the specialist's office, emphasis is given to a special part of the body or a special kind of complaint. This portion of the chapter will outline some pathology and techniques most commonly seen in these specialties, which are discussed in alphabetical order. Some diagnostic aids, such as x-rays and laboratory tests, will also be mentioned. There will be no attempt to introduce the reader to all the specialties, or to all the many procedures done, or to the pathology seen within one specialty.

Knowledge is increased and technical developments are discovered almost daily. The medical assistant is fortunate to be in an employment situation where the availability of these new findings may be learned, thereby offering continuing education. A member of the health team should never allow oneself to remain static in this rapidly changing medical world.

Allergy

This is the specialty of diagnosing and treating allergic conditions. It is difficult to separate allergy and immunology: to understand one it is necessary to have a degree of understanding of the other. In a normal immune reaction an antigen unites with an antibody and results in the elimination of the harmful antigen. An allergic reaction is the same, *but* the interaction of the antigen and the antibody is accompanied by a harmful effect on the body tissue and a substance called histamine is released in excess. This turn of events from the normal immune response is referred to as "hypersensitive reaction," and the diseases arising from it are called "diseases of hypersensitivity." Among such diseases are allergy, hay fever, serum sickness, and transfusion reactions. In short, the immune reaction can take two turns, a good turn or a bad turn.

Symptoms of an allergy can occur for the first time at any age. The substances that produce an allergic response can be eaten, inhaled, injected, or applied topically to the skin. The response to these antigens, or allergens, as the allergists prefer to call them, bears no relationship to the type of material involved. For example, foods may cause **eczema, rhinitis,** or **asthma.** Pollens may also cause any of these conditions. When rhinitis is caused by a pollen, it is given a special name, hay fever, although "hay" is not necessarily the causative agent.

An allergic reaction does not occur on the first contact with the allergen because the antibodies have not yet been produced by the body. It *may* occur on the second contact, when the antibodies have been released and are in reserve in the body tissues. The reaction may not occur until later in life, when contact with the allergen suddenly develops into a sensitivity. An allergy is said to be a reaction to a substance that ordinarily is harmless to the majority of persons. There are almost as many allergens, such as pollens, foods, plants, animal fur, insect bites, and chemicals, as there are substances. The reactions range from a mild sneezing to a more severe serum sickness or anaphylactic shock, which is serious and can be fatal unless immediate emergency measures are taken.

The diagnosis of an allergy is made by taking a very careful history from the patient, performing a careful and complete physical examination, and following this up with selected laboratory tests, which may include x-ray studies, blood and urine examination, and finally skin tests. This history and physical examination are always made by the physician, but the skin tests and laboratory tests are usually the responsibilities of a medical assistant or laboratory technician. Since skin tests are potentially very hazardous to perform, they should always be conducted under direct supervision of a physician. It should be emphasized that skin tests by themselves are not strictly diagnostic of an allergy but, when combined with a careful history and other factors, they are helpful in establishing the diagnosis. Skin tests are ordinarily performed by one or more of several methods: scratch, intradermal, ophthalmic, or patch.

SCRATCH TEST. The most common and possibly the least satisfactory is the scratch and puncture test. It is most popular because it is rapid and simple to perform. The tests may be performed on any smooth surface of the skin, but the arm and back are most popular. Of the two, the arm is safer (either the outer surface of the upper arm or the palmar surface of the lower arm, Fig. 28–5), since a serious reaction may be limited by the application of a tourniquet above the site. However, the back is favored in infants and in young children because of the large area of skin available and the possibility of immobilizing such a patient if necessary.

Scrub the skin well with alcohol or acetone and allow to dry. If several tests are to be given, use a definite pattern in order to facilitate accurate reading of reactions. Make a scratch on the skin with a needle or scarifier. It is not necessary to draw blood; in fact, it is inadvisable. Scratch only deep enough to permit the extract to enter the skin. The length of the scratch should be about one-eighth inch or less. If a scarifier is used, it should be placed on the skin and twirled with slight pressure. Then place one very small drop of the extract over the scratch area. Do not use too much, because the fluid may run into an adjoining scratch and the test will be of no value.

A reaction will usually occur within 10 to 30 minutes. If the reaction is positive, a **wheal (hive)** will be formed at the site of the scratch. The interpretation of the test should always be based on a comparison of this reaction with that of the control, which is a scratch with a plain base fluid free from any allergy-producing extract.

The interpretation or reading of the skin tests is performed by the physician. However, a few doctors delegate this step to the trained skin tester. Reactions are commonly graded from 2 to 4. No precise definition of a reaction can be given, and indeed the intensity may vary among individuals. However, as a general rule, a 2 reaction implies a wheal that is definitely larger than that of the control. A larger

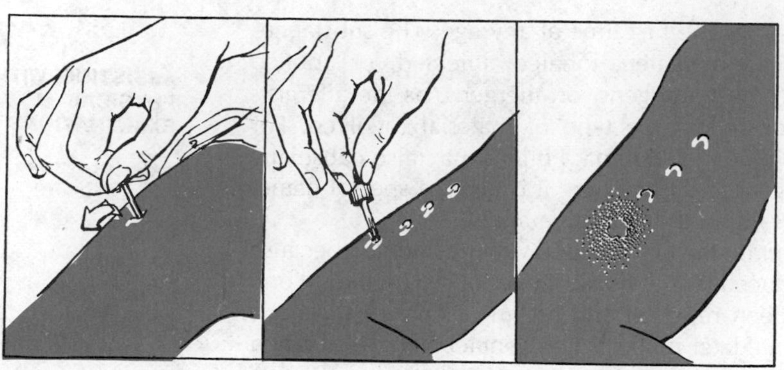

FIGURE 28–5 Technique of the scratch test.

wheal is interpreted as a 3, whereas the presence of **pseudopods** — fingerlike extensions around the periphery of the wheal — may be read as 4. It is advisable to carefully wipe off the extract to stop the reaction when a strong reaction is occurring. Erythema or reddening around the wheal is usually disregarded in the interpretations. Frequently the large or significant reactions are accompanied by local itching (Fig. 28–5).

INTRADERMAL (INTRACUTANEOUS) TEST. This method can be used if a patient has shown a questionable or negative reaction to the scratch method. This test is more sensitive than the scratch test. Extracts are injected into the skin, with usual sterile technique, in a dose of 0.01 to 0.02 cc. The reaction time is identical to that of the scratch test. The antigen, however, is more dilute. Remember the extract cannot be wiped off as in the scratch method. This method is always done on the patient's arm. This is a safety measure in case of a hypersensitivity. Apply a tourniquet immediately above the reaction area in order to retard absorption of the extract. Immediately prepare epinephrine to be administered on the physician's orders.

PATCH TEST. This method of testing is of some value in tracking down the cause of contact dermatitis. In the patch test the suspected material is placed on the skin — near the original lesion, if possible — covered with a small square of cellophane, and held down with strips of adhesive or transparent tape or even collodion. The reaction is read within one to four days (Fig. 28–6).

The tuberculin patch test is commonly used because of the ease in administering it. The tuberculin is incorporated into a small square of gauze, which is held in place on the skin for two days. A red spot on the skin at the place of application is read as a positive reaction.

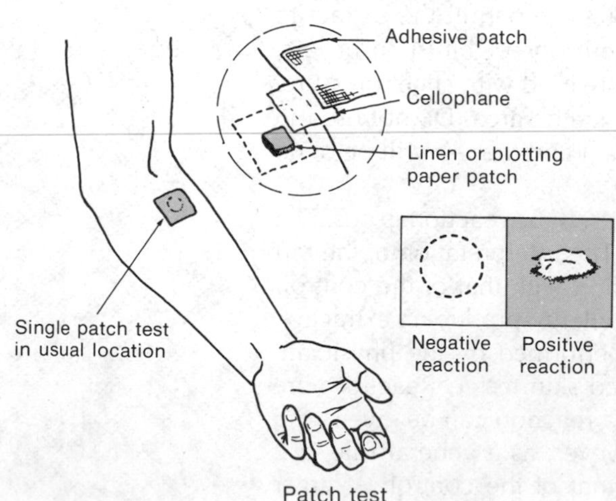

FIGURE 28–6 Patch test for skin allergies. (From Miller, B. F., and Keane, C. B.: *Encyclopedia and Dictionary of Medicine, Nursing, and Allied Health*. 2nd ed. Philadelphia, W. B. Saunders Co., 1978.)

OPHTHALMIC TEST. This test is less common. The testing extract is dropped into the conjunctiva of the eye. This procedure is rarely done and is mentioned only for the sake of completeness.

Considerable controversy exists as to the best way of performing skin tests. But the one item that seems to be overlooked even by professional allergists is the nature of the materials that are used for skin testing. In the hands of the finest skin tester, poor testing materials are without value. Unfortunately there is no standardization of testing materials, and the potency and specificity will vary from one supplier to another. Furthermore, the number of materials that are available for skin testing is frequently ludicrous. Under active investigation are methods that use the patient's blood directly. However, such methods are still experimental.

ENVIRONMENTAL CONTROL. Patients are encouraged and instructed in the various methods of making their surroundings as free as possible from the offending allergens. One could be the elimination of animals, feathers, and dust-collecting items within the house. The garden is checked for offending grasses and pollens. Foods that cause problems are best eliminated. Contacts such as soaps and cosmetics are avoided.

Anesthesiology

Anesthesiology is the branch of medicine concerned with the administration of anesthetics and maintenance of the patient while under anesthesia. An *anesthesiologist* is a specialist in this branch of medicine, and the term is usually reserved for the physician administering the anesthetic. An *anesthetist* is one who administers anesthetics; this may be a nurse-anesthetist or a physician-anesthetist. The word "anesthetic" was given to medicine by Dr. Oliver Wendell Holmes (1809–1894).

Clinical assisting duties in an anesthesiologist's office are extremely limited and usually confined to the scheduling of appointments for the doctor to administer an anesthetic at a hospital and to the keeping of accounts. Many anesthesiologists do not maintain an office, as we think of a physician's office, but are hospital-based and use the services of a secretary. But medical assistants should be familiar with a few terms and definitions that are applicable to this specialty of medicine.

Anesthetics seem to fall into one of two groups, *general* or *local*. There is considerable controversy regarding these two terms, but for convenience they will be used here. A general anesthetic implies a state of unconsciousness, insusceptibility to pain, and a degree of muscle relaxation. General anesthetics are classed according to the route of administration. The *inhalants* are gases or highly volatile liquids; *intravenous* and *rectal* anesthetics are the nonvolatile drugs. The term "local anesthetic" is used when loss of sensation is confined to a limited area. Other terms used for local anesthetic are *conduction anesthesia* and *regional anesthesia*. Local anesthetics are also often referred to as *tissue infiltration anesthetics*. This is because the immediate surrounding tissue is injected or infiltrated with a local anesthetic so each individual nerve ending is blocked. This method may be used to induce spinal or caudal blocks. The names of local anesthetics usually end with *-caine*. A *topical anesthetic* is a local anesthetic applied directly to a certain area of the skin or mucous membrane, such as a spray on the nasal mucosa.

Dermatology

The human skin, also called the integument or integumentary system, is the largest organ of the body. It has many different functions: it aids in controlling body temperature, is a barrier to most bacteria, furnishes a sensory system, and is an insulator against outside elements. Both the term "dermis" (Greek) and the term "cutis" (Latin) are used when referring to the skin. Dermatitis and cutitis are synonymous for inflammations of the skin, but dermatitis is by far the preferred term.

The skin has an outer layer, the epidermis, and an inner layer, the dermis or corium. Blood vessels and nerves as well as the sweat glands, hair roots, and the nail beds are located in the dermis (Figure 28–7). Normality of the skin depends on the person's age, sex, and physical and emotional health. The skin reflects both internal systemic conditions and external contact reactions.

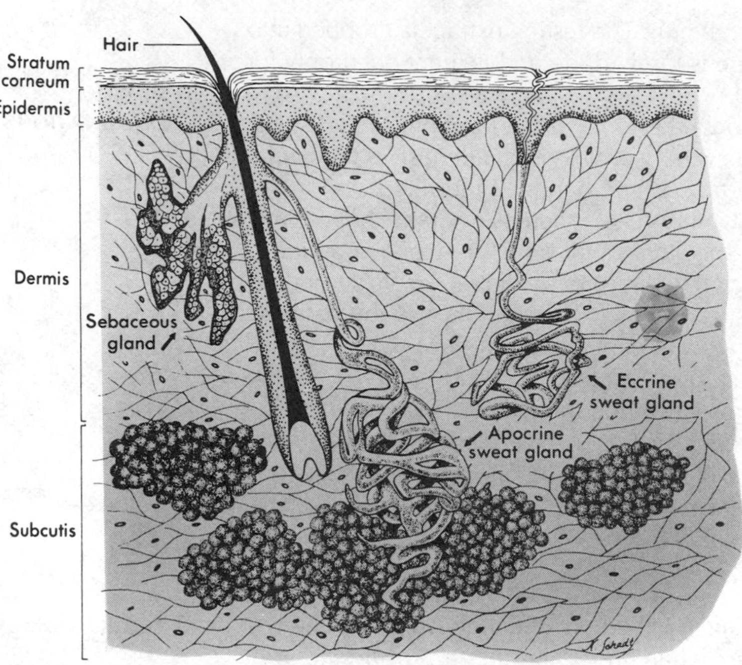

FIGURE 28–7 The histologic anatomy of the skin and its appendages. (From Prior, J. A., and Silberstein, J. S.: *Physical Diagnosis*. 4th ed. St. Louis, The C. V. Mosby Co., 1973.)

Examination of the skin is basically inspection followed with detailed examination by palpation, **diascopy**, and special tests. The **diascope** is a glass plate pressed against the skin to permit observation of changes produced in the underlying areas by the pressure. The impairments that most frequently bring a patient to the dermatologist's office are the cosmetic disfigurements caused by a skin disease, pain and **pruritus,** and interference with sensations or movements. The possibility that a skin lesion is the result of a systemic condition is sometimes a major concern.

Inspection of the skin may show color changes such as erythema, **leukoderma,** jaundice, or vitiligo. Localized red or purple changes may be the result of vascular neoplasms, birthmarks, or subcutaneous hemorrhages (**petechiae** and **ecchymoses**). Palpation is used to confirm and amplify findings seen by inspection. Inspection and palpation are interrelated in confirming diagnoses. Palpatory findings may be texture, elasticity, or edema.

One disorder of the skin is **seborrheic dermatitis**, a chronic inflammation of the scalp, commonly called dandruff. It may spread to face, neck and body. **Acne vulgaris** is also a disorder of the sebaceous glands and presents pustules, blackheads **(comedones)**, and cysts. **Furuncles** (boils) and **carbuncles** (extensions of a furuncle) are often seen.

Disorders of the skin may be divided into primary and secondary lesions. Primary lesions are those that appear immediately. **Macules, papules, plaques, nodules, comedones, cysts, wheals,** and **pustules** are all primary lesions. Secondary lesions never appear originally but are the result of alterations in a primary lesion. Examples of secondary lesions are scales, crusts, fissures, erosions, ulcerations, and scars. A burn gives a blister. The blister is the primary lesion; the blister breaks and an ulceration forms; then healing ends in a scar. The ulceration and the scar are secondary lesions (Fig. 28–8).

Materials needed:

- Good light
- Microscopic slides
- Ultraviolet light with Wood's filter
- #15 knife blade
- Comedo extractor
- Diascope
- Dropper bottle of 10 per cent potassium hydroxide.

Draping a patient for a skin examination depends on the area to be examined. Remember to expose the area adequately but protect the patient's privacy. Try to make the patient as comfortable as possible and offer support when it is needed.

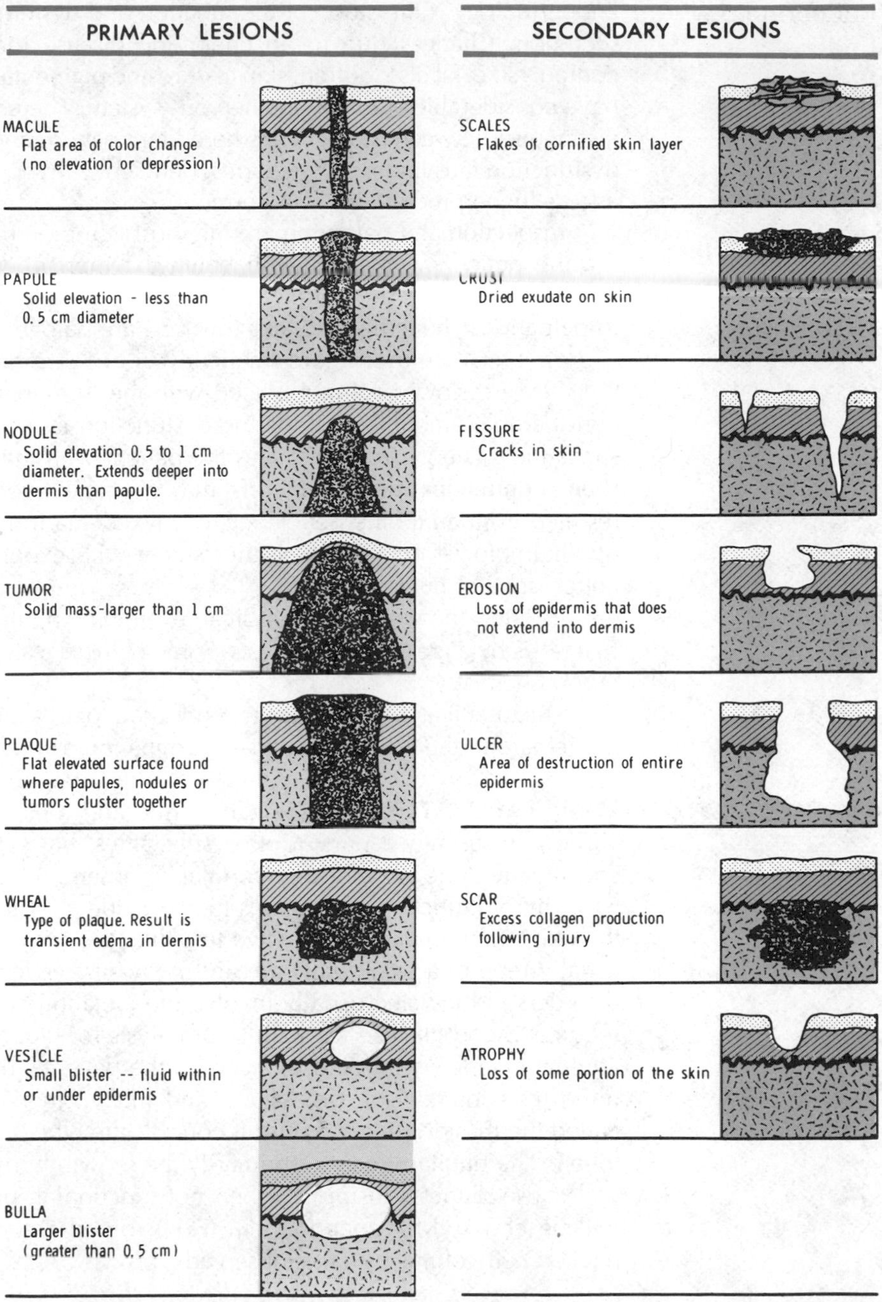

PRIMARY LESIONS

MACULE
Flat area of color change (no elevation or depression)

PAPULE
Solid elevation - less than 0.5 cm diameter

NODULE
Solid elevation 0.5 to 1 cm diameter. Extends deeper into dermis than papule.

TUMOR
Solid mass-larger than 1 cm

PLAQUE
Flat elevated surface found where papules, nodules or tumors cluster together

WHEAL
Type of plaque. Result is transient edema in dermis

VESICLE
Small blister -- fluid within or under epidermis

BULLA
Larger blister (greater than 0.5 cm)

SECONDARY LESIONS

SCALES
Flakes of cornified skin layer

CRUST
Dried exudate on skin

FISSURE
Cracks in skin

EROSION
Loss of epidermis that does not extend into dermis

ULCER
Area of destruction of entire epidermis

SCAR
Excess collagen production following injury

ATROPHY
Loss of some portion of the skin

FIGURE 28–8 **Characteristics of common skin lesions. (From Sana, J. M., and Judge, R. D. (eds.): *Physical Appraisal Methods in Nursing Practice*. Boston, Little, Brown, and Co., 1975.)**

SOME SPECIAL TESTS

Potassium hydroxide examination of the cornified surface of the skin, such as the palms and soles, is done by scraping a small amount off, placing it on a microscopic slide, mixing with the slightly warmed 10 per cent KOH solution, and placing it under the microscope. This is done in conjunction with a culture for fungi.

Gram's stain is done for bacterial organisms. Dark-field microscopy identifies the organism of syphilis.

Wood's light examination is a visual examination of the skin made in a darkened room with the ultraviolet lamp. Differences in the ultraviolet light absorption and fluorescence bring out characteristics of some skin diseases, such as **tinea capitis (ringworm).**

Endocrinology

Endocrinology is the study of the function and dysfunction of the glands of internal secretion. Changes due to an endocrine disease may cause alterations in body contour, size, fat distribution, skin texture and pigmentation, and circulation, and may have considerable effect on the nervous system. The endocrinologist must be able to distinguish between the patient's hereditary pattern and endocrine dysfunction. This dysfunction falls into two categories: deficiency (hypoproduction) of a hormone and excess (hyperproduction) of a hormone.

Inspection and palpation are the most common methods employed in examining the patient, with inspection being the more prevalent. Of the six endocrine glands in the body, the thyroid and the male gonads (testes) are the most accessible to palpation. The female gonads (ovaries) are palpable to a degree.

Eponyms are used more frequently in endocrinology than in other specialties, but they are slowly being replaced with the true anatomic or pathologic name. A considerable amount of endocrine dysfunction is included in the therapy in other specialties. The gynecologist sees the patient with the ovarian changes of **amenorrhea** and **menopause**. The internist may examine an enlarged thyroid gland that has resulted from an iodine deficiency, or myxedema from severe hypothyroidism. The ophthalmologist may examine the patient with exophthalmic goiter that gives the appearance of bulging eyes.

Besides the complete physical examination, the physician is aided in his diagnosis by a great variety of tests. Some of these tests are x-rays, radioisotopes, and blood chemistry.

The medical assistant in an endocrinologist's office will be called upon to participate in the routine physical examination as outlined earlier in this chapter.

SOME LABORATORY TESTS. Endocrine and metabolic disorders, as mentioned earlier, are usually a part of other specialties, but some of the following tests are specifically done for various glandular disorders.

Thyroid function evaluations may include a protein-bound iodine (PBI), serum thyroxine, and certain radioactive tests like the thyroid scan. The parathyroids will usually require a serum calcium and x-ray studies for skeletal changes. Pancreatic disorders in medicine usually involve the metabolic disease diabetes mellitus. This requires blood glucose tests and a urinalysis for glucose and acetone content. The adrenal glands warrant close check on the patient's blood pressure and blood and urine tests for cortisol, potassium, and many other levels. The pituitary gland is called the master gland because it controls the other endocrine glands. The anterior lobe of the pituitary secretes primarily the growth hormones, and the posterior lobe will cause diabetes insipidus when not functioning properly. A 24-hour urinalysis will be checked for gonadotropin (FSH); blood chloride levels, blood count, and packed cell volume are also observed.

GENERAL SURGERY

A surgeon's practice is what may be called a "referral specialty." That is, the patients are usually referred to the surgeon from other specialties or by the family physician. The procedure to be followed in the evaluation of the patient and the comprehensive preoperative examination requires teamwork between the surgeon and the referring physician. An effective working arrangement between these two physicians sometimes depends upon the cooperation of the medical assistant. The referring physician frequently takes care of the initial physical examination and basic preoperative laboratory tests. His knowledge of the patient's past medical and family history is shared with the surgeon. The surgeon will then have a clear understanding of the objectives of surgery and the patient's preoperative status. The surgeon may offer the patient a simple and understandable description of the operation, its rationale, and possible complications. (This is the basis of "informed consent.")

The psychological preparation of the patient is also shared by the referring physician and the surgeon. Anxieties of the patient are normal and inevitable and can be somewhat lessened by the attitude of a good medical assistant. The medical assistant in the surgeon's office can identify the patient with special needs. Families and relatives are anxious about the surgical patient. The medical assistant, with the surgeon's consent, can reduce some of these anxieties with simple explanations and reports.

Assisting the surgeon may include assisting with preoperative examinations and postoperative office visits. Physical examinations would follow the outline given previously in this chapter. The office postoperative care may include dressing changes and suture removal. These are described in Chapter 29, Assisting with Office Surgery.

Internal Medicine

Internal medicine is a nonsurgical specialty with several subspecialties, such as gastroenterology, **rheumatology**, cardiology, pulmonary diseases, and **bariatrics.** Internists are often known as the "diagnosticians of medicine" as well as frequently being considered to be the "family physicians." The physical examination frequently follows the outline given earlier in this chapter.

Each part of this general physical examination may be lessened or intensified, depending on the patient's medical history and complaints. Like the family physician, the internist often provides continuing care for the patient. Also like the family physician, the internist consults and cooperates with other specialties in the maintenance of the patient's total care. Dr. Robert E. Rakel says, "Family practice is a horizontal specialty that, like pediatrics and internal medicine, shares large areas of content with other clinical disciplines."

Gastroenterology

This specialty covers an extremely wide area that includes the stomach, the small intestines, and the bowel, down to the rectum. In other words, the gastroenterologist examines the digestive system with the exclusion of the lower bowel and rectum, which are areas for the proctologist.

A patient with a gastrointestinal (GI) problem may complain of such things as nausea, anorexia, or abdominal pain as well as numerous other symptoms. It may be difficult for the medical assistant to organize a patient's complaints when a patient first contacts the office by telephone for an appointment. The patient may say he has a "belly ache" when the discomfort is really in the stomach area; the "belly" is the central portion of the entire abdominal cavity. Or the patient may say he has a stomach ache when the discomfort is in the *hypo*gastric area and not in the *epi*gastric area. Careful questioning will guide the patient to a more precise description of the symptoms.

Emotional factors play an important part in many GI problems, often making the separation of functional disorders and organic disorders difficult. Abdominal pain may be classified as chronic or acute. The chronic abdomen, or chronic pain, may or may not be abdominal in origin, but may originate in the thoracic cavity or musculoskeletal system. The acute abdomen may demand immediate attention, as in acute appendicitis or acute gastritis with possible hemorrhage. Both may demand surgical therapy.

In order to isolate an abdominal problem it is frequently necessary for the physician to do a sigmoidoscopic examination as well as a pelvic examination on the female patient. The accessory organs of the digestive system play an important part. These are the liver, gallbladder, and pancreas. Jaundice is a sign of liver disease and may be the result of viral hepatitis, alcoholic liver disease, or obstructive jaundice due to **choledocholithiasis** (a calculus in the common bile duct). Acute pancreatitis will give diffuse pain and tenderness in the epigastrium.

Many of the diagnostic tests for GI symptoms are **noninvasive** in nature. The patient may be asked to have various **roentgenograms** of the digestive system. These would be a barium swallow, upper GI series, and barium enema. The gallbladder is viewed by **cholecystography**, and liver function is checked by various liver function tests done on the blood serum. The SGOT and SGPT are commonly done blood serum tests. The urine is tested for bilirubin and urinary amylase. The stool is tested for occult blood, intestinal parasites and organisms, fat excretion, and color.

Pulmonary Medicine

Those patients with respiratory problems may present themselves to the office with chronic or acute symptoms. A common complaint seen in this specialty, the *upper respiratory infection* (URI), may be, like the others, either chronic or acute. Other infections involving the so-called *lower respiratory system,* the lungs, also present as a chronic or acute problem. Many of the infections of the lungs are in the wide group of **pneumonias**. It is estimated that there are over 50 different causes of pneumonia ranging from bacterial, viral, and fungal to chemical irritants. The term **pneumonitis** is synonymous with pneumonia. The diagnosis *lobar pneumonia* refers to an infection involving a segment or lobe of the lung.

Diagnostic aids vary with the possible diagnosis. The most frequently used are chest x-rays, blood count, TB skin tests, and analysis of sputum. Arterial blood tests, pulmonary function tests, and lung scans are also done.

If a patient in the waiting room is coughing very much or if the cough is productive, it would be advisable to have this patient wait for the physician in an examining room. Provide this patient with ample tissues and show him where the waste receptacle is located.

Materials needed:

- X-rays in the viewing box
- Source of light
- Tongue depressors
- Cleansing tissues
- Stethoscopes
- Otoscope

Cardiology

Heart disease is the major cause of death in the United States as well as the cause of many chronic illnesses. People are concerned and apprehensive about their hearts. No physician would consider examining a patient without checking the patient's heart. Patients seem to derive some therapeutic value from just having a physician "listen to their heart." A heart attack or diagnosis of heart disease does not condemn a patient; in fact, if the physician's instructions are followed, the patient's life is often prolonged.

The topographical landmarks of the chest (see Fig. 28–2) are helpful in localizing and describing the heart's location and borders (Fig. 28–9). The heart is examined primarily by auscultation, but the other methods may also be employed. The examination of the heart is not limited to just listening to the heart and running an electrocardiogram but actually starts with observing the general appearance of the patient. The physician may notice a degree of cyanosis, facial edema, clubbing of the

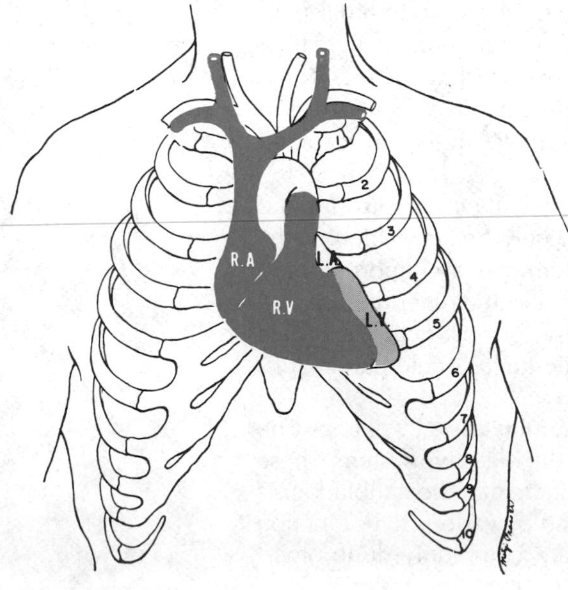

FIGURE 28–9 Topographic anatomy of the heart. R. A., Right atrium; R.V., Right ventricle; L.A., Left atrium; L.V., Left ventricle. (From Prior, J. A., and Silberstein, J. S.: *Physical Diagnosis*. 4th ed. St. Louis, The C. V. Mosby Co., 1973.)

fingertips, a cough, or shortness of breath. Cardiac disease has many symptoms and many etiologies; **hypertension, arteriosclerosis** of the coronary arteries, and **rheumatic fever** are the leading causes. *Congestive heart failure* is the inability of the heart to maintain sufficient circulation to meet the body's needs. **Arrhythmia** may or may not be associated with congestive heart failure. **Angina pectoris** is acute chest pain due to a decrease of blood supply to the heart muscles; it is not a disease but a symptom. These methods of examination are aided by x-rays and the electrocardiogram, both resting and exercise ECG such as the Master's two-step, or treadmill or bicycle **ergometer** test (an apparatus for measuring the amount of work done by the patient). The cardiologist will also use such tests as cardiac catheterization and angiocardiogram. Cardiac *catheterization* is accomplished by introducing a small flexible catheter into the vein of the arm, usually the left antecubital, under fluoroscopic guidance, and gently passing it into the right atrium, right ventricle, and on to the pulmonary artery. The pressure of the blood is measured in these vessels and heart chambers. Samples of the blood are also withdrawn from these areas to determine their oxygen content. The **angiocardiogram** is a special x-ray procedure using an opaque dye to show the heart and its major bloods vessels.

Occasionally the physician will mark the patient's chest where he wishes the electrocardiogram electrodes to be placed. The patient is disrobed to the waist and placed in a sitting position. To assist in attaining complete relaxation, ask the patient to void first. The room must be warm and the patient relaxed. Silence is a must while the physician is listening to the heart. If a cardiogram was done prior to the examination the medical assistant should have it ready for the physician along with any x-rays.

Neurology

As in other physical examinations, a careful history provides valuable clues in diagnosing neurologic malfunctions. These may be **seizures, syncope, diplopia, incontinence**, and subjective sensations. The patient's general health often complicates a neurologic diagnosis. The purposes of a neurologic examination are to determine whether a nervous system malfunction is present, discover its location, and identify its type and extent. During the history-taking the physician may determine the patient's emotional status, intellectual performance, and general behavior, which may be evident in the patient's grooming and mannerisms. The patient's ability to communicate is also observed at this time.

Each cranial nerve is checked. For example, the first cranial nerve, the olfactory nerve, is examined by the patient's ability to identify familiar odors, such as coffee, tobacco, or cloves. The fifth cranial nerve, the trigeminal nerve, is checked by the patient's differentiating between warm and cold objects held on his right and left cheeks.

The motor system is examined by observing the patient's muscular strength and movements. The diameters of the upper arms and the calves of the legs are measured for muscular atrophy. The sensory system is examined by noting the patient's ability to perceive superficial sensations, such as a wisp of cotton brushed on the skin, a light pinprick, or hot and cold touching on certain areas. Several reflexes, such as the patellar and Achilles, are examined. A stroke with a dull instrument on the lateral aspect of the sole of the foot may show the Babinski sign.

Some other tests may include skull x-rays, angiograms, myelograms, and brain scans. An electroencephalogram (EEG) will also be done. The medical assistant may wish to remind the female patient to wear a head scarf after the EEG because there may be some contact paste left on the scalp. Diseases could be a stroke (cerebral vascular accident [CVA]), cerebral aneurysm, a brain tumor or abscess, Parkinson's disease, or multiple sclerosis (MS), among others.

The patient is given a gown and disposable slippers, and asked to disrobe completely, except perhaps for brassiere and underpants. The patient is then seated on the edge of the examining table. The medical assistant will hand the physician the various items as they are needed. After she has gone through this examination a few times with the physician, she will know which item he needs at each point of the examination.

Materials needed:

- Neurologic hammer or percussion hammer
- Cotton
- Tongue depressor
- Finger cot
- Two test tubes for holding hot and cold water
- Small brush (paint brush type)
- Large pin
- Measuring tape
- Applicator stick
- Dropper vials of sugar water and salt water for tasting
- Vials of coffee, tobacco, and cloves for smelling

Obstetrics and Gynecology

Examination of the female reproductive system is done to assure normality of the reproductive organs or to diagnose and/or treat abnormalities of these organs. Because of the intimate nature of the examination, every consideration must be given to the patient.

A gynecologic history includes age at menarche; regularity of the menstrual cycle; amount and duration of the menstrual flow; menstrual disturbances such as **dysmenorrhea; intermenstrual** or **postmenstrual** bleeding; and the presence of vaginal discharges. Prenatal care is a major portion of the Ob/Gyn office's appointments. The first prenatal visit is rather extensive with a complete history and physical examination and a pelvic examination that includes pelvic measurements, serologic tests, and routine laboratory tests. Follow-up prenatal visits include urinalysis, weight, blood pressure, and advice on diet and health habits. The patient's questions are answered, and she is given assurance.

The examining room must be adequately equipped and the surroundings pleasant. A dressing area with an adjacent toilet should be provided. The dressing area should assure privacy and be equipped with tissues and sanitary protection items. Some offices provide a little "goodie box" with safety pins and sanitary belts. Disposable examination gowns are also placed in this room. Check the supplies frequently throughout the day.

The patient should be instructed to empty her bladder and rectum, completely disrobe, and put on a gown. Unless contraindicated, the patient should have been advised at the time her appointment was made that she should NOT douche or have sexual intercourse for 24 hours before the examination in order to properly evaluate vaginal discharges and to have a more satisfactory and accurate cytologic study.

The medical assistant should remain in the examining room to provide reassurance to the patient as well as offer legal protection to the physician. Furthermore, the patient should be given assistance in getting on and off the table. The lithotomy position is very awkward to get into unassisted and is embarrassing to the patient.

Dr. Allen C. Barnes, in *Physical Diagnosis: A Physiological Approach to Clinical Examination*, states: "For a woman in the lithotomy position on the examining table, this 'criterion of coverage,' interestingly enough, is most often the knee. There are said to be two principles of British Law: first, the trial must be fair; and secondly, the trial must give the illusion of being fair. The same might be said of draping the patient for gynecologic examination: she should be decently covered, and she should have the illusion of being decently covered. As long as she does not look up to see her knee exposed, this illusion is largely maintained."

The physician will first inspect the external genitalia and palpate the perineal body, Bartholin's and Skene's glands, and the urethral meatus. The patient may be asked to "bear down" in order to show any muscular weaknesses that may be the result of lacerations of the perineal body during childbirth. A third-degree laceration may have involved the rectal sphincter and cause rectal incontinence.

Next the vaginal speculum is inserted for examination of the cervix and vaginal canal (Fig. 28–10). The normal cervix points posteriorly and is smooth, pink-colored squamous epithelium. Abnormalities most frequently seen are ulcerations (erosions),

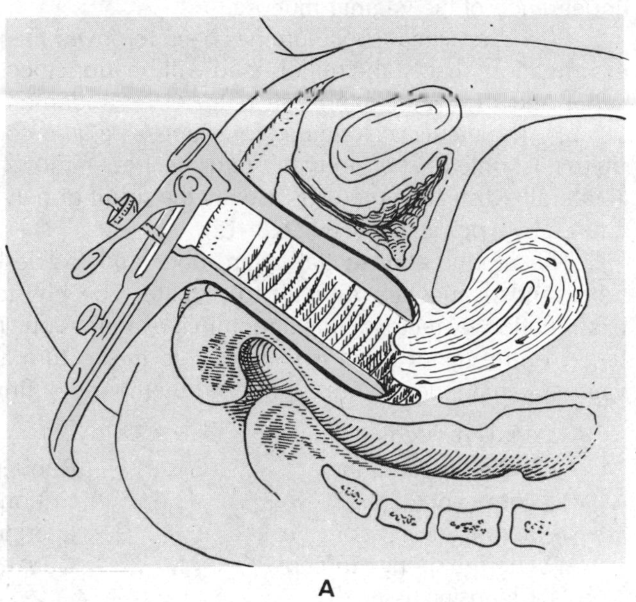

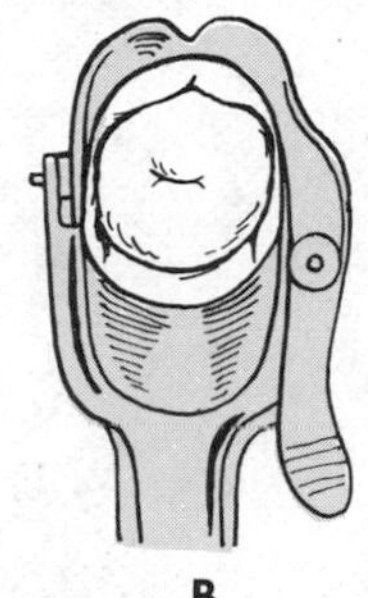

A B

FIGURE 28–10 *A,* Proper position of inserted speculum for examination of the cervix uteri. (From Dunphy, J. E., and Botsford, T. W.: *Physical Examination of the Surgical Patient: An Introduction to Clinical Surgery*. 4th ed. Philadelphia, W. B. Saunders Company, 1975; reprinted with permission.) *B,* Normal parous cervix as seen through a speculum. (From Luckmann, J., and Sorensen, K. C.: *Medical-Surgical Nursing: A Psychophysiologic Approach*. 2nd ed. Philadelphia, W. B. Saunders Co., 1980; reprinted with permission.)

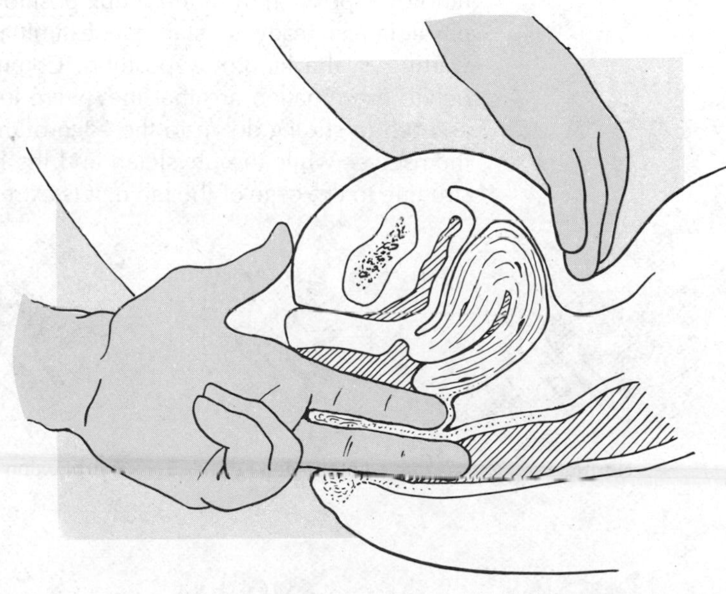

FIGURE 28–11 Bimanual pelvic examination. The hand on the abdomen brings more of the pelvic contents into contact with the inserted fingers. This technique provides a more adequate palpation of the pelvic viscera than can be accomplished by vaginal examination alone. (From Dunphy, J. E., and Botsford, T. W.: *Physical Examination of the Surgical Patient: An Introduction to Clinical Surgery*. 4th ed. Philadelphia, W. B. Saunders Co., 1975; reprinted with permission.)

nabothian cysts, and cervical polyps. Since erosions cannot be palpated, inspection is the only method of knowing their presence. Healed lacerations resulting from childbirth are common in the multiparous patient. Pregnancy increases the size of the cervix, and hormone deficiency will cause it to atrophy. The vaginal wall is reddish-pink and has a corrugated appearance. Vaginal infections will change the appearance of the vaginal mucosa.

After the vaginal speculum has been removed the physician will do a bimanual examination; that is, the minor hand will be lubricated and inserted into the vaginal canal and the major hand will palpate the abdomen over the pelvic organs (Fig. 28–11). The uterus is examined for shape, size, and consistency. The position of the uterus is noted. The normal uterus is freely movable with limited discomfort. A laterally displaced uterus is usually the result of pelvic adhesions or displacement caused by a pelvic tumor (Fig. 28–12).

The uterine **adnexa** (fallopian tubes and ovaries) are evaluated. The normal tubes and ovaries are difficult to palpate. The physician may now complete the examination by rectovaginal abdominal examination. This is done when the middle finger of the minor hand is inserted into the rectum and the index finger is in the vaginal canal. The rectum is checked by the index finger inserted into the rectum.

Materials needed:

- Vaginal speculum
- Lubricant
- Spot light
- Uterine sponge forceps
- Cleansing tissue
- Rubber gloves
- Cotton applicator sticks
- Uterine dressing forceps
- Gauze dressings or cotton balls

1. Greet the patient and briefly explain what examination is to be done.
2. Have the patient empty her bladder and save the specimen.
3. Have the patient disrobe completely (except for her shoes if heel stirrups are used) and put on a gown. Tell the patient the physician's preferences for the gown open in back or front.
4. Place a towel on the edge of the examining table and have the patient sit on the towel or use examining table paper. Some offices put the patient directly into the lithotomy position from the sitting position, but this should never be done unless the physician is ready to start the examination immediately. Never leave a patient waiting in the lithotomy position. Common complaints from women regarding a pelvic examination are that they were left waiting in the lithotomy position or not assisted in sliding down to the edge of the table but were told to "scoot down" by themselves while the physician and the medical assistant stood and watched them struggle to the edge of the table. It is extremely awkward and embarrassing to "scoot

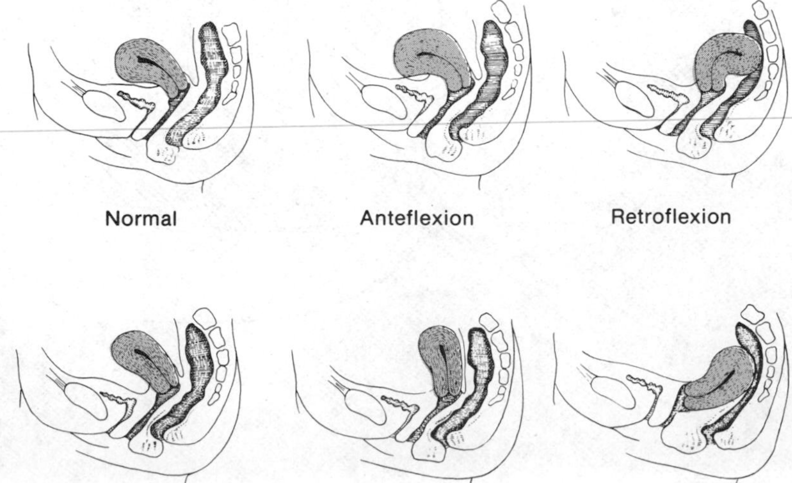

FIGURE 28–12 Positions of the uterus in sagittal section. (From Dunphy, J. E., and Botsford, T. W.: *Physical Examination of the Surgical Patient*. Philadelphia, W. B. Saunders Co., 1975.)

down" by oneself, especially if the stirrups are not far enough out or the patient is nearing full-term pregnancy. Please, medical assistants, assist the patient. This may be done simply by standing at the foot of the table and placing her heels in the stirrups. Next, lower or push in the foot board. Now reach up and grasp the patient's upper calf just below the knees and easily slide her down so the buttocks rest on the edge of the table. This can be done without looking under the drape sheet by watching the patient's face and talking to her. The physician will push the drape back when the examination starts. Patients greatly appreciate this extra care and consideration.

There are several methods of draping for the lithotomy position. One method is to use a small square sheet. The patient holds one corner over her chest. The corners adjacent to this are draped over each knee and the far corner hangs between her legs, covering the perineum, and can be pushed back by the physician.

Some offices use a small sheet cut especially for the lithotomy position. This sheet is approximately 25 in. wide and 40 in. long. It is slit lengthwise about 24 in. This drape does cover the knees but offers little protection from the side and, if made of disposable paper, tends to slide off easily.

Another method is to use a regular square sheet that has been folded into a triangle. The inside fold is placed over the patient's abdomen, the two adjacent corners go over the patient's knees, and the corner points are wrapped around the patient's ankles and tucked in place. The far corner from the fold hangs down over the perineum and can be pushed back by the physician.

Frequently a regular cot sheet is used and placed over the patient as a top sheet would be placed. Because there is ample sheet to drape the entire area, there is no need for special placement of the sheet. The physician may then push back the sheet between the patient's legs and over her abdomen, thus exposing the perineum.

No matter what drape is preferred, its size must be ample to give the patient a feeling of security. If the patient is afraid a flimsy disposable sheet will slide off or too many areas are exposed, she will not relax, and relaxation is essential in a pelvic examination.

5. Direct the light source so the light is focused into the vaginal speculum.
6. Assisting the physician may consist of:
   a. Warming the speculum under warm running water. (The newer examining tables have a warming drawer.)
   b. Assisting the physician with his gloves.
   c. Holding the microscopic slides or making the smear when he hands you the applicator. For easy identification of the source of the material to be smeared you can make a "V" for vaginal, "C" for cervical, and a "U" for urethral secretion.
   d. Handing the dressing forceps or sponge forceps with a sponge, handle first.
   e. Handing the sterile tenaculum for lifting the cervix to view the posterior vaginal fornix.
   f. Applying the lubricant to the physician's fingers. Be careful not to touch the lubricant tube to the physician's fingers. Apply about 1 to 2 in. of lubricant across the ends of his fingers.
   g. Placing the soiled instruments in a receiving basin.

7. Assist the patient to relax by having her breathe deeply and slowly. Instruct her to cross her hands over her chest. Sometimes a little conversation helps a patient to relax.

8. After the physician has completed the examination, *make certain the patient is pushed back on the table before sitting up*. Do not rush the patient. If there has been an extensive examination or treatment, it is best to slide the patient back on the table, raise the foot board and have the patient remain in a supine position for a few minutes. A patient may become dizzy when sitting up too rapidly after an examination, and there may be a tendency to fall forward. Records show some

lawsuits resulting from this type of injury that probably could have been easily prevented.

9. In offices where vaginal specula are frequently used, they are kept warm by placing an electric pad in the drawer of the examining table and leaving it at the lowest temperature.

10. The patient may now dress. Remember to give her instructions.

11. Clean up the room immediately.

SPECIAL DIAGNOSTIC TESTS AND PROCEDURES

PAPANICOLAOU SMEAR ("PAP" SMEAR). Perhaps the single most important test done in a physician's office today is the obtaining of cells from the cervical area for cytologic study. This is done for the early detection of cancer of the cervix. These smears are best obtained when the patient has not douched or had sexual intercourse for 24 hours prior to taking the specimen. It is done without the aid of any lubricating jelly or glove powder.

These cells are obtained by one of two methods: (1) the cells are scraped from the cervical os with a special cervical spatula or wooden tongue depressor and then spread on a glass microscopic slide, or (2) the cells may be obtained from secretions aspirated from the posterior fornix of the vagina by means of a glass cervical aspirator tube and bulb. Hold the slide firmly by the frosted end and hold at the physician's level. The slide is immediately immersed in a fixing solution of 50 per cent alcohol and 50 per cent ether for at least 30 minutes, or it may be sprayed with a commercial fixative. Use whichever the cytologist prefers. Make certain the slide or slide container is correctly identified. (See also Cytological Examinations in Chapter 31, and Fig. 31–8.)

Materials needed (other than the routine pelvic setup):

Cervical spatula
Cervical aspirator
Labels and laboratory forms already completed with patient's name, date, and source (C = cervical; V = vagina)
Microscopic slides (make two slides for each area the specimen is taken from)
Fixative solution (loosen jar lid before physician starts)

MATURATION INDEX. This test is done to measure the patient's **estrogen** level to determine whether the patient has an estrogen deficiency. The test results will aid in the diagnosis of endocrine disturbances such as are found in menopause or amenorrhea. The technique for obtaining the cells is the same as for other cytologic studies, such as the "Pap" smear. Be certain to mark the laboratory form for "Maturation Index" and last menstrual period (LMP).

TRICHOMONIASIS. This vaginal discharge is caused by the protozoa *Trichomonas vaginalis*. The discharge is frothy pale yellow or white and has a distinct odor. The patient complains of burning and itching. It is a moderately common vaginal discharge, and the patient must be assured it is *not* a venereal disease. The vaginal trichomonad is an actively motile organism and the diagnosis is confirmed by a wet smear (hanging drop). This is usually done in the physician's office since the organism is easily identified.

Materials needed:

Microscope
Cervical aspirator
Cotton applicators
Normal saline
Microscopic slide or hanging drop side

CANDIDIASIS. This is an infection caused by the fungi of the genus *Candida*. It was formerly known as moniliasis, caused by the fungi of the genus *Monilia*. It is a yeastlike fungus. The vaginal discharge is clear with a curdlike substance in it. The patient complains of burning and itching. The discharge is examined by a direct smear or by special culture media.

Materials needed:

Microscopic slides	Cotton applicators (sterile)
Culture media (especially for *Candida*)	10 per cent potassium hydroxide

ATROPHIC VAGINITIS. Also called senile or adhaesiva vaginitis, this vaginitis occurring in older women is marked by the formation of raw patches on the vaginal walls. There is frequently a clear watery discharge. The patient complains of some burning and itching, as well as dyspareunia. A **maturation index** is usually done to confirm the diagnosis.

BACTERIAL VAGINAL DISCHARGES. Vaginal discharges due to bacterial origin are usually divided into two classes, *specific* and *nonspecific*. Those in the *specific* class are caused by a specific organism, usually *Neisseria gonorrhoeae*. Gonorrhea is a highly infectious venereal disease. Diagnosis is confirmed by a smear made from the discharge found in the vagina and urethral meatus. Occasionally a culture may be taken, but the majority of times two microscopic smears are taken and sent to the laboratory. If smears are taken from several places they are identified by smearing the exudate in the form of a "V" for the vaginal discharge, a "C" for cervical, and a "U" for the urethral smear. These smears are then air dried, labeled, and sent to the laboratory. Take great care in handling the materials.

Materials needed:

Microscopic slides	Labels and laboratory forms
Cotton applicators (sterile)	Culture media or culturette applicator

The *nonspecific* bacterial discharge may be caused by several different organisms. Because the organism(s) are unknown, the physician may do both bacterial smears and cultures. It is best to check with the laboratory for the type of culture media preferred.

Ophthalmology

A complete examination of the eye is technical and requires expensive equipment, but the practitioner of general medicine does become involved with some examinations and treatments of the eye with the use of basic office equipment. The use of the ophthalmoscope to examine the retina of the eye is an essential part of every

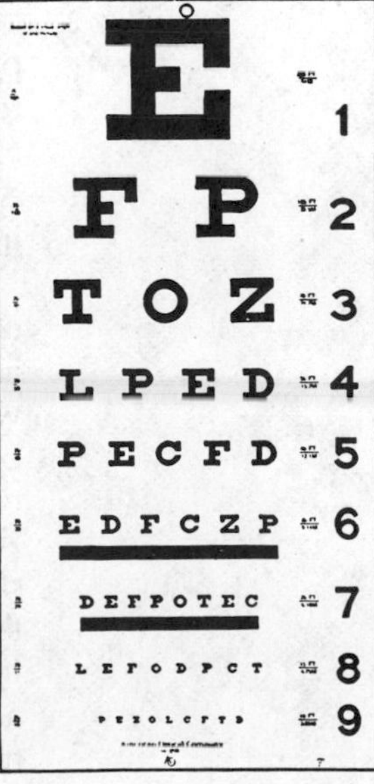

FIGURE 28–13 Snellen visual acuity chart. (From Harley, R. D. (ed.): *Pediatric Ophthalmology*. Philadelphia, W. B. Saunders Co., 1975.)

complete physical examination. The eye often reflects an individual's general health or may be involved in a systemic disease or injury. The eye may react to a systemic medication the patient is taking.

The most routine eye test, other than the use of the ophthalmoscope, is the distance acuity test, usually given with the *Snellen Chart* (Fig. 28–13). This test may be administered by the medical assistant. She may also be trained to check the patient's near vision with the *Near Vision Acuity Chart.* This is especially done on the patient past 40 years of age for possible **presbyopia.** Testing a patient's color vision is important, especially if the patient is in certain occupations. All children by the age of five years should be checked with the color vision charts.

The eyelids are examined for edema, which may be the result of nephrosis, heart failure, allergy, or thyroid deficiency. **Ptosis** of the eyelid may be an involvement of the third cranial nerve. Infections of the eyelids are frequently a **sty** (an infected eyelash follicle) that is painful or a **chalazion** (a beady nodule in the eyelid) that is usually not painful unless infected. If the lacrimal ducts are obstructed, the patient will have constant tearing known as **epiphora.** The conjunctiva of the eye is the delicate membrane covering the eyeball and lining the eyelids. Inflammation of the conjunctiva may be bacterial or viral, and there is a highly contagious **conjunctivitis** commonly called *pinkeye.*

The *corneal reflex* or corneal sensitivity is tested by touching the cornea of the eye quickly with a wisp of cotton. The patient will blink. The pupils of the eye are normally round and equal in size. Normal pupils will constrict rapidly in response to light and during accommodation. This is seen by shining a bright pinpoint light into one eye from the side of the patient's head. The pupil of the illuminated eye will constrict, and the pupil of the other eye will constrict equally. This test is called *light and accommodation* (L&A). An older patient's eyes do not accommodate as well as a younger person's. Each eye is checked this way. Then the patient is asked to look at the physician's finger as it is moved directly towards the patient's nose.

The *ophthalmoscope* is used for examining the interior of the eye. It projects a bright narrow beam of light which permits the physician to examine the interior parts of the eye and the retina through the lens of the eye. It is helpful in detecting possible disorders of the eyes as well as disorders of other organs, the conditions of which are reflected in the condition of the eyes.

Intraocular pressure has been checked by the ophthalmologist for many years, but nowadays many general practice physicians are also checking their patients (especially those past 35 years of age) for intraocular pressure. Elevated intraocular pressure, known as **glaucoma,** causes pressure on the nerve fibers and thus may possibly result in blindness. The *tonometer* is used to measure this intraocular pressure. The patient is placed in a reclining position or sitting with the head resting back on a support. A topical anesthetic is instilled in each eye. After a minute the patient is instructed to fix his vision on a spot on the ceiling. The physician will then touch the sterile footplate of the tonometer to the cornea of the eye (Fig. 28–14). The tonometer is an extremely delicate instrument requiring particular care and storage. After each use it must be sterilized and returned to its stand. Read the manufacturer's instructions and follow them carefully.

Strabismus, crossed eye, is seen predominantly in a small percentage of small children because it is diagnosed early in life and treated as early as possible. There are several problems that cause eyes to turn, but most commonly it is due to weakness of an extraocular muscle. Evaluation of patients with strabismus includes a cover test, measurement of visual acuity, and a careful ophthalmoscopic examination.

Special techniques used in the ophthalmologist's office include the use of a *slit-lamp biomicroscope.* This is used to see the fine details in the anterior segment of the eye. It is also used to view a corneal foreign body because it gives a well illuminated and highly magnified view of the area. The patient with **exophthalmia,** abnormal protrusion of the eye due possibly to overactive thyroid or a tumor behind the eyeball, is checked with the **exophthalmometer.** This instrument is designed to

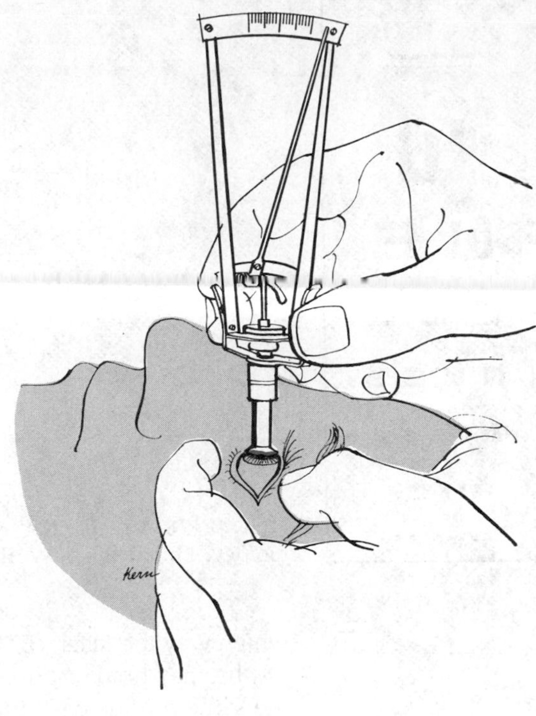

FIGURE 28–14 Application of a tonometer. (From Demorest, B. H. *In* Conn, H. F., Rakel, R. E., and Johnson, T. W. (eds.): *Family Practice*. 1st ed. Philadelphia, W. B. Saunders Co., 1973.)

measure the forward protrusion of the eye. The **ophthalmodynamometer** is used to measure the pressure of the central retinal artery. It is helpful in patients with circulatory disease because it measures the blood pressure in the retinal artery.

Materials needed:

- Distance acuity chart
- Color-vision charts
- Ophthalmic topical anesthetic for corneal anesthesia
- Tonometer (sterile)
- Near vision acuity chart
- Pencil flashlight
- Cotton (sterile)
- Ophthalmoscope

The patient is placed in a sitting position. There is no special draping. Hand the patient some paper tissues.

DISTANCE VISUAL ACUITY. Distance visual acuity is frequently part of a complete physical examination. It is widely used in schools and industry. To date it is the best single test available for visual screening. Many cases of **myopia, astigmatism,** or **hyperopia** have been detected by this routine test. The most common chart used is the Snellen Alphabetical or "E" chart. This chart has various letters of the alphabet for general use. If the office has patients with an English language handicap, then the "E" chart may be used (Figure 28–15). There is also a chart available that uses pictures as symbols (Fig. 28–16). This chart is also used for preschool patients, slow learners, or mentally retarded children who have not yet learned the English alphabet. The symbol on the top line of the chart can be read by persons of normal vision at 200 feet. In each of the succeeding rows, from the top down, the size of the symbols reduces to the point where a person with normal vision can see them at a distance of 100, 70, 50, 40, 30, and 20 feet.

The patient must not be allowed to study the chart before the test. The room or hall should be long enough that the 20 foot distance can be marked off accurately. The chart should be hung at eye level and with maximum light, without glare on the chart. The patient may be standing or sitting with the chart at eye level.

Most adults do not need the chart explained, but you must have the patient's cooperation. If the "E" chart is used, explain how you want the patient to tell you

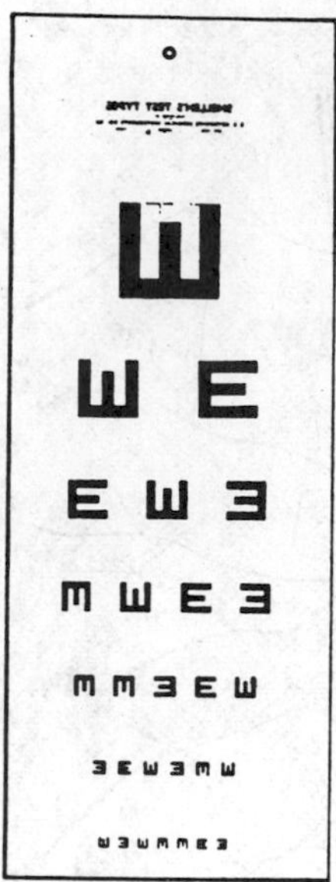

FIGURE 28–15 The "E" visual acuity chart. (From Harley, R. D. (ed.): *Pediatric Ophthalmology*. Philadelphia, W. B. Saunders Co., 1975.)

which way the letter "E" is facing. The patient may point up or down or right or left. Or, he may hold his three fingers in the same direction the letter "E" is facing. Use the same routine each time the patient is tested by starting with the right eye. If the patient is wearing glasses the physician may want him tested first with the glasses on and then without the glasses. Make certain you record the "with" and "without."

Test one eye at a time. Both eyes are to be kept open during the test, but the eye not being tested is to be covered with a paper cup or a piece of cardboard. The paper cup is best because a piece of paper should not touch the eye. Under no circumstances should the patient use his fingers to "hold the eye closed." Allow a moment between changing eyes. The medical assistant should stand beside the chart and point to the line to be read.

Start with the line having the larger symbols in order to help the patient develop confidence in himself; then proceed to the lower lines. If there is no apparent

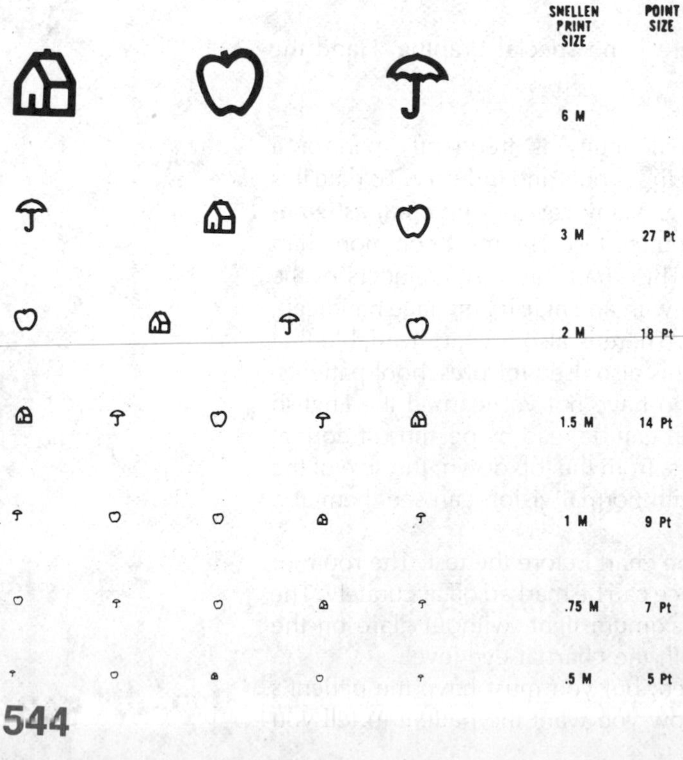

SNELLEN PRINT SIZE	POINT SIZE
6 M	
3 M	27 Pt
2 M	18 Pt
1.5 M	14 Pt
1 M	9 Pt
.75 M	7 Pt
.5 M	5 Pt

FIGURE 28–16 Picture visual acuity chart. (From Harley, R. D. (ed.): *Pediatric Ophthalmology*. Philadelphia, W. B. Saunders Co., 1975.)

difficulty, skip to the 50 line. If the patient responds rapidly, then skip to the 20 line. Have the patient try to read another line after he says he cannot read one.

Observe the patient's behavior during the test to see if he squints, leans forward and appears to strain, or the eyes fill with tears. Record the reactions. Record the responses of each eye separately. The response is recorded in the form of a fraction. The numerator (top number) is the distance of the patient from the chart, the denominator (lower number) is the lowest line read satisfactorily by the patient tested. Allow one mistake per line. For example, if the patient reads the 20 line at 20 feet, the fraction 20/20 is recorded for that eye tested. If the 40 line is the lowest line the patient can read, the fraction 20/40 is recorded for that eye. Make certain the record reads "right eye" (OD) and "left eye" (OS); the record may show OD 20/20 and OS 20/40.

Orthopedic Surgery

An orthopedist is concerned with the body's mobility and with diagnosing and treating diseases and abnormalities of the musculoskeletal system. A considerable part of this practice may be caring for fractures of the injured patient, especially in some resort areas. One orthopedist said the most common complaint heard in his office was the complaint of a "low back pain." Other diseases seen are **rheumatoid arthritis, osteoarthritis, gout,** and **bursitis.** Also, a considerable portion of the patients have traumatic conditions other than fractures. These are dislocations, strains, and ruptures.

Besides a careful history, the examination covers basically the back and the extremities. The physical examination of the musculoskeletal system is performed largely by inspection, but palpation and mensuration are done. The orthopedic physician wants to determine the condition of the muscles, joints and bones. A considerable amount of the examination is done to determine the direction and range of active and passive motion in the joints.

The first step is usually inspection of the patient's posture in standing, sitting, and supine positions. A lateral view of the patient in a standing position shows the position of the head in relation to the trunk of the body. Normal or rigid curves of the cervical, thoracic, and lumbar spine may be seen. Abnormalities such as kyphosis or lordosis are seen in this lateral inspection. A scoliosis is seen from the posterior view. To determine the patient's gait, the physician will ask him to walk. The physician may observe a limp, possibly due to ankylosis, or a scissor gait as seen in spastic paraplegia.

Each major joint of the body is inspected for range of motion. A goniometer is used for precise measurement of a joint's flexion and extension. Muscles are examined for hypertrophy or atrophy. The measurement of the circumference of an extremity at a given point. such as the calf of the leg or the biceps of the arm, is compared with the opposite side. The tendon reflexes are checked.

The spine, or vertebral column, is referred to in divisions. The first seven vertebrae are the cervical spine, the next twelve are the thoracic spine, and the next five are the lumbar spine. These are the 24 movable vertebrae. Below the lumbar vertebrae are the sacrum and coccyx. When referring to the movable spine the physician may say C-5, meaning the fifth cervical vertebra, or L-3, meaning the third lumbar vertebra.

In a considerable part of an orthopedic examination the patient looks as if he were doing various gymnastics with the physician's help or guidance. Physicians specializing in industrial medicine and worker's compensation cases have special terminology and methods for recording and measuring the musculoskeletal system. The American Academy of Orthopaedic Surgeons has published a guide called *Joint Motion: Method of Measuring and Recording.*

The medical assistant must be familiar with such terms as **extension,** which is a movement by which both parts are pulled as far apart as possible, such as a limb being in a straight condition. Opposite to this is **flexion,** which is the act of bending. The amount of bending is recorded in degrees (Fig. 28–17). Other terms

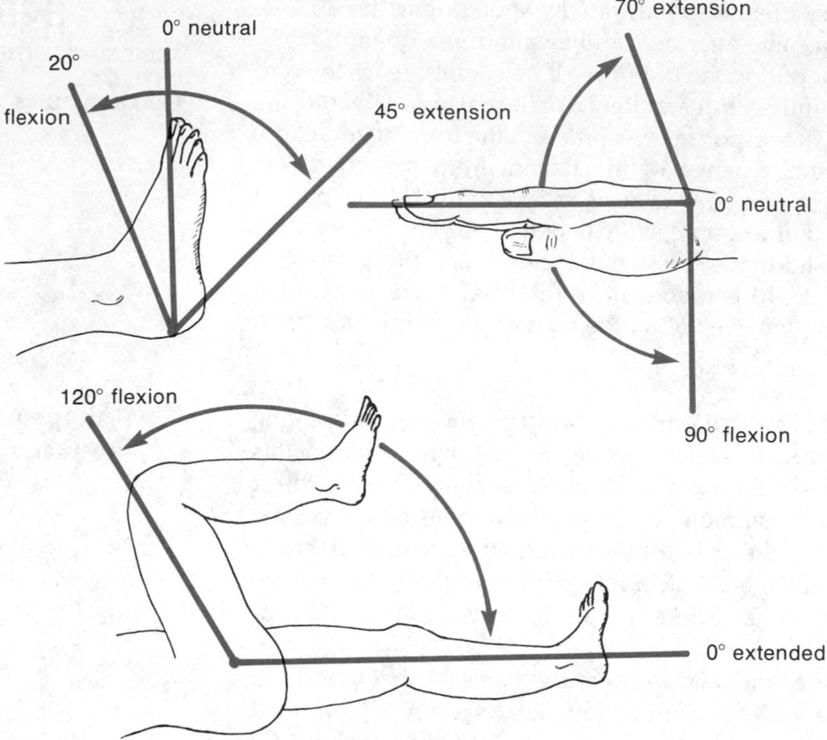

FIGURE 28–17 Flexion and extension in degrees.

used are **abduction,** meaning lateral movement *away* from the middle plane. **Adduction** is *toward* the middle plane. These terms are frequently used in preparing reports for Worker's Compensation.

Radiographs are the most common diagnostic aid used in the orthopedic office. Urinalysis and blood studies are also ordered when there is joint involvement or severe pain and swelling. Physical therapy and rehabilitation are also a major part of the therapy.

Materials needed:

- X-ray view box and x-rays
- Percussion hammer
- Tape measure
- Goniometer and dynamometer

In order for the physician to view the patient's entire back and the hip joints it is necessary for the patient to disrobe completely and be given a loin cloth type of garment. The female patient may also keep her brassiere on. Give the patient a gown and seat him on the edge of the examining table. Most physicians also prefer that the patient remove his shoes.

Otorhinolaryngology (Otolaryngology)

This is the medical specialty that deals with the ear, nose, and throat. It is frequently referred to as otolaryngology or even as a single specialty of otology or laryngology. Because the term otorhinolaryngology is difficult for the average person to understand, it is referred to simply as ear, nose, and throat (ENT). Where the ENT examination begins varies with the physician. Most of the involved area is visible to the physician, with the exception of the nasal accessory sinuses and the middle and inner ear. A large part of this examination consists of the inspection of the mucosa.

If the ears are examined first, the external auditory canal is viewed with an otoscope or a light and ear speculum. The normal external canal has a small amount of cerumen (wax) in it. An excessive amount may be removed by the physician with an ear spoon or curette or by irrigation. (See Chapter 29, Ear Irrigation.) The patient may be given a hearing test with an audiometer to disclose any hearing loss. There are three types of hearing loss: conductive, perceptive, and mixed. *Conductive* hearing loss is a disturbance in the conduction of sound as it passes through the ear canal, tympanic membrane, and the ossicular chain to the oval window and to the inner ear. *Perceptive* deafness is a disturbance anywhere in the inner ear or in the hearing center of the brain. *Mixed* hearing loss is a combination of both conductive and perceptive. The anatomic differences between the adult's and the child's eustachian tube (the tube from the middle ear to the pharynx) make children far more susceptible to middle ear infections **(otitis media).** Occasionally it may be necessary to do a **myringotomy** to drain the exudate from the middle ear.

The inner ear can be invaded by bacteria, especially as a complication of acute otitis media. Vertigo is the sensation of dizziness and may be a symptom of some diseases of the inner ear. Tinnitus, a ringing in the ears, is also a subjective symptom. It may be present in labyrinthitis, damage of the eighth cranial nerve, or cerebral **arteriosclerosis.**

Examination of the nasal cavity is mainly inspection of the mucous membrane. The common cold and allergies are the main causes of changes in the mucosa. Because the physician cannot see into the nasal sinuses, these are examined by palpation and transillumination. If the mucosa is swollen, it may be necessary to spray the area with a vasoconstrictor. The throat is the area that includes the larynx and pharynx and is viewed with the aid of a mirror and tongue depressor or piece of gauze to grasp the tongue (Fig. 28–18). In the nasopharynx the physician will look for enlarged adenoids (pharyngeal tonsil) and the orifice of the eustachian tubes. It may be necessary to grasp the tongue with the aid of a piece of gauze in order to view the laryngopharynx. Spraying the throat with a topical anesthetic helps with the gagging patient.

In the oral cavity the patient's teeth and gums are carefully examined. The palatine (faucial) tonsils (if present) are checked for size and the presence of crypts. The lingual tonsils are also checked. The salivary glands are palpated.

Materials needed:

- Laryngeal mirror
- Illuminated otoscope
- Tongue depressor (wooden or metal)
- Ear basin

List continued on following page

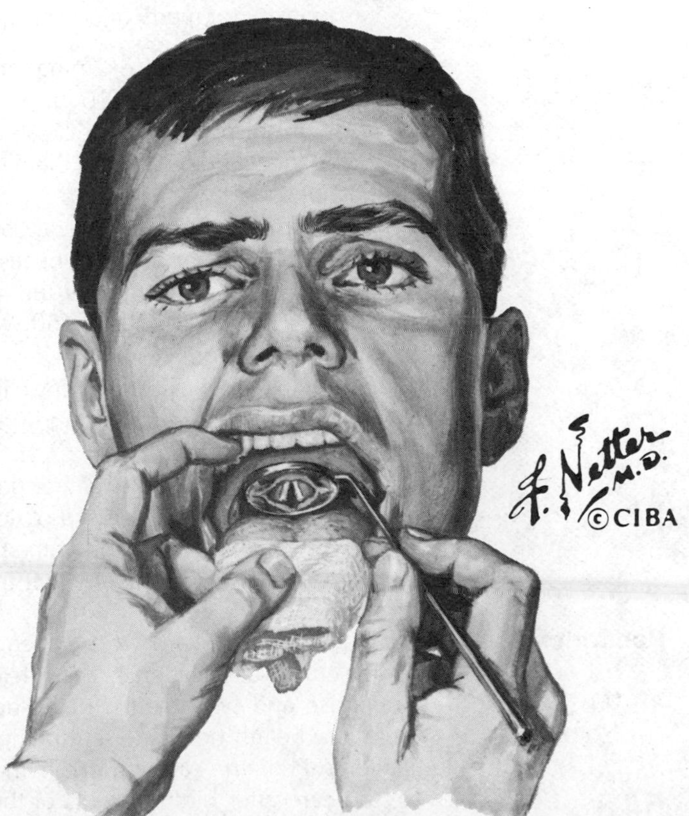

FIGURE 28–18 Examination of the larynx with a laryngeal mirror and a piece of gauze. © Copyright 1964 CIBA Pharmaceutical Company Division of CIBA-GEIGY Corporation. Reproduced, with permission, from the CLINICAL SYMPOSIA, illustrated by Frank H. Netter, M.D. All rights reserved.

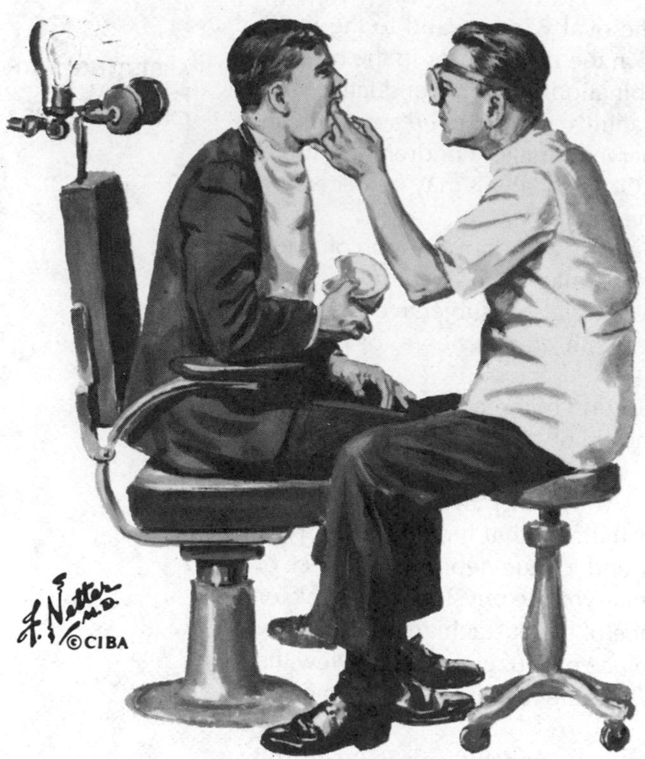

FIGURE 28–19 Position of physician and patient for an E.N.T. examination. © Copyright 1964 CIBA Pharmaceutical Company. Division of CIBA-GEIGY Corporation. Reproduced, with permission, from the CLINICAL SYMPOSIA, illustrated by Frank H. Netter, M.D. All rights reserved.

Materials needed (*continued*):

Nasal speculum	Ear speculum
Metal applicator	Bayonet dressing forceps
Ear curette or spoon	Head mirror and light
Gauze square (4 in by 4 in)	Cotton applicator sticks and cotton
Vasoconstrictor medication spray	Topical anesthetic spray

1. For a good ENT examination the patient is in an upright position, sitting very erect with the head about 10 in. from the back of the chair. The correct ENT position is not a restful position (Fig. 28–19).
2. Place a drape around the patient's neck. If medications are to be used, drape the patient's lap.
3. Hand the patient several tissues.
4. Hold the ear basin, if necessary.
5. Most specialists prefer the head mirror rather than illuminated instruments. The light source is usually a 150-watt light bulb placed directly behind and to the right of the patient.
6. If the laryngeal mirror fogs, it may have to be warmed. This can be done with a small alcohol lamp flame, under warm water, or by holding it in your hand for a few moments.
7. Specialists are also rather particular about the cotton applicator. They prefer a metal applicator with a wisp of cotton wrapped around the end of the applicator, leaving a small tuft of cotton at the tip. Be very careful that the metal tip is not at the very end but back about one-half inch.

Pediatrics

A large percentage of the patients in the pediatric office are "well-baby" or "well-child" care patients. The role of the physician and the medical office staff is to supervise and help maintain the health of the patients. An increasing number of auxiliary health personnel are being involved in the health services given to young patients. Pediatric care starts from the time of conception, but we are more conscious of the care after birth. Parents of these young patients must be involved with their care and development. The medical assistant can help a great deal in the communications between the patient, the parents, and the medical staff. The confidence a child develops in the care and the considerations received in the physician's office is the basis of good medical care.

The frequency of the well-child visits will vary with the physician and the community. It may follow this pattern: 2 weeks, 7 weeks, 4 months, 1 year, 2 years, 5 years, 10 years, and 15 years. Immunizations and illnesses will significantly increase the frequency of these visits.

As with any other physical examination, the medical history is an essential guide to the examination. With the infant, the physician is dependent on the parent for the history, but as the child gets older some history may be obtained from the child and clarified or amplified by the parent. Generally a child is extremely honest in the facts of his illness. Close observation will also give the physician considerable information. A wince may indicate tenderness, and the facial expression associated with nausea should alert the physician and his staff.

Explaining what is to be done and showing the child the instruments to be used will often contribute to his cooperation. The instruments and the examiner's hands should be warm. Quick "behind the back" moves will startle a child and make him suspicious. Small infants are usually undressed by the mother and examined while being held on the mother's lap. The duties of the medical assistant will be to weigh and measure the infant, record this information on the mother's records and on the office record, and check whether immunizations are due.

A child's vital signs differ somewhat from the adult's. Examples:

Age	Pulse	Respiration	B.P.
2–4 yr	80–120	20–30	85/60
6+	70–115	18–26	90/60
14+	60–110	15–20	110/68

The sequence of the examination will vary. This sequence is frequently adapted to the cooperation of the child, leaving until last the areas to which the patient may object the most and be the least cooperative. Sometimes a tongue depressor in each little hand will keep an infant from grabbing the stethoscope.

The physician will be concerned with the patient's growth and development. The child's alertness and responses will tell the physician a considerable amount. In infancy (birth to 2 years) and in the young child of preschool age (2 to 6 years) the child's eating, sleeping and elimination habits are closely questioned. The school age child (6 to 12 years or to puberty) is usually a little more cooperative during an examination and can answer most questions without parental assistance. The adolescent (onset of puberty to the cessation of growth or roughly 12 to 19 years of age) is in a difficult period of life. These patients are usually sensitive, embarrass easily, and are concerned about their health and appearance. More physicians are now specializing in adolescent medicine.

RESTRAINTS FOR CHILDREN. For routine examinations it is usually not advisable to use strong restraints. A small child may be held on an adult's lap, with the child's right arm tucked under the adult's left arm. The child's left arm may be held in place by the adult's right hand. The adult's left hand is then free to support the child's head. For eyes, ears, nose, and throat examinations and treatment, the child is placed on the examining table with the medical assistant at the child's head as shown in Figure 28–20*A*. When picking up an infant's legs to expose the buttocks, make certain you have your index finger between the ankles to prevent the infant's ankle bones from being pressed together. Frequently a child is crying from pain resulting from the restraining hold and not from the examination. If more extensive restraints are necessary you may place a child on a large sheet that has been folded lengthwise, the top of the sheet being even with the shoulders and the

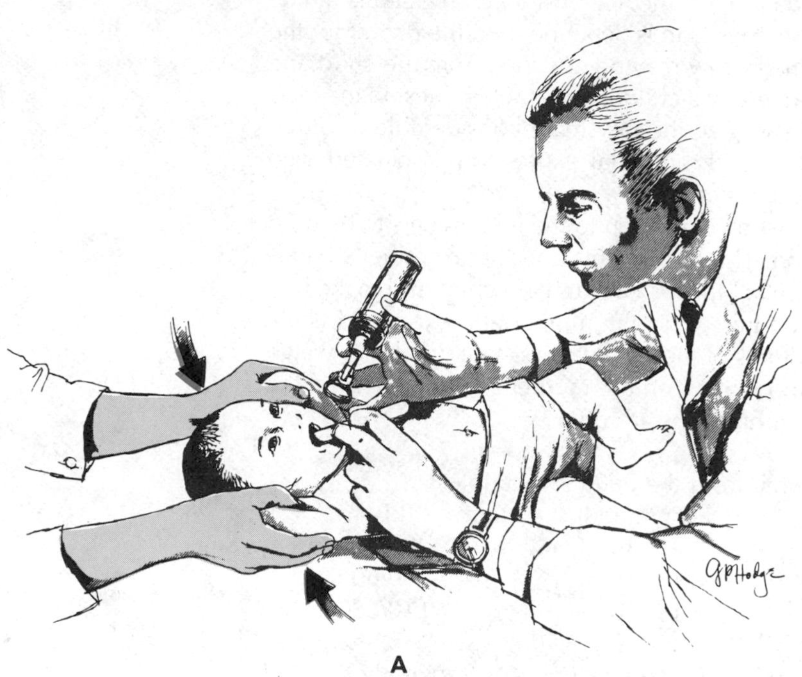

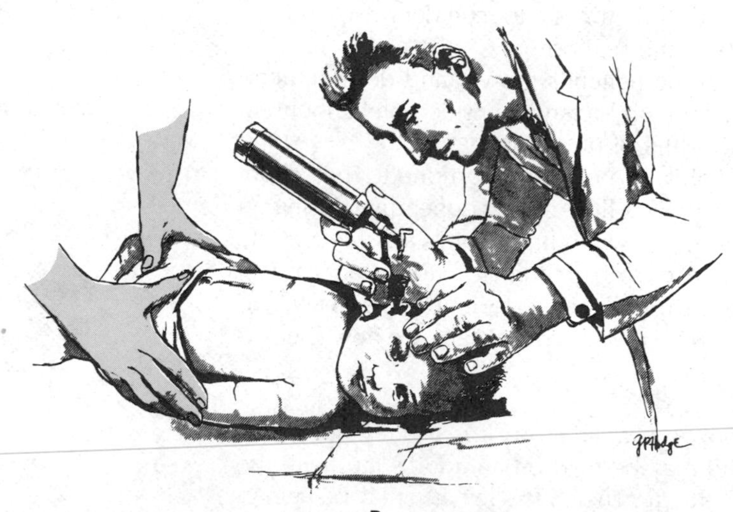

FIGURE 28–20 *A,* Examination of the throat in the young patient. Note that the child's head is held still by exerting pressure on his arms against the sides of the head. In this manner one person can immobilize the head and arms. *B,* Technique of ear examination in the young child. Note that the examiner's hand holding the otoscope rests on the patient's head, so that any sudden movement will be transferred to both the hand and instrument and prevent trauma to the ear canal. (From Judge, R. D., and Zuidema, G. D.: *Physical Diagnosis: A Physiological Approach to the Clinical Examination.* 2nd ed. Boston, Little, Brown & Co., 1968.)

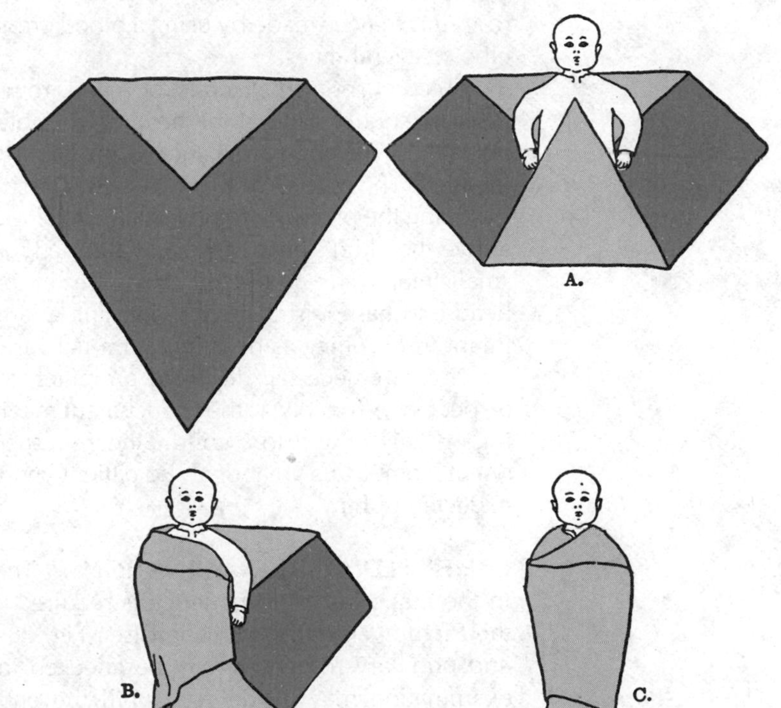

FIGURE 28–21 Mummy restraint for infant. (From Standard Nursing Procedures of the Department of Hospitals, City of New York, published by The Macmillan Company.)

bottom of the sheet just below the feet. Leave a greater portion of the sheet on the left side of the child. Now bring this longer side back *over* the left arm and *under* the body *and* right arm. Next, bring the sheet back *over* the right arm and *under* the body again. The two arms will be completely restrained, leaving the abdomen exposed. If you wish to restrain the entire body, bring the right portion of the sheet over the abdomen and tuck it securely under the entire back and out again on the right side.

Another method of restraint is the mummy style (Fig. 28–21). This is done by folding the sheet into a triangle and placing it on the examining table. The distance from the fold to the lower corner of the sheet should be twice the length of the child. Now place the child on the sheet with the fold slightly above the shoulders. Loosen any tight clothing and straighten the arms and legs of the child. Next, bring the lower corner of the sheet up over the child's body. Now the left corner is brought over the body and tucked under the body snugly, leaving the arm exposed. Next, bring the opposite corner over the exposed arm and under the child's body. This restraint is quick and easy to make and can be used to leave either arm exposed while securing the opposite arm and also the legs and body. It may be pinned if necessary. Elbow restraints may be made by using a blood pressure cuff or a towel wrapped around the elbow several times.

To prevent a small child or infant from rolling his head from side to side, the assistant should stand at the head of the table and support the child's head between her hands, making certain not to press on the ears or on the anterior or posterior fontanel. The reverse of this may be the assistant's restraining a child with her body by taking the place of the physician (Fig. 28–20*B*), and the physician's working from above the child's head. This may be used for an examination of the child's eyes. A small infant may be placed crosswise on the examining table which has both the head and base raised slightly, forming a large **V** in the table. This will prevent the infant from rolling as he might on a flat surface.

It is not necessary to drape an infant, but the older child's modesty should be respected. A friendly, rather nonchalant manner will help, but never be condescending or "talk down" to a child. Sincere respect and conversation at the child's level will accomplish a great deal. Be patient and wait for the child to understand what is expected of him.

OTHER PEDIATRIC EXAMINATIONS. The eyes are examined in the same way as in the adult, but more patience is required. The "E" Eye Chart (see Fig. 28–15) or the Picture Visual Acuity Chart (see Fig. 28–16) may be used. Ocular movements and pupillary responses may be checked in the infant. The ear, nose, and throat examination may be delayed until the end of the examination, because it may require restraints. The medical assistant can assist the physician by offering the child a distraction while the physician is examining the chest and abdomen. A rectal examination is important and may require a moderate restraint.

The neurologic examination is usually accomplished by game playing, such as grasping a toy or putting blocks together. How a baby sits and how it moves its legs are important. The gait of a child tells a physician a lot.

Materials needed:

Flashlight	Illuminated diagnostic set
Tongue depressor	Scales
Stethoscope	Finger cots
Tape measure	

Proctology

The proctosigmoidoscopic, or "procto," examination is the examination of the rectum and lower colon. It is an important part of a thorough physical examination. Since at least 70 per cent of cancers of the entire rectum and colon are anatomically within reach of the sigmoidoscope (25 cm or 10 in.), it is obvious why a "procto" examination is important. About 13 per cent of the malignancies are found within digital reach (8 cm or 3.2 in.). In past years the examination was done on the symptomatic patient, but because the examination is relatively simple and does not cause too much discomfort, it is fairly routine.

The most common complaint from patients is rectal bleeding. It is important for the physician to know the amount of bleeding, the color of the stool, when the bleeding occurs, and for how long. *Pruritus* is another frequently heard complaint. The physician will question the patient as to any change in his bowel habits. **Tenesmus** (ineffectual and painful straining during bowel movement) is important because this is a cardinal symptom of possible carcinoma.

Hemorrhoids are treated by various methods, ranging from conservative ones such as suppositories and avoidance methods of constipation, to the injecting of a sclerosing solution, the "rubber-band" ligation, or freezing, to surgical hemorrhoidectomy.

Diagnostic aids used are gastrointestinal x-ray series, barium enema, and gallbladder x-ray studies. A stool specimen is examined for occult blood, parasites, ova, or fungi. Pinworms and fungal infections are the most common.

Some physicians feel there is no need for special bowel preparation if the patient is examined after normal defecation. They believe the use of laxatives or enemas does not preserve the normal appearance of the intestinal mucosa. The day before the examination the patient should have a light diet of soft foods and after 6:00 PM, nothing solid but clear fluids only. On the day of exam, the patient should eat nothing, can have clear fluids only, and must take an enema. If only bowel preparation is desired, the patient is instructed to use a laxative or one of the commercial saline enemas during the latter part of the day prior to the examination. The medical assistant should know the physician's desires and instruct the patient properly.

The anal area is first inspected for evidence of lesions, external hemorrhoids, fissures, or fistulas. Next, a small amount of lubricant is applied to the physician's index finger and the anal sphincter is dilated. The rectal sphincter muscle will relax after a few moments of pressure. Internal hemorrhoids cannot be felt unless they are thrombosed. Physicians will vary as to whether they use the sigmoidoscope, anoscope, or rectal speculum next. Besides inspecting for the malignant lesions, the physician may observe polyps and/or abscesses.

Materials needed:

Sigmoidoscope	Anoscope
Rectal speculum	Insufflator
Suction pump	Probe with bulb tip
Gloves	Finger cots
Long cotton applicators	Lubricating jelly
Basin of water	

Before the examination starts be certain to check the illuminated instruments for light. See that the obturators are positioned correctly. Have a basin to receive the used instruments. The basin of water is to rinse out the suction pump immediately after each use. The pump tubing is very difficult to keep clean and free of odor.

1. Greet the patient and briefly explain the examination to be done. Patients are extremely apprehensive about this examination and will need extra assurance and consideration.
2. Have the patient empty his bladder and save the specimen.
3. It is best to have the patient disrobe completely and put on a gown.
4. Assist the patient into the correct position. Proper positioning is very important for the comfort of the patient and to insure accessibility of the rectum and sigmoid colon to the physician. An examining table that will adjust to the proctological position is far superior for both of the above reasons. With the

proctological table, the patient assumes the position of kneeling on the knee board with the trunk of the body over the bend of the table and the forearms and elbows resting on the headboard. The patient may then rest his head on his arms. The table is next tilted forward, and his body trunk is then adjusted so the hips, *not* the waist, are bent over the bend of the table. If correctly positioned the abdomen will hang forward and downward freely. This allows the **S** curve of the sigmoid colon to straighten out somewhat. Since many offices do not have a procto table (see Fig. 28–1*F*), other positions are used. The lift illustrated in Figure 28–1*G* (Hamilton board) gives the patient support, but remember, the trunk of the body must be forward with the patient bending at the hips and not at the waist. The knee-chest or knee-elbow position is frequently used (see Fig. 28–1*I*). In the correct knee-chest position the patient's back is in a "swayback" position. This is difficult to maintain, and many patients cannot get into a true knee-chest position. It may help if the medical assistant stands beside the table and offers support to the patient. The Sims' position is used for rectal examinations or for patients who cannot be placed in the other more advantageous positions. However, the physician is somewhat limited in the depth of the bowel he can examine.

5. A **fenestrated** drape is superior for this examination, but two small sheets may be used and clipped together at the sides, or one larger sheet may be draped around and clipped over the patient's back. A small towel is placed directly under the anus and over the perineal body.

6. The medical assistant should watch the patient for any undue reactions and offer assurance.

7. Have tissues ready for the physician to wipe his gloved finger. Take the used instruments and applicators from the physician by the handle or with a tissue to protect yourself. Have the long applicators ready to hand the physician and remember to rinse out the suction tubing after each use.

8. The used instruments are placed in a basin of disinfectant solution and removed from the room to be sanitized and sterilized later.

9. When the physician has finished, assist the patient off the table or into a supine position. Do not let patients rise too rapidly because they are frequently dizzy after this examination. It is best to level the table and have the patient remain there for a few minutes.

10. The patient may then dress after the resting period. Be sure to have cleansing tissue in the dressing area and don't forget to give the patient any instructions the physician wanted him to have.

Urology

The urologist treats diseases of the genitourinary tract of the male and the urinary tract of the female. Frequently the urologist works with the gynecologist to treat the female patient.

The upper urinary system (kidneys and ureters) is assessed mainly by abdominal palpation. The urinary bladder is palpable when distended, but this is very discomforting to the patient. A considerable part of a urinary survey is dependent on the patient's history, such as frequency, urgency, **dysuria,** or **incontinence. Cystitis** is the most common disorder of the bladder, especially in the female. Renal **calculi** are the most painful. A major part of the examination is urinalysis. The medical assistant must be able to instruct the patient, especially the female, in the collection of a clean-catch urine specimen, although a voided specimen is not always satisfactory, especially from the female. It is best to have the patient void in the physician's office so the specimen can be examined immediately. Most urologists prefer to examine a catheterized specimen.

Major complaints presented to the urologist involve changes in the frequency of urination. This is the symptom of several conditions such as cystitis, **diabetes mellitus,** and **diabetes insipidus** (increased volume) and renal failure and conditions with decreased volume. This symptom may or may not be accompanied by painful or difficult urination **(dysuria).** Urgency is another very annoying symptom since it is the inability to control the urine after the desire to urinate occurs. Similar to this is **incontinence,** the involuntary loss of urine. Stress incontinence is the loss of urine during physical stress, such as during coughing, sneezing, or laughing. This is commonly seen in the **multiparous** woman with a **cystocele** or **urethrocele.**

There are many diagnostic aids in urology, and the complete urinalysis is probably the most common. Renal function tests include determination of serum creatinine and blood urea nitrogen (BUN) levels. An excretory test is the phenosulfonphthalein (PSP) test. Radiographic studies are often the intravenous pyelogram (IVP) or the retrograde pyelogram. A film of the abdomen may show the kidneys, ureters, and bladder (KUB) for possible calculi. Radioisotopic studies as well as **sonography** are useful. Sonography is the use of ultrasound to detect masses in the urinary system. Some of these tests are discussed in Chapter 31.

Cystoscopy is the examination of the bladder by means of a cystoscope passed through the urethra and into the bladder. The cystoscope illuminates the bladder interior. By means of special lenses and mirrors the bladder mucosa is examined for inflammation, tumors, and calculi. A catheter can be passed through the cystoscope and on into the ureters and kidneys to obtain samples of urine or introduce an opaque substance for x-rays.

There is no special instrument setup for a routine urologic examination unless a special procedure, such as obtaining a catheterized urine specimen, is done. Most offices are now using the prepackaged disposable units for catheterization and for bladder irrigations.

Both male and female patients are disrobed and given a gown. The female patient is placed in a lithotomy position, as for a pelvic examination. The male patient is seated on the examining table and the physician will instruct the patient to do what is needed.

References

Conn, H. F., Rakel, R. E., and Johnson, T. W. (eds.): *Family Practice*. Philadelphia, W. B. Saunders Co., 1978.

Essentials of the Gynecological History and Examination. Smith, Kline & French Laboratories, 1965.

Essentials of the Neurological Examination. Smith, Kline & French Laboratories, 1968.

Judge, R. D., and Zuidema, G. D. (eds.): *Physical Diagnosis: A Physiological Approach to Clinical Examination.* 2nd ed., Boston, Little, Brown and Co., 1968.

Prior, J. A., and Silberstein, J. S.: *Physical Diagnosis,* St. Louis, The C. V. Mosby Company, 1977.

Proctosigmoidoscopy for the Detection of Asymptomatic Cancer. American Cancer Society, Inc., 1962.

Stein, H. A., and Slatt, B. J.: *The Ophthalmic Assistant: Fundamentals and Clinical Practice.* 2nd ed., St. Louis, The C. V. Mosby Co., 1971.

Sutton, A. L.: *Bedside Nursing Techniques in Medicine and Surgery*. Philadelphia, W. B. Saunders Co., 1969.

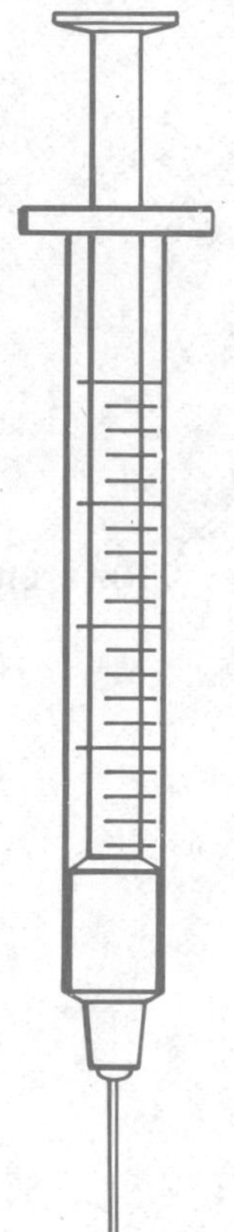

CHAPTER OUTLINE

Terminology of Wounds
Dressings and Bandages
Solutions and Medications
Sutures and Suture Needles
General Instructions
  Preoperative Instructions
  Postoperative Instructions
Positioning the Patient
Handwashing
Physician's Reference File
Preparing Sterile Packs
Observing Sterile Technique
Setting Up the Sterile Field
Preparing the Patient's Skin for Surgery
Basic Surgical Setups

BEHAVIORAL OBJECTIVES

The medical office assistant should be able to:

- **Instruct the surgical outpatient in preoperative and postoperative care and procedures.**
- **Prepare the patient both physically and emotionally for surgery.**
- **Practice aseptic technique around the operating field and in handling sterile supplies.**
- **Prepare the basic surgical setups for suturing, needle biopsy, gynecologic procedures, and so forth.**
- **Assist the surgeon in outpatient procedures for cyst removal, special irrigations, fracture casting, and so on.**
- **Apply and change dressings for incisions and wounds.**
- **Identify apparatus and materials routinely used in office surgery.**

29

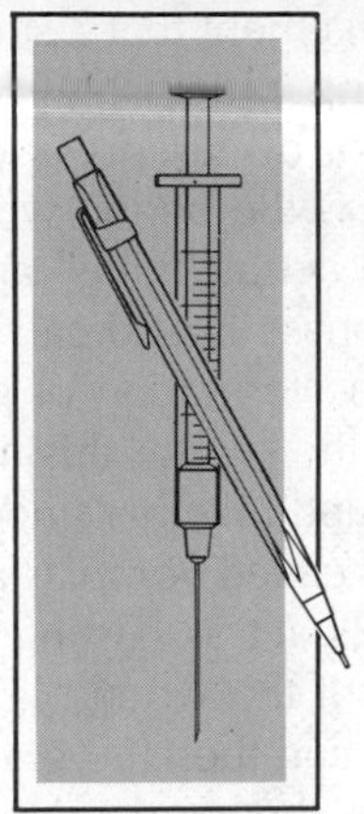

ASSISTING WITH OFFICE SURGERY

The amount of surgery performed in the physician's office often depends upon the location of the office. In an urban area where hospitals are more accessible, it is easier to use the hospital facilities on an outpatient basis, but many rural physicians find themselves doing more office surgery because of the greater distances to hospitals. As a rule a physician prefers to use hospital facilities if the patient is diabetic or has a heart condition or any blood **dyscrasia.** The removal of lesions and growths that may need immediate **histologic** or **cytologic** study presents a problem for office surgery. Performing office surgery is also difficult if the patient will be immobile after the procedure.

TERMINOLOGY OF WOUNDS

The medical office assistant, whether she assists the doctor with minor surgery or is merely responsible for transcribing dictation or writing insurance reports, needs a clear understanding of the terminology used in the surgical areas. The clinical assistant especially will need to understand the types of wounds and the healing phases of the patient undergoing treatment. The assistant who is responsible for stocking the supplies must have a thorough knowledge of the materials needed. The remainder of this chapter will be directed toward these needs.

A *wound* is any interruption in the continuity of the internal or external body tissue. It may be *accidental* or *intentional, open* or *closed*. A surgical incision is an intentional wound. It is clean, neat, and made under controlled conditions; an accidental wound is none of these. An open wound is one with an outward opening where the skin is broken and underlying tissue exposed. A closed wound does not have an outward opening, but the underlying tissue is damaged, as in a hematoma or bruise. It is usually the result of a contusion.

An **abrasion** is a *superficial wound.* The depth is compared to that of a second degree burn. It is usually the result of friction, such as a skinned knee, and is usually accidental. An abrasion is painful and easily infected. A **puncture** or **penetrating wound** is intentional when made by a trocar for draining purposes or by a hypodermic needle. It is accidental when the patient has stepped on a nail. A **laceration** is usually thought of as being accidental and having the appearance of a tear, but a surgical incision may also be classed as a laceration. A "clean" laceration presents the same problems and management that a surgical incision would present.

All wounds go through a **healing** process, which is the restoration of the structure and function of the injured or diseased tissue. This healing process takes place in three phases. The *first phase* is the period when the blood serum and red cells form a network in the wound to act as "glue" and form a clot that plugs the wound, resulting in a scab. This first phase is also called the *lag phase*. The *second phase* is the mending process with the formation of granulation tissue. The same materials that arrest bleeding prepare the site for this mending. These fibrin threads contract and pull the edges of the wound together under the clot or scab. Epithelial cells start to form. This second phase is called *fibroplasia,* the development of fibrous tissue in the wound. These repair cells act as basting stitches and are disposed of when the permanent cells are joined. If the wound is a clean surgical cut there is practically no loss of the normal cells, and there is very little scarring. Scarring takes place in the *third phase,* also known as the *contraction phase*. In this third phase, if the edges are uneven or if there is considerable damage to the tissue, it is difficult for the repair cells to pull the edges together and they must build a bridge over the gap and form connective tissue. This is not true skin, nor can it change into true skin — it is scar tissue. *Scar tissue* is usually very strong, but it cannot stand the tension of normal skin because of its loss of elasticity. It is also devoid of normal blood supply and nerves.

There are several factors that influence the healing process. Healing is assisted by youth, adequate nutrition, and rest to the area. Destruction or reinjury during the second phase can increase the scarring and delay healing. Wounds are susceptible to infection because the normal skin barrier does not exist and this may result in **necrotic** tissue, which in turn acts as a culture for the infection. This necrotic tissue must be removed. This removal is called **debridement**. Pus is often seen with necrotic tissue. It is a combination of necrotic tissue, bacteria, dead leukocytes, exudates, and other tissue breakdown products.

A *lesion* is any **pathologic** or **traumatic** alteration of tissue. This alteration may be intentional as in a surgical incision or unintentional, as seen in an abrasion. *Primary* lesions are those that appear as the immediate result of the causative factor. A *secondary* lesion is the result of alterations in the underlying primary lesion. Scars and scales are the result of a primary lesion and are therefore secondary lesions. See Figure 28–8 Primary and Secondary Lesions.

DRESSINGS AND BANDAGES

These terms are used in the broadest sense, since they may mean a roller bandage, a gauze pad, or even a medication. Before discussing the many different uses of dressings and bandages, let us consider the other viewpoint, that of no dressing on a wound. This is referred to as the "open wound" method of healing. Some of the advantages of no dressing are: (1) the wound will suffer no irritation or friction due to a dressing or bandage; (2) an open wound will stay dried and, therefore, will not be a medium for bacterial growth as is the moisture under a dressing; (3) sutures stay dry and hold together and there is less danger of infection around the stitches; (4) if the patient has been closely shaved before surgery, small dry nicks will heal faster than moist nicks; and (5) an existing infection may remain localized and not spread by a dressing. These are all good points, but there are also disadvantages to having no dressing.

A *wound dressing* will prevent outside infection from entering the wound, absorb secretions, hold edges together, protect against trauma, restrict movement and act as a splint, cover a disfigurement, may be used to apply cold packs or **fomentations,** and may act as a pressure dressing, which is important in the healing process.

Regardless of the type or material of the dressing a good dressing must be effective and comfortable, and remain in place. Dressings and bandages frequently appear easy and simple to apply, but a special skill is required to apply a good functional dressing that serves the purpose for which it was intended. To the patient a neat, comfortable dressing is a mark of competence. Care must be taken to apply the dressing properly so it will remain in place. It is distressing to the patient to have a dressing fall off before he reaches home.

ROLLER BANDAGES. Roller bandages are not applied directly over a wound. First, gauze squares are placed over the wound, making absolutely certain the sterile gauze square completely covers the wound; this may be anchored in place with tape. Under no circumstances should tape be touching or near the wound. Plain

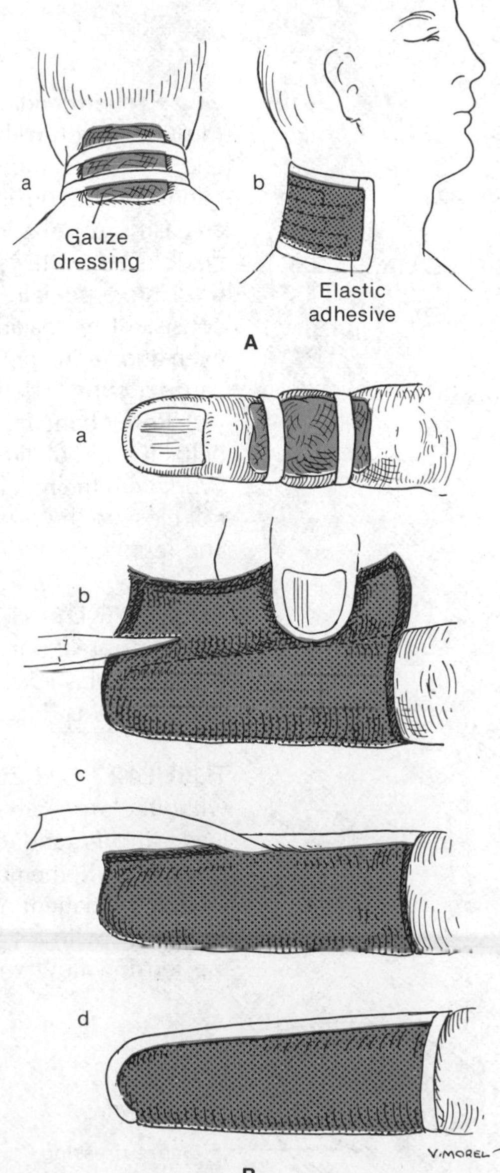

FIGURE 29–1 Elastic adhesive bandage used on the neck *(A)* and the finger *(B)*. (From Ochsner, A., and DeBakey, M. E.: *Christopher's Minor Surgery*. 8th ed. Philadelphia, W. B. Saunders Co., 1959.)

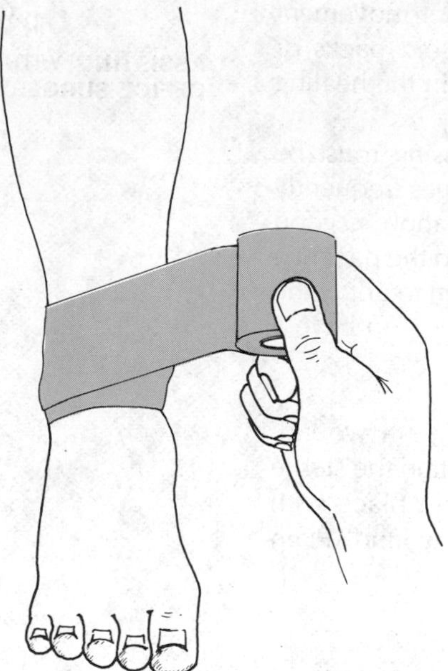

FIGURE 29–2 Applying a roller bandage. Start at the distal point. Keep the roll close to the patient with the roll upwards. Keep tension and spacing consistently even.

gauze roller bandage is almost a thing of the past. It is difficult to apply because it must be put on with reverse spiral turns if the area is uneven. It also has no elasticity and tends to bind. It does not adhere to itself and is more likely to slip. Elastic bandages or wrinkled-crepe type lend themselves to various shapes and do not slide as easily. An elastic bandage or patch with adhesive backing makes a secure but flexible cover (Fig. 29–1). When applying elastic roller bandages as a pressure dressing, especially to the lower limbs, it is absolutely essential to keep the bandage consistent in spacing and tension with an overall pressure over a large area. This even and gentle pressure stimulates circulation and healing, but any unevenness will cause a constriction point and may possibly create an ulcer.

Roller bandages are applied from the **distal** to the **proximal** part of the area. This helps the circulation. Elevation of the limb during bandaging is also advantageous. Work with the roller facing upward in your major hand. This enables you to keep the roll close to the patient's skin and you are more likely to keep the tension consistent and less likely to drop the roll (Fig. 29–2).

ADHESIVE DRESSINGS TO SMALL AREAS. Liquid adhesive dressings are useful for small areas that are difficult to bandage (Fig. 29–3). There are commercially prepared elastic adhesive bandages in various shapes that lend themselves to different spots (Fig. 29–4).

TUBULAR GAUZE BANDAGES. Seamless tubular gauze bandages, with or without elastic, are superior material for covering any round surfaces, such as arms, legs, fingers and toes. These tubular bandages are applied with a cage-like applicator. Remember to work with the cutting channel of the applicator facing in toward the patient. You may start in the middle of the area and anchor the dressing, if necessary, with a small piece of tape. Hold the applicator in both hands and control the tension flow with your fingers as the applicator is gradually rotated and the

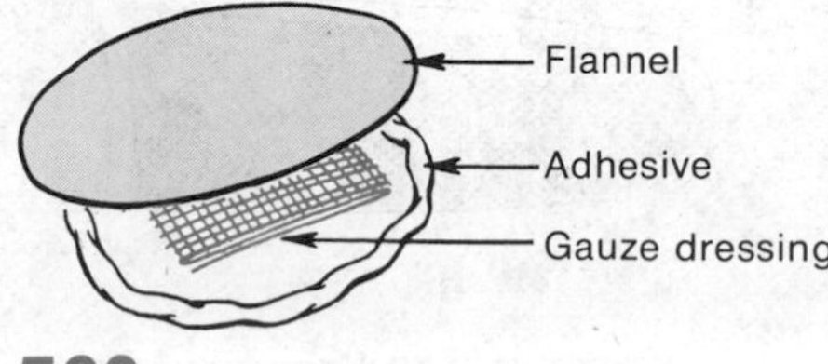

FIGURE 29–3 Liquid adhesive for spot dressing. (From Sutton, A. L.: *Bedside Nursing Techniques in Medicine and Surgery*. 2nd ed. Philadelphia, W. B. Saunders Co., 1969.)

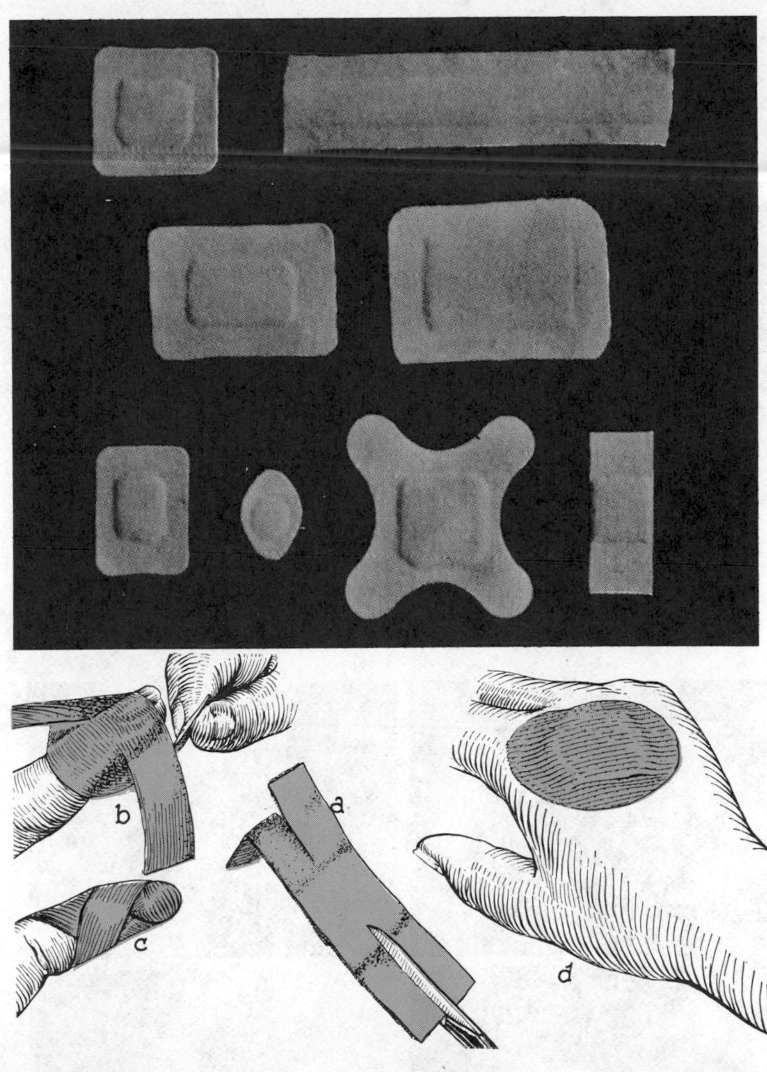

FIGURE 29–4 Commercial elastic adhesive spot bandages. (From Ochsner, A., and DeBakey, M. E.: *Christopher's Minor Surgery*. 8th ed. Philadelphia, W. B. Saunders Co., 1959.)

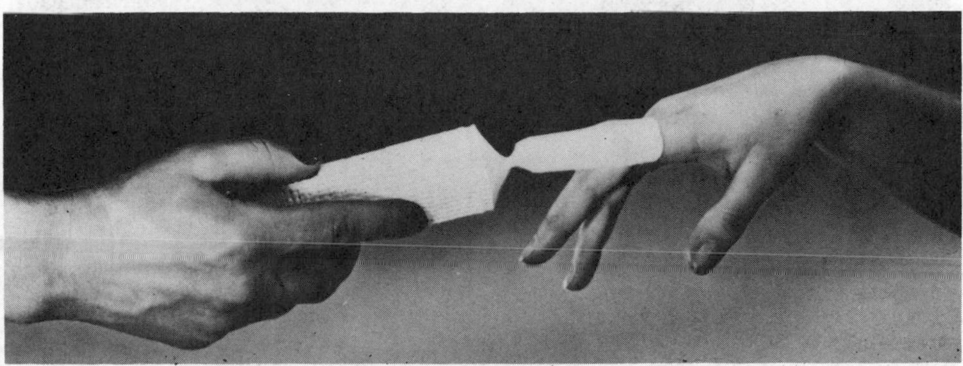

FIGURE 29–5 Tubegauz applied to a finger. (Courtesy of Scholl, Inc., Hospital Products Division.)

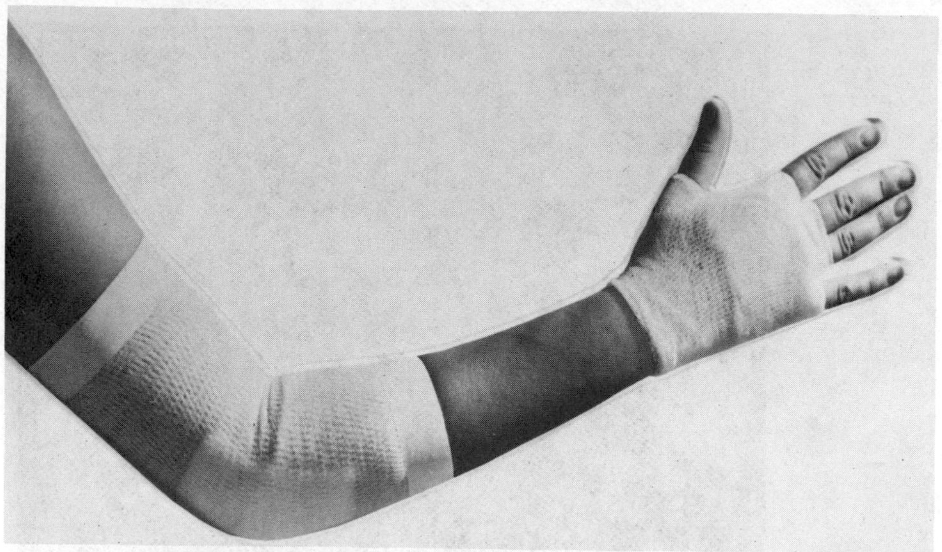

FIGURE 29–6 Tubegauz to elbow and hand. Courtesy of Scholl, Inc., Hospital Products Division.)

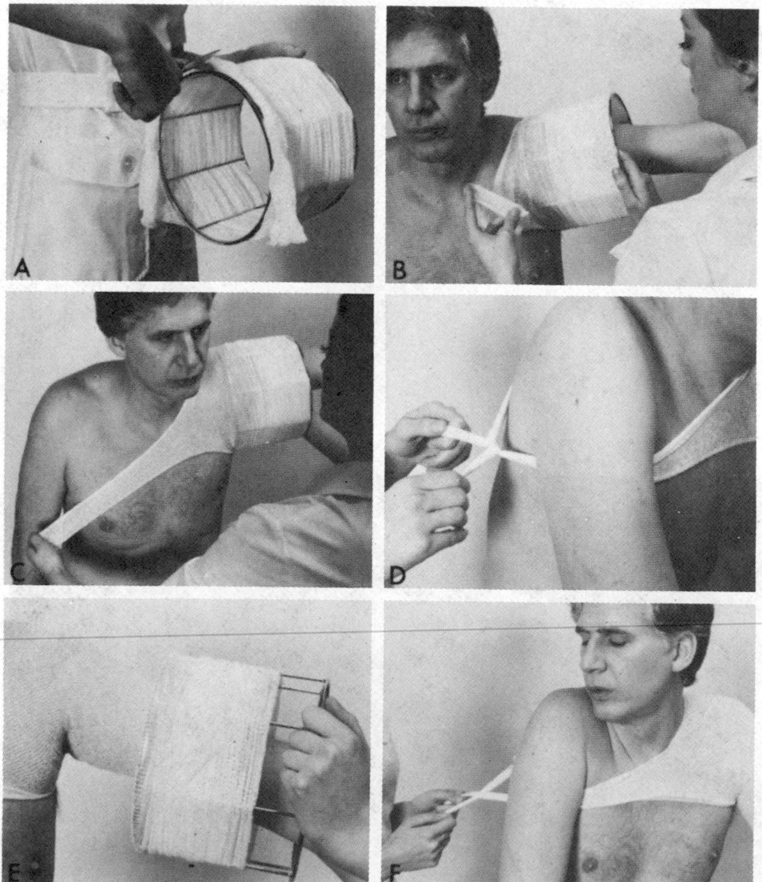

FIGURE 29–7 Shoulder bandaging with Tubegauz. *A,* With a loaded applicator, make two slits in the Tubegauz, one slit at the top and another at the bottom of the applicator. You'll need to make a longer slit at the bottom. *B,* Place the arm through the applicator up to the shoulder. *C,* Pull one tail of Tubegauz across the chest, the other across the back. *D,* Pulling the pieces taut, tie the two tails under the other arm. *E,* Bring applicator slightly down arm, and anchor, then move applicator to the shoulder. *F,* Cutting from the smooth-rim end, make two slits as before, bring tails across back and chest, and tie under arm. (Courtesy of Scholl, Inc., Hospital Products Division.)

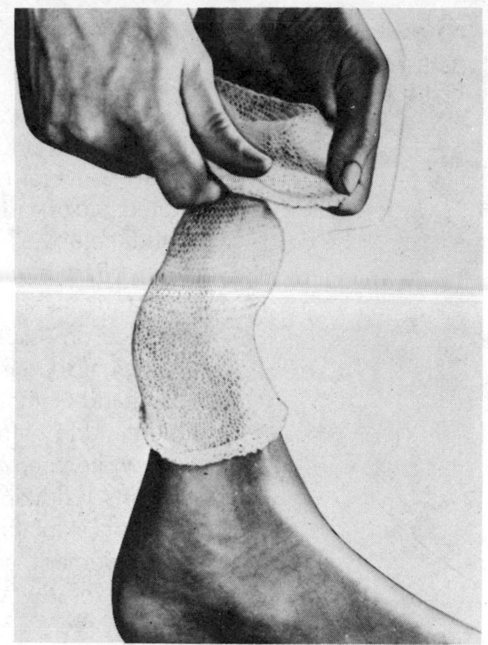

FIGURE 29–8 Tubegauz to toes. (Courtesy of Scholl, Inc., Hospital Products Division.)

material slides off. These tubular dressings may be applied with or without slight pressure. Beyond the tip of the bandaged part, give the applicator a full half-turn, place the applicator again over the part, and repeat the procedure. Be very careful not to create a tourniquet effect when you reverse the applicator. When the desired thickness of the bandage is reached, cut the gauze, and anchor the final dressing with tape. This lightweight tubular gauze is not stockinette for casting (Figs. 29–5 through 29–8).

Patients should be told to call the office if there is any problem with the dressing. Swelling may occur after a dressing is put on, and the patient may need a dressing change sooner than planned.

SOLUTIONS AND MEDICATIONS

Treatment room supplies include, in addition to the various types of dressings, some standard solutions and medications that are used in minor surgery and dressing changes. The solutions and medications listed here are basic, and every physician will have his preferred items and methods of applying them. Many of these items will be used by the medical assistant as directed by the physician. Others are used by the physician only, but the assistant should be familiar with their usage.

Sterile distilled water is kept in two forms. Multiple-dose vials are used for the injectable distilled water and as a diluent for medications. Larger containers of sterile distilled water are used for rinsing instruments that have been in a chemical disinfectant solution. These containers of rinsing water may be prepared in the office. (See Chapter 26 for Sterilization of Solutions.)

Sterile physiologic saline solution (0.85 per cent sodium chloride) is also stocked in two sizes. The smaller multiple-dose vials are used for injection (do not prepare these injectables in your office; purchase those commercially made). Larger containers of physiologic saline are used for rinsing and irrigating wounds.

Alcohol is usually 70 per cent isopropyl. It is used as a skin antiseptic, has moderate cidal power, is a fat solvent, and has wetting ability. Ethyl alcohol is also used and has the same properties as the isopropyl. It will not kill spores.

Zephiran chloride. The tincture of Zephiran is colored and used as a skin antiseptic. The 1:1000 aqueous solution is used as an instrument disinfectant. Do not mix or confuse these two solutions. Each has a definite and different use.

Tincture of merthiolate is also a skin antiseptic and is colored, as is *tincture of mercresin*. Because they are alcoholic preparations they will evaporate if left in open containers.

Iodine has always been one of the most effective disinfectants used. The newer iodine products do not cause the problems of the earlier tincture of iodine. Betadine is used in several different ways: swabs for skin preparation, surgical scrub soap, saturated gauze pads (3 in. by 9 in.) and topical ointment. This iodine preparation may be bandaged over.

Bard-Parker germicide is a popular instrument disinfectant and is used in the same manner as aqueous Zephiran chloride. The instruments must be rinsed off before being used on tissue.

Surgical soap is an important item in the medical office. Examples are pHisoHex, Septisol, and Gamophen. Surgical soaps are used for handwashing and for cleansing a patient's skin before the application of an antiseptic.

Hydrogen peroxide (H_2O_2) in a 3 per cent solution is used as a mild antiseptic. It kills by its oxidizing power. This oxidizing action creates minute bubbles when applied to a skin abrasion or wound and has cleansing action. It is used in irrigations and debridement, and is nonirritating.

Local anesthetics usually found in a physician's office are *Procaine, Xylocaine,* and many others. They may be plain or with epinephrine. These solutions are usually purchased in 30 to 50 cc multiple-dose vials.

Tincture of benzoin has many uses. It is used in inhalants and expectorants, but its main use in the office is as a protective coating over ulcers and abrasions. It is also used under adhesive tape to increase holding power and decrease skin sensitivity to tapes. It is supplied in spray cans as well as in solution for painting on the skin. Do not confuse tincture of benzoin with benzene (benzol), which is used as a cleaning solvent.

Ethyl chloride is a highly volatile liquid that is sprayed on the skin; it evaporates so quickly that the tissue is immediately cooled. It is used as a skin anesthetic. It is a topical anesthetic of very short duration, sometimes called "freezing."

Epinephrine 1:1000 (adrenalin) is a vasoconstrictor, used to check **hemorrhages, asthmatic paroxysms,** and **shock.** It prolongs the action of a local anesthetic. It is also used in allergic reactions. It is administered parenterally (injected), topically, and by inhalation.

Aromatic spirits of ammonia are usually found in small glass ampules covered with cotton and gauze that are easily crushed. Their most common use is for reviving persons who feel faint.

Collodion, sometimes called "new skin," is a flexible substance that acts as a local protector to the area when applied. It has a clear plastic appearance.

Formalin, 10 per cent solution, is used to preserve excised tissue, such as that taken in biopsy, for histologic study.

Lubricating jelly is used for the lubrication of instruments such as a vaginal speculum. It is packaged sterile in flexible tubes, like toothpaste. K-Y Jelly is a popular brand.

Vaseline (petroleum jelly or petrolatum) may be used plain as an ointment but is most frequently impregnated in gauze squares or strips.

Iodoform gauze strips are strips of gauze ¼ to ½ inch wide that are treated with iodoform, about 96 per cent iodine. They are used to pack into an abscess, acting as a wick to drain out the infection and also as a local antibacterial.

Ether is used in offices as an antiseptic and to cleanse the skin of skin oils.

Silver nitrate ($AgNO_3$) is found both in solution and on applicator sticks. It is a caustic and is applied topically. It must be kept in a lightproof brown container. The most commonly used solution is 20 per cent, but it also is used frequently in 10 and 50 per cent solutions. The applicator sticks are convenient for touching oral lesions.

SUTURES AND SUTURE NEEDLES

The word *suture* is used as both a noun and a verb. As a noun it refers to a surgical stitch or to the material used; as a verb it refers to the act of stitching. Sutures were used as long ago as 2000 BC. History does not record the first surgical operations and the use of sutures, but ancient medical writings do make references to the use of sinews and strings to tie off bleeding blood vessels. Hippocrates wrote of his use of sutures and Aesculapius was said to have used sutures during the Trojan War. Before Joseph Lister, infection and pus were inevitable when a wound was closed by sutures. Modern surgery and the use of sutures began in 1865 when Dr. Lister developed antisepsis and the disinfection of suture materials. Many kinds of materials have been used over the centuries, including precious metals, horsehair, animal tendons, and cotton and linen cord. Most of the improvement in suture materials and techniques has occurred in the last 50 years.

A *suture* may also be used as a *ligature*. This is a strand of suture material used to tie off a blood vessel or to constrict tissue. To *ligate* means to apply a ligature.

TYPES OF SUTURE MATERIALS. Suture material may be classed as either absorbable or nonabsorbable. The absorbable suture is one that is digested and absorbed by the tissue enzymes during the process of wound healing. It is referred to as surgical gut, sometimes incorrectly called "catgut." The name came from the use of sheep intestines as fiddle strings by the Arabs. The Arabic word for fiddle is "kit" and these "kitgut" strings were used by surgeons for suturing. Surgical gut is still made from sheep intestines.

If the surgical gut is untreated it will be digested and absorbed by the body in a few days, usually about five days. Plain gut is used when healing is fairly fast and the need for the stitch does not exceed the usual five days. Treated gut is slower to absorb. It is coated with soluble chromium salts, which delay absorption. The amount of coating controls the absorption from 20 to 40 days. This is somewhat dependent on the type of tissue it is in, the health of the patient, and the presence or absence of infection.

Nonabsorbable sutures are more frequently used in the medical office because a majority of suturing is superficial and in areas where sutures can be removed after healing has taken place. These removable sutures are made of many different materials. *Silk* is popular. It ties easily and can be autoclaved. It is twisted or braided and sometimes **impregnated** with wax or coated with silicone. It is usually black. Dermal silk is a protein-coated silk that resists body action and is usually blue. Surgical *cotton* is very tough and resistant. It may be used internally when no absorption is desired, such as in a ligation. Cotton is white or may be dyed. *Stainless steel* is very strong and fine. It is noncorrosive and well tolerated. It may be a little more difficult to handle than other materials. *Nylon* and *polyethylene* are very strong, have a degree of elasticity, and are relatively nonirritating to the tissue. They are supplied in a single strand (monofilament) or in braided strands (multifilament). These synthetics have replaced the horsehair or silkworm gut formerly used for very fine suturing needs. They are colorless, blue, or green. The sizes of suture material are standard as set by the United States Pharmacopeia. They range from 7–0 (the smallest) to 3 (the largest). The 2–0 to 4–0 is used most frequently in the medical office. These may also be referred to as 000 or 0000 for the 3–0 and the 4–0.

NEEDLES. These are chosen according to the area in which they are to be used and the depth and width of the desired stitch. They are classed according to their parts — eye or eyeless, straight or curved, cutting edge or noncutting (rounded) edge. Eyeless needles are much less traumatic because a single strand of suture is pulled through the tissue rather than the double strand of a threaded needle. Figure 29–9 illustrates the shape and edge of surgical needles as well as the atraumatic (eyeless) and traumatic (with an eye). The majority of suture materials used in the physician's office are presterilized and packaged ready for use.

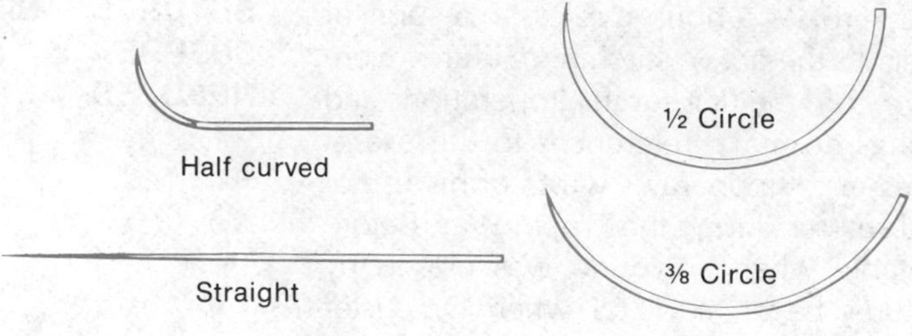

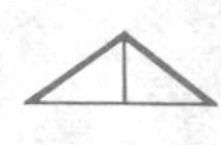

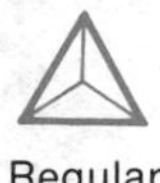

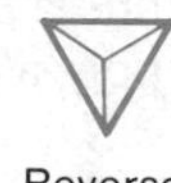

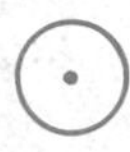
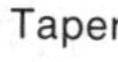

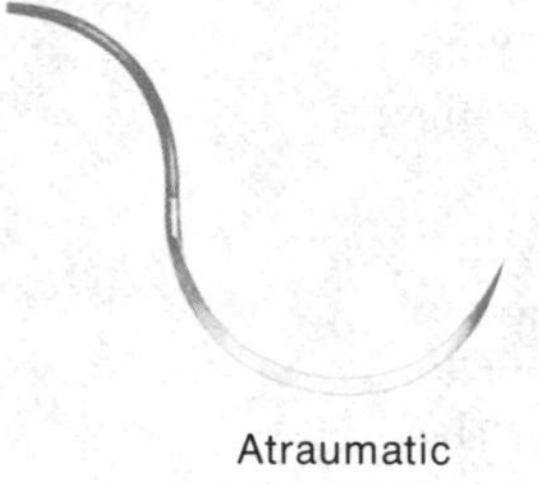

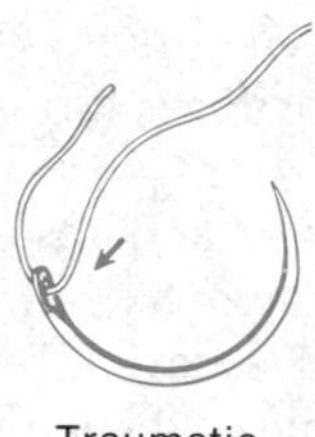

FIGURE 29–9 Types of surgical needles.

Techniques and types of skin closures vary greatly, and it would be impossible to describe or illustrate them. The majority of skin closures in an office are limited to superficial suturing by the interrupted and continuous (uninterrupted) techniques (Fig. 29–10).

GENERAL INSTRUCTIONS

PREOPERATIVE INSTRUCTIONS. When planning office surgery, the medical assistant should complete the following procedures before the time of the appointment:

1. Have the necessary consent forms ready to sign.
2. Give the patient all the necessary preoperative instructions such as medications to be used and special skin cleansing.
3. Ask the patient to arrange to have someone bring him to the office and take him home, if it will be necessary.

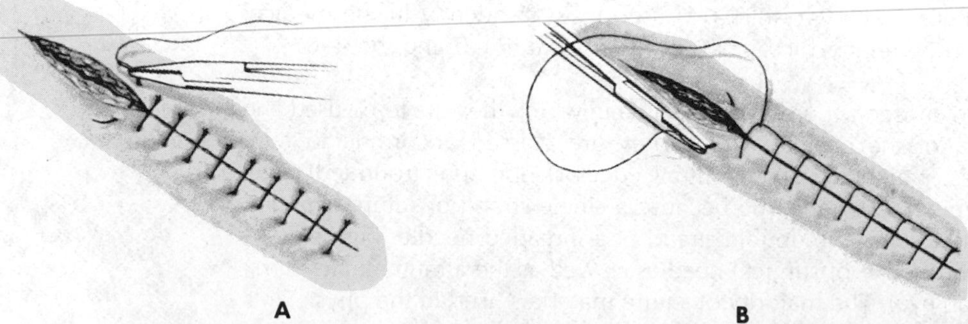

FIGURE 29–10 Types of skin closures. *A,* Interrupted technique. *B,* Continuous technique. (Courtesy of Ethicon, Inc.)

4. When appropriate, instruct the patient to wear special clothing that is easily removed and can be worn home over bulky dressings or a cast.

5. Always call the patient the day before the appointment to confirm special instructions.

POSTOPERATIVE INSTRUCTIONS. Consideration should be given to postoperative care, not only the immediate care but after the patient leaves the office.

1. Give the patient time to rest after the surgery. If a sedative was given, make certain the patient is sufficiently recovered to avoid injury to himself.

2. If the patient was given a topical or local anesthetic that will be wearing off, this should be explained to the patient. Check with the physician if a pain medication is to be prescribed.

3. Make certain the patient has all the necessary postoperative instructions. These instructions may include: (a) how to apply a compress, (b) elevation of a limb, (c) possibility of drainage if there is a drain in a wound, (d) the necessity of changing or not changing a dressing, and (e) taking any special medications. Complications could result from inadequate postoperative instructions.

4. Tell the patient when the physician wishes to see him again and make the next appointment.

5. Tell the patient the importance of calling the office if there are any changes or questions. If the patient does not call the office as requested, then the medical assistant should call the patient. Many patients will tend to "ride it out" or say they didn't want to bother you.

6. Never allow a patient to leave the office without the physician's knowledge.

POSITIONING THE PATIENT

Always remember to *have the patient disrobe sufficiently* to completely expose the area. There is too much risk of contamination in doing the procedure while either the medical assistant or the patient is holding back clothing that may slide over the area where the physician is working. Clothing held back may also act as a tourniquet or make it extremely difficult to apply a dressing or bandage properly. The patient's clothing may also be stained with the skin disinfecting solution, or prevent a very large area from being prepared properly.

It is equally important to *position the patient as comfortably as possible.* An uncomfortable position can be held for a limited time, and then the patient will have to move, often in the middle of a procedure. If bandaging is applied to an area with the patient in an awkward position, the bandage will bind or fit improperly when the patient assumes a normal position.

The medical assistant must *consider where the physician will be positioned* during the procedure, where the instruments will be placed, where the light source will be from, and where she will be positioned in order to assist the physician advantageously and observe the patient.

HANDWASHING

Washing the hands is the most effective means of preventing the spread of infection. The hands should be washed, using correct technique, before and after each patient. It is not necessary to do an extended scrub each time; only the first scrub in the morning is extensive. If a good surgical soap is used, it will leave a film of antiseptic that will last several hours on the skin, and a normal wash is sufficient during the remainder of the day, unless your hands become highly contaminated. It is not advisable to rinse your hands with alcohol because it will remove the residual antiseptic film left by the antiseptic soap, and alcohol is extremely drying to the skin. Buy good surgical soap that is gentle to the hands; the purchase of inexpensive surgical soaps is a false economy. Each sink in the office should be equipped with two dispensers; one with liquid surgical soap and the other with a good grade of hospital hand lotion. Dry cracked skin is a source of infection.

Running water and friction are the two main factors in proper hand washing;

surgical soap is of no value without these two. The water should be tepid, not hot. Water that is too hot or too cold is harmful to the skin and will cause chapping. Friction means the firm rubbing of *all* surfaces of the hands and forearms. The fingers should be interlaced and rubbed thoroughly. All jewelry except for a plain wedding band and engagement ring should be removed. Bracelets and costume jewelry are not worn in the medical office.

PROCEDURE. Wet the hands well and apply ample soap. Rub the soap around well with plenty of friction. Interlace the fingers and rub the finger sides well. Now start *up* the forearm by rubbing the wrists and on up the lower arm. Rinse well under running water by starting at the fingertips and working up the arms. Keep the hands held above the wrist level. If necessary, clean the fingernails with the blunt end of a toothpick. Repeat soaping and scrubbing. For general office procedure it is not necessary to scrub with a brush — good manual friction is sufficient. After the hands and arms have been rinsed well for the second time, blot them dry by starting at the hands and working upwards toward the elbows. Do not return down the arm. Use a fresh towel for each arm. Turn off the faucets with the used paper towel. It is advisable to use a good grade of paper towels that are gentle to the skin.

PHYSICIAN'S PREFERENCE FILE

It is advisable for the medical assistant to keep a file card for each special procedure done in the office. This is particularly necessary for seldom-done procedures or especially complicated ones. Even some routine procedures will require a card if there are several physicians in a medical group and each physician has a different preference for an instrument or numerous other considerations. These cards should be color-coded as patient's charts are often color-coded for the individual physicians in the group practice. A 5 by 8 card rather than the smaller 3 by 5 size is recommended. This file must be kept current. If, during a procedure, the physician changes a routine, make a note on the card after it has been discussed with the physician. It may be advisable to have the physician date and initial the change.

This card could contain such information as: special instruments used, medications, syringe and needle sizes, glove size, preoperative and postoperative instructions, and preferred time for follow-up check. With this card the medical assistant will not forget techniques and will not have to bother the physician for instructions each time.

PREPARING STERILE PACKS

Before making up a pack to be autoclaved, make absolutely certain you have checked and double checked all items needed. A file card for the procedure will be very helpful in this checking (See Physician's Preference File, as previously mentioned). If a rather complicated procedure is done often, a copy of this file card should be posted inside a cupboard door for quick reference. Wrap the contents according to the standard flap-back fold as shown in Figure 26–8. Label the contents, date, and initial. It is sometimes helpful to sterilize separately a pair of sterilizer forceps so a dry sterile instrument may be used to rearrange the instruments on the sterile field in the sequence they will be used. Towels that are to be used for drape are best autoclaved separately, usually one to a package. A limited amount of instruments may be autoclaved in the field drape towel, making the drape and instruments one package, but be careful when opening this pack not to contaminate it. Towels that are used for incision drapes may be autoclaved with two in a pack. Remember to fanfold all drapes so they may be opened with sterile technique.

It is often advantageous to use the presterilized disposable items whenever practical. Risks of cross-infection are minimal with these items. Most of the disposable drapes are made of a plastic material and are therefore nonabsorbable and are barrier drapes. Steri-Drapes* are available in several different materials and sizes, with and without apertures. They have the advantage over the fabric since they

*3-M, Medical Products Division, St. Paul, MN.

are more pliable and are nonabsorbable. The incisional drapes have an adhesive backing around the aperture to prevent slipping.

In many cases an entire setup may be autoclaved together such as the necessary instruments, sponges, dressings, suture materials, and syringe and needles. The only problem to this convenience is you must make certain all items are **thermostable**.

OBSERVING STERILE TECHNIQUE

Although the procedures outlined in this chapter are called minor surgery, all the sterile techniques of major surgery must be observed. The medical assistant must have a sound knowledge of sterility and sterile technique. The medical assistant should keep in mind the analogy that *everything sterile is white and everything that is nonsterile is black, and there is no gray*. It should be remembered that air currents carry bacteria, so body motions, coughing and talking over the area should be kept at a minimum. Hands and hair are the two greatest sources of contamination. Hands should be washed very carefully and often. Hair that is allowed to fall free over the shoulders and forward will give a cloud of bacteria; it must be held back. The habit of brushing hair off the face with your hands is a constant source of contamination.

With self-discipline, the medical assistant must learn what may be touched with the hands and what must be touched only with sterile forceps or sterile gloved hands. Sterile transfer forceps are used only to touch sterile items. Remember these transfer forceps must be kept sterile by proper use and by keeping the sterilizing solution fresh and the container filled. Never turn transfer forceps upside down; keep the tips pointing down. By turning them upside down the solution will run into a nonsterile area and then back down over the sterile tips, thus contaminating the forceps. Transfer forceps are wet so this offers a problem in some procedures. They may be dried by touching a piece of sterile gauze.

This moisture is another problem in sterile technique. Moisture acts as a capillary; that is, it is drawn up from underneath and brings along particles with it. This will happen when a sterile dry towel is placed on a surgical field where there is a drop of moisture. The towel surface is no longer sterile. It will remain sterile only as long as it is dry. This cannot happen when the sterile field drape is nonabsorbable. These *barrier* drapes are made of plastic or a plastic-backed nonabsorbable material.

Sterile field drapes as well as surgical drapes are fan-folded in order that they may be opened without touching the sterile surfaces that must remain sterile. When opening a pack be careful to lift each flap of the wrapper by reaching under the small folded back tab and therefore, not touching the contents or the inner surface. If the wrap does not have a tab then the flap is pulled back by pinching (Fig. 29–11).

Prepackaged sterile disposable items in the peel-apart packaging such as syringe and needles, suture needles, and suture material should be opened by pulling the flaps apart and dropping the contents in the sterile field from a distance of at least 12 in. Be careful you do not touch the contents. Packs that are not peel-apart but folded with the four flaps as shown in Figure 26–8 require that the first flap be opened away from you. The side flaps are each pulled away, while you make sure not to reach across the contents. This may be done by reaching under the pack or changing hands if you are holding the pack. The last flap is pulled toward you, exposing the contents. Take care the flaps do not touch the sterile field when the contents are dropped on the field. Do not open the packs over the field, but off to the side. If the pack is large, it may be best to place it on a clean dry surface and follow the same sequence to open the flaps. Handling sterile items requires a degree of dexterity and vigilance.

When lifting the lid off a jar containing sterile items, the lid is lifted straight up and then a little to one side, keeping the lid faced down. Do not turn the lid over. The contents are removed by reaching straight in and not touching the sides of the container (Fig. 29–12). If the lid *must* be placed on the counter then place it upside down, taking care not to touch the inside surface. Do not talk over an open container, and do not leave the container open for any length of time.

Important Steps	Key Points
8. Place the sterile item on a sterile field.	Be sure your hand is underneath the sterile wrapper so that the contents remain sterile when being transferred to a sterile field.

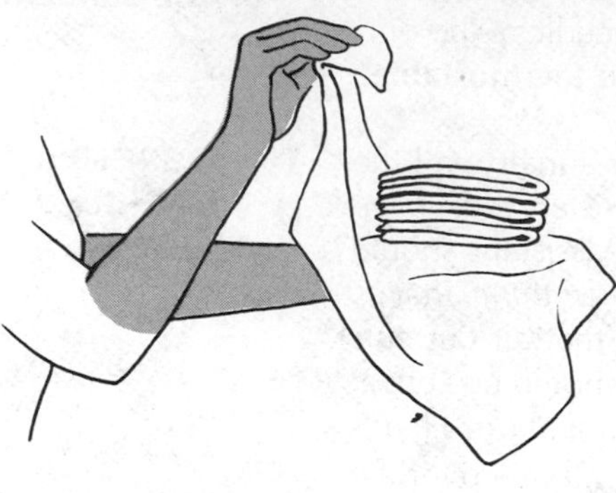

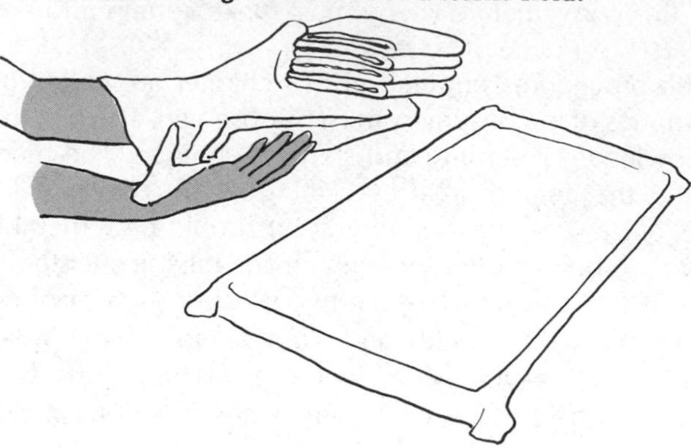

9. Or hand the item to someone in the sterile field.

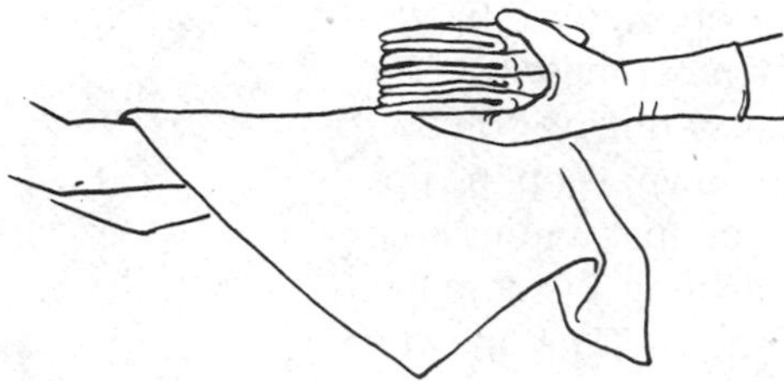

FIGURE 29–11 Holding open a sterile pack. (From Wood, L. A., and Rambo, B. J.: *Nursing Skills for Allied Health Services*, volume 3. Philadelphia, W. B. Saunders Co., 1980.)

When pouring from a bottle place your hand over the label and pour away from the label. If the container does not have a double cap as shown in Figure 26–10, then pour off a small amount of the solution into the sink in order to rinse the bottle lip and pour the amount desired into a sterile medicine glass or iodine cup. Pour directly above at least 8 in. Never rest the neck of a bottle on the rim of the container into which you are pouring the solution.

When handing sterile items to the physician, pick up the items with the sterile forceps so they may be handed to the physician with the handle first as shown in Figure 29–13.

Remember: *Sterile is white . . . non-sterile is black . . . and there is no gray.* Hands, hair, and air currents cause contamination. Never allow a sterile item to go

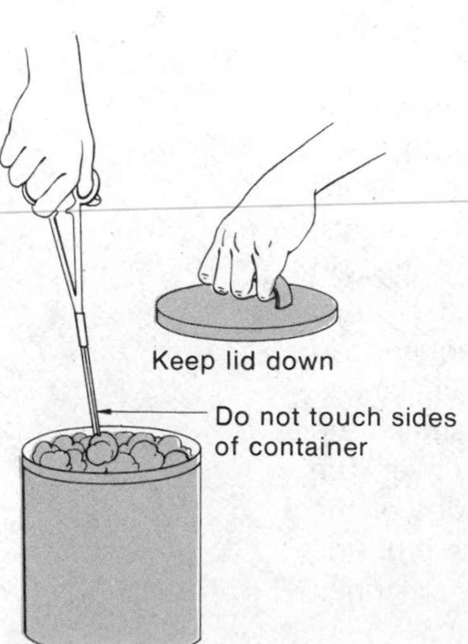

FIGURE 29–12 Entering sterile dressing jar with lid. (After Sutton, A. L.: *Bedside Nursing Techniques in Medicine and Surgery*. 2nd ed. Philadelphia, W. B. Saunders Co., 1969.)

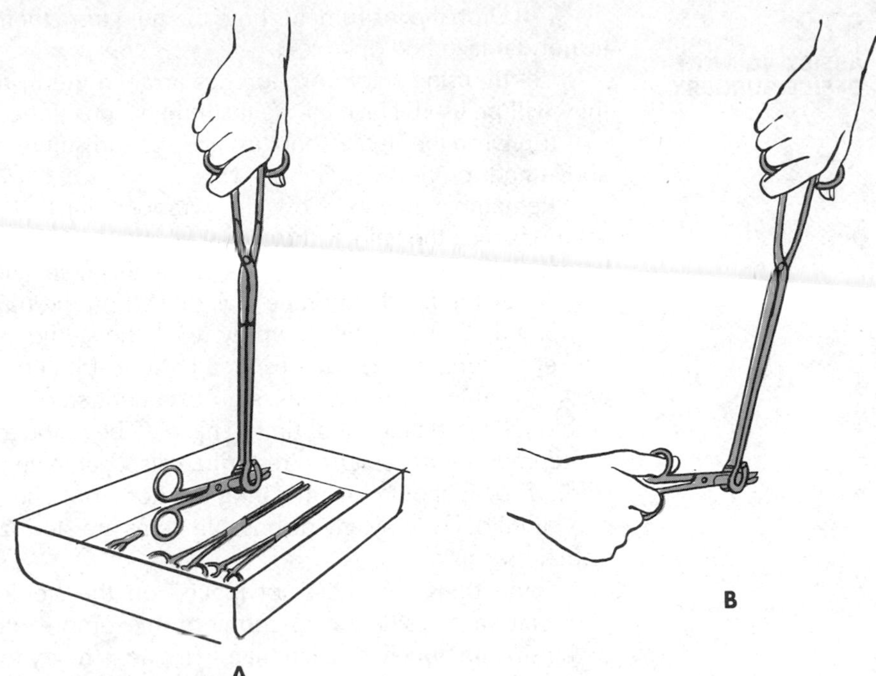

FIGURE 29–13 Handling sterile instruments with sterile forceps. (From Sutton, A. L.: *Bedside Nursing Techniques in Medicine and Surgery*. 2nd ed. Philadelphia, W. B. Saunders Co., 1969.)

below your waist level. Consider all opened or damaged packs as contaminated. There is no mystery about sterile technique; it is only a matter of reasoning and planning with self-discipline and honesty.

SETTING UP THE STERILE FIELD

This technique has such a wide range of possibilities that it is impossible to give every example, but common sense and reasoning are the guides for what will be needed for each procedure and how that particular setup will be done.

GENERAL PROCEDURE

(1) Clean the tray surface with a **germicide** and dry it thoroughly with a piece of sterile gauze or allow it to evaporate dry.

(2) Drop the sterile field drape from its wrapper on to the cleaned surface.

(3) Use a sterile forceps, or by touching the corners only, spread out the drape. Do not reach across the field. Do not touch the inner sterile area of the drape in any way.

29

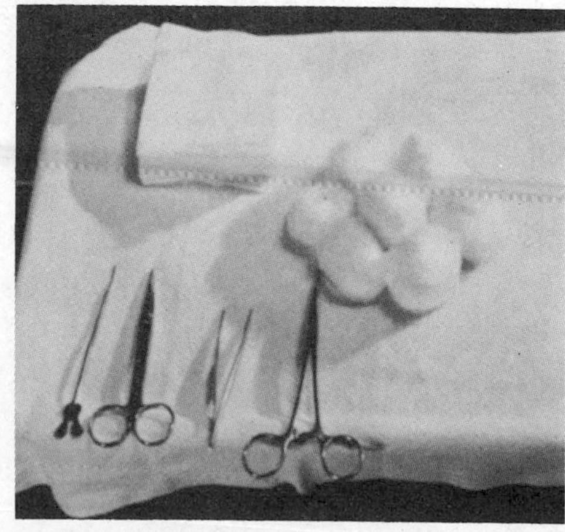

FIGURE 29–14 Sterile instruments and sponges on sterile field. (From Ochsner, A., and DeBakey, M. E.: *Christopher's Minor Surgery*. 8th ed. Philadelphia, W. B. Saunders Co., 1959.)

(4) Drop the instruments onto the field from their wrapper, handles first in order to not damage fine tips.

(5) By using sterile dry forceps arrange the instruments in the order in which they will be used. Have all the instruments positioned in one direction (Fig. 29–14).

(6) Drop the sterile sponges, gloves, and suture materials from peel-aparts from above and to one side (Fig. 29–15).

Remember not to allow the wrapper flaps to touch the field. Do not pour solutions over the field as there may be splashing of droplets. If there may be a delay before the procedure starts, then cover the field with a sterile drape in the same manner as the first field drape was placed on the tray.

Small fields may be set up by using the sterile inside of a wrapper, such as the packet of sterile gauze squares, or a basic instrument setup such as a suture removal pack. An autoclave tray makes an excellent sterile field if the setup is to be used within a limited amount of time. This may be autoclaved as shown in Figure 25–15. Sometimes it is necessary to resterilize disposable items in order to have them on the sterile field without contaminating the item, but check first that the disposable item can be autoclaved. Many disposable items are sterilized by gas and are not thermostable.

Some things are best not placed on the sterile field but are handed to the physician from a side tray or counter. An example may be sterile gloves placed next to the sink and opened when the physician is ready to don them. Extra dressings and sponges may be unopened but ready to be dropped on the field. If the physician is already gloved it is not possible for him to pick up a multiple dose vial and fill a syringe with a local anesthetic. This is best done by the medical assistant cleansing

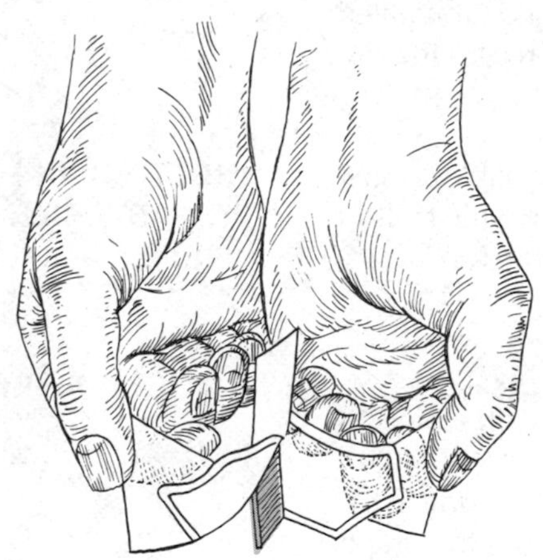

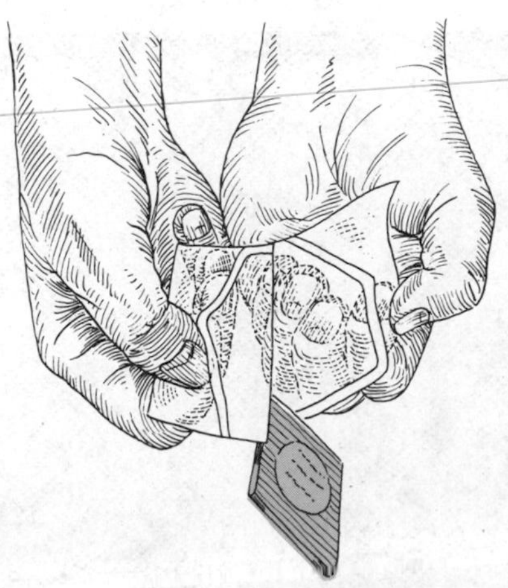

FIGURE 29–15 Dropping sterile suture from outer package onto the sterile field. Do not touch inner package.

the vial stopper, showing the physician the label, holding the bottle securely with both hands while the physician enters the vial and withdraws the desired amount of solution. With this technique the physician does not contaminate his gloves or the sterile syringe and needle that has been dropped on the field from a peel-apart package. The medical assistant may fill the syringe with the local anesthetic if the physician injects the anesthetic before the sterile gloves are donned.

Before the physician is notified that everything is ready, the medical assistant should quickly "walk through" the procedure with her imagination in order to make certain everything is available and ready.

PREPARING THE PATIENT'S SKIN FOR SURGERY

The human skin is a reservoir of bacteria. These bacteria are basically in one of two groups: *transit bacteria* that may be washed off with friction and running water and *resident bacteria,* sometimes called **commensal bacteri**, that reside in the pores and glands of the skin. These resident organisms canno be removed or completely destroyed, therefore, the *skin cannot be sterilized.* As a rule these resident organisms are not harmful to their host, whereas the transit bacteria may be harmful. It is because of these harmful bacteria that every care must be given to cleanse the patient's skin as thoroughly as possible. This procedure is called "skin prep." A good skin prep eliminates as much as possible the transference of harmful organisms to the incision site.

As mentioned earlier in preoperative instructions, some patients may have been instructed to cleanse the area with **bacteriostatic** or **antiseptic** soap several days before the surgery. Sometimes a patient may be asked to shave the area immediately before coming to the office.

Skin Preparation

Materials needed:
- Towels
- Basins
- Germicidal detergent
- Sterile gauze squares
- Sterile sponges
- Sponge forceps
- Skin disinfectant solution or presaturated pads
- Scissors or shaving equipment

Most of the above supplies will depend on the extent and the location of the procedure. Frequently, skin preparation items may be kept on the side counter and a field setup is not necessary. One of the dangers of skin preparation is not cleansing with sufficient friction and not covering a large enough area. A detergent is superior to a fatty base soap since it aids in the removal of the natural skin oils, thereby allowing the disinfecting solution to penetrate further into the skin. Friction rubbing will aid in the removal of the **desquamated cells**.

When the patient arrives at the office, check if the preoperative instructions were followed such as cleansing the area or taking a special medication. Have the patient void. After the patient has disrobed and been properly positioned, place sufficient toweling under the area and cleanse again, if indicated. If the area is to be shaved, this is done now. A wet shave is preferred because there is less danger of nicks and the moisture prevents the minute hairs from blowing around. Rinse the area again and blot dry with a sterile gauze. Some physicians prefer not rinsing but blotting off the soap with a sterile gauze. The residual soap film aids in the diffusion of the skin antiseptic next applied. Now paint the area with the skin disinfectant using cotton applicators, presaturated pads, or sponges. Starting in the center of the site circle outwards, not circling back over the area. If indicated, repeat the disinfection using fresh sponges and solution. Be sure to prepare a large enough area to go beyond the opening of the surgical drape that is next applied.

BASIC SURGICAL SETUPS

Since there are so many different office surgical procedures and setups and since each physician has individual preferences, this book will not attempt to list all the specific items for each specific technique. The following setups will not include the general instructions for preparation of the patient, such as disrobing, emptying the bladder, positioning, and skin preparation, unless there is something particular to that procedure. Nor will bandaging and dressing be explained unless there are unique needs. Remember to check the Physician's Preference File for unique needs and procedures.

Changing a Dressing

Materials needed:
- Sterile dressing forceps (2)
- Bandage scissors
- Gloves
- Towels
- Dressings
- Tape
- Bandages
- Medication
- Hydrogen peroxide

The above supplies must be handy, though it is not always necessary to set up a special field area. But remember, you cannot reach into a container or cupboard after you have touched a wound.

Check the patient's medical record and follow the physician's instructions carefully. Have the patient disrobe sufficiently to expose the area and place the patient in a comfortable position with the area to be dressed well supported. Arrange sufficient toweling under the area. If the wound is infectious, you should wear gloves to handle the contaminated dressings; otherwise, use the "no-touch technique" by using dressing forceps. Do not ask the patient to look at the wound. Be careful not to reveal any unpleasant reactions, either by your comments or facial expressions.

Cut off the bandage with bandage scissors; do not unwind a roller bandage unless it is a reusable elastic. When taking off a reusable elastic keep it gathered in your hands and close in to the patient; do not allow it to fly around. Do not return the bandage scissors to your pocket without disinfecting first. Cut tape next to the dressing. Always remove tape by pulling *toward* the wound. If the old dressing is adhered to the wound it may have to be soaked off with hydrogen peroxide or sterile saline. *Do not pull off a dressing that is stuck to a wound.* Sometimes it is advisable to leave old tape on, if it is adhering well, and place the new tape directly over the old. Frequent changes and pulling off tape can make a patient's skin very tender.

Place the removed dressing directly into a container or covered receptacle. Do not leave a soiled dressing on the dressing tray or countertop within view of the patient. It is contaminated material (Table 29–1). Cleanse the area and the wound by gently blotting with sterile gauze. It may be necessary to use hydrogen peroxide or sterile saline for cleansing. Surgical soap may also be used, if indicated. Avoid using cotton because it will adhere to **granulation tissue**.

If there is any question as to the type of fresh dressing to be used, consult the physician. Also, if the wound appears not to be healing properly or if there is any abnormal change, the physician should be consulted and his instructions carefully followed.

Work from a dressing tray or the counter where fresh supplies have been assembled. Apply any necessary medications, taking care that the wound is completely and evenly covered. Sprays and powders do not present a problem, but ointments are more difficult to apply if not in a presaturated gauze pad. Do not spread an ointment directly on a wound. Using a sterile tongue depressor, spread the ointment evenly on a sterile gauze square, being careful not to contaminate the dressing or the medication. Make certain you have covered a larger area than the wound. Secure the dressing with tape, and do not let the tape touch the wound in

TABLE 29–1 Contamination While Dressing a Wound

Sources	Prevention
Mechanical	
Hands and instruments	Dress one wound at a time Use instruments whenever possible to handle items Keep sterile items separate from contaminated items
Environmental	
Air currents from windows, moving drapes, and leaning over field	Keep moisture to a minimum Move drapes slowly and keep low over area Avoid passing over wound area; work from the side Avoid leaning over sterile field
Personal	
Talking, coughing, hair falling forward	Keep hair under control Avoid talking and coughing, or wear surgical mask

any way. Apply an outer dressing or bandage if necessary. Take great care that the dressing and bandages are even in pressure and that any splint or support does not cause needless pressure on one given area. An improper bandage can do considerable harm.

Be certain you recorded the dressing change accurately in the patient's medical record. In addition to the date, the entry should include how much discharge there was on the old dressing, the condition of the wound (**purulent** matter, granulation tissue, etc.), what medication was applied, and when the patient is to return.

Suture Setup

If an emergency patient arrives in the office with a pressure dressing over a laceration, do not remove the pressure dressing until the physician is ready to suture. If the patient's pressure cloth *must* be removed, have ample sterile dressings ready to apply immediately. Ask the patient the possible length, depth, and exact location of the laceration. Usually there is limited cleansing of a wound because of the bleeding. If not, let the physician instruct you on the necessary cleansing.

On the side:
- Local anesthetic
- Dressings and bandages
- Splints or guards
- Tape
- Drape

Sterile field:
- Gloves
- Syringe and needle
- Hemostats (3)
- Scissors
- Sponges
- Suture material and needle
- Tissue forceps or skin hook
- Needle holder

The needle and syringe used will depend on the area and depth to be injected for local anesthesia. This same factor will determine the size of the suture material and needle used. Frequently, clean lacerations in a moderately protected area will not be dressed but left open. The patient will be instructed to keep the area clean and dry. Some lacerations may be closed with adhesive strips. These are becoming increasingly popular, since they reduce the chance of infection and do not leave suture scars.

TO APPLY SUTURELESS CLOSURES (STERI-STRIPS — 3M COMPANY)

1. Clean and dry skin at least $2\frac{1}{2}$ inches around the wound, making sure to remove skin oil and exudates. A light spray of skin tackifier or tincture of benzoin may be applied (Fig. 29–16*A*).

2. Peel open the package of closures and remove the end tab to facilitate strip removal.

3. At midportion of the incision apply one-half (one side) up to the edge of the incision and press firmly into place. Now appose the skin edges exactly together using fingers or forceps. Now press the free half of the strip firmly into place (Fig. 29–16*B*).

4. On larger wounds the closures may be applied at alternate spaces (Fig. 29–16*C*) Always be very careful that the skin edges are smoothly approximated. Then return and apply strips in the spaces to give a smooth even closure. Strips should be about $\frac{1}{4}$ inch apart.

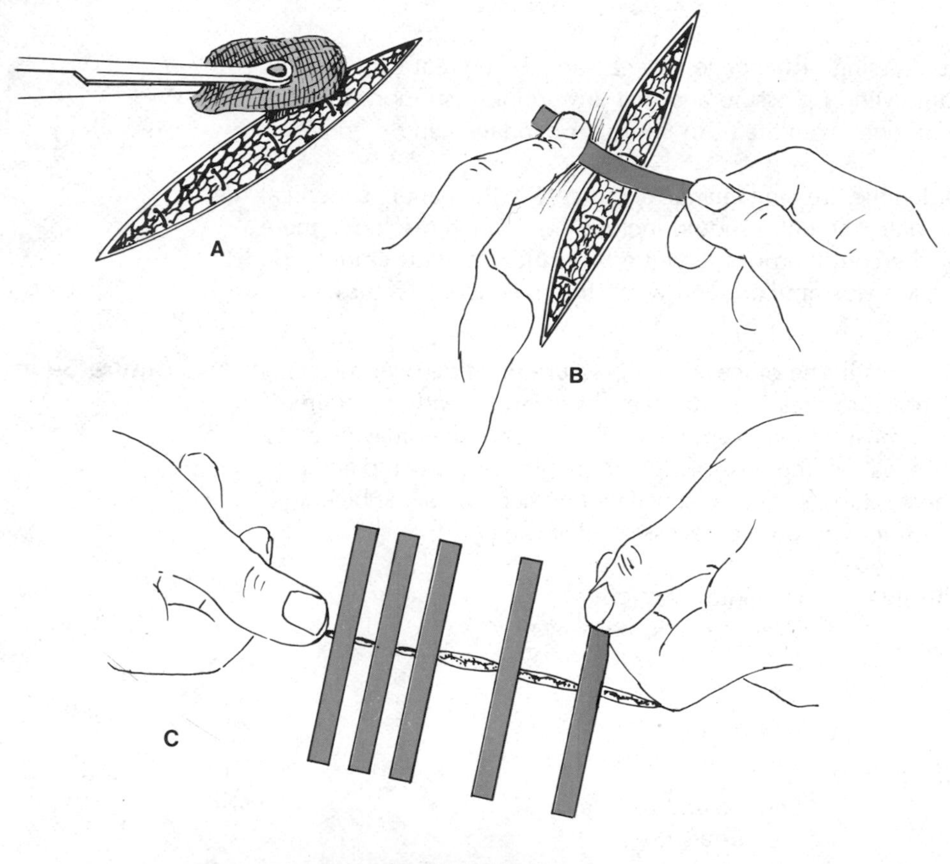

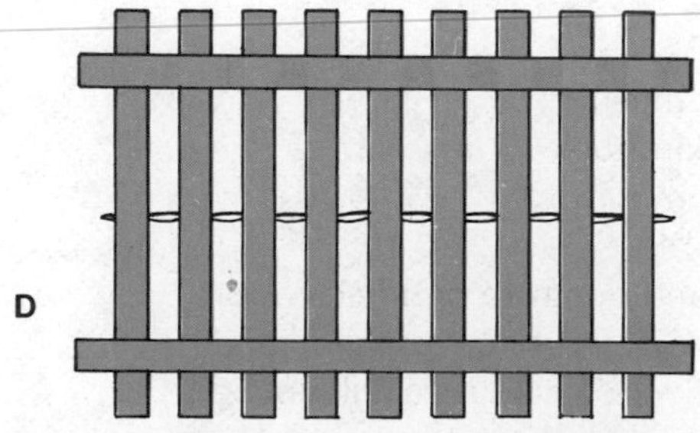

FIGURE 29–16 Steri-Strip skin closures. *A,* Cleansing the wound. *B,* Affixing Steri-Strip at midpoint of wound. *C,* Applying Steri-Strip on a larger wound, filling in spaces. *D,* Finishing with strips applied parallel to wound for strength.

5. Apply additional closures approximately ½ to ¾ inch parallel with the incision to give added strength (Fig. 29–16*D*).

Suture Removal

There is a great variety of cutting instruments used for suture removal. Some individuals prefer a plain Bard-Parker disposable blade, whereas others may use Littauer stitch scissors, iris scissors, or general operating scissors.

First remove the dressing carefully. If the dressing is stuck to the incision, *do not pull the dressing off*. Hydrogen peroxide may be used to soak the dressing off, but do not oversoak. Sometimes it is best to clip the dressing off as close as possible to the incision. The area may be disinfected and blotted dry immediately with a sterile gauze pad if it does not appear clean.

To remove a stitch, grasp the knot of the suture with the dressing forceps and cut the suture as nearly as possible at skin level. Now extract the stitch by *pulling toward* the incision. By pulling toward the incision there is not the danger of opening the incision and there is less discomfort to the patient. Butterflies or Steri-Strip closures may be placed over the incision area to give support and strength. When removing these tape closures later, always pull each end of the closure strip toward the incision line.

Materials needed:
- Dressing forceps (6 in.)
- Sterile cutting blade or scissors
- Skin antiseptic
- Sterile sponges
- Skin closures

The patient may be cautioned to keep the area clean and dry and to not place excess strain on the area.

Needle Biopsy

A biopsy is the examination of tissue removed from the living body. Biopsies are usually done to determine whether a growth or swelling is malignant or benign; however, it may be done as a diagnostic aid in other diseases or infections. A needle biopsy may be done by aspiration with a needle and syringe or by a special biopsy needle. The specimen is then sent to a pathologist for either a cytologic or histologic examination. (See Chapter 31 on Specimen Collection.)

On the side:
- Specimen bottle with sufficient fixative or preserving solution
- Laboratory form and label
- Local anesthetic

On the sterile field:
- Gloves
- Biopsy needle
- Syringe and needle
- Sponges

Usually there is no special dressing required after a needle biopsy. A Band-Aid is often sufficient.

Abdominal Paracentesis

This is the insertion of a trocar into the peritoneal cavity for the removal of excessive fluids. The patient is instructed to empty his bladder. With the lower abdomen exposed, the patient is placed in a well supported sitting position. The skin just below the umbilicus is cleansed, and a local anesthetic is injected. A small incision is made to aid in the insertion of the trocar. The amount and character of the fluid obtained is recorded and the fluid saved if the physician requests it. Use sufficient towels under the buttocks and catch-basin

On the side:	Measuring vessel Local anesthetic Extra sponges Skin antiseptic solution Specimen bottle with label Laboratory form
On the sterile field:	Gloves Trocar Drain tube for trocar Syringe and needle Sponges Knife with #11 or #15 blade

After the paracentesis, a small sterile dressing or a large Band-Aid is placed over the puncture site.

Cyst Removal

A sebaceous cyst is a benign retention cyst of a sebaceous gland containing fatty substance of the gland. It is also called a wen. They may occur any place on the body with the exception of the palms of the hands and the soles of the feet. They are more common on the neck and shoulder and because they are frequently the source of irritation, they are removed. Ordinarily the cyst is attached only to the skin and moves freely over the underlying tissue. For cosmetic reasons the physician will

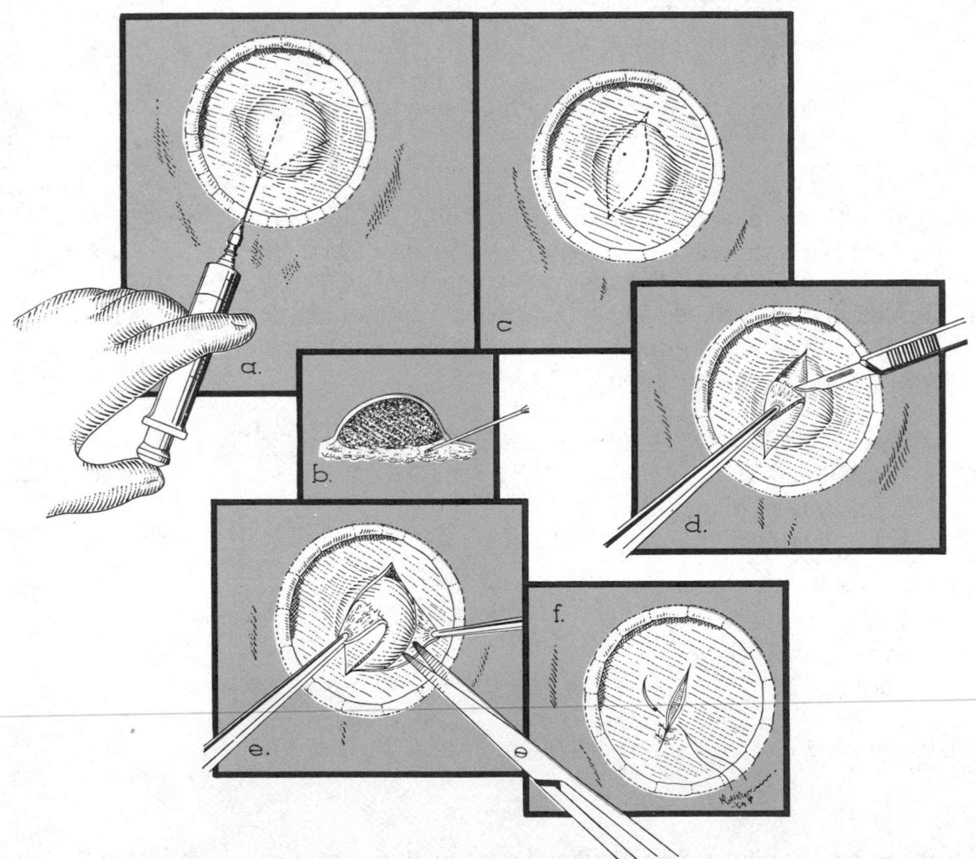

FIGURE 29–17 Drawing showing technique of excision of sebaceous cysts or wens. *a* and b, Infiltration of the tissues surrounding the cyst is performed with procaine hydrochloride 0.5 per cent solution. c and *d,* An elliptical incision is made over the cyst to remove a small segment of skin including the puncta. e, Using the attached ellipse of skin for traction purposes the cyst is removed intact if possible. *f,* Bleeding points are controlled with fine catgut ligatures, and the skin incision is closed with nonabsorbable sutures. (From Ochsner, A., and DeBakey, M. E.: *Christopher's Minor Surgery*. 8th ed. Philadelphia, W. B. Saunders Co., 1959.)

make the incision on the natural skin crease lines. Figure 29–17 illustrates the procedure.

On the side:	Local anesthetic Disinfectant (skin prep) Laboratory form Dressing, size depends on site
On the sterile field:	Gloves Drape Kelly hemostats: 2 str. and 2 cvd. Dressing forceps (2) Suture and needle Scissors s/s or s/b Dissector (physician's choice) Skin hook Syringe and needle Knife handle with blade #11 or #15 Tissue forceps (2) Allis forceps Needle holder Sponges Coagulant gel (physician's choice)

Draining an Abscess

An **abscess** is a localized collection of pus in a cavity formed by the disintegration of tissue. Abscesses may appear in any part of the body. **"Furuncle,"** "boil," and **"carbuncle"** are names applied to different types of abscesses. In most abscesses pyogenic cocci, usually staphylococci, are found, but it is not uncommon to find secondary organisms. The treatment for abscesses, other than those on the face, is usually incision and drainage. Because of the infectious organisms, extreme caution should be taken in handling the contaminated materials and instruments.

On the side:	Wax or plastic bag for contaminants Extra sponges Medications Skin antiseptic Bandages Ethyl chloride spray Extra applicators
On the sterile field:	Gloves Hemostats (2) Probe Scissors Abscess needle (physician's choice) Gauze stripping, iodoform Knife handle with blade #15 Dressing forceps (2) Sponges Dressing

The physician may choose to inject a local anesthetic if the abscess is deep rather than use the ethyl chloride to "freeze" the area. The medical assistant may cut the length of gauze stripping for packing at the physician's request. When dressing the area, several layers of gauze sponges should be placed over the abscess opening, especially if a drain has been inserted, and the gauze anchored with bandage. Frequently a patient is instructed to apply warm moist packs for a couple of days. Daily dressing changes may also be indicated because of the copious drainage.

Joint Aspiration and Injection

This procedure may be done in order to obtain synovial fluid for analysis or to inject an antiinflammatory medication. This fluid is obtained from any swollen joint such as a knee, elbow, hip, or shoulder. After aspiration the physician may remove the aspirating syringe and attach a syringe filled with a medication such as cortisone to be injected intraarticularly.

On the side:	Sterile specimen tubes with label and lab form Dressing (usually a Band-Aid is sufficient) Local anesthetic Ethyl chloride Medication Skin disinfectant
On the sterile field:	Syringe and needle for local anesthetic 20 cc aspirating syringe 18–20 g needle for aspirating (length depends on site) Syringe for medication (needle is removed after syringe is filled with medication) Drape Gauze dressings (3 in. by 3 in.)

Postoperative instructions to the patient may be complete rest of the limb, heat, and medication. The patient may have to be instructed on the use of crutches if a knee is involved.

Thrombotic Hemorrhoid Incision

Hemorrhoids are varicosities, enlarged veins, within or just outside the rectum. They are usually caused by straining during stool evacuation or pressure from internal organs, such as the uterus during pregnancy. Ideally the patient should be placed in the proctological position and well supported by the table or a Procto Board. If this is not possible, then the lateral Sims' position or the knee-chest (or knee-elbow) position may be used. If the latter is used, the patient must have assistance in maintaining this uncomfortable position. The anal area is thoroughly, and gently, cleansed with soap, water, and cotton and then dried and painted with an antiseptic solution. The buttocks may be spread apart with 3 in. bands of adhesive tape.

On the side:	Local anesthetic, injectable and topical
On the sterile field:	Gloves Coagulant foam or gel Knife handle with blade Ample sponges Hemostat, mosquito (2) str. and (2) cvd. Surgical gut for possible ligation Scissors Padding material rolled or small roll of crepe roller bandage

The physician may prefer to use electrosurgical **cautery** for the bleeding. After the blood clot is removed, the padding is placed against the anus and the buttocks are released and taped together.

Urethral Dilation

This is done for the purpose of expanding or enlarging the urethral meatus. The female patient is placed in the lithotomy position. The male patient is in a dorsal recumbent position. Check the patient's record for the size dilators needed.

On the side: Basin
Specimen bottle for urine
Topical anesthetic jelly or solution
Antiseptic solution
Laboratory form

On the sterile field: Gloves
Disposable catheter set
Sponges
Urethral sounds

Toenail Resection

Ingrown toenails are usually the result of incorrect footwear or too short hosiery. Cutting the toenail corners back too far also contributes to this very painful condition. Severely ingrown nail must be removed surgically. This is usually done in the hospital but can be done in the office. The patient is placed in a semi-sitting position with the back and foot well supported. The toe is shaved and thoroughly cleansed.

On the side: Extra sponges
Local anesthetic, injectable
Local anesthetic, topical

On the sterile field: Knife handle with #10 blade
Heavy hemostats (2) str.
Needle holder
Scissors s/s
Sterile rubber bands
Suture and needle
Gloves
Syringe and needle

A special nonadhesive dressing is used over the site. A silk or Teflon dressing is preferred along with petroleum gauze or topical anesthetic ointment. The patient may be instructed to keep the foot elevated for a couple of days.

Plaster Cast Application

The application of a plaster cast to set a simple fracture is frequently done in the medical office. The comfort of the patient and the skill of the physician are greatly dependent on the help of a competent medical assistant. It is essential that she follow the physician's directions exactly, especially in holding the patient in the exact position he requests. Do not hold up the limb by pulling on the stockinette as this will distort the stockinette and may cause a crease. She must also know the warning signs of a cast's becoming too tight so that proper care can be given before permanent damage is done.

Materials needed: Stockinette
Plaster roller bandages
Splint or guard
Adhesive tape
Marking pencil
Pail of tepid water 95 to 105° F
Sheet wadding or cast padding
Cast cutter
Cast knife
Bandage scissors
Felt or sponge padding
Patient's x-ray in viewer

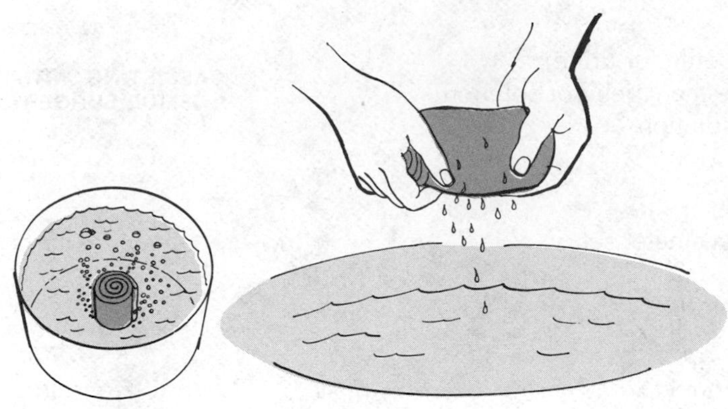

FIGURES 29–18 Wetting a plaster roll. (From Sutton, A. L.: *Bedside Nursing Techniques in Medicine and Surgery*. 2nd ed. Philadelphia, W. B. Saunders Co., 1969.)

The patient is placed in a comfortable position with the arm or leg completely exposed. Be very careful in moving the patient. If the clothing is cut off, try to cut on a seam so the garment can be repaired. Protect the patient with a sheet or plastic drape. Cleanse the area as the physician directs. This is important because a cast is usually on for some period of time, and skin rashes may occur. Measure the stockinette and allow at least two inches above AND below the needed length. If the physician instructs the medical assistant to dip the plaster rolls in water, they are dipped into the water vertically and then held horizontally. Bubbles will rise as the roll becomes saturated. (Instructions will be on the plaster roll package). The roll is then held horizontally between the palms of the two hands, and the excess water is expelled by a slight twist of the wrists (Fig. 29–18).

Unroll the end of the bandage about two inches and hand it to the physician. Because plaster starts to set very rapidly, the medical assistant must pace herself with the physician.

Plaster warms slightly as it sets, so tell the patient to anticipate this, but it will not get hot. The physician will trim the cast and turn the stockinette down over the edges and secure it with tape. He may date it and draw where the fracture is located. The cast should be supported with a pillow to prevent any strain and change in shape while it is drying. Instruct the patient to avoid any pressure on the cast for 24 hours. Do not hasten the drying by heat because the cast will dry from the outside inward with a resulting musty odor. When the cast is dry it will be white and shiny and will sound resonant when it is tapped.

The patient is instructed to watch for any signs of constricture such as numbness, tingling, heat or cold, and disturbances in the circulation such as undue swelling or change in color of the limb to white or bluish.

Some of the new porous honeycomb cast materials are much easier for the patient to care for. The patient may bathe and even go swimming with them because they dry quite readily but still give the same support as the plaster cast.

Cervical Biopsy

This is the examination of the tissue removed from the cervical area of the uterus. A biopsy is usually done to determine whether there is a **malignancy** present. It is also a diagnostic aid in diagnosing other diseases. If the Papanicolaou smear test is positive, it is usually confirmed by a cervical biopsy. The patient is placed in the lithotomy position with a towel under the buttocks.

On the side:
- Specimen bottle 10% formalin with label
- Laboratory form
- Skin antiseptic solution

On the sterile field:
- Gloves
- Vaginal speculum
- Uterine dressing forceps (2)
- Cervical biopsy punch
- Coagulant foam or gel
- Sponges
- Uterine tenaculum
- Vaginal tampon or packing

Since the cervix is devoid of nerve endings that would respond to cutting and burning stimuli, there is very little discomfort. Postbiopsy bleeding may be controlled by the application of a coagulant gel or foam, or the physician may choose to lightly cauterize the area. The physician may also choose to remove a piece of tissue by means of electrical conization.

Cervical **polyps** are frequently encountered, especially in women nearing menopause. They are **asymptomatic** and are usually removed in the medical office. The procedure is basically the same as for a cervical biopsy. The pedicle of the polyp is seized with a uterine sponge forceps and cut off with a blade or uterine polyp forceps. The removed polyp is then sent to the pathologist for a histologic examination.

CERVICAL CONIZATION. Electrosurgical therapy is used frequently in the gynecologist's office, especially for disorders of the cervix. The patient may be instructed to take daily douches for a specified period of time before the treatment. A **conization** is usually done about one week after menstruation in order to permit the cervix to heal before the onset of the next period.

The patient is placed in the lithotomy position and the instrument set-up is the same as for the routine pelvic examination. The physician may request the addition of plastic vaginal speculum, vaginal pack, or tampon, ¼ or ½ in. gauze stripping for packing, and a medication.

If the dispersing plate is used, it may be placed on the patient's abdomen and held in place with a sandbag or the patient's hands; frequently it is placed under the

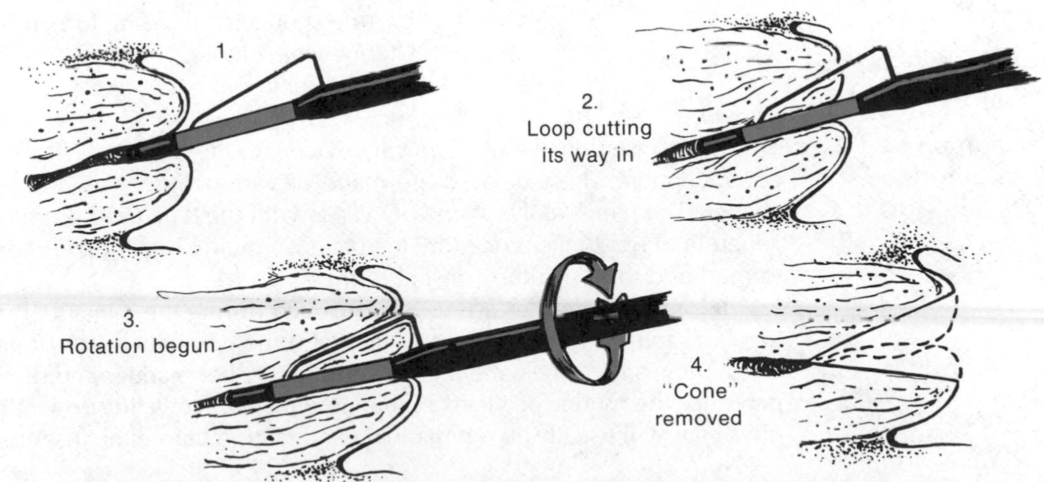

FIGURE 29–19 Cervical conization. (Drawn by Patric Claiborne, Courtesy of Medical Art Section, Medical Center of Washington, D.C.; from Otto, J. F., Jr. (ed.); *Principles of Minor Electrosurgery*. Liebel-Flarsheim Co., 1957.)

sacral area of the patient's back. A conductive or coupling gel is applied generously and evenly to the plate, and the patient's bare skin is contacted with the plate.

After the vaginal speculum is inserted the physician will cleanse the vaginal and cervical areas with a mild disinfectant. The cervical os must be free of any discharge or mucus. A topical or local anesthetic is sometimes used; a cocaine solution is the most commonly used. This solution is applied to the cervical area by soaking a cotton applicator with cocaine and leaving it in the cervical os for about ten minutes. Some patients may be given a mild sedation before coming to the office.

Postoperative care varies with the patient's needs and with the physician. Some physicians insert a vaginal tampon with or without a medication. Sometimes a gauze strip is packed into the cervical os and may be removed after 24 hours to a few days. The medical assistant should ask the physician before the procedure is done so the correct items are ready before the procedure. Antiseptic douches are sometimes prescribed after the packing and tampon have been removed. The patient is given an appointment in a week or two in order for the physician to pass a small uterine sound or dilator into the cervical os to check for **patency** of the cervical canal.

Gynecologic Pack

A pack is a dressing or similar material that is inserted into a body opening or cavity, usually to control bleeding and to hold medication in a given area. A cervical or gynecologic pack may be inserted following cervical surgery. The patient is in the lithotomy position with a towel under the buttocks. The routine pelvic examination instruments are ready for use with the addition of a vaginal pack or tampon, uterine dressing forceps, uterine sponge forceps, medication glass, and medication. Explain to the patient that a pack has been inserted and relay any instruction from the physician. These instructions may advise her when to remove the pack, and whether she is to take a specific type of douche. Remember to give the patient a sanitary pad if there is an excess of medication on the pack.

Insertion of Laminaria

This is the insertion of a small piece of dried seaweed (kelp) about the size of a matchstick. It is inserted into the cervical canal just prior to menses. As the laminaria absorbs moisture it will expand and thus dilate the cervix.

The patient is prepared for the routine pelvic examination with the usual setup. In addition to the routine instrument setup the following instruments are placed on a sterile field:

Sterile setup:
- Uterine sound
- Uterine dilator
- Uterine sponge or dressing forceps
- Uterine tenaculum
- Scissors, long, cvd.

Insertion of Intrauterine Device (IUD)

This is the insertion of a mechanical device into the uterine cavity for the purpose of contraception. These devices are made of various materials and come in various shapes. The effective life of an IUD varies with the type used, from one to two years generally. Prior to the procedure the patient should be given the information booklet to read and then sign the consent form.

Intrauterine devices are usually inserted during the menstrual period since the cervix is somewhat dilated at this time and the possibility of existing undetermined pregnancy is less. The patient is asked to empty her bladder and disrobe. She is prepared for the routine pelvic examination with extra toweling under the buttocks. The physician will usually do a bimanual examination before the insertion of the IUD.

On the side:
- Examining gloves
- Skin disinfecting solution
- Vaginal tampon

Sterile setup: IUD and inserter
Uterine tenaculum
Uterine sound
Uterine dilator
Scissors, long, cvd.
Uterine sponge or dressing forceps
Vaginal speculum
Sponges
Gloves

After the insertion of the device the patient may be instructed how to examine herself to feel the transcervical appendage, if that type of device is used. The patient should be instructed that there may be some cramping and excess bleeding for the next few menstrual periods. She should check the presence of the device at least monthly, usually after the menstrual period. The patient should call the office if: (1) the device has been expelled or she cannot feel it, (2) aspirin or other mild medication does not ease the cramping, or (3) there is a heavy vaginal discharge or unpleasant odor. The patient should be reexamined six weeks after the insertion of the IUD.

Removal of Intrauterine Device (IUD)

The removal of an IUD is usually a simple procedure. The patient is prepared for a routine pelvic examination with the usual setup. After the vaginal speculum is inserted the physician will grasp the string with a sterile sponge or dressing forceps and pull. It may be necessary to grasp the anterior lip of the cervix with a sterile tenaculum. A sterile vaginal tampon may be inserted following the removal.

Rubin's Test

This is a test for the **patency** (openness) of the uterine tubes, made by the transuterine insufflation of carbon dioxide. If the tubes are patent (open) the gas will enter the peritoneal cavity and may be seen by x-ray or fluoroscope. The patient will feel some pain in the shoulders because of the subphrenic pneumoperitoneal pressure. Besides the regular pelvic examination setup you will have ready:

On the side: Germicide solution
Carbon dioxide gas

On the sterile field: Sterile towels
Uterine tenaculum
Uterine sound
Tubal insufflator with cannula tip

Marshall-Marchetti Test

This is a urinary stress incontinence test. Incontinence is the inability to retain the urine under stress situations such as coughing and sneezing. It is involuntary escape of urine. The urinary bladder is filled with 200 to 300 cc of sterile water or saline, and the patient is asked to cough or suddenly strain, "bear down." If the water escapes, then there is a weakness of the bladder sphincter. The patient is in the lithotomy position with a basin and ample toweling under the buttocks. A routine pelvic examination is usually done before the test.

On the side: 500 cc sterile water or saline
Lubricating jelly
Germicide solution

On the sterile field: Catheter setup
Asepto syringe

Huhner Test (hoon'er)

The Huhner test involves the determination of the number and condition of spermatozoa in mucus aspirated from the vaginal canal within 2 hours after coitus and to what extent they have penetrated the cervical mucus. The patient is prepared as for a pelvic examination and with a pelvic examination setup. In addition, have ready a cervical aspirator and bulb and microscopic slides.

Amniocentesis

Amniocentesis is the transabdominal aspiration of **amniotic fluid** in order to obtain a specimen for diagnostic **cytogenic** studies for inherited disorders such as **Down's Syndrome, PKU, sickle cell anemia**, and **hemophilia**. Through biochemical analysis, such defects as **Tay-Sachs disease** can be determined.

This procedure is often performed on women with a medical history indicating a possible problem that is genetically linked or on pregnant women past the age of 40.

The patient is placed in a comfortable dorsal recumbent position and the abdomen is exposed. The routine skin preparation is done and sterile drapes placed.

On the side:
- Skin disinfectant
- Adhesive bandage/small dressing

On the sterile field:
- Surgical gloves
- Syringe and needle for local anesthetic (25 g, 1 in., 3 ml)
- Spinal needle (22 g, 5 in. with stylet in place)
- 10 ml syringe (to aspirate fluid)
- Test tube(s) (depending on number of tests)
- Sponges
- The local anesthetic may be placed on the field if it is in a sterile vial; otherwise, the bottle is held by the assistant.

Ultrasound is used to aid in guiding the specimen needle. This is possible after 13 weeks gestation. A TV screen is used so both the physician and the patient may view the abdomen. This method is also used to evaluate abdominal and pelvic tumors. It is particularly useful in obstetrics and gynecology to evaluate multiple fetuses as well as the size, maturity, and placement of the fetus.

Before letting the patient up from the table check for possible faintness, pain, or the onset of contractions.

Paracervical Block

Paracervical block is the injection of a local anesthetic into the cervical area. This may be done before the insertion or the removal of an IUD. The physician will use a syringe and needle unit; 10 ml syringe with an 18 or 20 gauge, 1½ in. needle. This will vary according to the physician's directions. A vial of local anesthetic (Carbocaine, Procaine, or xylocaine, as the physician requests), a skin disinfectant, and sterile sponges will be necessary.

Colposcopy

Colposcopy is done to determine visual changes in the cervix for possible malignancy. The cervix can be stained and the tissues examined in situ. It is designed to evaluate an abnormal "Pap" smear or an abnormal appearing cervix. With the use of the colposcope, which is a vaginal speculum with a magnifying lens, the physician can better examine the cervix.

On the side:
- Specimen jar with 10% formalin
- Laboratory form
- Medication
- Vaginal tampon
- Tissue disinfectant

On the sterile field:
- Colposcope
- Tenaculum
- Uterine dressing forceps
- Uterine sponge forceps
- Sponges
- Colposcopy punch or cervical biopsy punch
- Cotton applicators

It should be explained to the patient that there may be mild abdominal discomfort for a couple of days and that the tampon the physician has inserted may be removed the next day, or sooner if necessary. The patient should also be told that after several days there may be a light discharge but this is only temporary. The patient should be told not to douche or have intercourse during the next week. The patient is usually seen again in four weeks if there are no problems in the meantime.

Cryotherapy (Cryosurgery)

This is the process of freezing tissue for the purpose of destroying cells. This method is used in many different specialties but especially in dermatology and gynecology. In gynecology it may be applied if a patient shows an **atypical** or possible malignancy as seen in a Class 11 "Pap" smear. It is also used for chronic cervical infections and erosions since the offending organisms may be entrenched in the cervical cells and glands. Cryocautery destroys these infected areas and in the healing process new clean cells grow.

Liquid nitrogen is applied to the site until the tissue is frozen to approximately -20°C. As the site thaws the destroyed cells become gelatinous and slough out, then the healing starts. For use on the cervix cryotherapy is similar to electrocautery. The probe tip of the cryosurgery unit is applied to the site. Once the probe is in contact with the tissue, the cooling agent (liquid nitrogen, nitrous oxide, Freon, or carbon dioxide) flows through the probe. The time of application varies depending on the freezing agent used, but it is usually 30 to 45 seconds.

The patient should be told there will be a clear vaginal discharge for several weeks. Complete healing for a moderately extensive cryotherapy is about eight weeks. The patient is to be seen once or twice during the healing period. Instructions for douching and sexual relations will vary and the physician should be consulted.

In *dermatology* cryotherapy is used to treat small growths such as **verrucae** (warts) or **keratoses**, both benign and malignant. The freezing agent is applied to the top of the lesion until freezing occurs throughout the site that is being destroyed.

There is some discomfort but it is slight and lasts only a short time. A blister is formed within a few hours after treatment. The patient should be instructed to leave the blister as the roof of the blister serves to protect the healing tissue beneath. If the blister is extra tender it may be cleansed and punctured with a sterile needle on one edge. This should be kept clean and dry. A dressing is not recommended. The blister will usually heal within two weeks and the under tissue will appear reddish-purple. There is sometimes a little scarring where treated.

Frequently on the smaller sites of treatment there is no office follow-up. Occasionally a site may have to be treated more than once.

Hormone Pellet Implant

A preoperative diagnosis for this procedure may be hypoestrogenism with menopausal symptoms. The purpose of the procedure is to implant small pellets, usually three, into the subcutaneous tissue in the groin area of the patient. The hormones implanted are **estrogen** and **testosterone**. The patient is placed in a supine position and the groin area is exposed and prepared.

Materials needed: Local anesthetic
Syringe (2 cc) and needle 25 g 7/8″
Barton implanter, sterile
Dressing (Band-Aid is usually sufficient)

There are no particuar postoperative instructions for the patient.

Endometrial Curettage by Suction (Endometrial Lavage)

This is done for the purpose of obtaining a specimen of the lining of the uterus. There are differences of opinion as to the time during the menstrual cycle that this procedure should be done. The physician's orders should be given to the patient. Careful sterility must be maintained. Place patient in lithotomy position.

On the side: Laboratory form
Antiseptic solution
Lubricating gel

On the sterile field: Vaginal speculum
Uterine tenaculum
Uterine sound
Uterine dressing forceps
Uterine sponge forceps
Gloves
Sponges
Cotton swabs
Disposable endometrial lavage set (Gravlee or Vabra)

Have the patient remain in a dorsal position on the table for a few minutes after the procedure. Have a sanitary pad available. Send the specimen to the pathologist for examination immediately.

Ear Irrigation

An ear irrigation is usually done to remove excessive or impacted **cerumen** from the auditory meatus. Occasionally a patient will have a foreign body in the ear canal, such as a bug, bean, or wad of paper. The physician will examine the ear and remove the foreign body, but occasionally the medical assistant will do the ear irrigation on the physician's orders. Usually the patient has been given pretreatment instructions to place drops of cerumen-removal medication in the ear before coming to the office in order to soften the cerumen. Have the patient lie on his side, place a few drops in his ear, remain in this position for 15 minutes, and then repeat on the other ear. Instruct the patient to make absolutely no attempt to "clean out the ear." Sometimes the patient is instructed to use 3 per cent hydrogen peroxide drops in the ear just before coming to the office. Have the patient assume a sitting position with the back well supported. The hair should be pinned up and away from the ear and a terry towel placed over the patient's shoulder. A large plastic drape over the patient's shoulder and lap will give good protection.

Materials needed: Medicine droppers (2)
Metal applicator, str.
Medication and/or H_2O_2
Illuminated otoscope
Cotton
Cotton applicators
Ear basin (emesis basin)
Irrigating syringe (Reiner or Asepto)

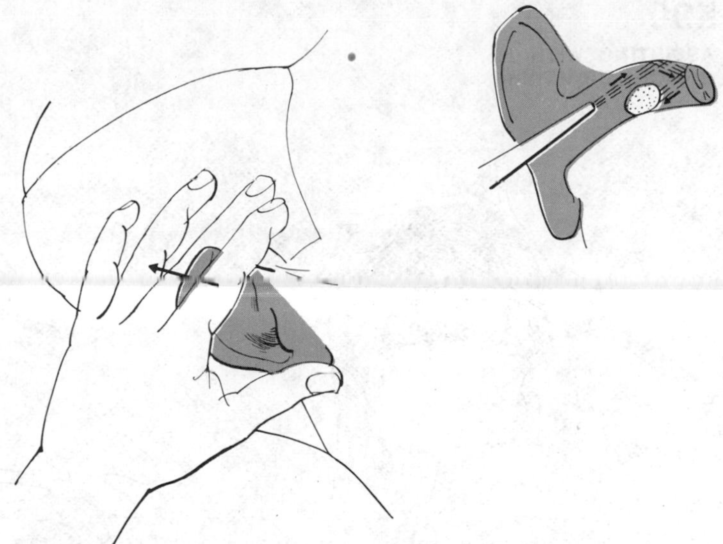

FIGURE 29–20 Holding the ear correctly for irrigation. (From Sutton, A. L.: *Bedside Nursing Techniques in Medicine and Surgery*. 2nd ed. Philadelphia, W. B. Saunders Co., 1969.)

Prepare a quart of mild soapy or plain water at 98.6°F. It is important that the water be body temperature. Grasp the ear between the middle and index fingers, leaving the thumb free to act as a rest for the syringe. Gently place the syringe tip inside the meatus and very gently direct the flow of water up and back (Fig. 29–20). Remember, do not force the water in and do not empty the syringe completely because the remaining bubbles will make a considerable roar in the ear that is quite annoying to the patient. It is necessary for the patient to hold the ear basin, but watch that it does not get too full and spill.

When the irrigation is completed, dry the external ear with gauze and gently dry the ear canal with a soft cotton applicator with a tuft on tip. Record in the patient's history what was done and the amount of cerumen removed.

Nose Drops and Nasal Pack

A nasal pack is inserted into the nasal cavity, usually for the purpose of stopping hemorrhage or for the application of medication. The patient is placed in a sitting position with the back well supported. Drape the front of the patient and give him some paper tissues.

On the side:
- Head mirror and light
- Emesis basin
- Medication
- Laryngeal mirror
- Tongue depressor (metal or wooden)
- Topical anesthetic

On the sterile field:
- Nasal speculum
- Cotton applicators
- Scissors
- Metal applicator, str. and cvd.
- Nasal packing with string (4″)
- Dressing forceps (bayonet)
- Hemostatic forceps, str.
- Medicine glass
- Nasal pack, 1 inch, plain or iodoform

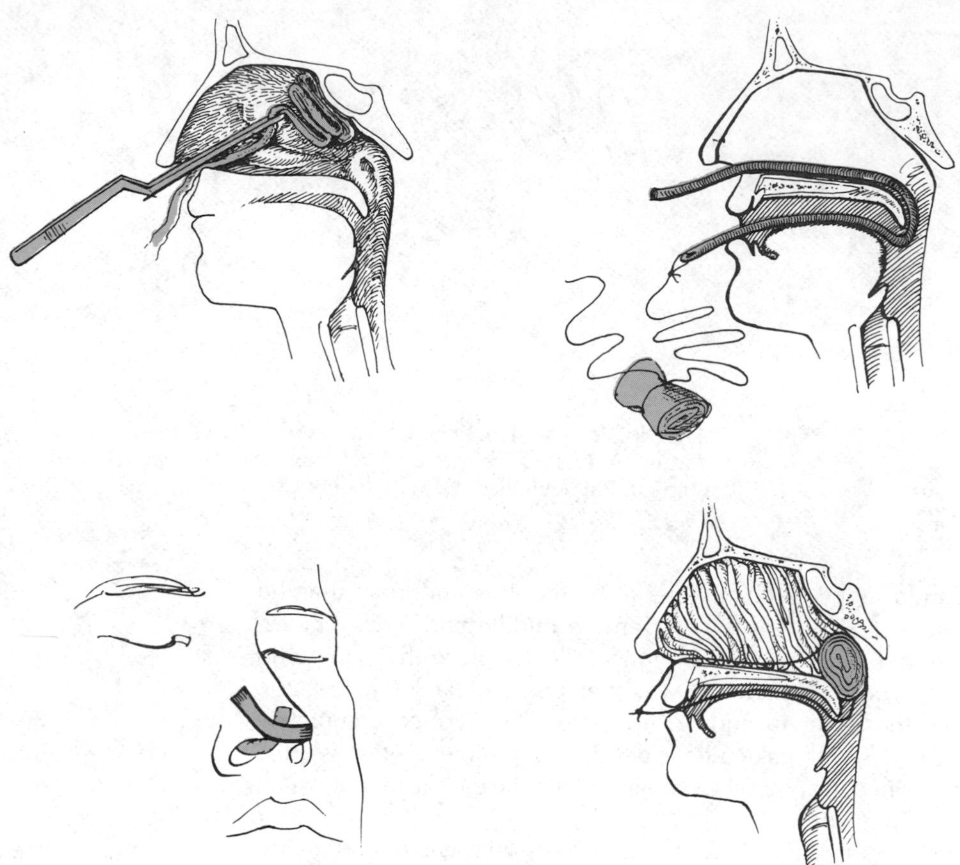

FIGURE 29–21 Nasal pack used after some types of nasal surgery and for uncontrollable epistaxis. (From Sutton, A. L.: *Bedside Nursing Techniques in Medicine and Surgery*. 2nd ed. Philadelphia, W. B. Saunders Co., 1969.)

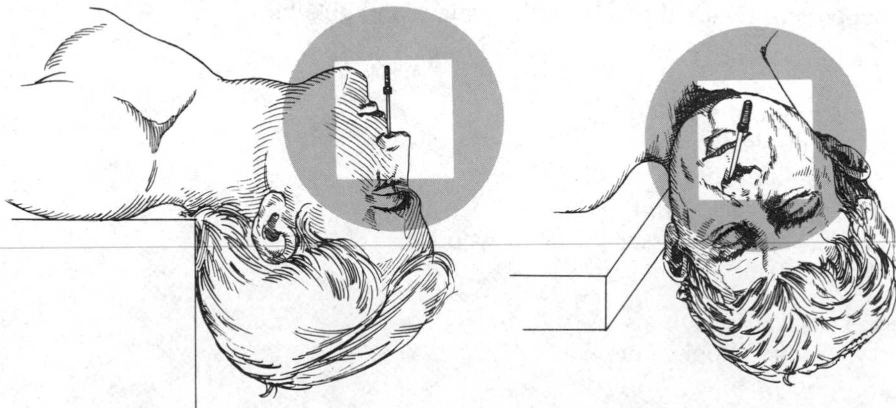

FIGURE 29–22 Instillation of nose drops.

See Figure 29–21 for the procedure. This is not usually a painful procedure, but it is uncomfortable, and the patient may require moral support.

If nose drops are to be administered, the patient is placed on his back with the head lower than the shoulders and turned to one side (Fig. 29–22). Draw sufficient medication into the dropper for both nostrils, turning the head for each side. Place the dropper about ⅓ of an inch inside the nostril. Instruct the patient to remain in this position for about 5 minutes. Provide the patient with a paper tissue. For infants and small children, it is best to use a rubber-tipped dropper. Hold the child's head by cupping your hand under his chin.

Eye Irrigation

Irrigation of the eye is done to cleanse it or apply a medication such as an irrigating solution. The sterile solution should be warmed to body temperature. The patient is placed on his side with the head turned to the side of the eye to be irrigated and the head held level by placing a pillow under the patient's neck as shown in Figure 29–23. A basin is placed under the temple. The patient may hold the basin, if necessary. Use a sterile syringe to moisten a cotton ball with solution to cleanse the eyelid and eyelashes of the affected eye. Be gentle. Instruct the patient to stare at a fixed spot during the irrigation. Place the sterile syringe filled with solution on the bridge of the nose parallel to the eye. The irrigating solution should move in a gentle, steady flow. Dry the eyelid with a sterile cotton ball or dressing.

On the side:	Emesis basin
On the sterile field:	Medicine droppers (one for each eye) or small Asepto syringes Cotton balls or gauze dressing squares Medication or irrigating solution

Check the physician's orders carefully for which eye requires care. Use the correct abbreviations when recording the procedure into the patient's chart:

OD — right eye
OS — left eye
OU — both eyes

Instillation of Eye Drops

This is done to introduce medication into the eye for examination or treatment of the eye. Always check an eye medication very carefully. Some medications are not stable, especially if exposed to the light. Improper use of the medicine dropper will cause contamination of the medication. DO NOT TILT THE MEDICINE DROPPER

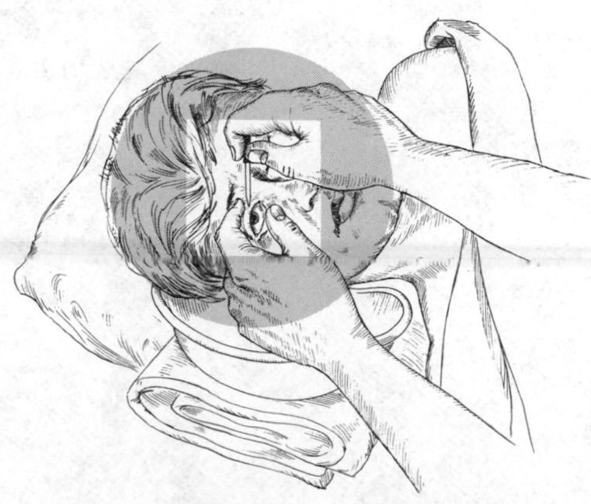

FIGURE 29–23 Eye irrigation.

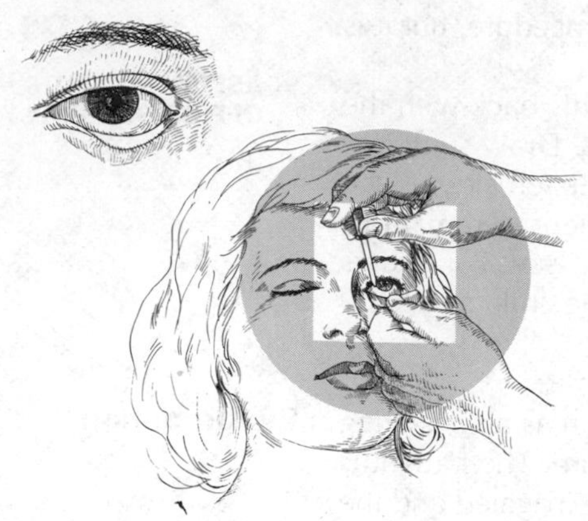

FIGURE 29–24 Instillation of eye drops.

SO THE MEDICATION ENTERS THE RUBBER BULB. This is a major source of contamination and cross mixing of medications. Each medication must have its own sterile dropper. The patient is usually in a sitting position but may be supine with the head tilted backward. Draw the medication into the sterile dropper, don't tilt, and place the required drop(s) just inside the inner surface of the lower eyelid near the center. To pull the lower eyelid down place your finger on the patient's cheek bone and gently pull downward (Fig. 29–24). Pressure over the lacrimal sac will prevent the medication from draining into the nasal cavity if the physician so requests. Do not touch the eyelid or eyelashes with the medicine dropper but hold it about ½ inch above the eye. Instruct the patient to stare at a fixed spot on the ceiling. Then have the patient close the eye and roll the eyeball a few times, unless the motion of the eye is contraindicated. Gently blot the excess medication with a gauze or cotton ball.

An ointment is applied by squeezing the tube from the bottom and applying a thin line of ointment into the lower eyelid cul-de-sac. Take great care to not touch the eye or eyelid with the tip of the tube. Have patient close the eye. Wipe off excess medication with tissue.

The general physician does not do minor surgery of the eye in his office but will refer the patient to an ophthalmologist. With adequate facilities and a specially trained assistant the following two procedures may be done in the ophthalmic office.

Surgical technique and sterility must be maintained as with any other type of surgery.

Chalazion Incision

A chalazion is an obstruction of a sebaceous gland in the eyelid. It is removed from under the eyelid through a vertical conjunctival incision or through the external surface of the skin.

On the side:
- Topical anesthetic
- Local anesthetic
- Antibiotic ointment
- Ophthalmic antiseptic solution

On the sterile field:
- Chalazion clamp
- Curette (3)
- Eye dressing forceps (3)
- Gauze dressings (3 in. by 3 in.)
- Knife (#11 blade and #7 handle)
- Small scissors, s/s, cvd
- Cotton applicators (6)
- Eye pad
- Syringe (2 cc) and needle (27 g ½″)

The patient is placed in the operating chair, and a drape is placed over the chest and lap. Hand the patient some tissues. **Hemostasis** is obtained by pressure directly over the site of the chalazion removal. After the ophthalmic antibiotic ointment has been applied, the eye patch is applied by folding the patch in half and fixing it firmly in place with tape. The tape should be placed in an overlapping fashion. Be careful not to have any of the patient's hair caught in the tape.

Removal of Foreign Bodies in the Eye

Because these are extremely uncomfortable to the patient, he will appreciate care as soon as possible. It must be immediately stressed to the patient that the eye must not be rubbed in any way. The patient is best placed in a supine position with a small pillow under the shoulders so the chin is tilted up. Many foreign particles can be removed from the eye with a small cotton applicator moistened with saline. If this method does not remove the object, a foreign body eye spud may have to be used.

Materials needed:
- Topical anesthetic
- Sterile cotton applicators
- Sterile saline solution for irrigation
- Hand lens
- Fluorescein (a **fluorescing** dye)
- Sterile eye spud
- Antibiotic ophthalmic solution

The physician will grasp the patient's eyelash with one hand and place an applicator stick horizontally on the middle portion of the eyelid and then pull upwards on the eyelid and downwards on the stick, thus flipping the eyelid exposing the under surface. This is not painful to the patient and facilitates a better view of the eyeball.

References

Brunner, L. S.: *The Lippincott Manual of Nursing Practice*. Philadelphia, J. P. Lippincott Co., 1974.

Hill, G. J.: *Outpatient Surgery*, 2nd ed. Philadelphia, W. B. Saunders Co., 1980.

Ochsner, A., and DeBakey, M. E.: *Christopher's Minor Surgery*, 8th ed. Philadelphia, W. B. Saunders Co., 1968.

Otto, J. F. Jr., (ed.): *Principles of Minor Electrosurgery*. Liebel-Flarsheim Co.

Rakel, R. E., and Conn, H. F.: *Family Practice*, 2nd ed. Philadelphia, W. B. Saunders Co., 1978.

Sutton, A. L.: *Bedside Nursing Techniques in Medicine and Surgery*, 2nd ed. Philadelphia, W. B. Saunders, 1969.

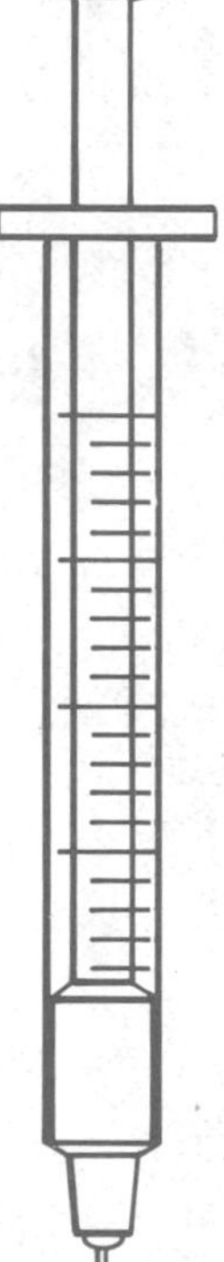

CHAPTER OUTLINE

Short Wave Diathermy
Radiation Therapy
  Infrared Therapy
  Ultraviolet Radiation
Ultrasonic Energy
Electromuscle Stimulators
Galvanic or Direct Current
Electrosurgery
Other Modalities
  Hydrotherapy
  Massage
  Cold Therapy

BEHAVIORAL OBJECTIVES

The medical office assistant should be able to:

- **Identify the major modalities used in office physical therapy and their applications.**
- **Identify indications and contraindications for use of short-wave diathermy, radiation therapy, ultrasonic therapy, and other therapies introduced in this chapter.**
- **Prepare the patient for physical therapy.**
- **Assist the physician in administration of the physical therapies introduced in this chapter.**

30

ASSISTING IN PHYSICAL THERAPY

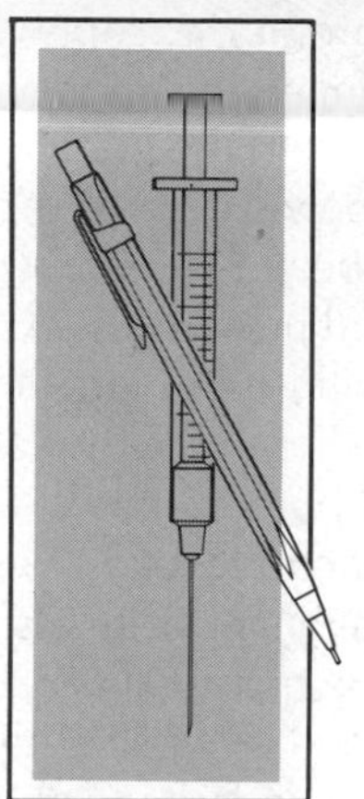

The duties of the medical assistant in physical therapy may be limited, and the authors recognize that it would be preferable if all medical offices employed graduate physical therapists to administer therapeutic treatment according to their employer's prescription. Since, however, there are a limited number of trained therapists, most of them being employed in hospitals and clinics, the medical assistant in the physician's office is almost universally required to learn to administer the various types of physical therapy treatments. Usually the physician himself administers the first treatment to the patient, directing and supervising subsequent treatments given by the medical assistant. This chapter is devoted simply to briefing the reader on the types of equipment employed and some suggestions on the use of these **modalities.**

Manufacturers of the various modalities provide materials that may be studied by the medical assistant to gain a better understanding of their nature and use. Manufacturers will frequently, on request, train the individual assistant in the proper handling of a given instrument so that the physician's orders may be carried out efficiently.

Mechanical and electrical modalities used in the office to treat the variety of conditions are considered **adjuncts.** Adjunctive therapy is an aid to another remedy or to the normal body functions in promoting a faster healing effect. This term is frequently applied to the various methods of physical therapy.

SHORT WAVE DIATHERMY

The use of short wave diathermy has been popular for many years and is used in some physician's offices. The short wave diathermy machine is designed to produce energy very similar to that emitted by a radio station. Applied to human tissue, this energy penetrates deep within the body tissues and is expended in the form of heat. It is simply called "heat within," or diathermy (dia = through, thermy = heat). The temperature rise is the "yardstick" of the rate of energy expended in the tissues. This radio frequency energy produces heat within the tissues that dilates the capillaries, veins, and arteries, and a temperature rise of a few degrees above normal will greatly increase the rate of blood flow through the heated area. Diathermy is therefore prescribed in cases in which the physician believes a materially increased blood supply is indicated. As a general rule, diathermy (heat) is indicated in all inflammatory processes (acute, subacute or chronic), except where there is encapsulated pus without drainage or where there is danger of hemorrhage. Diathermy treatments over the abdominal area are contraindicated in the pregnant patient. Caution should also be taken in applying heat over the pelvic area of a patient menstruating if there is danger of hemorrhage. Diathermy heat will also concentrate in any conductive materials such as surgical implants and prostheses. The patient should be asked if she has an intrauterine device. Patients with scars in the area to be treated should also be carefully questioned to make certain there is no implant beneath the area. Since scar tissue does not have the normal supply of blood vessels or nerves, precautions should be taken in applying the electrode pads over these areas. Areas that are suspected or known to be near a malignancy are also avoided. Be very cautious in cases where there is absence of or the possibility of impaired sensation. Infants and psychotic patients cannot always report excessive heat sensations. Erythema of the skin may be a possible indication of an underlying obstruction such as a blood clot in the vascular system. Other contraindications are cases of possible impairment in the cardiovascular and renal systems, respiratory diseases, and osteoporosis. Careful observation of the skin should be made for the possibility of blisters that may be the result of hot water bottles, heating pads, or skin ointments and salves that have been applied previously by the patient.

PATIENT PREPARATION. The patient should be disrobed and the area to be treated exposed and examined for scars, color changes of the skin, and any metals. Hearing aids and metal objects, such as rings, bra or underslip metal snaps, should be removed, because heat can concentrate in these objects. Do not place the patient on a metal table or permit him to come in contact with metal objects. Make certain the patient is comfortable before applying the electrodes (pads or drums). Possibly, this will prevent the patient from changing his position later to be more comfortable, resulting in the electrode's being moved to an incorrect position. For sanitary reasons and to collect perspiration, place a towel over the patient between the skin and the electrode. Excessive perspiration may cause a steam blister if it is allowed to pool on the skin.

After the diathermy applicator has been applied to the area to be treated, the dosage power should be adjusted so only a mild sensation of warmth is felt by the patient. Ask the patient to tell you when he feels the first sensation of warmth. At this point deep tissue heating will be at maximum, and the surface heating will be at minimum. Many patients feel that if a little warmth will produce results, more heat will produce greater results. This theory does not follow with short wave diathermy. DO NOT PERMIT THE PATIENT TO ASK FOR OR DEMAND MORE HEAT. NEVER INCREASE THE VOLUME OF ENERGY (HEAT) ABOVE THE INITIAL COMFORTABLE TOLERANCE OF THE PATIENT. The patient's receptor cells have become adjusted to the warmth; power has not been reduced. When the energy has been increased, it increases the temperature and the dose of treatment is increased. Remember that the patient cannot give you a true answer about what he feels because he does not know. DO NOT position the machine so the patient can reach it himself and turn up the energy. If the treatment temperature has been correct, the patient should receive benefit within 36 to 48 hours after the treatment has been administered. If the patient has been overtreated (too much heat), he may not receive these benefits but may have pain or discomfort afterwards from the excessive energy expended in the tissues. The correct amount of heat in the underlying tissue results in dilation of the blood vessels in the area, which promotes a favorable amount of blood supply to the area not only during the treatment time but lasting for an additional period during the cooling off time. The average underlying muscular tissue temperature will reach around 105° F.

Diathermy treatments may be administered on a daily basis or three times a week depending on the physician's instructions. The average duration of the treatment is 20 to 30 minutes. Do not let the patient demand more time beyond the prescribed treatment.

Read the manufacturer's instructions carefully. The machine must be kept clean. Do not permit the electrical cords to kink or have any pull on the connections. The cords or cables leading to the patient electrodes should not be permitted to cross each other or to touch the patient in any way. Electricity follows the path of least resistance and will flow from one cord to another or to the places it touches and the patient will not receive any energy, since the current will be flowing from cord to cord. Almost all machines will have spacers on these cords to prevent this. Some machines may require a "warm up" period.

RADIATION THERAPY

This is treatment by use of therapeutic rays. The two most used rays in the physician's office are the invisible infrared ray and the ultraviolet ray. The roentgen (x-ray) and radium emanations are akin to these but, because their use requires highly specialized training, they are not discussed in this book.

Infrared Therapy

This type of therapy is produced by the infrared lamp, which gives heat much the same as the diathermy machine. This heat, however, is generated by a metal coil element or a special heat-producing lamp. The beam from the infrared lamp is directed to the area of the patient's body needing treatment. The energy hits the skin surface, and since very shallow penetration occurs (the penetration is about 3 to 5 mm (or 0.1 to 0.2 in.); and is dependent on conduction to the lower tissues), this results in about one degree of temperature elevation in those tissues (Fig. 30–1). While not as effective as diathermy in producing a deep heat, the infrared lamp provides a very simple and fast superficial heat.

PATIENT PREPARATION. The area to be treated by this modality should be exposed and examined for scars, redness, or any condition that contraindicates applying heat to the area. The patient should be placed in a comfortable position, either lying on a treatment table or sitting in a chair. Do not let the patient contact any metal surface that may also be heated by the lamp. Remove any metal from the treatment area. The lamp is positioned about 24 to 36 in. from the patient; an

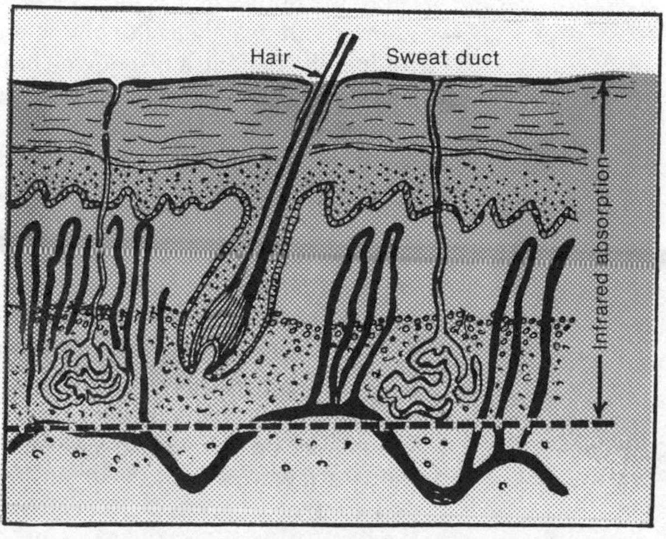

FIGURE 30–1 Depth of penetration of infrared rays.

average of 30 in. is frequently used. Radiation is usually of 20 to 45 minutes duration, according to the physician's instructions.

During the course of the treatment the patient's skin will become flushed and pink, but a sunburn does not occur. DO NOT PERMIT THE PATIENT TO "GRIT HIS TEETH" AND TOLERATE EXCESSIVE HEAT. A gentle mild heat is sufficient. Remember, the infrared lamp can bring about a surface burn in exactly the same manner as any other source of heat, such as a hot stove or iron.

Infrared rays are used to promote muscular relaxation, speed circulation, and aid in the localization of an inflammatory process. They are also helpful in maintaining heat in a moist dressing. The infrared rays have no germicidal power any more than other forms of similar heat.

Maintenance of the infrared lamp is simple. The heating element is best kept in a down position when not in use to prevent dust from accumulating on the element. The electrical connections should be checked and kept in good working condition.

Ultraviolet Radiation

This modality produces light energy in the same form as the rays from the sun that bring on the common sunburn. The portion of the sun's rays that we see is known as visible light; that portion we feel is heat, or infrared energy. Ultraviolet rays are themselves completely invisible, yet they bring about such a potent chemical reaction in the skin that in a few hours there follows the condition known as sunburn or erythema. Most of the sun's ultraviolet rays are absorbed or filtered out by the earth's dust and smoke. Ultraviolet rays are lethal to many microorganisms and, when applied in intense amounts to a localized area, are germicidal and effectively used in many skin diseases.

These rays are generated by different types of lamps. One way is to employ a high voltage, low current discharge through certain gases in a quartz tube, which produces intense ultraviolet rays with very little generation of heat; this is known as the cold quartz method and is the one most frequently used in the physician's office. Another method is by electrically heating a quantity of mercury within a quartz tube. This is known as the hot quartz method. Still another method is to burn the chemical contents of carbon rods; this is the carbon arc method.

Regardless of the method of generating the ultraviolet rays, great care must be employed in exposing the patient to this radiation. There are two types of cold quartz ultraviolet lamps used in the medical office. One type produces the long waves in the ultraviolet spectrum and is used for general body radiation. This energy is very potent and care must be taken to avoid tissue damage by overexposure. The physician personally should direct the assistant as to the exact number of seconds or minutes for the duration of the treatment in order to avoid an excessive burn. The distance from the burner unit to the patient is exceedingly important, and this, too, should be carried out exactly as the physician directs. At a distance of 36 in. from the burner unit to the patient, a first degree burn can be produced in 30 seconds to one minute, a second degree burn in one to two minutes, and a third degree burn in two to four minutes.

The patient should be disrobed and the area to be treated sufficiently exposed. Extra care should be taken in treating areas that have impaired circulation or areas that have not been exposed during previous treatments. Portions of the patient's body that are not to be treated, such as the genital area, should be protected with a clean towel. *Both the operator's and the patient's eyes should be protected with dark sun glasses to prevent the energy from entering the eyes.*

For general body radiation it was previously said that the lamp should be held 36 in. from the patient. There are two important facts to keep in mind when administering this treatment. First, if the distance from the patient to the lamp is decreased by one half, then strength of the radiation is increased four times (inverse square law). Second, the intensity of radiation striking the skin at right angles is greatest; at an angle of 30 degrees the intensity decreases to 80 per cent (Lambert's

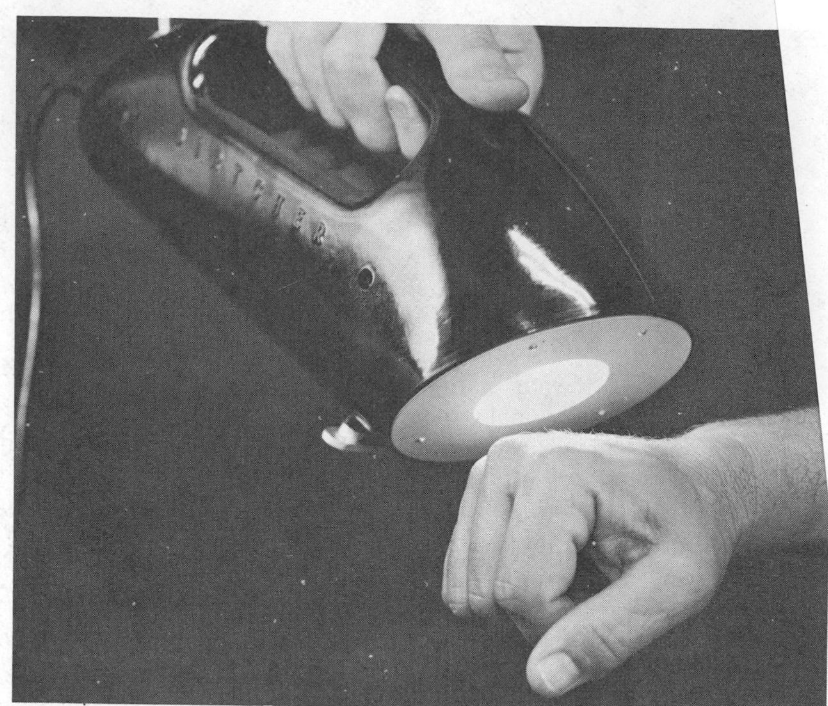

FIGURE 30–2 The Spot-Quartz, a portable cold quartz lamp. (Courtesy of the Birtcher Corporation.)

cosine law). Thus, it is important that the distance and the angle of the ultraviolet rays are the same for each treatment.

The size of the dose is usually governed by the erythematous response of the patient's skin. Treatments are generally given every other day, since 24 hours may not disclose the maximum erythematous response of the skin. The penetration of the rays is less than 0.1 mm. There is some tanning of the skin. The rays are considered to be carcinogenic if their use is prolonged for a considerable amount of time. Primary uses are for bactericidal and antirachitic therapy. Dermatologists may use this ray for the treatment of acne vulgaris. It causes capillary hyperemia and stimulates epithelial cell growth, and the vascular engorgement increases the skin's defenses against bacterial infections.

For small area therapy the hand-held portable quartz lamp can be very useful. This instrument, called the Spot-Quartz, is placed near or in contact with the area to be treated (Fig. 30–2). Since there is practically no heat generated in the lamp's coils, it will not burn the skin. The treatment time is from a few seconds to minutes, depending on the skin condition and the distance between patient and lamp. A masking adapter for small areas attaches to the face of the lamp, and a filter to eliminate the visible light (Wood's Filter) for diagnostic use is available. When not in use, the Spot-Quartz may be hung on the wall bracket supplied and is available for use after about one minute's warm-up of the quartz grid.

The glass coils of both the hand model and the larger lamp must be protected from breakage and kept free of dust and soil. They may be cleaned by carefully wiping with alcohol to remove oil.

ULTRASONIC ENERGY

This is the science of dealing with mechanical radiant energy. Since 1948 the use of ultrasonic energy as a therapeutic measure has been increasing. Early studies were first made in Europe, but the use of ultrasonic energy has advanced throughout the United States as well as other parts of the civilized world. Ultrasonic energy is simply sound energy, the same sort of energy that comes from a radio speaker or from the human voice. The customary sound with which we are familiar and which we hear is produced by sound waves vibrating at a rate of 100 to 12,000 cycles per second (frequency). A few exceptional people can hear sound waves vibrating at 15,000 cycles. Birds and dogs can hear frequencies of 25,000 cycles and more.

What is known as ultrasonics, as employed in therapeutic machines, is similar vibrating energy but at the rate of a million times per second. The mechanical energy at this frequency is created by an electronic machine that carries an electrical current up into an applicator or transducer. This electrical energy is fed to an element called a piezoelectric transducer. This material may be pure quartz or barium titanate. It is similar in size and shape to a half dollar coin. When activated by an electrical current it oscillates (vibrates) at a rate of one million times per second. The quartz crystal actually expands and contracts the same number of times per second as the frequency of the electrical current. When this crystal transducer is brought in contact with human tissue, the vibrating goes through the tissue. Though the frequency of this vibration is high, the total amount of energy is low. As measured by acoustical watts by engineers, the total energy administration to a patient is very small and is normally indicated on the output meter of the ultrasonic generator in total watts or watts per square centimeter of transducer element area. Acute ailments may be treated with the power as low as 0.5 to 1.0 watt per square centimeter as registered on the output meter on the generator. Chronic cases may be treated at a power output of 1.5 to 2.5 watts per square centimeter. The duration of a treatment will vary from 5 to 15 minutes, depending on the physician's instructions.

These ultrahigh frequency sound waves do not travel through air. The transducer (sound wave head or applicator) must be held snugly in contact with the body surface and aided in this contact by a coupling agent such as mineral oil. These sound waves do travel very well through water. Because of this, treatments are administered under water whenever it is convenient and that portion of the patient's anatomy needing treatment can be immersed. In deep body tissues that have a high water content, such as muscles, the ultrasonic waves penetrate better than the waves from the diathermy microwave; thus, absorption and heating are less. Ultrasound has less penetration and greater heating in tissues of low water content, such as bone. These minute sound waves bombard the tissues and cause the tissue to vibrate at the frequency rate. There is a small amount of heat generated in the tissue, but this is of limited importance. It is the extremely rapid vibrations that stimulate the circulation. One could say they cause the tissues to "flap" extremely rapidly. Results have been attributed to the vibrations causing the increase of blood flow, and this, in turn, creates a chemical action in the tissues that has a favorable effect in the body. All this takes place with little or no heat as experienced in the diathermy short wave and other heat modalities. The patient feels no sensation of pain and very little heat.

Ultrasonic therapy is used by orthopedic surgeons and neurosurgeons and is usually administered by a physical therapist on a physician's orders or prescription. Read the manufacturer's instructions carefully. Ultrasonic waves are also used for diagnostic purposes. This will be discussed with other imaging techniques in Chapter 31.

ELECTROMUSCLE STIMULATORS

These low voltage machines provide an electrical current similar to that coming from an ordinary wall outlet, except the machine controls the wave form, the frequency, and the intensity. These low voltage currents are useful for stimulation of motor and sensory nerves. It is said to be a passive way to exercise a muscle when a patient cannot activate the muscle himself. It is used to revitalize a muscle or to keep a muscle from atrophying.

There are various types of waves, or sine currents, used. These are basically: (1) pulsating; (2) spasmodic or twitching; (3) surging, that is, a slow steady tightening; and (4) tetanizing, which contracts rapidly and holds tight. The type of current is prescribed by the physician.

Small electrode pads are saturated with tap water to moisten them in order to increase the contact with the patient's skin. These pads are held by the technician or strapped in place. The electrical current and vibrations of the muscle or muscles, depending on the placement of the pad, are varied in frequency as prescribed. An interrupted current will stimulate denervated muscles and is used by physicians to

help maintain a nearly normal state of the muscle by frequent application, while awaiting reinnervation. Stimulation is also beneficial in retraining a patient to use a muscle or muscles. Various currents are used in electrodiagnosis.

Acute ailments are treated with a tetanizing effect which contracts the muscle and holds it in contraction for a period of time. This causes the muscle to fatigue and allows the blood to flow through the area again with resulting pain. Chronic ailments are treated with a slow alternating muscle vibration for a period of 15 to 20 minutes, which promotes blood flow and encourages relief of pain. Proper use of this modality produces spectacular results and will often demonstrate to a patient that a muscle is not "dead" but can be revitalized.

GALVANIC OR DIRECT CURRENT

The current found in some offices requires a machine to change the quality of the current supply from the wall outlet to one that flows continuously in the same direction, known as a direct or galvanic current. Sometimes the physician may have a machine that simply employs batteries for the electrical supply source. The direct or galvanic current has a chemical action. Exactly like the process of nickel-plating or silver-plating electrically in industry, certain drugs can be conducted into the human tissue by the use of direct or galvanic current. In some types of disorders this method is considered extremely effective. This process is sometimes referred to as "iontophoresis" or medical ionization. This treatment is usually employed by the physician himself. The assistant need only prepare the equipment for her employer's use.

ELECTROSURGERY

The use of electrosurgical modalities is an important part of the office practice of many physicians. It is a therapeutic modality with great versatility. Although considerable major surgery is accomplished in the hospital by use of the electrical surgical machines, in the physician's office only minor surgery is done by this means. The dermatologist will use this method for the removal of warts, moles, skin tags, and various skin blemishes. Some skin cancers, **senile keratoses,** seborrheic keratoses, spider nevi and hemangiomas are also treated. An **otolaryngologic** practice may use electrosurgery for the treatment of tonsil tags, shrinking inferior turbinates, and nasal polyps, and the control of **epistaxis. Proctologic** techniques may include coagulation of **condylomata,** removal of polyps and the control of bleeding after a biopsy. A **gynecologist** is one of the most frequent users of office electrosurgery for cervical coagulation of **erosions,** removal of cervical polyps, and treatment of **skenitis** and **bartholinitis** by coagulation.

The chief reasons that this modality is used in medical offices are the great versatility of the units themselves and the range of electrode tips that may be employed (Fig. 30–3). The technique can be used for incision, excision, tissue destruction, or a combination of these. The cutting current may be used instead of a knife or curet; the coagulation current is used for effects similar, but often superior, to thermal cautery, carbon dioxide snow, or sclerosing injections. Certain types of high frequency electrical current will actually cut tissue when guided through tissue by an ordinary wire or the point of a needle. An electrosurgical unit, when set in a "pure cut" mode, produces a steady, uninterrupted high frequency current. Therefore, tissue is divided cleanly with little or no bleeding. The cutting is faster than with a sharp surgical blade. This cutting current minutely explodes the tissue cells as it passes through and seals the cells, thus sealing off vascular bleeding and oozing. The area is sterilized by the heat generated, and the shape of the wire loop or blade defines the shape of the cut (see Fig. 29–19).

These modalities are sometimes referred to as the "Bovie"* machine, or it is said to be a "Bovie" procedure. In 1925 Dr. Harvey Cushing, the famous neurosurgeon, became interested in electrosurgery and enlisted the aid of Dr. W. T.

*"Bovie" trademark identifies every model of electrosurgical unit manufactured by Ritter Company, Sybron Corporation, Rochester, NY 14603

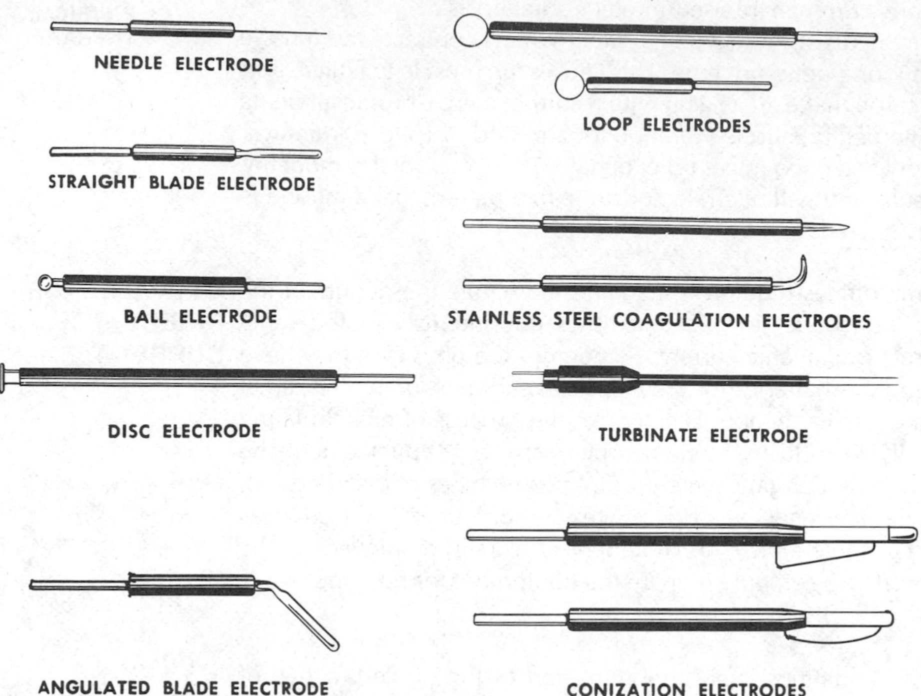

FIGURE 30–3 Types of electrodes used for electrosurgery. (From Otto, J. F., Jr., M.D. (ed.): *Principles of Minor Electrosurgery*. Liebel-Flarsheim Co., 1957.)

Bovie, a physicist at Harvard University, to develop a unit that would provide a cutting modality with suitable **hemostasis.**

An electric current proceeds from the machine through the output cable into the active **electrode** tip, which is hand-held and activated by the physician. From the tip or the cutting edge of the active electrode, the current continues through the patient's body, seeking an exit route that offers the least resistance to its flow. It seeks the dispersing plate or pad that is attached to the patient's body, sometimes called the indifferent plate. If a biterminal electrode is used, a dispersing plate may not be used. All the power concentrates in the electrode tip and surges through this tip held by the physician; it then seeks a pathway to the ground.

TYPES OF CURRENTS USED

The types of currents used differ with the needs: **coagulation, desiccation, fulguration,** and **epilation** (Fig. 30–4).

Electrocoagulation. This means to clot by means of an electrical current, sometimes referred to as "to cook." This is accomplished by the biterminal method, that is, a dispersing plate is used or a biterminal tip is used. Coagulation tends to produce more **necrosis** than desiccation, but this current is often advantageous in the treatment of larger or deeper growths. The amount of destruction depends on the size of the current and the length of time applied. Coagulation takes place only between and immediately around the tips if a bipolar (biterminal) electrode is used. The destruction will cause the tissue to turn a grayish-white. Depending on the depth and the size of the area treated, the tissue will slough between 5 and 15 days. When the slough has completely separated, healthy tissue appears beneath. The patient undergoing cervical coagulation should be told there will be a slight grayish discharge

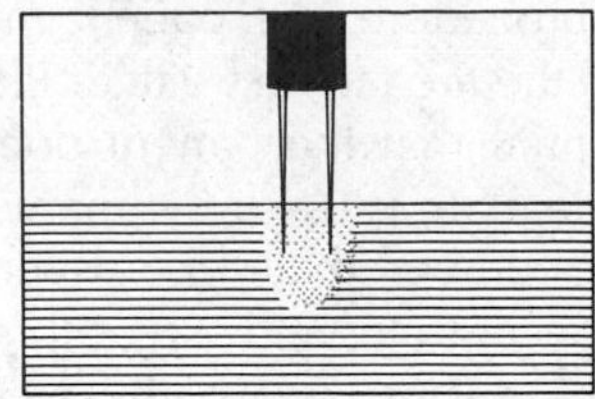
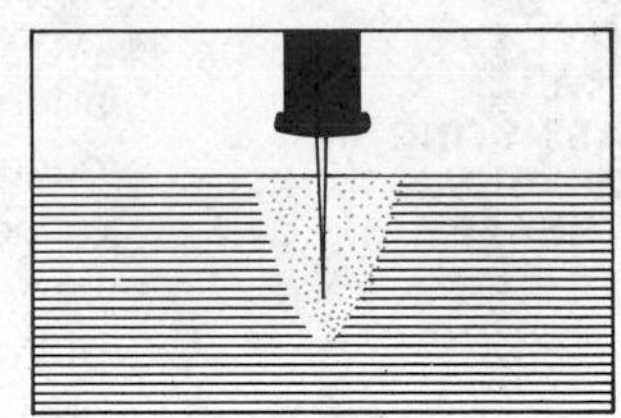
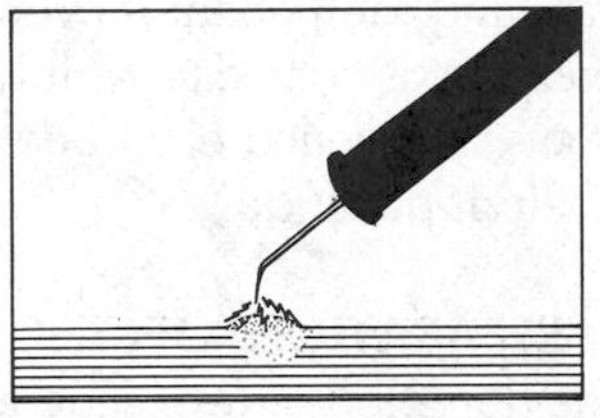
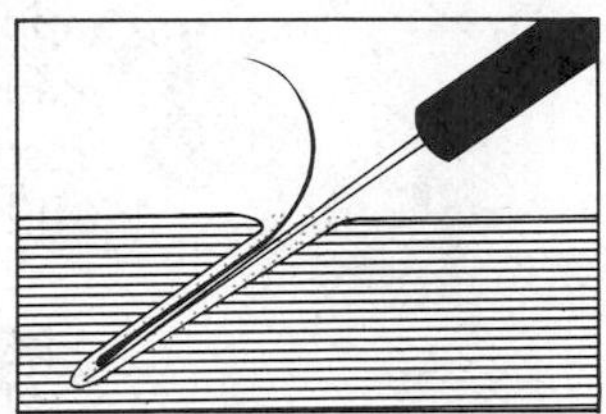
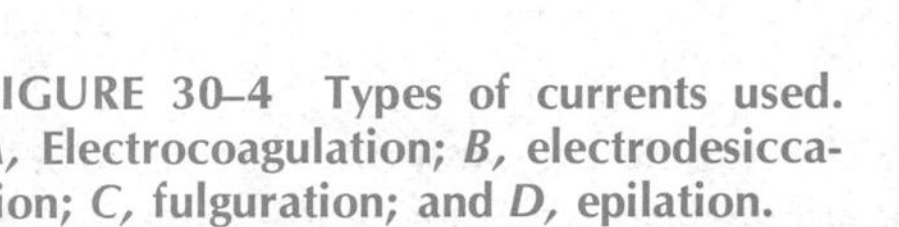
FIGURE 30–4 Types of currents used. *A,* Electrocoagulation; *B,* electrodesiccation; *C,* fulguration; and *D,* epilation.

from the area. A topical antibiotic may be given but is usually not necessary because the electrical current itself creates a sterile area (Fig. 30–5*A*).

Electrodesiccation. This means the destructive drying of cells and tissue by means of short, high frequency electrical sparks. This is done by means of a monoterminal electrode, that is, no dispersing plate is used, which somewhat limits its effectiveness in elevated or deep growths. Monoterminal desiccation, like fulguration, may be used in destroying granulations and small **polypoid** recurrences. It is sometimes used to destroy the stem of a **pedunculated** growth after the growth has been removed by a cold snare, in order to provide hemostasis and to minimize growth (Fig. 30–5*B*.).

Fulguration. This term is taken from the Latin "fulgurare" meaning lightning or spark. It is the destruction of tissue by means of electric sparks. It is usually monoterminal, using the same electrode tip as desiccation *but* the needle tip is not inserted into the tissue (Fig. 30–5*C*). It is held about 1 or 2 mm away from the surface of the site, allowing the current to spark to the tissue being treated. A grayish-white **coagulum** is formed on the surface and, depending on the mass, will slough in a few hours to a few days. Small superficial growths will carbonize when touched with the electrical spark and may be lifted off immediately with no surface evidence.

Epilation. This procedure is not frequently done in the physician's office because of the time involved. The word is taken from *epi* meaning upon and *pilus* meaning hair. It is the art of the extraction and destruction of hair follicles. A very fine steel monoterminal needle is inserted into the hair follicle beside the hair. These needles are very fragile and bend easily. The patient should be instructed to not shave or cut the hair in any manner for at least two to three weeks before the treatment. It is necessary for the hair to be grasped while the needle is inserted into the follicle (Fig. 30–5*D*).

PREPARATION OF THE PATIENT. The patient should be questioned regarding any surgical implants that may be disturbed by high frequency voltage. The dispersing plate should not be placed over hair, scar tissue, bony protuberances, or highly irregular contours that would make even contact difficult to maintain. Also be very careful the patient is not placed in a position where contact may be made with metal of the treatment table.

As with any procedure, the patient must be sufficiently disrobed in order to adequately expose the area to be treated. Place the patient in a comfortable position because it is essential that the patient does not move during the procedure. If a dispersing electrode plate is used, the medical assistant must follow the instructions very carefully. Remember that this dispersing plate is the same as the ground plate. All power concentrates and surges through the small tip of the active electrode and then seeks the easiest exit pathway or ground. This is the purpose of the dispersing plate. If the ground plate is bent, wrinkled, applied to bony prominences of the body, or not evenly coated with the conductive medium (coupling gel), the current will concentrate and "hot spots" or "cuts" can occur. The corners of these dispersing electrode plates are rounded to avoid a tendency for electron build-up on the clearly defined edges of square corners. The coupling gel must be uniformly applied to the plate and the patient, covering the entire surface. Missed spots may cause burns, whereas areas coated too thinly may dry out during a lengthy procedure, resulting in hot spots. Pre-gelled electrodes make application easier, but care must still be taken in their application.

PREOPERATIVE PREPARATION OF THE SKIN. Skin preparation will vary greatly with the procedure done, but a few general suggestions may be made to guide the medical assistant in assisting the physician. The area of skin to be treated is usually cleansed with surgical soap and rinsed. It is then painted with a skin disinfectant. If an alcohol-base disinfectant is used, be careful that it has been completely dried before using any type of treatment that may form a spark. This is especially important when working on the scalp or other hairy regions. Local anesthetics may or may not be used, depending on the method of treatment and the age and sensitivity of the patient. If a local anesthetic is injected the physician may use a limited amount in order to not place too much liquid in the tissue. Freezing with ethyl chloride is sometimes done, but care should be taken using this substance near an electric spark.

The physician may need tissue forceps to hold the growth steady during the procedure and surgical scissors to trim off carbonized tissue.

POSTOPERATIVE CARE. The after-care is simply to prevent trauma and infection. The crust remaining after desiccation is sterile, and the postoperative application of any antiseptic solution is usually not necessary, nor is a dressing required if the treatment area is small and superficial. A small, dry gauze dressing or Band-Aid may be applied to protect the area from trauma or for esthetic reasons. Dressings are not often advisable since the crust **in situ** should be kept dry, and a dressing may become moist or hold the natural skin moisture in. The patient should be told to return to the office in a few days so the area may be examined. Further treatm nt may be done in two to six weeks if necessary.

CARE OF ELECTROSURGICAL EQUIPMENT. Protection of the patient is a major concern of both the physician and the medical assistant, and the assistant is responsible for the maintenance of the equipment as faulty equipment may cause considerable damage. As with all electrical appliances the electric cords must not be allowed to kink or become loose in their attachments. The wires inside the attachments are fragile and easily broken if they are mistreated. The medical assistant should become familiar with the various electrodes used in electrosurgery. Usually the electrodes do not have to be sterilized because they sterilize themselves by means of the electric current, but they must be kept clean and polished. A fine piece of steel wool or emery paper may be used for polishing the metal tips. The handles and cords may be wiped with alcohol or another germicide. Read the manufacturer's instructions for care of the equipment.

OTHER MODALITIES

HYDROTHERAPY. This is the use of water in a tank. It provides buoyancy and moist heat. It also has a cleansing action that may be used for debridement of wounds. Special equipment, such as the Hubbard tank and the whirlpool baths, have agitated water that provides a gentle massage. Warm water is a very useful medium for exercise. The temperature is usually kept approximately at 110° F to 115° F.

FOMENTATIONS. Fomentations are the application of warm moist packs. The term is also used for the substance applied as with a poultice.

FEVER THERAPY. Fever therapy is the induction of high body temperature by physical means or by a bacterial or fever-producing vaccine. A therapeutic fever is known as **pyretotherapy.**

MASSAGE. Massage is the systematic therapeutic stroking or kneading of the body or a body part. A medical assistant is usually not asked to apply therapeutic massages to a patient, but she should be familiar with the terminology used. **Effleurage** is a stroking movement. In natural childbirth, a light circular stroke of the lower abdomen is done in a rhythm with controlled breathing, to aid in the relaxation of the abdominal muscles. **Petrissage** is a kneading or rolling type of massage while pressing. This is also called **foulage.** A vibratory massage is a rapidly repeated light percussion done with the side of the hands or with a vibratory instrument or sound.

COLD THERAPY. Also called induced hypothermia, this is a method in which the body temperature is deliberately lowered and held to below 90° F (32° C). This form of therapy is used during some types of heart surgery. This type of body cooling does not have any seriously harmful effects on the body. Applications of cold act as a vasoconstrictor and cause contraction of the involuntary muscles of the skin, thus reducing the blood supply to the skin. Extensive use of this topical application of cold may cause tissue damage because of the decreased blood supply. Cold is used to reduce tissue action to trauma and may be used to check an inflammatory process or control bleeding. It inhibits swelling and relieves pain and loss of motion in an inflamed area. It also slows down bacterial growth in a local infection. Cool sponge baths consisting of water and alcohol are used to reduce body temperature when a fever is present. Methods of cold application are by cold packs, cold water baths, ethyl chloride, and carbon dioxide. Dermatologists use carbon dioxide (CO_2) for the removal of certain skin growths. The terms **cryotherapy** and **cryosurgery** are also used.

PARAFFIN BATH. A paraffin bath is especially useful in chronic joint diseases. A mixture of seven parts paraffin and one part mineral oil is heated to melting at about 126° F. The patient's hand or foot is dipped into the warm paraffin mixture, removed, and dipped again until a thick coat is formed on the part. This is left on for about 30 minutes and is then peeled off. It leaves the skin soft, warm, and pliable, with a slight erythema. Patients are usually very fond of this form of treatment.

PSAMMOTHERAPY. Psammotherapy is similar to paraffin baths except that hot sand is used instead of paraffin. This is useful for treatment of the hands, although the entire body may be treated by this method.

CONTRAST BATH. A contrast bath utilizes two tanks. The patient's appendages are alternately immersed in hot and then cold water to enhance the flow of blood and stimulate the body's circulation.

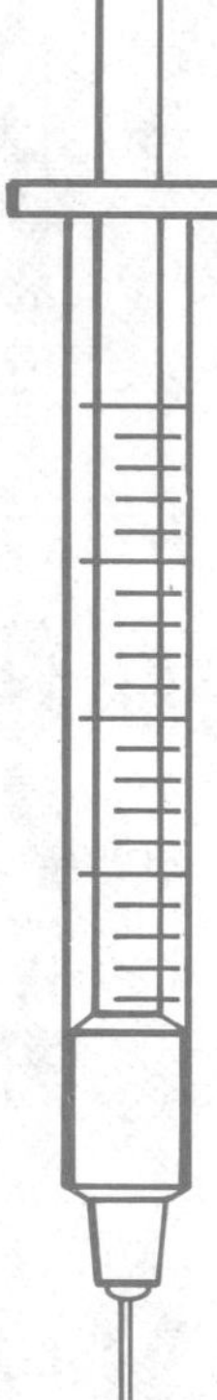

CHAPTER OUTLINE

Specimen Collection
- Labeling of Specimens

Urine
- Collection of Urine Specimens
- Routine Urinalysis
- Special Urine Tests

Blood
- Collection of Blood Specimens
- Special Blood Tests: Chemical, Serologic

Sputum

Feces
- Collection of Feces Specimen
- Special Tests on Feces

Collection of Semen

Mycology Tests

Ectoparasites
- Body Fluids: Exudates, Transudates, Synovial Fluids

Cytologic Examinations

Histologic Examinations

Cerebrospinal Fluid

Electroencephalogram

Radiologic Examinations
- Special Roentgenographic Procedures
- Radioactive Isotopes
- Other Imaging Systems

BEHAVIORAL OBJECTIVES

The medical office assistant should be able to:

- **Identify the need for accuracy and care in collecting, labeling, and handling of specimens in the medical office.**
- **Describe routine procedures involved in the examination and testing of urine, blood, sputum, feces, and other laboratory specimens.**
- **Identify the variety of radiographic techniques introduced in this chapter, as well as the indications for their use in special circumstances.**

31

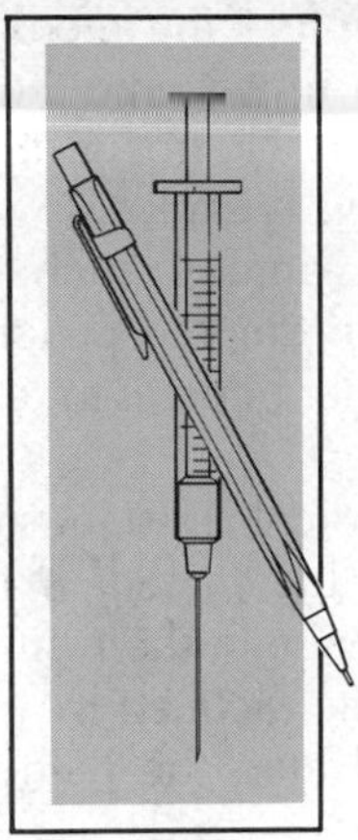

DIAGNOSTIC LABORATORY PROCEDURES AND INSTRUCTIONS

Because laboratory tests and x-rays are an essential part of a medical diagnosis, and aid to treatment, and frequently a control of medication, it is important that the medical assistant have an understanding of these **auxiliary** services. This understanding should include the various tests available for the special needs of the physician, the preparations the patient should be instructed to follow, and how the specimens are collected and sent to the laboratory.

There must be good communication between the patient, the physician's office, and the x-ray or laboratory departments. This communication can exist only with the understanding of the needs of each area in aiding the others with better patient care and testing. Remember, the medical assistant is usually the link among these services, and her knowledge and accuracy are essential.

It is frequently the medical assistant's attitude toward these services that determines whether the patient realizes the importance of cooperating and carefully following instructions in preparation for the tests. It can be helpful if the medical assistant has a basic knowledge of the equipment used or of the steps of the particular procedure in order to ease the patient's apprehensions or fears. To a degree, she will be called upon to teach the patient in preparation for some tests; therefore, she must be informed in order to be accurate in her teaching.

As well as possessing knowledge of the various tests requested by the physician, the medical assistant should know the normal ranges for these tests. This is essential when an abnormal report that should be brought to the physician's attention immediately is received in the office. No report should be filed in a patient's medical record until it has been shown to the physician. It may be a good idea to have the physician initial each report *before* it is filed. Many pathologists and roentgenologists will telephone the referring physician if there is an abnormal result that may require immediate care. These calls should be put through to the physician immediately.

Accuracy in reporting cannot be stressed enough. It is a dangerous practice to retype or copy a report onto the patient's medical record. Most offices have some method of entering the laboratory or x-ray form directly in the patient's file. An illustration of laboratory forms in a patient's record is shown in Figure 11–2 in Chapter 11, "The Patient Record." Most laboratories require the technicians to sign or initial their reports. This practice is helpful if the referring physician has any questions. If it is necessary to retype or copy a report onto the patient's record, then be very careful to copy it exactly as it is written. Do not destroy the original report; but file it with other reports from the laboratory. A carelessly misplaced decimal point could be extremely dangerous, and so could an error such as typing "gm" for "mg." Some medical assistants will underline with colored pencil any abnormal results. This is helpful if the forms are small and rather difficult to read. This can also be done with lengthy x-ray reports or summaries.

If the physician requests, the medical assistant should note on the laboratory or x-ray request form any medication the patient may be taking that could make changes or cause a possible interference in the results. A clinician's interpretations may also be sharpened by a brief note dictated by the physician or taken from the patient's medical record that would alert the pathologist or roentgenologist to a possible or tentative diagnosis.

No attempt is made in this book to give detailed instructions for the techniques of doing the tests but only to alert the medical assistant to the various tests requested by the physician. She must know how to collect the specimens, know what special instructions to give to the patient, and know the normal ranges for these tests. With this knowledge, she can enhance patient care and increase her value to the clinical laboratory and radiology departments. This knowledge will also enable her to answer some of the questions from patients and to alert the physician if time is an important factor.

SPECIMEN COLLECTION

The importance of accurate specimen collection cannot be overemphasized. If this is not done correctly it can easily lead to inaccurate results. Be careful while collecting and handling a specimen in order to prevent **contamination** of the specimen or of yourself.

Use only the correct containers. Never use a preservative or disinfectant unless you have been so instructed. Check whether the specimen needs to be kept warm or cool.

LABELING OF SPECIMENS. All specimens must be labeled accurately and neatly. It is best to type a label whenever possible. If it must be handwritten, then use a ballpoint pen and write legibly and firmly enough to be read through all carbon copies. Include the following information:

1. Patient's full name, surname first.
2. Patient's age and sex.
3. Patient's address. This is important if the specimen is sent out of the office or if the results may be reportable, such as for a **contagious** disease or a venereal disease.
4. The physician's full name. This is important if the specimen is sent to an outside laboratory or if there are several physicians in the office.
5. The date the specimen was collected as well as the date it was sent to the laboratory. Some specimens may require the hour of the day they were collected; time is important in many tests.
6. Source of the specimen. Many times it is not obvious whether it is a sputum or a gastric specimen, an exudate from an abscess, or a throat smear.
7. The specific test requested. There are many different tests that can be done on a urine specimen alone. State whether the physician wants a routine urinalysis, bacteriologic examination, special chemistry test, and so forth. Be specific.

8. Possible diagnosis. Many times this is only a tentative diagnosis, but it will give the pathologist or technologist a lead and alert him to watch for specifics.

9. Any other information that may be of importance, such as whether the patient has had any special medication or treatment that may interfere with the test. It is very important, in some cases, to state whether it is a new diagnosis or a treated case.

URINE EXAMINATION

COLLECTION OF URINE SPECIMEN. A specimen for a routine urinalysis should be collected in a clean, dry container, and the specimen should be fresh. A specimen over two hours old may not give accurate test results. If it is necessary to keep a urine specimen over two hours, it should then be refrigerated and the time of collection written on the label. It is best to collect the specimen in the office or the laboratory for immediate examination. Provide the patient with a wide-mouthed container that has a secure lid and is properly labeled. If the specimen is collected at home, the patient is instructed to bring it to the laboratory as soon as possible after voiding. It is advisable to provide the patient with a container that can be used at home. Do not allow the patient to use a container which has had perfume, hair oil, or any other contaminants in it, because these interfere with the examination. There are two ways to collect a urine specimen — a freely voided specimen and a catheterized specimen. The freely voided specimen is the most frequently used and is satisfactory if correctly collected. Catheterization is necessary for some bacteriologic cultures, but is an unpleasant procedure for the patient and does involve some degree of risk.

The first voiding in the morning is usually used because it is more concentrated, except in possible **diabetes mellitus** or **orthostatic** albuminuria. A freely voided specimen in the male is easy, but a specimen from the female may present a problem, especially if the patient has a vaginal discharge. The medical assistant should instruct her in the collection of an uncontaminated voided specimen.

Clean Catch

Instructions for the female patient. This technique is especially necessary during menstruation. If the menstrual flow is heavy, a tampon should be inserted in the vagina and the area cleansed very carefully.

1. Clean the entire vulvar area with soap and water, then follow with a thorough cleansing with a commercial disinfectant towelette (Zephiran chloride). If the Zephiran towelettes are used, instruct the patient to use several.
2. With the labia still held apart, have the patient void forcibly a small amount and then collect the midstream in a sterile bottle.
3. Cap the bottle immediately with a sterile cap.
4. Take the specimen directly to the laboratory.

Instructions for the male patient.

1. Clean the urethral meatus and glans well with soap and water and follow with a commercial disinfectant towelette (Zephiran chloride).
2. Have the patient void a small amount. Then collect the midstream portion of the urine in a sterile bottle.
3. Cap with sterile cap and take immediately to the laboratory.

Collecting Urine Specimens From Infants. The male infant presents very few problems because a pediatric urine collector may be lightly taped over the penis. This collector may also be used for the female infant.

ROUTINE URINALYSIS. This includes several tests.

Appearance. The color of the specimen may be influenced by various drugs, foods, and diseases. The clarity or turbidity is also influenced by these.

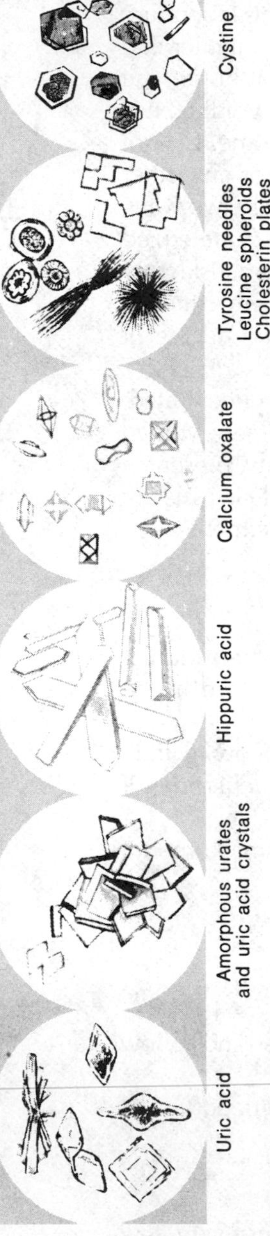

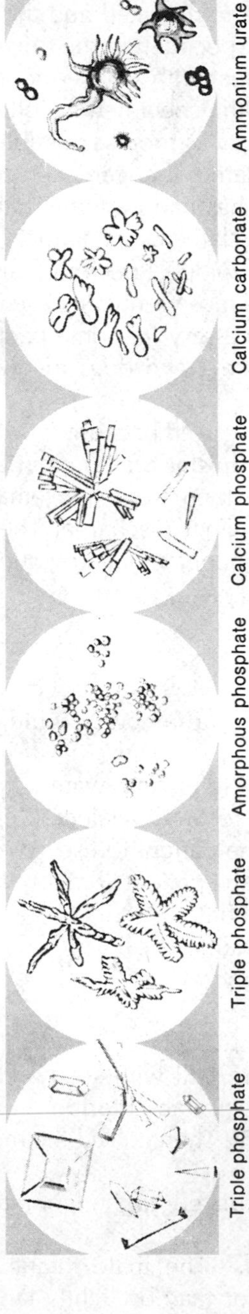

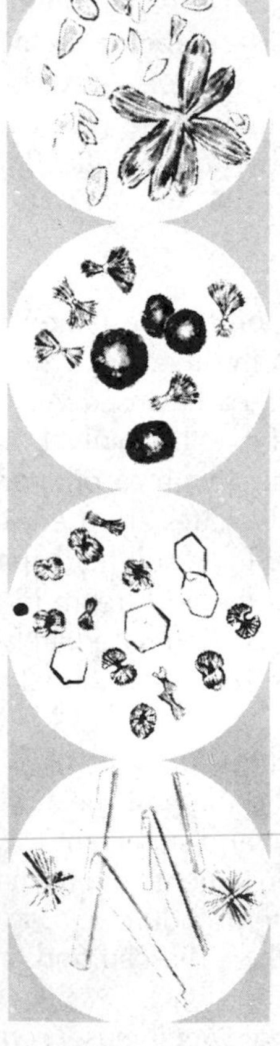

FIGURE 31–1 Ames Atlas of Urine Sediment. (Courtesy of Ames Company, Inc., Elkhart, Indiana.)

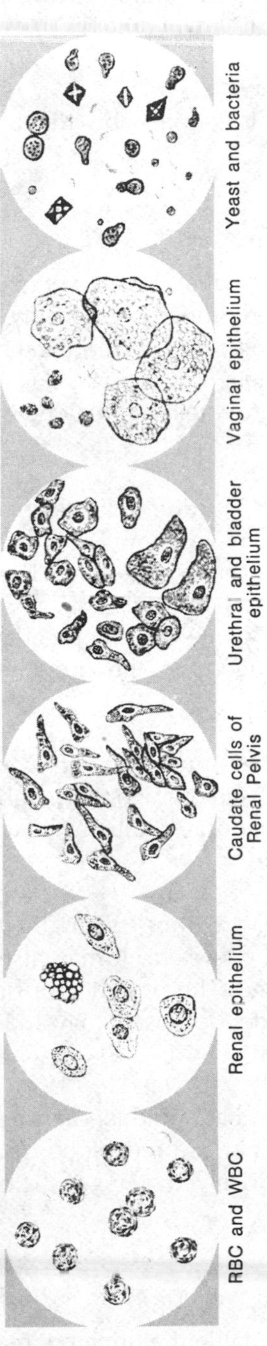

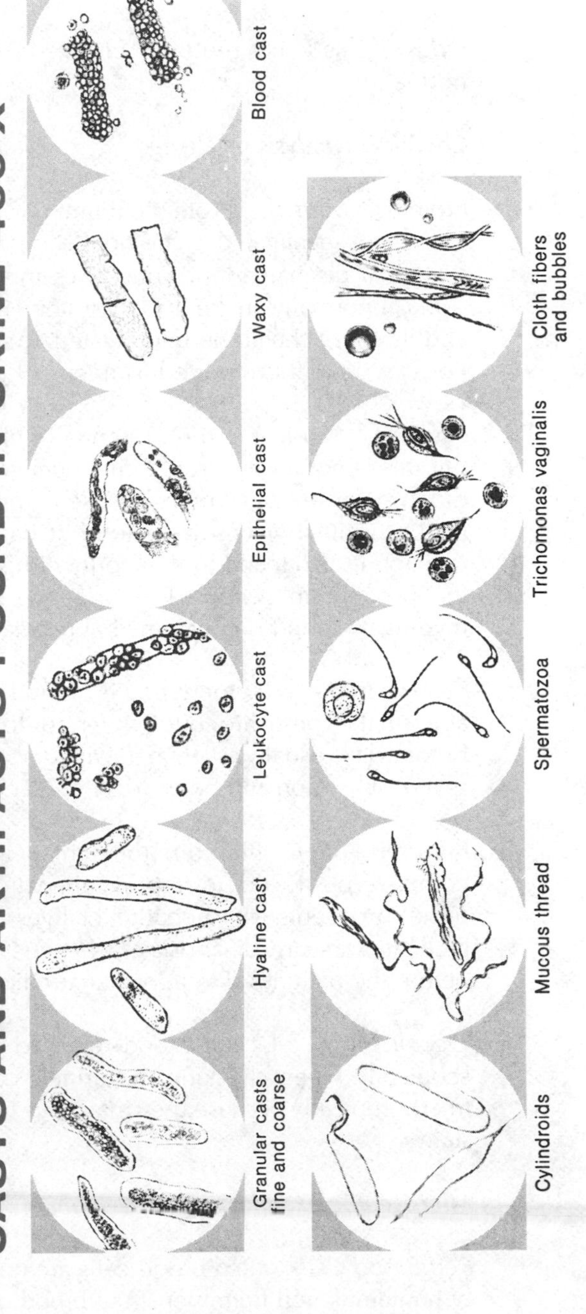

FIGURE 31–1 *Continued*

pH (Acidity or Alkalinity). This information is important only if the specimen is freshly voided. The pH determines whether certain elements are preserved or destroyed for microscopic examination. An example of this would be urinary casts that are highly diagnostic and are destroyed in an alkaline pH. Normal urine has a pH range of 4.5 to 7.5, slightly acidic to neutral.

Specific Gravity. Specific gravity is the weight of a substance or a liquid. It is a convenient way to measure the dilution or concentration of the urine. A highly concentrated urine may imply that the patient is dehydrated. The normal range is 1.010 to 1.025. (Distilled water has a specific gravity of 1.000.)

Odor. This is not routinely checked unless it is noticeably different from that of normal urine.

Chemical Analysis of Urine

Protein (Albumin). Protein (albumin) is not a normal constituent in urine. It may be found in a specimen that has not been collected properly, especially in women with a vaginal discharge, and thus gives misleading results. True **proteinuria** indicates some abnormality in the urinary system. Persistent proteinuria is due to renal disease, and its cause should be investigated. Transient proteinuria may be of little account. Positive protein is reported as trace, 1+, 2+, 3+, and 4+.

Glucose. Ordinarily the presence of glucose in urine indicates diabetes mellitus, but this is not always true. Some persons may have a low renal threshold, i.e., the blood sugar level at which glucose is spilled over into the urine. These persons will give a positive glucose reaction but have no **intrinsic** disease. A positive glucose reaction is also found in a majority of healthy women during pregnancy and during the postpartum period. The presence of glucose in the urine warrants further investigation and is considered abnormal.

Ketone Bodies. Ketone bodies found in the urine are also considered to be abnormal. These are often referred to as "acetone" on the laboratory forms. **Ketonuria** is usually associated with diabetic acidosis, but it may be found in cases of severe starvation and body wasting **(cachexia)**.

Bilirubin (Bile). Bilirubin (bile) may appear in urine when there is partial or complete obstruction of the extrahepatic biliary system. It may also appear in the urine in patients with hepatitis or liver damage. The presence of bile in the urine facilitates an early diagnosis of a hepatic disorder because it may appear in the urine before the patient's skin appears jaundiced.

Occult Blood. Occult blood refers to blood that is hidden and not seen macroscopically when checking the urine's color; nor are red blood cells always seen microscopically because they may have been dissolved owing to the urine hypotonic state.

Microscopic Examination of Urine

Red Blood Cells. Red blood cells are not normal in the urine but may be the result of contamination from menstrual blood or a slight injury to the tissue during catheterization.

White Blood Cells. White blood cells, sometimes called "pus cells" on the laboratory forms, are usually present in voided specimens, especially in the female. They are reported by how many are seen per high-power field on the microscope.

Normally 0 to 5 cells may be found. An excess of this number is usually checked to make certain it is not from external contamination of a voided specimen.

Epithelial Cells. Epithelial cells are also found in the urine. They are usually of three types: renal cells that are found in excess if there is renal damage; transitional cells that are from the pelvis of the kidney, ureters, and bladder and are present when pathologic conditions exist in these areas; and squamous cells that are from the urethra and vagina. Squamous cells are the most numerous and are continually being sloughed off from time to time; they are not considered pathologic. Cells are reported by how many there are per low-power field on the microscope. If there are too many to count, then they are reported from 1+ to 4+.

Urinary Casts. As mentioned earlier, urinary casts are highly diagnostic. They are molds of the urinary tubules and are made up of protein-plasma gel and/or cells. They are seen in urines with a pH of 6.0 or less and with a high salt concentration (hypertonic). Casts are named usually for the element contained in them, such as pus casts, blood casts, and granular (containing crystals) casts. Hyaline casts are seen in cases of renal disease, heart failure, high fevers, shock, or excessive exercise. Casts are reported by how many are seen per field under the microscope.

Crystals. Crystals are often seen in urinary sediment but are of limited diagnostic interest unless associated with the administration of drugs, such as sulfonamides, or with protein breakdown. Crystals are noted if there is a tendency to form renal calculi. Crystals commonly seen are classed by the pH of the urine. The acid urine crystals are amorphous urates, uric acid, and calcium oxalate. Those seen in the alkaline urine are amorphous phosphates, triple phosphates, calcium diphosphates, and ammonium biurate crystals.

Other Features. Other elements such as cotton fibers (lint) are not reported and are from clothing or container contamination. Bacteria seen are of limited value, especially in a voided specimen or one that is not fresh. In a catheterized specimen, bacteria are significant and should be reported and further investigated. Spermatozoa are seen in the urine and are not highly significant but are reported. Parasites, such as *Trichomonas vaginalis*, may be present and are also reported. These are from vaginal secretions.

SOME SPECIAL URINE EXAMINATIONS

Addis Count. This is done to find the patient's urinary output for a given period of time, 12 or 24 hours (Table 31–1). During the time of the test, the patient is allowed no fluids and he is to collect all the urine voided. The volume of the output is measured and examined for protein. The amount of fluid taken in for approximately 16 hours prior to the test is restricted or eliminated. This test is a diagnostic and prognostic aid in the treatment of renal disease.

Pregnancy Tests. There are many types of pregnancy tests now available. The most common ones are based on measuring the chorionic gonadotropin hormone present. There are two types of tests used: the biologic tests in which animals (rabbits and frogs) are used and the immunologic tests that are based on antigen-antibody reactions involving agglutination. Some of the biologic tests are Ascheim-Zondek, Friedman, Wiltberger-Miller, Hogben, and Magnini. The immunologic tests include Pregnosticon (Organon, Inc.), UCG (Wampole Laboratories), and Gravindex (Ortho Pharmaceutical Co.).

Fluids are avoided after the evening meal, and the morning urine specimen is collected. It should be collected without vaginal contamination. At least 2 ounces is required. The specimen is delivered to the laboratory as soon as possible after

TABLE 31–1 Recommended Patient Instructions for 24-Hour Urine Collection (Written instructions to be provided to patient with specified laboratory collection container. Supplement these instructions by discussing them with patient and explaining why the test and collection procedure are required)

TO THE PATIENT: Follow these instructions in collecting your 24-hour urine specimen.

You will find it more convenient to void (urinate) into the smaller container provided and transfer the urine into the larger collection bottle. DO NOT ADD ANYTHING but urine to the bottle, and do not pour out any liquid or powder that may already be in the collection bottle.

The collection bottle should be kept refrigerated throughout the collection period.

1. Upon rising in the morning, urinate into the toilet, emptying your bladder completely. *Do not collect this specimen.* Note the exact time and *write it down* on the container label.
2. Collect all urine voided after this time for 24 hours in the container provided by the physician. *All* urine passed during the 24-hour time period (*day and night*) must be saved.
3. Refrigerate the collected urine between all voidings or keep in a cool place.
4. At *exactly* the same time the following morning, void completely again (first time after awakening) and add this sample to the collection container. This completes your 24-hour collection.
5. Take the entire 24-hour specimen to the physician's office or laboratory as soon as possible, maintaining the cool temperature in transit by placing the specimen in a portable cooler or insulated bag.

---

collection. The patient should be instructed to discontinue any sedatives or analgesics for 24 hours prior to the test if an animal test is to be done, because they may kill the animal. The following criteria should be met in order to obtain the best results: (1) At least 41 days must have passed since the beginning of the patient's last menstrual period; (2) The specimen must have a specific gravity of at least 1.010. For this reason, an early morning concentrated specimen is preferred. The patient's blood may also be used for some pregnancy tests; about 1.5 to 2 cc serum is needed.

Routine Bacteriologic Urine Cultures. If a urine specimen is to be sent to the laboratory for a bacteriologic culture, it must be collected and handled with sterile technique. Of course, a catheterized specimen is preferred, but this is not always possible or advisable. A voided specimen can be used for culturing if the patient follows the instructions carefully.

BLOOD TESTS

Collecting blood from a patient consists of more than just inserting a needle into the patient's vein or puncturing the finger for a few drops of blood. It is important that the medical assistant considers this as the first step in obtaining test results for the physician, being no less important than the actual running of the test. If a specimen is incorrectly collected, the results will be altered and may lead to an incorrect interpretation. It is therefore essential that all specimens are collected and handled according to directions. Several hematologic tests, as with the urinalysis, are done routinely in medical offices. New patients, as well as returning patients, are given tests as part of a routine physical examination, to aid and confirm a diagnosis and to assist the physician in the administration and control of medications. Designating a test as "routine" does not minimize its importance. On the contrary, a physician can obtain valuable information from these tests. Tests performed on the blood are so numerous that they fill volumes of books. Only a few basic and routine tests will be mentioned here.

Generally there are two sources of blood for laboratory testing, **capillary** (also called **peripheral** blood) and venous blood. (Arterial blood is also used for some tests but not usually collected by the medical assistant.) Capillary blood is usually obtained from the finger and sometimes the ear lobe. The quantity of blood from this source is limited to a few drops but is sufficient for such tests as a complete blood count (CBC), hematocrit, some bleeding and coagulation times, and many chemical and agglutination tests. These often carry the term *micro-* as their designation. If several tests are done or if a greater amount of blood is needed, then venous blood must be drawn by the intravenous method. This is called *IV blood*.

Persons in the medical profession must keep in mind that the average person is apprehensive, if not frightened, at having blood drawn by any method. Because medical personnel often appear heartless to a frightened patient, they must remember to be calm and sympathetic, and give a brief explanation to the patient of the procedure to be done. If these procedures are done correctly there is very little discomfort. To a patient, several tubes or 10 cc of blood withdrawn appears to be a great deal of "blood loss." The patient can be assured that this is only a "little more than a few tablespoonsful" and that the body replenishes the loss almost immediately. It may be advisable to use the term "blood test" carefully, since many people associate this with a test for syphilis. A brief explanation of the kinds of tests will clarify this misunderstanding. Be careful about telling a patient what test is being done for him, since the physician may prefer that the patient not be informed.

Remember when collecting blood that you are an important part in the diagnosis and care of that patient. You may be the only direct contact the patient has with the laboratory. By your attitude and technique you must impress on the patient that everything will be done to make the procedure as comfortable as possible.

Capillary blood is usually obtained from the ring or great finger of the adult or older child. The great toe may be used for an infant, and the posterior-curved portion of the heel for a newborn child. If the fingers are extremely rough or calloused, then the ear lobe may be used. It may also be advisable to use the ear lobe if the patient will be immediately handling contaminated material. Actually the ear lobe puncture is painless, but patients are apprehensive about this. Venous blood is obtained from the veins found in the anterior cubitus (inner bend of the elbow) area of the arm (Fig. 31–2). This blood is called venous blood. The new vacuum needle and syringe units, such as the Vacutainer,* make this procedure practically painless if the correct technique is employed. The term **venipuncture** is used when a vein is punctured for

*Becton-Dickinson Co.,

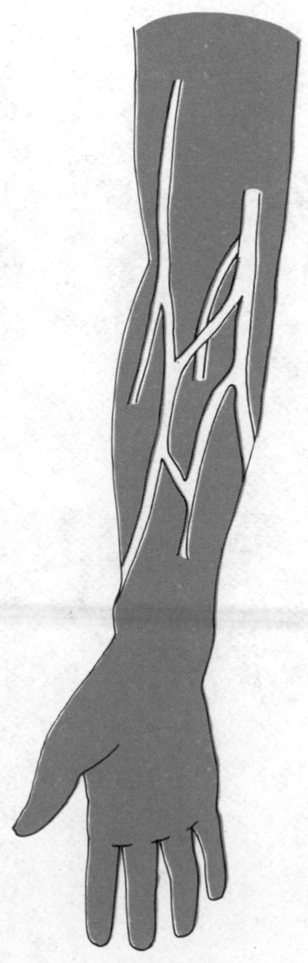

FIGURE 31–2 Veins in the anterior cubitus of the arm, a common site for withdrawal of venous blood.

any purpose, whether to withdraw blood or to administer a medication into the vein and circulatory system.

Because so many different tests other than the ones termed hematologic are performed on the blood, it is necessary to handle these specimens, especially venous blood, in different ways. Blood is sent to the laboratory in one of two ways: either the blood is prevented from clotting, or it is allowed to coagulate and form a clot, thus leaving a clot and **serum**. Speaking very generally the majority of blood chemistry tests and blood cell counts are done on *whole blood* to which an anticoagulant has been added to prevent a clot from forming. Blood may be prevented from forming a clot if it is shaken rather vigorously or agitated with glass beads in the tube. Never add an anticoagulating agent unless instructed. There are several different agents used, and it is very important that the correct one be used. If this anticoagulated blood were centrifuged, the cells would be spun to the bottom of the tube leaving **plasma** at the top. Plasma is the fluid portion of the blood from which the cells have been suspended, or forced to the bottom, by centrifuging.

The other method of handling blood is withdrawing the blood and allowing a clot to form. Nothing is added to the blood, and it is not shaken or chilled. In a moderately short time, normal blood will form a clot, leaving a fluid called *blood serum*, which does not contain any cells or fibrin. This fluid is used for blood **serologic** tests, such as for syphilis or antigen-antibody reactions.

Venipuncture Technique

EQUIPMENT NEEDED

Vacuum blood collecting unit such as a Vacutainer (Fig. 31–3):
- Glass tube(s) with rubber stopper
- Plastic holder with guide line
- Double-pointed needle with sheath

Tourniquet
Skin disinfectant swabs
Sterile dry cotton balls
Elastic bandage strips
Labels and laboratory forms

The tourniquet should be a thin, flat-walled rubber tubing such as a Penrose tube. There are several tourniquets on the market that are about 1 in. wide and have Velcro closures. A blood pressure cuff may also be used if the patient is extra sensitive to pain. The cuff is inflated to about 40 mm Hg. A small rubber tube such as the blood pipette tubing is not recommended as the best to use. Be careful not to pinch the skin with the half bow.

If the syringe technique is used for the venipuncture, then you would need in place of the vacuum tube unit:

Syringe, 10 cc or 20 cc (must be sterile and dry)
Needle, 19–21 gauge, 1–1½ in. (smaller gauge should not be used as it may damage the cells.)
Collection tube(s) with rubber stopper
Labels and laboratory forms

If a disposable syringe is used, then loosen the plunger by moving it back and forth a few times. Attach the needle securely, and loosen the sheath on the needle. Remove the needle *before* placing the blood in the tube(s), and inject the blood slowly into the tube(s). Invert the anticoagulant tubes 10 to 12 times.

VEIN SELECTION. Intravenous blood is usually drawn from a vein in the antecubital area of the arm (inner bend of the elbow). Ask the patient if he is right- or left-handed and, if possible, select the minor arm, but both arms should be checked for the best site. A vein does not have to be visible to be a good selection, but it must be carefully **palpated** to assure the technician it is a good selection. Superficial veins are not usually best to use, especially the large ones that roll easily.

A

how to assemble

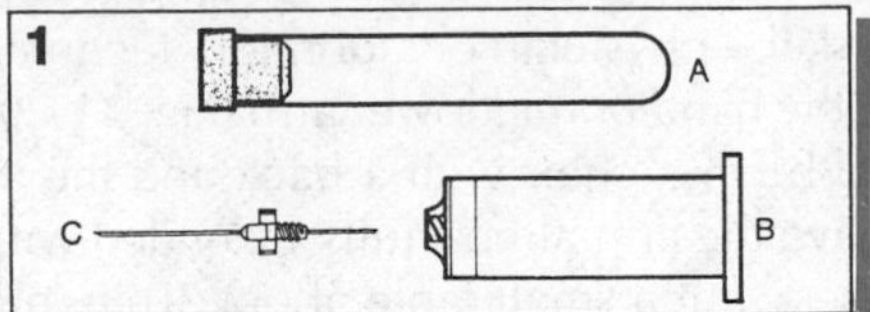

Description of parts:
A. Evacuated Glass Tube with Rubber Stopper
B. Plastic Holder with Guide Line
C. Double-Pointed Needle

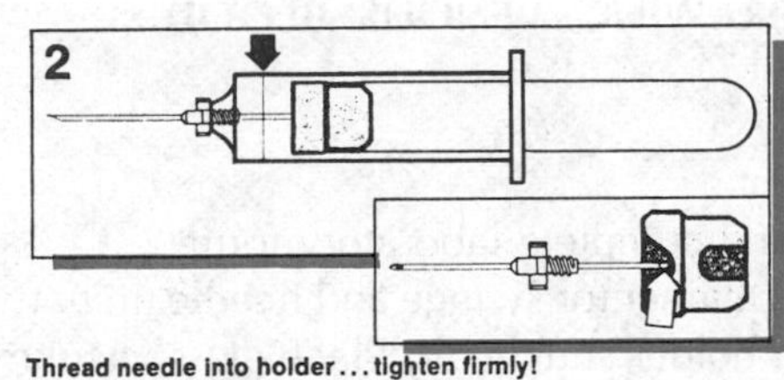

Thread needle into holder . . . tighten firmly!
Place tube in holder with needle touching stopper.

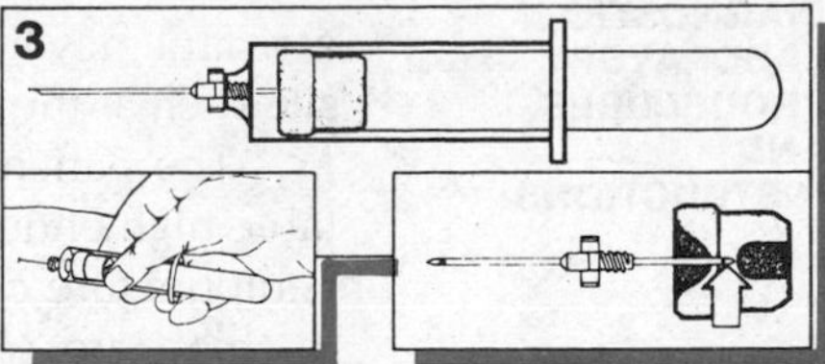

Push tube forward until top of stopper meets guide line. Let go. Tube stopper will retract below guide line—leave it in that position.
At this stage, the full point of the needle is embedded in the stopper (see cross section) thus avoiding blood leakage upon venipuncture and preventing premature loss of vacuum.

Alternate Method
If needle and adapter are used, follow these instructions in place of steps 1 and 2.

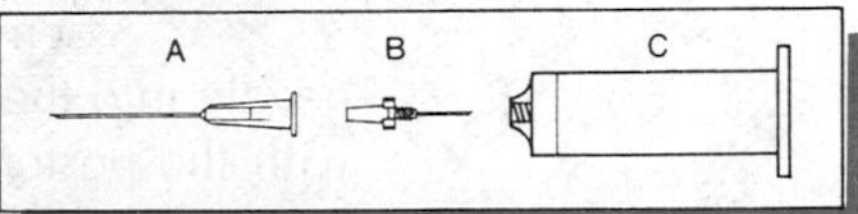

Description of parts:
A. Luer Hub Needle
B. VACUTAINER Adapter
C. Plastic Holder
Thread adapter into holder . . . tighten firmly!
Attach Luer Needle to Adaptor slip as you would needle to a syringe. Place tube in holder with needle touching stopper, then proceed to step 3, above.

B

how to use

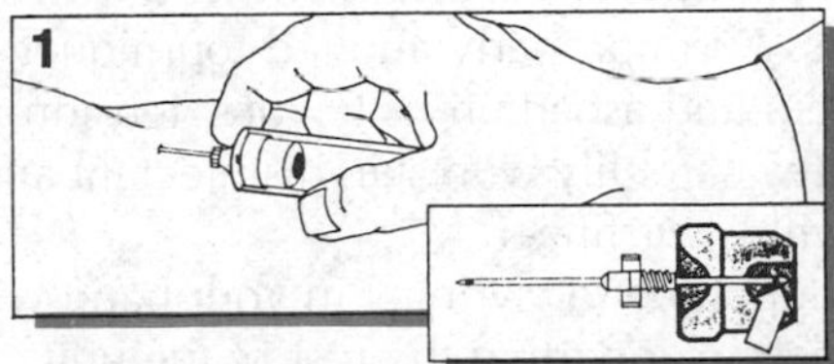

With rear point embedded in stopper, enter tissue—and immediately on tissue entry complete puncture of diaphragm.

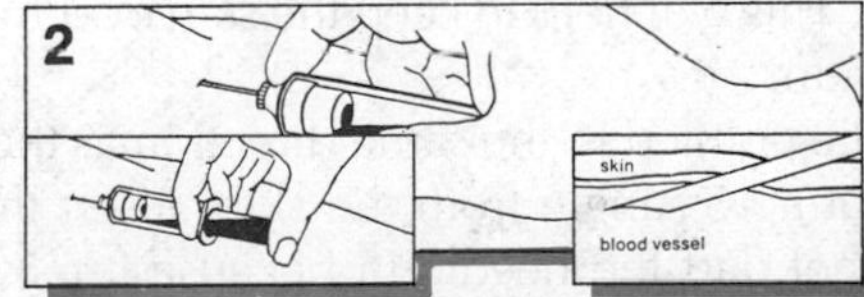

If in vein—blood flows immediately. Note: Technologist with small hands, proceed as you would with a hypodermic syringe. Holder provides finger grip and tube acts as plunger (see inset).

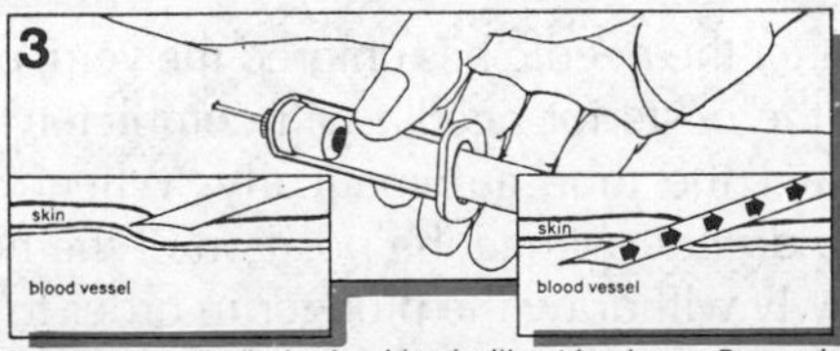

If in tissue instead of vein—blood will not be drawn. Proceed until venipuncture is signaled by intake of blood into VACUTAINER Tube, as shown.

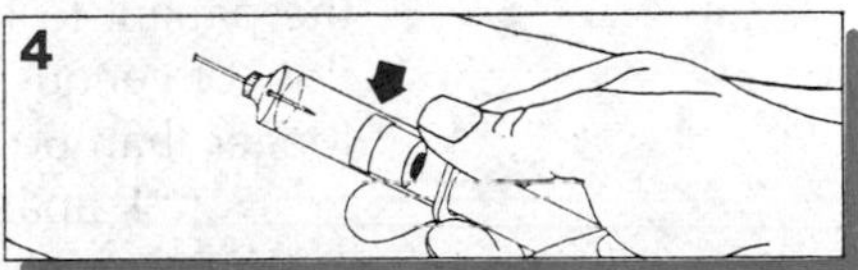

Where vein cannot be located—to conserve vacuum—remove tube from rear cannula (see arrow) before withdrawing needle from tissue.

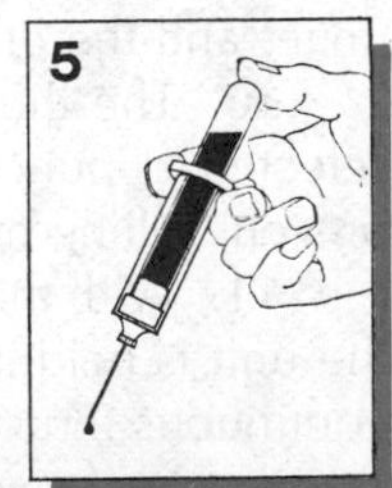

How to obtain blood drops for red and white cell counts, blood smears, etc. After tube is filled—grasp holder as illustrated and press firmly on bottom of tube. After each drop, release pressure and repeat for successive drops.

Additional Information
Incomplete Venipuncture, which may cause the tube to fill slowly or partially, may be corrected by deeper vein entry.
Transfixing of the vein may be corrected by pulling back slowly with needle until flow of blood indicates vein lumen re-entry.
Multiple Specimens (2, 3 or more) may be taken with one venipuncture and without loss of blood by releasing tourniquet while first tube is filling, and switching tubes while needle remains in vein.
Vein occlusion can be minimized by using VACUTAINER Adapter and smaller gauge needles (23, 24 or 25 gauge), thus slowing up flow of blood.
Proper degree of vacuum in each VACUTAINER Tube is doubly assured by the B-D Can Pack.

FIGURE 31–3 **B-D Vacutainer method of making a venipuncture.** ***A,*** **How to assemble B-D Vacutainer.** ***B,*** **How to use B-D Vacutainer. (Courtesy of Becton, Dickinson and Company.)**

Have the patient extend the arm and support it on a rolled towel, or the patient may place his other fist under the elbow for support. Before applying the tourniquet, gently palpate over the area and select the best vein. A vein has a spongy feeling very much like a small rubber tube. Tissue feels entirely different and does not feel "hollow" or have the bounce that a vein has. A tendon has a solid firmness and, of course, an artery is pulsating.

The median basilic vein and the median cephalic vein are the most commonly used. It may be very difficult to locate a vein on an **obese** person, and the medical assistant may have to ask the physician or laboratory technician to select an alternate site such as the back of the hand or mid lower arm (Fig. 31–2).

The patient should be in a chair with a back and the arm well-supported on a table high enough to have the arm almost fully extended with only a slight flexion. A venipuncture chair is best, but a small table about 30 in. high and a chair about 16 in. high are satisfactory. Make certain the patient will not fall off if he should faint.

PROCEDURE FOR DRAWING VENOUS BLOOD

1. Wash hands.
2. Identify patient.
3. Label tubes and complete laboratory form.
4. Assemble Vacutainer (or syringe and needle unit). *Vacutainer*: (a) Screw the needle into the plastic holder snugly. (b) Place glass vacuum tube in plastic holder with the posterior tip of the needle just touching the stopper. (c) Push the needle forward until the rubber stopper reaches the guide line. (d) Release the tube. It will fall back slightly below the guide line and should remain in position. *Syringe and needle*: Place needle snugly on syringe and loosen needle sheath.
5. Place patient's arm in correct position and select vein.
6. Apply tourniquet to about 2 to 3 in. above the bend of the elbow and ask the patient to make a fist. The tourniquet tension should be enough to impede the flow of venous blood but not obstruct arterial flow. DO NOT leave a tourniquet on longer than 60 seconds. An improperly applied tourniquet can be painful.
7. Palpate the vein and ascertain its texture, tension, and position.
8. Cleanse the area carefully with skin disinfectant and allow it to dry. Do not touch the area again with your finger.
9. Hold the vacuum tube (or syringe) in your hand with the thumb and index finger and the other fingers supporting the rest of the unit.
10. The thumb of the other hand is placed about 1½ to 2 in. below the site selected for puncturing. This will help to keep the skin over the vein taut and possibly prevent rolling of the vein.
11. With the needle pointed in the same direction as the vein and the bevel up, the unit is held at about a 15° angle from the skin. Insert the needle with a steady continuous thrust. Do not dart the needle in because it may penetrate through the vein's posterior wall. A slight "pop" may be felt as the needle penetrates the vein.
12. Level the needle angle with the vein and insert about ¼ in. into the lumen of the vein.
13. Immediately after the needle has entered the vein, push the glass tube of the Vacutainer forward so the posterior needle will completely enter the vacuum tube. Blood will begin to enter the tube automatically. When you push the glass tube forward, be careful you do not change the position of the needle in the vein. If you are using a syringe, slowly withdraw the plunger in order to create a suction and fill the syringe. DO NOT push on the plunger in any way. If the blood flow is slow, leave the tourniquet on a little longer.

15. After a sufficient quantity of blood has been withdrawn, release the tourniquet and ask the patient to unclench his fist.
16. Place a sterile dry cotton ball over the site of the needle insertion and withdraw the needle moderately slowly.
17. Immediately apply firm pressure over the puncture site and hold for a few moments. The patient may help by elevating the arm and holding the cotton ball firmly. Sometimes a patient is asked to bend the arm in order to stop the bleeding, but this does not cause pressure over the lateral veins, and bleeding from a large deep vein will not stop if the arm is only bent. Pressure directly over the site is the best

method for preventing formation of a hematoma. Inspect the site, and if the bleeding has stopped, apply a pressure bandage strip with a large dry cotton ball. Do not let the patient leave without making certain that the bleeding has stopped.

18. Check the labels and forms for completeness. Inspect the anticoagulant tubes to see that they were thoroughly mixed.

19. Destroy the needles and disposable equipment.

Points to Remember

1. If the puncture is incomplete and the needle withdrawn from the tissue in order to locate another site, the needle should be discarded and another unit used.
2. If blood starts to flow but immediately stops, the needle may have penetrated through both vein walls and entered the tissue behind the vein. Withdraw the needle slightly until the flow of blood starts again.
3. If blood flow into the tube is slow, this may be corrected by repositioning the needle slightly or penetrating a bit deeper.
4. On very rare occasions, the vacuum may be gone from the tube and another tube will have to be used.
5. If the vein has collapsed, it may help to apply pressure above the puncture site with two fingers and then release. This will help the vein fill up and should start the flow again.
6. If the patient has been seriously ill or is an elderly person, it may be difficult to complete a venipuncture. It may be best for the medical assistant to ask the physician or laboratory technician to find an alternate site.
7. When using a standard type of syringe with a plunger, do not pull too fast or too hard on the plunger. This can cause a vein to collapse.
8. If possible, avoid using a site that has had frequent punctures. The vein may be scarred in this area and will be difficult to puncture.
9. Learn the difference between the feel of a vein and a tendon. It is quite painful for the patient if a tendon rather than a vein is punctured.

THE DIFFICULT PATIENT. If at all possible, you should try to persuade the patient to permit you to proceed. This is best done by talking to the patient and explaining that the physician wants this done because he thinks it is necessary. Do not get into a discussion with the patient regarding the importance of or reason for the test. Emphasize that the physician has requested it. If this does not work, then the physician will have to be notified. Sometimes the difficulty is not that the patient does not cooperate but that the vein is impossible to find. This may happen with the obese patient or if the patient has very small delicate veins. Patients who have been severely ill and have been given considerable intravenous fluids may also have troublesome veins. It is advisable that a patient not be stuck more than two times. It is probably best for the medical assistant to call the physician or the laboratory technician, and they may wish to use an alternate vein such as on a hand. Sometimes puncture of a finger will offer sufficient blood for a test.

CHOICE OF ANTICOAGULANT. An anticoagulant is an agent that is added to blood to prevent the formation of a clot. As with all blood specimens, it must be handled gently and instructions must be carefully followed. Blood cells are fragile, and mishandling may cause destruction of the cells and possibly lead to inaccurate test results.

If blood is transferred from a syringe and needle unit to a tube, the needle must be removed first and the blood expelled into the tube gently and without any air bubbles forming. The stopper is replaced and if an anticoagulant is added, the tube is inverted 10 to 12 times. DO NOT SHAKE. If a vacuum tube is used, the tube is inverted in the same manner.

The choice of anticoagulant used is determined by the test to be performed. You must use the recommended agent because otherwise test results could be altered. Check with the laboratory instructions or the laboratory technician for the proper directions.

EDTA. This agent does not destroy blood cells and is often the preferred anticoagulant, especially when there is to be a cell study.

Heparin. This agent does not kill blood cells and is used mainly for electrolytes.

Oxalates. Potassium oxalate and ammonium oxalate, when used separately, will damage blood cells but in combination do not affect a hematocrit.

Citrates. These are used primarily for coagulant studies.

For a serologic test, about 2½ times the amount needed for the test is collected; that is, 10 ml of blood yields approximately 4 ml of serum. Do not shake or chill the blood but replace the stopper and set the tube in an upright position. A clot will form within 30 to 60 minutes. Most laboratories prefer that the physician's office not "ring" the blood or attempt to remove the clot. Handle the specimen carefully and send it to the laboratory as soon as possible.

COMPLETE BLOOD COUNT (CBC). This is the most frequently done blood test. It usually consists of a *white blood cell count (wbc)*, also called *leukocyte* count; a *red blood cell count (rbc),* also called *erythrocyte* count; a *hemoglobin determination (hgb);* and a *white cell differential count (diff.)*. Frequently a **hematocrit** *(Hct)* is also done with the complete blood count, or the physician may request a white blood cell count, a differential, and a hematocrit. There is some variance in the so-called routine complete blood count, depending on the physician's wishes. These tests are usually done on capillary blood but can be done on venous blood. There is no special patient preparation for these tests.

The *red cell count* is the number of red blood cells in one cubic millimeter of blood. The normal range is 4.8 to 5.5 million per cu mm for men and 4.4 to 5.0 million per cu mm for women. These may be written out in full, such as 4,400,000 to 5,000,000. An increase in erythrocytes is referred to as **polycythemia** and a decrease is called **anemia**. Technically, an anemia is a laboratory finding and not a diagnosis. For example, a normocytic normochromic anemia is a *finding* in malnutrition; malnutrition is the *diagnosis*. There are many different types and causes for an anemia.

The *white cell count* is the number of white blood cells in one cubic millimeter of blood. The normal range varies with hematologists, but the *average is 5,000 to 10,000 per cu mm*. The white blood cell count is very diagnostic and can fluctuate fairly rapidly. In some diseases the count rises, and in other diseases the count falls. The rise and fall has been compared to a barometer that indicates the course of a disease or the progress of an infection. Leukocytes also play some role in the repair of injured tissue, but their chief function is to protect the body against microorganisms causing disease.

Hemoglobin Determination. Hemoglobin is contained within the red blood cells. It is composed of heme (an organic compound of iron) and globin (a simple protein). The normal ranges are 14.5 to 16.0 gm per 100 ml of blood for men and 13.0 to 15.5 gm per 100 ml of blood for women. Hemoglobin is the essential carrier of oxygen in the body. The hemoglobin and red cell counts do not always rise and fall together, but there is generally some correlation between the two. In hemorrhage both the number of red cells and the level of hemoglobin fall, but in an iron deficiency anemia the hemoglobin is reduced more than the red cells are. In pernicious anemia or in a polychromasia, the red cells are reduced more than the hemoglobin.

Differential White Cell Count. There are several different white blood cells that can be identified microscopically when the blood is smeared on a microscopic slide

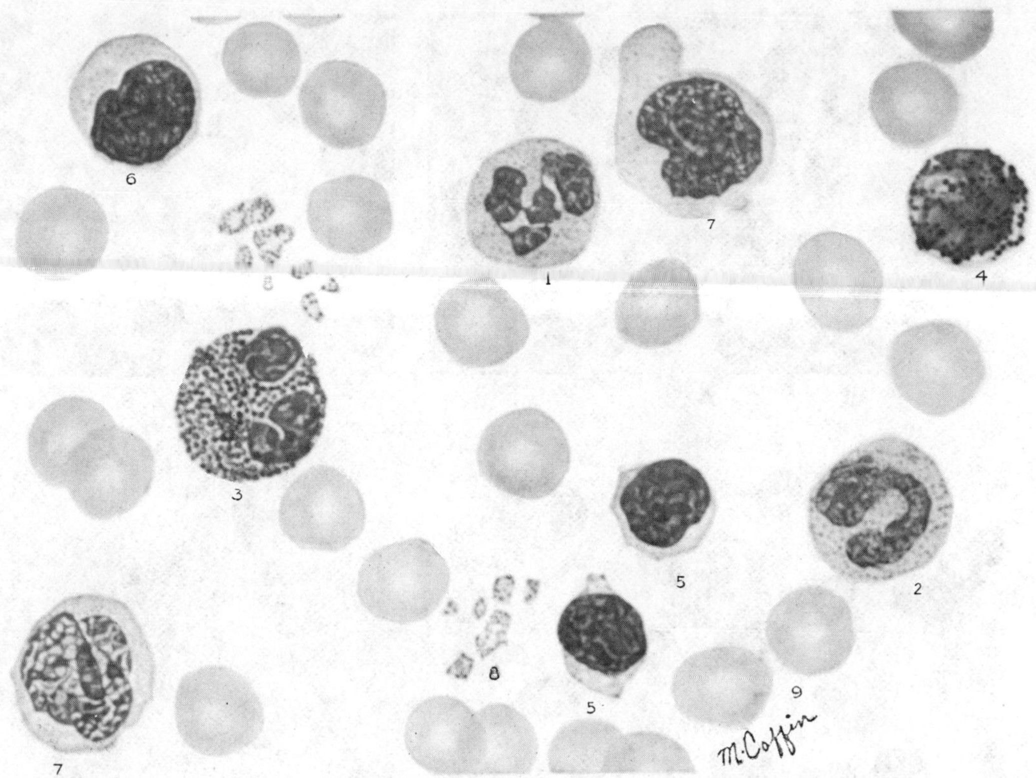

FIGURE 31–4 **Normal cellular constituents of adult human blood. I, Segmented (polymorphonuclear) neutrophil; 2, Band (stab) neutrophil; 3, Segmented eosinophil; 4, Basophil; 5, Small lymphocytes; 6, Large lymphocyte; 7, Monocytes; 8, Thrombocytes; and 9, Erythrocytes. (From Custer, R. P. (ed.):** ***An Atlas of the Blood and Bone Marrow*****. 2nd ed. Philadelphia, W. B. Saunders Co., 1974.)**

and stained (Fig. 31–4). It is very helpful to the physician to know whether the normal percentage range of these cells has changed. This change may indicate the progress or direction of a disease or infection. Because this change is so important, it should always be a part of a complete blood count. The number of white blood cells in the complete blood count does not tell which one of the various white cells has increased or decreased. These leukocytes are divided into five types: lymphocytes, monocytes, neutrophils, eosinophils, and basophils. The last three are often referred to as granulocytes. A change in these cells is extremely important, and especially so when considered with the white blood count and the patient's condition or diagnosis. An example of this is an increase in eosinophils often seen in some parasitic diseases and some allergic conditions. A marked increase of younger, immature neutrophils is called a "left shift" and can be prognostic to the physician. Frequently the progress of a disease will appear in the blood "picture" before the patient shows any clinical signs or symptoms. Normal ranges for these leukocytes are:

Neutrophils	54 to 62 per cent
Eosinophils	1 to 3 per cent
Basophils	0 to 1 per cent
Lymphocytes	25 to 33 per cent
Monocytes	0 to 9 per cent

While the hematologist is counting and studying the white blood cells, she is also examining the red blood cells seen on the slide. These erythrocytes, as they are correctly called, are examined for size and shape, for how they have taken the stain, or for any abnormality that may be seen (Fig. 31–5).

Hematocrit (Hct). This test measures the relative volume of cells and plasma in the blood. It is often done in combination with the red cell count and the hemoglobin, or

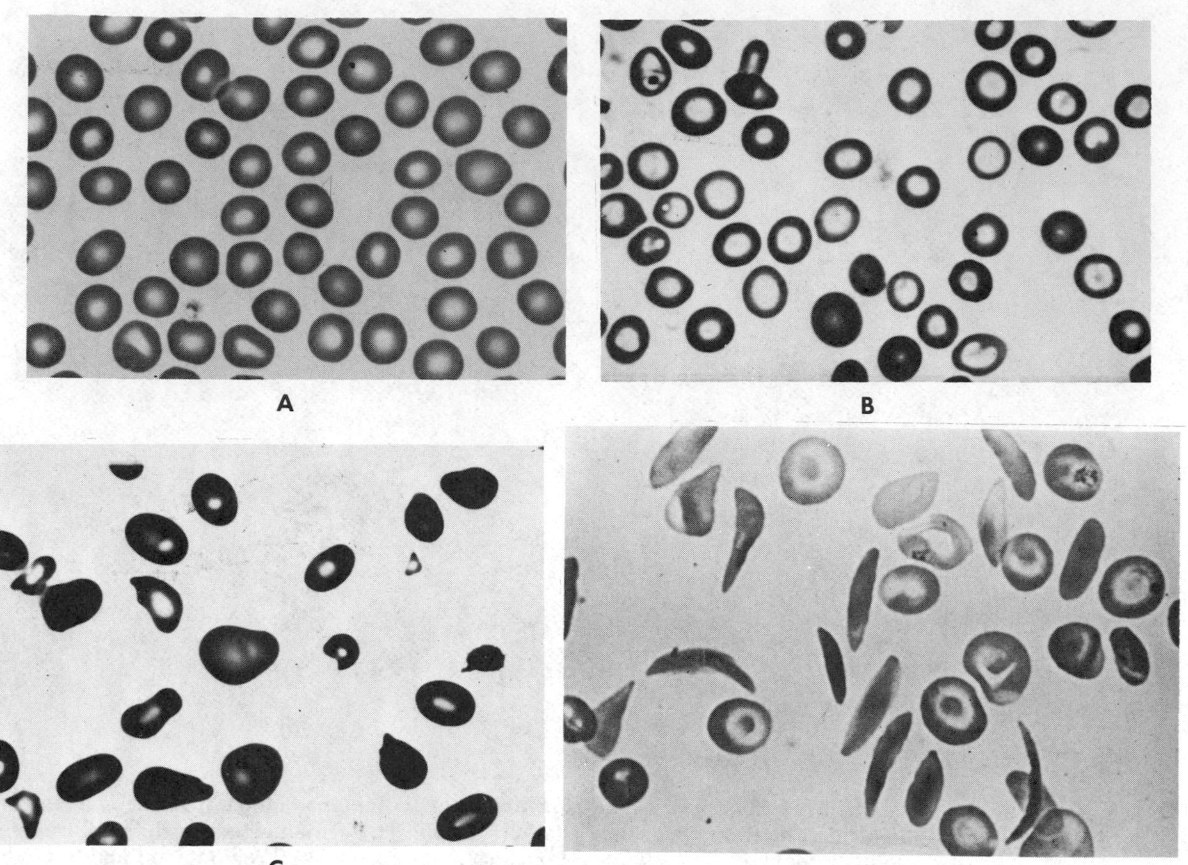

FIGURE 31–5 A comparison of red blood cells. *A,* Normal blood. *B,* Iron deficiency anemia. Note lack of color (hypochromia), smaller size (microcythemia), and elliptical cells. *C,* Megaloblastic anemia. Note varying size of cells (anisocytosis) and large cells (macrocytosis). (All from Henry, J.: *Clinical Diagnosis and Management by Laboratory Procedures.* 16th ed. Philadelphia, W. B. Saunders Co., 1979.) *D,* Sickle cell anemia, showing sickle-shaped cells and target cells. (From Raphael, S. S.: *Lynch's Medical Laboratory Technology*. 3rd ed. Philadelphia, W. B. Saunders Co., 1976.)

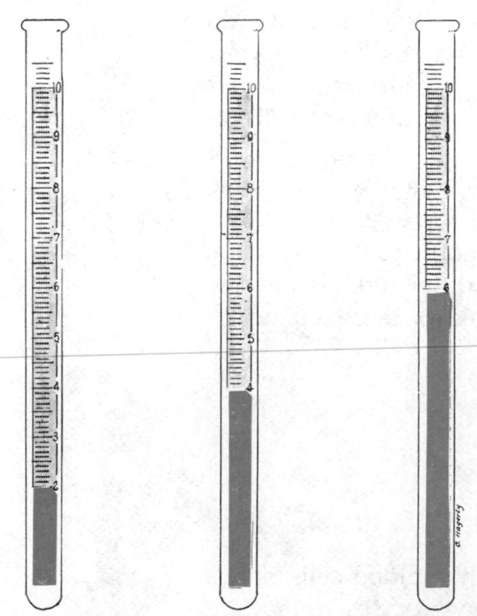

FIGURE 31–6 High and low hematocrit readings (Wintrobe tubes). (From Seiverd, C. E.: *Hematology for Medical Technologists*. 4th ed. Philadelphia, Lea and Febiger, 1972.)

in place of the hemoglobin. In anemias and after a hemorrhage the hematocrit reading is lower than normal, while in dehydration and polycythemia the reading is higher. Both capillary and venous blood are used. If the test is done with capillary blood it is then called "microhematocrit." There is no special preparation for the patient. The blood must be prevented from coagulating. If venous blood is used, an anticoagulant is added to the blood. Special capillary tubes containing an anti-coagulant are used for the micro method (Fig. 31–6).

The results are expressed in cubic millimeters per 100 ml of blood, or in volumes per 100 ml. Normal ranges are 45 to 50 vol per 100 ml for men and 40 to 45 vol per 100 ml for women.

Erythrocyte Sedimentation Rate (SR, ESR, or Sed Rate). When red blood cells are allowed to settle out of their plasma, the speed of their fall in a given length of time is known as the *sedimentation rate*. This rate has been found to depend, to some degree, on changes in the blood proteins. There are several different methods for running this test, and the normal ranges vary with each method. The laboratory will usually list the normal range for the method used. There are also differences of opinion as to the reliability of the test. It was once said that "it doesn't tell where the fire is, but does tell how hot it is." It is used as a rough index of the progress or presence of an inflammatory disease such as rheumatoid arthritis, rheumatic fever, or respiratory disease. Both capillary and venous blood are used. It is prevented from coagulating so that the cells can settle. There is no patient preparation for a sedimentation rate. Women tend to have a higher reading than men, especially during menstruation. Some samples of normal ranges are (Fig. 31–7):

	Men	*Women*
Cutler Method	0–8	0–10
Wintrobe Method	0–6.5	0–15
Westergren Method	0–15	0–20

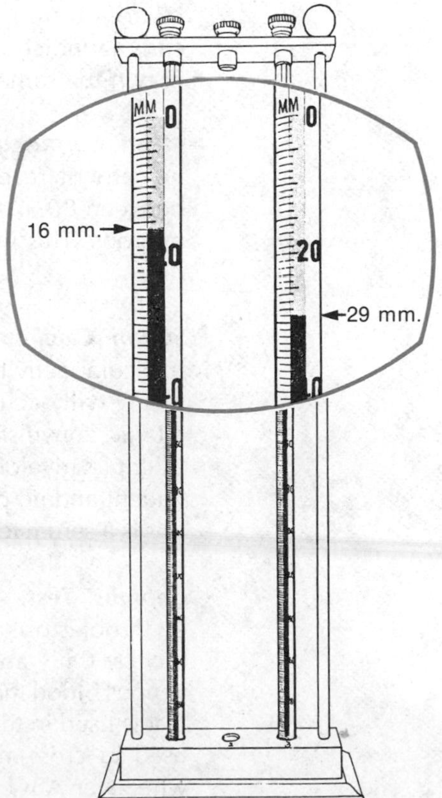

FIGURE 31–7 ESR, Erythrocyte sedimentation rate. Reading the sedimentation rate in a Westergren tube. In the circled inset, the upper very light portion of each tube is plasma. The lower darker portion is red cells. Normal rates are: males, 1-15 mm/hr and females, 1-20 mm/hr. Both patients' blood illustrated here are below normal. (From Seiverd, C. E.: *Hematology for Medical Technologists*. 4th ed. Philadelphia, Lea and Febiger, 1972.)

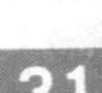

Prothrombin Time (pro Time or PT). This is a test to measure the clotting ability of the blood. It is an essential test in establishing and maintaining anticoagulation therapy, such as the administration of Dicumarol and other similar drugs. This test may also be done daily during acute stages of myocardial infarction. Prothrombin content of the blood is often low in liver diseases, vitamin K deficiency, and thrombinemia in infants. Venous blood is used and mixed with a special solution. Certain medications such as barbiturates may interfere with accurate results; otherwise there is no special patient preparation. Normal ranges depend on the specific type of test done, but the usual range is from 11 to 18 seconds.

Heterophil. Basically, this is a test used to confirm a clinical diagnosis of infectious mononucleosis, but it is also used in the diagnosis of serum sickness. It is an agglutination reaction between the patient's blood serum and washed sheep cells. A series of dilutions is made in test tubes, then incubated. The greatest dilution that agglutinates the erythrocytes is noted. There are no special restrictions or instructions for the patient. Venous blood is drawn and allowed to coagulate to obtain the blood serum. Normal range is near 1:28. A reading of 1:56 is considered diagnostic.

Tests for the Presence of Bile (Bilirubin) in the Blood

Bilirubin (van den Bergh Method). This is to determine the presence of free bilirubin that is broken down from hemoglobin. It is an important liver function test and is also done on newborn infants to determine the possibility of performing an exchange transfusion. There are several drugs and some foods, when taken in excess, that can interfere with an accurate reading. It may be best to check with the laboratory if there is a question. It is preferred that fasting venous blood be used, but this is not absolutely necessary. The blood is allowed to coagulate and the serum is used. Normal range is from 0.1 to 1.0 mg per 100 ml of serum.

Icterus Index. This is a simple test to determine the amount of bilirubin in blood serum, but it does not differentiate between bilirubin due to hemolysis or due to a biliary obstruction, so this test does have limitations. It is useful in discovering an early jaundice condition before it is visible to the physician. The patient's serum is drawn the same as in the above bilirubin test. Normal range is 4 to 6 units.

Mean Corpuscular Volume (MCV). This is a measurement calculated from the hematocrit reading and the red blood cell count. The MCV in normal adults is between 80 and 90 microns. In some microcytic anemias it may go as high as 150 microns. This index is not valid unless the red blood cell count is absolutely accurate.

Serum Calcium (Ca). Calcium is essential in the formation of bone tissue, in muscular activity, and in blood coagulation. When there is a deficiency of calcium, tetany will occur. This condition is characterized by a twitching of muscle fibers and tetanic convulsions. An increase of blood calcium is found in hyperparathyroidism, multiple myeloma, and some respiratory diseases. There is no preparation of the patient and no patient restrictions. Venous blood is drawn and allowed to clot, since this is a serum test. Normal range is 8 to 11 mg per 100 ml of serum.

Coombs' Test. This test is done basically on newborn infants for the diagnosis of erythroblastosis fetalis. In many hospitals it is done routinely on all umbilical cord blocks. Only about 2 cc of blood is needed and is taken directly from the cord, or venous blood may be drawn. Normally the results are negative. The indirect Coombs' test is used in the detection of various minor blood type factors, including Rh, and is used in cross-matching blood for blood transfusions. Rh typing is done routinely whenever ABO blood typing is done. The test determines whether the Rh factor is present (Rh-positive) or absent (Rh-negative) in the patient's or the donor's blood. Normal reading is negative.

Blood Urea Nitrogen (BUN). This is a kidney function test. Normally the kidneys excrete urea, a major product of the kidneys, the end product of protein metabolism. In some kidney diseases this may be impaired and the kidneys do not excrete urea sufficiently, so the urea nitrogen in the blood increases. This test gives essentially the same information as the nonprotein nitrogen (NPN) but is more accurate. There is no preparation of the patient nor any food restrictions. Venous blood is drawn, and an anticoagulant is added. Normal range is 8 to 28 mg per 100 ml of blood.

Uric Acid. This test is used basically to aid in the diagnosis of gout, a **metabolic** disease marked by acute arthritis and inflammation of the joints. Uric acid is the end product of purine (a protein) metabolism. An increase of uric acid is also seen in severe kidney damage and **toxemias** of pregnancy. There is no preparation of the patient or dietary restriction. Venous blood is used and an anticoagulant added. Normal range is 3.0 to 5.0 mg per 100 ml of blood.

Protein-Bound Iodine (PBL). Since iodine is used by the thyroid gland to manufacture thyroxin, and since iodine is also stored in the thyroid gland, this test is basically a thyroid function test. Iodine in the blood serum is bound, or attached, to the protein molecule and is not free iodine in the blood, thus the name protein-bound iodine. Hypothyroidism will give a low reading, whereas hyperthyroidism produces an increased reading. There is no preparation of the patient, but this test is affected by many medications and by any radiographic contrast media. Some radiopaque iodine-containing injectable media can produce a falsely high PBI reading for several months, or even years. The patient's history must be carefully checked. Venous blood is used and allowed to clot, since this is a serum test. Normal range is 5 to 8 micrograms per 100 ml of serum.

Thyroxine Iodine or Butanol-Extractable Iodine (BEI). These tests are for thyroid function and have a distinct advantage over the PBI because radiographic contrast media do not interfere. It is generally preferred that the patient's diet be iodine-free for three days before the test. Venous blood is drawn and allowed to clot, since the test is done on blood serum. Normal range is 3.5 to 6.5 micrograms per 100 ml of serum.

Blood Glucose or Blood Sugar (Bl S). This is one of the most frequently performed blood chemistry tests. It is used in the diagnosis of diabetes and as an aid in the control of diabetic patients. This test is requested by a wide range of specialists in the medical profession. The ophthalmologist sees patients with blurred vision and the podiatrist sees patients with foot ulcers that are not healing normally. Each of these conditions may be seen in diabetic patients.

An increase in the blood sugar is called **hyperglycemia** and a decrease is called **hypoglycemia.** Because "fasting blood" is used, patients are instructed to eat or drink nothing, except water, for 12 hours before the test is done. Diabetic patients should not take their dose of insulin until after the blood has been drawn. Occasionally a physician will want to know a patient's response to food intake, and he will order a blood sugar test at a specific time after a meal. In this case the time of the meal and the time the blood is drawn must be noted. It is usually done two hours after the meal. The laboratory will usually ask the patient for a urine specimen at the time the blood is drawn. Venous blood is used and an anticoagulant is added. Normal range for fasting blood is 80 to 120 mg per 100 ml.

Glucose Tolerance or Sugar Tolerance. These tests are done to determine a patient's response to a standard amount of glucose. The patient reports to the laboratory in a fasting state the same as for a regular blood glucose. Fasting blood is drawn and a urine specimen requested. The patient is then given a rather large dose of glucose, usually in one of various flavors of a soda pop-type mixture that the patient drinks. At regular intervals thereafter, blood is drawn and a urine sample requested. These tests determine how the patient's body handles the added glucose. These tests are valuable in ruling out diabetes mellitus and in diagnosing a possible hyperinsulinism. The patient should be told that it will be necessary to stay at the laboratory for three to five hours, depending on the physician's request. Blood is drawn and an anticoagulant is added for each interval test. The normal response to the oral glucose intake is that the blood sugar peaks not more than 150 mg per 100 ml and returns to the fasting state within two hours. Very elderly patients may reach a slightly higher peak.

Cholesterol (Chol). Cholesterol is normally found in the blood, but some disease states will raise or decrease the cholesterol concentration. An elevated reading may aid in the diagnosis of liver function, hypothyroidism, and a possibility of **atherosclerosis,** although these findings on the last condition are still in the research state. A decrease is found in hyperthyroidism, anemias, cachexia, and acute infections. The patient is often asked to avoid high cholesterol foods for a period of time before the test, or some physicians and laboratories want fasting blood used for the test. It is advisable to check with the physician and/or the laboratory before instructing the patient. The blood is drawn and allowed to coagulate. The normal range is 150 to 250 mg per 100 ml.

Serum Triglycerides. Elevated serum triglycerides are best interpreted in association with serum cholesterol levels and lipoprotein electrophoreses. Triglyceride levels are often elevated in patients with coronary artery disease, diabetes mellitus, **nephrotic syndrome,** hyperthyroidism, and hepatic disease. The values are most reliable after 24-hour fasting. The normal range is 40 to 150 mg per 100 ml.

Serologic Test for Syphilis (STS). This test may also be referred to as a test for Venereal Disease, Syphilis (VDS) or Venereal Disease Research Laboratory test (VDRL). There are several varieties of tests for this disease, and there are too many to list here. Often the medical office is not concerned with the specific type of test run but with the results of the test. There are several factors that interfere with the results of various tests. The interpretation requires skill and experience, as well as correlation with the clinical findings and patient's medical history. All the questions on the laboratory request form must be answered, such as whether it is a new case or treated case. Solomon Garb, M.D., in *Laboratory Tests in Common Use,* has written: "In early primary syphilis the serology is negative. In late, adequately treated syphilis, the serology may be fixed at a high positive titer although the patient is, in effect, cured. In late, improperly treated syphilis, the serology may be negative even though the patient is not cured and is developing central nervous system involvement."

Many physicians' offices and most hospitals now require a routine STS on all patients. Most states have legal requirements for syphilitic testing before marriage and before the birth of a baby. These are the required "premarital" and "prenatal" tests.

There is no special patient preparation or restriction. Since the test is a serologic test, the blood is drawn and allowed to coagulate. Normally the reaction is negative. A faintly positive reaction usually warrants further testing and study because it may indicate some other disorder.

EXAMINATION OF SPUTUM

Sputum is the secretion from the lungs, bronchi, and trachea which is ejected through the mouth and is usually obtained by deep coughing. Sputum must not be confused with saliva and postnasal secretions. Saliva and postnasal secretions are considered contaminants in a sputum specimen and complicate or interfere with accurate sputum examinations. Sputum is examined primarily for agents causing infectious diseases such as tuberculosis, pneumonia, and candidiasis (one of the many fungal infections found in the lungs). The Papanicolaou stain is also done on cells found in sputum to determine cancer. For the detection of pulmonary carcinoma the sputum is collected in a 95 per cent alcohol solution for 72 consecutive hours.

Special containers should be provided to the patient. These are about two-ounce wide-mouthed sterile jars or waxed paper cardboard containers. The caps should fit snugly. Most laboratories and public health department laboratories will furnish these containers. Instruct the patient to give only sputum and not saliva. Many patients have their most productive cough the first thing in the morning. Tell the patient to be very careful, not to contaminate the outside of the container, and not to fill it more than half full. If the specimen cannot be taken to the laboratory within the next few hours, or a 24-hour or three days' specimen is requested, then the container should be refrigerated.

EXAMINATION OF FECES (STOOL) SPECIMENS

If you compare feces to blood or urine, there are relatively few tests done on feces. However, these few tests are important to both the patient's health and as an aid to the physician's diagnosis. Perhaps the infrequency with which the tests are performed is the reason for considerable mishandling of these specimens. It is very important that the medical assistant instruct the patient correctly, and that the specimen be taken to the laboratory as instructed. The laboratory technicians will appreciate this. Technicians say that of all the specimens brought into the laboratory, the feces specimen is the most mishandled, thus making it difficult for them to examine or causing them to instruct the patient and request another specimen. No one would appreciate repeating this procedure unless necessary for further testing and certainly not because of mishandling or poor instructions.

Because defecation does not take place at will, as urination does, the patient cannot be sent to the lavatory to get a specimen at any time. When a patient is told to bring a specimen to the laboratory he is usually embarrassed and somewhat confused as to how this procedure will have to take place. The medical assistant can ease the patient by simple matter-of-fact instructions. Remember to remind the patient that time is very often important, and that the feces must NOT be contaminated with urine. This is especially important when instructing the female patient. The patient must NOT take a laxative unless specifically instructed to do so, and then it is to be only a mild saline laxative and never one containing oil or a harsh chemical, which would interfere with the tests.

Furnish the patient with a wide-mouthed container, the same type used for collection of sputum. The patient may void into a plastic bag or onto a paper plate, then transfer a small amount, about the size of a walnut, into the container provided. Give the patient a few wooden tongue depressors to use for this transfer. This small amount is sufficient for most tests, unless otherwise specified.

SOME SPECIFIC TESTS AND THEIR COLLECTION. Specimens for *viral culture* must be taken to the laboratory immediately. It would be best to have the patient void while at the laboratory. If there is a delay between collecting the specimen and culturing it, then it must be kept very cold, even frozen, if necessary. *Bacterial culturing* also requires immediate examination. If the feces is diarrheal, a sterile cotton swab dipped into the specimen and placed in a sterile test tube is sufficient. The swab is best dipped into an area of the specimen that appears purulent. If *dysentery bacilli* are suspected, the physician will probably take a swab from the rectal or lower bowel area by holding the anus open with an anoscope. Place the swab in a sterile test tube and deliver to the laboratory immediately.

A patient may be furnished with a container of enriched broth. In this he places a piece of stool the size of a pea and immediately takes it to the laboratory. In some cases, a sterile swab may be inserted into the rectum and then placed in the broth. This method is used to detect Salmonella carriers.

Examination for Parasites. Loose, fluid stools to be examined for *intestinal amebae* and other *flagellates* are to be kept at body temperature and examined within 30 minutes. Well-formed stools to be examined for *ova* or *cystic forms of parasites* do not have to be kept warm and can be taken to the laboratory within a few hours. A small amount is sufficient for both examinations. If there is a possibility of a *tapeworm* the specimen may first be examined for diagnosis by the examination of a small amount to find the ova of the tapeworm, but if a purgative medication was given, the patient must then bring in the *entire* feces so the laboratory can search for the head (scolex) of the tapeworm. This is important, since the patient must be given another purgative unless the head is found. A plastic bag or large jar is used.

Pinworms inhabit the lower intestinal tract and are diagnosed by the presence of the ova. The female pinworm migrates to the anus during periods of rest, particularly at night, and deposits her eggs (ova). The most satisfactory means of confirming this diagnosis is to use a piece of transparent tape. The sticky side of the tape is pressed gently into the anal folds and then with the sticky side down the tape is placed on a microscopic glass slide and sent to the laboratory. There are also commercially prepared collecting applicators that may be used. This specimen should be taken immediately upon awakening, before any excess movement or going to the bathroom.

Occult Blood. The patient is instructed to eat no meat, including fish and poultry, for three days before a specimen is examined. Otherwise, false positive results may occur from the meat residue. Only a small amount of feces is needed.

Chemical Analysis. This requires the entire specimen defecated, since the amounts of the substances tested are reported and calculated on the basis of daily output. It would be advisable to keep the specimen cool to prevent excess bacterial growth.

Large amounts of undigested food in the stool may indicate abnormalities in digestion. Since this may be both a microscopic and macroscopic examination the amount needed may vary. It is best to check with the physician and the laboratory. A clay-colored stool may indicate a lack of the normal amounts of bile and will assist the physician in diagnosing a biliary obstruction. A small amount of specimen would be needed for testing for urobilin, also called stercobilin.

COLLECTION OF SEMEN

Semen (sperm) analysis is usually done for fertility studies, especially after vasectomies in order to establish the effectiveness of the vasectomy. The patient is asked to refrain from intercourse for two to four days before the sample is collected. The specimen is collected by masturbation or intercourse, with ejaculation into a clean sterile glass vial. Condoms (prophylactics) must not be used since they contain a spermicide powder. Semen taken from the vaginal canal may also be altered by vaginal secretions. The cap of the vial must be tightly closed, with the patient's name, date, and time of ejaculation written on the label. The specimen should be kept at body temperature and taken to the office or laboratory as soon as possible, preferably within 30 to 60 minutes. Several tests are usually done before any definite conclusions are given.

If a condom is used it must be carefully washed, rinsed, and thoroughly dried before using.

MYCOLOGY

Mycology is the study of fungus diseases. These vegetable cellular organisms are very numerous in the air, water and soil, but a few of them are capable of causing disease. Fungus diseases are often slow to appear and sometimes are difficult to diagnose and treat. Although many are resistant to treatment, only a very few are fatal. Among some fungus infections are histoplasmosis, coccidioidomycosis, ringworm, athlete's foot, and thrush.

Histoplasmosis is a disease caused by the inhalation of dust or decayed fowl and bird droppings containing the offending fungi. It begins in the lungs and then becomes systemic. It is not contagious between humans. It first appears as an influenza and resembles tuberculosis when x-rayed. A sputum specimen is collected and tested to aid in this diagnosis.

Coccidioidomycosis is also a fungal disease affecting the respiratory tract, but it can be superficial as well as systemic. The fungus is found in the dust in dry, hot southwestern areas of the United States and Mexico. It is called *desert fever* or *San Joaquin Valley fever.* It first appears as a respiratory, influenza-type disease. It is diagnosed by sputum examination, gastric washings, and skin scrapings, if the infection is superficial.

Ringworm (microsporum) causes some of the various dermatomycoses — diseases of the skin and hair. These are included in the large group of collagen diseases, and are diagnosed by scrapings of the skin, hair, and nails, and by Wood's light examination. In the Wood's examination the infected area is viewed in a darkened room under ultraviolet light filtered through a Wood's glass. Different fungi will show characteristic fluorescent colors, a bright green, pink, or gold. *Athlete's foot* is also a dermatomycosis and may be caused by several different fungi.

Thrush is caused by *Candida albicans*. It involves mucous membranes of the mouth, anus, and vagina (see Chapter 28, "Assisting With Physical Examinations," Obstetrics and Gynecology). Heavy antibiotic therapy may decrease the normal bacterial flora of these areas and thus allow *Candida* to flourish. It is found more frequently in babies, obese persons, and those who sweat profusely. It is diagnosed by direct examination and skin scrapings for microscopic slides and cultures. Because fungal infections can be diagnosed with a high degree of accuracy by microscopic examination of skin scrapings, this method of examination is frequently used. The scrapings are placed on a microscopic slide with a solution of 10 per cent potassium hydroxide (KOH) and gently warmed. The potassium hydroxide will digest normal skin cells and debris without destroying the long, stringy, hairlike hyphae of which the fungus is composed. Sometimes it is necessary to culture a specimen. A special medium for anaerobic culture may be used, for instance, for a deep chronic pulmonary disease. Culture of a superficial fungal disease sometimes will show a positive result when the skin scraping for a microscopic slide examination is negative. The student is referred to Chapter 22 for techniques of preparing and mounting slides for microscopic examination.

ECTOPARASITES

These are parasites attached to, or living on, the outer surface of the body or immediately beneath the skin. The most common of these is the well-known *itch mite* that causes *scabies*. It is highly contagious and holds no respect for its victim's pedigree or socioeconomic position. It usually infects the entire family. Schools will send a child home in haste if the mite is found. Patients are frequently shocked by this diagnosis. Examination of the skin is made with the aid of a magnifying lens to obtain skin scrapings for the mite and its eggs, also called *nits*.

The three lice that are found on man are identified by the area of the body they inhabit. They are: *Pediculus humanus capitis,* found in the hairs of the head by examining the hair for the eggs and the adult insect; *Pediculus humanus corporis,* the so-called body louse that lives in the clothing but migrates to the body to feed; its eggs are found in the seams and folds of clothing; and *Phthirus pubis (Pediculus pubis),* the pubic louse found in the hairs of the pubic region, which is also diagnosed by examining the pubic hairs for the presence of eggs.

BODY FLUIDS

Transudates are fluids that accumulate in body cavities, such as the abdominal or pericardial spaces. These fluids are not the result of an inflammation but are the result of edema and congestion. They are clear and light yellow in appearance. They are low in protein, contain very few white cells, and have no bacteria. Laboratory examinations include appearance, specific gravity, cell count, and protein determination. A Papanicolaou stain is done on the sediment for the possibility of malignancy. These fluids are taken from the body cavity by sterile puncture and draining technique.

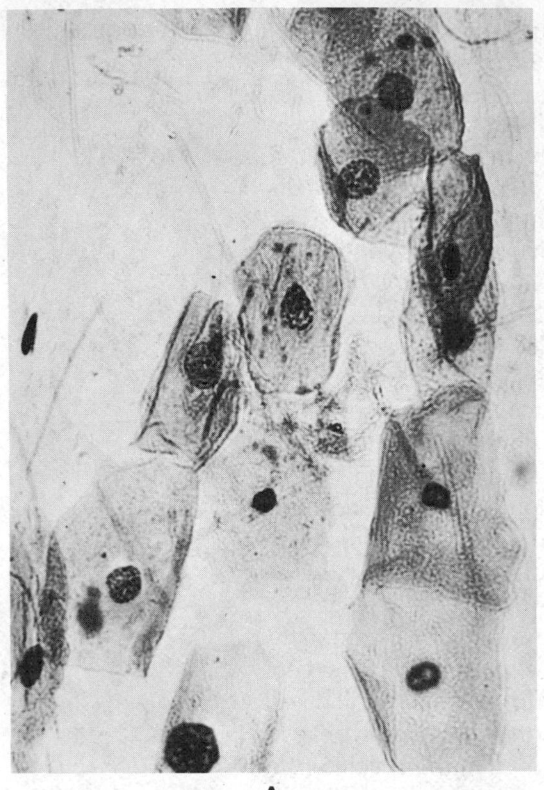

A

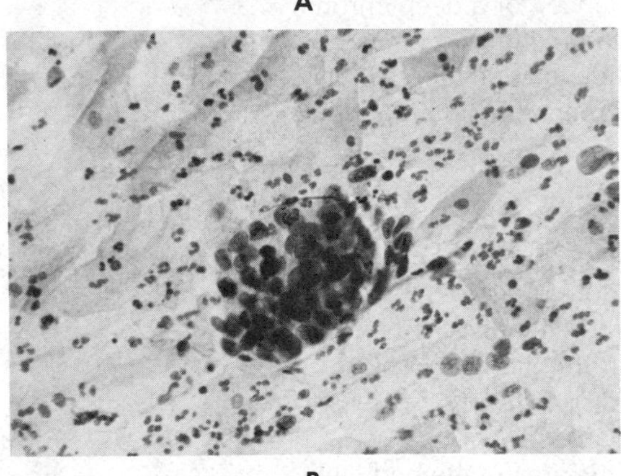

B

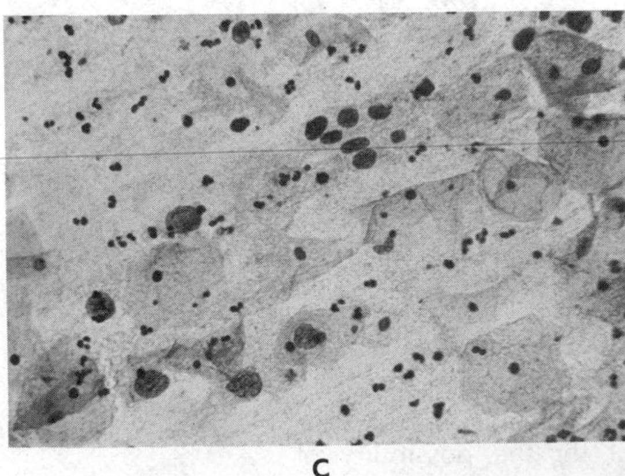

C

FIGURE 31–8 *A,* Exfoliative cell smear showing normal biologic flora of the genital tract. Cells are largely flattened surface squamous epithelial cells. (From Robbins, S. L., and Cotran, R. S.: *Pathologic Basis of Disease*. 2nd ed. Philadelphia, W. B. Saunders Co., 1979.) *B,* Malignant tumor cells in a vaginal smear (so-called class V Papanicolaou smear). *C,* Atypical cells consistent with tumor cells (class V or class IV, depending on opinion of the cytologist). (From Parsons, L., and Sommers, S. C.: *Gynecology*. 2nd ed. Philadelphia, W. B. Saunders Co., 1978.)

Exudates are the product of an inflammatory condition. They may be found in a body cavity or in the tissues. They are usually cloudy, deeper yellow, and much thicker in appearance. They contain many blood cells, red and white, and usually bacteria are present. This fluid is also drained by sterile technique, but it frequently is obtained by a draining abscess or open wound. Bacterial cultures and stained smears are made from exudates; a "Pap" stain may also be done, but not as frequently as with a transudate.

Synovial fluids are obtained from a bursa, joint, or tendon sheath. A cell count is done, or it may be cultured or smeared for bacteria. The fluid is usually obtained by sterile puncture technique.

See Chapter 29, "Assisting with Office Surgery," for collection of these body fluid specimens.

CYTOLOGIC EXAMINATIONS

Exfoliated cells are cells that have sloughed off from both normal and malignant epithelial tissue. These exfoliated cells that lend themselves well to the Papanicolaou method of staining may be obtained from vaginal and cervical scrapings and secretions, bronchial secretions and washings, urinary sediment, pleural and peritoneal fluid sediments, and discharges from the mammary glands.

To insure accuracy of the "Pap smear," it should be fixed immediately after smearing on the microscopic slide in a solution of 50 per cent ether and 50 per cent ethyl alcohol. The slide should remain in this fixing solution for at least 30 minutes and then be removed and placed on end to air dry. Label with the patient's name and send to the laboratory for the cytotechnician or the pathologist to examine (Fig. 31–8).

Papanicolaou smears are reported on a 5-point scale as follows:

Grade I	Absence of **atypical** or abnormal cells
Grade II	Atypical cytology but no evidence of malignancy
Grade III	Cytology suggestive but not conclusive for malignancy
Grade IV	Strongly suggestive of malignancy
Grade V	Conclusive for malignancy

See Chapter 28, "Assisting with Physical Examinations," for the procedure to obtain a cervical and vaginal cytologic smear.

HISTOLOGIC EXAMINATION

Histology is the microscopic study of the form and structure of the various tissues of the body. This differs from cytology, which is the study of the exfoliated cells themselves, not in relation to other cells. Specimens for histologic study must be *fixed* as soon as possible. Fixation refers to arresting the life processes of the tissue cells. It also stops any dehydration, bacterial growth, or enzymatic activity. Tissue specimens are obtained by biopsy. The usual recommended fixative solution is 80 per cent alcohol and 10 per cent formalin with the ratio of the solution to the specimen being ten to one. The specimen must be completely immersed and free from any side pressure. It is best to have it floating free.

The laboratory will then specially treat the tissue, so that it can be sliced microscopically thin and mounted on slides to be passed through a series of stains. It is then studied by the pathologist. The container must be properly labeled with the patient's full name, physician's name, the date, and the nature of the specimen. The possible diagnosis is sometimes included.

See Chapter 29, "Assisting with Office Surgery," for obtaining a specimen by biopsy.

CEREBROSPINAL FLUID (CSF)

The procedure to obtain cerebrospinal fluid, sometimes called spinal fluid, is usually done in a hospital on an outpatient basis, but occasionally, a physician will do a spinal puncture in the office. It is considered a minor surgical procedure.

Normally it is a clear, colorless fluid found in the ventricles of the brain and the central canal of the spinal cord. Approximately 100 cc of fluid is present normally, and usually that amount is produced and reabsorbed daily. This fluid is obtained by a lumbar puncture, and about 2 to 3 cc is allowed to drip into a series of small sterile vials. Three vials are usually taken; these vials are to be numbered 1, 2, and 3 in the sequence taken. A lumbar puncture is not too painful for the patient, but because of the reduced volume of fluid in the spine and ventricles, the patient is advised to remain flat for a few hours in order to prevent a severe headache. There is no special diet restriction or patient preparation for this procedure. It is also required in some institutions that the patient sign a permission form for a lumbar puncture to be performed.

Some tests done on this cerebrospinal fluid are the following. A white *cell count* often indicates the presence of an infection. This should be done immediately after the fluid has been obtained. A high cell count is found in most cases of meningitis. A *serologic test* is done to discover the presence of neurosyphilis and the involvement of this disease in the central nervous system. A *Colloidal-Gold* test aids in the diagnosis of multiple sclerosis. The *total protein* is increased in several diseases of the central nervous system, especially in meningitis, subarachnoid hemorrhage, or a spinal block due to a tumor.

ELECTROENCEPHALOGRAM (EEG)

This is a tracing of the electrical waves produced by the brain. This is usually done when the brain is at rest, the patient's eyes are closed, the mind is not concentrating, and there are no distractions. Under these circumstances most people's brains will show fairly regular rhythms. These microvolts from the brain are amplified one million times by the electroencephalogram machine and recorded.

Either very fine needles are inserted a fraction of an inch into the scalp or small silver discs are pasted on the scalp in order to pick up these waves and record them on paper. In no way can the machine give any information about a person's thoughts. It can usually tell if the patient is awake or asleep, or if the patient is concentrating on something, but it cannot tell the subject matter of this concentration.

Because a **coupling** paste is used to secure the discs to the scalp, female patients will appreciate being reminded that they may wish to bring a head scarf to wear home.

RADIOLOGIC EXAMINATIONS

In 1895, Wilhelm Konrad Roëntgen discovered that rays emitted from a cathode ray tube could pass through solid objects like a book, wood, and his hand. Since that time, the x-ray, the name Roëntgen gave to this unknown phenomenon, has served as an important aid in the diagnosis and treatment of disease. Great advances in the knowledge of these rays have continued to be made since their first discovery. Increased knowledge has brought more safety in the use of radiation. Early workers did not fully appreciate the dangers of this force, but nowadays, concentrated efforts are being made to insure more precise handling of radiation equipment.

The term *x-ray* will, no doubt, be used for many years, but these rays have now been named *roentgen* rays in honor of their discoverer. Two terms used to describe the study of radiation should not be confused. The term **roentgenology** is limited to the science of the roentgen ray, while **radiology** is the study of all forms of radiation including the roentgen ray, radioactive substances, and other forms of radiant energy.

Many states prohibit medical assistants from using radiologic equipment unless they are specifically trained and certified. However, you may be responsible for informing patients about various procedures, filling out request forms for radiography in the hospital, filing film records, or otherwise assisting the physician or radiologic technologist in positioning the patient or developing film. It is therefore important to know some basics of radiologic examinations.

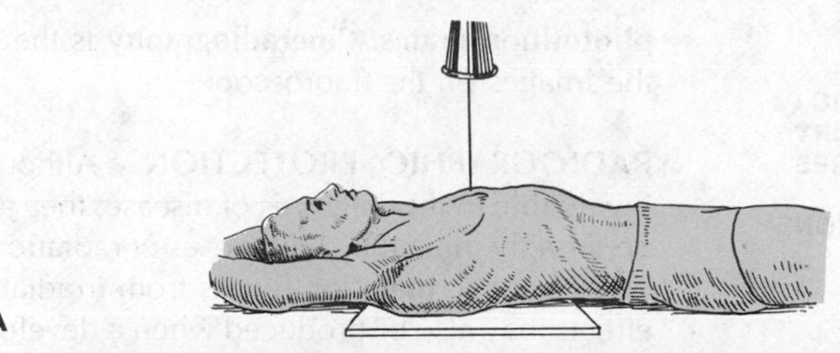

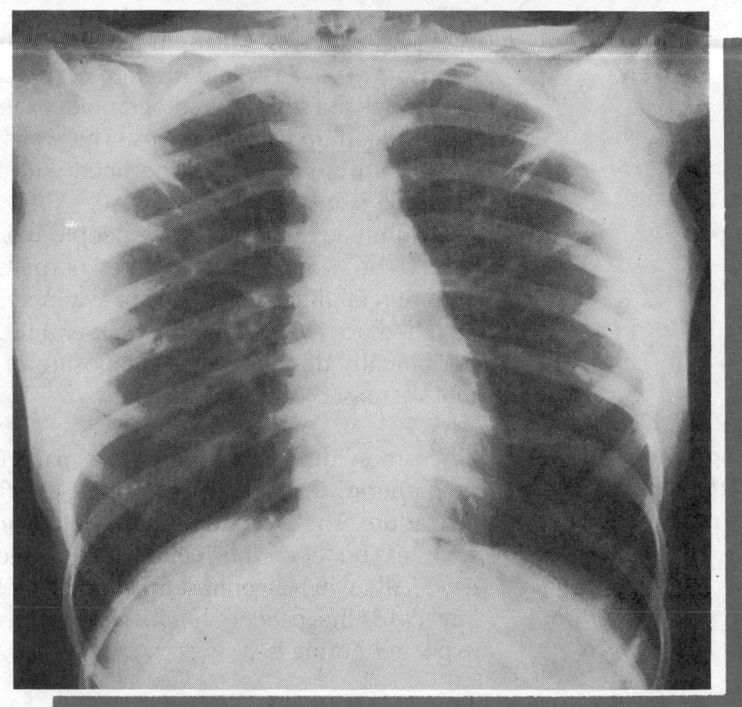

FIGURE 31–9 Anteroposterior recumbent study of chest. *A,* Positioning of patient. *B,* Radiograph. (From Meschan, L.: *Radiographic Positioning and Related Anatomy*. Philadelphia, W. B. Saunders Co., 1968.)

RADIOGRAMS, CONTRAST MEDIA, AND FLUOROSCOPY. Roentgen rays, which can be produced by high-velocity electrons in a vacuum tube, can expose (turn black) a photographic plate. They can also be absorbed by substances, to a degree relative to the density of the substance. Thus, if part of the body is positioned on a photographic plate and roentgen rays are directed through it, the rays will be absorbed or scattered by the various substances in the body and will expose the plate in varying degrees. The resulting image will show the pattern of substances inside the body. Air, for instance, is least dense and will appear as black areas, while water, fat, and metal appear increasingly white. This image is called a *roentgenogram* or *radiogram* (Fig. 31–9).

Contrast media are sometimes used to increase the difference in densities between areas and make them easier to distinguish visually. Contrast media may be gases (air, oxygen, CO_2), heavy metals (barium sulfate, bismuth, carbonate), organic iodides, and others. Some of these concentrate in particular body organs, such as the gallbladder. These are called **radiopaque** dyes and can be administered orally, intravenously, or directly into the area. Other contrast media are used in body cavities and passages, such as the digestive tract, urinary tract, ventricles, bronchial tree, uterus, fallopian tubes, and spaces in the brain.

The image can also be directed on a fluorescent screen. This is called **fluoroscopy.** Motion of a body part can be viewed on the screen. Contrast media are also used in this method. Thus, a physician can observe the action of the esophagus and stomach when a patient under the fluoroscope swallows a barium mixture. The image on the fluoroscope can be recorded on photographic film to produce

photofluorograms. Cineradiography is the technique of making motion pictures of the images on the fluoroscope.

RADIOGRAPHIC PROTECTION. Although roentgen rays have proven to be invaluable in the diagnosis of disease, they are hazardous to living tissue. Tissues can be directly injured by high doses of radiation, and future generations can be affected when genetic **mutation** results from irradiation of the reproductive organs. Harmful effects may also be produced when a developing embryo or fetus is exposed to radiation.

Lead absorbs radiation and can therefore protect parts of the body from exposure. A lead shield should be placed over every patient's **gonads.** Medical personnel assisting in radiographic examinations and positioning should always wear a lead apron and gloves. The walls of the x-ray room and any windows and doors into the room must be lined with lead. The door must be closed while the machine is in operation.

Film badges are worn by people working with radiographic equipment. These should be worn on the pocket or belt, as close to the gonads as possible. If commercial film badges are not available, a small piece of dental film may be used, attached to clothing with a paper clip. The film is exposed by x-rays and is periodically developed. Overexposure of the worker to x-rays can be detected, so that increased care must be exerted.

Special Roentgenographic Procedures

Since individual radiologists have particular methods and preferences for patient preparation, it is advisable to check with them before instructing a patient on a procedure. The procedures given below are generally applicable. In some instances, such as bone or lung studies, no special preparation is necessary. In others, especially when a contrast medium is used, preparation of the patient is essential. In any case, the patient should be informed of the procedure and what should be expected during it.

Cleansing Enema Instructions. Gas and feces in the intestinal tract have densities that will not allow x-rays to fully penetrate. These substances must be completely eliminated for a successful diagnostic film to be taken. The intestinal tract must also be free from gas and fecal material for a clean film of the ureters and kidneys, since these organs are posterior to the intestines.

Since this cleansing of the intestines is so important, the physician's office may be supplied with printed instructions to be given to the patient. Most preparation instructions include dietary and/or fluid restrictions or bowel cleansing procedures. The success of an x-ray examination depends largely on how conscientiously a patient is given instructions and how carefully they are followed.

The taking of an enema is often misunderstood, and poor results ensue. The patient should be instructed to take one quart of plain warm water, about 100° F or a little warmer than body temperature. The patient should lie down, with the enema can or bag about three feet above head level. The first third of the enema should be taken lying on the left side, the middle third lying flat on the back, and the final third lying on the right side. The liquid should be held for several minutes before evacuating.

INTRAVENOUS PYELOGRAM (IVP). This is the study of the ureters and kidneys after a contrast medium has been introduced intravenously. As mentioned above, gas and fecal material must be removed from the intestinal tract. This may be done by the administration of castor oil and a cleansing enema. The evening meal the night before the test should be light, consisting of toast, tea, and fruit. There must be no food or fluids after 9:00 PM that evening or in the morning before the test. The contrast medium is then injected intravenously on the morning of the test at designated intervals, and the x-ray films are taken at given intervals to observe the rate of excretion, the concentration of the contrast medium in the kidney calices and pelves, the outline of the ureters, and the urinary bladder. The patient should be told there will probably be two venipunctures and that the test will take about one hour. He may have breakfast after the test.

RETROGRADE PYELOGRAM. This test is the same as the intravenous pyelogram except that the contrast medium is introduced into the kidneys by means of a ureteral catheter through a cystoscope. The excretory procedure is not viewed adequately because the catheter is obstructing the ureters. This method is done when special studies of certain parts of the urinary tract are indicated or when adequate concentration of the contrast medium cannot be achieved by the intravenous method.

CHOLECYSTOGRAM. This is an examination of the gallbladder, showing function, the presence of any gallstones, or anomalies. The intestinal tract must be cleared as instructed. The patient should eat a fat-free light meal the night before examination; he may usually have lean meat, vegetables, fruit, dry toast, tea, or coffee. Dye tablets (usually six or nine) are swallowed with the meal at regular intervals; specific instructions are issued with the tablets. Small amounts of water may be taken during the evening until bedtime. Patients should be warned that they may have some diarrhea and nausea after taking the tablets, but not to be alarmed. Many times after the first films are taken the patient may be instructed to eat a fatty meal, to stimulate functioning of the gallbladder, and then return for more films to be taken. This examination usually takes about one hour, including the fatty meal.

CHOLANGIOGRAM. This is done to view the cystic, hepatic and common bile ducts by using a **radiopaque** dye. In the intravenous method the dye is excreted by the liver into the bile ducts. X-ray films are taken at ten minute intervals. The procedure takes about four hours. The patient is instructed to restrict fluid intake in order to concentrate the dye. The evening meal the night before the test is fat-free, and the intestines must be cleared by castor oil and an enema.

A postoperative cholangiogram utilizes the drainage tube left in place at surgery. The dye is injected through the drain tube and the series of films is started immediately.

BARIUM ENEMA. This is valuable in viewing the colon (Fig. 31–10). Obviously, the colon must be cleared of fecal material and gas. The day before the examination the patient is instructed to take castor oil and an enema. A light supper is eaten. Some radiologists prefer that the patient be placed on a low-residue diet for 24 hours before the examination. Nothing is taken by mouth after 9 PM the evening before or the morning of the test. Tell the patient he will be given an enema of an opaque substance (barium sulfate) while on the table. He will be moved from the left side, to the back, and to the right side to completely fill the colon. He is then fluoroscoped, and films are taken before he may evacuate the barium. The barium is then evacuated in the lavatory. If the physician requests, air is injected into the colon after the barium has been evacuated. The air is a contrast medium that gives a contrast to the barium coating the mucosa of the colon. This technique is done to better visualize polypoid masses. A barium enema will take from 15 to 30 minutes.

GASTROINTESTINAL SERIES. This is also sometimes called a Barium Meal, GI Series, or an Upper GI. This is an x-ray series of the stomach and/or small intestine, depending on the physician's request. The radiologist observes by fluoroscope the filling of the stomach as the patient drinks a suspension of barium sulfate. Films are made during the filling or immediately after the fluoroscopic examination. This takes about 30 minutes. A physician may request more pictures be taken at a six hour period and/or at a 24 hour period. Patients are instructed to eat a light supper and take nothing by mouth after midnight the evening before the test. A patient may eat

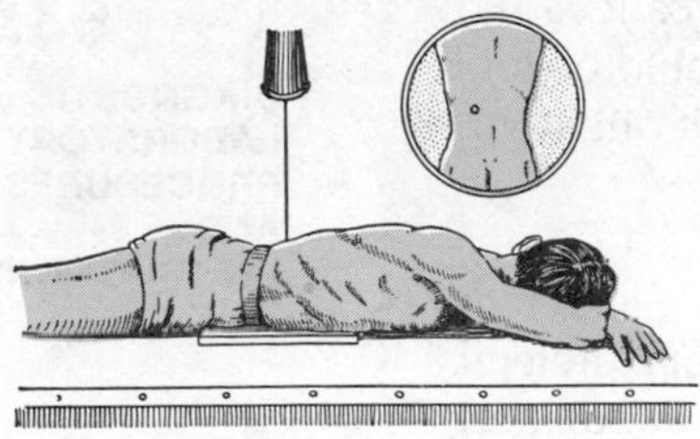

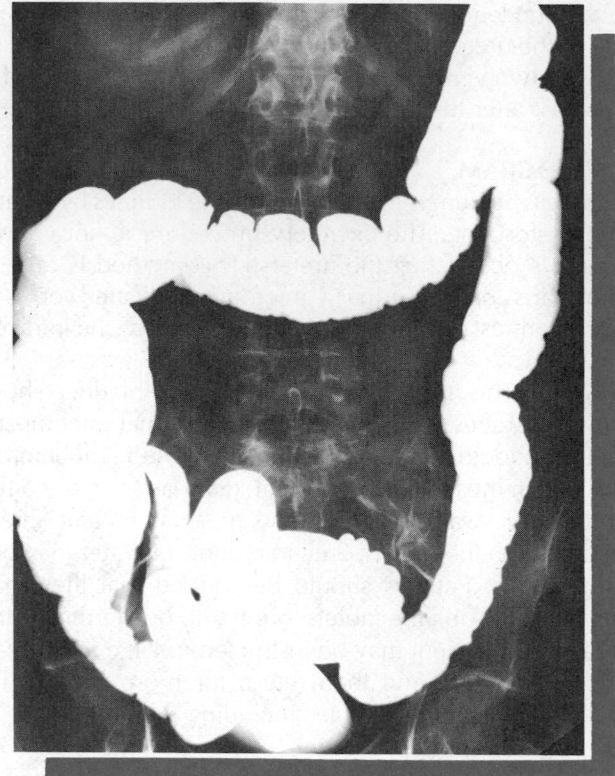

B

FIGURE 31–10 Colon distended with barium. *A,* Positioning of patient. *B,* Radiograph. (From Meschan, I.: *Radiographic Positioning and Related Anatomy*. Philadelphia, W. B. Saunders Co., 1968.)

breakfast after the first series of films is taken. The patient may be requested to prepare the bowel with castor oil and/or an enema, if the barium is to be followed through more than the upper gastrointestinal area. The patient should be told that his stool may be light in color after the examination because of the barium passing. Some patients may need a cathartic or enema after all the films are taken if they have had difficulty with normal bowel movements.

BRONCHOGRAMS. These are x-ray pictures of the bronchial tree. Small amounts of iodized oil are introduced by atomizer in order to visualize the outlines of the tubes and their branches. The films are taken immediately after the contrast medium has been introduced. A topical anesthetic is sprayed into the nose and throat to prevent coughing and gagging when the instrument is inserted to introduce the medium.

The patient is given nothing by mouth following this procedure until the anesthetic has worn off. The contrast medium is drained off by means of postural drainage. This is done by placing the patient in a prone position with the head and trunk of the body lower than the buttocks and legs.

HYSTEROSALPINGOGRAM. This procedure is also known as *uterosalpingogram.* A contrast medium is injected slowly through the cervical canal into the endometrium of the uterus and fallopian tubes. This is done to aid in the diagnosis of endometrial polyps, submucous fibroids, and tubal and uterine **anomalies.** Tubal patency (openness) and obstructions are also demonstrated. The patient may be instructed to clear the lower intestines and bowel by taking castor oil and an enema, but this is not always indicated. Otherwise, there are no special instructions to the patient.

MAMMOGRAPHY. These are x-ray pictures taken of the breast tissue with or without an opaque medium introduced into the mammary ducts. A *simple mammography* is without the use of an opaque medium.

New films and exposure techniques, as well as the skill of the x-ray technician, now make it possible to view this soft tissue. This is an important aid to diagnosis but is not considered to be a substitute for biopsy. It is used to differentiate **fibrocystic** disease and can help in the early detection of lesions too small to produce symptoms. It is used as a follow-up procedure in patients who have had a mastectomy. Periodic examinations can help detect early lesions in the remaining breast.

XERORADIOGRAPHY. In xeroradiography, the x-ray images are processed on specially treated xerox paper instead of x-ray film. The process takes only 90 seconds and permits visualization of soft tissues. For this reason, it is most often used to detect lesions or calcifications in the soft tissue of the breast (Fig. 31–11).

COMPUTED TOMOGRAPHY. This is a relatively new technique that enables visualization of cross-sections of the body. It is most useful in detecting tumors of the brain and abdomen. Computed **tomography** equipment is extremely expensive and is available in only some hospitals. Scheduling a patient for a procedure is very important, as the relatively few machines are in high demand. The patient's head or torso is placed inside an opening in the machine. Roentgen rays are directed in an arc of 180°, and the information given by the passage of each ray through the body is processed in the computer to produce a cross-sectional image. Several of these "slices" will be taken at different levels. The amount of radiographic exposure is not more than in a conventional radiograph. The whole examination takes a few minutes, and the patient need not be hospitalized as with many **invasive** methods (Fig. 31–12).

Radioactive Isotopes (Radioisotopes) and Nuclear Medicine

A radioactive isotope is a chemical element with an unstable nucleus that emits radiation in the form of beta rays (electrons) and gamma rays (light). Each radioisotope disintegrates at a fixed rate. This is measured as the amount of time necessary for half of a quantity of the radioisotope to disintegrate and is called the half-life. This amount can range from a split-second to thousands of years. Radioisotopes used in medicine usually have a half-life of one or two days. Gold-198, for instance, has a half-life of two days (one-half of an amount of gold-198 will disintegrate in two days) and is a good choice in some diagnostic procedures.

In diagnostic nuclear medicine, a radioisotope is administered intravenously or orally. The isotope will be absorbed by particular tissues, in amounts measured by a counter, scintiscanner, or gamma camera. Tests of the thyroid gland provide a good example. Iodine-131 (radioiodine), with a half-life of eight days, is given to the

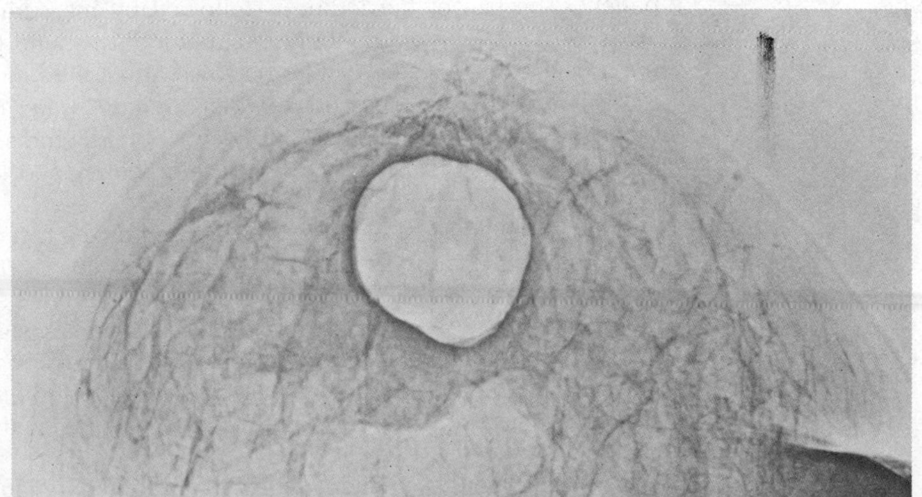

FIGURE 31–11 Cyst of the breast as seen in a xeroradiograph. (From Scherrd, L. et al.: *Atlas of Xeroradiography*. Philadelphia, W. B. Saunders Co., 1977.)

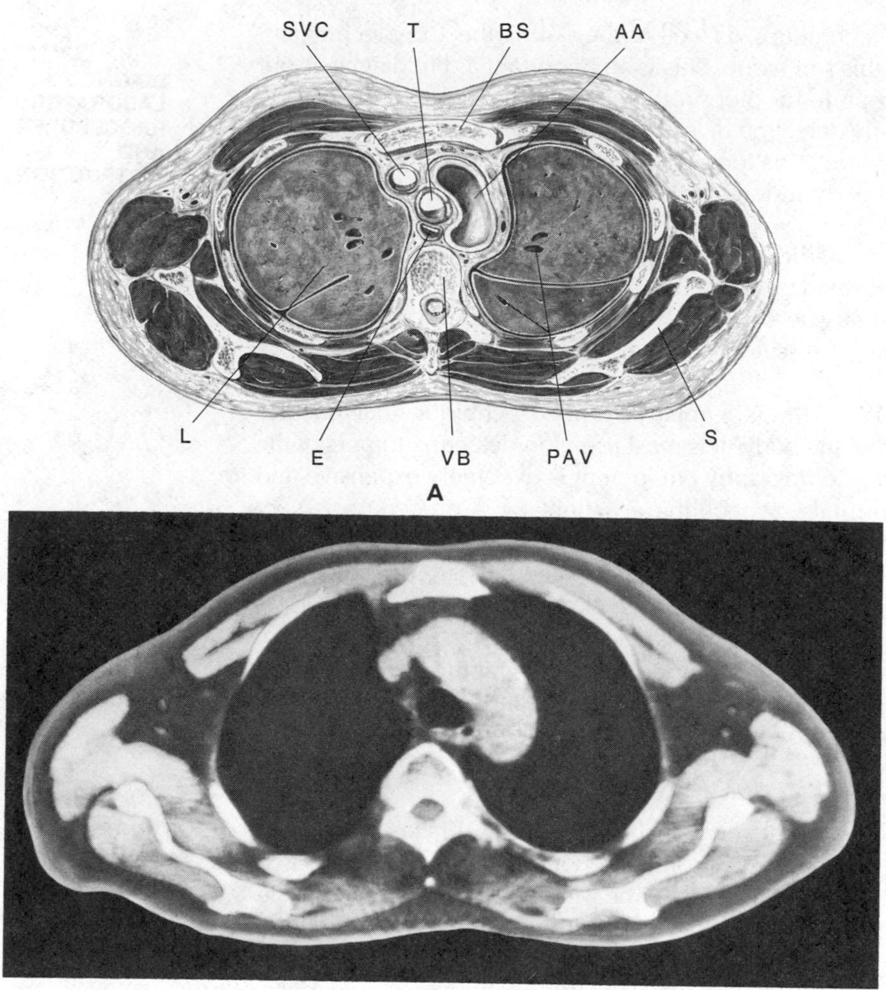

FIGURE 31–12 A computed tomograph through the aortic arch level. Lungs, bone, spine, and blood vessels can be visualized and compared with anatomic drawings. T = trachea, SVC = superior vena cava, L = lung, E = esophagus, BS = body of sternum, AA = aortic arch, S = scapula, PAV = pulmonary arteries and veins, VB = vertebral body. (From Meschan, I.: *Synopsis of Radiologic Anatomy with Computed Tomography*. Philadelphia, W. B. Saunders Co., 1980.)

patient. The fate of the iodine is followed by measuring concentration in three areas — the thyroid gland, the urine, and iodine bound to protein in the blood. A good deal of information can be obtained about the function of the thyroid gland. Other radioactive isotopes used in diagnostic tests are iron-52, strontium-85, and technetium-99m. These are used to identify brain tumors, intraocular tumors, bone tumors, pernicious anemia, and to perform kidney and liver scans and other procedures.

Therapeutic use of radioisotopes is based on the fact that activity of diseased or cancerous tissue can be suppressed by radioactivity. Treatment is aimed at effective destruction of malignancies without harming normal tissue. Since beta rays can penetrate only a few millimeters of tissue and gamma rays (produced by radium, for instance) penetrate deeply, radioisotopes that produce mostly beta rays will be less harmful to surrounding tissues. Thus, beta-rays from iodine-131 are able to destroy cancerous thyroid tissue, where the isotope collects, without harming the parathyroids.

Radioisotopes used internally are administered in liquid or solid form. The ideal half-life for such radioisotopes is from 12 hours to 12 days, to permit effective

A

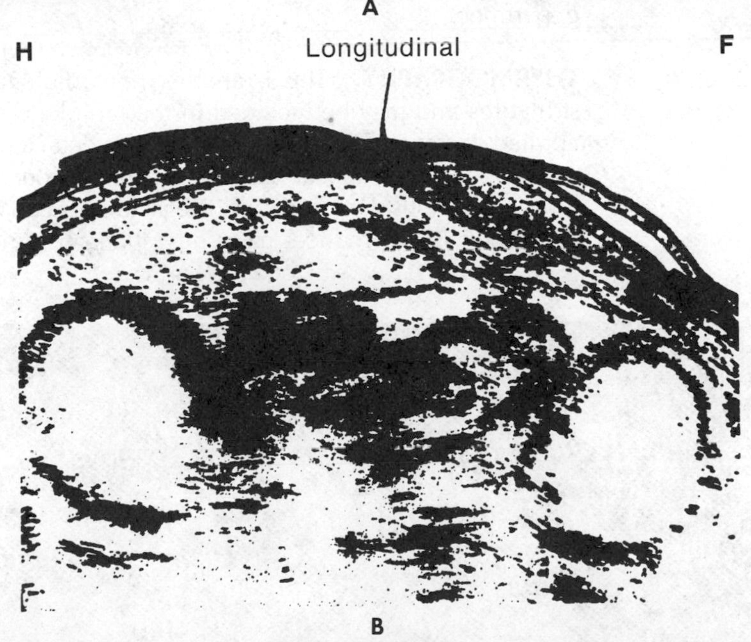

B

FIGURE 31–13 *A,* Early pregnancy. The fetus is seen in the gestation sac. The crown-rump length (CRL) is 3.3 cm, which is the average for 10 weeks of gestation. (From Beischer, N. A., and Mackay, E. V.: *Obstetrics and the Newborn.* Philadelphia, W. B. Saunders Co., 1977.) *B,* The heads of a pair of twins can be seen in this sonograph taken at nine months. Experienced sonographers can determine the infants' positions. (From Gosink, B. B., and Squire, L. F.: *Diagnostic Ultrasound.* Philadelphia, W. B. Saunders Co., 1976.)

exposure of diseased tissue without undue radiation to the rest of the body. Some examples of these radioisotopes are phosphorus-32, gold-198, and iodine-131. Some radioisotopes that emit mostly gamma rays or have a long half-life (cobalt-60 and cesium-137) are directed toward the tumor from a shielded unit outside the body.

Side effects often occur after treatment with radiation. These include nausea, loss of hair, and bone marrow suppression leading to anemia. A patient undergoing treatment should be cautioned about possible effects and followed carefully during the treatment process.

Other Imaging Systems

ULTRASOUND. This procedure is not technically a radiographic procedure, but it too permits visualization of internal structures and is usually performed in a hospital's radiology department. Sound waves are directed through the patient's body, and the echoes made when the waves are reflected off internal structures are detected, processed, and converted to a visual image on an **oscilloscope.** The body may be immersed in water or covered with oil or gel to ensure good transmission of the waves between the skin and the **transducer.** Because sound waves do not have the hazards of roentgen rays when used at low energy levels, ultrasound is ideal for observing the developing fetus and determining multiple births (Fig. 31–13). It is also used to detect tumors or lesions in the brain, eye, abdomen, reproductive organs, and breasts.

ECHOCARDIOGRAPHY. Echocardiography uses the principles of ultrasound to produce an image of the action of the heart over a period of time. This procedure may be performed in the cardiology unit of the hospital rather than in the radiology department.

THERMOGRAPHY. This is another nonradiologic technique that reveals internal structures and may be included in the radiology department. No physical agent is applied. Instead, the body's heat energy is detected and converted to a visual image, so that cool areas appear dark, warm areas appear light, and intermediate temperatures are various shades of gray. Breast tumors can be identified in this method, since the tumor tissue produces more heat than surrounding normal tissue (Fig. 31–14).

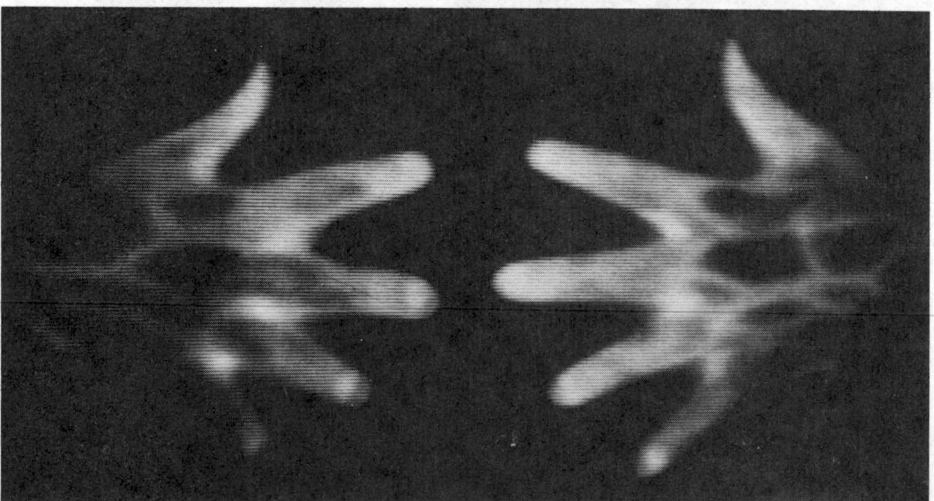

FIGURE 31–14 **Normal hand thermogram. Note that the region of the fingertips is warmer than the remainder of the hand, but the change in warmth is gradual. Vascular structures along the dorsum of the hand are visualized as white streaks. (Courtesy of Dr. W. Reynolds, Henry Ford Hospital, Detroit, Michigan; from Poznanski, A. K.: *The Hand in Radiologic Diagnosis.* Philadelphia, W. B. Saunders Co., 1974.)**

French, R. M.: The Nurse's Guide to Diagnostic Procedures. 3rd Ed. New York, McGraw-Hill Book Co., 1971.
Garb, S.: Laboratory Tests in Common Use. 5th Ed. New York, Springer Publishing Co., Inc., 1971.
Garnet, T., and Barbata, J.: Laboratory Specimens. Totowa, N.J., Littlefield, 1964.
Kark, R. M., et al.: Primer of Urinalysis. 2nd Ed. New York, Harper & Row, 1963.
Lynch, M. J., et al.: Medical Laboratory Technology and Clinical Pathology. 2nd Ed., Philadelphia, W. B. Saunders Co., 1969.

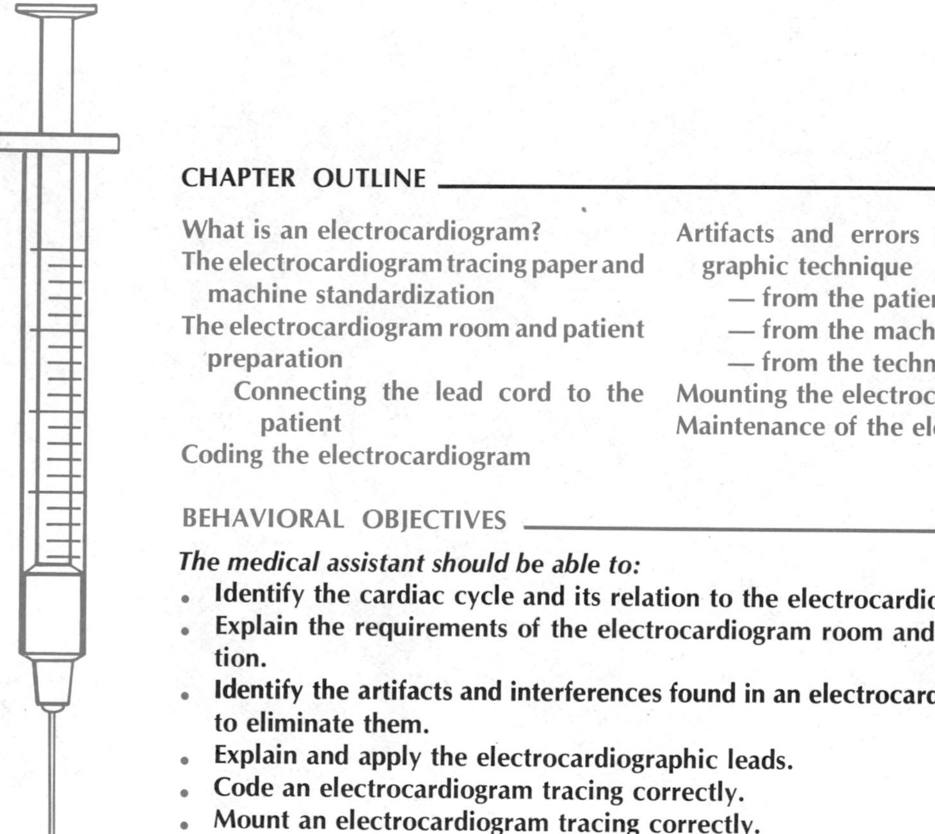

CHAPTER OUTLINE

BEHAVIORAL OBJECTIVES

The medical assistant should be able to:

- **Identify the cardiac cycle and its relation to the electrocardiogram tracing.**
- **Explain the requirements of the electrocardiogram room and patient preparation.**
- **Identify the artifacts and interferences found in an electrocardiogram and how to eliminate them.**
- **Explain and apply the electrocardiographic leads.**
- **Code an electrocardiogram tracing correctly.**
- **Mount an electrocardiogram tracing correctly.**

32

ELECTROCARDIOGRAPHY

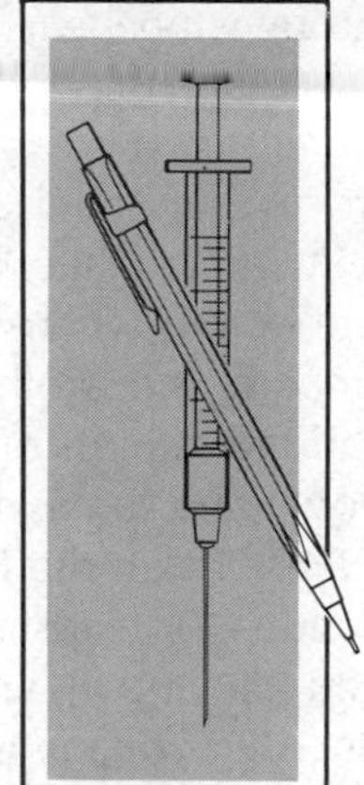

The electrocardiogram (ECG or EKG) is a graphic recording from the body surface of the potential of electric currents generated by the heart and magnified 3000 times onto a tracing paper moving at a designated speed. The pattern of the heart waves is traced on the paper, indicating the heart's rhythm and other actions.

The electrocardiogram is a valuable diagnostic aid that is often part of a complete physical examination. It has some limitations in that it does not necessarily predict heart disease, but it is useful in recording arrhythmia and some damages inflicted on the heart muscles. It may also aid in recording the progress of a heart condition and the effects of some medications.

The mechanics of operating an electrocardiograph are relatively simple, but it is essential that the technician doing the procedure for the physician have a basic knowledge of what is happening when the heart beats and the machine records this heartbeat on the tracing paper. Because the machine is very delicate and sensitive, the medical assistant must be able to recognize sources of error and **artifacts** and be able to eliminate them. Good standardization technique should be followed each time a test is run. The standardization must be consistently accurate because most patients do not have a single tracing but rather several tracings taken over a period of time, which must be compared. Constant vigilance will help one to develop the ability to minimize artifacts and interferences, thus giving the physician a clearly readable electrocardiogram.

The electrocardiographs in physicians' offices are basically the same, but each machine has some variation particular to its manufacturer. We will not attempt to discuss specific machines but will discuss general rules that are applicable to the running of an electrocardiograph in general. If you do not find the manufacturer's instruction manual for the machine in your office then write to the manufacturer and request the one for your particular model.

WHAT IS AN ELECTROCARDIOGRAM?

The electrocardiogram (ECG) is a recording of the electrical impulses from the heart and is used to detect the rhythmic disturbances of the heart and to distinguish types of **myocardial** disorders. The electrocardiograph (or the electrocardiogram machine) is an extremely sensitive machine that records a "picture" of the passage of electrical currents through the heart from various angles. Figure 32–1 illustrates these angles. The recording, or tracing, represents the amount of voltage that travels through the heart as shown by the vertical deflections of the tracing forming the PQRST waves and by the time required for the voltage to travel through the heart as shown in the horizontal movement of the paper. The graphic picture depends on the various connections between the machine and the patient.

The position of the heart is not fixed; it may vary in individuals. It depends on the person's respiration, height of the diaphragm, body type, and age. In some cases the physician may outline the patient's heart and indicate exactly where the leads are to be placed. Routinely the placement of the leads is standard unless otherwise indicated. The heart is one-third on the right side of the chest and two-thirds on the left side. The base of the heart is at the top and the apex points down and somewhat forward to the left. The heart's beat is **myogenic,** that is, it originates within the heart itself.

There are many combinations of these connections, or leads as they are called. For the routine ECG there are twelve leads: limb lead I, II, and III, and the augmented leads AVR, AVL, and AVF. The AV stands for **augmented** voltage and the R for right arm, L for left arm, and F for foot. The chest leads, also called precordial leads, are V1, V2, V3, V4, V5, and V6. Each of these numbers signifies the position of the electrode on the anterior chest.

The cardiac complex, also known as the cycle or beat, is designated by a series of waves called PQRST and sometimes U. These letters were arbitrarily selected to signify the various parts of the complex. This beat is the result of a minute electrical

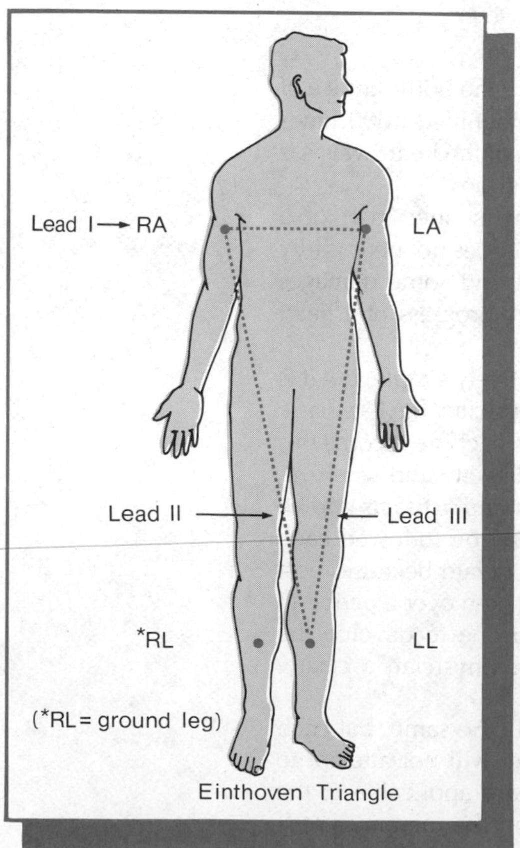

FIGURE 32–1 Einthoven triangle and picture of the heart.

impulse that is conducted through the atrium by the sinoatrial node (SA node), thus making the P wave. This SA node is the spark plug of the heart and is sometimes also called the cardiac pacemaker. This electrical impulse travels down the right atrium to the atrioventricular node (AV node) into the bundle branches known as the bundle of His. These right and left bundle branches travel through the center septum that divides the right and left ventricles of the heart and cause the contraction that is recorded as the QRS wave. This is where the blood is pumped out of the heart and into the body. The ST segment of the complex is a transitional movement from the end of the ventricular depolarization to the repolarization of the ventricles. The last wave seen in the tracing is the P wave, when the heart relaxes until another excitation is started from the SA node and the PQRST complex starts over again. The T wave attracts a great deal of attention in heart disease because it is sensitive to disease and medication. The U wave is a small wave that is very seldom seen. In potassium depletion, the U wave may be seen but a specific myocardial function has not yet been discovered. Figure 32–2 illustrates the path of the PQRST complex through the heart in relation to the tracing on the paper.

THE ECG TRACING PAPER AND MACHINE STANDARDIZATION

Before you start taking a patient's tracing you must make certain the machine is correctly standardized (Fig. 32–3*A*). This is usually done at the start of every recording. Some physicians request one or two standardizations to appear within the patient's tracing. These are shown at the heart's resting state usually in limb lead I and chest lead V1. The resting place is the straight baseline between each complex (Fig. 32–3*B*). Check with the physician for his preferences.

When the STD button is depressed with a quick pecking motion releasing one millivolt of electricity, the recording stylus should deflect *exactly* 1 cm (10 mm) (Fig. 32–4*A*). The manufacturer's manual will tell you the method of adjustment to get a perfect standardization.

If the amplitude of the QRS wave is too high and records off the tracing paper, that is, it cannot be recorded in its entirety, the machine should be put on ½ sensitivity. If that is necessary, make certain you have shown a ½ STD (0.5 cm or 5 mm) on the tracing for the physician to note, as seen in Fig. 32–4*B*.

If the patient's heart rate is very rapid or when certain parts of the complex are too close together, it may be necessary to adjust the paper run to 50 rather than the standard 25 run. This will double the speed of the paper run and extend the recording to twice its normal width. Again, make certain this is noted on the tracing for the physician (Fig. 32–5*A* and *B*).

Because the complex picture differs with the various leads it may be necessary to adjust the position of the recording stylus in order to have the whole complex (not just the baseline) appearing in the center of the paper. No part of the complex should touch either the top or bottom of the paper. Remember that mounting may take off some of the chart near the top or bottom of the paper.

One roll of paper is usually sufficient for 20 or more electrocardigram tracings, depending on the number of leads and the type of mount used.

THE ECG ROOM AND PATIENT PREPARATION

The ECG room should be quiet and free from interruptions. It should be warm and the treatment table comfortable, away from other electrical equipment such as x-ray, short-wave diathermy, and electrical appliances. Electric fans, refrigerators, and air conditioners may also cause AC interferences. An ECG will record any kind of electrical voltage within its area, either AC or **somatic.**

The cot or treatment table used should be wide enough so the patient can relax his shoulders and not have to hold his arms close to his body. The patient may tuck his thumbs with the palms down under the buttocks to secure the arms on the table and allow the shoulders to relax. Remember that any tense muscle may record as somatic

Text continued on page 651

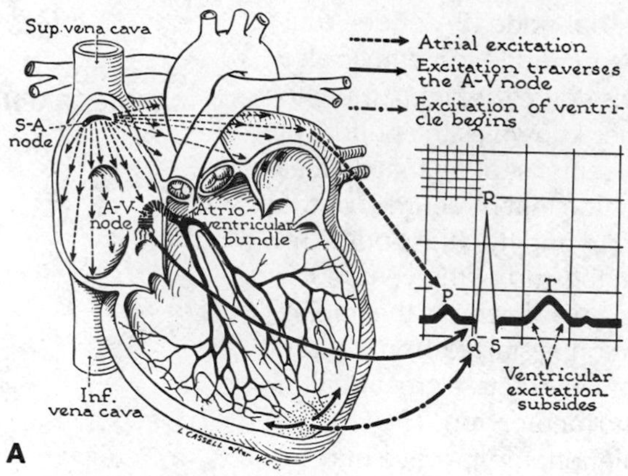

A

FIGURE 32–2 *A,* Electrocardiogram complex showing the complete cardiac cycle. (From Sutton, A. L.: *Bedside Nursing Techniques in Medicine and Surgery*. 2nd edition. Philadelphia, W. B. Saunders Company, 1969.) Components of the electrocardiogram complex as they relate to the electrical activity of the heart during one beat. *B–D,* Spread of electrical current through the atria (atrial depolarization), making the P wave.

Illustration continued on opposite page

Atrial Depolarization

Electrocardiographic Representation

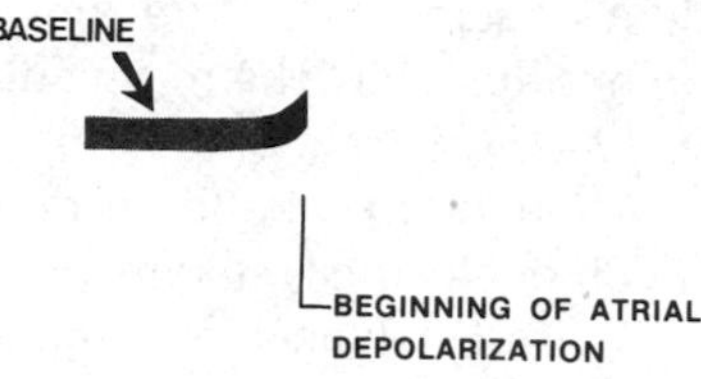

B

C

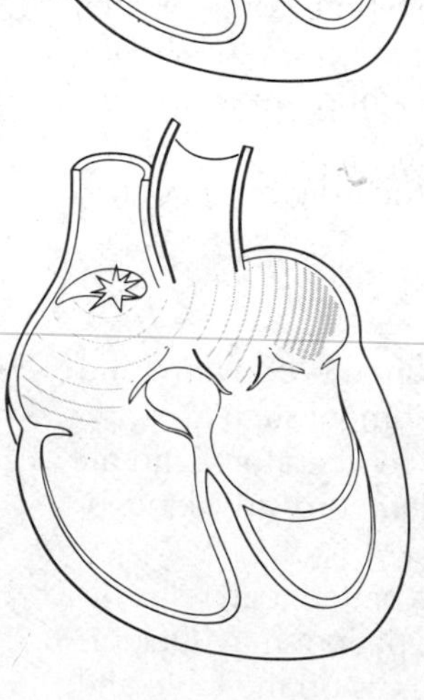

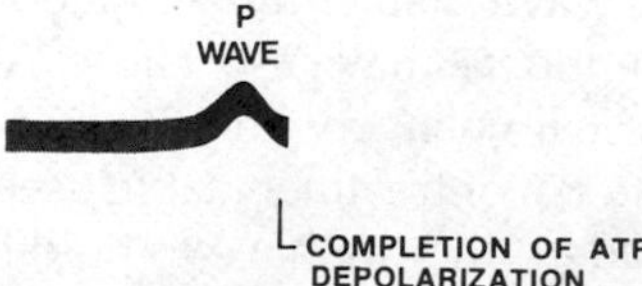

D

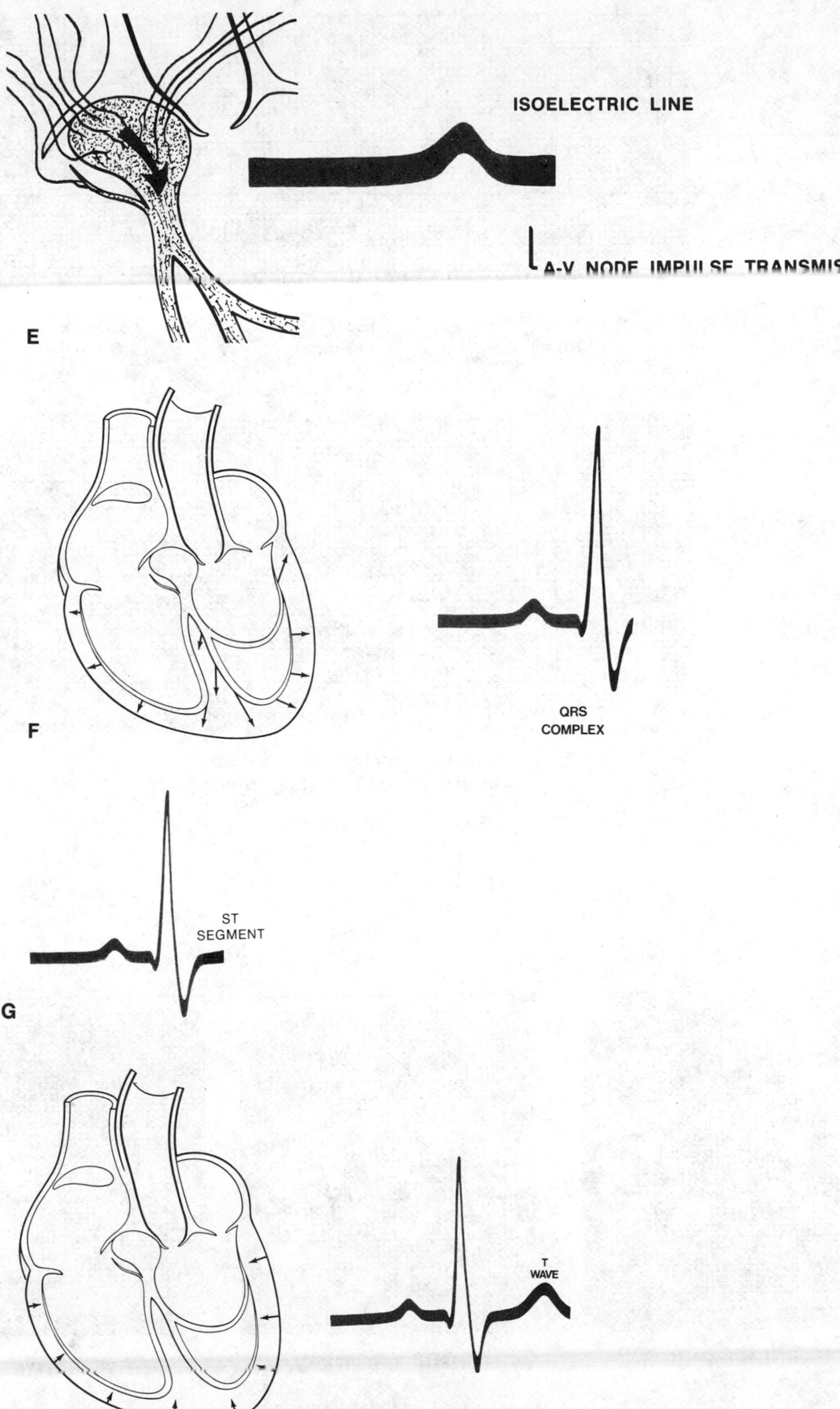

FIGURE 32–2 *Continued* *E,* Atrioventricular (A-V) node depolarizes, relaying the impulse from the atria to the ventricles. *F,* Impulse activates the ventricles, which records as the QRS wave. *G,* ST segment, a transitional moment. *H,* Ventricles repolarize (return to previous state), and the cycle is ready to begin again (T wave). (From Phillips, R. E., and Feeney, M. K.: *The Cardiac Rhythms: A Systematic Approach to Interpretation.* 2nd ed. Philadelphia, W. B. Saunders Co., 1980.)

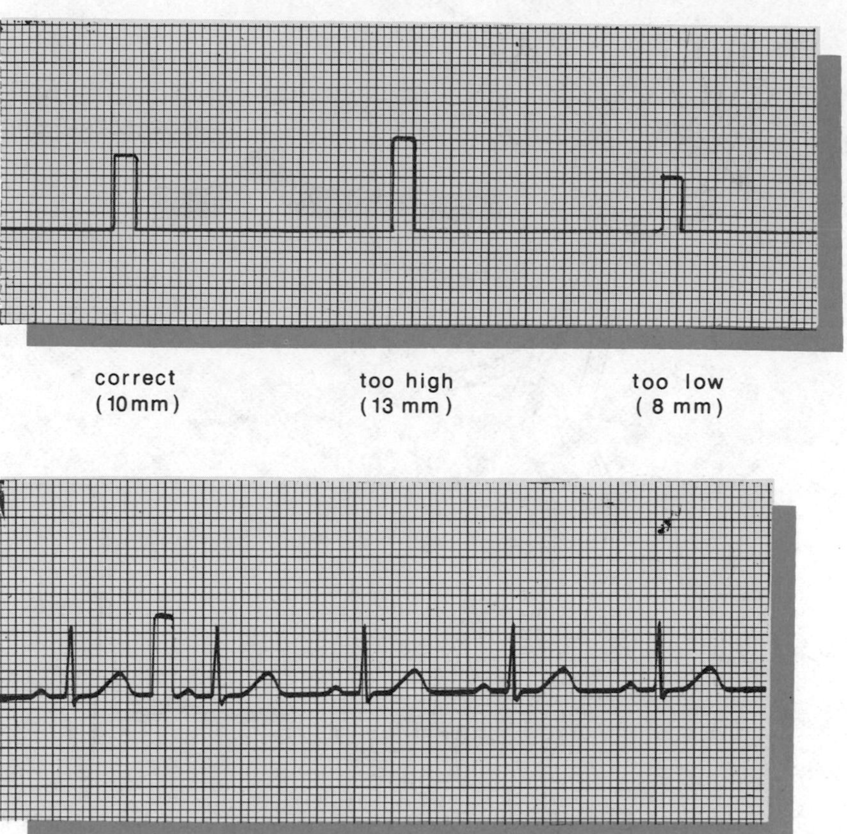

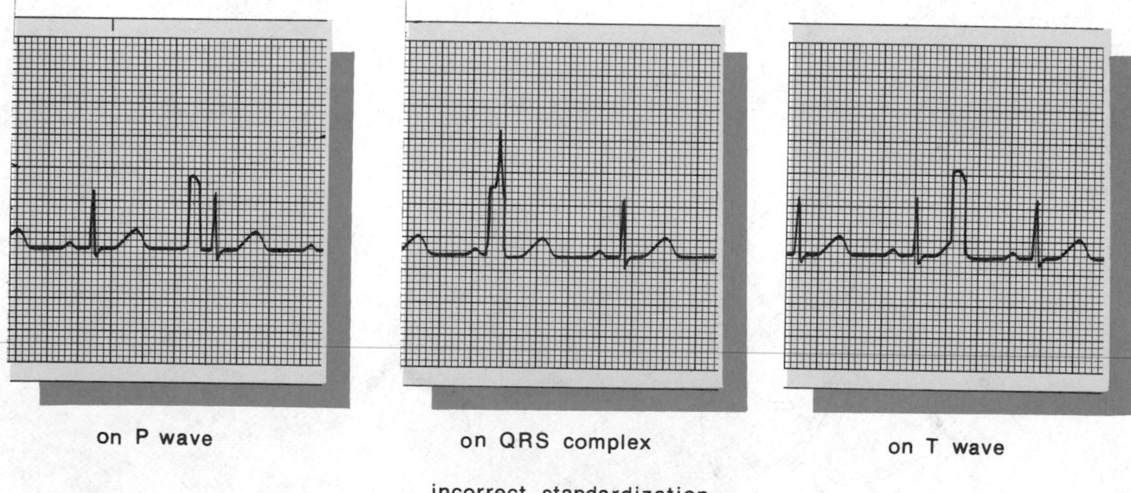

FIGURE 32–3. *A,* Standardization: Correct (10 mm), Too high (13 mm), too low (8 mm). *B,* Correct standardization within a lead at heart's resting stage. *C,* Incorrect standardizations within the complex.

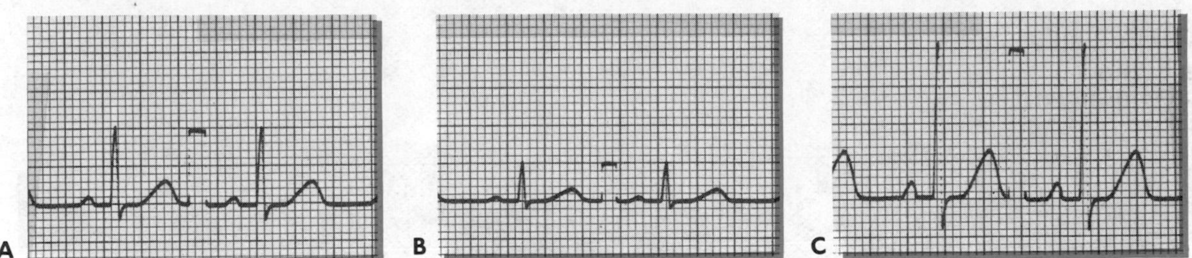

FIGURE 32–4 Sensitivity control. *A,* Correct standardization of 1 cm (10 mm). *B,* ½ is at half sensitivity of 0.5 cm (5 mm). *C,* 2 is double the sensitivity of 2 cm (20 mm). (From *Electrocardiography: A Better Way*. Milton, Wisconsin, The Burdick Corp., 1976.)

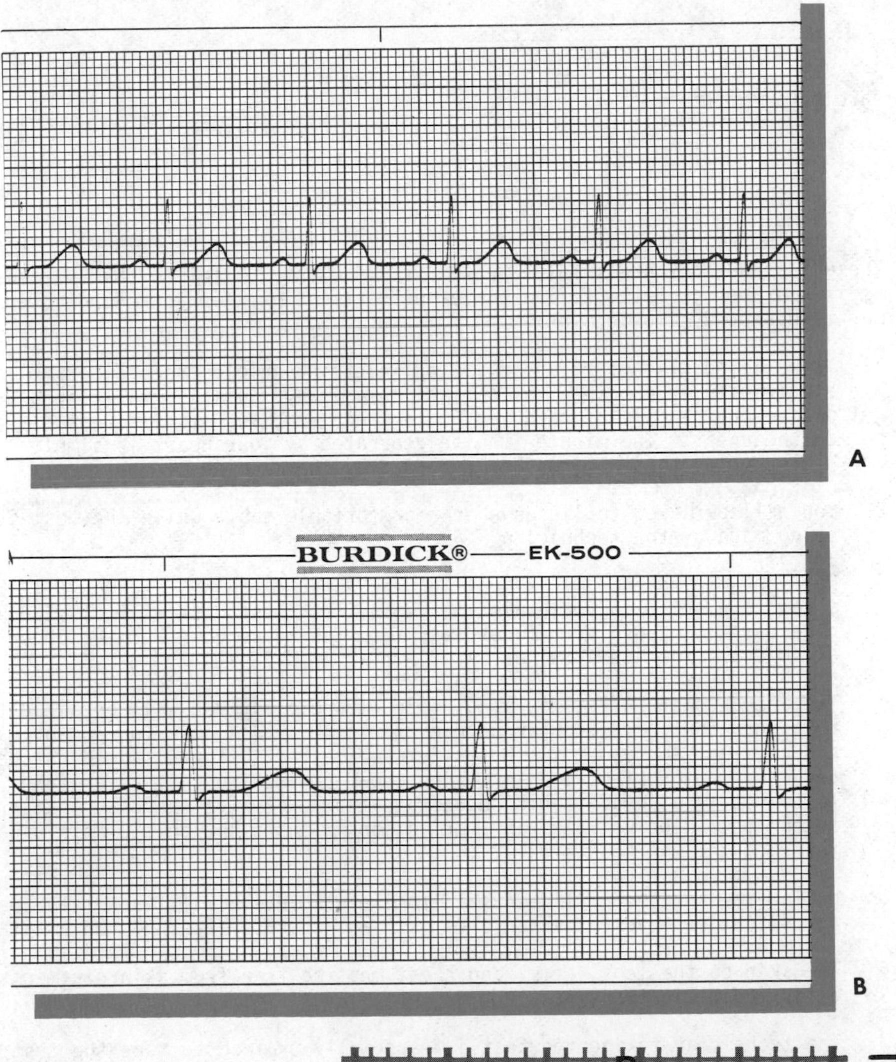

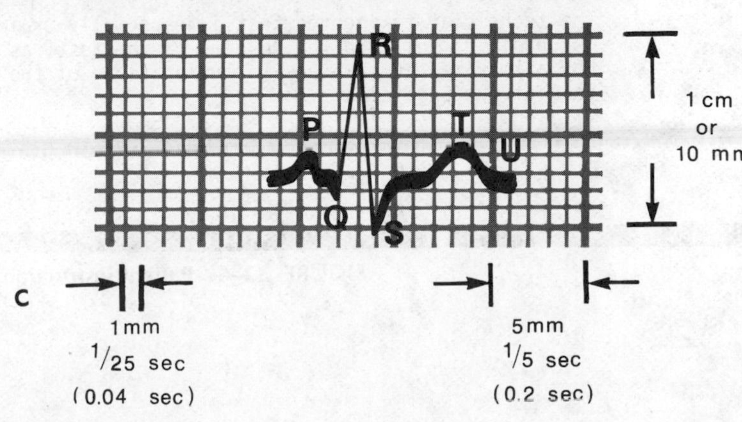

FIGURE 32–5 Paper Run. *A,* Run 25 is the normal speed for recording, 25 mm per second. *B,* Run 50 makes the paper run at double speed, 50 mm per second. It is used when the heart rate is very rapid and the complexes are too close together. This extends the complexes twice as far apart. *C,* Enlarged section of record.

INSTRUCTIONS FOR PATIENT BEFORE TAKING AN ELECTROCARDIOGRAM

Name: ______________________________

Your cardiogram appointment is ______________, ________________ at __________ a.m./p.m.
Day Date Time

These instructions are simple, but it is important you follow them. Please call us if you are unable to follow these instructions or keep your appointment so we may make another appointment.

1. There is no discomfort or sensation in taking an electrocardiogram. No electricity is put into the patient in any way. Small metal plates are placed on the calf of each leg and on each arm, and at different places on the chest. The minute impulse generated by your heart is simply picked up by these plates and recorded by the machine.

2. You will be asked to lie down on a comfortable table while the test is being made by the technician.

3. For your convenience it is best to wear loose clothing, and you will be asked to disrobe to your waist to expose the chest. It will also be necessary to expose your lower legs from the knees down and the upper arms just below the shoulders.

4. The actual test only takes about five minutes, but you will be asked to rest for about half an hour before the test. It is best you do not have a heavy meal for about two hours before the test. There should not be any consumption of cold drinks, ice cream or smoking just before the test. It is also advisable to refrain from excessive exercise just prior to the test. Do not take any medications without the physician's usual instructions and knowledge.

5. During the test you will be asked to lie absolutely still and relax, as the slightest movement interferes with an accurate tracing. Do not talk.

6. The skin on the legs, arms, and chest must be free from skin ointments, oils, and medications.

7. The technician taking the test is especially trained to take the test but is unable to tell you the results of the test, as she is neither trained nor authorized to make any interpretations of the cardiogram. This is the task of the physician.

FIGURE 32–6 Patient instructions.

interference. The table should be wood or have some form of insulation between metal legs and the surface. It is best to have the table positioned so the technician is working from the patient's left side. Small pillows are helpful in aiding a patient to relax. One pillow may be used under the patient's head but should not be pressing down on or elevating the patient's shoulders. A small pillow under the patient's knees may also help him to relax. The patient should be flat on his back. If this is not possible, the patient may be placed in a semi-Fowler's position or be seated on a wooden chair. In the sitting position the patient's feet should be on the floor on a rubber mat or on a wooden footstool or a stack of books. The legs must not hang free nor should there by any pressure on the back of the legs just above the knees. If the patient is in a sitting position or a semi-Fowler's position it is necessary to make a note of this in the patient's recording.

The patient must be completely relaxed. The legs should not be touching each other. The patient is disrobed to the waist and the lower legs are exposed. Cover a woman's breasts until you are ready to run the chest leads. Wristwatches, necklaces, and all metals near the leads should be removed. Loosen all tight clothing.

It is best to have the patient rest for at least ten minutes before the test. Ask the patient if he was able to follow instructions (Fig. 32–6) on the appointment sheet he was given. It should be noted on the patient's chart if he has taken any medication that the physician may not be aware of.

Connecting the Patient Lead Cord

It is nice to chat with the patient while preparing him for the test. Most patients are a little apprehensive, especially on their first test, when the technician starts dabbing paste, rubbing it in, and then hooking up a lot of wires and straps. You may hear the comment, "Just like the electric chair," which shows a degree of apprehension. Friendly smiles and simple explanations will assure the patient that it is a simple, harmless test but that his cooperation is necessary.

Place the **electrodes,** also called **sensors,** in the standard places unless you have been instructed otherwise. The limb electrodes are most frequently placed on the upper outer arm, and the lower limb electrodes are best on the outer midcalf. Some physicians prefer to place the leg electrode over the bone of the lower leg, whereas others prefer to place it over a fleshy area. Care must be taken that the electrode plates are flat over the area they are placed. Do not allow an electrode to be tilted.

There are several types of contact or electrolytic materials available. It may be necessary for your office to have more than one type. There are times when a salty paste may be necessary, while often the thinner ones are sufficient. The purpose of the contact material is to reduce the skin's resistance and increase the sensitivity of the electrodes to the minute current sent by the patient's heart. If the patient's skin is extra dry or highly pigmented, it will require rubbing the skin's surface until a slight **erythema** appears. Make certain you have the same amount of contact medium for each lead. Wipe off the excess material. Do not allow your hands to carry the material from the patient to the equipment. Be neat with the contact media. Unequal amounts and "contamination" on the wires and equipment can cause artifacts and a poor recording. Presaturated pads are good in that they assure equal amounts of electrolyte for each lead. You may use the pad to prepare the patient by briskly rubbing the skin with the edge of the electrode, with the pad folded over the edge. Do not let the pad wrinkle under the electrode plate.

Place the electrodes with the lead connectors pointing toward the feet. Place the strap around the limb until the hole just meets the hook, then move one hole tighter and fasten. This should provide the correct tension. An accurate tracing cannot be made if the straps are too tight or too loose. Figure 32–7 shows the artifacts frequently found as a result of poor electrode hookups. Now insert the tip of the patient's lead cord into the lead connector holes by placing the tip of the cable over the electrode plate of the legs and around into the tip of the arm electrodes (Fig. 32–8). This will help keep the electrode plate flat and in place. Check to make certain you have con-

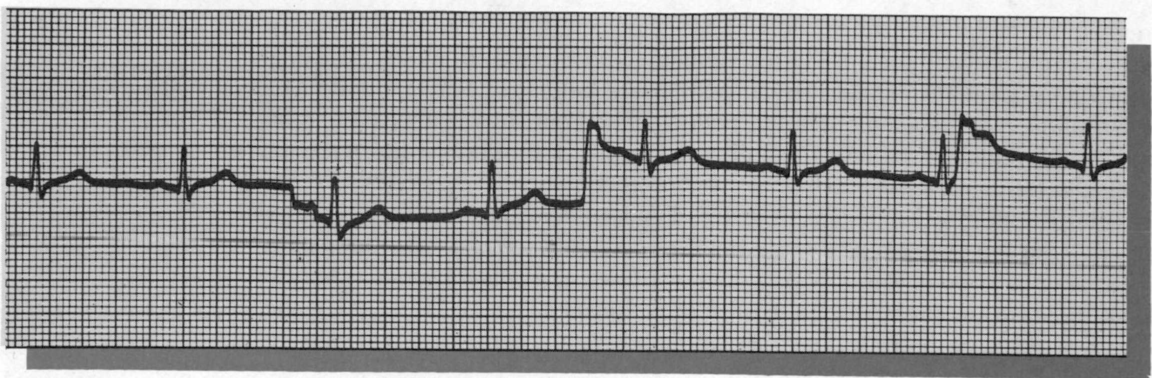

FIGURE 32–7 Artifacts. Baseline shifts resulting from electrodes that are too tight or too loose.

nected the correct lead terminal into the corresponding electrode. These are color-coded, but it is still easy to confuse the patient's right and left sides. Rest the lead cable on the patient's abdomen in order to prevent any pull on the cable that would cause an electrode plate to tilt. Give each lead cord terminal a gentle pull after you have secured it. PULL ON THE WIRE ONLY BY THE THICKENED END because these wires are extremely delicate. The placement of the chest leads is also standard. If you are uncertain about the placement of the chest electrodes it may be best to mark the patient's chest with a skin marker and have the physician check them for correct placement. The chest electrode may be held in place with tape if it is difficult to keep in place. Any variations from the standard lead placements should be indicated on the record. Figure 32–9*A* and *B* will show the six standard chest lead placements:

V1 — fourth intercostal space at the right margin of the sternum
V2 — fourth intercostal space at the left margin of the sternum
V3 — midway between V2 and V4
V4 — fifth intercostal space at junction of left midclavicular line
V5 — at horizontal level of position 4 at left anterior axillary line
V6 — at horizontal level of position 4 at left midaxillary line

Remember that V4, V5, and V6 are all on the same line and directly down from the midclavicular, anterior axillary fold and the midaxilla. It is usually advisable that the contact medium not be applied to the chest until you are ready to run the chest leads. Remember V1 and V4 are extremely important. If these two leads are incorrect the other chest leads will probably be incorrect also. (Refer to Fig. 28–2, Topography of the Chest, in Chapter 28, Physical Examinations.)

CODING

Some ECG machines will automatically code the various leads as they are recorded, but many machines do not. Therefore, it is necessary to mark each lead with a code that is internationally recognized. Without this coding it would be very difficult to

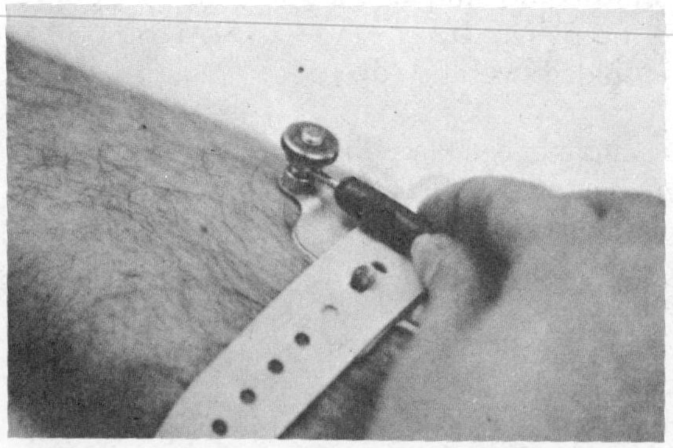

FIGURE 32–8 Electrode hook-up on patient's leg. (From *Electrocardiography: A Better Way*. Milton, Wisconsin, The Burdick Corp., 1976.)

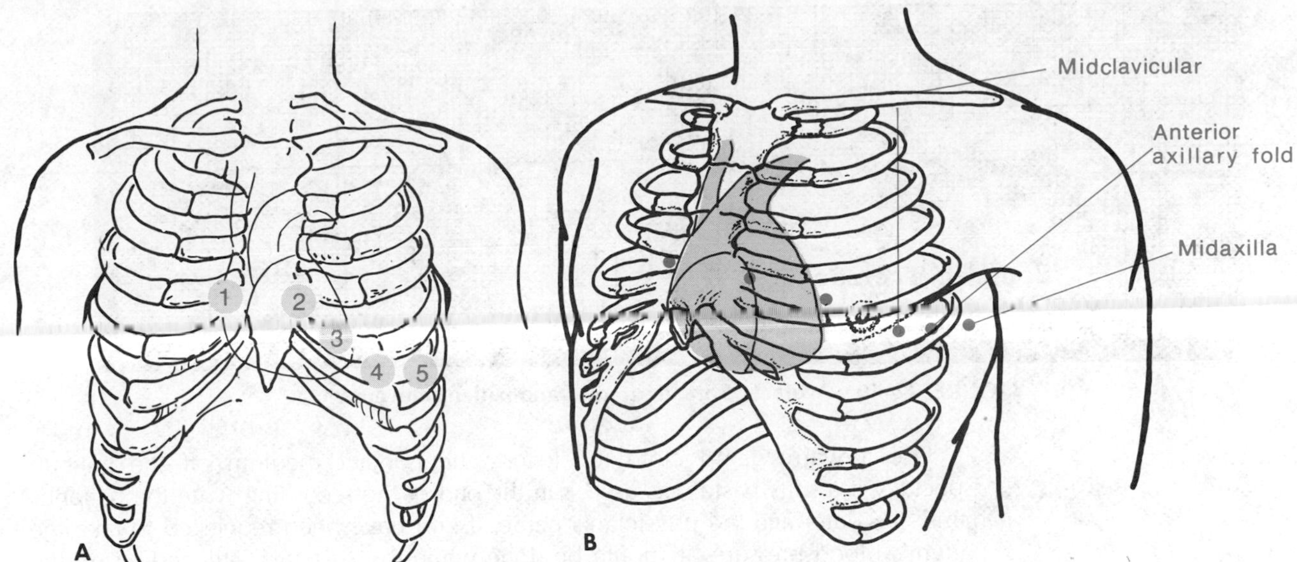

FIGURE 32–9 Chest lead placement. ***A,*** **Anterior view;** ***B,*** **lateral view.**

mount a tracing accurately. It also allows the technician to go back and rerun a specific lead that has been discovered to have artifacts or otherwise be unsatisfactory. It is simple and easy to check the tracing before the patient is disconnected and rerun any leads needing retracing.

Standard Marking Code

• = limb lead I
•• = limb lead II
••• = limb lead III

— = AVR
— — = AVL
— — — = AVF

— • = V1
— •• = V2
— ••• = V3
— •••• = V4
— ••••• = V5
— •••••• = V6

Keep the code dots and dashes close together. Make the dot appear as a dot and the dash as a short dash (as shown above).

The physician may request the medical assistant to run an extra long lead for the purpose of studying the patient's heart rhythm. This is called a "rhythm strip" and is usually limb lead II. This is usually run for about 20 inches.

If a patient has lost a limb then apply the electrode to the remaining portion of the limb, or if the entire limb has been amputated attach the electrode with tape to the site of the amputation. If the patient's chest is exceptionally small, use the infant size chest electrode. Use only a small amount of electrolyte and apply each time individually, being very careful not to let any run over into another lead site. This will cause a double exposure type of complex. Be consistent with the electrolyte.

It may be necessary on some machines to protect the recording stylus from violent movement by turning off the AMP switch each time a chest electrode is moved to another position. After you have completed the twelve leads and before you unhook the patient, check back over the tracing for any artifacts or errors. Rerun a lead if it is not accurate and readable, and make certain you code this lead correctly because it will be out of sequence.

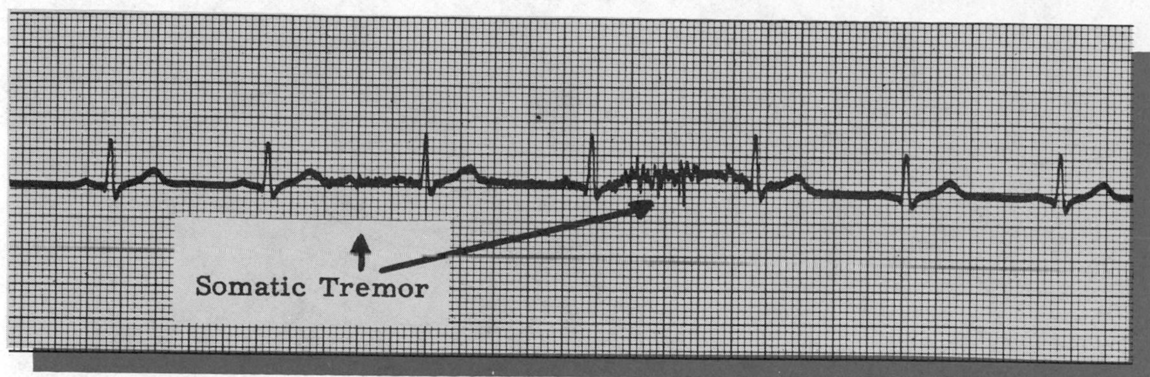

FIGURE 32–10 Artifacts. Somatic tremor and patient movement.

Use a warm damp cloth to cleanse the contact medium off the patient, especially if a salty paste was used. On the end of the recording write the patient's name, the date, and the physician's name. If you have been requested to take the patient's blood pressure, it should be done while the patient is still resting on the table. Record the blood pressure on the tracing with the other information.

Roll the tracing loosely with the tracing on the inside and place a small paper clip on the very edge. Do not roll tightly and do not put the paper clip all the way on. Tracings scratch easily and should be carefully handled. Some physicians wish to check the tracing before it is mounted and placed in the patient's medical record.

SOME TIPS TO KEEP IN MIND. Keep the electrodes polished. Do *not* use steel wool or any metal base polish as it will interfere with the tracing and cause artifacts. Use only a fine grade of scouring powder. Regardless of the contact medium used, it is necessary to polish the electrode regularly. Always rinse well and dry before storing. Use an applicator to clean the connecting holes and the inside of the suction-type chest electrode. If corrosion should occur, use only an extra fine grade of sand paper to polish. Electrodes must be kept polished and should be cleaned as soon as possible after each use. They cannot conduct properly if they are dirty or corroded.

Be certain to condition the skin properly with a little friction rubbing. Almost all skins take a little rubbing but especially those that are dry and highly suntanned. Keep the contact paste tube clean, and do not let dried paste collect. Dried paste particles can cause lumps, which cause artifacts and poor contact. Saturated pads must be flat and smooth.

ARTIFACTS AND ERRORS IN ELECTROCARDIOGRAPHIC TECHNIQUE

FROM THE PATIENT

1. The patient may have a pathologic condition causing muscular movement, resulting in somatic **tremor** (Fig. 32–10).
2. The patient may not be able to relax, is chilled, uncomfortable, or frightened.

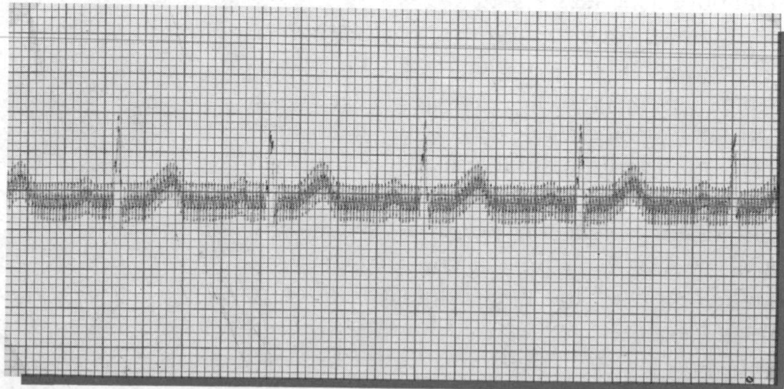

FIGURE 32–11 Electrical (AC) interference is a constant pattern in the tracing. It may be heavy (as shown) or very slight. It is not uneven as in somatic interference (shown in Figure 32–10).

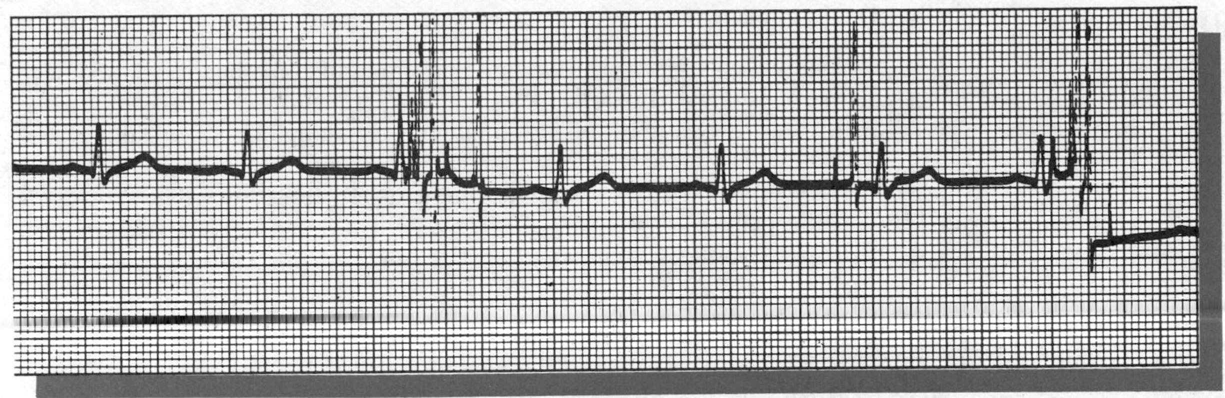

FIGURE 32–12 **Artifacts possibly due to a break in the patient's lead cord or a loosened wire. This cannot usually be repaired but must be replaced.**

Make the patient comfortable; use small pillows or a blanket. Allow the patient to slightly change position by moving an electrode.

3. Minute particles of metal may be embedded in a metal worker's skin. Move the electrode to the upper *inner* part of the arm and prepare the skin carefully. Use a paste rather than one of the lighter solutions.

4. An extremely nervous patient may have to be sedated by the physician's orders. An uncooperative child may have to undergo a trial run to prove there is no discomfort.

FROM THE MACHINE

1. Jarring the machine may cause a deflection. Keep the machine away from the table and the patient. Do not lean on the machine. Move the machine away from the patient 12 inches or so.

2. Incorrect standardization will cause an incorrect deflection. Make certain the STD is exactly 1 cm (10 mm) high.

3. Excessive heat or too cool a recording stylus will obscure a deflection and not show a clear tracing. Excessive heat will also shorten the life of the stylus.

4. AC interference (Fig. 32–11) will cause an artifact and obscure a deflection. Check the manufacturer's manual for grounding instructions. There may be an electrical appliance nearby. Change to another wall plug, if possible. Check that the electrical power cord is not near or crossing the patient's lead cord. These two cords should not be near each other.

5. A break in a wire in the patient's lead cord will cause artifacts. These wires are very delicate and should be handled carefully (Fig. 32–12).

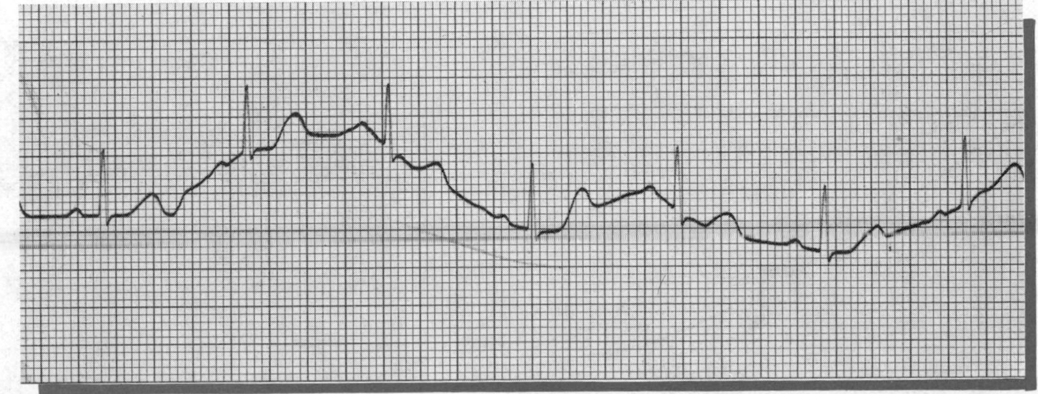

FIGURE 32–13 **Shifting or wandering baseline due to a loose electrode or connection. If resting place of baseline is smooth, a shifting baseline could be normal respiration in the chest leads.**

FROM THE TECHNICIAN

1. Static electricity from a synthetic uniform and clothing, especially with nonconductive rubber soled shoes.
2. Static electricity in nylon and synthetic carpeting. Use nonstatic carpet spray.
3. Improperly applied electrodes: too tight or too loose; not flat but slightly tilted by a cable pull.
4. Improperly applied electrolyte, lumpy paste, wrinkled pads.

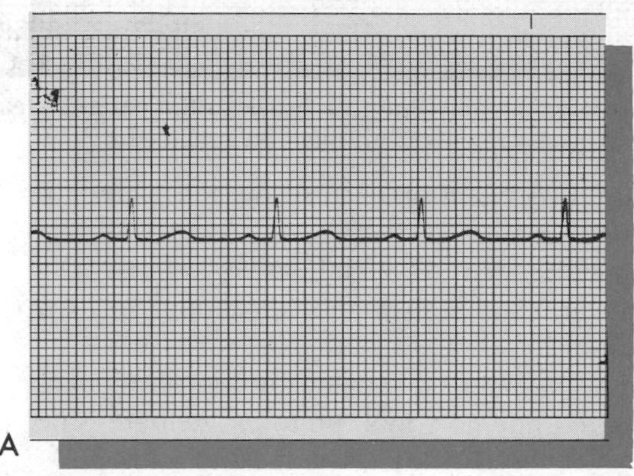

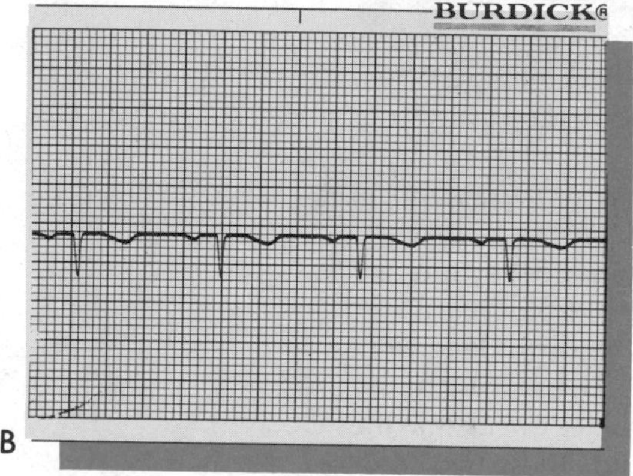

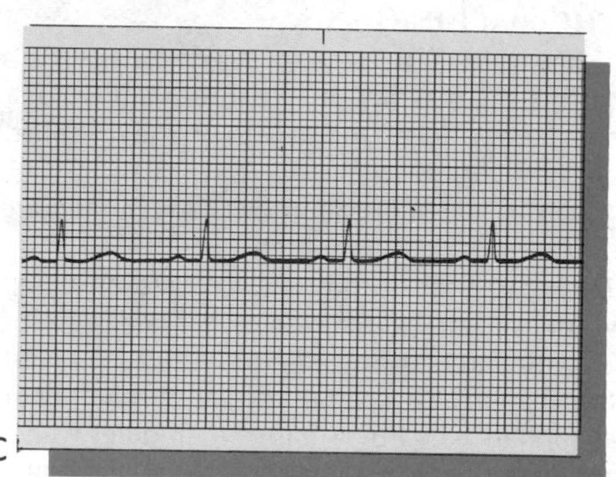

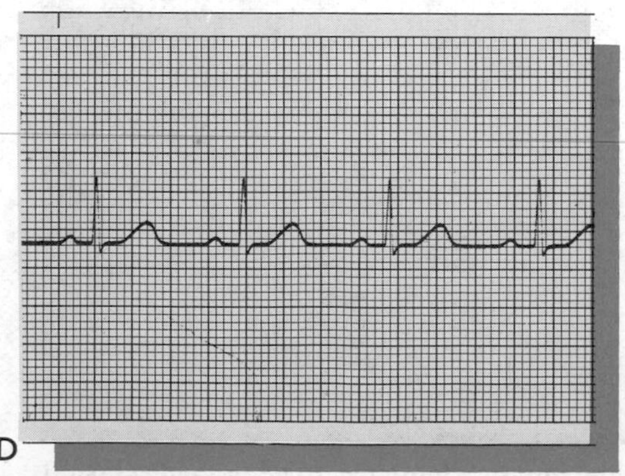

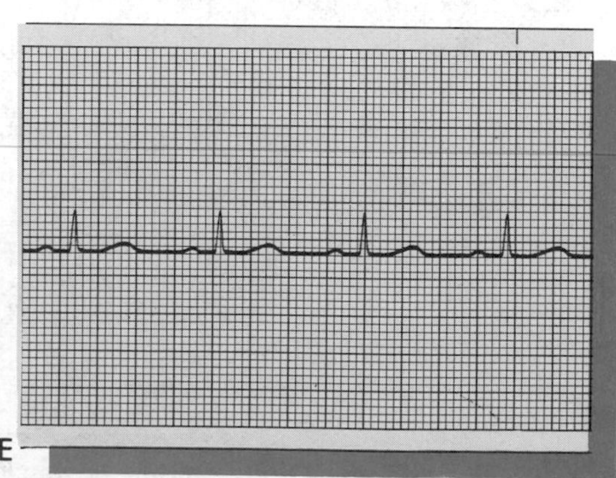

FIGURE 32–14 Cords of limb lead I crossed up. *A,* Correct; *B,* RA and LA crossed; *C,* LL and RL crossed; *D,* LL and LA crossed; *E,* RA and RL crossed.

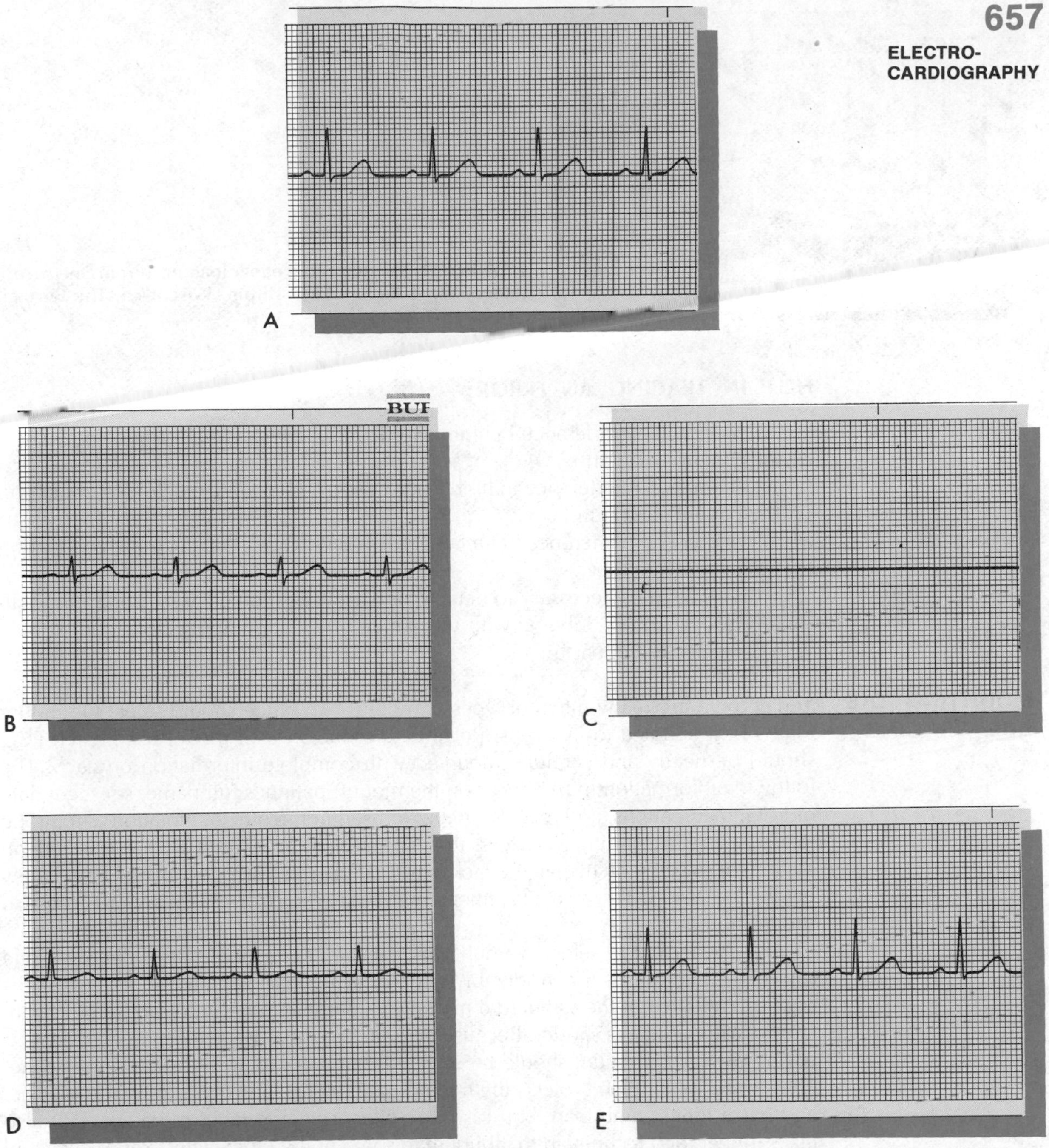

A

B

C

D

E

FIGURE 32–15 Cords of limb lead II crossed up. *A*, Correct; *B*, RA and LA crossed; *C*, LL and RL crossed; *D*, LL and LA crossed; *E*, RA and RL crossed.

5. Chest electrode not flat or not snug enough (Fig. 32–13).

6. Lead wires mixed: right and left sides crossed, arm leads on the leg electrodes (Figs. 32–14 and 32–15, especially 32–14*B* and 32–15C).

7. Dirty and corroded electrodes. Steel wool may have been used in error.

8. Improper mounting: wrong lead in wrong place or upside down. Special care must be taken in mounting.

9. Incorrect coding of the leads.

10. Room uncomfortable: cold, noisy, interruptions, etc.

11. Technician's nervous movements, surprised expressions, misunderstood comments about the tracing and/or the patient.

12. Incorrect paper loading (Fig. 32–16).

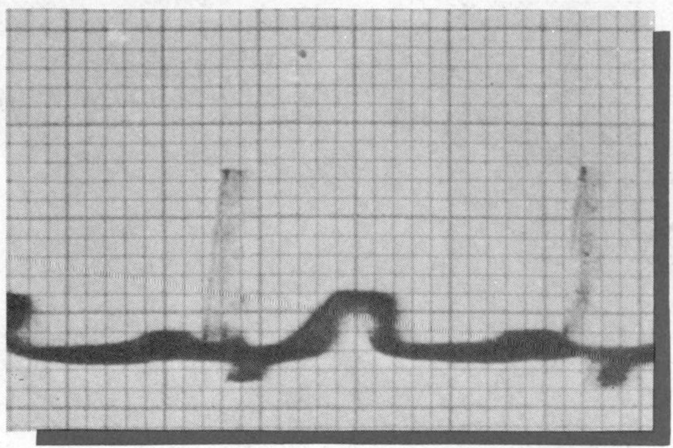

FIGURE 32–16 Improper paper loading. (From *Electrocardiography: A Better Way*. Milton, Wisconsin, The Burdick Corp., 1976.)

HELP IN TRACING AN ERROR

1. If there is interference in limb leads I and II, check the electrode connection on the patient's right arm.

2. If there is interference in limb leads I and III, check the electrode connection on the patient's left arm.

3. If there is interference in limb leads II and III, check the electrode connection on the patient's left leg.

It is sometimes necessary to detach the electrode momentarily, abrase the skin slightly with vigorous rubbing with wet gauze or a cotton applicator, then reapply with new electrolyte paste.

MOUNTING THE ECG TRACING

Today there are many different types of mounts. An office should select the mount that is best adapted to its needs. Regardless of the style of mount used, each ECG should be neatly and carefully mounted with complete information on each. The following information must appear on the mount: patient's full name, sex, age, date of ECG, medications, and record number (if used in the office). Notations should be made if there is anything that differs from the routine, such as a very nervous patient, a different position of the patient, lack of rest before the test, or smoking immediately before the test. If the lead placements were different from the standard this also should be noted.

It is advisable to select a mount that can be easily read in its entirety on one surface, which makes it considerably easier for the physician. The three limb leads are best mounted in the standard 6 in. lengths. Some mount limb lead II in the 6 in. length, with all others shorter. Because tracings are usually a series of records over a period of years, a mount should be selected that will last with the passing of time. The slotted folder type protects the tracings, can all be seen on one surface at once, and has a longer limb lead, but it is more expensive and takes more space. It also takes longer for a technician to mount than some of the other styles. Paper clips and staples should not be used because they will scratch a tracing. Clear tape can be used, but some become sticky or yellow with time. The new copy machines help with making a copy of tracing on a single sheet without fear of damaging the record; this also takes less space.

Extreme care should be taken in mounting as incorrect mounting is a common source of error. Do not allow the desk to become cluttered with tracing trimmings. Discard the trimmings into a waste container as you trim them off. Do not cut off the lead coding until you are ready to mount that particular lead. Double-check each lead code with the mount placement. Mounts vary in that some have the precordial leads horizontal, whereas others have them vertical. Take great care not to mount a lead upside down. If you have been requested to show the STD in a lead then do not cut it off. Do not hide the tip of the QRS waves in the slot-type of mount. Most tracings are easily scratched, so be wary of scratching with rings or sleeve buttons. Do not stack other items on top of the open-faced type of mount.

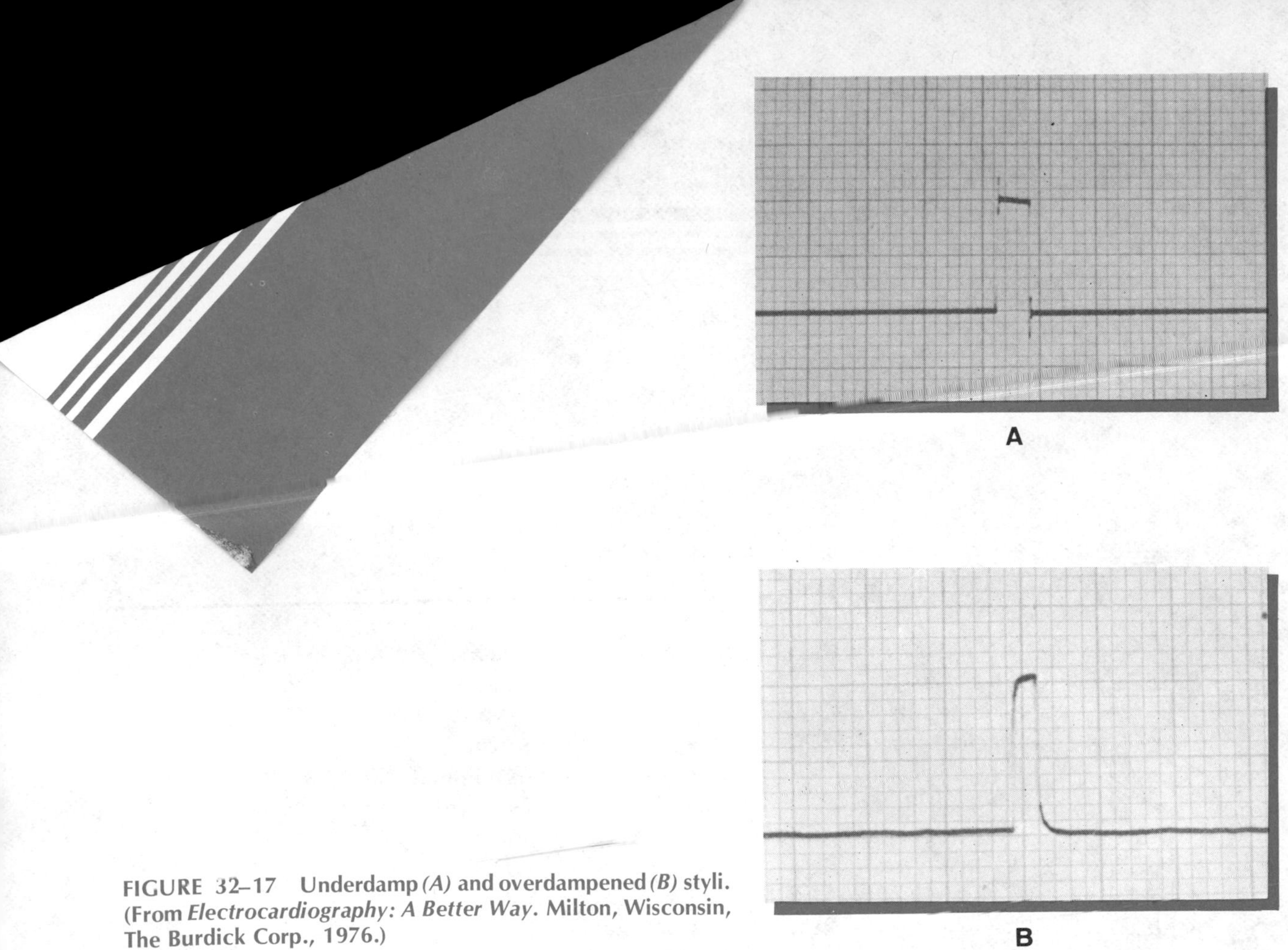

FIGURE 32–17 Underdamp *(A)* and overdampened *(B)* styli. (From *Electrocardiography: A Better Way*. Milton, Wisconsin, The Burdick Corp., 1976.)

Place the mounted ECG tracing on the physician's desk with the patient's medical record and previous ECG tracings for evaluation.

MAINTENANCE OF THE MACHINE

The manufacturer's manual will explain the general care of your machine. It is relatively easy to maintain if you remember it is a delicate instrument. An occasional adjustment of the recording stylus may be necessary on some machines that have a tendency to have an over-sensitive or under-sensitive stylus (Fig. 32–17). Proper adjustment is essential because it is reflected in the beat complex. An over-sensitive stylus can over-respond to the QRS waves and give a false voltage reading. If it is under-sensitive it will reduce the height of the R wave and distort the S-T portion of the complex. Follow the manufacturer's instructions carefully, or have an expert service person service the machine. It is important for the physician to receive an accurate picture of the patient's heart.

References

Burch, G., and Winsor, T.: *A Primer of Electrocardiography*. 6th ed. Philadelphia, Lea & Febiger, 1972.

Burdick Corp.: *Electrocardiography — A Better Way*. Milton, Wisc., The Burdick Corp., 1976.

Butler, H. H.: *How to Read an Electrocardiogram*. Oradell, NJ, Medical Economics Co., 1973.

Conover, M. H., and Zabis, E. G.: *Understanding Electrocardiography: Physical and Interpretative Concepts*. 2nd ed. St. Louis, C. V. Mosby Co., 1976.

Schnitzer, K.: *Electrocardiographic Technique*. 2nd ed. New York, Grune and Stratton, 1960.

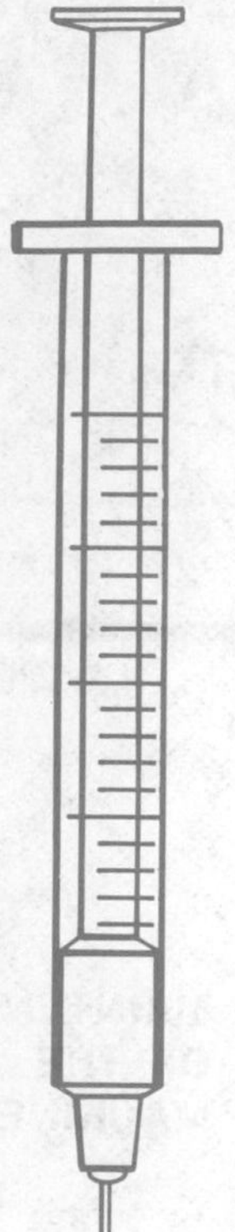

CHAPTER OUTLINE

Accident-Proof the Office
Plan Ahead
Community Emergency Services
Accidents and Children
Crash Tray
General Rules
Some Specific Problems
- Fainting
- Choking and the Heimlich Maneuver
- Emergency Respiratory Resuscitation
- Cardiopulmonary Resuscitation
- Chest Pain
- Cerebrovascular Accident (CVA)
- Poisoning
- Insect Stings
- Anaphylaxis (Anaphylactic Reactions)
- Shock
- Asthma
- Seizures
- Abdominal Pain
- Obstetric Emergencies
- Sprains
- Fractures
- Burns
- Lacerations
- Animal Bites
- Nosebleeds
- Hemorrhages
- Head Injuries
- Foreign Body in the Eye

BEHAVIORAL OBJECTIVES

The medical office assistant should be able to:

- **Accident-proof the physician's office to minimize risk of injury to visitors.**
- **Familiarize herself with local emergency services so that the severely ill or injured can be transferred quickly for critical care.**
- **Prepare and maintain a "crash tray" of essential drugs and equipment for emergency use.**
- **Apply first aid in common presenting conditions such as poisoning, hemorrhaging, fractures, and burns.**

33

FIRST AID AND MEDICAL EMERGENCIES

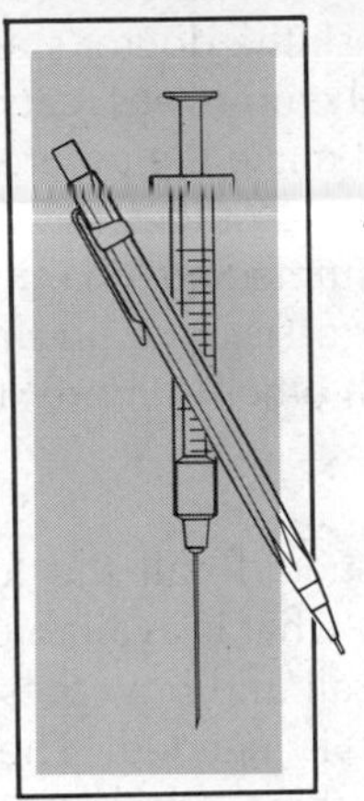

There are many different approaches to the manner of emergency care, but this discussion will attempt to remain within general principles. Each medical assistant should consult with her physician-employer for the preferences in handling emergencies in that particular practice. Each medical assistant should enroll in an American Red Cross First Aid course and obtain an advanced certificate. A refresher course should be taken every few years. It is also strongly recommended that medical assistants encourage their local chapters of the AAMA to have workshops conducted by their local physicians and the emergency facilities in their community.

In a true emergency, the law permits anyone to do whatever is reasonably necessary, provided that the care given is within the scope and skill of the first aider's competence. The law holds persons giving emergency care to be responsible for any injury that they cause owing to their negligence or failure to exercise reasonable care.

Some medical emergencies may require the medical assistant to make an immediate decision that comes rather close to making a medical diagnosis. The obvious injury of spurting blood does not present this problem, but the ashen-faced patient gasping for breath and in obvious pain calls for medical knowledge in order to make a decision. The medical assistant must remember her limitations and never forget that her employer may be held liable for her mistakes.

ACCIDENT-PROOF THE OFFICE

It is usually the medical assistant's responsibility to accident-proof the office as much as possible. Do not use scatter rugs, delicate chairs, or have slippery floors. Keep cupboard doors and drawers closed. Wipe up any spills immediately and pick up dropped objects. All medications should be kept out of sight; dangerous drugs should be kept in locked cupboards. If there are children in the office, keep all sharp objects out of reach. NEVER give a child a disposable syringe and needle for a toy or as a reward for being good. These items are not toys and should be destroyed and carefully discarded. Never leave a seriously ill patient or a restless, depressed, or unconscious patient unattended.

PLAN AHEAD

The office staff should discuss possible emergencies that may occur in that office or area. Local industries, for instance, may present unique problems that call for very specialized care. Plan for these, and ask the doctor's advice on what procedure he wants you to follow. If there are several employees, each should be assigned specific duties. Organization and planning will make the difference between organized care for the patient and complete chaos. Some offices have set up the "buddy system." This system allows one person to take immediate charge of the patient while another obtains needed materials and calls for assistance. In this way the patient is not left unattended. They can also relieve each other in more strenuous work like resuscitation and external heart massage.

COMMUNITY EMERGENCY SERVICES

In every area, the medical assistant should call the local fire department, police department, or rescue squad and know what is available to her and the patients. She should learn ahead what numbers to call and how these calls are handled. Usually one call will send all the help that is needed. These emergency services are extremely well coordinated in dispatching resuscitators, ambulances, and other emergency care.

Every office should have a list of emergency numbers posted. This list should include the Poison Control Center, the local rescue squad, and fire and police department. The list should be in plain sight and known to all office personnel. Check if your area has the 911 emergency number. When in doubt, dial "0" for operator. A fire department emergency rescue squad captain once told a group of medical assistants that the rescue squad made almost as many calls to physicians' offices as they did to private homes. Remember, the fact that you are in a medical office does not mean you can handle all emergencies. Neither is the doctor always in the office when you are there.

ACCIDENTS AND CHILDREN

Accidents are the leading cause of death for children under 15 years of age. The Children's Bureau of the Department of Health, Education, and Welfare has published pamphlets on helpful tips on preventing accidents. Martin Green in *A Sigh of Relief** shows how to buy safe toys, bikes, and camping equipment. He also tells how to "childproof" your home. These publications should be of special interest to medical assistants, especially in pediatrics and family practice.

CRASH TRAY

The *emergency* or *crash tray* that is made up in your office should be kept in an easily accessible place known to all personnel in the office. A firm rule must be made that *no one* borrows *any* item from the tray. It should be checked periodically and all medications kept fresh and ready for use. The contents of the tray will vary to some degree according to the type of emergencies your office will possibly encounter. A household cleaners tray is excellent. It has a handle and several divided sections and is brightly colored. Listed below are some basic items found in crash trays.

Epinephrine (adrenalin), injectable
Apomorphine hydrochloride, injectable (a narcotic.)
Antihistamine, injectable and oral
Ipecac, oral
Isuprel, aerosol spray (isoproterenol hydrochloride)
Sterile dressings
Tourniquet (not often recommended)

*Bantam

Disposable syringe and needle units
Adhesive tape
Airways of various sizes
"Instant" type of hot and cold packs

The *epinephrine* should be a ready-to-use cartridge syringe and needle unit. These are supplied in one cc cartridges. Then, in case of an insect sting, 0.5 cc may be given immediately at the site of the sting and 0.5 cc may be given in the opposite arm. Epinephrine is also used to check hemorrhage and relieve asthmatic **paroxysm** and **shock.** It is a **vasoconstrictor** and cardiac stimulant and relaxes the bronchioles.

Other drugs that may be found in this section are *atropine, Lanoxin,* and *Xylocaine. Atropine* decreases secretions, increases respiration and heart rates, and is a smooth muscle relaxant. It will dilate the pupil of the eye and is a general cerebral stimulant. It gives relief of gastrointestinal cramps and hypermotility. It may also be used to relieve pain locally. *Lanoxin* is a trade-name for digoxin, a cardiotonic. It is used to treat congestive heart failure. It is good for emergency use because it has a relatively rapid action. *Xylocaine* is a trade-name for lidocaine and is used as both a local and topical anesthetic. It is also used in cardiac arrhythmias and is effective in 3 to 5 minutes.

Apomorphine hydrochloride is a prompt and effective emetic and is used in cases of poisoning when a stomach pump cannot be employed. *Ipecac* is also an emetic and many physicians are recommending that mothers keep it on hand at home for use in cases of emergency. Antihistamine counteracts the effect of histamine and is used in the treatment of allergic reactions and anaphylaxis. Isoproterenol hydrochloride is an antispasmodic and is used in bronchial spasm; it is also a cardiac stimulant. Some trade names for this product are *Isuprel* (Winthrop), *Medihaler-Iso* (Riker), and *Norisodrine* (Abbott). Other medications found useful in a crash tray are *Aramine* for severe shock, *amytal sodium* and *Valium* for convulsions and as sedatives, dextrose and insulin to treat diabetics, and *Lasix* for congestive heart failure. *Glucagon* is used primarily to counteract severe hypoglycemic reactions in diabetic patients taking insulin.

Many physicians and others involved in emergency care do not recommend the use of a tourniquet except in cases of insect or snake bites on the arms or legs because there is considerable danger from the *incorrect* use of a tourniquet. It should be used very cautiously. It is much better in cases of bleeding to apply pressure directly over the bleeding area. In cases of insect or snake bites, the tourniquet is applied just above the bite area, or just above the place where the offending medication was administered in the case of an error in injection of a medication.

Small cans, with pull tab openers, of orange juice are handy for quick sugar administration.

If bottles of intravenous solutions are kept in the crash tray, it has been suggested that a hammer and large nail also be kept in the tray. A nail quickly driven into the wall may relieve some person from having to hold the bottle above the patient. One can find oneself quite often without a place to hang a bottle or irrigation bag, and one small nail hole is well justified by the great convenience it affords.

Another good suggestion is to have cards in the tray that have the emergency numbers on them. By doing so, the person in charge can hand the correct number to a specific person with instructions to call that number. This may save a few moments searching for a number.

GENERAL RULES

Make the patient as comfortable as possible. Do not leave an ill or emergency patient in the reception room. The first and most important rule is to KEEP CALM. Stop for 30 seconds, survey the situation, and recognize what is the actual emergency. A decision must be made as to whether the need is immediate or nonimmediate. This decision may call for some medical knowledge and calm judgment. After you have surveyed the situation, calmly but firmly give specific instructions to the patient and the other office personnel. Never say "Will someone call the doctor?" Say, "YOU call the doctor," "YOU get a blanket," and "YOU get the emergency tray." After the emergency is under control, make certain that all the events and medications used are recorded accurately. Be precise when recording. It is a good idea to have statements of how the accident happened or what events just preceded the emergency. If the patient is one of your employer's regular patients, make sure the patient's medical chart is flagged with this pertinent information. If the patient is not a regular patient in your office, he should be given any necessary information that he can take with him to prevent a possible recurrence of the emergency.

Whenever a patient is being sent to a hospital for an emergency that may require an anesthetic, it is advisable to instruct the patient not to take anything by mouth. Food in the stomach can present quite a problem when a patient is receiving a general anesthetic.

SOME SPECIFIC PROBLEMS

Fainting

One of the most common emergency problems to confront the medical assistant is a patient's fainting or feeling faint. Fainting is usually caused by a lack of oxygen in the blood with a consequent lack of oxygen to the brain. If a patient faints, or even says, "I feel faint," if his face becomes pale, or if perspiration becomes profuse, especially on the forehead, the patient should be positioned with the head lower than or on the same level as the heart. If the patient is placed on the treatment table, turn his head to one side and loosen all tight clothing. Give aromatic spirits of ammonia; be careful not to hold the ammonia directly under the patient's nostrils but pass it back and forth about six inches from the nose. Cold water lightly sprinkled on the face will help. Take the patient's pulse, respiration, and blood pressure; then report to the physician. Keep the patient in a supine position for at least ten minutes after he has regained consciousness.

If it is not possible to get the patient onto a bed, place him in a sitting position and lower his head between his knees. If the patient cannot sit or lie down, tell him to kneel on one knee as if tying a shoelace; this gets the head lower than the heart. Never try to hold up a patient who faints but ease him gently to the floor if he cannot be assisted to a bed. On the floor, he is placed in a level position. After the patient has regained consciousness he may be given some tea or coffee. Recovery usually occurs within five minutes. If it does not, a physician should be called.

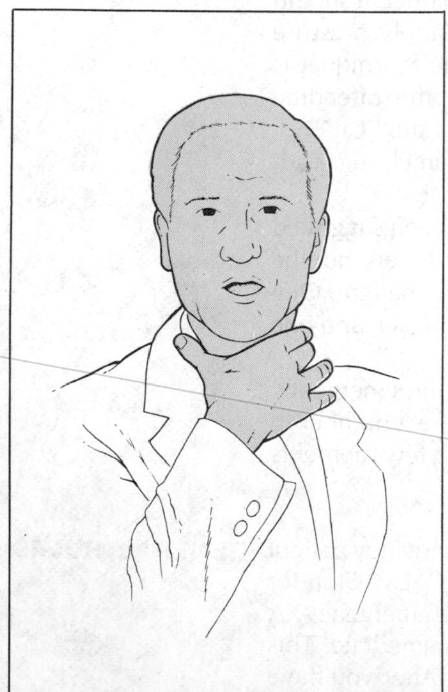

FIGURE 33–1 The choking sign. (From Heimlich, H. J.: The Heimlich maneuver: Where it stands today. Emerg. Med., July 1978.)

Choking and the Heimlich Maneuver

Choking is caused by a foreign object, usually food, lodged in the upper airway. Exhalation can often take place, but inhalation is blocked, so that the lungs quickly empty. The patient may hold his neck in the "choking sign" (Figure 33–1) or may turn blue in the face and neck.

There is some controversy over the best method for immediate care of the choking person, but the Heimlich maneuver is widely used at present (Fig. 33–2*A–D*). DO NOT give the victim soft bread, a drink of water, or anything else by mouth.

If the victim is a child, simply turn the child upside down or across your lap with the entire trunk of the body hanging down. Firm taps on the back may help. Since this could lodge the object in another spot, it should be attempted only as a last resort.

It may be necessary to search for the object in the victim's throat. Do not probe without looking. Use a light and work with your fingers. Extreme care must be taken in retrieving the object with an instrument. If the object cannot be immediately removed, then medical help must be gotten immediately. Time is of the essence with the choking person.

Sometimes air can pass around the object, and the person can be given mouth-to-mouth resuscitation. Start **resuscitation** if initial attempts to clear the airway have proven unsuccessful.

Emergency Respiratory Resuscitation

Breathing may suddenly cease for a variety of reasons, including shock, disease, and trauma. The most obvious sign that breathing has stopped is if the chest is no longer moving. Artificial respiration must be begun immediately, since death will follow within minutes.

Resuscitation techniques should be studied and practiced in courses directed to this purpose, but we will present the basics here as an introduction or a reference. The airway must first be opened by positioning the patient on his back and relieving possible obstruction of the air passage by the tongue (Fig. 33–3). Extreme caution must be used if there is any chance that the patient has suffered a cervical neck injury, as should be assumed in any accident. If neck injury is not suspected, the head is tilted by downward pressure on the forehead and upward pressure under the neck or chin. If neck injury may be present, grasp the angles of the victim's lower jaw without extending the neck.

Mouth-to-mouth resuscitation is begun if breathing does not follow opening of the airway (Fig. 33–4). Position yourself on the side of the patient's head. One hand should continue pressing on the forehead and should also be turned so that the fingers can hold the nose shut. The other should continue lifting the chin up. Place your mouth over the mouth of the victim and give four quick breaths, then continue ventilating the lungs every five seconds until the patient is breathing spontaneously or help arrives.

Artificial airways may be inserted by trained personnel to establish or maintain breathing (Fig. 33–5). Airways of various types and sizes should be kept ready on the emergency tray.

Cardiopulmonary Resuscitation

Loss of breathing may be accompanied by cessation of the heart beat, or cardiac arrest, identified by the lack of pulse. Artificial respiration must then be accompanied by external (closed) cardiac massage. This is called cardiopulmonary resuscitation (CPR). Cardiopulmonary resuscitation must be begun immediately to attempt to prevent death or permanent damage to body organs, especially the brain.

Since CPR may also cause injuries to the ribs, heart, liver, lungs, and blood vessels, it should be used only if you are certain that the heart has stopped and if you are trained in this procedure.

In CPR, the heart is compressed by downward pressure on the sternum, which should cause the blood to circulate. The proper position is for the heel of one hand to be placed on the sternum, two finger widths above the lower notch where the ribs

Text continued on page 670

The basic technique

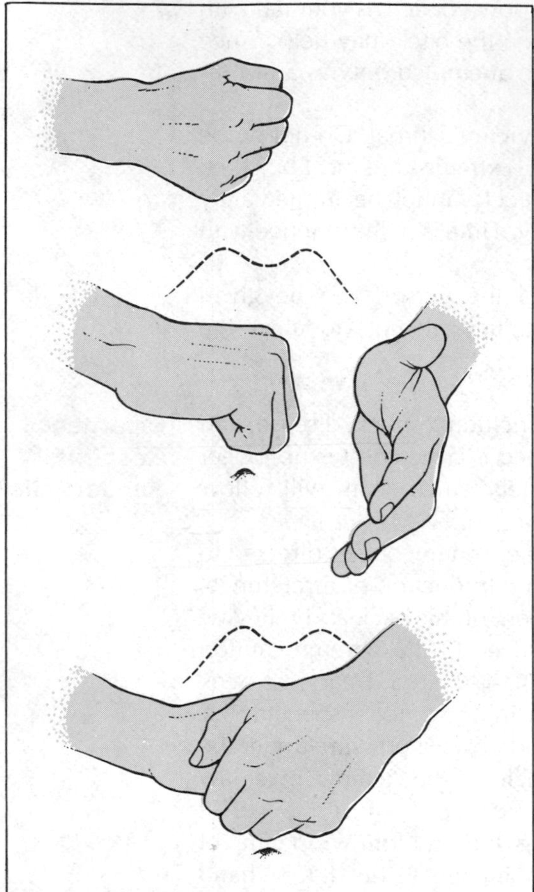

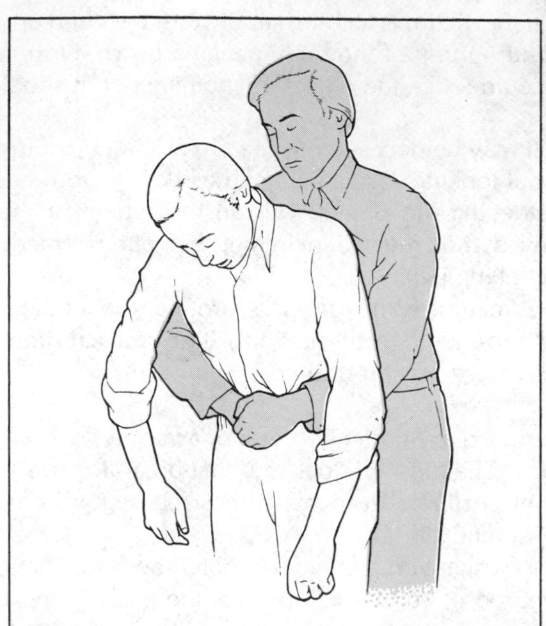

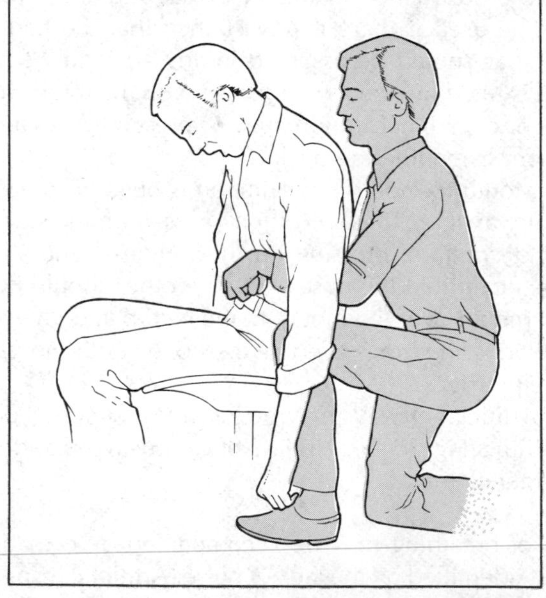

The Heimlich maneuver uses air in the lungs to force an obstruction out of the airway. To move the air you have to apply sudden pressure below the rib cage, which forces the diaphragm up and compresses the lungs. The basic technique (above) begins with a fist. Note the knob formed by the thumb and index finger—that's what helps push the diaphragm upward. Place your fist thumbside against the abdomen, slightly above the navel and below the rib cage. Then grasp your fist with your free hand and press into the abdomen with a quick upward thrust. Do this while standing or kneeling behind a standing or sitting victim with your arms wrapped around his waist (right). Repeat this procedure several times if necessary.

A

FIGURE 33–2 *A,* Basic technique for the Heimlich maneuver. The Heimlich maneuver for the fallen victim.

Illustration continued on opposite page

The fallen victim

When the victim is on the floor or too big for you to handle standing up, get him flat out on his back, face up, and kneel astride his hips. Place the heel of one hand on the abdomen slightly above the navel and below the rib cage and cover it with the other hand. Press into the victim's abdomen with a quick upward thrust and repeat if necessary.

B

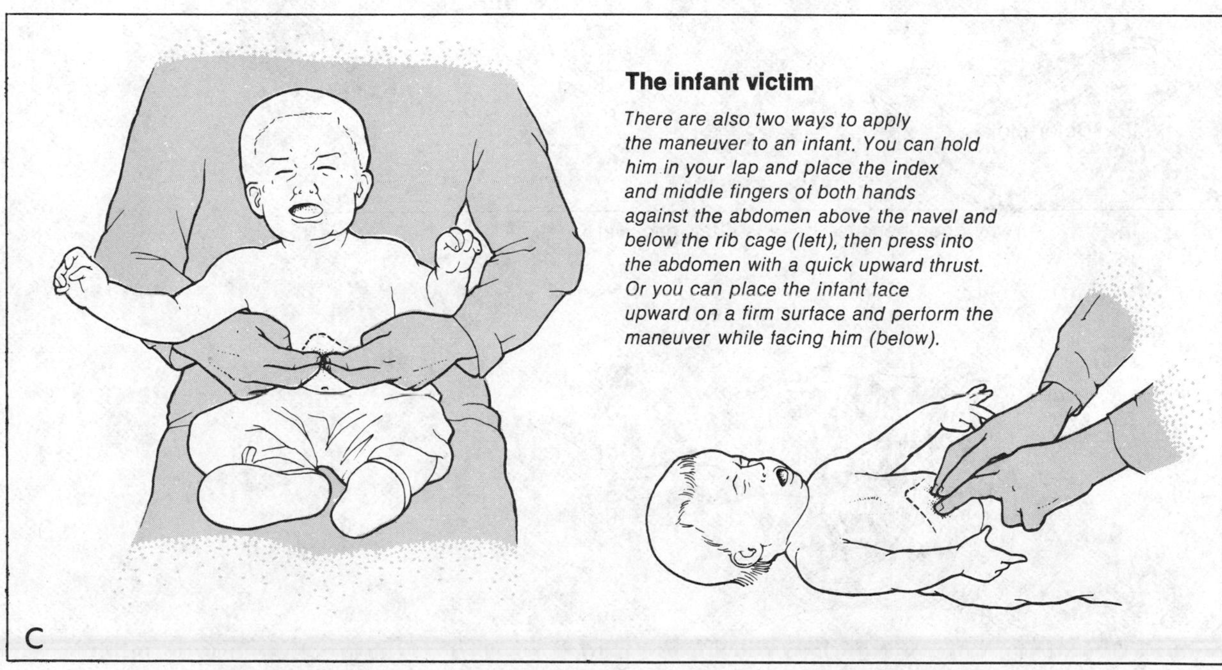

FIGURE 33–2 *Continued* (B) and for the infant victim *(C)*.

Illustration continued on following page

Four don'ts

1. Don't slap the victim's back.
2. Don't squeeze or compress the chest.
3. Don't kneel alongside the victim when performing the maneuver supine.
4. Don't turn the supine victim's head to the side.

D

FIGURE 33–2 *Continued* *D,* Precautions. (From Heimlich, H. J.: The Heimlich maneuver: Where it stands today. Emerg. Med., July 1978.)

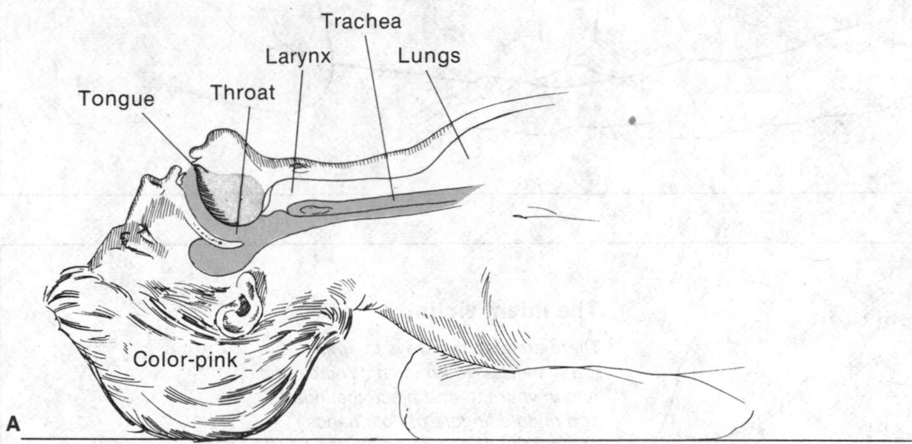

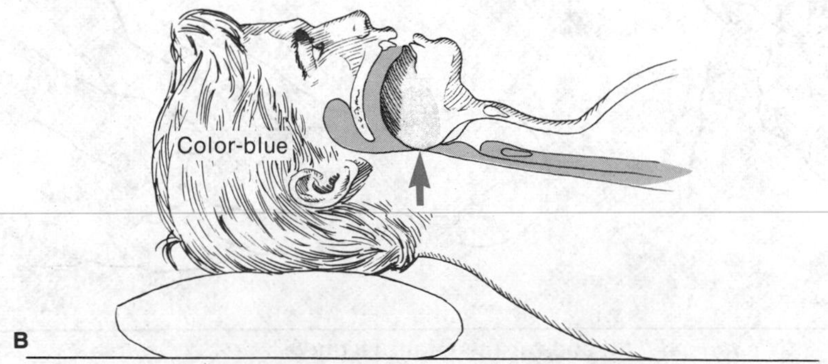

FIGURE 33–3 Position of head for mouth-to-mouth resuscitation.

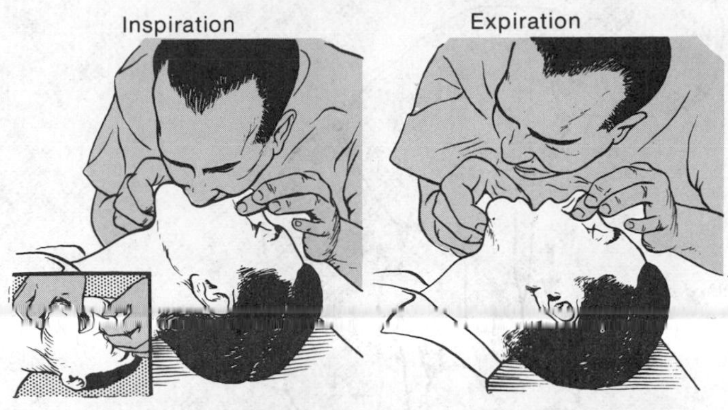

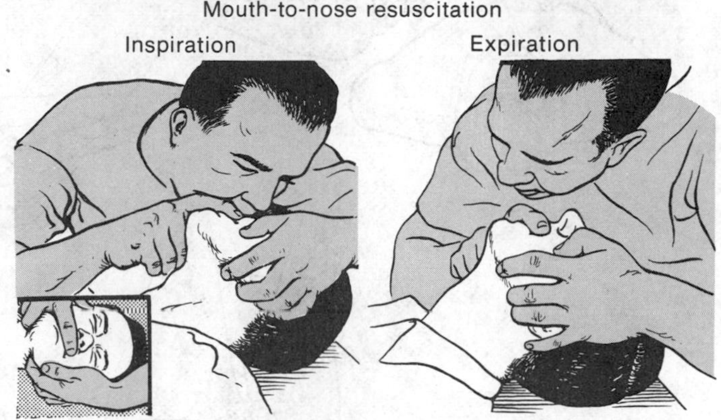

FIGURE 33–4 *Mouth-to-mouth*. 1. Remove any obstructions from the mouth. 2. Hyperextend the patient's neck. 3. With your thumb hold the jaw open. 4. Pinch patient's nostrils closed. 5. Take a deep breath then breathe directly between the patient's lips, forming an air-tight seal with your mouth. 6. Allow the patient to exhale. 7. Repeat every 4 or 5 seconds in the adult, slightly faster for a child. 8. For the small child the resuscitator's mouth may cover the patient's nose and mouth. *Mouth-to-nose*. Same procedure, except the patient's mouth is held closed and air is breathed into the nostrils. (From Gordon, A. S., et al.: J.A.M.A., *167*:320, 1958).

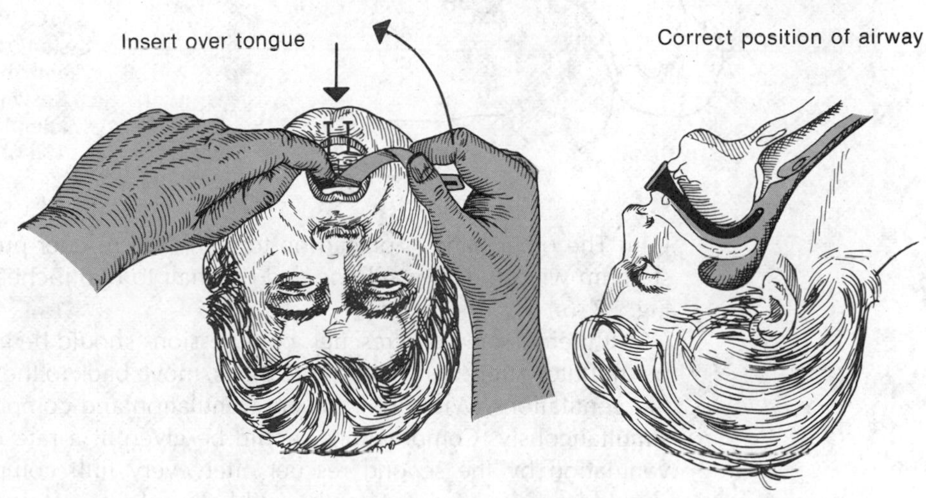

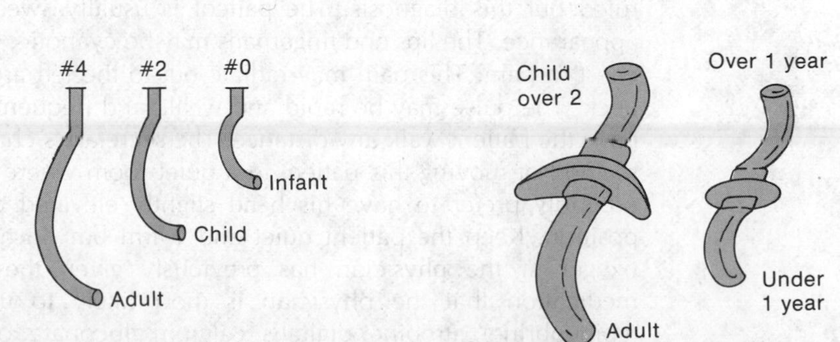

FIGURE 33–5 Proper placement of an artificial airway device.

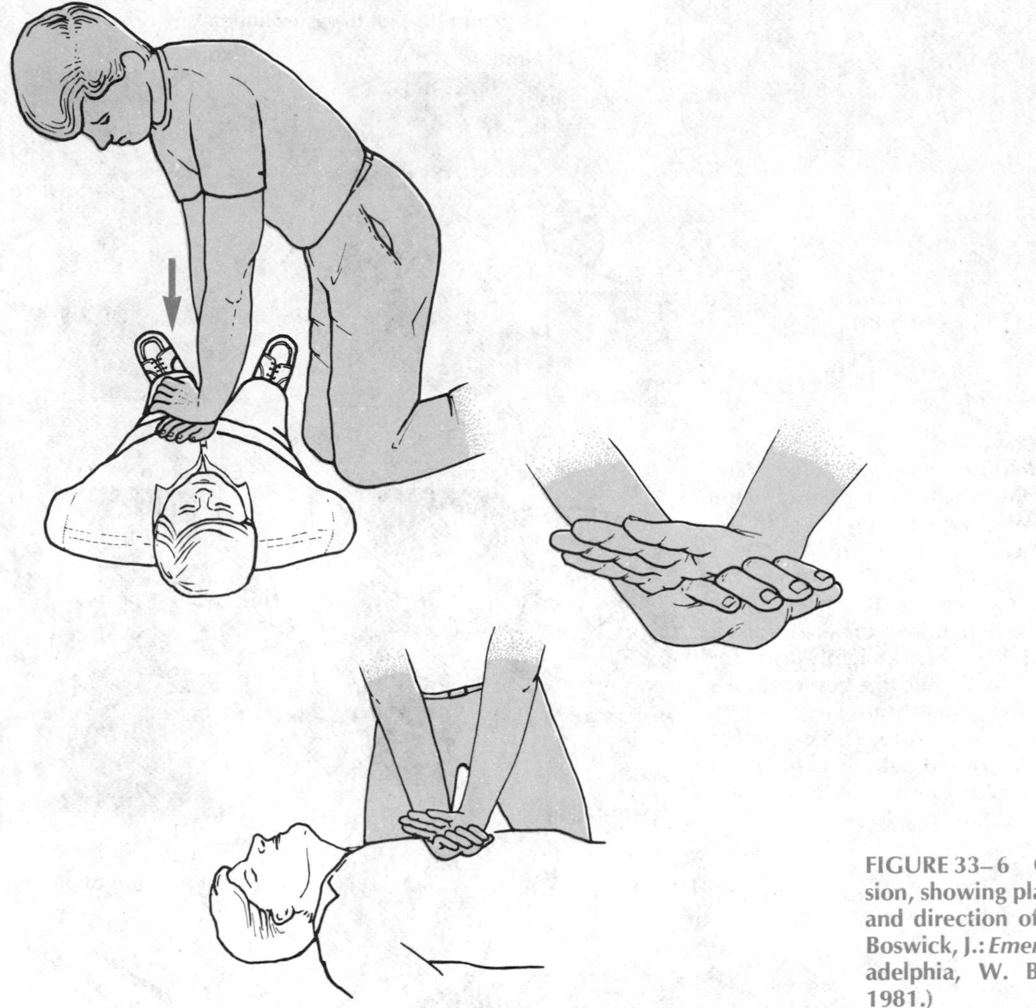

FIGURE 33–6 Cardiac compression, showing placement of hands and direction of pressure. (From Boswick, J.: *Emergency Care*. Philadelphia, W. B. Saunders Co., 1981.)

join. The other hand is placed on top, and the rescuer presses straight down. (The sternum will be depressed one and one-half to two inches with sufficient pressure; Fig. 33–6.)

If there is only one rescuer, compressions should be given at a rate of 80 times per minute. After every 15 compressions, move back to the mouth to give two quick, full ventilations. With two rescuers, ventilation and compression can be performed simultaneously. Compressions should be given at a rate of 60 per minute, with a ventilation by the second rescuer after every fifth compression. This procedure should be performed constantly until help arrives.

Chest Pain

All patients with chest pain are treated as cardiac emergencies until a physician has ruled out this diagnosis. The patient is usually sweating and has a gray, ashen appearance. The lips and fingernails may be cyanotic. He is frequently clutching his chest in pain. This pain may radiate out to the left arm and up the left side of the neck. The pulse may be rapid and weak, and frequently there is nausea. DO NOT have the patient walk any distance. The secretary's chair with rollers is an excellent method of moving this patient to a quiet room where he can rest. The patient will probably prefer to have his head slightly elevated or even be in a semi-sitting position. Keep the patient quiet and warm but do not overheat him. Administer oxygen if the physician has previously given these instructions. Prepare the medication that the physician is most likely to use. This may be adrenalin (epinephrine), atropine, digitalis, calcium gluconate, or morphine.

If the physician cannot be reached, call the local emergency squad at the police or fire department. It may be necessary to start mouth-to-mouth resuscitation if the patient is unconscious and there is no evidence of breathing. Loosen all tight clothing. Some physicians may give you permission to give the patient some aspirin if the patient is fully conscious. DO NOT give the patient anything such as alcohol, food, or water by mouth without the physician's permission. If the patient is conscious, ask him if he has any medication with him. This medication is usually nitroglycerine tablets that are administered sublingually. The patient will tell you what to do. DO NOT give any smelling salts.

If the physician is in the office or immediately on his way in, connect the patient to the electrocardiograph and make some tracings. Limb lead II is usually considered to be the monitoring lead. It is extremely important that the office staff remain calm, since all heart patients are extremely frightened persons and will need assurance.

Only a physician can tell the difference between a heart attack and a case of acute indigestion.

If chest pain progresses to cardiac arrest, CPR must be performed.

Cerebrovascular Accident

Cerebrovascular accident (CVA) is a disorder of the blood vessels serving the cerebrum, resulting in an impairment of the blood supply to a part of the brain. The term "stroke" is often applied to this problem. The result of this blood deficiency is neurologic damage. These accidents, or attacks, may be so minor that there is no perceivable residual damage to the brain. On the other hand, a CVA may be so severe that there is considerable injury done, with extensive residual damage to the brain.

The patient's clothing especially around the neck, should be loosened. Turn the patient's head to one side to prevent choking on the excess saliva. The patient may be raised to a Fowler's position or have the head raised in order to lessen the blood pressure in the head. Do everything to keep the patient calm and quiet. If needed, keep the patient's airway open for adequate intake of oxygen. If the patient has a **convulsion,** guide his movements to prevent his injuring himself. Have an ambulance take the patient to the hospital as soon as possible. Vital signs should be taken at regular intervals and recorded for the physician.

Poisoning

Each office should have the telephone number of the local Poison Control Center. This center is often located in the largest local hospital or the county hospital. When a patient calls to report a poisoning, ask him the name of the poison taken, how long ago it was taken, and how much was taken. Tell him to bring the poison with him to the office or to the hospital.

If the name of the poison is unknown, then ask what type is was, that is, was it a pill like aspirin or a fluid like kerosene. It is always best to send poison cases to the hospital, especially if it has a Poison Control Center. You should know the location of the center well enough to instruct the patient on how to get there. Unless the antidote is written on the label of the poison, be cautious about advising the patient to take an emetic, although it is generally safe to try to dilute the poison with water or milk. Milk is frequently preferred. Then induce vomiting. Save the vomitus for analysis. Remember, DO NOT induce vomiting if the patient has ingested a strong alkali, acid, kerosene, or gasoline. If ipecac is not available, large amounts of tepid water may be given. The universal antidote is one part strong tea, one part milk of magnesia, and two slices of crumbled burnt toast. This last item, however, is usually not readily available. Some first-aiders recommend using lots of milk with egg white in it. It may be necessary to make the patient gag to start the vomiting. The gag reflex is started by touching the back of the tongue lightly.

Insect Stings

If the insect's stinger is still in the skin, it should be removed by brushing it off or by using a fine tweezer. Be very careful not to squeeze the stinger and further inject more venom into the skin but place a tweezer as close to the skin as possible, *not over the stinger sac,* and gently remove the stinger. Apply ice over the area. If the sting is on the arm or leg, a broad, flat tourniquet may be applied above the site of the sting. Release the tourniquet every ten minutes for about one minute. To relieve itching, a paste of baking soda or a compress of ammonia water may be applied. Do not give the patient any stimulants or alcohol. Keep the patient's activities at a minimum in order to limit circulation. If the patient gives a history of allergies, especially to insect venom, then the patient should be taken to the nearest medical facility for immediate care. This patient will experience dyspnea and a decrease in blood pressure. Sometimes there is edema of the lips and face. When the patient is in acute anaphylactic shock from the sting, death may occur within one hour if proper measures are not taken.

Anaphylaxis

This is an acute allergic reaction characterized by **urticaria** (the appearance of itching, swelling, or wheal), respiratory distress, vascular collapse, and occasionally vomiting, abdominal cramps and diarrhea. It occurs in a person who receives a foreign substance (antigen) to which he is specifically sensitive. This reaction has an extremely broad range of reactions, ranging from a mild itching to true **anaphylactic** shock. It is the anaphylactic shock that presents a true emergency, and timing is crucial. The patient will have severe dyspnea, be cyanotic (with bluish skin), and may sometimes have **convulsions.** Epinephrine and oxygen should be ready for immediate administration on the physician's orders. The patient will appear flushed and have a rapid pulse as a result of the administration of the epinephrine, and he should be assured that this is a side effect of the medication and not to be alarmed. In severe cases of respiratory reaction a patient may not respond to epinephrine and the physician may order intravenous administration of aminophylline. Severe cases may also involve the cardiovascular system, causing the patient to have severe hypotension and vasomotor collapse. Antihistamines may be used as well as cortisone, but these are considerably slower in action than epinephrine.

Shock

In this state, the patient's peripheral blood circulation is impaired. Shock is the result of a **traumatic** condition, such as hemorrhage, injury, pain, or fear. It may follow the changing of a surgical dressing or the administration of a medication by injection. It may be immediate or delayed, severe or mild. The patient is pale, clammy feeling, often has dilated pupils, weak and rapid pulse, low blood pressure, and complains of thirst and feels **lethargic** and faint. He may have labored breathing. Place the patient on his back with the legs elevated, loosen all tight clothing, and keep the patient warm. Do not give the patient any stimulants. If medical care will arrive within about 20 minutes, it is best not to give the patient anything by mouth. Tea or coffee may be given later if there is no evidence of internal hemorrhage or head injury. Because there are so many different causes of shock, it is advisable to administer only basic first aid care and get immediate medical help.

Asthma

Since only a physician can treat asthma, the medical assistant should give the patient all the assurance she can. Have the respiratory medication ready for the physician's orders. Some asthmatic patients will carry a respiratory inhalator with them. In this case, you can assist them in using this inhalator. A bronchodilator such as epinephrine or aminophylline may be ordered by the physician. Other medications are used to thin the mucus in the air passages so the patient may clear his lungs more easily. Emotions play a very important part in the severe asthmatic, and he must be assured and kept calm.

Seizures

Seizures are frightening to witness, but the patient is not usually suffering, nor is he in great danger. Tranquility is usually an essential component of such care. Loosen the clothing, but do not attempt to restrain the patient's movements except to protect him from injuring himself. Move anything that might be in the way and cause the patient injury. Give neither fluids nor medication by mouth. If the patient remains unconscious after the jerking has subsided, turn his face to one side because there is frequently considerable saliva. Many physicians do not recommend attempting to place anything between the patient's teeth during the convulsion, unless there is evidence that the patient is chewing his tongue. In this case, a piece of gauze wrapped around two tongue depressors may be placed in the mouth between the teeth. Do not use your fingers.

If the patient has not regained consciousness within 10 to 15 minutes, it may be advisable to call a physician. After the seizure is over, let the patient rest or sleep in a quiet room. If the seizure has occurred in an inconvenient place for the patient to rest, he may be moved to a quiet place after he has regained consciousness and can tell you his name and where he is. This way you will know he is sufficiently oriented.

Abdominal Pain

If a patient is vomiting, place him on his side or keep his head and upper torso elevated so that he is in a semi-sitting position. Have the emesis basin available. If possible, place the patient in a room near a toilet. Keep him warm and quiet. Give him nothing by mouth. You may allow him to rinse his mouth out after vomiting if he is fully conscious. DO NOT apply heat to the abdomen unless the physician instructs you to do so. If the patient is not vomiting, he may have a few sips of water occasionally, but give him nothing else by mouth. Abdominal pain may be due to the ingestion of a food or drug, heat exhaustion, gallstones, diarrhea, or many other causes. Severe and persistent abdominal pain should have medical attention as soon as possible, but all abdominal pain should be considered. Appendicitis does not always present as severe pain. Gentle pressure over the abdomen will determine if the muscles are rigid. If they are "hard as a board," there may be a peritoneal irritation. Take the patient's temperature.

Obstetrical Emergencies

An obstetrical office presents problems that are unique to this specialty. Every medical assistant employed in this specialty or any office where the physician delivers babies should be trained to handle the emergencies. The majority of these problems will be presented to you over the telephone. Of course, if the physician is in the office the call should be transferred to him immediately.

If a pregnant patient calls in to report vaginal bleeding, you must ask some specific questions. Is the bleeding like a menstrual flow or is it a gushing type of hemorrhage? Is it painful or without any pain? If the bleeding is gushing, then the patient must be told to lie down immediately while you send for an ambulance. It takes only a few minutes for both mother and baby to bleed to death from a ruptured uterus. If the bleeding is like a normal menstrual flow, have the patient go to bed with the foot of the bed elevated and tell her you will report this to the physician immediately.

If the tissue passed is liverlike, it may possibly be a blood clot; white tissue may be the fetus. No matter what the tissue appears to be, have the patient save it, if possible, and take it with her to the hospital.

Sprains

A sprain is an injury to a ligamentous structure surrounding a joint and is usually caused by twisting or wrenching of the part. The most accepted first aid today is the immediate application of ice. There is considerable advantage if the ice is applied within 20 to 30 minutes after the injury. The ice should remain on the part for 24 hours with the injured area elevated. After 24 to 36 hours, application of mild heat is usually indicated. The patient may be advised to demobilize the part.

Fractures

Many kinds of fractures can result from trauma or bone-weakening disease (Fig. 33–7). When a patient with a fracture is brought into the office, there is little the medical assistant can do other than make the patient comfortable, support the fractured area, and keep the patient quiet. Have the patient lie down in a position

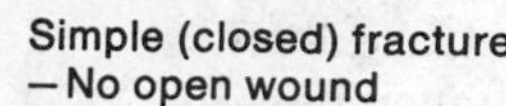

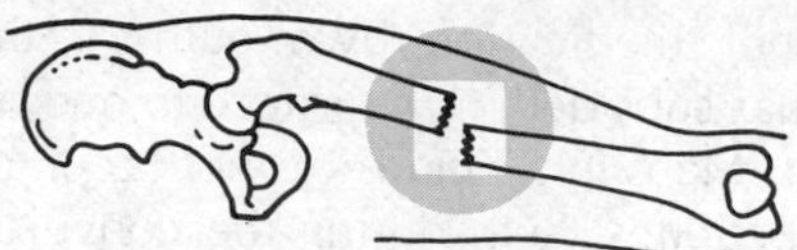

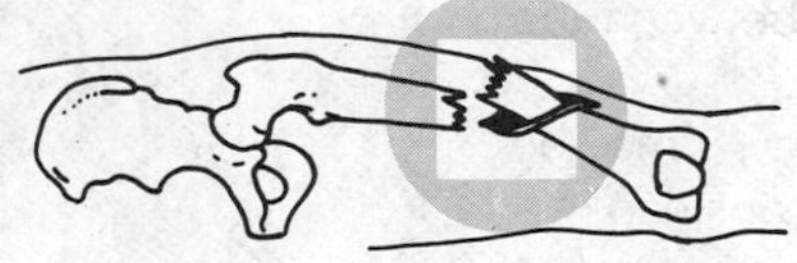

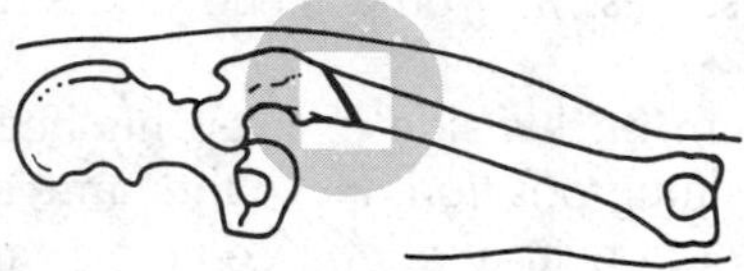

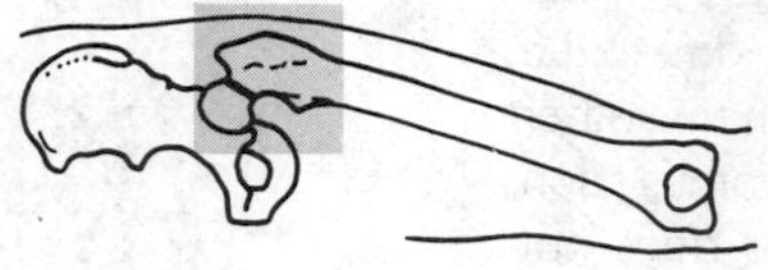

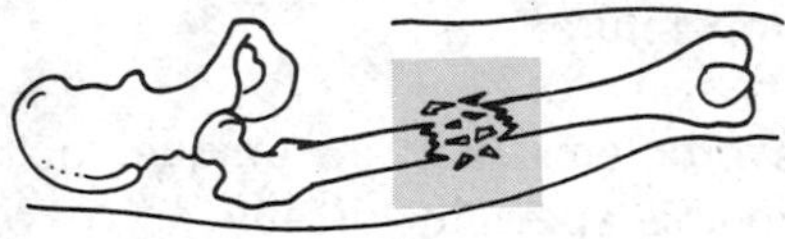

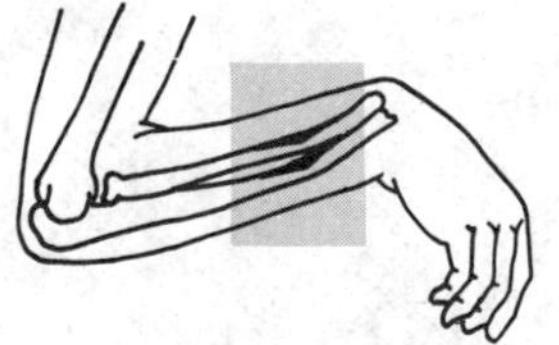

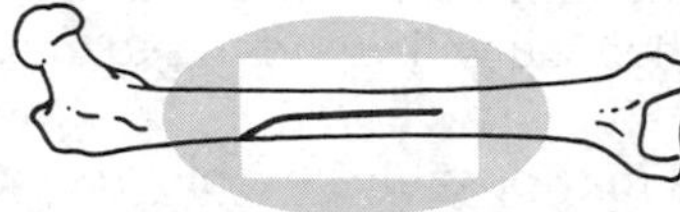

FIGURE 33–7 Types of fractures. (From Ethicon, Inc.: *Nursing Care of the Patient in the O.R.*, 1973.)
Illustration continued on opposite page

that will not place a strain on the area and that will prevent any movement. If there is an abrasion or bleeding, place a sterile dressing over the area. Do not apply too much pressure on the bleeding area if there is a fracture beneath. Be gentle. DO NOT ATTEMPT TO STRAIGHTEN THE FRACTURE or move it in any way. If the patient must be moved, then give support to the fractured area before moving. If possible, an x-ray of the area should be ready when the physician arrives.

Burns

Burns are extremely painful and dangerous. There is always the danger of infection from contamination because the burned tissue acts as a culture medium for bacteria and there is no circulation through this tissue to carry medication such as an antibiotic. Burns may be classed as thermal, chemical, or electrical. Each of these may be superficial to very deep and reported as first, second, third, and fourth degree burns (Figure 33–8). The most frequently recommended first aid for a burn is to

Transverse fracture–Break runs across bone

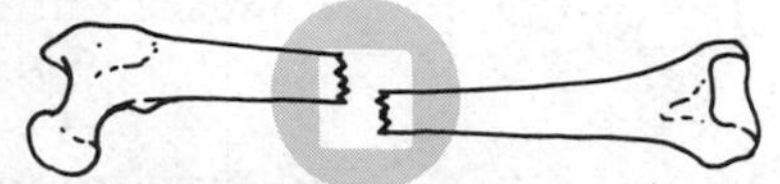

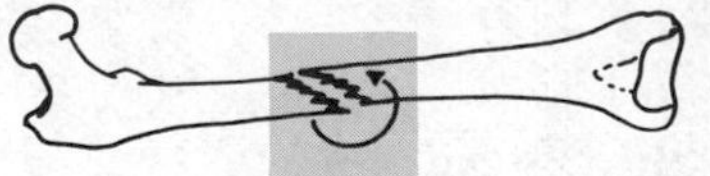

Oblique fracture–Break runs in slanting direction on bone

Spiral fracture–Break coils around bone

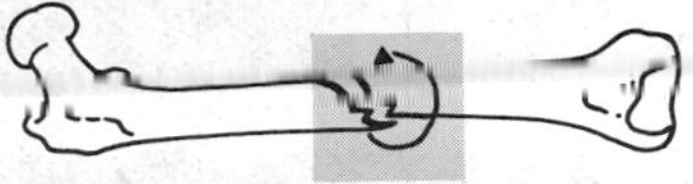

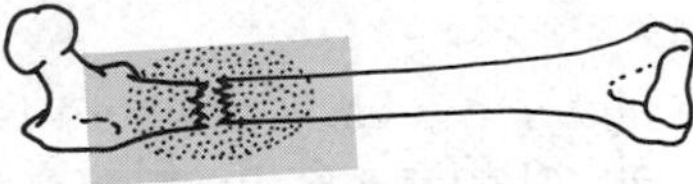

Pathologic fracture–Break is at site of bone disease

Impacted fracture–Bone broken and wedged into other break

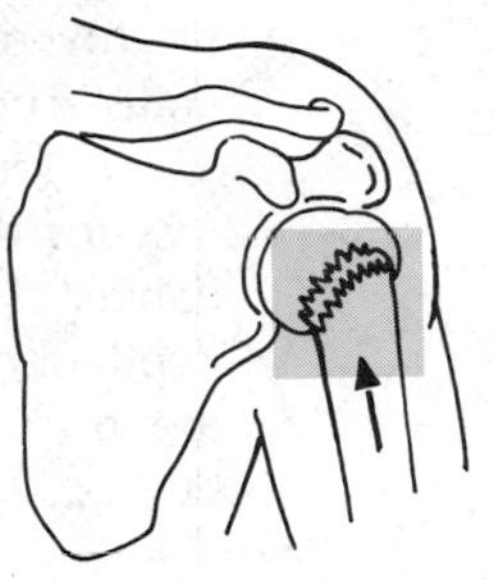

Fracture dislocation–Break complicated by bone out of joint

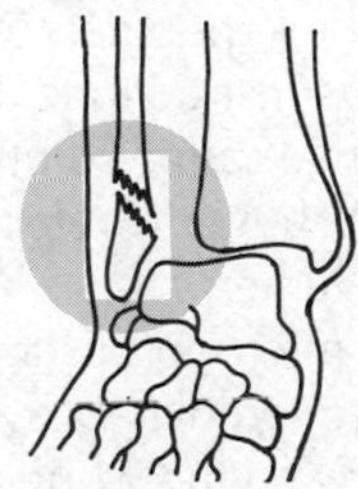

Depressed fracture–Broken skull bone driven inward

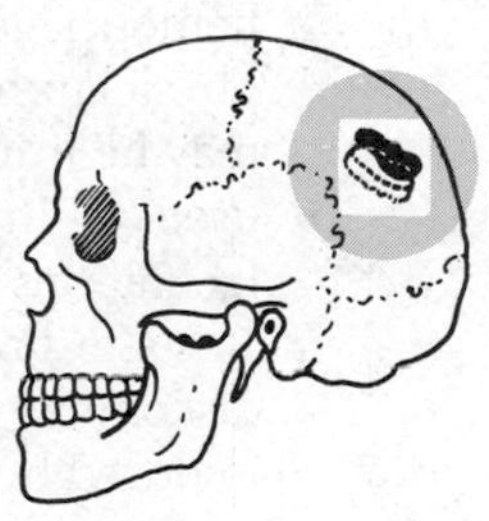

FIGURE 33–7 *continued*

immerse it immediately in cool water. This will give immediate relief from the pain. The other danger that a burned patient has is the possibility of shock, which can be very serious. If immersion in water is not possible, then apply sterile wet compresses to the area. DO NOT apply any medications or ointments unless instructed to do so by a physician. If the burn is over a large area, wrap a clean towel (sterile, if possible) over the area and get the patient to the hospital as soon as possible. If clothing is to be removed, do not pull it off; cut it away carefully. DO NOT open blisters. Chemical burns should be thoroughly rinsed with plenty of water and covered with a sterile moist dressing.

A *first degree burn* shows erythema of the epidermis only. The tissue destruction is superficial without blistering. There is little or no pain.

A *second degree burn* includes the entire epidermal layer and varying depths of the dermis. Blisters are usually formed, and there is some pain. There is also danger

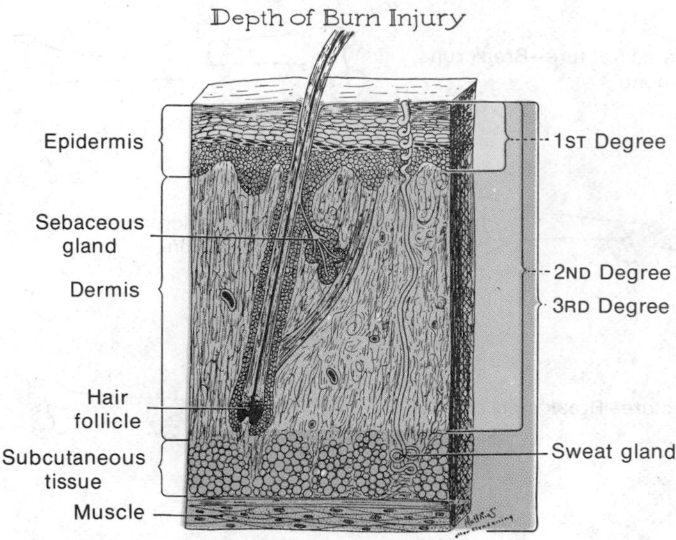

FIGURE 33–8 (From Haynes, Jr., B. W., Ochsner, A., and DeBakey, M. E. (eds.): *Christopher's Minor Surgery*. 8th ed. Philadelphia, W. B. Saunders Co., 1959.)

of infection in the blistered area. If the burn is deep enough there may be some destruction of the hair follicles and the sebaceous glands.

A *third degree burn* is the destruction of all the epithelial structure. The destroyed skin will slough off, leaving a raw area. It may be necessary to have skin grafts. There is great pain and danger of infection.

A *fourth degree burn* is sometimes known as a "charred burn." This burn reaches the underlying muscular tissue and is extremely painful. There is great danger of infection. Grafts and plastic surgery are usually necessary. Diagnosis of the depth or degree of a burn differs because skin varies in depth in different locations of the body. A burn is usually mixed in degrees in the different areas that are burned.

Lacerations

Lacerations are a common presentation in general practice and pediatrics. Have the patient lie down and cover the injured area with a sterile dressing. Use enough thicknesses to absorb the bleeding. If the bleeding persists or is profuse, apply pressure to the dressing and also to the area just above the wound. For any type of hemorrhage, the patient should be kept quiet. Do not use any disinfectant unless the physician has given you previous instructions. If the laceration is extremely dirty, it may be irrigated with sterile normal saline solution. Hydrogen peroxide is frequently used to irrigate small areas. A butterfly closure strip may be used over small lacerations to hold the edges together.

Closure of a wound with microporous tape (see Fig. 31–16) eliminates the discomfort of suturing and suture removal, as well as some of the risks of infection imposed by sutures. First the skin and the wound, if necessary, should be cleansed to assure a clean dry skin. The tape in ¼ or ½ inch widths is placed at approximately ¼ inch intervals until the wound is closed. Generally, closure is started near one end, but a longer wound could be brought together in quarters and then the intervening spaces closed next. A dry dressing may be placed over the area although it is usually not necessary.

Animal Bites

Any animal bite that breaks the skin should be seen by a physician and reported to the authorities. The animal must be identified and confined for quarantine. The animal should not be killed because a positive rabies identification is almost impossible to make if the animal has been dead for awhile. Many pet owners will not admit their pet has bitten a person because they fear the animal will be killed. Assure them the Health Department authorities only want to confine the animal for observation. The bite should be washed thoroughly with soap and water and treated as any other wound would be. The victim should be seen by a physician.

Nosebleeds

If the patient is cooperative, bleeding from the nose may be controlled by inserting a ball of cotton into the bleeding nostril and then applying external pressure to the side of the offending nostril. Sometimes a cotton ball placed between the upper lip and teeth, with outside pressure over this area, will help. Cold compresses to the face may also be of value. The patient's head should be elevated.

Until a physician is seen another method of control may be to have the patient hold the nostrils closed for at least 15 minutes. This MUST be a steady hold and cannot be released for a single moment. **Epistaxis** is the term usually used in reference to a hemorrhage from the nose.

Hemorrhages

Bleeding may be external or internal. First-aiders can do little about internal bleeding, except to keep the patient very quiet and warm to prevent shock. Get medical help immediately.

External bleeding is not as complex as internal bleeding. You can frequently see the source of the bleeding. There are three practical ways to control bleeding. First, use direct pressure over the area by applying a sterile pad. Do not press too hard, especially if there is the possibility of a fracture beneath the bleeding area. The second method is to apply pressure over the nearest pressure point between the bleeding area and the heart. The third method is to apply a tourniquet, but only as a last resort. A broad, flat tourniquet is best, and a pad should be used under the area of the tie. Gently tighten the tourniquet until the bleeding is stopped. Do not make it any tighter, since the tissues beyond the tourniquet can die without blood circulation. Do not release the tourniquet every 20 minutes, but get medical help within that period of time. Most physicians recommend the first method of direct pressure over the bleeding area. If a sterile dressing is available it, of course, is best to use; otherwise, use the cleanest material available. With the newer antibiotics the threat of infection is not so great as in the past.

Head Injuries

Head injury may cause the patient to be dizzy, have a severe headache, or even be unconscious. The loss of consciousness may be brief or prolonged; it may appear immediately or be delayed for as long as a half hour, but any loss of consciousness is diagnostic. The pupils of the eyes may be unequal. If the patient is unconscious, do not attempt to arouse him. If the face if flushed, raise the head and shoulders slightly. If the face is gray and ashen, keep the patient flat. If there are signs of vomiting, place him on his side. Do not give any stimulants. Use extreme caution in moving the patient. Watch the pupils of the eyes and record any changes. Also record the blood pressure. Report the time of any changes in the eyes and blood pressure. Check the ears for any bleeding in the canals. Keep the patient warm and quiet; *do not allow him to move about.* All head injuries must be considered serious and in need of medical care. There may be bleeding around the brain even when there is no evidence of external bleeding or injury and the patient says he feels fine.

Foreign Body in the Eye

This kind of emergency is most uncomfortable, and it is often extremely difficult to keep the patient from rubbing the eye. However, he must be instructed not to touch the eye in any way. If the doctor has given you prior permission, you may put a few drops of ophthalmic topical anesthetic in the eye. The patient will greatly appreciate this and will experience almost immediate relief. Unless the foreign object is clearly visible, do not attempt to search for it or remove it. The patient should be placed in a darkened room to wait. Have plenty of tissues available. If there is a contusion and swelling, cold wet compresses will help. If you have been trained to turn an upper eyelid out, then do so gently and search for the foreign body. Be very careful not to place any pressure on the eye. If the foreign body cannot be found, then ask the patient to close his eye normally, place a pad over the eye, and hold it in place with a strip of tape. Get medical care.

Appendix 1

SUGGESTED READINGS AND REFERENCE BOOKS FOR MEDICAL ASSISTANTS

American Medical Association: The Business Side of Medical Practice. Chicago, American Medical Association, 1979.

American Medical Association: Judicial Council Opinions and Reports. Chicago, American Medical Association, latest edition.

American Medical Association: Medicolegal Forms with Legal Analysis. Chicago, American Medical Association, latest edition.

American Medical Association: The Wonderful Human Machine. Chicago, American Medical Association, latest edition.

American Medical Association: X-ray Examinations—Guide to Good Practice. Chicago, American Medical Association, latest edition.

Anthony, C. P.: Structure and Function of the Body, 5th ed. St. Louis, C. V. Mosby Company, 1976.

Aurner, R. R., and Wolf, M. P.: Effective Communication in Business, 6th ed. Cincinnati, South-Western Publishing, 1974.

Beck, L. C.: The Physician's Office. Princeton, Excerpta Medica, 1977.

Bonewit, K.: Clinical Procedures for Medical Assistants. Philadelphia, W. B. Saunders Company, 1979.

Bryan, A. H.: Bacteriology: Principles and Practice, 6th ed. New York, Barnes & Noble, 1962.

Burke, S. R.: The Composition and Functions of Body Fluids, 3rd ed. St. Louis, C. V. Mosby Company, 1980.

Burton, G.: Personal, Impersonal and Interpersonal Relations—A Guide for Nurses, 4th ed. New York, Springer Publishing Company, 1977.

Carson, A. B., Carlson, A. E., and Burnet, M. E.: Accounting Essentials for Career Secretaries, 3rd ed. Cincinnati, South-Western Publishing Company, 1972.

Carvel, F. J.: Human Relations in Business, 3rd ed. New York, MacMillan Publishing Company, 1980.

Chabner, D.-E.: The Language of Medicine, 2nd ed. Philadelphia, W. B. Saunders Company, 1981.

Clement, J. E.: Medical Assistants Examination Review. New York, Arco, 1980.

Cooper, M., and Bredow, M.: The Medical Assistant, 4th ed. New York, McGraw-Hill Book Company, 1978.

Cotton, H.: Medical Practice Management, 2nd ed. Westwood, Medical Economics, 1977.

Cotton, H., and Martin, N.: Aid for the Medical Assistant: Managing the Doctor's Office. Westwood, Medical Economics, 1975.

Creighton, H.: Law Every Nurse Should Know, 4th ed. Philadelphia, W. B. Saunders Company, 1981.

Dennis, L.: Psychology of Human Behavior for Nurses, 3rd ed. Philadelphia, W. B. Saunders Company, 1967.

Diehl, M. O., and Fordney, M. T.: Medical Transcribing: Techniques & Procedures. Philadelphia, W. B. Saunders Company, 1979.

Dienhart, C. M.: Basic Human Anatomy and Physiology, 3rd ed. Philadelphia, W. B. Saunders Company, 1979.

Dorland's Pocket Medical Dictionary, 22nd ed. Philadelphia, W. B. Saunders Company, 1977.

Doyle, J. M., and Dennis, R. L.: The Complete Handbook for Medical Secretaries and Assistants, 2nd ed. Boston, Little, Brown & Co., 1978.

Fordney, M. T.: Insurance Handbook for the Medical Office, 2nd ed. Philadelphia, W. B. Saunders Company, 1981.

Frenay, Sister Agnes Clare: Understanding Medical Terminology, 6th ed. St. Louis, Catholic Hospital Association, 1977.

French, R. M.: Guide to Diagnostic Procedures, 4th ed. New York, McGraw-Hill Book Company, 1980.

Garb, S.: Abbreviations and Acronyms in Medicine and Nursing. New York, Springer Publishing Co., 1976.

Garb, S.: Laboratory Tests in Common Use, 6th ed. New York, Springer Publishing Co., 1976.

Gross, V. E.: The Structure of Medical Terms, revised 2nd edition. North Hollywood, Halls of Ivy Press, 1973.

Gross, V. E.: Mastering Medical Terminology, 5th ed. North Hollywood, Halls of Ivy Press, 1978.

Gross, V. E.: Illustrated Programmed Gross Anatomy. North Hollywood, Halls of Ivy Press, 1973.

Hardy, C. and Martin, N.: Your Roles as a Medical Assistant. Westwood, Medical Economics, 1974.

Hill, G. J. II: Outpatient Surgery, 2nd ed. Philadelphia, W. B. Saunders Company, 1980.

Hutchinson, L.: Standard Handbook for Secretaries, 8th ed. New York, McGraw-Hill Book Company, 1971.

Jacob, S. W., and Francone, C. A.: Structure and Function in Man, 4th ed. Philadelphia, W. B. Saunders Company, 1978.

JeHarned, R. N.: Medical Terminology Made Easy, 2nd ed. Chicago, Physicians Record Company, 1968.

Johnson, M. A.: Developing the Art of Understanding, 2nd ed. New York, Springer Publishing Company, 1972.

Kalish, R. A., and Johnson, A. I.: The Psychology of Human Behavior, 4th ed. Monterey, California, Brooks/Cole Publishing Company, 1977.

Kinn, M. E.: Review of Medical Terminology. New York, Brian C. Decker Division, Thieme-Stratton, Inc., 1980.

Klein, A. E.: New World Concise Secretarial Handbook. Cleveland, World Publishing Company, 1973.

Krueger, E. A.: The Hypodermic Injection. Philadelphia, J. B. Lippincott Company, 1965.

Laird, D. A., and Laird, E. C.: Psychology: Human Relations and Motivations, 5th ed. New York, McGraw-Hill Book Company, 1975.

Lane, Marc J.: The Doctor's Law Guide: Essentials of Practice Management. Philadelphia, W. B. Saunders Company, 1979.

Langley, L. L., Cheraskin, E., and Sleeper, R.: Dynamic Anatomy and Physiology, 5th ed. New York, McGraw-Hill Book Company, 1980.

Maedke, W., Robek, M. F., and Brown, G.: Information and Records Management. Beverly Hills, Glencoe Press, 1974.

Mager, N. H., and Mager, S. K.: The Office Encyclopedia, 9th ed. New York, Pocket Books, 1975.

Miller, B. F., and Keane, C.: Encyclopedia and Dictionary of Medicine and Nursing, Philadelphia, W. B. Saunders Company, 1978.

Morgan, J. A.: The Art and Science of Medical Radiography, 5th ed. St. Louis, Catholic Hospital Association, 1977.

Moritz, A. R., and Morris, R. C.: Handbook of Legal Medicine, 4th ed. St. Louis, C. V. Mosby Company, 1975.

Nanassy, L. C., Selden, W., and Lee, J.: Reference Manual for Office Workers. Beverly Hills, Glencoe Press, 1977.

Purtilo, R.: Health Professional-Patient Interaction, 2nd ed. Philadelphia, W. B. Saunders Company, 1978.

Sabin, W. A.: The Gregg Reference Manual, 5th ed. New York, Gregg Division/McGraw-Hill Book Company, 1977.

Seedor, M. M.: Introduction to Asepsis. New York, Teachers College Press, 1979.

Steen, E.: Abbreviations in Medicine, 4th ed. Philadelphia, F. A. Davis Company, 1978.

Stehli, G.: Microscope and How to Use It. New York, Sterling Publishing Company, 1970.

Strand, H. R.: An Illustrated Guide to Medical Terminology. Baltimore, Williams & Wilkins Company, 1968.

Strunk, W. Jr., and White, E. B.: The Elements of Style, 3rd ed. New York, Macmillan Publishing Company, 1978.

Thomas, C. L.: Taber's Cyclopedic Medical Dictionary, 13th ed. Philadelphia, F. A. Davis Company, 1977.

Tokay, E.: Fundamentals of Physiology: The Human Body and How It Works. New York, Barnes & Noble, 1970.

Waltz, J. R., and Inbau, F. E.: Medical Jurisprudence. New York, Macmillan Publishing Company, 1971.

Webster's Medical Office Handbook. Springfield, G. & C. Merriam Company, 1979.

Widmann, F. K.: Goodale's Clinical Interpretation of Laboratory Tests, 8th ed. Philadelphia, F. A. Davis Company, 1979.

Young, C. G., and Austrin, M. G.: Learning Medical Terminology Step by Step, 4th ed. St. Louis, C. V. Mosby Company, 1979.

Appendix 2

COMBINING FORMS IN MEDICAL TERMINOLOGY*

The following is a list of combining forms encountered frequently in the vocabulary of medicine. A dash or dashes are appended to indicate whether the form usually precedes (as *ante-*) or follows (as *-agra*) the other elements of the compound or usually appears between the other elements (as *-em-*). Following each combining form, the first item of information is the Greek or Latin word, or both a Greek and a Latin word, from which it is derived. Those words that are not printed in Greek characters are Latin. Information necessary to an understanding of the form appears next in parentheses. Then the meaning or meanings of the word are given, followed where appropriate by reference to a synonymous combining form. Finally, an example is given to illustrate the use of the combining form in a compound English derivative.

a- — *α-* (*n* is added before words beginning with a vowel) negative prefix. Cf. in-[3]. *a*metria

ab- — *ab* away from. Cf. apo-. *ab*ducent

abdomin- — *abdomen, abdominis*. *abdomi*noscopy

ac- — See ad-. *ac*cretion

acet- — *acetum* vinegar. *acet*ometer

acid- — *acidus* sour. *acid*uric

acou- — ἀκούω hear. *acou*esthesia. (Also spelled acu-)

acr- — ἄκρον extremity, peak. *acro*megaly

act- — *ago, actus* do, drive, act. re*act*ion

actin- — ἀκτίς, ἀκτῖνος ray, radius. Cf. radi-. *actin*ogenesis

acu- — See acou-. osteo*acu*sis

ad- — *ad* (*d* changes to *c, f, g, p, s,* or *t* before words beginning with those consonants) to. *ad*renal

aden- — ἀδήν gland. Cf. gland-. *aden*oma

adip- — *adeps, adipis* fat. Cf. lip- and stear-. *adip*ocellular

aer- — ἀήρ air. an*aer*obiosis

aesthe- — See esthe-. *aesthe*sioneurosis

af- — See ad-. *af*ferent

ag- — See ad-. *ag*glutinant

-agogue — ἀγωγός leading, inducing. galact*agogue*

-agra — ἄγρα catching, seizure. pod*agra*

alb- — *albus* white. Cf. leuk-. *albo*cinereous

alg- — ἄλγος pain. neur*alg*ia

all- — ἄλλος other, different. *all*ergy

alve- — *alveus* trough, channel, cavity. *alve*olar

amph- — See amphi-. *amph*eclexis

amphi- — ἀμφί (*i* is dropped before words beginning with a vowel) both, doubly. *amphi*celous

amyl- — ἄμυλον starch. *amyl*osynthesis

an-[1] — See ana-. *an*agogic

an-[2] — See a-. *an*omalous

ana- — ἀνά (final *a* is dropped before words beginning with a vowel) up, positive. *ana*phoresis

ancyl- — See ankyl-. *ancyl*ostomiasis

andr- — ἀνήρ, ἀνδρός man. gyn*andr*oid

angi- — ἀγγεῖον vessel. Cf. vas-. *angi*emphraxis

ankyl- — ἀγκύλος crooked, looped. *ankyl*odactylia. (Also spelled ancyl-)

ant- — See anti-. *ant*ophthalmic

ante- — *ante* before. *ante*flexion

anti- — ἀντί (*i* is dropped before words beginning with a vowel) against, counter. Cf. contra-. *anti*pyogenic

antr- — ἄντρον cavern. *antr*odynia

ap-[1] — See apo-. *ap*heter

ap-[2] — See ad-. *ap*pend

-aph- — ἅπτω, ἀφ- touch. dys*aph*ia. (See also hapt-)

apo- — ἀπό (*o* is dropped before words beginning with a vowel) away from, detached. Cf. ab-. *apo*physis

arachn- — ἀράχνη spider. *arachn*odactyly

arch- — ἀρχή beginning, origin. *arch*enteron

arter(i)- — ἀρτηρία elevator (?), artery. *arteri*osclerosis, peri*arter*itis

arthr- — ἄρθρον joint. Cf. articul-. syn*arthr*osis

articul- — *articulus* joint. Cf. arthr-. dis*articul*ation

*Compiled by Lloyd W. Daly, A. M., Ph.D., Litt. D., Allen Memorial Professor of Greek, University of Pennsylvania. *In* Dorland's Pocket Medical Dictionary, 21st Ed., Philadelphia, W. B. Saunders Co., 1968.

as- See ad-. *as*similation

at- See ad-. *at*trition

aur- *auris* ear. Cf. ot-. *aur*inasal

aux- αὔξω increase. enter*aux*e

ax- ἄξων or *axis* axis. *ax*ofugal

axon ἄξων axis. *axon*ometer

ba- βαίνω, βα- go, walk, stand. hypno*ba*tia

bacill- *bacillus* small staff, rod. Cf. bacter-. actino*bacill*osis

bacter- βακτήριον small staff, rod. Cf. bacill-. *bacter*iophage

ball- βάλλω, βολ- throw. *ball*istics. (See also bol-)

bar- βάρος weight. pedo*bar*ometer

bi-[1] βίος life. Cf. vit-. aero*bi*c

bi-[2] *bi-* two (see also di-[1]). *bi*lobate

bil- *bilis* bile. Cf. chol-. *bil*iary

blast- βλαστός bud, child, a growing thing in its early stages. Cf. germ-. *blast*oma, zygoto*blast*.

blep- βλέπω look, see. hemia*bleps*ia

blephar- βλέφαρον (from βλέπω; see blep-) eyelid. Cf. cili-. *blephar*oncus

bol- See ball-. em*bol*ism

brachi- βραχίων arm. *brachi*ocephalic

brachy- βραχύς short. *brachy*cephalic

brady- βραδύς slow. *brady*cardia

brom- βρῶμος stench. podo*brom*idrosis

bronch- βρόγχος windpipe. *bronch*oscopy

bry- βρύω be full of life. em*bry*onic

bucc- *bucca* cheek. disto*bucc*al

cac- κακός bad, abnormal. Cf. mal-. *cac*odontia, arthro*cac*e. (See also dys-)

calc-[1] *calx, calcis* stone (cf. lith-), limestone, lime. *calc*ipexy

calc-[2] *calx, calcis* heel. *calc*aneotibial

calor- *calor* heat. Cf. therm-. *calor*imeter

cancr- *cancer, cancri* crab, cancer. Cf. carcin-. *cancr*ology. (Also spelled chancr-)

capit- *caput, capitis* head. Cf. cephal-. de*capit*ator

caps- *capsa* (from *capio;* see cept-) container. en*caps*ulation

carbo(n)- *carbo, carbonis* coal, charcoal. *carbo*hydrate, *carbon*uria

carcin- καρκίνος crab, cancer. Cf. cancr-. *carcin*oma

cardi- καρδία heart. lipo*cardi*ac

cary- See kary-. *cary*okinesis

cat- See cata-. *cat*hode

cata- κατά (final *a* is dropped before words beginning with a vowel) down, negative. *cata*batic

caud- *cauda* tail. *caud*ad

cav- *cavus* hollow. Cf. coel-. con*cav*e

cec- *caecus* blind. Cf. typhl-. *cec*opexy

cel-[1] See coel-. amphi*cel*ous

cel-[2] See -cele. *cel*ectome

-cele κήλη tumor, hernia. gastro*cele*

cell- *cella* room, cell. Cf. cyt-. *cell*iferous

cen- κοινός common. *cen*esthesia

cent- *centum* hundred. Cf. hect-. Indicates fraction in metric system. [This exemplifies the custom in the metric system of identifying fractions of units by stems from the Latin, as centimeter, decimeter, millimeter, and multiples of units by the similar stems from the Greek, as hectometer, decameter, and kilometer.] *cent*imeter, *centi*pede

cente- κεντέω puncture. Cf. punct-. entero*cente*sis

centr- κέντρον or *centrum* point, center. neuro*centr*al

cephal- κεφαλή head. Cf. capit-. en*cephal*itis

cept- *capio, -cipientis, -ceptus* take, receive. re*cept*or

cer- κηρός or *cera* wax. *cer*oplasty, *cer*omel

cerat- See kerat-. a*cerat*osis

cerebr- *cerebrum*. *cerebr*ospinal

cervic- *cervix, cervicis* neck. Cf. trachel-. *cervic*itis

chancr- See cancr-. *chancr*iform

cheil- χεῖλος lip. Cf. labi-. *cheil*oschisis

cheir- χείρ hand. Cf. man-. macro*cheir*ia. (Also spelled chir-)

chir- See cheir-. *chir*omegaly

chlor- χλωρός green. a*chlor*opsia

chol- χολή bile. Cf. bil-. hepato*chol*angeitis

chondr- χόνδρος cartilage. *chondr*omalacia

chord- χορδή string, cord. peri*chord*al

chori- χόριον protective fetal membrane. endo*chori*on

chro- χρώς color. poly*chro*matic

chron- χρόνος time. syn*chron*ous

chy- χέω, χυ- pour. ec*chy*mosis

-cid(e) *caedo, -cisus* cut, kill. infanti*cide*, germi*cid*al

cili- *cilium* eyelid. Cf. blephar-. super*cili*ary

cine- See kine-. auto*cine*sis

-cipient See cept-. in*cipient*

circum- *circum* around. Cf. peri-. *circum*ferential

-cis- *caedo, -cisus* cut, kill. ex*cis*ion

clas- κλάω, κλασ- break. cranio*clast*

clin- κλίνω bend, incline, make lie down. *clin*ometer

clus- *claudo, -clusus* shut. Maloc*clus*ion

co- See con-. *co*hesion

cocc- κόκκος seed, pill. gono*cocc*us

coel- κοῖλος hollow. Cf. cav-. *coel*enteron. (Also spelled cel-)

col-[1] See colon-. *col*ic

col-[2] See con-. *col*lapse

colon- κόλον lower intestine. *colon*ic

colp- κόλπος hollow, vagina. Cf. sin-. endo*colp*itis

com- See con-. *com*masculation

con- *con-* (becomes co- before vowels or *h;* col- before *l;* com- before *b, m,* or *p;* cor- before *r*) with, together. Cf. syn-. *con*traction

contra- *contra* against, counter. Cf. anti-. *contra*indication

copr- κόπρος dung. Cf. sterco-. *copr*oma

cor-[1] κόρη doll, little image, pupil. iso*cor*ia

cor-[2] See con-. *cor*rugator

corpor- *corpus, corporis* body. Cf. somat-. intra*corpor*al

cortic- *cortex, corticis* bark, rind. *cortic*osterone

cost- *costa* rib. Cf. pleur-. inter*cost*al

crani- κρανίον or *cranium* skull. peri*crani*um

creat- κρέας, κρεατ- meat, flesh. *creat*orrhea

-crescent *cresco, crescentis, cretus* grow. ex*crescent*

cret-[1] *cerno, cretus* distinguish, separate off. Cf. crin-. dis*crete*

cret-[2] See -crescent. ac*cret*ion

crin- κρίνω distinguish, separate off. Cf. cret-[1]. endo*crin*ology

crur- *crus, cruris* shin, leg. brachio*crur*al

cry- κρύος cold. *cry*esthesia

crypt- κρύπτω hide, conceal. *crypt*orchism

cult- *colo, cultus* tend, cultivate. *cult*ure

cune- *cuneus* wedge. Cf. sphen-. *cune*iform

cut- *cutis* skin. Cf. derm(at)-. sub*cut*aneous

cyan- κύανος blue. antho*cyan*in

cycl- κύκλος circle, cycle. *cycl*ophoria

cyst- κύστις bladder. Cf. vesic-. nephro*cyst*itis

cyt- κύτος cell. Cf. cell-. plasmo*cyt*oma

dacry- δάκρυ tear. *dacry*ocyst

dactyl- δάκτυλος finger, toe. Cf. digit-. hexa*dactyl*ism

de- *de* down from. *de*composition

dec-[1] δέκα ten. Indicates multiple in metric system. Cf. dec-[2]. *dec*agram

dec-[2] *decem* ten. Indicates fraction in metric system. Cf. dec-[1]. *dec*ipara, *dec*imeter

dendr- δένδρον tree. neuro*dendr*ite

dent- *dens, dentis* tooth. Cf. odont-. inter*dent*al

derm(at)- δέρμα, δέρματος skin. Cf. cut-. endo*derm*, *dermat*itis

desm- δεσμός band, ligament. syn*desm*opexy

dextr- *dexter, dextr-* right-hand. ambi*dextr*ous

di-[1] *di-* two. *di*morphic. (See also bi-[2])

di-[2] See dia-. *di*uresis.

di-[3] See dis-. *di*vergent.

dia- διά (*a* is dropped before words beginning with a vowel) through, apart. Cf. per-. *dia*gnosis

didym- δίδυμος twin. Cf. gemin-. epi*didym*al

digit- *digitus* finger, toe. Cf. dactyl-. *digiti*grade

diplo- διπλόος double. *diplo*myelia

dis- *dis-* (*s* may be dropped before a word beginning with a consonant) apart, away from. *dis*location

disc- δίσκος or *discus* disk. *disco*placenta

dors- *dorsum* back. ventro*dors*al

drom- δρόμος course. hemo*dromo*meter

-ducent See duct-. ad*ducent*

duct- *duco, ducentis, ductus* lead, conduct. ovi*duct*

dur- *durus* hard. Cf. scler-. in*dura*tion

dynam(i)- δύναμις power. *dynam*oneure, neuro*dynamic*

dys- δυσ- bad, improper. Cf. mal-. *dys*trophic. (See also cac-)

e- *e* out from. Cf. ec- and ex-. *e*mission

ec- ἐκ out of. Cf. e- *e*ccentric

-ech- ἔχω have, hold, be. syn*ech*otomy

ect- ἐκτός outside. Cf. extra-. *ecto*plasm

ede- οἰδέω swell. *ede*matous

ef- See ex-. *ef*florescent

-elc- ἕλκος sore, ulcer. enter*elc*osis. (See also *helc*-)

electr- ἤλεκτρον amber. *electro*therapy

em- See en-. *em*bolism, *em*pathy, *em*phlysis

-em- αἷμα blood. an*emia*. (See also hem(at)-)

en- ἐν (*n* changes to *m* before *b, p,* or *ph*) in, on. Cf. in-[2]. *en*celitis

end- ἔνδον inside. Cf. intra-. *end*angium.

enter- ἔντερον intestine. dys*entery*

ep- See epi-. *ep*axial

epi- ἐπί (*i* is dropped before words beginning with a vowel) upon, after, in addition. *epi*glottis

erg- ἔργον work, deed. en*erg*y

erythr- ἐρυθρός red. Cf. rub(r)-. *eryth*rochromia

eso- ἔσω inside. Cf. intra-. *eso*phylactic

esthe- αἰσθάνομαι, αἰσθη- perceive, feel. Cf. sens-. an*esthe*sia

eu- εὖ good, normal. *eu*pepsia

ex- ἐξ or *ex* out of. Cf. e-. *ex*cretion

exo- ἔξω outside. Cf. extra-. *exo*pathic

extra- *extra* outside of, beyond. Cf. ect- and exo-. *extra*cellular

faci- *facies* face. Cf. prosop-. brachio*facio*lingual

-facient *facio, facientis, factus, -fectus* make. Cf. poie-. cale*facient*

-fact- See facient-. arte*fact*

fasci- *fascia* band. *fasci*orrhaphy

febr- *febris* fever. Cf. pyr-. *febr*icide

-fect- See -facient. de*fect*ive

-ferent *fero, ferentis, latus* bear, carry. Cf. phor-. ef*ferent*

ferr- *ferrum* iron. *ferro*protein

fibr- *fibra* fibre. Cf. in-[1]. chondro*fibr*oma

fil- *filum* thread. *fili*form

fiss- *findo, fissus* split. Cf. schis-. *fiss*ion

flagell- *flagellum* whip. *flagell*ation

flav- *flavus* yellow. Cf. xanth-. ribo*flav*in

-flect- *flecto, flexus* bend, divert. de*flect*ion

-flex- See -flect-. re*flex*ometer

flu- *fluo, fluxus* flow. Cf. rhe-. *flu*id

flux- See flu-. af*flux*ion

for- *foris* door, opening. per*for*ated

-form *forma* shape. Cf. -oid. ossi*form*

fract- *frango, fractus* break. re*fract*ive

front- *frons, frontis* forehead, front. naso*front*al

-fug(e) *fugio* flee, avoid. vermi*fuge*, centri*fug*al

funct- *fungor, functus* perform, serve, function. mal*function*

fund- *fundo, fusus* pour. in*fund*ibulum

fus- See fund-. dif*fus*ible

galact- γάλα, γάλακτος milk. Cf. lact-. dys*galact*ia

gam- γάμος marriage, reproductive union. a*gam*ont

gangli- γάγγλιον swelling, plexus. neuro*gangli*itis

gastr- γαστήρ, γαστρός stomach. cholangio*gastr*ostomy

gelat- *gelo, gelatus* freeze, congeal. *gelat*in

gemin- *geminus* twin, double. Cf. didym-. quadri*gemin*al

gen- γίγνομαι, γεν-, γον- become, be produced, originate, or γεννάω produce, originate. cyto*gen*ic

germ- *germen, germinis* bud, a growing thing in its early stages. Cf. blast-. *germ*inal, ovi*germ*

gest- *gero, gerentis, gestus* bear, carry. con*gest*ion

gland- *glans, glandis* acorn. Cf. aden-. intra*gland*ular

-glia γλία glue. neuro*glia*

gloss- γλῶσσα tongue. Cf. lingu-. tricho*gloss*ia

glott- γλῶττα tongue, language. *glott*ic

gluc- See glyc(y)-. *gluc*ophenetidin

glutin- *gluten, glutinis* glue. ag*glutin*ation

glyc(y)- γλυκύς sweet. *glyc*emia, *glycy*rrhizin. (Also spelled gluc-)

gnath- γνάθος jaw. ortho*gnath*ous

gno- γιγνώσκω, γνω- know, discern. dia*gno*sis

gon- See gen-. amphi*gon*y

grad- *gradior* walk, take steps. retro*grad*e

-gram γράφω, γραφ- + -μα scratch, write, record. cardio*gram*

gran- *granum* grain, particle. lipo*gran*uloma

graph- γράφω scratch, write, record. histo*graph*y

grav- *gravis* heavy. multi*grav*ida

gyn(ec)- γυνή, γυναικός woman, wife. andro*gyn*y, *gynec*ologic

gyr- γῦρος ring, circle. *gyro*spasm

haem(at)- See hem(at)-. *haem*orrhagia, *haemat*oxylon

hapt- ἅπτω touch. *hapt*ometer

hect- ἑκτ- hundred. Cf. cent-. Indicates multiple in metric system. *hect*ometer

helc- ἕλκος sore, ulcer. *helc*osis

hem(at)- αἷμα, αἵματος blood. Cf. sanguin-. *hem*angioma, *hemato*cyturia. (See also -em-)

hemi- ἡμι- half. Cf. semi-. *hemi*ageusia

hen- εἷς, ἑνός one. Cf. un-. *hen*ogenesis

hepat- ἧπαρ, ἥπατος liver. gastro*hepat*ic

hept(a)- ἑπτά seven. Cf. sept-[2]. *hept*atomic, *hepta*valent

hered- *heres, heredis* heir. *hered*oimmunity

hex-[1] ἕξ six. Cf. sex-. *hex*yl-. An *a* is added in some combinations.

hex-[2] ἔχω, ἐχ- (added to σ becomes ἑξ-) have, hold, be. cac*hex*y

hexa- See hex-[1]. *hexa*chromic

hidr- ἱδρώς sweat. hyper*hidr*osis

hist- ἱστός web, tissue. *hist*odialysis

hod- ὁδός road, path. *hod*oneuromere. (See also od- and -ode[1])

hom- ὁμός common, same. *homo*morphic

horm- ὁρμή impetus, impulse. *horm*one

hydat- ὕδωρ, ὕδατος water. *hydat*ism

hydr- ὕδωρ, ὑδρ- water. Cf. lymph-. achlor*hydr*ia

hyp- See hypo-. *hyp*axial

hyper- ὑπέρ above, beyond, extreme. Cf. super-. *hyper*trophy

hypn- ὕπνος sleep. *hypn*otic

hypo- ὑπό (*o* is dropped before words beginning with a vowel) under, below. Cf. sub-. *hypo*metabolism

hyster- ὑστέρα womb. colpo*hyster*opexy

iatr- ἰατρός physician. pedi*atr*ics

idi-	ἴδιος peculiar, separate, distinct. *idi*osyncrasy
il-	See in-[2, 3]. *il*linition (in, on), *il*legible (negative prefix)
ile-	See ili- [ile- is commonly used to refer to the portion of the intestines known as the ileum]. *ile*ostomy
ili-	*ilium* (*ileum*) lower abdomen, intestines [ili- is commonly used to refer to the flaring part of the hip bone known as the ilium]. *ili*osacral
im-	See in-[2, 3]. *im*mersion (in, on), *im*perforation (negative prefix)
in-[1]	ἴς, ἰνός fiber. Cf. fibr-. *in*osteatoma
in-[2]	*in* (*n* changes to *l*, *m*, or *r* before words beginning with those consonants) in, on. Cf. en-. *in*sertion
in-[3]	*in*- (*n* changes to *l*, *m*, or *r* before words beginning with those consonants) negative prefix. Cf. a-. *in*valid
infra-	*infra* beneath. *infra*orbital
insul-	*insula* island. *insul*in
inter-	*inter* among, between. *inter*carpal
intra-	*intra* inside. Cf. end- and eso-. *intra*venous
ir-	See in-[2, 3]. *ir*radiation (in, on), *ir*reducible (negative prefix)
irid-	ἶρις, ἴριδος rainbow, colored circle. kerato*irid*ocyclitis
is-	ἴσος equal. *is*otope
ischi-	ἰσχίον hip, haunch. *ischi*opubic
jact-	*iacio*, *iactus* throw. *jact*itation
ject-	*iacio*, *-iectus* throw. in*ject*ion
jejun-	*ieiunus* hungry, not partaking of food. gastro*jejun*ostomy
jug-	*iugum* yoke. con*jug*ation
junct-	*iungo*, *iunctus* yoke, join. con*junct*iva
kary-	κάρυον nut, kernel, nucleus. Cf. nucle-. mega*kary*ocyte. (Also spelled cary-)
kerat-	κέρας, κέρατος horn. *kerat*olysis. (Also spelled cerat-)
kil-	χίλιοι one thousand. Cf. mill-. Indicates multiple in metric system. *kil*ogram
kine-	κινέω move. *kine*matograph. (Also spelled cine-)
labi-	*labium* lip. Cf. cheil-. gingivo*labi*al
lact-	*lac*, *lactis* milk. Cf. galact-. gluco*lact*one
lal-	λαλέω talk, babble. glosso*lal*ia
lapar-	λαπάρα flank. *lapar*otomy
laryng-	λάρυγξ, λάρυγγος windpipe. *laryng*endoscope
lat-	*fero*, *latus* bear, carry. See -ferent. trans*lat*ion
later-	*latus*, *lateris* side. ventro*later*al
lent-	*lens*, *lentis* lentil. Cf. phac-. *lent*iconus
lep-	λαμβάνω, ληπ- take, seize. cata*lep*tic
leuc-	See leuk-. *leuc*inuria
leuk-	λευκός white. Cf. alb-. *leuk*orrhea. (Also spelled leuc-)
lien-	*lien* spleen. Cf. splen-. *lien*ocele
lig-	*ligo* tie, bind. *lig*ate
lingu-	*lingua* tongue. Cf. gloss-. sub*lingu*al
lip-	λίπος fat. Cf. adip-. glyco*lip*in
lith-	λίθος stone. Cf. calc-[1]. nephro*lith*otomy
loc-	*locus* place. Cf. top-. *loc*omotion
log-	λέγω, λογ- speak, give an account. *log*orrhea, embry*olog*y
lumb-	*lumbus* loin. dorso*lumb*ar
lute-	*luteus* yellow. Cf. xanth-. *lute*oma
ly-	λύω loose, dissolve. Cf. solut-. kerato*ly*sis
lymph-	*lympha* water. Cf. hydr-. *lymph*adenosis
macr-	μακρός long, large. *macr*omyeloblast
mal-	*malus* bad, abnormal. Cf. cac- and dys-. *mal*function
malac-	μαλακός soft. osteo*malac*ia
mamm-	*mamma* breast. Cf. mast-. sub*mamm*ary
man-	*manus* hand. Cf. cheir-. *man*iphalanx
mani-	μανία mental aberration. *mani*graphy, klepto*mani*a
mast-	μαστός breast. Cf. mamm-. hyper*mast*ia
medi-	*medius* middle. Cf. mes-. *medi*frontal
mega-	μέγας great, large. Also indicates multiple (1,000,000) in metric system. *mega*colon, *mega*dyne. (See also megal-)
megal-	μέγας, μεγάλου great, large. acro*megal*y
mel-	μέλος limb, member. sym*mel*ia
melan-	μέλας, μέλανος black. hippo*melan*in
men-	μήν month. dys*men*orrhea
mening-	μῆνιγξ, μήνιγγος membrane. encephalo*mening*itis
ment-	*mens*, *mentis* mind. Cf. phren-, psych- and thym-. de*ment*ia
mer-	μέρος part. poly*mer*ic
mes-	μέσος middle. Cf. medi-. *mes*oderm
met-	See meta-. *met*allergy
meta-	μετά (*a* is dropped before words beginning with a vowel) after, beyond, accompanying. *meta*carpal
metr-[1]	μέτρον measure. stereo*metr*y
metr-[2]	μήτρα womb. endo*metr*itis
micr-	μικρός small. photo*micr*ograph
mill-	*mille* one thousand. Cf. kil-. Indicates fraction in metric system. *mill*igram, *mill*ipede
miss-	See -mittent. intro*miss*ion
-mittent	*mitto*, *mittentis*, *missus* send. inter*mittent*
mne-	μιμνήσκω, μνη- remember. pseudo*mne*sia
mon-	μόνος only, sole. *mon*oplegia
morph-	μορφή form, shape. poly*morph*onuclear
mot-	*moveo*, *motus* move. vaso*mot*or
my-	μῦς, μυός muscle. inoleio*my*oma
-myces	μύκης, μύκητος fungus. myelo*myces*
myc(et)-	See -myces. asco*mycet*es, strepto*myc*in
myel-	μυελός marrow. polio*myel*itis
myx-	μύξα mucus. *myx*edema
narc-	νάρκη numbness. topo*narc*osis
nas-	*nasus* nose. Cf. rhin-. palato*nas*al
ne-	νέος new, young. *ne*ocyte
necr-	νεκρός corpse. *necr*ocytosis
nephr-	νεφρός kidney. Cf. ren-. para*nephr*ic
neur-	νεῦρον nerve. esthesio*neur*e
nod-	*nodus* knot. *nod*osity
nom-	νόμος (from νέμω deal out, distribute) law, custom. tax*onom*y
non-	*nona* nine. *non*acosane
nos-	νόσος disease. *nos*ology
nucle-	*nucleus* (from *nux*, *nucis* nut) kernel. Cf. kary-. *nucle*ide
nutri-	*nutrio* nourish. mal*nutri*tion
ob-	*ob* (*b* changes to *c* before words beginning with that consonant) against, toward, etc. *ob*tuse
oc-	See ob-. *oc*clude.
ocul-	*oculus* eye. Cf. ophthalm-. *ocul*omotor
-od-	See -ode[1]. peri*od*ic
-ode[1]	ὁδός road, path. cath*ode*. (See also hod-)
-ode[2]	See -oid. nemat*ode*
odont-	ὀδούς, ὀδόντος tooth. Cf. dent-. orth*odont*ia
-odyn-	ὀδύνη pain, distress. gastr*odyn*ia
-oid	εἶδος form. Cf. -form. hy*oid*
-ol	See ole-. choleste*rol*
ole-	*oleum* oil. *ole*oresin
olig-	ὀλίγος few, small. *olig*ospermia
omphal-	ὀμφαλός navel. peri*omphal*ic
onc-	ὄγκος bulk, mass. hemat*on*cometry
onych-	ὄνυξ, ὄνυχος claw, nail. an*onych*ia
oo-	ᾠόν egg. Cf. ov-. peri*oo*thecitis
op-	ὁράω, ὀπ- see. erythr*op*sia
ophthalm-	ὀφθαλμός eye. Cf. ocul-. ex*ophthalm*ic

or- *os, oris* mouth. Cf. stom(at)-. intra*or*al

orb- *orbis* circle. sub*orb*ital

orchi- ὄρχις testicle. Cf. test-. *orchi*opathy

organ- ὄργανον implement, instrument. *organ*oleptic

orth- ὀρθός straight, right, normal. *ortho*pedics

oss- *os, ossis* bone. Cf. ost(e)-. *oss*iphone

ost(e)- ὀστέον bone. Cf. oss-. en*ost*osis, *oste*anaphysis

ot- οὖς, ὠτός ear. Cf. aur-. par*ot*id

ov- *ovum* egg. Cf. oo-. syn*ov*ia

oxy- ὀξύς sharp. *oxy*cephalic

pachy(n)- παχύνω thicken. *pachy*derma, myo*pachyn*sis

pag- πήγνυμι, παγ- fix, make fast. thoraco*pag*us

par-[1] *pario* bear, give birth to. primi*par*ous

par-[2] See para-. *par*epigastric

para- παρά (final *a* is dropped before words beginning with a vowel) beside, beyond. *para*mastoid

part- *pario, partus* bear, give birth to. *part*urition

path- πάθος that which one undergoes, sickness. psycho*path*ic

pec- πήγνυμι, πηγ- (πηκ- before τ) fix, make fast. sym*pec*tothiene. (See also pex-)

ped- παῖς, παιδός child. ortho*ped*ic

pell- *pellis* skin, hide. *pell*agra

-pellent *pello, pellentis, pulsus* drive. re*pellent*

pen- πένομαι need, lack. erythrocyto*pen*ia

pend- *pendeo* hang down. ap*pend*ix

pent(a)- πέντε five. Cf. quinque-. *pen*tose, *penta*ploid

peps- πέπτω, πεψ- (before σ) digest brady*peps*ia

pept- πέπτω digest. dys*pept*ic

per- *per* through. Cf. dia-. *per*nasal

peri- περί around. Cf. circum-. *peri*phery

pet- *peto* seek, tend toward. centri*pet*al

pex- πήγνυμι, πηγ- (added to σ becomes πηξ-) fix, make fast. hepato*pex*y

pha- φημί, φα- say, speak. dys*pha*sia

phac- φακός lentil, lens. Cf. lent-. *phac*osclerosis. (Also spelled phak-)

phag- φαγεῖν eat. lipo*phag*ic

phak- See phac-. *phak*itis

phan- See phen-. dia*phan*oscopy

pharmac- φάρμακον drug. *pharmac*ognosy

pharyng- φάρυγξ, φαρυγγ- throat. glosso*pharyng*eal

phen- φαίνω, φαν- show, be seen. phos*phen*e

pher- φέρω, φορ- bear, support. peri*pher*y

phil- φιλέω like, have affinity for. eosino*phil*ia

phleb- φλέψ, φλεβός vein. peri*phleb*itis

phleg- φλέγω, φλογ- burn, inflame. adeno*phleg*mon

phlog- See phleg-. anti*phlog*istic

phob- φόβος fear, dread. claustro*phob*ia

phon- φωνή sound. echo*phon*y

phor- See pher-. Cf. -ferent. exo*phor*ia

phos- See phot-. *phos*phorus

phot- φῶς, φωτός light. *phot*erythrous

phrag- φράσσω, φραγ- fence, wall off, stop up. Cf. sept-[1]. dia*phrag*m

phrax- φράσσω, φραγ- (added to σ becomes φραξ-) fence, wall off, stop up. em*phrax*is

phren- φρήν mind, midriff. Cf. ment-. meta*phren*ia, meta*phren*on

phthi- φθίνω decay, waste away. ophthalmo*phthi*sis

phy- φύω beget, bring forth, produce, be by nature. noso*phy*te

phyl- φῦλον tribe, kind. *phyl*ogeny

-phyll φύλλον leaf. xantho*phyll*

phylac- φύλαξ guard. pro*phylac*tic

phys(a)- φυσάω blow, inflate. *phys*ocele, *phys*alis

physe- φυσάω, φυση- blow, inflate. em*physe*ma

pil- *pilus* hair. e*pil*ation

pituit- *pituita* phlegm, rheum. *pituit*ous

placent- *placenta* (from πλακοῦς) cake. extra*placent*al

plas- πλάσσω mold, shape. cine*plas*ty

platy- πλατύς broad, flat. *platy*rrhine

pleg- πλήσσω, πληγ- strike. di*pleg*ia

plet- *pleo, -pletus* fill. de*plet*ion

pleur- πλευρά rib, side. Cf. cost-. peri*pleur*al

plex- πλήσσω, πληγ- (added to σ becomes πληξ-) strike. apo*plex*y

plic- *plico* fold. com*plic*ation

pne- πνοιά breathing. traumato*pne*a

pneum(at)- πνεῦμα, πνεύματος breath, air. *pneum*odynamics, *pneumato*thorax

pneumo(n)- πνεύμων lung. Cf. pulmo(n)-. *pneumo*centesis, *pneumon*otomy

pod- πούς, ποδός foot. *pod*iatry

poie- ποιέω make, produce. Cf. -facient. sarco*poie*tic

pol- πόλος axis of a sphere. peri*pol*ar

poly- πολύς much, many. *poly*spermia

pont- *pons, pontis* bridge. *ponto*cerebellar

por-[1] πόρος passage. myelo*por*e

por-[2] πῶρος callus. *por*ocele

posit- *pono, positus* put, place. re*posit*or

post- *post* after, behind in time or place. *post*natal, *post*oral

pre- *prae* before in time or place. *pre*natal, *pre*vesical

press- *premo, pressus* press. *press*oreceptive

pro- πρό or *pro* before in time or place. *pro*gamous, *pro*cheilon, *pro*lapse

proct- πρωκτός anus. entero*proct*ia

prosop- πρόσωπον face. Cf. faci-. di*prosop*us

pseud- ψευδής false. *pseudo*paraplegia

psych- ψυχή soul, mind. Cf. ment-. *psych*osomatic

pto- πίπτω, πτω- fall. nephro*pto*sis

pub- *pubes* & *puber, puberis* adult. ischio*pub*ic. (See also puber-)

puber- *puber* adult. *puber*ty

pulmo(n)- *pulmo, pulmonis* lung. Cf. pneumo(n)-. *pulmo*lith, cardio*pulmon*ary

puls- *pello, pellentis, pulsus* drive. pro*puls*ion

punct- *pungo, punctus* prick, pierce. Cf. cente-. *punct*iform

pur- *pus, puris* pus. Cf. py-. sup*pur*ation

py- πύον pus. Cf. pur-. nephro*py*osis

pyel- πύελος trough, basin, pelvis. nephro*pyel*itis

pyl- πύλη door, orifice. *pyl*ephlebitis

pyr- πῦρ fire. Cf. febr-. galacto*pyr*a

quadr- *quadr-* four. Cf. tetra-. *quadri*geminal

quinque- *quinque* five. Cf. pent(a)-. *quinque*cuspid

rachi- ῥάχις spine. Cf. spin-. encephalo*rachi*dian

radi- *radius* ray. Cf. actin-. ir*radi*ation

re- *re-* back, again. *re*traction

ren- *renes* kidneys. Cf. nephr-. ad*ren*al

ret- *rete* net. *ret*othelium

retro- *retro* backwards. *retro*deviation

rhag- ῥήγνυμι, ῥαγ- break, burst. hemor*rhag*ic

rhaph- ῥαφή suture. gastror*rhaph*y

rhe- ῥέω flow. Cf. flu-. diar*rhe*al

rhex- ῥήγνυμι, ῥηγ- (added to σ becomes ῥηξ-) break, burst. metror*rhex*is

rhin- ῥίς, ῥινός nose. Cf. nas-. basi*rhin*al

rot- *rota* wheel. *rot*ator

rub(r)- *ruber, rubri* red. Cf. erythr-. bili*rub*in, *rubr*ospinal

salping- σάλπιγξ, σάλπιγγος tube, trumpet. *salping*itis

sanguin- *sanguis, sanguinis* blood. Cf. hem(at)-. *sanguin*eous

sarc- σάρξ, σαρκός flesh. *sarc*oma

schis- σχίζω, σχιδ- (before τ or added to σ becomes σχισ-) split.

Cf. fiss-. *schisto*rachis, rachi*schisis*

scler- σκληρός hard. Cf. dur-. *sclero*sis

scop- σκοπέω look at, observe. endo*scope*

sect- *seco, sectus* cut. Cf. tom-. *sect*ile

semi- *semi-* half. Cf. hemi-. *semi*flexion

sens- *sentio, sensus* perceive, feel. Cf. esthe-. *sens*ory

sep- σήπω rot, decay. *sep*sis

sept-[1] *saepio, saeptus* fence, wall off, stop up. Cf. phrag-. naso*sept*al

sept-[2] *septem* seven. Cf. hept(a)-. *sept*an

ser- *serum* whey, watery substance. *ser*osynovitis

sex- *sex* six. Cf. hex-[1]. *sex*digitate

sial- σίαλον saliva. poly*sial*ia

sin- *sinus* hollow, fold. Cf. colp-. *sin*obronchitis

sit- σῖτος food. para*sit*ic

solut- *solvo, solventis, solutus* loose, dissolve, set free. Cf. ly-. dis*solut*ion

-solvent See solut-. dis*solvent*

somat- σῶμα, σώματος body. Cf. corpor-. psycho*somat*ic

-some See somat-. dictyo*some*

spas- σπάω, σπασ- draw, pull. *spas*m, *spas*tic

spectr- *spectrum* appearance, what is seen. micro*spectr*oscope

sperm(at)- σπέρμα, σπέρματος seed. *sperm*acrasia, *spermat*ozoon

spers- *spargo, -spersus* scatter. dis*pers*ion

sphen- σφήν wedge. Cf. cune-. *sphen*oid

spher- σφαῖρα ball. hemi*spher*e

sphygm- σφυγμός pulsation. *sphygm*omanometer

spin- *spina* spine. Cf. rachi-. cerebro*spin*al

spirat- *spiro, spiratus* breathe. in*spirat*ory

splanchn- σπλάγχνα entrails, viscera. neuro*splanchn*ic

splen- σπλήν spleen. Cf. lien-. *splen*omegaly

spor- σπόρος seed. *spor*ophyte, zygo*spor*e

squam- *squama* scale. de*squam*ation

sta- ἵστημι, στα- make stand, stop. genesi*sta*sis

stal- στέλλω, σταλ- send. peri*stal*sis. (See also stol-)

staphyl- σταφυλή bunch of grapes, uvula. *staphyl*ococcus, *staphyl*ectomy

stear- στέαρ, στέατος fat. Cf. adip-. *stear*odermia

steat- See stear-. *steat*opygous

sten- στενός narrow, compressed. *sten*ocardia

ster- στερεός solid. chole*ster*ol

sterc- *stercus* dung. Cf. copr-. *sterc*oporphyrin

sthen- σθένος strength. a*sthen*ia

stol- στέλλω, στολ- send. dia*stol*e

stom(at)- στόμα, στόματος mouth, orifice. Cf. or-. ana*stom*osis, *stomat*ogastric

strep(h)- στρέφω, στρεπ- (before τ) twist. Cf. tors-. *streph*osymbolia, *strep*tomycin. (See also stroph-)

strict- *stringo, stringentis, strictus* draw tight, compress, cause pain. con*strict*ion

-stringent See strict-. a*stringent*

stroph- στρέφω, στροφ- twist. ana*stroph*ic. (See also strep(h)-)

struct- *struo, structus* pile up (against). ob*struct*ion

sub- *sub* (*b* changes to *f* or *p* before words beginning with those consonants) under, below. Cf. hypo-. *sub*lumbar

suf- See sub-. *suf*fusion

sup- See sub-. *sup*pository

super- *super* above, beyond, extreme. Cf. hyper-. *super*motility

sy- See syn-. *sy*stole

syl- See syn-. *syl*lepsiology

sym- See syn-. *sym*biosis, *sym*metry, *sym*pathetic, *sym*physis

syn- σύν (*n* disappears before *s*, changes to *l* before *l*, and changes to *m* before *b*, *m*, *p*, and *ph*) with, together. Cf. con-. myo*syn*izesis

ta- See ton-. ec*ta*sis

tac- τάσσω, ταγ- (τακ- before τ) order, arrange. a*tac*tic

tact- *tango, tactus* touch. con*tact*

tax- τάσσω, ταγ- (added to σ becomes ταξ-) order, arrange. a*tax*ia

tect- See teg-. pro*tect*ive

teg- *tego, tectus* cover. in*teg*ument

tel- τέλος end. *tel*osynapsis

tele- τῆλε at a distance. *tele*ceptor

tempor- *tempus, temporis* time, timely or fatal spot, temple. *tempor*omalar

ten(ont)- τένων, τένοντος (from τείνω stretch) tight stretched band. *ten*odynia, *tenon*titis, *tenon*tagra

tens- *tendo, tensus* stretch. Cf. ton-. ex*tens*or

test- *testis* testicle. Cf. orchi-. *test*itis

tetra- τετρα- four. Cf. quadr-. *tetra*genous

the- τίθημι, θη- put, place. syn*the*sis

thec- θήκη repository, case. *thec*ostegnosis

thel- θηλή teat, nipple. *thel*erethism

therap- θεραπεία treatment. hydro*therap*y

therm- θέρμη heat. Cf. calor-. dia*therm*y

thi- θεῖον sulfur. *thi*ogenic

thorac- θώραξ, θώρακος chest. *thorac*oplasty

thromb- θρόμβος lump, clot. *thromb*openia

thym- θυμός spirit. Cf. ment-. dys*thym*ia

thyr- θυρεός shield (shaped like a door θύρα). *thyr*oid

tme- τέμνω, τμη- cut. axono*tme*sis

toc- τόκος childbirth. dys*toc*ia

tom- τέμνω, τομ- cut. Cf. sect-. appendec*tom*y

ton- τείνω, τον- stretch, put under tension. Cf. tens-. peri*ton*eum

top- τόπος place. Cf. loc-. *top*esthesia

tors- *torqueo, torsus* twist. Cf. strep-. ex*tors*ion

tox- τοξικόν (from τόξον bow) arrow poison, poison. *tox*emia

trache- τραχεῖα windpipe. *trache*otomy

trachel- τράχηλος neck. Cf. cervic-. *trachel*opexy

tract- *traho, tractus* draw, drag. pro*tract*ion

traumat- τραῦμα, τραύματος wound. *traumat*ic

tri- τρεῖς, τρία or *tri-* three. *tri*gonid

trich- θρίξ, τριχός hair. *trich*oid

trip- τρίβω rub. en*trip*sis

trop- τρέπω, τροπ- turn, react. sito*trop*ism

troph- τρέφω, τροφ- nurture. a*troph*y

tuber- *tuber* swelling, node. *tuber*cle

typ- τύπος (from τύπτω strike) type. a*typ*ical

typh- τῦφος fog, stupor. adeno*typh*us

typhl- τυφλός blind. Cf. cec-. *typhl*ectasis

un- *unus* one. Cf. hen-. *un*ioval

ur- οὖρον urine. poly*ur*ia

vacc- *vacca* cow. *vacc*ine

vagin- *vagina* sheath. in*vagin*ated

vas- *vas* vessel. Cf. angi-. *vas*cular

vers- See vert-. in*vers*ion

vert- *verto, versus* turn. di*vert*iculum

vesic- *vesica* bladder. Cf. cyst-. *vesic*ovaginal

vit- *vita* life. Cf. bi-[1]. de*vit*alize

vuls- *vello, vulsus* pull, twitch. con*vuls*ion

xanth- ξανθός yellow, blond. Cf. flav- and lute-. *xanth*ophyll

-yl- ὕλη substance. cacod*yl*

zo- ζωή life, ζῷον animal. micro*zo*aria

zyg- ζυγόν yoke, union. *zyg*odactyly

zym- ζύμη ferment. en*zym*e

Appendix 3
COMMON ABBREVIATIONS, ACRONYMS, AND SYMBOLS

abd abdomen
a.c. before meals
ad lib as desired
$AgNO_3$ silver nitrate
A/KA above knee amputation
Anesth anesthesia
A & P anterior and posterior, auscultation and percussion
ASCVD arteriosclerotic cardiovascular disease
ASHD arteriosclerotic heart disease
A & W alive and well

BE barium enema
BID twice a day
B/KA below knee amputation
BM bowel movement
BMR basal metabolic rate
BP blood pressure
BPH benign prostatic hypertrophy
BUN blood urea nitrogen
Bx biopsy

C centigrade
Ca calcium
CA carcinoma
cal calorie
CBC complete blood count
cc cubic centimeter
CCU Coronary Care Unit
CHF congestive heart failure
cm centimeter
CNS central nervous system
CO_2 carbon dioxide
COPD chronic obstructive pulmonary disease
CPR cardiopulmonary resuscitation
C/S cesarean section
CSF cerebrospinal fluid
CVA cerebrovascular accident
cysto cystoscopy

D & C dilatation and curettage
disch discharge
DJD degenerative joint disease
DM diabetes mellitus
DNA deoxyribonucleic acid
DOA dead on arrival
DOB date of birth
DPT diphtheria, pertussis, tetanus
DR delivery room
Dx diagnosis

EDC estimated date of confinement
EEG electroencephalogram
EENT eye, ear, nose, and throat
EKG electrocardiogram
ENT ear, nose, and throat
EOM extraocular movements
ER emergency room
EUA examination under anesthesia
expl lap exploratory laparotomy

F female
Fa or F Fahrenheit

FB	foreign body
FBS	fasting blood sugar
FH	family history
FHT	fetal heart tones
FS	frozen section
FTG	full thickness graft
FU	follow up
FUO	fever of unknown origin
Fx	fracture
GB	gallbladder
GE	gastroenterology
GI	gastrointestinal
gm	gram
GP	general practitioner
GTT	glucose tolerance test
gtt	drops
GU	genitourinary
GYN	gynecology
HCl	hydrochloric acid
HCVD	hypertensive cardiovascular disease
Hgb	hemoglobin
hs	at bedtime
Hx	history
ICU	Intensive Care Unit
I & D	incision and drainage
IM	intramuscular
inj	injection
int & ext	internal and external
I & O	intake and output
IP	inpatient
IPPB	intermittent positive pressure breathing
IT	inhalation therapy
IUD	intrauterine device
IV	intravenous
IVP	intravenous pyelogram
K	potassium
KJ	knee jerk
KUB	kidney, ureter, and bladder
L	left
L & A	light and accommodation
lat	lateral
LLQ	left lower quadrant
LMP	last menstrual period
LOM	limitation of motion
LUQ	left upper quadrant
M	male
MH	marital history
MS	multiple sclerosis
NB	newborn
NP	neuropsychiatric
NPN	nonprotein nitrogen
N.P.O.	nothing by mouth
N & V	nausea and vomiting
OB	obstetrics
O.C.	oral contraceptive
OD	overdose
O.D.	right eye
OP	outpatient
O.R.	operating room
O.S.	left eye
O.U.	both eyes
Path	pathology
PBI	protein bound iodine
p.c.	after meals
PCCU	Postcoronary Care Unit
Peds	pediatrics
PERRLA	pupils equal, round, regular, react to light and accommodation
PFT	pulmonary function test
PH	past history
PID	pelvic inflammatory disease
PKU	phenylketonuria
PMR	Paramedic run
PND	paroxysmal nocturnal dyspnea
PO	by mouth (per os)
PROM	premature rupture of membranes
pro time	prothrombin time
prn	when needed
Psych	psychiatry
pt	patient
PT	physical therapy
PU	peptic ulcer
Px	physical examination
q	every
qd	every day
qh	every hour
QID	four times a day
qn	every night
qns	quantity not sufficient
R	right
Ra	radium
R.A.	rheumatoid arthritis
RBC	red blood cell
REM	rapid eye movement
RHD	rheumatic heart disease
R/O	rule out
ROS	review of systems

R.R.	recovery room
Rx	prescription
SH	social history
sig	directions
SMR	submucous resection
SOB	shortness of breath
stat	immediately
STG	split thickness graft
subq	subcutaneous
SWD	short wave diathermy
T	temperature
T & A	tonsillectomy & adenoidectomy
tab	tablet
TB	tuberculosis
TIA	transient ischemic attack
TID	three times a day
TPR	temperature, pulse, respiration
TUR	transurethral resection
UA	urinalysis
UCHD	usual childhood diseases
UR	utilization review
URI	upper respiratory infection
UTI	urinary tract infection
VA	visual acuity
VD	venereal disease
VDRL	Venereal Disease Research Laboratory
VS	vital signs
Wass	Wassermann
WBC	white blood cell
WDWN	well developed and well nourished
WF	white female
WM	white male
WNL	within normal limits

Symbols

$\bar{a}$	before
$\overline{aa}$	of each
$\bar{c}$	with
$\bar{p}$	after
$\bar{s}$	without
↓	decreased
↑	increased
>	greater than
<	less than
✲	birth
—	negative
+	positive
±	negative or positive (indefinite)
♂	male
♀	female
μ	micron
†	death

GLOSSARY

abduction the act of drawing away or being drawn away from the median plane (the imaginary plane passing longitudinally through the body from front to back and dividing it into right and left halves). Opposite of adduction.
abortion premature expulsion of the human fetus.
abrasion a wound caused by rubbing or scraping the skin.
abscess a localized collection of pus in a cavity formed by the disintegration of tissue and microorganisms.
acne vulgaris a chronic inflammatory disease of the sebaceous gland and surrounding tissues. Small, pink papules (sometimes surrounding comedones) or pustules form on the face, chest, or back.
acromegaly abnormal enlargement of the extremities of the skeleton (nose, jaws, hands and feet) resulting from hypersecretion of the pituitary gland's growth hormone.
adduction the act of being drawn toward a median line. Opposite of abduction.
adipose fatty.
adjunct something joined or added to another thing but not essentially a part of it.
administer to instill a drug into the body of a patient.
adnexa appendages; accessory organs.
agar a medium for the culture of microorganisms. It is a protein gel to which nutrients are added.
agent a person authorized by another to act for him; one entrusted with another's business.
aggression a tendency to attempt to dominate.
allergen a substance capable of inducing an allergic reaction or hypersensitivity.
allergic reaction bodily response brought about by a hypersensitivity to certain irritating substances.
Allis, Oscar Huntington, M.D. Philadelphia surgeon, 1833-1921.
alopecia areata loss of hair; baldness.
ambulatory walking or able to walk; not confined to bed.
ameba (pl., amebae) a minute, one-celled protozoan.
amenorrhea absence of the menses.
amicably in a friendly manner.
amino acid any one of a class of organic compounds containing the amino group (NH_2) and the carboxyl group (COOH). They form the structure of proteins, and several are essential in human nutrition.
amniocentesis surgical transabdominal perforation of the uterus to obtain amniotic fluid.
amniotic pertaining to the amnion. *amniotic fluid*, fluid in which the fetus is bathed. *amniotic sac*, the sac enclosing the fetus.
anaerobic growing in the absence of oxygen.
anaphylactic shock a serious and profound state of shock brought about by anaphylaxis to an allergen.
anaphylaxis an exaggerated reaction to a foreign protein; hypersensitivity.
anemia reduction below the normal number of erythrocytes, the quantity of hemoglobin, or the volume of packed red cells in the blood, any of which affects the oxygen-carrying potential of the blood.
angina pectoris acute pain in the chest, resulting from decreased blood supply to the heart muscles.
angiocardiogram a radiologic procedure that uses an opaque dye to show the heart and its major blood vessels.
anomalies marked deviations from the normal standard, especially as a result of congenital or hereditary defects.
annotate to furnish with notes, which are usually critical or explanatory.
antibiotic destructive of life.

antibody protein substances developed by the body, usually in response to the presence of an antigen that has entered the body.
antigen a substance that induces the formation of antibodies.
antiseptic preventing sepsis (contamination; presence of pathogenic organisms).
aperture an opening.
aphasia defect or loss either of the power of expression by speech, writing, or signs or of the comprehension of spoken or written language.
aphonia loss of voice, inability to produce vocal sound.
apnea temporary cessation of breathing.
arbitration the hearing and determination of a cause in controversy by a person or persons either chosen by the parties involved or appointed.
arbitrator a neutral person chosen by both sides to decide disputed issues.
armamentarium the equipment of a practitioner or institution, including books, instruments, medicines, and surgical appliances.
arrhythmia a variation from normal rhythm, especially of the heartbeat.
arteriosclerosis an arterial disease characterized by thickening and loss of elasticity of the arterial walls; popularly called "hardening of the arteries."
arthritis inflammation of a joint
arthrospore a bacterial spore formed by segmentation.
artifact a structure or appearance that is not natural but is due to manipulation (man-made).
artificial insemination the introduction of semen into the vagina or cervix by artificial means.
ascites the abnormal accumulation of serous fluid in the peritoneal cavity.
aspirate to withdraw fluid by negative pressure, or suction. Also, the fluid derived by such means.
aspiration the act of inhaling foreign matter into the lungs. Also, the removal of substances from a cavity by suction.
assault an intentional, unlawful attempt of bodily injury to another by force.
asthma a condition marked by recurrent attacks of dyspnea, with wheezing due to spasmodic constriction of the bronchi.
asthmatic paroxysm seizure with labored or difficult breathing and wheezing, due to spasmodic constriction of the bronchi.
astigmatism in vision, an error of refraction in which a ray of light is not sharply focused on the retina but is spread over a more or less diffuse area.
asymmetry a lack or absence of symmetry (corresponding likeness of both sides).
asymptomatic showing no symptoms.
ataxic lacking muscular coordination resulting in irregular muscular action.
atherosclerosis a form of arteriosclerosis in which atheromas (yellow plaques containing cholesterol) are formed on the innermost surfaces of the large or medium-sized arteries.
atrophy decrease in size from a normally developed organ or tissue; wasting.
atypical irregular; not conforming to the type.
augmented enlarged or increased in size, amount, or degree; made bigger.
autoimmune disease a disease such as rheumatoid arthritis or systemic lupus erythematosus, in which an individual produces antibodies to his own tissues.
autonomous self-governing; without outside control.
auxiliary affording aid.
avocational pertaining to a subordinate occupation or a hobby.
bacteriostatic arresting the growth or multiplication of bacteria. Also, an agent that so acts.
bacterium (pl., bacteria) a one-celled microscopic organism. Bacteria are classified in three basic groups, according to their shape. Rod-shaped bacteria are called bacilli; spiral-shaped bacteria, spirilla; and dot-shaped bacteria, cocci.
bariatrics a field of medicine encompassing the study of overweight, its cause, prevention, and treatment.
bartholinitis inflammation of the Bartholin gland located on each side of the vaginal orifice.
battery a willful and unlawful use of force or violence upon the person of another.
benign not recurrent or progressive. Opposite of *malignant*.
beri-beri a disease caused by a deficiency of thiamine (vitamin B_1). It may cause heart failure, edema, or paralysis and atrophy of muscles.
bilirubin a bile pigment formed in the breakdown of hemoglobin.
biologic pertaining to biology or life processes.
biopsy removal and examination, usually with a microscope, of tissue from the living body.
blasé appearing unable to enjoy, or disinterested in things that appeal to most people.

blood agar plate a mixture of blood and nutrient agar in a Petri dish, used as a culture medium for growing certain microorganisms.
bradypnea abnormal slowness of breathing.
bruit a sound or murmur heard in auscultation, especially an abnormal one.
buccal pertaining to the cheek or mouth.
bursa (pl., bursae) a padlike fluid-filled sac or cavity found in connecting tissue, usually in the vicinity of joints (where friction would otherwise occur).
bursal pertaining to a bursa.
bursitis inflammation of a bursa, often accompanied by a calcium deposit.
cachexia a profound and marked state of constitutional disorder; general ill health and malnutrition.
calculus (pl., calculi) a stone, gallstone, or kidney stone. An abnormal concretion of mineral salts occurring within the body, chiefly in the hollow organs or their passage.
calorie a unit of heat, the amount required to raise one gram of water one degree Celsius. A kilocalorie (Calorie or large calorie), the amount of heat required to raise one kilogram of water one degree Celsius, is used to describe energy found in food substances.
cannula a tube for insertion into a duct or cavity.
capillary any one of the minute vessels that connect the arterioles and venules.
carbuncle a necrotizing infection of skin or subcutaneous tissue, composed of a cluster of boils and usually due to *Staphylococcus aureus*.
carcinoma a malignant new growth of epithelial cells, tending to infiltrate surrounding tissue.
cardinal of primary or preeminent importance.
caries decay of bone or teeth.
carotene a yellow or red pigment found in foods such as carrots, sweet potatoes and milk fat. It can be converted by the body to vitamin A.
catalyst a substance that speeds up the rate of a chemical reaction without itself being permanently altered in the reaction.
cataract an opacity of the lens of the eye or its capsule.
catheterize to pass or introduce a catheter (a tube) into a body cavity for withdrawal of fluids from (or introduction into) the cavity.
causative effective or responsible as a cause or agent.
cautery application of a caustic agent, a hot iron, an electric current, or a chemical in order to destroy tissue.
celiac pertaining to the abdomen.
cellulose a carbohydrate forming the supporting framework of plants. Ordinarily it is not chemically changed or absorbed in digestion.
censure act of blaming or condemning sternly.
cerebral thrombosis the formation, development, or presence of a blood clot in a vessel of the brain.
cerumen a waxy secretion of the glands of the external ear canal; ear wax.
CEU continuing education unit, generally leading to renewal of a certificate or license.
chalazion a small eyelid mass resulting from chronic inflammation of the meibomian gland. Also called meibomian cyst.
chemotherapy the treatment of disease by chemical agents.
Cheyne-Stokes respiration breathing characterized by rhythmic waxing and waning of the depth of respiration; the patient breathes deeply for a short time and then breathes very slightly or stops breathing altogether. The pattern occurs repeatedly every 45 seconds to 3 minutes. It is caused by disease affecting the respiratory centers, usually heart failure or brain damage, and usually is considered a serious sign.
chlamydia a genus of microorganisms that cause a wide variety of diseases in humans and animals.
chocolated blood agar a nutrient agar to which fresh whole blood has been added; when heated, the blood changes to a chocolate-brown color
cholecystography roentgenography of the gallbladder.
choledocholithiasis the presence of gallstones.
cholesterol a white, waxy crystalline organic alcohol, present in all animal fats and oils.
chronologic in the order of time.
cicatrization the formation of a scar; scarring.
ciliate having hair.
cineradiography the making of a motion picture record of the successive images appearing on a fluoroscopic screen.
civil liability liability under civil law, as distinguished from criminal law.
coagulable susceptible to solidification or forming a clot.
coagulate to cause to clot; to become clotted.
coagulation the formation of a clot.

coagulum a blood clot.
collaborative working or acting jointly to attain a common goal.
colposcope a speculum for examination of the vagina and cervix by means of a magnifying lens.
comedo (pl., comedones) a blackhead; a plug of keratin and sebum within a secretory duct of the skin.
commensal bacteria living on or within another organism without harming the host. These are the same as resident bacteria on the skin.
commensurate equal in measure or extent.
competence the quality of answering all the requirements.
compound to put together, as elements or parts, to form a whole.
compulsory obligatory; enforced.
condylomata (sing., condyloma) a wartlike growth of the skin, usually seen on the external genitalia or near the anus.
confidentiality the condition of being confidential; the keeping of secrets.
conization excision of a cone of tissue, as of the mucous membrane of the cervix.
conjunctiva the delicate membrane lining the eyelids and covering the eyeball.
conjunctivitis an inflammation of the conjunctiva. The infectious form is highly contagious.
contagious capable of being transmitted from one person to another.
contamination the act of soiling, staining, or polluting, especially the introduction of infectious materials or germs that produce disease.
contract an agreement, especially one legally enforceable, between two or more persons to do or forbear something.
contrast bath the immersion of a part of the body alternately into hot water and cold water.
convulsion an involuntary contraction or a series of contractions of voluntary muscles.
corporeal pertaining to the body.
criteria (sing., criterion) standards on which a judgment or decision may be based.
coupling a pairing or joining. A coupling agent is a substance used to increase contact between two surfaces.
cretinism a condition that results from a deficiency of thyroid hormone during early infancy and is characterized by stunted growth, apathy, distended abdomen, and arrested mental development.
cryosurgery the destruction of tissue by application of extreme cold.
cryotherapy the therapeutic use of cold.
Cushing, Harvey Williams, M.D. Boston surgeon, 1869–1939.
cutaneous angioma a benign tumor of the skin made up of blood and lymph vessels.
cyanosis a bluish discoloration of the skin and mucous membranes, due to excessive concentration of reduced hemoglobin in the blood.
cyst a closed epithelium-lined sac or capsule, containing a liquid or semisolid substance.
cystitis inflammation of the urinary bladder.
cystocele herniation of the urinary bladder into the vagina.
cytogenic pertaining to the origin and development of the cell.
cytology the study of the origin, structure, function, and pathology of cells.
cytopathogenic effect capable of producing pathologic changes in cells.
debridement the removal of all foreign material and all contaminated and devitalized tissues from a traumatic or infected lesion until healthy tissue is exposed.
decimated destroyed a large part of.
deficiency the state of being insufficient, a lack or shortage.
delayed hypersensitivity a slowly developing allergic reaction to a specific antigen mediated by, or involving, T-cells.
depleted reduced in number or quantity so as to interfere with functioning.
depreciated having diminished in value.
depressant an agent that will depress a body function or nerve activity.
dereliction abandonment; a failure in duty
derivative something that is not original or fundamental; in chemistry, a compound obtained from other substances.
dermatology the science that deals with the structure, functions, and diseases of the skin.
desiccation the act of drying out.
desquamate to shed or scale off the surface epithelium (skin).
deviation a noticeable or marked departure from accepted norms of behavior.
diabetes insipidus a metabolic disorder resulting from decreased activity of the posterior lobe of the pituitary gland.
diabetes mellitus a disorder of carbohydrate metabolism due to faulty pancreatic activity and disturbance of the normal insulin mechanism.
diagnose to make a determination of the nature of a disease.

diagnostic a mark or symptom that aids in recognizing a disease or condition.

diaphoresis perspiration, especially profuse perspiration.

diascope a glass plate pressed against the skin to permit observation of changes produced in underlying skin after blood vessels are emptied and skin is blanched.

diascopy examination with a diascope.

diction art or manner of speaking.

dietetics the study of diet in relation to health and disease.

dietitian a specialist in dietetics, the science of diet and nutrition.

digestion the act or process of converting food into chemical substances that can be absorbed into the blood and utilized by the body tissues.

dilation expansion of an orifice with a dilating instrument.

diligence quality of persevering.

diplomate one who has passed the boards for a medical specialty.

diplopia the perception of two images of a single object; double vision.

disbursements funds paid out.

discretion quality of being discreet; Cautious reserve, especially in speech.

discrimination a distinction, as in treatment; especially an unfair or injurious distinction.

disease a definite morbid process having a characteristic train of symptoms; may affect the whole body or any part of it.

disinfection the removal or killing of pathogenic organisms.

dispense to deal out in portions; to put up a prescription or medicine.

disruption a breaking down or upset.

dissect to cut apart or separate.

disseminated disease a disease that is scattered or distributed over a considerable area.

distal remote; farther from point of reference. Opposite of proximal.

diuretic increasing urine excretion or the amount of urine.

dorsal directed toward or situated on the back surface. Opposite of *ventral*.

Down's syndrome congenital condition characterized by physical malformations and some degree of mental retardation. It is caused by the presence of an extra chromosome in the cells of affected individuals. Formerly known as mongolism.

dyscrasia a morbid condition.
blood dyscrasia, any abnormal or pathologic condition of the blood.

dysmenorrhea painful menstruation.

dyspepsia impairment in the power or function of digestion

dysphagia difficulty in swallowing.

dysphasia impairment of speech through lack of coordination and failure to arrange words in their proper order.

dyspnea labored or difficult breathing.

dysuria painful or difficult urination.

ecchymosis (pl., ecchymoses) a small nonelevated purplish patch, larger than a petechia, caused by hemorrhage.

E. coli *Escherichia coli,* a rod-shaped bacterium that normally inhabits the human intestinal tract. It may produce infection in other parts of the body, especially the genitourinary tract.

eczema a general term for any superficial inflammatory process involving primarily the epidermis.

edema the abnormal accumulation of fluid in the intercellular spaces of the body.

EEG electroencephalogram; a recording of electric currents developed in the brain.

effleurage stroking movement in massage.

effusive excessively demonstrative.

electrode either the positive or negative connection to an electrical system, such as the terminals of a battery or the leads of an electrocardiograph.

electroencephalograph an apparatus for detecting and recording brain waves.

electrolyte a substance that dissociates into ions when fused or in solution, thus becoming capable of conducting electricity. Electrolytes play an essential role in the workings of the cell and in maintaining fluid balance and normal acid-base balance.

elliptical pertaining to the shape of an ellipse; an oval-like shape. An elliptical incision permits excising a section of skin.

emancipated minor a person under legal age who is self-supporting and living apart from parents or guardian.

empathy imaginative projection of one's own consciousness into another being.

emphysema a pathologic accumulation of air in tissues or organs. Pulmonary emphysema is a lung disorder in which terminal bronchioles become plugged with mucus and eventually lose elasticity.

encephalitis inflammation of the brain.

endogenous produced within or caused by factors within the organism or body; growing from within.

endorsement act of writing on the back of a check or other written instrument; sanction or approval.
enunciation the act of pronouncing with distinction or articulation.
enzyme a protein secreted by the body, which acts as a catalyst by promoting or accelerating a chemical change in other substances while remaining unchanged in the process.
epidemiology the study that is concerned with defining and explaining the interrelationships of the host, agent, and environment in causing disease.
epilation the removal of hair by the roots.
epiphora an abnormal overflow of tears down the cheek, mainly due to stricture of the lacrimal passages.
epistaxis hemorrhages from the nose; a nosebleed.
eradicated plucked out by the roots; exterminated.
ergometer an apparatus for measuring the muscular, metabolic, and respiratory effects of exercise.
erosion an eating away of tissue; a kind of ulceration.
erythema redness of the skin.
estrogen generic name for the female sex hormones.
ethical the term used to refer to matters involving (1) moral principles or practices, (2) customs and usages of the medical profession, and (3) matters of policy not necessarily involving issues of morality in the practice of medicine.
ethics that branch of moral science that treats of the duties a member of the profession owes to the public, his colleagues, and his patient or client.
etiologic pertaining to the cause(s) of disease.
eugenics the science of improving the physical and mental qualities of human beings through control of the heredity factors.
euthanasia the act or practice of painlessly putting to death a person suffering from incurable and distressing disease.
exfoliation a falling off in scales or layers.
exogenous originating outside or caused by factors outside the organism or body.
exophthalmia abnormal protrusion of the eye. Also called exophthalmos.
exophthalmometer an instrument for measuring the extent of protrusion of the eyeball.
exophthalmos abnormal protrusion of the eye.
exploitation selfish or unfair utilization.
expulsion act of expelling or forcing out.
extension the movement that increases the angle between adjoining bones.
extracurricular relating to those activities that form part of the life of students but are not part of the courses of study.
exudate a fluid with a high content of protein and cellular debris that has escaped from blood vessels and has been deposited in or on tissues, usually as a result of inflammation.
fallopian tube one of a pair of tubes in the female that carries the egg from the ovary to the uterus.
feasible capable of being done or carried out.
fee splitting the sharing by two or more persons, without the knowledge of the patient or his representative, of a fee that has been given by the patient supposedly as payment for the services of one person alone.
fenestrated pierced with one or more openings, as a drape.
fenestration the act of perforating, or the condition of being perforated.
fermentation a chemical decomposition induced in a carbohydrate by a ferment, or enzyme, such as yeast.
fiber an elongated threadlike structure; that which gives texture or substance.
fibrocystic characterized by an overgrowth of fibrous tissue and the development of cystic spaces, especially in a gland.
fissure a narrow slit or cleft; a groove or crack.
fistula any abnormal, tubelike passage within body tissue.
flagellate any microorganism having at least one flagellum, a whiplike process.
flatulence excessive formation of gases in the stomach or intestine.
flexion the act of bending or the condition of being bent.
flora plant life.
fluke (parasitic) common name for species of flatworms (Trematoda), especially the parasitic variety.
fluorescing capable of causing fluorescence, the emission of radiation, or a visible glow or light.
fluoroscopy examination by means of a fluoroscope, a screen that reveals the shadows of x-rays passing through the body.
fomentation treatment by warm, moist applications; also, the substance thus applied.
format shape, size, and general make-up of a publication.
fornix an archlike structure or the vaultlike space created by such a structure. Often applied to the space between the vaginal wall and the vaginal part of the cervix of the uterus.

foulage kneading and pressing of a muscle in massage. Also called petrissage.

fremitus a vibration perceptible on palpation or auscultation.

frivolity inappropriate gaiety or lack of seriousness.

fulguration destruction of living tissue by an electric spark generated by a high-frequency current.

functional affecting the function but not the structure.
functional disease, a disease involving body functions but without detectable tissue changes.

fungi a general term used to denote a group of plantlike organisms that includes yeasts and molds.

furuncle a focal suppurative inflammation of the skin and subcutaneous tissues. Also called a boil.

generic pertaining to the origin; nonproprietary; a drug name not protected by trademark, sometimes called "public name."

germicide an agent that destroys pathogenic microorganisms.

ghost surgery a situation in which a patient has consented to have surgery done by surgeon A, but without the patient's knowledge or consent the surgery is actually performed by surgeon B.

glaucoma a group of diseases of the eye characterized by increased intraocular pressure.

gliadin any of various simple proteins obtained from wheat and rye. Also called gluten.

glycogen the form in which carbohydrate is stored in the body, especially in the liver and muscles.

goiter enlargement of the thyroid gland.

gonad a sex gland; the ovary in the female and the testis in the male.

gonadal pertaining to the gonads, or sexual glands (the ovaries and testes).

Good Samaritan acts the acts of law that protect the physician and others from liability for any civil damages as a result of rendering emergency care.

gout a hereditary form of arthritis in which uric acid appears in excessive quantities in the blood and may be deposited in the joints and other tissues.

Gram's stain a method used to classify bacteria based on the ability of the organisms to retain a basic dye (crystal violet). Those bacteria retaining the violet stain are called *gram-positive,* and those that do not retain it are *gram-negative.*

granulation tissue newly formed vascular tissue normally produced in the healing of soft tissue wounds.

gynecologist a physician who specializes in diseases that affect women.

hallucinogenic producing a sense perception without a source in the external world.

healing a process of cure; a restoration.

heat-labile easily altered or decomposed by heat.

helminth any animal, living free or parasitic, belonging to a kingdom of worms. Examples include flatworms, roundworms, and segmented worms.

hematocrit the volume percentage of erythrocytes in whole blood. Abbrev., Hct. Also called packed cell volume.

hematology the branch of medical science that treats diseases of the blood and blood-forming tissues.

hematoma a localized collection of escaped blood in an organ, space, or tissue. Bruises and black eyes are familiar forms of a hematoma.

hemophilia a hereditary hemorrhagic disease due to the deficiency of a coagulation factor.

hemorrhage a bleeding; the escape of blood from a ruptured vessel. It can be external, internal, or into the skin or other tissues.

hemostasis the arrest of the escape of blood by either natural (clot) or artificial (compression or ligation) means.

hemostatic pertaining to an agent that checks the flow of blood.

hermetically in an airtight manner.

histamine a substance normally present in the body tissues. It dilates capillaries, constricts bronchial muscles, and increases gastric secretion.

histology the study of anatomy that deals with the minute structure, composition, and function of the tissues.

hives urticaria, or a skin reaction marked by the temporary appearance of smooth, slightly elevated patches either redder or paler than the surrounding skin, and often accompanied by severe itching.

hydrocele a painless swelling of the scrotum caused by a collection of fluid in the tunica vaginalis testis.

hydrogenate to combine an unsaturated compound with hydrogen.

hyperglycemia excessive glucose in the blood.

hyperopia farsightedness.

hyperpnea abnormal increase in the depth and rate of respiration.

hypersensitivity abnormal sensitivity to a stimulus of any kind.

hypertension persistently high pressure of the blood against the arterial walls.

hyperventilation increase of air in the lungs above the normal amount; abnormally prolonged and deep breathing.

hypha (pl., hyphae) one of the many filaments or threads of a fungus.

hypocalcemia a marked reduction of calcium in the blood.

hypodermical pertaining to application or administration beneath the skin.

hypoglycemia an abnormally low level of glucose in the blood.

hypotension a consistently low blood pressure with a systolic pressure lower than 100 mm of mercury.

immediate hypersensitivity a rapid allergic reaction caused by antibodies already circulating in the blood of an individual who has previously been sensitized to the antigen. Also called anaphylaxis.

immunocompromised referring to patients who have deficiency in immune response.

immunoglobulin a protein of animal origin with known antibody activity.

immunology that branch of biomedical science concerned with the response of the organism to antigenic challenge.

impregnated rendered pregnant; saturated or charged with.

incontinence the inability to control excretory functions.

indirect (filing system) one in which another source must be consulted in order to locate the file.

infectious caused by or capable of being communicated by infection.

informed consent a consent in which there is understanding of what is to be done and of the risks involved, why it should be done, and alternative methods of treatment available and their attendant risks. The alternatives include the failure to treat and the attendant risk.

inhalation therapist a technician specializing in treatment aimed at restoring toward normal any pathophysiologic alterations of gas exchange in the cardiopulmonary system.

inoculum material used in inoculation.

in situ in the natural or normal place; confined to the site of origin without invasion of neighboring tissues.

integral essential; being an indispensable part of a whole.

intercom an intercommunication system; a direct telephone line from one station to another.

intermenstrual occurring between menstrual periods.

intermittent coming and going at intervals.

internal medicine that branch of medicine that deals especially with the diagnosis and medical treatment of diseases and disorders of the internal structures of the human body.

interpretation explanation, construction, or sense given by an interpreter.

intramuscular pertaining to within a muscle.

intravascular within a vessel or vessels.

intrinsic situated entirely within, or pertaining exclusively to, a part.

invasive having a tendency to spread through tissue. Also applies to procedures in which the body is entered.

inventory an itemized list of goods.

jaundice yellowness of skin, sclerae, and excretions due to hyperbilirubinemia (high levels of bilirubin in the blood) and deposition of bile pigments. Also called icterus.

judgment the official decision of a court of justice upon the respective rights and claims of the parties to an action or suit therein litigated and submitted to its determination.

keratosis (pl., keratoses) any horny growth, such as a wart.

ketonuria an excess of ketone bodies (metabolic products of lipids) in the urine, often seen in diabetes.

Koplik's spot small, irregular, bright red spots on the buccal (cheek) and lingual (tongue) mucosa with a minute bluish-white speck in its center.

kyphosis abnormally increased convexity in the curvature of the thoracic spine as viewed from the side. Also called hunchback.

laceration a wound produced by the tearing of body tissue, as distinguished from a cut or incision.

lateral denoting a position farther from the median plane; pertaining to the side.

lethargic pertaining to a condition of drowsiness or indifference.

leukoderma an acquired condition with localized loss of pigmentation of the skin.

liability state or quality of being liable; that for which one is liable, such as debts.

liable bound or obligated in law or equity; responsible; chargeable; answerable; compellable to make satisfaction, compensation, or restitution.

lien a charge upon real or personal property for the satisfaction of some debt or duty ordinarily arising by operation of law.

lipid any group of organic substances, including fatty acids, neutral fats, waxes, steroids, and phosphatides, which are insoluble in water but soluble in alcohol, ether, and other fat solvents.

litigation contest in a court of justice for the purpose of enforcing a right.

lordosis a forward curvature of the lumbar spine. Also known as swayback.

macrophage any of the highly phagocytic cells in the wall of blood vessels and in loose connective tissue.

macule a stain, spot, or thickening; an area distinguishable from its surroundings by color or some other way.

malaise a feeling of uneasiness or indisposition.

malignancy tendency to become worse and to result in death; a malignant neoplasm.

malpractice professional misconduct, improper discharge of professional duties, or a failure to meet the standard of care by a professional, resulting in harm to another.

matrix that in which anything originates, develops, takes shape, or is contained.

maturation the stage or process of attaining maximal development.

mediastinum the mass of tissues and organs separating the sternum in front and the vertical column behind, containing the heart and its large vessels, trachea, esophagus, thymus, lymph nodes, and other structures and tissues.

medium (pl., media) *culture medium*, a substance used to support the growth of microorganisms or other cells.

contrast medium, a radiopaque substance used in roentgenography.

melanin a dark pigment normally found in the hair, skin, ciliary body, choroid of the eye, pigment layer of the retina, and certain nerve cells.

meniscus something crescent-shaped, as a convex or concave surface of a column of liquid in a pipet or cylinder.

menopause the span of time during which the menstrual cycle wanes and eventually stops.

menses menstruation.

menstruation the periodic discharge from the vagina of blood and tissues from a nonpregnant uterus; the culmination of the menstrual cycle.

metabolic pertaining to the nature of metabolism.

metabolic disease a disease caused by some defect in the chemical reactions of the cells of the body.

metabolism the sum of the physical and chemical processes by which a living organized substance is produced or energy is made available.

metabolized subjected to or transformed by metabolism.

meticulous excessively careful of small details.

microbe a microorganism, especially a pathogenic bacterium.

modality a method of application, or the employment of any therapeutic agent; limited usually to physical agents.

Monilia fungi belonging to the genus now called Candida. Though they normally inhabit parts of the body, they often cause infection, especially in the genital area (yeast infection).

monitor to check by means of listening through a receiver the conversation being transmitted by telephone.

mortality death rate, or proportion of deaths to population.

mucocutaneous pertaining to mucous membranes and skin.

mucopeptide a polymer of high molecular weight that forms the tough, rigid structure of bacterial cell walls.

multigravida a woman pregnant for the third, or more, time.

multipara a woman who has had two or more pregnancies resulting in viable offspring.

multiparous having had two or more pregnancies resulting in viable offspring.

multiple sclerosis a chronic disorder of the nervous system. Abbrev., MS.

muscular dystrophy one of several genetically determined diseases in which muscles degenerate without involvement of the nervous system.

mutation a change in form, quality, or other characteristics. Genetic mutation is a change in chromosomal structure that may produce major alteration in body structure or function.

mycoplasma a genus of microorganisms including the pleuropneumonialike organisms.

mycotic pertaining to or caused by fungi.

myocardial pertaining to the muscular tissue of the heart.

myopia nearsightedness.

myringotomy incision of the tympanic membrane (eardrum).

myxedema a condition resulting from advanced hypothyroidism, characterized by a dry, waxy type of swelling with deposits of mucin in the skin and other tissues.

narcotic drugs drugs that in moderate doses allay sensibility, relieve pain, and produce profound sleep; in poisonous doses, they produce stupor, coma, or convulsions.

necrosis death of individual cells or a group of cells.

necrotic pertaining to or characterized by the death of the tissues.

negligence the omission of an act that would be done by a reasonable person guided by those considerations which ordinarily regulate human affairs; the doing of something which a reasonable and prudent person would not do.

negotiable legally transferable to another party.
nephrotic syndrome a condition characterized by massive edema, heavy proteinuria, hypoalbuminemia, and peculiar susceptibility to intercurrent infections. Also called nephrosis.
nodule a small solid node that can be detected by touch.
noninvasive not having the tendency to spread or invade tissues.
nonproprietary not owned by a private individual; not protected by trademark.
nutrient a substance that affects the metabolic processes of the body, or is nourishing.
nutrition the sum total of the processes involved in the taking in and utilization of food substances for growth, repair, and maintenance of the body.
obese excessively fat.
obesity excessive accumulation of fat in the body; increase in weight beyond that considered desirable with regard to age, height, and bone structure.
objective
(adj.) perceivable by external senses. Objective signs are also called physical signs.
(n.) an aim or end of action.
obstetrics the science or art of assisting women in the management of pregnancy and labor.
obturator an object that closes an opening. When used with a cannula, an obturator plugs the lumen (channel or opening) of the tube to make insertion easier.
Ochsner, Albert John surgeon in Chicago, 1858–1925.
opaque neither reflecting nor emitting light.
ophthalmodynamometer an instrument for measuring the retinal arterial pressure, to determine the near point of convergence.
oral hygiene the proper care of the mouth and teeth for the maintenance of health and prevention of disease.
orthopnea difficult breathing except in an upright position.
orthostatic pertaining to or caused by standing erect.
orthostatic albuminuria the presence of serum albumin in the urine due to the sudden arising from a recumbent to an upright position.
orthostatic hypotension hypotension occurring upon suddenly arising from a recumbent position or from standing still.
oscilloscope an instrument that displays a visual picture of an electrical current.
osteoarthritis a degenerative joint disease occurring chiefly in older persons.
otitis media inflammation of the middle ear.
otolaryngologic pertaining to the branch of medicine that deals with the ear, nose, and throat.
pallor paleness; absence of skin coloration.
palpate to examine by pressure of the hand; to feel.
papule a small, circumscribed, superficial, solid elevation of the skin.
paracentesis a surgical puncture of a cavity for the purpose of aspirating fluid.
paracervical the area beside, accessory to, apart from, or against the cervix.
paraffin bath the application of heated liquid wax to a part of the body and permitting the wax to solidify. Also, the immersion of a part of the body in heated liquid wax maintained at a constant temperature.
paraphrase a restatement of a passage or work, giving the meaning in another form.
parenteral taken into the body not through the alimentary canal but rather by injection into skin, muscle, blood vessel, or some other route.
paroxysm a sudden recurrence or intensification of symptoms; a spasm or seizure.
patency condition of being wide open; freely open.
pathogen any disease-producing agent or microorganism.
pathologic pertaining to pathology, a branch of medicine concerned with disease; due to a disease.
pediatrics the medical science that treats of the hygiene and diseases of children.
peduncle a stemlike connecting part, like the stalk that attaches a tumor to normal tissue.
pedunculated having a peduncle.
pellagra a disease or syndrome due to the deficiency of niacin. The nervous system is affected with various mental disturbances, and diarrhea and dermatitis occur.
penal pertaining to punishment or penalties.
penetrating wound a deep opening into the skin.
periodontitis inflammatory reaction of the tissues surrounding a tooth, usually resulting in gingivitis.
peripheral pertaining to or situated near the outward part, or the surface.
peritoneal pertaining to the peritoneum (the thin and watery membrane that lines the walls of the abdominal and pelvic cavities and invests their large organs).
perjured testimony telling what is false when sworn to tell the truth.
petechia (pl., petechiae) a pinpoint, nonraised, round, purplish-red spot caused by intradermal or submucosal hemorrhage.

petrissage kneading and pressing of a muscle in massage. Also called foulage.
pH abbreviation for the power of hydrogen; the degree of acidity or alkalinity. A solution of pH 7.0 is neutral; values below indicate acidity and values above indicate alkalinity.
phagocytosis ingestion of foreign or other particles by certain cells (phagocytes).
pharmaceutical relating to pharmacy or a pharmaceutical product (drug).
phonetic of or pertaining to the voice, or its use.
photofluorogram the film produced by fluoroscopic images on small films, using a fast lens.
physical pertaining to the body, or material things, or to physics.
PKU phenylketonuria, a metabolic disorder caused by deficiency of an enzyme, resulting in mental retardation, light pigmentation, epilepsy, and microcephaly (small head).
placenta the organ on the wall of the uterus to which the embryo is attached by the umbilical cord.
plaque any patch or flat area.
plasma the fluid portion of the blood in which the corpuscles are suspended.
pleural pertaining to the serous membrane lining the thoracic walls and investing the lungs.
pneumatic pertaining to air or respiration.
pneumonia inflammation of the lungs with consolidation and exudation.
pneumonitis inflammation of the lungs.
polycythemia an increase in the total red cell mass of the body.
polyp any growth or mass protruding from mucous membrane. Polyps attached with a thin stalk are called *pedunculated* polyps. If they have a broad base, they are known as *sessile* polyps.
polypoid resembling a polyp.
postmenstrual the time immediately following cessation of the menstrual flow.
precipitin band in a precipitation test, the region where there is equal concentration of antigen and antibody, which permits them to bind together in a large lattice, forming a visible precipitate.
prepartum (prepartal) occurring before, or just previous to, labor.
prerogative an exclusive and unquestionable right belonging to a person or body of persons.
presbyopia hyperopia and impairment of vision due to advancing years or to old age.
prescribe to issue a prescription for the patient; to direct, designate, or order use of a remedy.
probate official proof, especially of an instrument offered as the last will and testament of a person deceased.
proctologic pertaining to the branch of medicine concerned with the rectum or anus.
professional courtesy the traditional practice of physicians caring for the medical needs of their colleagues and their dependents without charge.
prognosis (pl., prognoses) forecast of the course of a disease.
pronunciation act or manner of pronouncing words.
proprietary of or belonging to a proprietor; subject to exclusive ownership.
propriety the character or quality of being proper.
protein any of a group of complex nitrogenous substances that contain amino acids as their fundamental structural units.
proteinuria the presence of an excess of serum proteins in the urine.
prothrombin a plasma protein that is converted into thrombin during the second stage of blood coagulation.
protozoa a group of the simplest forms of the animal kingdom, consisting of unicellular organisms.
proximal nearest or closest to any point of reference. Opposite of *distal.*
prudent capable of directing or conducting oneself wisely and judiciously.
pruritus itching.
psammotherapy treatment of disease by sand bath. Also called ammotherapy.
pseudopod a temporary protrusion of the cytoplasm of an ameba; a false foot. The term can also describe the appearance of the circumference of a wheal.
psychiatry the medical science and specialty that deals with the origins, diagnosis, prevention, and treatment of mental and emotional disorders.
psychologic directed toward the mind or will.
ptosis prolapse of an organ, or part; a drooping or sagging.
public domain the realm embracing property rights that belong to the community at large and are subject to appropriation by anyone.
puerpera a woman who has just given birth to an infant.
pulmonary edema an effusion of fluid into the air sacs and interstitial tissue of the lungs, producing severe dyspnea.
puncture a wound made by piercing the skin with a pointed object or instrument.
puree food that has been rubbed through a strainer.

purulent consisting of or containing pus; associated with the formation of or caused by pus.
pustule a visible collection of pus within or beneath the epidermis, often in the hair follicle or sweat pore.
pyorrhea a discharge of pus.
pyretotherapy treatment by artificially increasing the patient's body temperature.
quackery pretense of medical skill.
radical mastectomy surgical removal of a breast, pectoral muscles, axillary lymph nodes, and associated skin, performed in the treatment of breast cancer.
radiology that branch of medical science that deals with the use of radiant energy in the diagnosis and treatment of disease.
radiopaque quality or property of obstructing the passage of radiant energy, such as x-rays.
rales abnormal respiratory sounds heard in auscultation and indicating some pathologic condition.
ratchet a hinged catch with sloping teeth to permit motion only in one direction.
rebate a return of a portion of a payment.
reciprocity an obligation under which something is done or given by each of two to the other.
recumbent lying down.
reflex an involuntary response to a stimulus.
regimen a systematic course of action or therapy.
repel cause aversion or rejection.
respondeat superior "Let the master answer." This maxim means that a master is liable in certain cases for the wrongful acts of his servant, and a principal for those of his agent.
resume a summing up; an abridgment or summary, as of one's education and employment record.
resuscitation the restoration to life or consciousness of one apparently dead.
reticuloendothelial system a network of cells and tissues found throughout the body, especially in blood, general connective tissue, spleen, liver, lungs, bone marrow and lymph nodes.
revocation the act of annulling by recalling or taking back.
rheumatic fever a disease caused by hemolytic streptococci (organisms that rupture red blood cells and cause release of hemoglobin into the plasma) and characterized by fever and pain in the joints similar to that of rheumatism.
rheumatism any of a variety of disorders marked by inflammation, degeneration, or metabolic derangement of the connective tissue structures of the body, especially the joints.
rheumatoid resembling rheumatism.
rheumatology the science of rheumatism and disorders of the connective tissue structures of the body, especially joints.
rhinitis inflammation of the mucous membranes of the nose.
rhythmic pertaining to a measured time or movement; occurring with regularity.
rickettsiae a genus of small, rod-shaped to round microorganisms found in the cytoplasm of tissue cells of lice, fleas, ticks, and mites, and transmitted to man by their bites.
roentgen the international unit of x- or y-radiation; named for its discoverer, Wilhelm Conrad Röntgen, German physicist, 1845–1923.
roentgenogram a film produced by roentgen ray photography.
roentgenology the science of applying roentgen rays (x-rays) for diagnostic or therapeutic purposes.
Salmonella carrier an individual who harbors in his body the Salmonella (typhoid fever) organism without manifesting symptoms, and thus is a carrier of the infection.
sanitization the process of making clean.
scientific basis systematic pursuit of knowledge involving as necessary conditions the recognition and formulation of a problem, the collection of data through observation and if possible experiment, the formulation of hypotheses, and the testing and confirmation of the hypotheses formulated.
scleroderma a chronic disorder of unknown etiology, characterized by progressive thickening and hardening of the dermis.
sclerosing causing or developing a sclerosis (a hardening).
scoliosis a lateral curvature of the spine.
screen to shield from observation or annoyance with or as with a screen.
scrupulous careful; exact.
scurvy a nutritional deficiency disease resulting from the lack of vitamin C (ascorbic acid).
seborrheic dermatitis chronic inflammatory skin disease characterized by redness, dry, moist, or greasy scaling, and yellow crusted patches, especially in the scalp. Also called seborrhea.

seizure the sudden attack or recurrence of a disease; an attack of epilepsy.
semen a viscid secretion carrying spermatozoa, discharged from the male urethra at the climax of sexual excitement.
senescence the process or condition of growing old.
senile pertaining to old age.
senile keratosis a sharply outlined growth or wart that may develop into a horn on the skin and may become malignant. It usually occurs in middle-aged or elderly persons and is due to excessive exposure to the sun. Also called actinic or solar keratosis.
sensor a device that can detect and transmit impulses. In electrocardiography, an electrode is applied to the skin, where it detects electrical impulses released in the functioning pulse.
serologic pertaining to the study of sera, usually in reference to blood serum tests and antigen-antibody reactions.
serration a formation of a series of teeth or notches like those of a saw.
serum the clear, straw-colored liquid that separates in the clotting of blood from the clot and corpuscles. It does not contain fibrinogen or cells but may contain antibodies.
sheath a covering protective structure.
shock a severe physiologic reaction to bodily trauma.
sickle cell anemia an inherited anemia, mostly among Negroes, characterized by abnormal hemoglobin and sickle-shaped erythrocytes. Attacks of fever and pain occur, and the increased viscosity of the blood may produce convulsions and paralysis.
sigmoidoscopy visual inspection of the sigmoid colon, with the aid of special instruments.
sign any objective evidence of a disease or dysfunction.
Sims, James Marion New York gynecologist, 1813–1883.
skenitis inflamed condition of the Skene's glands located just inside the female urethra.
solicitation an attempt to obtain patients by persuasion or influence.
somatic pertaining to or characteristic of the body.
sonography a diagnostic aid in which high frequency sound waves are used to detect the presence of pregnancy or pelvic tumors or to locate the placenta.
stain a substance used to impart color to tissues or cells, to facilitate microscopic study and identification.
Staphylococcus a genus of microorganisms that are spherical, tend to form masses of cells, and often cause infection.
STAT report an immediate report (from the Latin, *statim* meaning *at once*).
statute an act of the legislature declaring, commanding, or prohibiting something. This word is used to designate the written law, in contradistinction to the unwritten law.
stem cell a generalized mother cell whose descendants specialize.
sterilization the process of destroying all microorganisms and their pathogenic products. Also, the process of rendering an individual incapable of reproduction.
sterilize to render sterile or free from live microorganisms; to render incapable of procreation.
stimulant anything, particularly a drug, that accelerates the activity of the body or a part of the body.
strabismus a visual disorder in which one eye cannot focus with the other eye.
strain a group of organisms within a species or variety, characterized by some particular quality, as rough or smooth strains of bacteria.
striae thin stripes or bands, often found in groups in parallel.
stridor a shrill, harsh sound, especially the respiratory sound heard during inspiration in laryngeal obstruction.
stylet a wire run through a catheter or cannula to stiffen it or to remove debris from its lumen (channel or cavity).
subcutaneously pertaining to beneath the skin, or in the subcutaneous tissue.
subjective perceived only by the affected individual and not by the examiner.
substantive law pertaining to or constituting the essential part or principles of the law.
suit a proceeding in a court of law in which a plaintiff demands the recovery of a right or the redress of a wrong.
surgery the branch of medical science that relates to bodily injuries, deformities, and diseased conditions requiring treatment by operative procedures, with or without instruments.
suspend to interrupt; to discontinue temporarily, but with an expectation or purpose of resumption.
suture the operation of uniting the edges of a cut or wound by or as by stitching; the thread, silver wire, or other material used in this operation; the interlocking of two bones at their edges, as in the skull.
symmetry correspondence in size, form, and arrangement of parts on opposite sides of a plane.
symptom any indication of a disease perceived by the patient.

syncope a temporary suspension of consciousness due to cerebral anemia; fainting.
syndrome a combination of symptoms resulting in a single cause or so commonly occurring together as to constitute a distinct clinical picture.
synovial fluid the transparent, sticky fluid secreted by the inner membrane (synovial membrane) that lines certain joint cavities, usually those joints permitting more or less free movement.
synthesize to combine to produce a complex compound from simpler ones.
systemic pertaining to or affecting the body as a whole.
tachypnea very rapid respiration; a respiratory neurosis marked by quick shallow breathing.
Tay-Sachs disease an inherited condition producing blindness, mental retardation, and premature death, chiefly affecting Jewish infants. Also called cerebral sphingolipidosis.
tenesmus a painful ineffectual straining to urinate or defecate.
testosterone one of the male sex hormones produced by the testes.
tetany continuous tonic spasm of a muscle, which may be caused by inadequate amounts of calcium in the blood.
therapeutic of or relating to the treatment of disease or disorders by remedial agents or methods.
thermostable not affected by heat.
thrombotic related to, caused by, or of the nature of, a thrombus (clot).
thymus a ductless glandlike body lying in the upper mediastinum beneath the sternum. It plays an immunologic role during life.
tickler (file) a chronologic file used as a reminder that something must be taken care of on a certain date.
tinea capitis a fungus skin disease, especially ringworm, of the scalp.
tinea pedis chronic fungal infection of the skin of the foot; athlete's foot.
tinnitus a noise in the ears, as ringing, buzzing or roaring.
tomography the roentgenography of several selected levels of the body while blurring structures at all other levels.
topography a description of an anatomic region or a special part.
torticollis wryneck, a contracted state of cervical muscles producing twisting of the neck.
toxemia a condition caused by the presence in the blood of poisonous products (toxins) of bacteria formed at a local site of infection.
toxic poisonous.
tranquilizer a drug that allays anxiety and calms the patient.
transducer a device that converts one form of energy to another.
transudate a fluid substance that has passed through a membrane or has been extruded from a tissue.
trauma a wound or injury, especially damage produced by external force.
traumatic pertaining to, resulting from, or causing physical injury or emotional shock.
tremor an involuntary trembling of the body or limbs.
trespass to exceed the bounds of what is lawful, right, or just.
Trichomonas a genus of protozoa bearing flagella that are parasites in the urogenital tract. One species produces vaginal discharge.
trophozoite the active, motile feeding stage of a sporozoan parasite.
tryptophan a naturally occurring amino acid, existing in proteins and essential for human metabolism.
tubal ligation sterilization of the female by constricting the uterine tubes by means of ligatures.
tympanic membrane the thin layer of tissue separating the middle from the external ear.
unethical term used to refer to conduct that fails to conform to the professional standards, customs and usages, or policies, as interpreted by the American Medical Association.
uremia retention in the blood of substances that are ordinarily eliminated in the urine.
urethrocele prolapse of the female urethra through the urinary meatus.
urticaria a vascular reaction of the skin marked by transient appearance of slightly elevated patches (wheals) that are redder or paler than surrounding skin. Also called hives.
vaccine a suspension of attenuated or killed microorganisms administered for prevention or treatment of infectious diseases.
vacuole a space or cavity in the protoplasm of certain unicellular organisms.
vagina the canal in the female that extends from the vulva to the cervix uteri.
vasectomy surgical removal of the vas deferens or a portion of it.
vasoactive exerting an effect on the caliber of blood vessels.
vasoconstrictor causing constriction of the blood vessels; a vasoconstrictive agent.
venereal due to or propagated by sexual intercourse.
venipuncture puncture of a vein, as when administering an intravenous injection.
verruca (pl., verrucae) a wart.
vertigo a sensation of rotation or movement of self, or of one's surroundings; dizziness.

vesicular composed of or relating to small, saclike bodies; pertaining to or made up of vesicles (blisters) on the skin.
viable able to maintain an independent existence; able to live after birth.
virus a minute infectious agent, smaller than a bacterium, which is able to replicate only within a living host cell.
viscosity state of thickness; being sticky or gummy.
vital relating to life, contributing to or essential to life.
vitamin an organic substance found in foods and essential in small quantities for growth, health, and the preservaton of life.
vitiligo sharply demarcated, milky-white patches on the skin. Also called acquired leukoderma.
wheal a round or ridgelike transitory swelling on the skin.
xanthelasma a form of xanthoma (slightly raised, yellow skin plaque) occurring on the eyelids.
xerophthalmia abnormal dryness and thickening of the surfaces of the conjunctiva and cornea due either to a deficiency of vitamin A or to a local disease.

INDEX

Page numbers in *italics* indicate illustrations.
Page numbers followed by a t indicate a table.

INDEX

INDEX

INDEX

INDEX